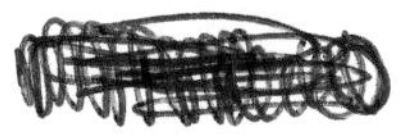

# RHEUMATOLOGY SECRETS

**Second Edition**

# RHEUMATOLOGY SECRETS

## Second Edition

**STERLING G. WEST, MD, FACP, FACR**

Professor
Department of Medicine, Division of Rheumatology
University of Colorado Health Sciences Center
Denver, Colorado

HANLEY & BELFUS, INC. / Philadelphia

Publisher: HANLEY & BELFUS, INC.
Medical Publishers
210 South 13th Street
Philadelphia, PA 19107
(215) 546-7293; 800-962-1892
FAX (215) 790-9330
Web site: http://www.hanleyandbelfus.com

*Note to the reader*: Although the information in this book has been carefully reviewed for correctness of dosage and indications, neither the authors nor the editor nor the publisher can accept any legal responsibility for any errors or omissions that may be made. Neither the publisher nor the editor makes any warranty, expressed or implied, with respect to the material contained herein. Before prescribing any drug, the reader must review the manufacturer's current product information (package inserts) for accepted indications, absolute dosage recommendations, and other information pertinent to the safe and effective use of the product described.

Library of Congress Cataloging-in-Publication Data

Rheumatology secrets / [edited by] Sterling West.—2nd ed.
p. ; cm.—(The Secrets Series®)
Includes bibliographical references and index.
ISBN 1-56053-474-5 (alk. paper)
1. Rheumatism—Miscellanea. I. West, Sterling G., 1950– II. Series.
[DNLM: 1. Rheumatic Diseases—Examination Questions. WE 18.2 R472 2002]
RC927.R487 2002
616.7'23'0076—dc21

2002024355

**RHEUMATOLOGY SECRETS, 2nd edition** ISBN 1-56053-474-5



Last digit is the print number: 9 8 7 6 5 4 3 2

# CONTENTS

## IV. SYSTEMIC CONNECTIVE TISSUE DISEASES



## V. THE VASCULITIDES AND RELATED DISORDERS

## VI. SERONEGATIVE SPONDYLOARTHROPATHIES



## VII. ARTHRITIS ASSOCIATED WITH INFECTIOUS AGENTS



## VIII. RHEUMATIC DISORDERS ASSOCIATED WITH METABOLIC, ENDOCRINE AND HEMATOLOGIC DISEASES



## IX. BONE AND CARTILAGE DISORDERS

# CONTRIBUTORS

**Ramon A. Arroyo, MD, FACR**
Assistant Professor of Medicine, Department of Medicine and Rheumatology Flight Commander, Uniformed Services University of the Health Sciences, Bethesda, Maryland; Wilford Hall Medical Center, San Antonio, Texas

**Daniel F. Battafarano, DO, FACP, FACR**
Director, Medical Education, Department of Medical Education, Brooke Army Medical Center, San Antonio, Texas; Adjunct Associate Professor, Department of Medicine, F. Edward Hebert School of Medicine, Bethesda, Maryland; Clinical Assistant Professor, Department of Medicine, University of Texas Health Science Center, San Antonio, Texas

**Kristin Bird, MD**
Rheumatology Fellow, Medical University of South Carolina, Charleston, South Carolina

**Vance J. Bray, MD**
Assistant Clinical Professor, Rheumatology, University of Colorado Health Sciences Center; Denver Arthritis Clinic, Denver, Colorado

**Amy Cannella, MD**
Rheumatology Fellow, University of Utah Medical Center, Salt Lake City, Utah

**Matthew T. Carpenter, MD, FACR**
Assistant Professor of Clinical Medicine, Uniformed Services University of the Health Sciences, Bethesda, Maryland; Program Director, Internal Medicine Clinic, Keesler Medical Center, Keesler Air Force Base, Mississippi

**Marc D. Cohen, MD**
Professor of Medicine, Rheumatology, Mayo Clinic Jacksonville; St. Luke's Hospital, Jacksonville, Florida

**David H. Collier, MD, FACR**
Associate Professor, Department of Medicine, University of Colorado Health Sciences Center; Chief, Rheumatology, Denver Health Medical Center, Denver, Colorado

**Carolyn Anne Coyle, MD, FACR**
Staff Rheumatologist, Rheumatology Department, Providence Portland Arthritis Center; Providence Portland Medical Center and Providence Milwaukee Hospital, Portland, Oregon

**Randy Q. Cron, MD, PhD, FACR**
Assistant Professor, Department of Pediatrics, Division of Rheumatology, Children's Hospital of Philadelphia/University of Pennsylvania; Attending Physician, Children's Hospital of Philadelphia, Philadelphia, Pennsylvania

**Gregory J. Dennis, MD, FACP, FACR**
Associate Professor, Department of Medicine, F. Edward Hebert School of Medicine; Uniformed Services University of the Health Sciences; Director of Clinical Program and Training, National Institute of Arthritis, Musculoskeletal, and Skin Diseases, Bethesda, Maryland

**Donald G. Eckhoff, MD, MS, FACS**
Professor, Department of Orthopedic Surgery, University of Colorado Health Sciences Center, Denver, Colorado

**Jennifer Rae Elliott, MD**
House Officer, Internal Medicine, University of Nebraska Medical Center, Omaha, Nebraska

**Raymond J. Enzenauer, MD, FACP, FACR**
Associate Professor of Medicine, Rheumatology Service, Department of Medicine, University of Tennessee College of Medicine-Chattanooga Unit; Erlanger Hospital, Chattanooga, Tennessee

**Alan R. Erickson, MD, FACR**
North Mississippi Medical Center, Tupelo, Mississippi

**David R. Finger, MD, FACP, FACR**
Chief, Rheumatology Service, Tripler Army Medical Center, Honolulu, Hawaii

**Terri H. Finkel, MD, PhD, FACR**
Associate Professor, Division Chief, Pediatric Rheumatology, Children's Hospital of Philadelphia/University of Pennsylvania, Philadelphia, Pennsylvania

**William R. Gilliland, MD, FACR**
Associate Professor, Department of Medicine, Uniformed Services University of the Health Sciences, Bethesda, Maryland

**Luis Gonzalez, MD**
Director, Department of Radiology, Northern Dutchess Hospital, Rhinebeck, New York

**Cliff A. Gronseth, MD**
Assistant Professor, Department of Rehabilitation Medicine, University of Colorado Health Sciences Center, Denver, Colorado

**Karen E. Hansen, MD, FACR**
Assistant Professor of Medicine, Rheumatology, University of Wisconsin; University of Wisconsin Hospital and Clinics; Chief of Rheumatology, William S. Middleton Memorial Veterans Affairs Hospital, Madison, Wisconsin

**Robert A. Hawkins, MD, FACP, FACR**
Associate Professor of Medicine, Department of Medicine, Wright State University School of Medicine, Dayton, Ohio; Kettering Medical Center, Kettering, Ohio

**Kathryn Hobbs, MD, FACR**
Assistant Clinical Professor of Medicine, Division of Rheumatology, Division of Allergy and Clinical Immunology, University of Colorado Health Sciences Center, Denver, Colorado

**V. Michael Holers, MD, FACR**
Professor of Medicine, University of Colorado Health Sciences Center; Attending Physician, University of Colorado Hospital, Denver, Colorado

**J. Roger Hollister, MD, FACR**
Professor, Department of Pediatrics, University of Colorado Health Sciences Center, Denver, Colorado

**Edmund H. Hornstein, DO, FACR**
Assistant Professor of Medicine, Chief, Rheumatology Division, Berkshire Medical Center; University of Massachusetts Medical School, Pittsfield, Massachusetts

**Robert W. Janson, MD, FACR**
Associate Professor of Medicine, Department of Medicine, Division of Rheumatology, University of Colorado Health Sciences Center; Chief, Rheumatology Section, Denver Veterans Affairs Medical Center, Denver, Colorado

**Mark Jarek, MD, FACP, FACR**
Cox Hospital, Springfield, Missouri

**John Keith Jenkins, MD, FACR**
Assistant Professor of Medicine, Division of Rheumatology/Molecular Immunology, University of Mississippi Medical Center, Jackson, Mississippi

**Brian L. Kotzin, MD, FACR**
Professor of Medicine and Immunology, Co-Head, Division of Clinical Immunology, University of Colorado Health Sciences Center, Denver, Colorado

**Elizabeth Kozora, PhD, ABPP**
Associate Professor, Departments of Medicine and Psychiatry, University of Colorado Health Sciences Center; National Jewish Medical and Research Center, Denver, Colorado

**James S. Louie, MD**
Professor of Medicine, UCLA School of Medicine; Chief, Division of Rheumatology, Harbor-UCLA Medical Center, Torrance, California

**Mark Malyak, MD, FACR**
Assistant Professor, Department of Medicine, Division of Rheumatology, University of Colorado Health Sciences Center, Denver, Colorado; Denver Arthritis Center, Denver, Colorado

**Kimberly P. May, MD, FACR**
Assistant Professor, F. Edward Hebert School of Medicine, Uniformed Services University of the Health Sciences, Bethesda, Maryland; Chief of Hospital Services, US Air Force Academy Hospital, Colorado Springs, Colorado

**Michael T. McDermott, MD, FACP**
Professor of Medicine, Division of Endocrinology, Metabolism and Diabetes, University of Colorado Health Sciences Center; University of Colorado Hospital and Denver Veterans Administration Medical Center, Denver, Colorado

**Richard T. Meehan, MD, FACP, FACR**
Chief of Rheumatology, Associate Professor of Medicine, National Jewish Medical Research Center, Denver, Colorado

**Michael O'Connell, MD, FAAI**
Assistant Clinical Professor, Department of Medicine, Division of Allergy and Clinical Immunology, University of Colorado Health Sciences Center, Denver, Colorado

**James R. O'Dell, MD, FACP, FACR**
Professor of Internal Medicine, Rheumatology, University of Nebraska Medical Center, Omaha, Nebraska

**Kevin M. Rak, MD**
Chief of Radiology, Department of Radiology, Divine Savior Hospital, Portage, Wisconsin

**James Singleton, MD, FACR**
Assistant Clinical Professor, Department of Medicine, University of Colorado Health Sciences Center, Denver, Colorado; South Denver Medicine Associates, Englewood, Colorado

**Robert T. Spencer, MD, FACR**
Assistant Clinical Professor of Medicine, Department of Medicine, Division of Rheumatology, University of Colorado Health Sciences Center; Swedish Medical Center and Porter Hospital, Denver, Colorado

**Scott Vogelgesang, MD, FACP, FACR**
Associate Professor, Division of Rheumatology, Department of Internal Medicine, University of Iowa, Iowa City, Iowa

**Sterling G. West, MD, FACP, FACR**
Professor, Department of Medicine, Division of Rheumatology, University of Colorado Health Sciences Center, Denver, Colorado

# DEDICATION

The Editor wishes to dedicate this book:

To my wife, Brenda, my best friend.

To my children, Dace and Matthew, the joys of my life.

To my sister, Karen, in heaven above. I love you.

To my parents, Patricia and Curtis, who taught me to pursue my dreams because all things are possible.

Their love, support, and encouragement make everything worthwhile.

# PREFACE

*In the past year, we have been so extensively authorized, approved, inspected, renovated, elevated, visited, consulted, circularized, informed; and have completed so many forms, orders, questionnaires, and reports that no medical progress has been made.*

Rudolf Virchow
Berlin, 1865

Notwithstanding Virchow's lament, there has indeed been progress in the field since the publication of the first edition of *Rheumatology Secrets*, and this is evidenced by the growth of the second edition by over 100 additional pages. Each chapter in the book has been extensively reviewed and updated, and a new chapter on the important area of pain management has been added.

As in the first edition, *Rheumatology Secrets, 2nd Edition*, is presented in the Socratic question and answer format that is the hallmark of *The Secrets Series*.® The chapters are organized into 16 sections, each with a common theme emphasized by an introductory quotation. Common and uncommon rheumatic disease problems that we encounter in clinical practice, discuss during teaching rounds, and find on board examinations are covered. Each chapter reviews basic immunology and pathophysiology, important disease manifestations, and practical management issues. The book also contains a wealth of mnemonics, lists, tables, and illustrations. We hope that the reader will find *Rheumatology Secrets, 2nd Edition*, both enjoyable and practically useful.

Sterling West, M.D.

## ACKNOWLEDGMENTS

As Editor, I want to thank:

All the contributors for their time and effort in writing their chapters,

Mrs. Helen Martinez for her exceptional administrative assistance throughout the preparation of this book,

The staff at Hanley & Belfus for their help and patience, and for giving me the opportunity to edit *Rheumatology Secrets*,

My patients, teachers, and students for what they have taught me.

# I. General Concepts

*The rheumatism is a common name for many aches and pains, which have yet no peculiar appellation, though owing to very different causes.*
William Heberden (1710–1801)
*Commentaries on the History and Cure of Diseases, ch. 79.*

## 1. CLASSIFICATION AND HEALTH IMPACT OF THE RHEUMATIC DISEASES

Sterling G. West, M.D.

**1. What is rheumatology?**
A medical science devoted to the study of rheumatic diseases and musculoskeletal disorders.

**2. What are the roots of rheumatology?**

| | |
|---|---|
| 1st century AD | The term *rheuma* first appears in the literature. *Rheuma* refers to "a substance that flows" and probably was derived from *phlegm*, an ancient primary humor, which was believed to originate from the brain and flow to various parts of the body causing ailments. |
| 1642 | The word *rheumatism* is introduced into the literature by the French physician Dr. G. Baillou, who emphasized that arthritis could be a systemic disorder. |
| 1928 | The American Committee for the Control of Rheumatism is established in the United States by Dr. R. Pemberton. Renamed American Association for the Study and Control of Rheumatic Disease (1934), then American Rheumatism Association (1937), and finally, American College of Rheumatology (ACR) (1988). |
| 1940s | The terms *rheumatology* and *rheumatologist* are first coined by Drs. Hollander and Comroe, respectively. |

**3. How many rheumatic/musculoskeletal disorders are there?**
Over 120.

**4. How have these rheumatic/musculoskeletal disorders been classified over the years?**

| | |
|---|---|
| 1904 | Dr. Goldthwaite, an orthopedic surgeon, makes the first attempt to classify the arthritides. He had five categories: gout, infectious arthritis, hypertrophic arthritis (probably osteoarthritis), atrophic arthritis (probably rheumatoid arthritis). and chronic villous arthritis (probably traumatic arthritis). |
| 1964 | American Rheumatism Association (ARA) classification |
| 1983 | The ARA classification is revised based on plans to revise the 9th edition of the *International Classification of Disease (ICD 9). ICD 10* is at present being developed. |

**5. The 1983 ARA classification is overwhelming. Is there a simpler outline to remember?**
Most of the rheumatic diseases can be grouped into 10 major categories:

I. Systemic connective tissue diseases
II. Vasculitides and related disorders
III. Seronegative spondyloarthropathies
IV. Arthritis associated with infectious agents
V. Rheumatic disorders associated with metabolic, endocrine, and hematologic disease
VI. Bone and cartilage disorders
VII. Hereditary, congenital, and inborn errors of metabolism associated with rheumatic syndromes
VIII. Nonarticular and regional musculoskeletal disorders
IX. Neoplasms and tumorlike lesions
X. Miscellaneous rheumatic disorders

**6. What is the origin and difference between a collagen-vascular disease and a connective tissue disease?**

1942 Dr. Klemperer introduces the term *diffuse collagen disease* based on his pathologic studies of systemic lupus erythematosus (SLE) and scleroderma.

1946 Dr. Rich coins the term *collagen-vascular disease* based on his pathologic studies in vasculitis indicating that the primary lesion involved the vascular endothelium.

1952 Dr. Ehrich suggests the term *connective tissue diseases*, which has gradually replaced the term *collagen-vascular diseases*.

In summary, the two terms are used synonymously, although the purist would say that the heritable collagen disorders (Chapter 59) are the only true "diffuse collagen diseases."

**7. How common are rheumatic/musculoskeletal disorders in the general population?**

Approximately 30% of the population has symptoms of arthritis and/or back pain. Only two thirds of these patients (i.e., 20% of the population) have symptoms severe enough to cause them to seek medical care. The prevalence of musculoskeletal disorders increases with the age of the patient population.

**8. What is the estimated prevalence for the various rheumatic/musculoskeletal disorders in the general population?**

*Estimated Prevalence of Rheumatic/Musculoskeletal Disorders in the U.S. Population*

| | PREVALENCE | NUMBER OF PATIENTS |
|---|---|---|
| All musculoskeletal disorders | 15–20% | 54 million |
| Arthropathies | | |
| Osteoarthritis | 12% | 21 million |
| Rheumatoid arthritis | 1% | 2.1 million |
| Juvenile rheumatoid arthritis | < .1% | 50,000 |
| Crystalline arthritis | 1% | 2–3 million |
| Spondyloarthropathies | .25% | 400,000 |
| Connective tissue disease | | |
| SLE | < .1% | 240,000 |
| Scleroderma | < .01% | 50,000 |
| Back/neck pain—frequent | 15% | 32 million |
| Soft tissue rheumatism | 3–5% | 5–10 million |
| Fibromyalgia | 2% | 3.7 million |

Overall 2% of the population have an inflammatory auotimmune disease with 50% of these patients having rheumatoid arthritis. For comparison, about 20 million people in the general population are being treated for hypertension, and 5 million people have diabetes mellitus.

**9. How often are one of the rheumatic/musculoskeletal disorders likely to be seen in an average primary care practice?**

About 1 out of every 5–10 office visits to a primary care provider is for a musculoskeletal disorder. Interestingly, 66% of these patients are < 65 years old. The most common problems are osteoarthritis, back pain, gout, fibromyalgia, and tendinitis/bursitis.

**10. How many rheumatologists are there in the United States?**

There are approximately 4000 board-certified rheumatologists. This number is projected to decrease over the next 10 years. This is why the delay to see a rheumatologist is so long.

**11. Discuss the impact of the rheumatic/musculoskeletal diseases on the general population in terms of morbidity and mortality.**

*Morbidity and Mortality of Rheumatic/Musculoskeletal Diseases*

| | PERCENT OF POPULATION |
|---|---|
| Symptoms of arthritis | 30% |
| Symptoms requiring medical therapy | 20% |
| Disability due to arthritis | 5–10% |
| Totally disabled from arthritis | 0.5% |
| Mortality from rheumatic disease | 0.02% |

Arthritis/back pain is the second leading cause of acute disability (behind respiratory illness) and is the number one cause of chronic disability in the general population. Ten percent of all surgical procedures are for disabilities related to arthritis.

**12. What is the economic impact of the rheumatic/musculoskeletal diseases?**

The 54 million patients (20% of U.S. population) with chronic musculoskeletal disorders cost the economy 193 billion dollars (2.5% of GNP) a year in direct health care expenditures for their musculoskeletal and nonmusculoskeletal conditions. The largest components of this cost are hospitalizations (37%), physician visits (23%), and prescriptions (16%). Overall, patients with musculoskeletal disorders incur 38% of all medical expenditures, which is 75% greater than any other chronic medical condition. The incremental cost for just the musculoskeletal conditions alone is 39 billion dollars (.5% of GNP).

Approximately 30% of working-age persons age (18–64) with arthritis are unable to work or cannot work in their usual occupation due to their disease. Consequently, 77 billion dollars in indirect costs due to lost wages needs to be added to the total direct medical costs in order to appreciate the full economic impact of musculoskeletal conditions.

## BIBLIOGRAPHY


1. Benedek TG: A century of American rheumatology. Ann Intern Med 106:304–312, 1987.
2. Bradley EM: The provision of rheumatologic services. In Klippel JH, Dieppe PA (eds): Rheumatology, London, Mosby, 1994, pp 1-9.1–1-9.10.
3. Decker JL, Glossary Subcommittee of the ARA Committee on Rheumatologic Practice: American Rheumatism Association nomenclature and classification of arthritis and rheumatism. Arthritis Rheum 26:1029–1032, 1983.
4. Reynolds MD: Origins of the concept of collagen—vascular diseases. Semin Arthritis Rheum 15:127–131, 1985.
5. Yelin E, Callahan LF: The economic cost and social and psychological impact of musculoskeletal conditions. Arthritis Rheum 38:1351–1362, 1995.
6. Lawrence RC, Helmick CG, Arnett FC, et al: Estimates of the prevalence of arthritis and selected musculoskeletal disorders in the United States. Arthritis Rheum 41:778–799, 1998.
7. Yelin E, Herrndorf A, Trupin L, Sonneborn D: A national study of medical care expenditures for musculoskeletal conditions. Arthritis Rheum 44:1160–1169, 2001.

# 2. RHEUMATOLOGY'S TEN GOLDEN RULES

Sterling G. West, M.D.

*A physician is judged by the three A's—ability, availability, and affability.*
Paul Reznihoff
*Aphorism*

Rheumatology can be confusing to many physicians during their housestaff training (and beyond!). Although nothing in medicine is 100%, I have found the following "golden rules" valuable when evaluating a patient with a rheumatic/musculoskeletal problem. I have limited the rules to 10, but certainly many others could be added:

1. A good **history** and **physical examination**, coupled with knowledge of musculoskeletal anatomy, is most important when evaluating a patient with a rheumatic disorder. You have to examine the patient!
2. Don't order a **laboratory test** unless you know why you're ordering it and what you will do if it comes back abnormal.
3. Patients with an acute inflammatory monoarticular arthritis need a **joint aspiration** to rule out septic arthritis and crystalline arthropathy.
4. Most patients with a chronic inflammatory monoarticular arthritis of > 8 weeks' duration, whose evaluation has failed to define an etiology for the arthritis, need **a synovial biopsy**.
5. **Gout** usually does not occur in premenopausal women or affect joints close to the spine.
6. Most **shoulder pain** is periarticular (i.e., a bursitis or tendinitis), and most **low-back pain** is nonsurgical.
7. Patients with **osteoarthritis** affecting joints not normally affected by primary osteoarthritis (i.e., metacarpophalangeals, wrists, elbows, shoulder, ankles) need to be evaluated for secondary causes of osteoarthritis (i.e., metabolic diseases, others).
8. Primary **fibromyalgia** does not occur for the first time in patients after the age of 55 years, nor is it likely to be the correct diagnosis in patients with musculoskeletal pain who also have abnormal laboratory values.
9. All patients with a positive **rheumatoid factor** do not have rheumatoid arthritis, and all patients with a positive **antinuclear antibody** do not have systemic lupus erythematosus.
10. In a patient with a known systemic rheumatic disease who presents with fever or multisystem complaints, rule out **infection** and possibly other nonrheumatic etiologies before attributing the symptoms and signs to the underlying rheumatic disease. Clearly, infection causes death of rheumatic disease patients more often than underlying rheumatic disease does.

Remember, nothing is 100%!

# 3. ANATOMY AND PHYSIOLOGY OF THE MUSCULOSKELETAL SYSTEM

*Sterling G. West, M.D.*

**1. Name two major functions of the musculoskeletal system.**

Structural support and purposeful motion. The activities of the human body depend on the effective interaction between joints and the neuromuscular units that move them.

**2. Name the five components of the musculoskeletal system.**

(1) Muscles, (2) Tendons, (3) Ligaments, (4) Cartilage, (5) Bone. All of these structures contribute to the formation of a functional and mobile joint.

**3. The different connective tissues differ in their composition of macromolecules. List the macromolecular "building blocks" of connective tissue.**

Collagen, elastin and adhesins, and proteoglycans.

## COLLAGEN

**4. How many types of collagen are there? In which tissues is each type most commonly found?**

The collagens are the most abundant body proteins and account for 20–30% of the total body mass. There are at least 19 different types of collagen divided into seven subclasses. The unique properties and organization of each collagen type enable that specific collagen to contribute to the function of the tissue of which it is the principal structural component.

*Collagen Types, Tissue Distribution, and Diseases Caused by Mutations*

| CLASSES | TISSUE DISTRIBUTION | DISEASE |
|---|---|---|
| **Fibril-forming (interstitial) collagens** | | |
| Type I | Bone, tendon, skin, joint capsule/synovium | OI, ED |
| Type II | Hyaline cartilage, disk, vitreous humor | CD, Stickler's |
| Type III | Blood vessels, skin, lung | ED, type IV |
| Type V | Same as type I | ED, types I & II |
| Type XI | Same as type II | SED |
| **Network-forming collagens** | | |
| Type IV | Basement membrane | Alport's |
| Type VIII | Endothelium | |
| Type X | Growth plate cartilage | MD |
| **FACIT collagens** | | |
| Type IX | Same as type II, cornea | MED |
| Type XII | Same as type I | |
| Type XIV | Same as type I | |
| Type XVI | Several tissues | |
| Type XIX | Rhabdomyosarcoma cells | |
| **Beaded filament-forming collagen** | | |
| Type VI | Most connective tissues | |
| **Collagen of anchoring fibrils** | | |
| Type VII | Dermoepidermal, cornea, oral mucosa | Epidermolysis bullosa |

(*Table continued on next page.*)

*Collagen Types, Tissue Distribution, and Diseases Caused by Mutations (cont.)*

| CLASSES | TISSUE DISTRIBUTION | DISEASE |
|---|---|---|
| **Collagen with a transmembrane domain** | | |
| Type XIII | Endomysium, placenta, meninges | |
| Type XVII | Skin, cornea | |
| **Other collagen** | | |
| Type XV | Many tissues, especially muscle | |
| Type XVIII | Many tissues | |

OI = osteogenesis imperfecta; ED = Ehlers-Danlos; CD = chondrodysplasia; SED = spondyloepiphyseal dysplasia; MED = multiple epiphyseal dysplasia; MD = metaphyseal dysplasia.

**5. Discuss the structural features common to all collagen molecules.**

The definitive structural feature of all collagen molecules is the **triple helix**. This unique conformation is due to three polypeptide chains (α-chains) twisted around each other into a right-handed major helix. Extending from the amino and carboxyl terminal ends of both helical domains of the α-chains are nonhelical components called telopeptides. In the major interstitial collagens, the helical domains are continuous, whereas in the other collagen classes the helical domains may be interrupted by 1 to 12 nonhelical segments.

The primary structure of the helical domain of the α-chain is characterized by the repeating triplet Gly-*X*-*Y*. *X* and *Y* can be any amino acid but are most frequently proline and hydroxyproline, respectively. Overall, approximately 25% of the residues in the triple helical domains consist of proline and hydroxyproline. Hydroxylysine is also commonly found. In the most abundant interstitial collagens (i.e., type I, II), the triple helical region contains about 1000 amino acid residues, $(\text{Gly-}X\text{-Y})_{333}$.

Diagram of interstitial (fibrillar) collagen molecule demonstrating triple helix configuration with terminal telopeptides.

**6. Identify the major collagen classes and the types of collagen included in each class.**

- Fibril-forming (interstitial)—types I, II, III, V, XI. The most abundant collagen class, these collagens form the extracellular fabric of the major connective tissues. They have the same tensile strength as steel wire.
- Fibril-associated collagens with interrupted triple helices (FACIT)—types IX, XII, XIV. XVI, XIX. These collagens are associated with the interstitial (fibrillar) collagens and occur in the same tissues.
- Collagens with specialized structures or functions:
  Basement membrane collagen—type IV
  Nonfibrillar collagens—types VI, VII, XIII, XV, XVII, XVIII
  Short-chain collagens—types VIII, X

**7. How are the fibril-forming (interstitial) collagens synthesized?**

1. There are at least 20 distinct genes encoding the various collagen chains. The collagen genes studied thus far contain coding sequences (exons) interrupted by large, noncoding sequences (introns). The DNA is transcribed to form a precursor mRNA, which is processed to functional mRNA by excising and splicing, which remove mRNA coded by introns. The

processed mRNAs leave the nucleus and are transported to the polyribosomal apparatus in the rough endoplasmic reticulum for translation into polypeptide chains.

2. The polypeptide chains are hydroxylated by prolyl hydroxylase and lysine hydroxylase. These enzymes require $O_2$ $Fe^{2+}$, α-ketoglutarate, and ascorbic acid (vitamin C) as cofactors. Hydroxyproline is critical to the stable formation of the triple helix. A decrease in hydroxyproline content as seen in scurvy (ascorbic acid deficiency) results in unstable molecules that lose their structures and are broken down by proteases.

3. Glycosylation of hydroxylysine residues, which is important for secretion of procollagen monomers (molecules).

4. Formation of interchain disulfide links, followed by procollagen triple-helix formation.

5. Secretion of procollagen into the extracellular space.

6. Proteolysis by procollagen peptidase of amino and carboxyl terminal telopeptides, resulting in conversion of procollagen to collagen.

7. Assembly of collagen monomers (molecules) into fibrils (microfibrils) by quarter-stagger shift, followed by cross-linking of fibrils.

8. End-to-end and lateral aggregation of fibrils to form collagen fiber.

Each collagen molecule is 300 nm in length and 1.5 nm in width and has five charged regions 68 nm apart. The charged regions align in a straight line when the fibrils are formed, even though the individual molecules themselves are staggered a quarter of their lengths in relation to each other. One can easily see that there are multiple steps where defects in collagen biosynthesis could result in abnormalities leading to disease (see also Chapter 59).

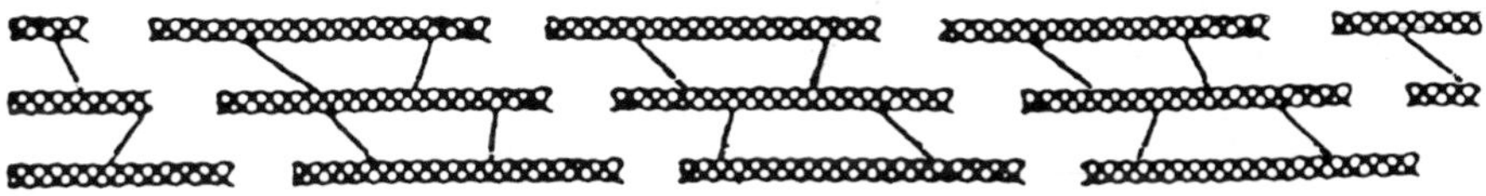

Self-assembly of collagen molecules into fibrils with cross-linking.

**8. Which enzymes are important in collagen degradation? How are they regulated?**

The most important collagenolytic enzymes responsible for cleavage of type I collagen belong to the **matrix metalloproteinase (MMP) group**. The collagenases are secreted in latent form and, when activated, cleave the collagen molecule at a single specific site 75% from the amino terminal end (between residues 775–776 of α1[I] chain). Gelatinases and stromelysins degrade the unfolded fragments.

Both α-macroglobulin and tissue inhibitors of metalloproteases (TIMPs) are capable of inhibiting collagenase activity. It is likely that other collagen types have type-specific collagenases capable of degrading them. Serum procollagen peptides, urinary hydroxyproline, urinary pyridinoline/deoxypyridinoline cross-links, and serum and urinary *N*-telopeptides are used as measures of collagen turnover.

## ELASTIN AND ADHESINS

**9. What is elastin, and where is it located?**

Elastin fibers are connective tissues that can stretch when hydrated and return to their original length after being stretched. They comprise a significant portion of the dry weight of ligaments (up to 70–80%), lungs, larger blood vessels such as aorta (30–60%), and skin (2–5%). Elastin is a polymer of tropoelastin monomers, which contain 850 amino acids, predominantly valine, proline, glycine, and alanine. When tropoelastin molecules associate to form a fiber, lysine residues cross-link by forming desmosine and isodesmosine, which are unique to elastin. Mutations in the elastin gene can cause cutis laxa and supravalvular aortic stenosis. Elastases, which are serine proteases, are capable of degrading elastase. Elastases are located in tissues, macrophages, leukocytes, and platelets. Such elastases may contribute to blood vessel wall damage and aneurysm formation in the vasculitides. Urinary desmosine levels are used as a measure of elastin degradation.

**10. What are fibrillin-1 and fibrillin-2?**

These fibrillins are large glycoproteins coded for by a gene located on chromosome 15 (fibrillin-1) and chromosome 5 (fibrillin-2). They function as part of the microfibrillar proteins, which are associated with an elastin core. Fibrillin can also be found as isolated bundles of microfibrils in skin, blood vessels, and several other tissues. Abnormalities in fibrillin-1 are thought to cause Marfan's syndrome (see also Chapter 59), while abnormalities in fibrillin-2 cause contractural arachnodactyly.

**11. List the important adhesins (cell-binding glycoproteins) that can be present in intracellular matrices and basement membranes.**

Fibronectin—connective tissue
Laminin—basement membrane
Chondroadherin—cartilage
Osteoadherin—bone

These glycoproteins have specific adhesive and other important properties. They bind cells by attaching to integrins on cells. Some have the classical arginine-glycine-aspartic acid (RGD) cell-binding sequence.

## PROTEOGLYCANS

**12. How do a proteoglycan and a glycosaminoglycan differ?**

**Proteoglycans** are glycoproteins that contain one or more sulfated glycosaminoglycan (GAG) chains. They are classified according to their core protein, which is coded for by distinct genes.

**GAGs** are usually classified into five types: chondroitin sulfate, dermatan sulfate, heparan sulfate, heparin, and keratan sulfate. GAGs make up part of proteoglycans.

**13. How are proteoglycans distributed?**

Proteoglycans are synthesized by all connective tissue cells. They can remain associated with these cells on their cell surface (syndecan, betaglycan), intracellularly (serglycin), or in the basement membrane (perlecan). These cell-associated proteoglycans commonly contain heparin/heparan sulfate or chondroitin sulfate as their major GAGs. Alternatively, proteoglycans can be secreted into the extracellular matrix (aggrecan, decorin, biglycan, fibromodulin, lumican). These matrix proteoglycans usually contain chondroitin sulfate, dermatan sulfate, or keratan sulfate as their major GAGs. Decorin helps bind type II collagen fibers together in cartilage, while fibromodulin and lumican bind type II collagen to type IX.

**14. How are proteoglycans metabolized in the body?**

Proteoglycans are degraded by proteinases, which release the GAGs. The GAGs are taken up by cells by endocytosis, where they are degraded in lysosomes by a series of glycosidases and sulfatases. Defects in these degradative enzymes can lead to diseases called **mucopolysaccharidoses**.

## MUSCULOSKELETAL SYSTEM

**15. Discuss the classification of joints.**

- **Synarthrosis**: Suture lines of the skull where adjoining cranial plates are separated by thin fibrous tissue.
- **Amphiarthroses**: Adjacent bones are bound by flexible fibrocartilage that permits limited motion to occur. Examples include the pubic symphysis, part of the sacroiliac joint, and intervertebral discs.

- **Diarthroses** (synovial joints): These are the most common and most mobile joints. All have a synovial lining. They are subclassified into ball and socket (hip), hinge (interphalangeal), saddle (first carpometacarpal), and plane (patellofemoral) joints.

**16. What major tissues comprise a diarthroidal (synovial) joint?**

A diarthroidal joint consists of **hyaline cartilage** covering the surfaces of two or more opposing bones. These articular tissues are surrounded by a **capsule** that is lined by **synovium**. Some joints contain **menisci**, which are made of fibrocartilage. Note that the joint cavity is a potential space. The pressure within normal joints is negative (–5.7 cm $H_2O$) compared with ambient atmospheric pressure.

**17. Describe the microanatomy of normal synovium.**

Normal synovium contains synovial lining cells that are 1–3 cells deep. Synovium lines all intracapsular structures except the contact areas of articular cartilage. The synovial lining cells reside in a matrix rich in type I collagen and proteoglycans.

There are two main types of synovial lining cells, but these can be differentiated only by electron microscopy. **Type A** cells are macrophage-like and have primarily a phagocytic function. **Type B** cells are fibroblast-like and produce hyaluronate, which accounts for the increased viscosity of synovial fluid.

Other cells found in the synovium include antigen-presenting cells called dendritic cells and mast cells. The synovium does not have a limiting basement membrane. Synovial tissue also contains fat and lymphatic vessels, fenestrated microvessels, and nerve fibers derived from the capsule and periarticular tissues.

**18. Why is synovial fluid viscous?**

Hyaluronic acid, synthesized by synovial lining cells (type B), is secreted into the synovial fluid, making the fluid viscous. Synovia means "like egg white," which describes the normal viscosity of synovial fluid.

**19. What are the physical characteristics of normal synovial fluid from the knee joint?**

Color—colorless and transparent
Amount—thin film covering surfaces of synovium and cartilage within joint space
Cell count—$< 200/mm^3$ with $< 25\%$ neutrophils
Protein—1.3–1.7 g/dl (20% of normal plasma protein)
Glucose—within 20 mg/dl of the serum glucose level after 6 hours of fasting
Temperature—32°C (peripheral joints are cooler than core body temperature)
String sign (measure of viscosity)—1–2 inches
pH—7.4

**20. What is the function, structure, and composition of articular cartilage?**

Articular cartilage is **avascular** and **aneural**. It serves as a load-bearing connective tissue that can absorb impact and withstand shearing forces. Its ability to do this relates to the unique composition and structure of its extracellular matrix.

Normal cartilage is composed of a sparse population of specialized cells called **chondrocytes** that are responsible for the synthesis and replenishment of extracellular matrix. This matrix consists mainly of collagen and proteoglycans. Most of the collagen is type II (> 90%), which makes up 50–60% of the *dry* weight of cartilage. Collagen forms a fiber network that provides shape and form to the cartilage tissue.

Proteoglycans comprise the second largest portion of articular cartilage. The proteoglycan monomers (aggrecan) are large (MW = 2–3 million) and contain mostly keratan sulfate and chondroitin sulfate GAGs. The proteoglycans are arranged into supramolecular aggregates consisting of a central hyaluronic acid filament to which multiple proteoglycan monomers are noncovalently attached and stabilized by a link protein.

The entire structure looks like a large "bottle brush" and has a MW of 200 million. These proteoglycans are stuffed into the collagen framework. The negative charge of the proteoglycans causes them to spread out until the elastic forces are balanced by the tensile forces of the collagen. Note that other collagens (types V, VI, IX, X, XI), proteins (chondroadherin, others), and lipid are also in cartilage.

Water is the most abundant component of articular cartilage and accounts for 80% of the tissue wet weight. Water is held in cartilage by its interaction with matrix proteoglycan aggregates.

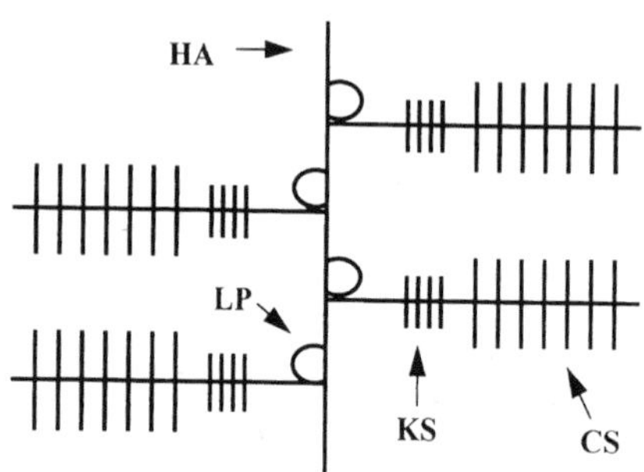


Diagram of proteoglycan aggregate in articular cartilage. Hyaluronate (HA) is the backbone of the aggregate. Proteoglycan monomers (aggrecan) arise at intervals from either side of the hyaluronate core. LP = link protein; KS = keratan sulfate; CS = chondroitin sulfate.

**21. What are the four zones of cartilage?**

The different molecular components of cartilage are highly organized into a structure that varies with the depth of cartilage. From top to bottom, these four zones include:

1. **Superficial (tangential) zone** (10%)—smallest zone. Collagen fibers are thin and are oriented horizontally to subchondral bone. Low GAG content. This zone is called the **lamina splendens**.
2. **Middle (transitional) zone** (50%)—largest zone. Collagen fibers are thicker and start to be arranged into radial bundles. High proteoglycan and water content.
3. **Deep (radial) zone** (20%)—largest collagen fibers arranged radially (perpendicular) to subchondral bone. Many chondrocytes.
4. **Calcified zone**—separates cartilage from subchondral bone. Collagen fibers penetrate into this zone and anchor the cartilage to the bone.

**22. Since cartilage doesn't have a blood supply, how do chondrocytes obtain nutrition?**

Adult cartilage is avascular, and chondrocytes obtain nutrients through diffusion. The nutrients are derived from the synovial fluid. Diffusion is facilitated during joint loading. With joint loading, some of the water in the cartilage is squeezed out into the synovial space. When the joint is unloaded, the hydrophilic properties of the cartilage proteoglycans cause the water to be sucked back into the cartilage. As the water returns to the cartilage, diffusion of nutrients from the synovial fluid is facilitated.

**23. If cartilage is not innervated, why do patients with osteoarthritis have pain?**

Patients experience pain due to irritation of the subchondral bone, which is exposed as the cartilage degenerates. Additionally, accumulation of synovial fluid can cause pain through distention of the innervated joint capsule and synovium. Mild synovial inflammation also causes pain.

**24. Describe the lubrication of diarthroidal joints.**

Diarthroidal (synovial) joints serve as mechanical bearings with coefficients of friction lower than the friction an ice skate generates as it glides over ice. Their three major sources of lubrication are:

- Hydrodynamic lubrication: Loading of the articular cartilage causes compression that forces water out of the cartilage. This fluid forms an aqueous layer that separates and protects the opposing cartilage surfaces.
- Boundary layer lubrication: A small glycoprotein called **lubricin**, which is produced by synovial lining cells, binds to articular cartilage where it retains a protective layer of water molecules.
- Hyaluronic acid: Produced by synovial lining cells, this molecule lubricates the contact surface between synovium and cartilage. It does not contribute to cartilage on cartilage lubrication.

**25. Discuss the normal matrix turnover of articular cartilage.**

In normal articular cartilage, chondrocytes rarely divide. Chondrocytes synthesize and replace the extracellular matrix components. Proteoglycans have a faster turnover rate ($t^1/_2$ of weeks) compared with collagen ($t^1/_2$ of months). The degradation of these macromolecules is accomplished by proteolytic enzymes. Metalloproteases, such as collagenases (MMP-1, 8, 13), stromelysins (MMP-3, 10), and gelatinases (MMP-2, 9), are the most important. Cytokines such as interleukin-1 and tumor necrosis factor-α can upregulate the degradative process, while transforming growth factor-β and insulin-like growth factor-1 have an anabolic effect on chondrocyte metabolism. Assays using monoclonal antibodies to measure type II collagen and proteoglycans (keratan sulfate, COMP) in bodily fluids have been used to detect cartilage breakdown.

**26. What is the difference between a ligament and a tendon?**

A **ligament** is a specialized form of connective tissue attaching one bone to another. It frequently reinforces the joint capsule and provides stability to the joint. A **tendon** attaches a muscle to a bone. Both are comprised mostly of type I collagen.

**27. Discuss the types and composition of bone.**

Bone is a mineralized connective tissue. It is comprised of two subtypes: **cortical** (or compact) bone and **cancellous** (or trabecular) bone. Cortical bone comprises 80% of the skeleton and is increased in long bone shafts. Cancellous bone is in contact with bone marrow cells and is enriched in the vertebral bodies, pelvis, and proximal ends of femora, all of which are subject to osteoporosis and fractures.

Bone is comprised mainly of type I collagen and contains three cell types: **osteoclasts**, which resorb mineralized bone; **osteoblasts**, which synthesize the proteins of the bone matrix; and **osteocytes**, which are probably osteoblasts that have secreted bone matrix and become buried within it. Osteocytes communicate with each other through a canalicular system. The skeleton contains 99% of the total body calcium, 80–85% of the phosphorus, and 66% of the magnesium.

**28. What is RANKL?**

RANKL (receptor activator of NF-κ B ligand) is a member of the tumor necrosis factor (TNF) superfamily. RANKL is a cell membrane–bound ligand on osteoblasts and activated T cells. It binds RANK on osteoclast precursors, which causes the osteoclast to differentiate and become activated. Osteoprotegrin (OPG) is a soluble, secreted member of the TNF receptor family that competitively binds RANKL and prevents its binding to RANK, thus inhibiting osteoclastogenesis. Expression of RANKL on osteoblasts is stimulated through vitamin D receptor (1,25 OH vitamin $D_3$), protein kinase A ($PGE_2$, parathyroid hormone), and gp 130 (IL-11). The periarticular osteoporosis seen on radiographs of individuals with inflammatory arthritis may be through local production of $PGE_2$ and interleukins (TNFα, IL-1), causing up regulation of RANKL on osteoblasts and T cells leading to osteoclast activation. Conversely, OPG may be a useful therapy for osteoporosis in the future. (See figure, top of next page.)

**29. How many muscles are in the human body?**

Approximately 640. Muscles constitute up to 40% of the adult body mass.

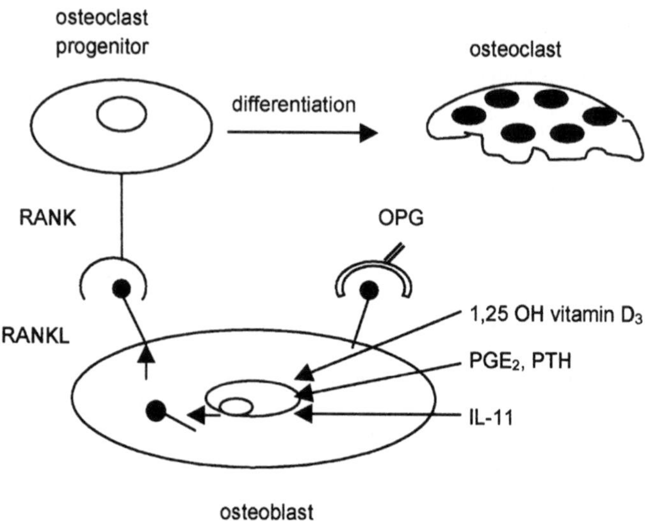


RANKL–RANK-OPG system.

**30. Discuss the morphology of muscle.**

Skeletal muscle consists of cells called **fibers**. Fibers are grouped into **fascicles**.

Muscle fibers are part of **motor units** that consist of a lower motor neuron originating from a spinal cord anterior horn cell and all the muscle fibers it innervates. All muscle fibers within a motor unit are of the same type. Different fibers within a single fascicle are innervated by different motor neurons.

Muscle fibers are divided into three types based on their metabolism and response to stimuli: types 1, 2a, and 2b. Fiber type can be altered by reinnervation with a different motor neuron type, physical training (controversial), or disease processes. However, heredity is the most important determinant of fiber type distribution. On average, muscle contains 40% type 1 and 60% type 2 fibers.

Each muscle fiber is surrounded by a plasma membrane called a **sarcolemma**. Fibers contain **myofilaments** called actin, troponin, tropomyosin, and myosin, which are contractile proteins. The myofilaments are bathed in sarcoplasm and organized into **fibrils**, which are enveloped by the sarcoplasmic reticulum. Communication between the sarcolemma and sarcoplasmic reticulum occurs through a channel network called the **T-tubule system**.

**31. Describe the characteristics of the three types of muscle fibers.**

- **Type 1** (slow twitch, oxidative fibers) (red fiber): Respond to electrical stimuli slowly. Fatigue-resistant with repeated stimulation. Many mitochondria and higher lipid content. Endurance training (long-distance running) enhances metabolism of these fibers.
- **Type 2a** (fast twitch, oxidative-glycolytic fibers): Properties intermediate between type 1 and type 2b.
- **Type 2b** (fast twitch, glycolytic fibers) (white fiber): Respond rapidly and with greater force of contraction but fatigue rapidly. These fibers contain more glycogen and have higher myophosphorylase and myoadenylate deaminase activity. Strength training (weight-lifting, sprinters, jumpers) leads to hypertrophy of these fibers.

**32. How does muscle contraction and relaxation occur?**

Muscle contraction occurs by shortening of myofilaments within muscle fibers. Stimulation causes an **action potential** to be transmitted along the sarcolemma, then through the T-tubule system to the sarcoplasmic reticulum. This causes release of calcium into the sarcoplasm. As the calcium concentration increases, **actin** is released from a state of inhibition, allowing actin-myosin cross-linkage and shortening of the myofilaments. The muscle fiber shortens until calcium is actively pumped back into the sarcoplasmic reticulum, which breaks the cross-links causing the fiber to relax. ATP, electrolytes (Na, K, Ca, Mg) and three ATPase proteins contribute to normal fiber contraction and relaxation. (See also Chapter 76.)

## BIBLIOGRAPHY

1. The musculoskeletal system. In Klippel JH (ed): Primer on the Rheumatic Diseases, 11th ed. Atlanta, Arthritis Foundation, 1997, pp 10–27.
2. Ala-Kokko L, Prockop DJ: Collagen and elastin. In Ruddy S, Harris ED, Sledge CB (eds): Kelley's Textbook of Rheumatology, 6th ed., Philadelphia, WB Saunders, 2001, pp 27–40.
3. Heinegard D, Lorenzo P, Saxne T: Matrix glycoproteins, proteoglycans, and cartilage. In Ruddy S, Harris ED, Sledge CB (eds): Kelley's Textbook of Rheumatology, 6th ed. Philadelphia, WB Saunders, 2001, pp 41–54.
4. Okada Y: Proteinases and matrix degradation. In Ruddy S, Harris ED, Sledge CB (eds): Kelley's Textbook of Rheumatology, 6th ed. Philadelphia, WB Saunders, 2001, pp 55–72.

# II. Scientific Basis of the Rheumatic Diseases

*The origin of all science is in the desire to know causes.*
William Hazlitt, 1829

*Science has been seriously retarded by the study of what is not worth knowing, and what is not knowable.*
Johann Wolfgang von Goethe, 1825

## 4. OVERVIEW OF THE IMMUNE RESPONSE

Michael O'Connell, M.D.

**1. What are the two broad categories of immunity involved in host defense?**

*Categories of Immunity*

| | NATURAL (INNATE) IMMUNITY | ACQUIRED (SPECIFIC/ADAPTIVE) IMMUNITY |
|---|---|---|
| Physical barriers | Skin, mucous membranes | Mucosal immune systems |
| Circulating factors | Complement, CRP, MBL | Antibody |
| Cells | Macrophages, neutrophils, NK | Lymphocytes |
| Cell-derived mediators | Monokines (IL-1, TNF, IL-12, interferons) | Lymphokines (interleukins) |

CRP = C-reactive protein; MBL = mannose-binding lectin; NK = natural killer

**2. What is the function of the innate immune system (IIS)?**

The IIS is phylogenetically older than the acquired (specific/adaptive) immune system. Since clonal expansion of lymphocytes in the acquired immune system takes 3–5 days to differentiate into effector cells, there needs to be a system capable of controlling a pathogen during that time so it doesn't damage the host. The effector mechanism of the IIS is activated immediately and can rapidly control the replication of the infecting pathogens until the lymphocytes can deal with it. Furthermore, the IIS can interact with and control the adaptive immune responses. Failure to do this may contribute to the development of autoimmune disease.

**3. What are the mechanisms that the innate immune system uses to recognize that an invading pathogen is foreign?**

The strategy of the IIS is to recognize a few highly conserved structures present in large groups of organisms. These structures are called pathogen-associated molecular patterns (PAMP), and the receptors of the IIS that recognize them are called pattern-recognition receptors. PAMPs are produced only by microbial pathogens and not by the host. Examples of PAMPs include bacterial lipopolysaccharides, peptidoglycan, mannans, and bacterial DNA/RNA.

Once the macrophages interact with PAMPs, they release cytokines (IL-1, TNFα, IL-8) that recruit and activate neutrophils and other leukocytes. Other cytokines that are released enhance microbial activities of phagocytes (interferon γ) and stimulate natural killer (IL-15) and Th1 cell-mediated immune responses (IL-12, IL-18).

**4. Name the pattern-recognition receptors that recognize PAMPs.**

- Mannan-binding lectin—this receptor is synthesized in the liver and secreted into the serum as part of the acute-phase response. It binds to microbial carbohydrates to initiate the lectin pathway of complement activation. The mannan-binding lectin has associated proteases that function like Clr and Cls to activate the classical complement pathway.

- Mannose receptor—a receptor on the surface of macrophages that recognizes mannoses on microorganisms and mediates their phagocytosis by macrophages.
- Toll-like receptors—there are at least ten mammalian toll-like receptors. They are on cell surfaces and recognize many of the PAMPs. Once stimulated, these receptors lead to activation of cell signaling pathways like NF-κ B pathway. This results in induction of inflammatory and immune response genes with subsequent elaboration of cytokines.

**5. How does the innate immune system interact with the acquired immune system?**

Pattern recognition receptors on antigen-presenting cells (APC) (example: mannose receptors) of the innate immune system bind pathogens, which are endocytosed. The phagocytized pathogen can then be processed and presented to T cells in the context of MHC class II molecules. Furthermore, binding of PAMPs to toll-like receptors signals the APC to upregulate CD80 (B7-1)/CD86 (B7-2) costimulatory molecules on the surface of the APC. Only when the APC presents both class II molecules with antigen to the T cell receptor and CD80 (B7-1) or CD86 (B7-2) to CD28 on the T cell can the T cell be activated resulting in stimulation of the acquired immune system.

Note that self antigens are not recognized by receptors of the innate immune system and therefore do not induce CD80 (B7-1) or CD86 (B7-2) molecules. This mechanism ensures that only pathogen-specific T cells are activated. However, it is conceivable that mutations in toll-like receptors could lead to abnormalities resulting in chronic stimulation of the immune system resulting in autoimmune disease.

**6. Acquired immune (adaptive/specific) responses can be active or passive. Describe and differentiate the two.**

**Active immunity** is so named because the host plays an active role in responding to the foreign antigen. The best example of active immunity is **immunization**, whereby a vaccine containing a foreign antigen is administered to a nonimmune host, resulting in active production of specific antibody and lymphocyte-based memory.

**Passive immunity** refers to transfer of soluble factors (either antibodies or cells) from an immune individual to a nonimmune host. This process confers immunity passively, without the recipient needing prior exposure to the antigen. A good example of passive immunity is parenteral administration of immune serum globulin to travelers as preexposure **prophylaxis** against unusual infections.

**7. What are the two main types of lymphocytes? How are they differentiated?**

- **T lymphocytes**, or T cells, are **T**hymus-derived and express the T cell receptor on their surface. They can be separated from other lymphocytes by use of monoclonal antibodies that recognize CD3, a component of the T cell receptor. The majority of circulating lymphocytes in the bloodstream are T cells.
- **B lymphocytes**, or B cells, are **B**one marrow–derived antibody-secreting cells that express surface immunoglobulin on their surfaces.

**8. Specific immune responses can be differentiated into two major categories based on whether B or T cells are primarily involved. What are these two categories?**

1. **Humoral immunity** refers to immune responses involving antibody that is produced by mature B cells and plasma cells (terminally differentiated B cells).
2. **Cellular immunity** is mediated by T cells that secrete cytokines and signal effector cells to direct an overall cell-mediated immune response.

**9. What is the difference between B1 and B2 populations of B cells?**

- B1—develop earliest during ontogeny. Most express CD5. They are the source of "natural" antibodies. These antibodies are low affinity, IgM, and polyreactive, recognizing both common pathogens and autoantigens.

- B2—develop later in ontogeny and lack CD5 surface marker. Before encountering antigen, mature B2 cells coexpress IgM and IgD antibodies on their surfaces. With antigen stimulation, they secrete highly specific antibody (IgM, IgG, IgA, or IgE) within the secondary lymphoid tissue.

**10. How does antibody participate in immune and inflammatory responses?**

There are three main ways in which antibody is immunologically active:

1. Antibody can coat and neutralize invading organisms, not allowing the organism access to the host.
2. Two classes of antibody (IgM and IgG) activate ("fix") complement, resulting in cell chemotaxis, increased vascular permeability, and target cell lysis.
3. Antibody coats foreign particles (opsonization), increasing the efficiency of phagocytosis by cells that contain surface immunoglobulin receptors (neutrophils and macrophages).

**11. Humoral (antibody-mediated) immunity is most important in host defense against which type of infectious organisms?**

Bacteria, especially those with a polysaccharide capsule. Patients with severe antibody deficiency (hypogammaglobulinemia) suffer from recurrent sinopulmonary infections, especially with encapsulated organisms (e.g., *Pneumococcus*, *Haemophilus influenzae*).

**12. Name the four major classes of antibodies. What specific role does each play in humoral immunity?**

The mnemonic is GAME:

**G—IgG—** Highest concentration in serum and excellent penetration into tissues. Can cross the placenta by week 16 of pregnancy. Fixes complement.

**A—IgA—** Most important antibody for host defense at mucosal surfaces (sites of antigen entry). Produced locally and often present in a modified form in secretions such as tears and saliva (secretory IgA). Secretory IgA is more resistant to enzymatic degradation.

**M—IgM—** The first class of antibody made in the primary response to antigen. Vigorously fixes complement and is very important in host defense against blood-borne antigens.

**E—IgE—** Binds to the surface of mast cells and basophils, and when cross-linked, results in release of granular contents (primarily histamine). Important in allergic diseases and host defense against parasites.

**Pearl**: Antibody (immunoglobulin) is also called gamma globulin because it is contained primarily in the gamma fraction when serum proteins are electrophoresed on a gel.

**13. What are the different types of T cells? How are they differentiated?**

- Classically, T cells can be functionally classified into helper/inducer, suppressor, and cytotoxic subsets.
- Most helper/inducer T cells express the CD4 cell-surface marker.
- The majority of cytotoxic T cells express the CD8 cell-surface marker.
- Suppressor T cells also classically express the CD8 cell-surface marker, but their existence as a separate distinct T-cell subtype is controversial.

**14. What is the difference between Th1 and Th2 helper T cells?**

The $CD4^+$ helper T cells can be divided into two types:

- Th1—secrete IL-2 and interferon γ. These cytokines are important in cell-mediated immunity including stimulating $CD8^+$ cytotoxic T cells to attack virally infected cells and stimulating macrophage function and granuloma formation. Tumor necrosis factor is also secreted promoting inflammation. IL-12 secretion by phagocytic cells is important for initial induction of the Th1 response. Interferon γ inhibits Th2 subset responses. Therapies that inhibit certain Th1 cytokines (anti TNFα) are used in Th1-mediated diseases (rheumatoid arthritis).

- Th2—secrete IL-4, IL-5, IL-6, IL-10, and IL-13. These cytokines are important in humoral immunity. IL-4 promotes immunoglobulin class switching to IgE, IL-5 activates eosinophils, and IL-6 promotes B cell maturation into a plasma cell. Il-4, IL-10, and IL-13 inhibit macrophage activation and TNF-mediated inflammation. IL-10 has been used to treat Th1 diseases (rheumatoid arthritis), and antibodies against IL-10 have been used to treat Th2 disease (SLE).

**15. What is the difference between α/β T cells and γ/δ T cells?**

- α/β T cells—these are $CD4^+$ and $CD8^+$ T cells that express a T cell receptor with α and β chains. Most T cells have this type of receptor, which can recognize antigen presented in association with major histocompatibility complex (MHC) on the surface of APC and other cells.
- γ/δ T cells—these are phylogenetically older T cells comprising up to 15% of the T cell population in certain epithelial tissues such as skin and gut. These T cells express T cell receptors with γ and δ chains. These T cell receptors can't recognize antigen in context with MHC. They can recognize antigen directly or in association with MHC class I–like molecules such as CD1 (binds glycolipid antigens) and MICA/MICB in the gut. Heat shock proteins can directly activate these cells.

**16. Cellular immunity (T cell mediated) is most important in host defense against which infectious organisms?**

Virus, parasites, fungi, and mycobacteria. AIDS patients have a severe dysfunction of T cell–mediated immunity and suffer from recurrent infections with these agents.

**17. What are NK cells, and how are they identified?**

NK cells are **natural killer** cells, so named because they are potent cytotoxic cells whose targets are not MHC-restricted (i.e., they are not antigen-specific). They make up 5–10% of the recirculating lymphocyte population. They are activated by IL-15. They have the appearance on light microscopy of large lymphocytes with numerous cytoplasmic granules and are sometimes called large granular lymphocytes. The granules contain substances that facilitate target cell lysis including perforin (a pore-forming protein) and granzymes. They classically express the CD16 and CD56 cell-surface markers. NK cells attack virus-infected or abnormal cells expressing low levels of class I MHC molecules, while $CD8^+$ T cells are MHC-restricted and attack cells with high levels of class I MHC complexed to antigen. NK cells insert perforin into the cells they are attacking and secrete granzymes through the pore. Granzymes attack the cell causing apoptosis.

NK cells can also kill cells through antibody-dependent cellular cytotoxicity where IgG bound to target cells interacts with Fc receptors (CD16) on NK cells causing release of lytic enzymes. NK cells are numerous in skin biopsies of patients with graft versus host disease following bone marrow transplant. They are also expanded in large granular lymphocyte (LGL) syndrome and in some patients with Felty's syndrome.

**18. Using the classification developed by Gel and Coombs, immune responses can be segregated into four main types. Name them.**

**Type I**—IgE-mediated immediate hypersensitivity (e.g., allergic rhinitis or hayfever)

**Type II**—Antibody-mediated tissue injury, (e.g., autoimmune hemolytic anemia)

**Type III**—Immune complex (antigen-antibody) formation (e.g., serum sickness, Arthus skin reaction)

**Type IV**—Delayed-type hypersensitivity (e.g., immune response to mycobacterial antigens, positive PPD skin test)

**19. What are MHC molecules, and on which cells are they found?**

MHC stands for **major histocompatibility complex**, a group of genes located on human chromosome 6. The products of MHC gene loci can be classified into two categories—class I and class II MHC molecules:

- Class I MHC molecules are expressed on the surface of all nucleated cells.
- Class II MHC molecules are found mostly on specialized cells called antigen-presenting cells.

**20. How do T cells recognize antigen to initiate a specific immune response?**

a. Unlike macrophages, neutrophils, and B cells, T cells classically cannot recognize free soluble antigen.

b. T cells can only "see" antigen via their surface T cell receptor, which will only bind to antigen bound to ("presented by") an MHC molecule on the surface of a cell.

c. T cells "see" only pieces of large antigens because the antigen-binding groove in a MHC molecule can only accommodate a small peptide. Large protein antigens are digested ("processed") prior to insertion in the groove.

d. An exception to the above involves stimulation of T cells by superantigens. A superantigen is typically a molecule of bacterial or viral origin that directly interacts with MHC class II molecules outside of the antigen-binding groove and then with the $V_\beta$ region in the T cell receptor. The result is direct T cell activation of large amounts of T cells, all of which contain a specific $V_\beta$ region in the T cell receptor. Therefore, the systemic host response to a superantigen can be dramatic. Examples include toxic shock syndrome caused by a staphylococcal exotoxin that acts as a T cell superantigen.

**21. Which cells are specialized antigen-presenting cells? Where are they found?**

*Antigen Presenting Cells*

| CELL TYPE | LOCATION |
|---|---|
| Macrophages | |
| Histiocyte | Connective tissue |
| Monocyte | Blood |
| Alveolar macrophage | Lung |
| Kupffer cell | Liver |
| Microglia | CNS |
| Osteoclast | Bone |
| Dendritic cells | Skin, lymph nodes, synovium |
| Langerhans cells | Skin |
| B lymphocytes | Lymph nodes |

**22. Which type of T cells do antigen-presenting cells (APCs) present antigen to?**

- APCs are cells that express surface MHC class II molecules.
- MHC class II molecules preferentially bind to T cell receptors associated with the CD4 surface molecule.
- Thus, APCs present antigen to the $CD4^+$ T cells, the helper/inducer subset.

**23. Which type of T cell recognizes antigen presented by class I MHC molecules?**

Class I MHC molecules preferentially bind to T cell receptors associated with the CD8 surface molecule. Thus, antigen presented in the groove of MHC class I molecules would interact with $CD8^+$ T cells, the cytotoxic/suppressor subset. Class I MHC molecules are present on the surface of all nucleated cells, thus allowing cells to present their internal antigens to cytotoxic T cells. This mechanism is critically important in host defense against intracellular pathogens such as viruses.

**24. How do T cells become activated?**

T-cell activation requires two signals:

- Engagement of the T-cell receptor by the antigen/MHC complex
- A second signal, usually transduced by direct cognate interaction ("touching") between costimulatory cell surface molecules on the APC and T cell

T-cell activation resulting from the two signals leads to production of cytoplasmic and nuclear factors, resulting in gene activation and new DNA synthesis.

**25. What are the important costimulatory molecules involved in second signaling of T cells that are interacting with MHC-peptide complexes on the surface of an APC?**

| T cell | APC |
|---|---|
| CD28 | B7-1 (CD80)<br>B7-2 (CD86) |
| CD 40 ligand (CD154) | CD40 |
| CD2 (LFA-2) | CD58 |
| CD45 | CD22 (proposed) |
| CTLA-4 | B7-1/B7-2 |

All the above help activate T cells except CTLA-4/B7 interaction, which downregulates T cells. CTLA-4 binds with much higher affinity than CD28 to B7. Biologics are being developed to interfere with these interactions in order to treat autoimmune diseases.

**26. If the T cell receptor is engaged by an antigen/MHC complex, but the second signal is not given, what happens?**

Typically, the T cell is tolerized (made unresponsive) to that antigen or the cell dies by undergoing apoptosis.

**27. What pathways lead to cellular apoptosis?**

Multiple triggers can lead to a cell undergoing apoptosis by one of two major pathways:

- Death receptors [Fas (CD95), TNFR1, TRAIL]—these receptors all have a homologous intracellular region "death domain." These death domains bind to adaptor protein (Fas binds to FADD, TNFR1 to TRADD). These adaptor proteins can activate the cysteine protease, procaspase 8. This can be inhibited by FLIP. The activated caspase 8 activates the executioner caspases (3, 6, and 7), which in turn activate an endonuclease called caspase-activated DNAse as well as others. These endonucleases cleave DNA causing fragmentation and cell death. Caspases also activate proteases that act on actin microfilaments leading to blebbing of the membrane.
- Mitochondria—cellular stress causes Bax, Bak, and/or Bid to bind to mitochondria. This displaces Bcl-2 and Bcl-x, which are normally on the outer mitochondrial membrane and inhibit apoptosis. When this happens, cytochrome c is released from the mitochondria. Cytochrome c activates the adaptor protein, Apaf-1, which is in the cytosol. Apaf-1 activates procaspase-9, which activates caspases 3 and 7 causing apoptosis (see above). Akt inhibits this pathway. Many tumors have chronically activated Akt, so the tumor cell doesn't undergo apoptosis.
- Others—(1) cytotoxic cells (T and NK cells) inject granzyme B, which activates caspases 3 and 7. (2) DNA damage is detected by p53, resulting in activation of apoptosis. Defective p53 can be found in some tumors and also synoviocytes in rheumatoid arthritis, perhaps contributing to their proliferation.

Abnormalities in cellular apoptosis can lead to cancer and autoimmune disease. Apoptotic bodies can serve as source of nuclear autoantigens for autoimmune diseases (SLE).

**28. What is the role of neutrophils in the immune response?**

Neutrophils are critically important in phagocytosing and digesting foreign particles at sites of inflammation and antigen entry. Neutrophils kill and dissolve microbes by release of enzymes and bactericidal products from their intracytoplasmic granules and by generation of toxic oxygen radicals and hypohalous acids. Clinical deficiency of leukocytes manifests as recurrent skin and soft tissue infections with pyogenic organisms and sepsis (as seen in cancer patients receiving toxic chemotherapy).

**29. What are the important adhesion molecules involved in the influx of neutrophils and mononuclear cells into blood vessel walls resulting in vasculitis?**

| TIME TO ACTIVATION | LEUKOCYTE | ACTIVATED ENDOTHELIUM |
|---|---|---|
| < 2 hours | L-selectin | Sialomucin (CD34) |
| | PSGL-1 (unactivated neutrophil) | P-selectin (Weibel-Palade bodies) |
| < 4 hours | ESL-1 | E-selectin (ELAM-1) |
| < 12 hours | LFA-1 (B2 integrin) (activated neutrophil) | ICAM-1 (CD54) |
| < 24 hours | Mac-1 (B2 integrin) (monocytes) | ICAM-1 |
| < 48 hours | VLA-4 (B1 integrin) (lymphocytes, monocytes adhesion molecules) | VCAM-1 |

Note that CD34, PSGL-1, and ESL-1 all contain sialylated carbohydrate determinants related to Sialyl-Lewis (CD15). The time to adhesion molecule activation explains why neutrophils enter inflammatory site first (acute inflammation) while mononuclear cells enter later (chronic inflammation). Biologic therapy to interfere with these interactions has been used in some cases of vasculitis (anti CD54).

**30. What is the role of eosinophils in the immune response?**

Eosinophils are active in immunity against parasites, especially helminths. Eosinophils are specialized leukocytes whose granules contain numerous toxic products, including major basic protein, eosinophil peroxidase, and eosinophil cationic protein. These products are especially toxic to helminths. Activated eosinophils also produce large quantities of leukotriene C4 ($LTC_4$) and TGF-β that promote increased venular permeability and fibroblast-dependent fibrosis, respectively.

**31. What is the role of complement in the immune response?**

Complement components have immunologic activity both individually and in an activation cascade leading to a polymer formed by C5, C6, C7, C8, and C9 (the membrane attack complex, or MAC), which results in lysis of target cell membranes (see figure). Early classic complement components (especially C3 products) act as opsonins and assist in the phagocytosis of bacterial particles by neutrophils and macrophages. Certain complement split products (C3a and C5a) are chemotactic for phagocytic neutrophils and also act as "anaphylatoxins," which directly stimulate mast cells and basophils to release histamine resulting in increased vascular permeability. Deficiency of early complement components is associated with increased pyogenic infections (C3 deficiency) and an increased incidence of autoimmune diseases (C1, 4, and 2 deficiency), possibly owing to impaired clearance of immune complexes. The MAC appears especially important in host defense against *Neisseria* infection. Deficiency of any one of the terminal complement components can result in recurrent infections with *Neisseria.*

**32. What activates the complement system?**

The complement system can be activated by three pathways:

Classical—IgM and IgG binding to antigen forming immune complexes that can bind Clq activating Clr and Cls to cleave C4. Other proteins including C-reactive protein (binds Clq), serum amyloid P, and C4 nephritic factor can activate this pathway.

Alternative—activated by lipopolysaccharide on microbial cell surfaces in the absence of antibody. C3 and factor B bind to cell surface forming C3bBb, which functions to cleave more C3 molecules. This is part of the innate immune system. IgA complexes and C3 nephritic factor can also activate this pathway.

Lectin—mannan-binding lectin is secreted by the liver and binds to microbial ligands. This activates mannan-binding lectin-associated proteases that are related to Clr and Cls and can cleave C4 resulting in complement activation.

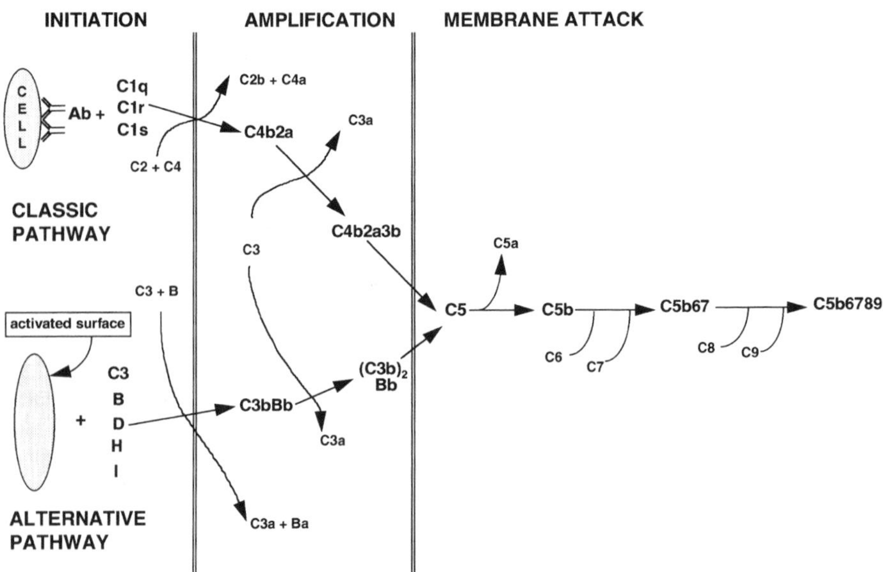


Overview of the classic and alternative complement cascades.

**33. Summarize the cellular interactions and cytokines involved in the immune response.**

Please see figure on opposite page.

## BIBLIOGRAPHY


1. Abbas AK, Lichtman AH, Pober JS: Cellular and Molecular Immunology, 4th ed. Philadelphia, WB Saunders, 2000.
2. Arend WP: The innate immune system in rheumatoid arthritis. Arthritis Rheum 44:2224–2234, 2001.
3. Delves PJ, Roitt IM: The immune system: First of two parts. New Engl J Med 343:37–49, 2000.
4. Delves PJ, Roitt IM: The immune system: Second of two parts. New Engl J Med 343:108–117, 2000.
5. Goodman JW: The immune response. In Stites DP, Terr AI, Parslow TG (eds): Basic and Clinical Immunology, 8th ed. Norwalk, CT, Appleton & Lange, 1994, pp 40–49.
6. Green DR: Apoptotic pathways: The roads to ruin. Cell 94:695–698, 1998.
7. Johnston RB: The complement system in host defense and inflammation: The cutting edges of a double-edged sword. Pediatr Infect Dis J 12:933–941, 1993.
8. Keller R: The macrophage response to infectious agents: Mechanisms of macrophage activation and tumor cell killing. Res Immunol 144:271–273, 1993.
9. Medzhitov R, Janeway C: Innate immunity. N Engl J Med 343:338–344, 2000.
10. Roitt I, Brostoff J, Male D: Immunology, 5th ed. England, Gower Medical Publishing, 1998.

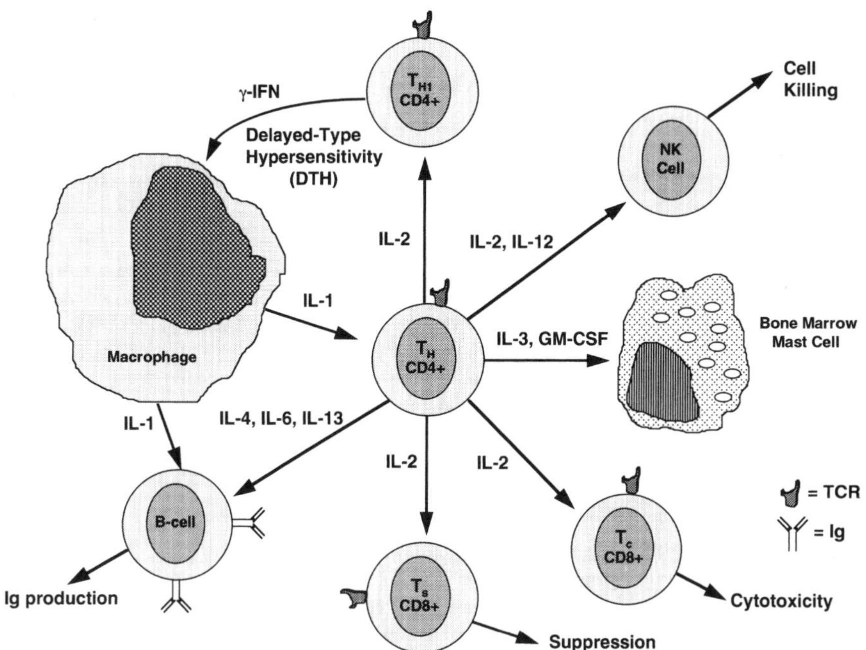


Overview of the framework of cellular immunity, illustrating the central role of the CD4+ T-helper cell. (IL, interleukin; TCR, T cell receptor; Ig, immunoglobulin; NK, natural killer; IFN, interferon; GM-CSF, granulocyte-macrophage colony-stimulating factor.)

# 5. OVERVIEW OF THE INFLAMMATORY RESPONSE

*Michael O'Connell, M.D.*

**1. Name the four cardinal signs of inflammation.**
Pain, swelling, warmth, and erythema (redness).

**2. What are the underlying mechanisms responsible for the signs of inflammation?**
Local arteriolar dilation produces the redness and warmth. Permeability increases in the postcapillary venules, allowing vascular fluid to leak into the surrounding tissue to produce swelling (edema). Pain is a result of the action of numerous inflammatory mediators and inflammatory cell-derived products on local nerves.

**3. Inflammatory responses can be either detrimental or beneficial to the host. Give examples of each.**

**Detrimental**

- Allergic diseases in which IgE-mediated (type 1) inflammatory reactions resulting from exposure to an allergen cause significant symptoms (e.g., rhinitis, anaphylaxis) despite the fact that the inciting agent is often of no threat to the host (e.g., pollen).

- Autoimmune diseases in which immunologically mediated inflammation is misdirected against host tissues, resulting in injury and destruction.

**Beneficial**

- In infection by foreign microorganisms, increased vascular permeability enhances the ability of immune defensive cells (e.g., neutrophils, lymphocytes) to egress the bloodstream and enter tissues invaded by foreign pathogens.
- In infection, increased local blood flow enhances delivery of oxygen to stressed tissues.

**4. What three types of inflammatory cells are involved in the majority of inflammatory reactions?**

Neutrophils, macrophages, and lymphocytes. Neutrophils predominate in acute inflammatory reactions, whereas lymphocytes are the key cell in chronic inflammatory processes. Other inflammatory cells are critically important in special types of inflammatory responses. Mast cells and basophils are the principal cells involved in IgE-mediated hypersensitivity (allergic) reactions. Eosinophils play a principal role in the host response to parasitic infection.

**5. What advantageous properties of neutrophils allow them to play a critical role in acute inflammatory responses to a foreign pathogen?**

Neutrophils are attracted by several types of chemotactic stimuli to sites of tissue injury, regardless of its cause. This property permits a rapid cellular response to many different types of injury, including infection, trauma, foreign body penetration, and burns. Additionally, since large numbers of neutrophils are constantly circulating in the blood, large numbers of cells can be mobilized quickly in response to an injury. These properties make neutrophils the cellular "first line of defense."

**6. How do neutrophils attack foreign substances that enter the body?**

Neutrophils are active phagocytic cells that can engulf foreign particles efficiently. Their cell membranes contain receptors for antibody and complement fragments, dramatically increasing the efficiency of phagocytosis of opsonized particles. Once the foreign particle is engulfed, neutrophils release granular contents, including degradative enzymes and microbicidal products. This results in killing/degradation of the foreign particle and local remodeling of the tissues—the first step in wound healing.

**7. Macrophages are also potent phagocytic cells. How is their role unique in the inflammatory response from that of the neutrophil?**

Macrophages possess three key properties that distinguish them from neutrophils:

1. They express MHC class II on their cell surface and function as antigen-presenting cells.
2. They produce/secrete a number of important proinflammatory and costimulatory cytokines, including tumor necrosis factor (TNF), interleukin 1 (IL-1), IL-6, and IL-8, which drive the so-called acute phase response.
3. Macrophages respond to certain cytokines (notable gamma-interferon derived from T cells) that cause their activation, dramatically increasing their phagocytic capacity and causing aggregation into granulomas and multinucleated giant cells.

**8. How do lymphocytes participate in chronic inflammatory responses?**

T lymphocytes are the master controllers of the specific immune response. After antigen stimulation via antigen-presenting cells, T cells secrete cytokines that (1) direct and activate effector cells (e.g., macrophages) in a specific fashion, and/or (2) direct B cells to produce antigen-specific antibody. These processes are long-lived, owing to the nature of the cells involved and the fact that certain T and B cells differentiate into memory cells with extremely long lifespans.

**9. What are the major classes of inflammatory mediators?**

**Vasoactive mediators**
- Histamine
- Arachidonic acid products
  - Prostaglandins
  - Leukotrienes
- Platelet-activating factor (PAF)
- Kinins

**Enzymes**
- Tryptase
- Chymase

**Chemotactic factors**
- Complement products (C3a, C5a)
- Leukotriene $B_4$
- Platelet-activating factor
- Cytokines (IL-8)

**Proinflammatory cytokines**
- Interleukins 1, 6, and 8
- Tumor necrosis factor
- Gamma-interferon

**10. How does histamine promote inflammation?**

Histamine is a preformed mediator rapidly released from mast cell and basophil granules after activation. Histamine interacts with specific cellular receptors (called H1, H2, and H3), resulting in increased vascular permeability, smooth muscle contraction, and increased glandular mucous secretion. This results clinically in sneezing, wheezing, itching, and edema. Antihistamine drugs block the receptors and limit or prevent symptom development.

**11. How are prostaglandins and leukotrienes formed?**

Unlike histamine (which is a preformed and stored mediator), prostaglandins and leukotrienes require active synthesis. The initial source molecule is arachidonic acid, which is liberated from cell membrane phospholipids by phospholipase $A_2$ that is bound to the cell membrane. Once formed, arachidonic acid can be metabolized by either of two enzyme pathways (see figure):

1. Cyclo-oxygenase pathway—results in prostaglandins
2. Lipoxygenase pathway—results in leukotrienes

**12. How do prostaglandins and leukotrienes promote inflammation?**

Prostaglandins (especially prostaglandin $D_2$) induce local vasodilation and increased vascular permeability. Leukotrienes (LT) fall into two classes: $LTC_4$, $LTD_4$, and $LTE_4$ induce smooth muscle contraction, bronchoconstriction, and mucous secretion. They were once collectively called slow reacting substance of anaphylaxis (SRS-A). $LTB_4$ has none of the above properties but is a potent chemotactic factor for leukocytes.

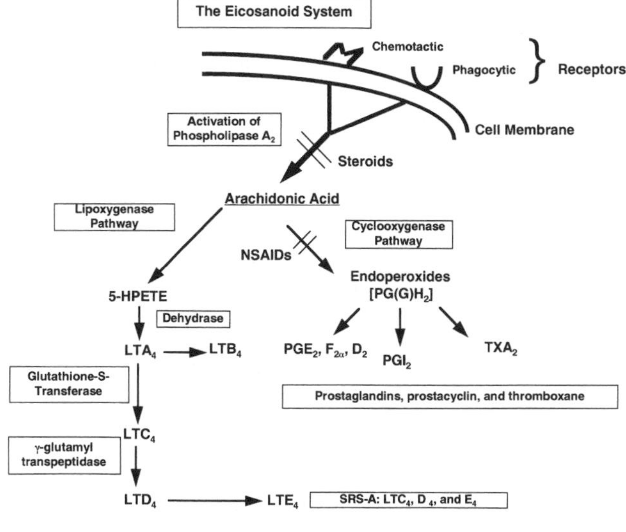


Eicosanoid pathways.

**13. By what mechanism are the anti-inflammatory effects of aspirin and NSAIDs mediated?**

- Both aspirin and NSAIDs block the activity of cyclo-oxygenase, resulting in decreased synthesis of prostaglandins.
- Drugs that block leukotriene synthesis (zileuton) and cellular leukotriene receptors (zafirlukast and montelukast) are currently used clinically to treat asthma.

**14. What is the acute phase response? What blood proteins are involved?**

The acute phase response is a complex cascade of primarily liver-synthesized proteins that rise in response to a variety of infectious or immunologic stimuli. This response results in multiple metabolic and cellular alterations that contribute to host defense and a return to homeostasis.

**Major acute phase proteins** include alpha-1-antitrypsin, C3, ceruloplasmin, C-reactive protein, fibrinogen, haptoglobin, and serum amyloid A. The liver synthesizes these proteins at the expense of albumin, which frequently decreases during acute inflammation.

**15. What mechanisms are involved in the initiation of an acute phase response?**

Macrophages and monocytes appear to be the principal cells involved (though T cells may also play a role). When activated by antigen or other stimuli, macrophages secrete IL-1, IL-6, and TNF. IL-6 is a potent hepatocyte-stimulating factor resulting in increased synthesis of acute phase proteins. IL-1 generally enhances the effects of IL-6 on hepatocytes.

**16. What is the difference between necrosis and apoptosis?**

- Necrosis—the pathologic death of one or more cells due to inflammation resulting in rupture and fragmentation of the nucleus and cell. The cellular debris released further contributes to the inflammatory reaction.
- Apoptosis—an orderly process of cell death in which activation of caspases results in chromatin condensation, membrane blebbing, and fragmentation of cell and nucleus into smaller membrane-bound apoptotic bodies. These are rapidly cleared by phagocytosis and do not trigger an inflammatory response.

**17. Describe the initial events in chronologic order resulting in an inflammatory response against a microbial pathogen.**

- Invading microbe breaches epithelial barrier.
- Innate immune system responds—alternate complement pathway activated by C3 and factor B binding to microbial membrane. Classical pathway activated by C-reactive protein and mannan-binding lectin pathway.
- *N*-Formylmethionyl peptides from microbe stimulate seven $\alpha$-helical transmembrane receptors on neutrophils and macrophages. These peptides are chemoattractants and activators of the neutrophils, so they upregulate integrins for binding to endothelium and produce reactive oxygen intermediates to kill microbes.
- Local macrophages phagocytize microbe by mannose and scavenger receptors and complement receptors as a result of complement opsonized microbe. Other plasma proteins and natural antibodies can also opsonize microbe to facilitate phagocytosis.
- Activation of macrophage toll-like receptors signal cytokine (IL-1, IL-6, IL-8, TNF) release.
- Prostaglandins and leukotrienes are released in response to cytokines (IL-1, TNF$\alpha$) and other stimuli. IL-6 stimulates liver to synthesize more acute phase proteins.
- Il-1 and TNF upregulate endothelial cell adhesion molecules to facilitate influx of neutrophils, monocytes, and lymphocytes into area. (See Chapter 4.)
- Complement activation products (C5a), IL-8, leukotriene B4, and platelet activating factor are chemoattractant for neutrophils and circulating monocytes. Monocytes enter inflammatory site and become macrophages.
- Neutrophils phagocytize microbes. Specific granules filled with degradative enzymes (lysozyme, collagenase, elastase) and azurophilic granules (lysosomes) destroy the phagocytized microbe. Neutrophils die at inflammatory site, contributing to inflammation.

- Monocytes and macrophages become dominant effector cells 24–48 hours into inflammation. Phagocytize opsonized microbe and release further inflammatory mediators.
- Inflammatory mediators released throughout this process contribute to cardinal signs of inflammation.
  Prostaglandin $E_2$: vasodilation (redness, warmth), increased vascular permeability (swelling), and increased pain sensitivity to bradykinin.
  Prostacyclin ($PGI_2$): vasodilation.
  Thromboxane $A_2$: platelet activation.
  Platelet-activating factor: vasodilation, increased vascular permeability, platelet activation.
  Bradykinin: activate nerve fibers (pain).
- Antigen presenting cells present antigen bound to MHC molecules to activate acquired (adaptive) immune system (T and B lymphocytes). Occurs 3–5 days after microbial invasion.

**18. How are cells in the inflammatory and immune response activated?**

- Signals—multiple signals can activate different cells. Examples include antigen, immune complexes and antibodies (Fc portion), cell ligands (example: CD28 and B7-1), cytokines and growth factors, and stress (heat, reactive oxygen metabolites, others).
- Receptors—signals act through receptors on cell surface.
  Immunoglobulin superfamily of receptors—examples include immunoglobulin on B cell surface, T cell receptor, class I and II MHC molecules, cell ligands (CD28, etc.), Fc receptor, IL-1, platelet-derived growth factor receptors.
  Cytokine receptors—hematopoietic growth factor/interleukin receptors, TNF receptors, interferon receptors, TGFβ receptors, and chemokine receptors (IL-8).
- Second messengers—stimulated receptors activate second messengers.
  Phospholipase C: acts on membrane phospholipids to form diacylglycerol (DAG) and inositol triphosphates (IP3).
  1. DAG activates protein kinase C pathways, which phosphorylate proteins that enter nucleus to regulate gene transcription.
  2. IP3 causes calcium release by endoplasmic reticulum. Calcium binds to calmodulin, which activates calcineurin which dephosphorylates proteins (example: NFAT = nuclear factor of activated T cells), which can then enter the nucleus to regulate IL-2 and other gene transcription in association with AP-1.

  Small G proteins (Ras, Rho, Rab)—activated directly or through protein kinase C after receptor binds to its ligand (i.e., signal).
- Mitogen-activated (MAP) kinases—activate small G proteins (GTPases) activate MAP kinase pathways (ERK, JNK, p38, NIK, JAK).
- Transcription factors—activated MAP kinases activate nuclear transcription factors that enter nucleus to regulate gene transcription by binding to nuclear response elements.
  1. AP-1 (Jun/Fos)/ATF-2—activated by ERK, JNK, p38 pathways and regulate matrix metalloproteinases, IL-1, IL-2, ICAM-1, and other genes.
  2. NF-κ B—activated by NIK pathways and regulates genes for cyclooxygenase-2, chemokines, multiple interleukins, TNF, adhesion molecules, others.
  3. STAT—activated by JAK, which is tyrosine kinase bound to many cytokine receptors. STAT regulates genes for adhesion molecules and plays role in Th1/Th2 differentiation and proliferation.

An understanding of these pathways is important because MAP kinase (and other) inhibitors are being developed to treat autoimmune diseases. Furthermore, this is how some of our medications work, such as cyclosporine (inhibits calcineurin) and corticosteroids (block activated NF-κ B binding to nuclear response element).

## BIBLIOGRAPHY

1. Dinarello CA, Wolff SM: The role of interleukin-1 in disease. N Engl J Med 328:106–113, 1993.

2. Firestein GS, Manning AM: Signal transduction and transcription factors in rheumatic disease. Arthritis Rheum 42:609–621, 1999.
3. Gabay C, Kushner I: Acute phase proteins and other systemic responses to inflammation. N Engl J Med 340:448–454, 1999.
4. Green DR: Apoptotic pathways: The roads to ruin. Cell 94:695–698, 1998.
5. Keller R: The macrophage response to infectious agents: Mechanisms of macrophage activation and tumor cell killing. Res Immunol 144:271–273, 1993.
6. Terr AI: Inflammation. In Stites DP, Terr AI, Parslow TG (eds): Basic and Clinical Immunology, 8th ed. Norwalk, CT, Appleton & Lange, 1994, pp 137–150.
7. Zurier RB: Prostaglandins, leukotrienes, and related compounds. In Ruddy S, Harris ED, Sledge CB (eds): Kelley's Textbook of Rheumatology, 6th ed. Philadelphia, WB Saunders, 2001, pp 211–224.

# 6. IMMUNOGENETICS OF RHEUMATIC DISEASES

V. *Michael Holers*, M.D.

**1. What types of molecules enable the immune system to bind specific antigens?**

Immunoglobulins [B-cell receptors (BCR)], T-cell receptors (TCRs), and major histocompatibility complex class I and II molecules (MHC I and II) are molecules from the adaptive immune system that bind specific antigens. In addition to these adaptive immune system molecules, a large number of other proteins that are part of the innate immune system, including C-reactive protein (CRP) and mannose-binding protein (MBP), are capable of binding with relatively high specificity to determinants such as repeating carbohydrates on foreign antigens. In combination, proteins from the innate and adaptive immune system are capable of recognizing essentially all foreign antigens. Importantly, each of these classes of proteins displays unique associations with and roles in rheumatic diseases. In particular, the associations between certain autoimmune diseases and the expression of specific MHC class I, II, and III genes, as well as the appearance of autoimmune diseases in the setting of deficiencies of innate immune proteins such as complement C1, provide insights into disease susceptibility and pathogenesis.

**2. What is the MHC, and what does it do?**

The major histocompatibility complex (MHC) is located on the short arm of chromosome 6 in a region stretching approximately 4 million base pairs. This entire region has been sequenced using current DNA technologies, so we know a lot about this area of the human genome. Within the MHC, there are three regions that encode for three different classes of proteins that have traditionally been defined—MHC Classes I, II, and III (see figure, top of next page).

The largest stretch, approximately 2 million base pairs, encodes the MHC Class I molecules, while a shorter stretch, approximately 1 million base pairs, encodes Class II molecules. The role of these two classes of molecules is to enable presentation of peptide antigens to T cells. There are many polymorphisms of Class I and II molecules that are found in the population. The remainder of the MHC complex stretches between the Class I and II regions and encodes various proteins that are not capable of presenting antigen. However, many of these MHC Class III proteins are involved in the regulation of the immune response, and some have rheumatic disease associations. These include C2, C4, and factor B of the complement system; tumor necrosis factors (TNF) $\alpha$ and $\beta$; and some of the heat-shock proteins. Both MHC Class I and II molecules are dimers. While the MHC encodes both the $\alpha$- and $\beta$-chains of the Class II molecules, it encodes only the MHC Class I $\alpha$-chain. $\beta_2$-microglobulin, the $\beta$-chain shared by all MHC Class I molecules, is encoded by a relatively invariant allele on chromosome 15.

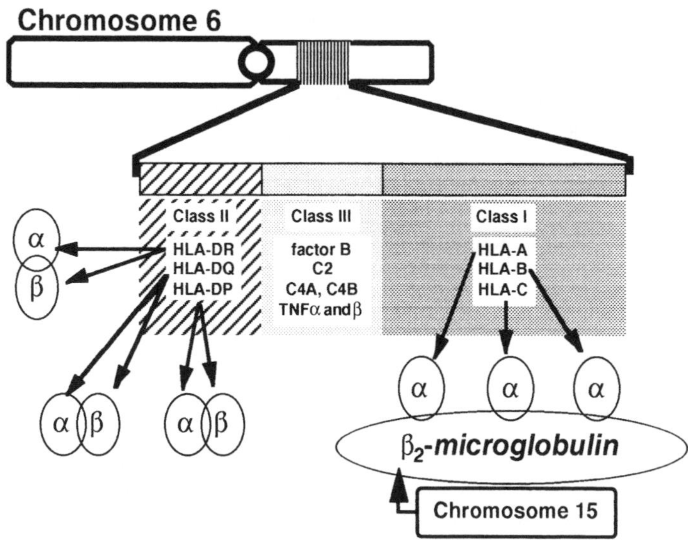


The major histocompatibility complex.

**3. Is there a difference between MHC and HLA?**

For many practical purposes, MHC and HLA (human leukocyte antigen) are used as interchangeable terms. However, technically, they are different. MHC specifically refers to the genes located on chromosome 6. The MHC genes encode HLA molecules. In other words, HLA molecules are the cell-surface proteins that are encoded by the different MHC genetic loci. Because these proteins are highly polymorphic in the human population and can be specifically recognized as foreign by other individuals, they are defined as antigens. Since these proteins were first described on human white blood cells as products recognized by sera from other individuals previously exposed to human cells from genetically different persons (such as by pregnancy), they are referred to as human leukocyte antigens (HLA). We now know that their distribution is considerably broader than leukocytes as, for instance, MHC Class I molecules are expressed on almost all cells.

**4. Why is the MHC complex so unusual when compared with the rest of our genome?**

The diversity enabled by the MHC is unparalleled in the remainder of the genome. There are a variety of factors responsible for this diversity, but the major effect is to allow both individuals and the population as a whole to recognize a very broad range of pathogens. In addition, the codominant pattern of expression of functional genes increases this diversity. Finally, the MHC manifests an unusually high level of linkage disequilibrium.

**5. What does polymorphism mean?**

An allele is one of the alternative forms of a gene that can be inherited at a specific locus. The prevalence of allelic alternatives for most of the MHC Class I and II gene loci exceeds the frequency that is either expected or observed to occur secondary to mutation alone in non-MHC proteins. Furthermore, unlike the single residue allelic differences that characterize other proteins, MHC allelic polymorphism is characterized by differences at multiple residues that occur at several dispersed sites along the primary sequence but that are also found within the same functional domain in the three-dimensional structure of the protein. So, instead of a protein gene product that differs by one or two amino acids at just one site, MHC molecules may differ by 10% of their amino acids. These differences primarily occur in several areas of MHC molecules called hypervariable regions 1, 2, and 3. These areas are responsible for the specific binding of the peptide fragments to be presented. This genetic polymorphism is the result of selection forces occurring over eons, the effect of which is to help us survive against the multiple antigens to which humans are constantly exposed.

Examples of MHC polymorphisms include the HLA-A α-chain locus, for which approximately 50 different alleles have been identified; HLA-B locus, 200 alleles; HLA-C locus, 35 alleles; HLA-DRβ chain locus, 200 alleles; HLA DQ and DP, over 25 alleles each. Each individual, however, inherits only two alleles for each locus, one from the mother and one from the father.

**6. What is the significance of linkage disequilibrium?**

The combination of alleles on a single chromosome is called a **haplotype**. Two combinations of chromosome 6 alleles, i.e., two haplotypes, are inherited by an individual, one maternal and one paternal. Analysis of MHC haplotypes shows linkage disequilibrium, i.e., certain combinations of alleles in the MHC are inherited with a strikingly high frequency, substantially greater than their chance inheritance based on the individual allele frequencies in the population and the expected multiple crossovers that would occur over time within the region during meiosis.

Linkage disequilibrium complicates genetic analysis and interferes with the ability to assign effects to single genes within the haplotype. As an example, many diseases are associated with HLA-DR3; however, there are a number of alleles in linkage disequilibrium with HLA-DR3. For example, Caucasian HLA-DR3 haplotypes contain the same HLA-DQA1 and HLA-DQB2 alleles as well as identical Class III alleles. Therefore, if we identify an HLA-DR3 association with a disease, the gene most responsible for the association may be either the DR3 allele itself or any of a number of genes that are commonly in linkage disequilibrium with HLA-DR3.

**7. What is the significance of codominant inheritance?**

For each locus along the MHC, an individual receives a paternal and maternal allele. Rather than one alternative or the other being expressed, both alleles are expressed. This again increases the number of possible combinations of MHC molecules. The effects of each of the molecules expressed appear to be dominant. Therefore, a person who has two particular disease-associated HLA molecules likely has an even higher vulnerability to that disease.

**8. What do the letters appearing with HLA mean—e.g., HLA-A, HLA-B, etc.?**

When you have HLA followed by a hyphen and one letter, such as HLA-A, it describes the specific gene location (region) within the MHC that codes for a particular HLA molecule. For example, HLA-A, HLA-B, and HLA-C describe the most important individual MHC I gene regions.

**9. Why does HLA-D get the extra letters—R, P, Q?**

The letter D describes the entire MHC Class II region, not just a single gene locus. Therefore, to describe an actual gene locus, you need more letters. For example, HLA-DP, -DQ, and -DR get you closer to the gene loci that code for the most important Class II molecules. To make matters worse, each MHC Class II molecule consists of two separate polypeptide chains, designated α and β. So, when you see HLA-DRA or HLA-DRB, it is describing the locus for the HLA-DR α- or β-chain, respectively.

**10. How do I know which letters (regions)—A, B, C, D, etc.—belong to which MHC class?**

*Major MHC Class I and II Molecules*

| MHC CLASS I | MHC CLASS II |
|---|---|
| HLA-A | HLA-DR |
| HLA-B | HLA-DQ |
| HLA-C | HLA-DP |

HLA-A, -B, and -C are the most important MHC Class I molecules. All HLA-D molecules are MHC Class II molecules, and HLA-DP, -DQ, and -DR, are the most important ones. There are other letters such as E, F, G, H, J, X; however, these are all Class I molecules of less currently known importance to the genetics of rheumatic diseases. HLA-DM and DO are Class II molecules expressed intracellularly and involved in peptide binding to Class II surface molecules by facilitating or inhibiting the removal of the invariant chain.

**11. How does the HLA protein bind its peptide antigen?**

Each peptide binding site has a similar configuration. It consists of a groove, the walls of which are α-helical structures. A series of anti-parallel strands of the molecule form the floor of the groove, a β-pleated sheet. In TCR and MHC II, this configuration is formed by the interaction between the amino termini of both the α and the β-chains. For immunoglobulins, the antigen-binding site is formed by the interaction of the amino termini of the heavy and light chains. MHC I differs in that the antigen-binding site is formed by the interaction between the two amino terminal domains of the same chain, the α-chain.

The antigen binds at points on both the α-helical walls and the β-pleated floor. When the TCR binds the MHC-peptide complex, it recognizes the unique conformation and charge of the antigen peptide and α-helices. Unlike the antigen, the TCR cannot "see" the unique determinants of the β-pleated floor.

The three areas of greatest genetic diversity (hypervariable regions) are expressed in segments of each of the α-helices and the β-pleated sheet. This genetic variation very specifically affects, or "selects," which antigens can bind to specific molecules. In addition, it specifically "selects" which TCRs can interact with specific combinations of MHC-antigen complex, often referred to as the trimolecular interaction.

These same areas correlate with the predisposition to certain diseases. In rheumatoid arthritis, for example, a specific sequence of amino acids in the hypervariable region is strongly associated with disease susceptibility—between amino acids from position 67–74 of the HLA-DR β-chain.

Antigen binding site.

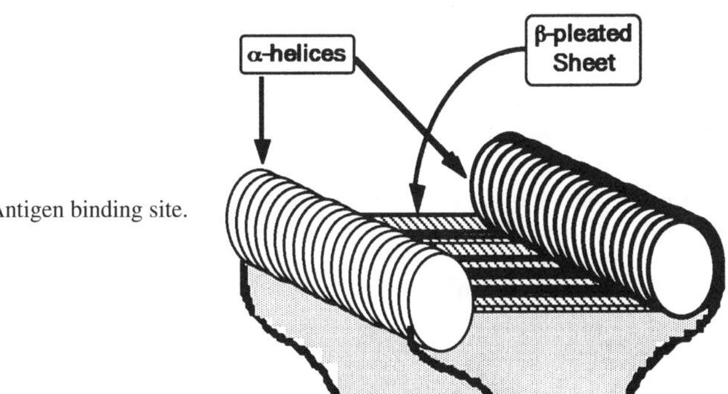


**12. How are the four molecules that specifically recognize antigen constructed?**

Immunoglobulins (BCR), TCR, and MHC Class I and Class II molecules all are expressed as transmembrane, cell-surface molecules (see figure). Each has two associated chains, which means each is expressed as a "dimer," in addition to many other proteins that co-associate with the complex. Each of the chains is based on a similar repeating structure that is derived from a common primordial gene known as the "immunoglobulin supergene." For each molecule, the furthest extracellular extension is the **amino terminus**; the intracellular end is the **carboxy terminus** (COOH). The site of antigen binding is located near the amino terminus of each molecule. In each of these molecules, the genes encode for extraordinary diversity at the **antigen-binding site**. More specifically, most of the diversity occurs in three **hypervariable regions** (HVRs 1, 2, and 3) near the amino terminus, with the greatest diversity occurring in HVR3. In contrast to these regions of marked diversity, the remainder of the structure is remarkably conserved to facilitate antigen binding and, in the case of the MHC and TCR molecules, MHC-TCR recognition.

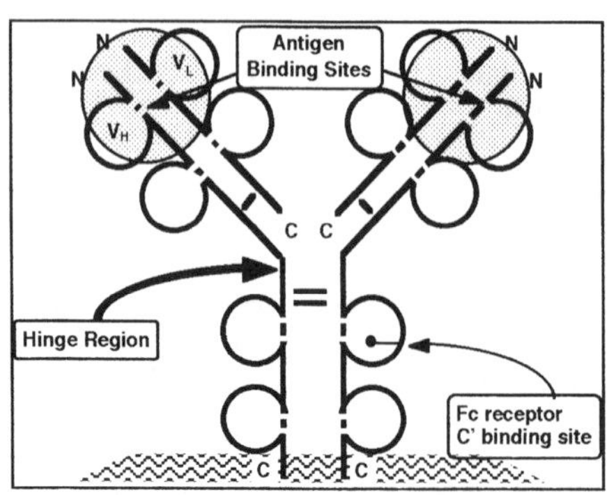


Surface Immunoglobulin

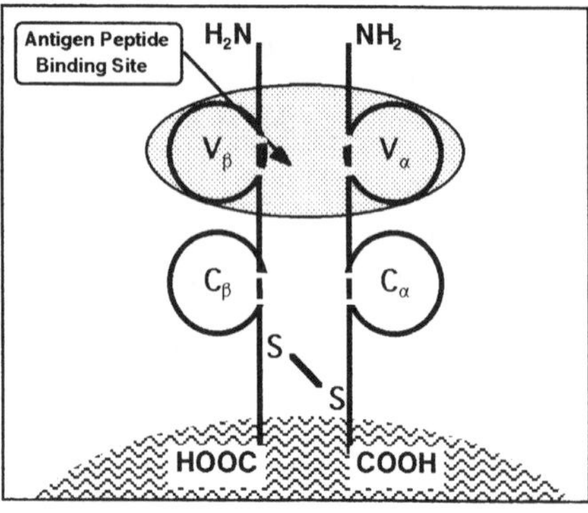


T Cell Receptor

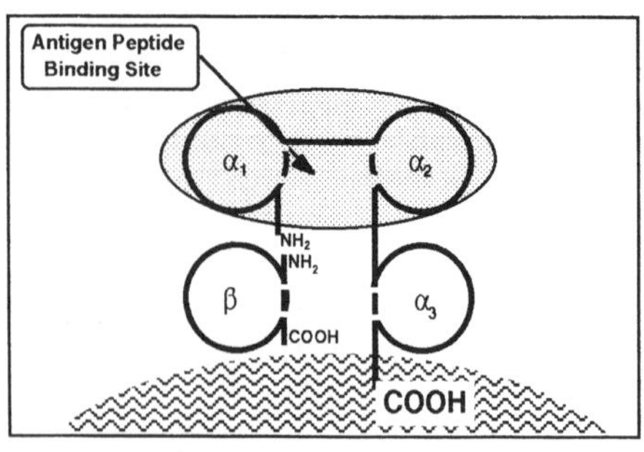


MHC Class I

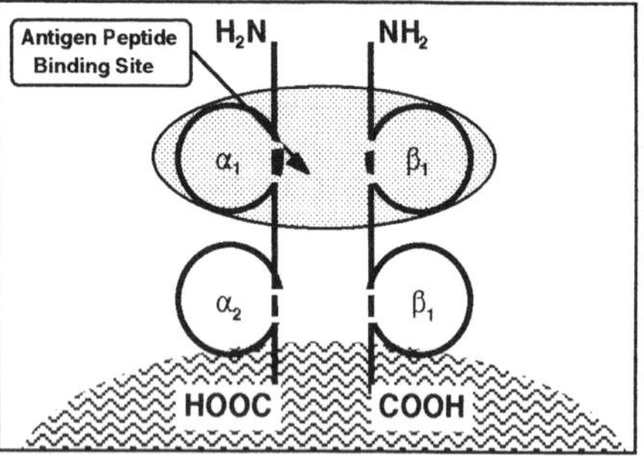


MHC Class II

**13. If the MHC Class I and II molecules share so much in common, why are they classified separately?**

While both are dimeric cell surface molecules, MHC Class II proteins show more diversity than MHC Class I proteins. Both the α- and β-chains of the MHC Class II are encoded by the Class II region of the MHC. However, while the α-chains of the MHC Class I molecules are encoded by MHC Class I alleles, they all share a common β-chain, $\beta_2$-microglobulin.

**14. How do the MHC Class I and II molecules differ in function?**

They differ in their cellular distribution, the antigenic peptide fragments they present, and the type of T cell that recognizes and responds to the complex they present.

*Function of MHC Class I and II Molecules*

| | MHC CLASS I | MHC CLASS II |
|---|---|---|
| Cellular distribution | All nucleated cells and platelets | Certain immune system cells, particularly if they serve as "professional" antigen presenting cells:<br>B cells<br>Monocytes/macrophages<br>Dendritic cells<br>Thymic epithelial cells<br>Some activated T cells<br>Some cells in which MHC Class II expression can be induced, particularly |

*(Table continued on next page.)*

*Function of MHC Class I and II Molecules (cont.)*

| | MHC CLASS I | MHC CLASS II |
|---|---|---|
| | | during chronic inflammatory processes: Endothelial cells Synovial cells |
| Antigen size | 8–13 amino acids in length | 13–25 amino acids in length |
| Antigen type | Antigenic peptide fragment endogenous to the cytoplasm or nucleus of the cell that is expressing the MHC molecule (e.g., endogenous or "self"-peptides; peptides of obligate intracellular pathogens such as viruses and chlamydia; tumor antigens) | Antigenic peptide fragment present in lysosomal compartments as a result of phagocytosis or receptor-mediated endocytosis (e.g., exogenous or foreign infectious material [bacteria]) |
| T-cell recognition | $CD8^+$ T cell | $CD4^+$ T cell |
| Resultant T-cell response | Cell-mediated killing or suppression of the MHC Class I–presenting cell | T cell–coordinated phagocytic and/or antibody response to eradicate the antigen that was presented |

**15. Is the total number of your potential and actual MHC Class II molecules greater than the total number of MHC Class I molecules?**

Yes. The possibilities of HLA-A and HLA-B MHC molecules approximate 50 and 100, respectively; the number of HLA-C possibilities is almost 40. However, even in an individual heterozygous at each MHC Class I β-chain allele, the total number of MHC Class I molecules expressed will be 6: 3 from Mom, 3 from Dad (see figure).

For MHC II, only the HLA-DR α-chain alleles are limited in variation. However, the polymorphism at the HLA-DP and -DQ α-chain loci and the HLA-DP, -DQ, and -DR β-chain loci is extraordinary. As a result, the number of possible combinations is staggering. Individuals with the greatest diversity will express 2 HLA-DR, 4 HLA-DP, and 4 HLA-DQ molecules. That is, with different alleles at each MHC Class II locus, except the HLA-DR α-locus, which is relatively invariant, a total of 10 types of MHC Class II molecules can be expressed. In addition, cross-pairing of α-and β-chains has also been described, which increases the diversity.

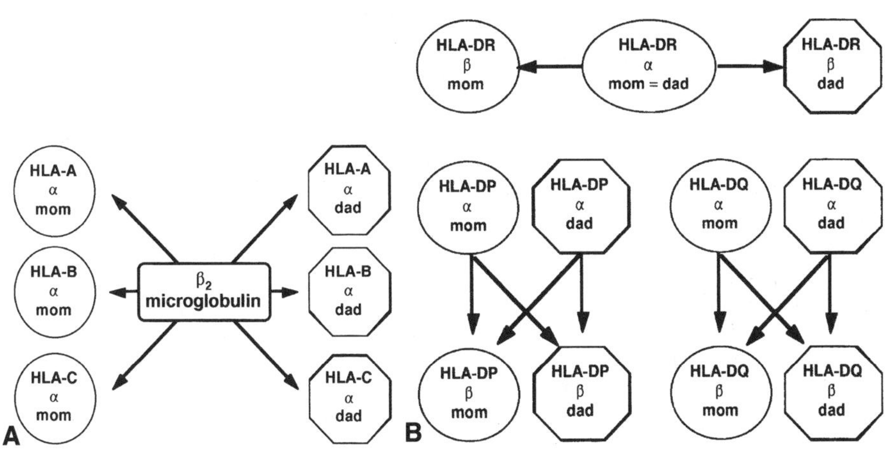


*A*, Inherited MHC I molecule possibilities in a given individual. *B*, Inherited MHC possibilities in a given individual.

**16. What are some of the commonly recognized associations of MHC molecules with diseases?**

*HLA-Antigen Associations*

| | | | |
|---|---|---|---|
| HLA-A29 | Birdshot choroidretinitis | HLA-DR4 | Rheumatoid arthritis |
| HLA-B5 | Behçet's disease | | Pemphigus vulgaris (Jews) |
| | Ulcerative colitis | | Insulin-dependent diabetes mellitus (Type I) |
| | Polycystic kidney disease | | IgA nephropathy |
| HLA-B27 | Seronegative spondyloarthropathies | HLA-DR5 | Pauciarticular juvenile rheumatoid arthritis |
| HLA-B38 | Psoriatic arthritis | | Pernicious anemia |
| HLA-DR1 | Rheumatoid arthritis | | Hashimoto's thyroiditis |
| HLA-DR2 | Narcolepsy | HLA-DR7 | Congenital adrenal hyperplasia |
| | Multiple sclerosis | HLA-DQ | Polymorphisms associated with various autoantibodies produced in SLE patients |
| | Goodpasture's syndrome | HLA-DQ3.2 | Insulin-dependent diabetes mellitus (type I) |
| HLA-DR3 | Systemic lupus erythematosus | | |
| | Sjögren's syndrome (primary) | | |
| | Gluten-sensitive enteropathy | | |
| | Chronic active hepatitis | | |
| | Dermatitis herpetiformis | | |
| | Graves' disease | | |
| | Insulin-dependent diabetes mellitus (type I) | | |
| | Idiopathic membranous glomerulonephritis | | |

**17. If T cells coordinate chronic inflammatory responses, what role do MHC molecules play in predisposing to the development of rheumatic diseases?**

First, MHC molecules are pivotal in the process by which the immune system decides whether naive developing T cells are allowed to survive in the thymus and develop or whether they must die. Second, MHC molecules control what T cells can see because T cells cannot recognize antigens alone but must do so when the antigen is physically associated with these proteins, a process termed "T-cell recognition in the context of MHC." The agents that T cells can normally specifically recognize, and therefore respond to, are predominantely MHC-peptide complexes.

**18. How do the MHC molecules control what the T cells see?**

They do this in two ways. First, the sequence of amino acids in an MHC molecule determines which antigenic peptide fragments can bind to that molecule. Only those "selected" antigenic peptides that can bind to one of an individual's MHC molecules have the potential to be specifically recognized. Second, not all T cells can see all the MHC molecules. The peptides presented in the context of MHC Class I molecules can only be seen by T cells that have CD8 molecules associated with their TCR, while the peptides presented in the context of MHC Class II molecules can only be seen by T cells that have CD4 molecules associated with their TCR.

**19. So a person inheriting HLA-DR4 will develop rheumatoid arthritis, just like with other hereditary diseases. Right?**

No. Unlike many diseases in which autosomal dominant or recessive genes actually transmit or cause the diseases with which they are associated (e.g., an absent or mutant gene might result in deficient production of a vital enzyme), most HLA-associated diseases cannot be explained in that way. Certainly, none of the rheumatic disease associations fits such an explanation. In addition, some HLA molecules may not cause or confer susceptibility to the disease with which they are associated, but instead they are associated just because they are commonly inherited in association with another gene that actually confers susceptibility to the disease, which is termed **linkage disequilibrium**. In several instances, however, particular HLA molecules do appear to confer susceptibility to the diseases with which they are associated.

**20. If a gene for an HLA molecule is not actually causing a disease, then maybe there is simply another gene that directly causes the disease? How can we tell?**

Identical twin studies provide us with the clearest response to this question. If an inherited gene directly caused the disease under study, identical twins would always suffer from the disease. It is clear that identical twins who express HLA-DR4, which is genetically associated with rheumatoid arthritis, both have a significantly higher, but not 100%, risk of developing rheumatoid arthritis. This suggests that additional factors, such as environmental exposures or stochastic events during development of the immune system, play major roles.

However, other studies compel us to believe that many of the HLA molecules are more than inherited "bystanders." In looking at penetrance of disease in heterozygotes versus homozygotes, we know that HLA molecules are "dominant" in their effects, because even heterozygotes display enhanced disease rates. Individuals who are homozygous for a particular gene are generally more vulnerable to the development of a particular disease than heterozygotes. Such studies of MHC **codominant expression** reinforce the belief that HLA associations are important in the pathophysiology of autoimmune diseases. Finally, "designer" rats may provide the most compelling information supporting a true immunopathogenetic relationship between HLA and disease. These rats, transgenic for human HLA-B27, are genetically designed to express HLA-B27 on their cells. As a consequence, they spontaneously develop gut, skin, nail, joint, urethra, and spine problems, some of which are dependent upon the presence of bacterial flora. The disease in rats is similar in many ways to the seronegative spondyloarthropathies associated with HLA-B27 in humans, supporting a direct role for B27 rather than a linked gene in humans.

**21. Why should we believe that a gene associated with a rheumatic disease does not cause the disease but does confer susceptibility?**

Although we know that some HLA molecules are associated with particular diseases, clearly not everyone who expresses that HLA molecule necessarily develops the disease. Thus, certain genes may confer susceptibility to certain diseases, even though they do not independently cause them. We also know that nongenetic factors, such as infections, have been clearly associated with the development of some HLA-associated diseases. Thus, there appear to be other factors, involving the host and its environment, in addition to chance alone that may result in the development of a disease in a person who is genetically susceptible.

**22. By what mechanism do MHC genes confer susceptibility?**

The answer to this question is unknown. However, the three most commonly discussed possibilities are that they bind pathogenic organisms in some fashion, control T-cell development in the thymus in such a fashion that is important for tolerance, or bind particular peptides that are "pathogenic." Certainly this is a centrally important question that many investigators are studying.

**23. How do you determine the strength of these associations? How susceptible to diseases are people with HLA associations?**

The risk of patients developing an HLA-associated disease is conventionally expressed as their relative risk. For example, relative risk describes the odds that an HLA-DR4–positive person will get rheumatoid arthritis compared with a person who is not HLA-DR4–positive:

$$\text{Relative risk} = \frac{(\%\text{antigen-positive patients})\ (\%\text{antigen-negative controls})}{(\%\text{antigen-negative patients})\ (\%\text{antigen-positive controls})}$$

The relative risk estimates vary somewhat based on the ethnicity of the population studied. For example, the relative risk of rheumatoid arthritis in HLA-DR4–positive whites of Northern European extraction is much greater than that in HLA-DR4–positive Jewish or black people.

**24. How do you determine a person's HLA type?**

HLA-DR3 or HLA-DR4 specificities are referred to as "serologic" specificities. These are determined by using transplantation or pregnancy sera in which the antibodies against MHC molecules have previously been identified. There are sera, for example, that contain antibodies only against HLA-DR2, HLA-DR3, or HLA-DR4. Combinations of these sera are then used to "type" or characterize an individual's MHC molecules. While this method has been extremely valuable over the years, especially in transplantation biology, more specific genetically based typing methods are now available to characterize the MHC identity of individuals and so investigate immunogenetic associations with diseases.

**25. Does serologic cross-reactivity correlate with disease susceptibility?**

Antibodies obtained from human sera that are directed against HLA molecules can bind to molecules that are very similar, but not identical. When serologic specificities were developed, the antibodies against the MHC molecules were not defined as being specific for that small area of the molecule that predisposes to autoimmune disease. If most but not all HLA-DR4 molecules are identical at the particular site that enhances the susceptibility to rheumatoid arthritis (RA), then most but not all HLA-DR4–positive individuals would have enhanced susceptibility to RA. In contrast, two individuals, one HLA-DR4–positive and the other HLA-DR1–positive, might both have enhanced susceptibility to RA if they share the site that enhances susceptibility to RA, even though their serologic specificities differ.

**26. Is it really this confusing? Can there really be people who are HLA-DR4–positive who are not predisposed to rheumatoid arthritis? Can there be people who are HLA-DR4–negative, but HLA-DR1–, DR6–, or DR10–positive, who are predisposed?**

Yes. This cross-reactivity, and therefore compromised specificity of serotyping, clarified the need for more genetically pure typing. Because of this, techniques have been developed that can define the nucleotide sequences of the MHC genetic loci designated, for example, by DRB*0402. They can be more specific for that special area of the HLA molecule that predisposes to the disease, such as a region called the "**shared epitope**." These methods provide improved estimates of relative risk.

The issue of cross-reactivity has created significant confusion in the study of RA. In different ethnic groups, HLA-DR1, -DR4, -DR6, and -DR10 molecules have been associated with RA. HLA-DR4 molecules share marked homology in the first and second hypervariable regions (HVRs), which align them according to serologic typing (note the striking homology in the HVRs 1 and 2 that characterize the upper four sequences in the figure on the next page). Some HLA-DR4, -DR1, -DR6, and -DR10 alleles, while very different in HVRs 1 and 2, share crucial amino acid homology in the HVR3 (see the homology in the HVR3 regions of the lower six sequences in the figure). This "shared epitope" in HVR3 appears to predispose to RA. In contrast, the HLA-DRB*0402 sequence (top sequence in the figure) does not predispose to RA. In the DRB*0402 allele, there are the amino acids isoleucine (I), aspartic acid (D), and glutamic acid (E) at positions 67, 70, and 71, respectively. The predisposition to RA seems to require a leucine (L) at position 67, glutamine (Q) or arginine (R) at position 70; arginine (R) or lysine (K) at position 71; and alanine (A) at position 74.

**27. How will the Human Genome Project and the revolution in genetic analysis techniques improve our understanding of the genetic predisposition to developing an autoimmune disease?**

The Human Genome Project has sequenced all 3.2 billion base pairs in the human genome. It is now recognized that there are 30,000–40,000 functional genes among the 46 chromosomes and 20 genes (inherited from the mother) in the mitochrondria. Yet individuals differ only .1% or 3 million base pairs over the entire genome. However, these polymorphisms account for our diversity as well as our predisposition to autoimmune diseases. Linkage analysis has enabled geneticists to identify genes causing rheumatic diseases inherited as autosomal or sex linked dominant or recessive traits. Examples include the HFE gene in hemochromatosis on the short arm

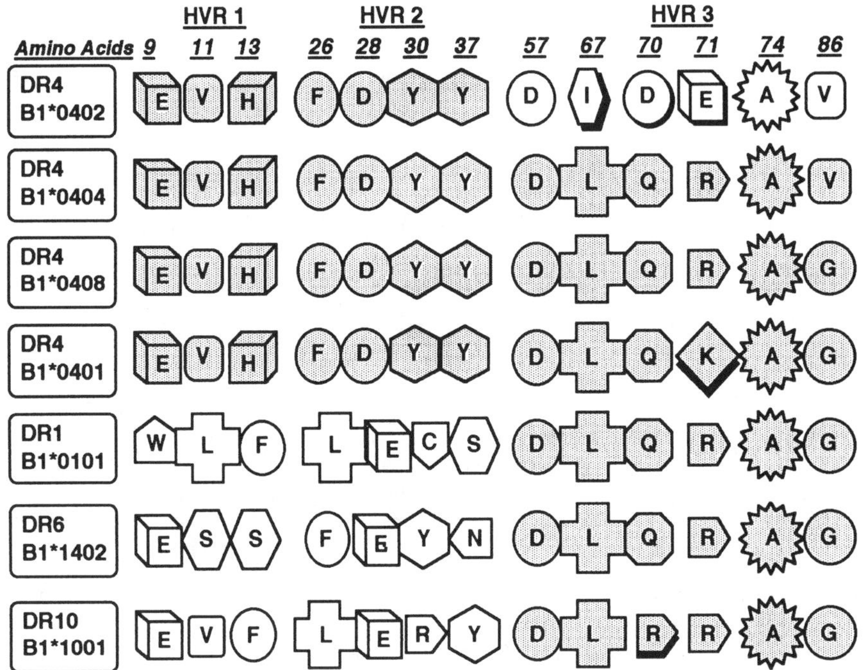


Amino acid sequence in the three hypervariable regions (HVR) of several different allelic forms of the HLA-DRβ chain.

of chromosome 6, the pyrin/marenostrin gene associated with familial Mediterranean fever on chromosome 16, and the P55 tumor necrosis factor receptor gene on chromosome 12 associated with an hereditary periodic fever syndrome. However, diseases with complex genetic traits such as RA and SLE require family studies such as analysis of allele sharing between affected sibling pairs. Microsatellite markers are used in this analysis to scan the genome looking for linkage between the marker and a candidate gene in an affected sibling pair. However, there are several limitations of genetic analysis identifying a gene as the cause of a rheumatic disease. Indeed, environmental influences, stochastic responses, effect of other genes on the candidate gene (i.e. epistasis), and posttranslational modifications of the gene product (i.e. protein phosphorylation) may all affect whether a certain gene contributes to the risk of developing an autoimmune disease.

## BIBLIOGRAPHY


1. Centola M, Aksentijevich I, Kastner DL: The hereditary periodic fever syndromes: Molecular analysis of a new family of inflammatory diseases. Human Molec Genet 7(10):1581–1588, 1998.
2. Gregersen PK: Genetics of rheumatic diseases. In Ruddy S, Harris ED, Sledge CB (eds): Kelley's Textbook of Rheumatology, 6th ed. Philadelphia, W.B. Saunders, 2001, pp 95–112. 8. Tan FK, Arnett FC: The genetics of lupus. Curr Opin Rheumatol 10(5):399–408, 1998.
3. Harley JB, Moser KL, Gaffney PM, Behrens TW: The genetics of human systemic lupus erythematosus. Curr Opin Immunol 10(6):690–696, 1998.
4. Klein J, Sato A: The HLA system (in two parts). N Engl J Med 343:702–709, 782–786, 2000.
5. Li H, Llera A, Malchiodi BL, Mariuzza RA: The structural basis of T cell activation by superantigens. Annu Rev Immunol 17:435–466, 1999.
6. Nepom GT: Major histocompatibility complex–directed susceptibility to rheumatoid arthritis. Adv Immunol 68:315–332, 1998.
7. Seldin MF, Amos CT, Ward R, Gregersen PK: The genetics revolution and the assault on rheumatoid arthritis. Arthritis Rheumatism 42(6):1071–1079, 1999.

8. Tan FK, Arnett FC: The genetics of lupus. Curr Opin Rheumatol 10(5):399–408, 1998.
9. Vyse TJ, Kotzin BL: Genetic susceptibility to systemic lupus erythematosus. Annu Rev Immunol 16:261–292, 1998.
10. Weyand CM, Goronzy JJ: HLA polymorphisms and T cells in rheumatoid arthritis. Internat Rev Immunol 18(1–2):37–59, 1999.

# 7. TOLERANCE AND AUTOIMMUNITY

V. Michael Holers, M.D.

**1. What is the primary goal of the immune system?**

The main objective of a healthy immune system is to distinguish pathogenic, dangerous non-self organisms and substances at the same time as remaining non-responsive to self tissues. The processes by which these two opposing forces are normally controlled and become dysregulated in disease are at the heart of the pathogenesis of rheumatic disease. The immune system is divided into the innate system (consisting of complement, scavenger receptors, Toll proteins, etc.) and the acquired immune system (in which B- and T-cell receptors function).

**2. What is tolerance?**

**Tolerance** is the term used to describe the phenomenon of **antigen-specific unresponsiveness**. In other words, the immune system encounters certain antigens to which it is programmed specifically to not respond and, therefore, not eradicate.

**3. Is tolerance innate or acquired?**

The phenomenon of tolerance is present in both the innate and acquired immune systems. We are protected from the innate immune system by specific mechanisms that block its activities, such as membrane complement regulatory proteins that protect self tissues from the alternative pathway. The adaptive immune system "learns" to be tolerant of some specific antigens, such as self tissues, just as it learns to be "intolerant" of many foreign antigens. When discussing autoimmune disorders, we often narrow our perspective to the tolerance of **autoantigens**, such as an individual's own nucleoproteins or cell-surface molecules, by the adaptive immune system. However, the phenomenon of tolerance is not limited to autoantigens. In fact, tolerance to **exogenous antigens**, such as dietary proteins, is just as crucial for the survival of an individual as "self tolerance." Valuable insights into the development and loss of tolerance in autoimmune disorders, as well as creative therapeutic approaches, are emerging from our understanding of tolerance to all forms of exogenous antigens, both protein and non–protein based. In addition, we now know that both the innate and acquired immune systems function in a linked fashion such that alterations of tolerance in one can affect the other. For example, alterations of tolerance in the innate immune system, such as deficiency states, can lead to a break of tolerance in the acquired immune system.

**4. What is autoimmunity?**

The term *autoimmunity* is commonly employed to describe conditions in which self tolerance is broken and an individual becomes the victim of his or her own immune response. Just like immunity to foreign antigens, autoimmune disorders are antigen-driven processes that are characterized by specificity, high affinity, and memory. However, an autoimmune process involves the immune system's recognition of an antigen, either foreign or self, that is then followed by an assault on its own self antigens (i.e., autoantigens). Typically, these processes develop in an individual who previously displayed tolerance to the same antigens that are now targeted by the immune response. Therefore, most autoimmune processes are better described not simply as an absence of tolerance but as a **loss of previously established tolerance**.

**5. If autoimmune processes involve a loss or absence of tolerance that leads to a chronic antigen-driven immune response against autoantigens, shouldn't the key to their control involve preventing the loss of tolerance or re-establishing tolerance?**

Many investigators believe this. However, effective implementation of this hypothesis presumes an understanding of the development and maintenance of tolerance. We have many observations confirming that tolerance is, indeed, developed, maintained, and can be pathologically lost. Unfortunately, our understanding of these processes is still limited. Therefore, current therapies for these disorders are often empiric and based on historical usage patterns. However, newer strategies directed at components of the process are in clinical trials or in pre-clinical phases of development.

**6. What are the major factors that influence the development of specific immune responses?**

- Characteristics of the antigen involved in the specific immunologic response
- Presence of sufficient and appropriate engagement of the innate immune system
- Characteristics of the accessory cells that initially interact with the antigen and process it
- Nature of the responding lymphocytes and the cytokines that they produce

**7. How can the characteristics of the antigen favor the development of tolerance rather than autoimmunity?**

The immune system will respond to an individual antigen in different manners based on its **chemical composition**, the initial **amount** to which an individual is exposed, the initial **route** by which the antigen is introduced to the immune system, and the type of **milieu** within which the antigen encounters the immune system. Two important aspects of that milieu include the level of development of the immune system at the time of initial antigen presentation and the presence or absence of surrounding inflammation at the site where the antigen is presented.

| TOLERANCE | IMMUNE RESPONSE |
|---|---|
| Intravenous or oral route | Subcutaneous or intradermal route |
| Monomeric antigen | Aggregated or polymeric antigen |
| Large dose | Small dose |
| Immunologic immaturity | Surrounding inflammation |

For example, small subcutaneous (SC) or intradermal (ID) doses of aggregated antigen are more likely to evoke an immune response than large intravenous (IV) or oral doses of the same monomeric antigen. If an inflammatory response is generated in the same locale as an antigen is introduced (e.g., by employing an adjuvant to activate the innate immune system), an antigen-specific response is more likely to develop. If, on the other hand, no inflammation is present or the exposed immune cells are immature at the time of antigen presentation, tolerance is relatively favored.

**8. Discuss T cell:B cell cooperation in the development of autoimmune disease.**

The majority of antigens targeted in autoimmune diseases are proteins. Antigen-specific memory responses to proteins are coordinated by B and T cells. T cells can only recognize protein antigens presented to them in the context of MHC molecules as peptides on antigen presenting cells. MHC molecules on B cells can present antigens to T cells very effectively, especially if the surface immunoglobulin is specific for the antigen and uptake and processing to peptides are thus promoted. The activated T cells then provide signals that also amplify B cell responses. This places B cell:T cell cooperation at the crux of the development of an immune response to both self and non-self antigens. The interactions of B and T cells require cell surface proteins on one cell type that specifically bind proteins on the other cell type in a receptor:counter-receptor system. These systems include B7-1/B7-2 with CD28, and CD40 with CD40 ligand. Blocking of these cell:cell interaction mechanisms is a major new therapeutic strategy currently being tested in various rheumatic diseases.

**9. How do variations in an antigen's amino acid sequence influence the development of autoimmune disease?**

It is not simply that antigens are proteins, but also the sequence of their amino acids that is important. When MHC Class I and II molecules present peptide to T cells, only a small peptide generated by intracellular proteolyic processing mechanisms fits in the antigen-binding cleft: 8–13 amino acids for MHC Class I and 13–25 amino acids for MHC Class II. It is also clear that individual amino acid positions in the MHC molecules are crucial for the binding of certain complementary peptide amino acid sequences, and these positions are typically in polymorphic regions.

**10. How can the primary structure of an antigen lead to a loss of tolerance?**

First, the peptide sequence of a foreign antigen may resemble a self antigen. If that happens, untoward sequelae may develop. Rheumatic heart disease is the classic example of such a situation. The myocardial autoantigens, myosin and sarcolemmal membrane proteins, resemble the streptococcal M protein structure. Part of the pathogenesis, supported by autoantibodies, may be secondary to innocent myocardial tissue becoming the target of immune response products evoked by M protein. Subsequently, the myocardial autoantigens could continue to drive the process.

In another example, there are peptides derived from some pathogens that have stretches of amino acids whose sequence is identical to the sequences in the antigen-binding cleft of certain MHC molecules themselves, For example, a string of five amino acids in a plasmid-derived peptide of *Shigella flexneri* has been found that is identical to a sequence within HLA-B27 from bacteria infecting patients with dysentery and Reiter's syndrome. Similar homology has been shown or predicted to exist for a number of other pathogen-derived products.

These are two examples of cross-reactivity in which the products of the immune response to a foreign antigen might inappropriately engage an individual's own antigens. This pathologic confusion is commonly referred to as **molecular mimicry**. The T- and B-cell clones that were initially activated by the foreign antigen might continue to be stimulated by the cross-reactive autoantigens. The likelihood of this happening may be increased by certain deficiency states, such as early components of the complement classical pathway like C1q, where autoantibodies commonly appear that are reactive with self antigens and clinical syndromes similar to SLE are found. It is conceivable that autoantigen-driven immune responses might persist long after the foreign antigen that initiated the process has been eliminated, thus complicating the search for etiologic agents.

**11. Discuss therapeutic strategies using the amount and route of antigen exposure to induce tolerance.**

Large doses of either protein or polysaccharide antigens in experimental situations have been shown to promote T- or B-cell tolerance, respectively. In the appropriate context, low-dose peptide presentation may evoke T-cell tolerance.

Recently, investigators have also attempted therapeutic trials that employ oral doses of an antigen in an effort to induce tolerance to endogenous antigens. For example, in experimental allergic encephalomyelitis, an animal model similar to multiple sclerosis, myelin basic protein (MBP) is the target autoantigen. Pre-treatment with oral MBP prior to injection of MBP in adjuvant systemically in these animals has reduced the severity of their disease. As a consequence, human therapeutic trials with oral doses of MBP, perhaps the autoantigen in multiple sclerosis, have been undertaken, as has oral collagen administration in patients with rheumatoid arthritis, in an attempt to take advantage of the same tolerogenic phenomenon. Unfortunately, convincing positive results have not been found. This outcome may relate to the observation in animals that pre-treatment orally can lead to tolerance, but there is no effect of the oral toleragen once the immune response has been initiated.

**12. What are superantigens? Do these lead to autoimmunity?**

Superantigens are foreign antigens, particularly of bacterial or viral origin, that are capable of binding to the T-cell receptor (TCR) and MHC Class II molecule outside the antigen-binding groove and, in turn, bind the two together (see figure). B cell superantigens also exist that bind to regions of surface immunoglobulin that are common to various sub-types. These kinds of antigens are not as restricted in their effects as typical antigens. In the case of T cells, superantigens do not need to be processed and subsequently presented in the antigen-binding cleft of MHC molecules in order to stimulate T-cell activation. The superantigen is specific for a segment in the variable (V) region of the TCR β-chain, the Vβ region. Up to 10% of T cells may share a common Vβ region for which the superantigen is specific. This results in the activation of extremely large numbers of different antigen-specific clones of T cells. B cell superantigens such as staphylococcal protein A appear to play a similar role in B cells. Although they are implicated in the pathology of toxic shock syndrome, T-cell superantigens do not appear to mediate the classic rheumatic diseases. However, studies are still ongoing to discern the exact role that these potent antigens play.

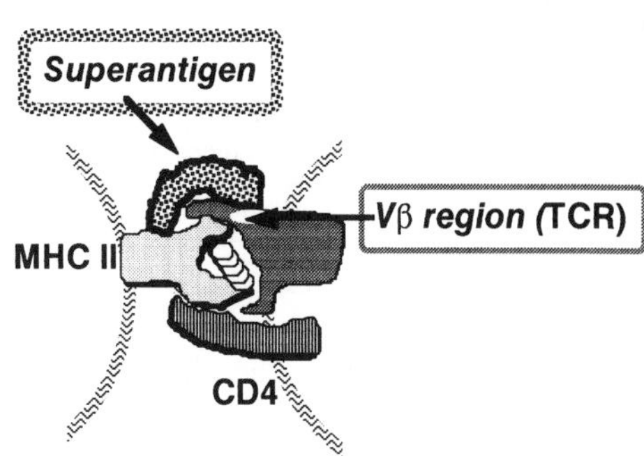


Superantigen specificity for the TCR Vβ region external to the conventional MHC-peptide antigen-binding cleft.

**13. How does the milieu affect the development of immunologic responses?**

It has long been recognized that the effectiveness of immunization can be enhanced by the use of adjuvants. The major role of adjuvants appears to be their ability to activate innate immune system components such as Toll receptors and complement. It may be that autoantigens to which an individual previously has been tolerant are sometimes "innocently" presented to lymphocytes in an area where inflammation is already established. This can be the result of enhanced and aberrant presentation of autoantigens because of cytokine stimulation of antigen-presenting cells. Such an event can lead to a loss of tolerance. This might then be followed by an autoantigen-driven specific immune response that persists long after the trigger of the initial inflammatory process has been eliminated.

**14. What is determinant (epitope) spreading?**

Determinant spreading describes the loss of tolerance and the generation of an active, ongoing, autoantigen-driven specific immune response to many epitopes of a single antigen, or to several physically associated antigens, following the initiation of a response to a single epitope of an antigen. An example is the linked autoantibody response to Sm and RNP antigens that appears to be initiated by the response to a single epitope of one of the antigens. The process that drives this is T- and B-cell dependent, and evidence of determinant, or epitope, spreading is found in both cell types. It may be that determinant spreading is promoted in the milieu of acute and chronic inflammation. The best evidence that this is important comes from studies that show evidence of maturing autoreactive T- and B-cell–mediated responses to a variety of autoantigens during the course of chronic autoimmune disease such as SLE.

**15. What is meant by the term "hidden antigens"?**

Hidden antigens are potential antigens for which an individual may never have developed specific recognition or tolerance. Therefore, these particular antigens have the potential to evoke an aggressive response from the immune system. Examples of this are antigens in the eye, thyroid, or cartilage to which the immune system has never been exposed. Physical damage may release these antigens and thus result in further immune mediated injury.

**16. How can accessory cells favor the development of tolerance rather than autoimmunity?**

Antigen-presenting cells (APCs) are often referred to as "accessory cells"—i.e., these cells are looked upon as being supportive to the lymphocytes. The cells both present antigen and elaborate signals that result in a process called **costimulation**. Costimulation is primarily mediated by surface proteins such as B7 molecules that interact with CD28 on T cells. This interaction is necessary for T cells to be activated, and to reciprocally activate B cells, and thus this is a target of new therapeutics such as CTLA-4-Ig, which physically blocks B7 interactions with T cells. APCs play a major role in the selection of the T-cell repertoire and the lifelong maintenance of tolerance. They influence this via their methods and choice of processing and presenting antigens, the MHC context within which they present it, the intensity within which they present it, and the costimulatory signals they provide. If APCs do not function properly, autoimmunity may be enhanced.

**17. Summarize the potential roles of MHC molecules in autoimmune processes.**

There are many postulated mechanisms. No one mechanism alone explains autoimmunity.

*Potential Roles of MHC Molecules in Autoimmune Disorders*

| ROLE IN AUTOIMMUNITY | EXPLANATION |
|---|---|
| T-cell selection bias | The T-cell population that is selected via the inherited disease-associated MHC molecules may include more autoreactive T cells or disease-specific autoreactive T cells. |
| Pathogenic receptor function | Certain disease-associated MHC molecules may function as a receptor for certain pathogens that cause autoimmune disease. |
| Unique peptide presentation | Disease-associated MHC molecules may be uniquely capable of presenting certain peptides that evoke the autoimmune response. This is supported by the shared epitope hypothesis. |
| Molecular mimicry | A foreign antigen or another MHC + foreign peptide may resemble the disease-associated MHC molecule, with or without bound peptide.<br>This may be followed by:<br>• An appropriate immunologic response followed by pathologic autoreactivity,<br>or<br>• The immune system, tolerized to its own MHC molecule with or without bound peptide, cannot mount an appropriate response to the cross-reactive foreign antigen. That foreign antigen may go on to cause the chronic disease. |
| Inappropriate peptide presentation | Presentation of self-antigens when the APC is also expressing costimulating molecules or when the cytokine presentation milieu will stimulate a response.<br>Presentation of improperly processed peptides.<br>Increased presentation of peptides that do not require a response may result from APC activation by cytokine stimulation. |

**18. What is clonal deletion?**

Clones of T lymphocytes are not useful if they cannot recognize "self MHC" or if they recognize but then try to eradicate it. In other words, the recognition by the T-cell receptor (TCR) for the MHC-peptide complex during development in the thymus cannot be either too high or too low of an affinity and must fall within a specified range. If not, T cells are instructed to kill themselves during development. **Clonal deletion** refers to this intrathymic process during which immature T cells are functionally deleted from the repertoire.

**19. How are T cells selected to survive or die in the thymus?**

Current observations are consistent with the existence of at least two processes:

1. The cells must be **positively selected**. That is, the TCR must recognize "self MHC plus peptide" enough to be able to respond when necessary. Those whose TCRs do recognize the MHC + peptide survive; if not, they die by undergoing apoptosis.

2. T cells must be **negatively selected**. That is, they must not have such a strong affinity for the MHC that they respond by eradicating self-MHC plus peptide. Those whose interaction is of too high an affinity have to be either deleted or inactivated.

**20. How can cells be activated to kill themselves? If they don't kill themselves on command, does that result in autoimmune disease?**

Recent investigations strongly support the notion that autoreactive T cells may not be eliminated because they cannot be effectively commanded to commit suicide. One mechanism by which this programmed cell death, termed **apoptosis**, can be initiated is by cross-linking of a cell-surface molecule called Fas/APO1 (CD95). A defect in Fas-mediated apoptosis appears to be the genetic defect in a murine model of SLE, the MRL-*lpr/lpr* mouse. Aberrant Fas-mediated apoptosis appears to also be the cause of rare cases of a human autoimmune disease resembling SLE.

**21. What is clonal anergy?**

We know that thymic T-cell selection and education are not absolutely correct. Because of this, there are a lot of potentially autoreactive T cells out in the circulation and secondary lymphoid tissues. **Clonal anergy** refers to the processes, implemented either centrally in the thymus or in the peripheral tissues, whereby autoreactive T cells are functionally inactivated but not destroyed. Clonal anergy is then the process by which these autoreactive T cells are inactivated such that they cannot respond to antigen.

**22. How does clonal anergy happen?**

Most cell activation responses, especially antigen-specific responses, require more than one signal. Evidence suggests that some anergy processes include an interaction of the MHC-peptide complex with an autoreactive TCR during which costimulatory signals are ***not*** provided to the autoreactive T cell.

**23. Does the term "suppressor T cell" describe some form of T-cell tolerance?**

The concept of the suppressor T cell is a controversial one surrounding the issue of whether there is a unique type of T cell that mediates ***only*** antigen-specific suppressor functions. Antigen-specific T-cell–suppressive effects, perhaps via release of TGF-β, may well modify autoreactivity. It appears that this effect is due to a unique T-cell subset that responds to antigens in the right context by secreting immunosuppressive substances such as TGF-β. This cytokine may inhibit responses to other antigen-specific T cells in the local milieu. Thus, while "suppressor T cell" may not be the correct term, there is clearly active suppression of immune responses by some T-cell types.

**24. Is there such a thing as B-cell tolerance?**

Yes, B-cell tolerance definitely exists using a mechanism acting both centrally and peripherally and leading to either deletion or functional inactivation of cells. Current evidence suggests that immature B cells that are specific for self antigen are likely to be deleted by apoptosis or inactivated and circulate in an "anergic" form. Encounter with antigen in the absence of specific T-cell help, particularly during early development, may be responsible for some B-cell tolerance. It has recently been proposed that loss of B-cell tolerance may occur without direct T-cell help.

**25. Where do autoantibodies fit into the picture?**

The normal presence of potentially autoreactive lymphocytes, B cells as well as T cells, is well recognized. It is also common for the production of very low affinity autoantibodies (rheumatoid factors and antinuclear antibodies) to increase transiently in the face of immune activation. This up-regulation appears to be a relatively normal phenomenon and is mediated by CD5+ B cells. With increasing age, autoantibody production increases, perhaps reflecting some loss in the maintenance of tolerance. This increase does parallel the increased prevalence of autoimmune diseases with advancing age but does not implicate autoantibodies in the pathogenesis of all autoimmune diseases.

**26. Describe some diseases in which autoantibodies appear to play a major pathogenic role.**

- Autoantibodies appear to deliver the major cytopathic lesion in some hemolytic anemias and autoimmune thrombocytopenias.
- In insulin-resistant diabetes mellitus, myasthenia gravis, and pernicious anemia, autoantibodies directed against cellular receptors directly lead to pathologic cellular responses.
- In Goodpasture's syndrome and bullous pemphigoid, antibodies directed against basement membrane components result in the major pathologic lesions of those diseases.
- In SLE and post-streptococcal glomerulonephritis, immune complexes involving autoantibodies appear to be responsible for glomerular damage.
- In other diseases, the association of certain autoantibodies with specific diseases or particular manifestations of diseases may indirectly lead to the pathology by promoting antigen presentation and pathogenic T-cell activation.

## BIBLIOGRAPHY

1. Bar-Or A, Oliveira EM, Anderson DE, Hafler DA: Molecular pathogenesis of multiple sclerosis. J Neuroimmunol 100(1–2):252–259, 1999.
2. Eisenberg R: Mechanisms of systemic autoimmunity in murine models of SLE. Immunol Res 17(1–2):41–47, 1998.
3. Kotzin BL: Autoimmunity. In Ruddy S, Harris ED, Sledge CB (eds): Kelley's Textbook of Rheumatology, 6th ed. Philadelphia, W.B. Saunders, 2001, pp 305–320.
4. Kumar V, Sercarz E: Distinct levels of regulation in organ-specific autoimmune diseases. Life Sci 65(15):1523–1530, 1999.
5. Marrack P, Kappler J: Positive selection of thymocytes bearing αβ T cell receptors. Curr Opin Immunol 9(2):250–255, 1997.
6. Medzhitov R, Janeway CA Jr: Innate immune recognition and control of adaptive immune responses. Semin Immunol 10(5):351–353, 1998.
7. Monroe JG: Balancing signals for negative selection and activation of developing B lymphocytes. Clin Immunol 95(1 Pt 2):S8–13, 2000.
8. Nemazee D, Weigert M: Revising B cell receptors. J Exp Med 191(11):1813–1817, 2000.
9. Fearon DT, Carroll MC: Regulation of B lymphocyte responses to foreign and self-antigens by the CD19/CD21 complex. Annu Rev Immunol 18:393–422, 2000.
10. Ridgway WM, Fathman CG: MHC structure and autoimmune T cell repertoire development. Curr Opin Immunol. 11(6):638–642, 1999.
11. Townsend SE, Weintraub BC, Goodnow CC: Growing up on the streets: Why B-cell development differs from T-cell development. Immunol Today 20(5):217–220, 1999.

# *III. Evaluation of the Patient with Rheumatic Symptoms*

*Specialism is a natural and necessary result of the growth of accurate knowledge, inseparably connected with the multiplication and perfection of instruments of precision. It has its drawbacks, absurdities even. . . . A few years ago a recent graduate and ex-hospital intern asked me, apparently seriously, to give him the name of a specialist in rheumatism. We can afford to laugh at these things . . .*

Frederick Shattuck, 1897
Professor of Medicine
Harvard Medical School

# 8. HISTORY AND PHYSICAL EXAMINATION

Richard T. Meehan, M.D.

**1. What symptoms or signs should your history include when interviewing a patient for connective tissue disease?**

A chronological history of symptom progression should include which joints have been involved (pain and or swelling) and identify any precipitating factors such as new drugs, recent infections, diet, activity, or recent trauma. Determine responsiveness to prior therapeutic modalities. Has the joint involvement been episodic, additive, mono, oligo, or polyarticular and/or in a symmetrical distribution? Identify any constitutional symptoms that suggest systemic illness, vasculitis, or paraneoplastic disease such as fever, weight loss, or fatigue. A complete review of systems is necessary to determine which organ systems may be involved such as: skin (malar rash, photosensitivity, alopecia, sclerodactyly, Raynaud's, digital ulcers, psoriasis, mucosal ulceration, purpura, nodules, ulcerations, genital lesions, or sicca symptoms), cardio-respiratory (dyspnea, cough, hemoptysis, pleurisy or pericardial pain, edema, or pulmonary emboli), gastrointestinal (reflux, dysphagia, abdominal pain, diarrhea, hematochezia, or jaundice), renal (prior proteinuria, or nephrolithiasis), hematologic (leukopenia, thrombocytopenia, anemia, fetal loss, unexplained DVT or PE or abnormal serologies), neurologic symptoms (neuropathies, weakness, TIA, strokes seizures, psychosis, cognitive deficits, or temporal headaches). Finally determine if there is underlying depression or risk factors for HIV, hepatitis B or C.

**2. What historical symptoms enable you to categorize a rheumatic disorder as inflammatory or mechanical (degenerative)?**

| FEATURE | INFLAMMATORY | MECHANICAL |
|---|---|---|
| Morning stiffness | >1 hr | ≤ 30 min |
| Fatigue | Significant | Minimal |
| Activity | May improve symptoms | May worsen symptoms |
| Rest | May worsen symptoms | May improve symptoms |
| Systemic involvement | Yes | No |
| Corticosteroid responsiveness | Yes | No |

**3. List the five cardinal signs of inflammation.**

Swelling (*tumor*)
Warmth (*calor*)
Erythema (*rubor*)
Tenderness (*dolor*)
Loss of function (*functio laesa*)

**4. In a patient with inflammatory arthritis, what history is useful in assessing disease activity?**

**Duration of morning stiffness, night pain, severity of constitutional symptoms such as fatigue, joint swelling, or new joint involvement** are more helpful than the severity of pain, which is too subjective.

**5. Which signs of inflammation are suggestive of acute synovitis in a joint?**

In the absence of corticosteroids, most joints affected by an inflammatory arthritis exhibit synovial distention, warmth, and limitation of range. The best indicator of synovitis is a distended joint capsule especially if accompanied by warmth. Swelling due to joint effusions may occur in the noninflammatory arthritides (e.g., osteoarthritis). Most inflamed joints are not typically erythematous, with exception of acute septic and crystalline arthritis. If you encounter red, hot joints, particularly in a monarticular distribution, your first thought should be "where's the needle?" This is needed in order to perform a joint aspiration.

**6. How much pressure should you apply when palpating a joint for synovitis?**

A good "rule of thumb" is to palpate with enough pressure to blanche your thumbnail (4 kg/cm$^2$). This standardizes the joint exam and ensures that adequate pressure is being applied to detect synovitis. Obviously, with overtly inflamed joints, this degree of pressure may be excessive. The tender points characteristic of fibromyalgia may be similarly palpated.

**7. How do you determine if joint pain is originating from intra-articular or extra-articular structures?**

"Stressing" a joint is easily accomplished by gentle passive range of motion of the joint by the examiner. In contrast, pain during attempted active ROM (performed by the patient) against a joint held immobile by the examiner suggests pathology in the surrounding tendons. Local tenderness by direct palpation of periarticular structures such as bursa may also indicate that the origin of pain is extra-articular.

**8. Describe the STWL system for recording the degree of arthritic involvement of a joint.**

The STWL system records the degree of **Swelling**, **Tenderness**, **Warmth**, and **Limitation** of motion in a joint based on a quantitative estimate of severity. A score of 0 (normal), 1 (mild), 2 (moderate), or 3 (severe) can be assigned to the S, T, and W categories. Limitation of motion is scored as 0 (normal), 1 (25% loss of motion), 2 (50% loss), 3 (75% loss), or 4 (ankylosis) or report the ROM of a joint in degrees. For example, Rt. 2nd MCP S2T2W1L2 means the right second MCP joint has moderate synovitis, moderate tenderness, mild warmth, and a 50% loss of normal range of motion. One should evaluate for joint instability and describe deformities such as swan-neck, ulnar drift, genu varus, etc.

**9. What is crepitus? What does it signify?**

Crepitus is an audible or palpable "grating" sensation felt during joint motion. The **fine** crepitus of inflamed synovium is of uniform intensity and perceptible only with a stethoscope. In contrast, **coarse** crepitus is easily detected, of variable intensity, and transmitted from damaged cartilage and/or bone. Crepitus may be elicited by compressing a joint throughout its range of motion.

**10. Which joints are included in a joint count?**

**Peripheral joints**

| | |
|---|---|
| Hand | Foot |
| Distal interphalangeal (DIP) | Interphalangeal |
| Proximal interphalangeal (PIP) | Metatarsophalangeal (MTP) |
| Metacarpophalangeal (MCP) | Talocalcaneal (subtalar) |
| Thumb carpometacarpal (CMC) | Ankle |
| Wrist | Knee |
| Elbow | |

**Axial joints**

| | |
|---|---|
| Shoulder | Spine |
| Glenohumeral | Cervical |
| Acromioclavicular | Thoracic |
| Sternoclavicular | Lumbar |
| Hip | Temporomandibular |
| Sacroiliac | |

**11. How do tender points and trigger points differ?**

| FEATURE | TENDER POINT | TRIGGER POINT |
|---|---|---|
| Disorder | Fibromyalgia | Myofascial pain syndrome |
| Distribution | Widespread | Regional |
| Abnormal tissue | No | ± |
| Tenderness | Focal | Focal |
| Referred pain | No | Yes |

**12. Define photosensitivity and photophobia.**

Photosensitivity refers to the development of a **rash following less than 30 minutes of sun exposure** (typically ultraviolet-B light). This feature is noted among 30–60% of patients with cutaneous lupus (discoid, or subacute cutaneous lupus), systemic lupus erythematosus, and dermatomyositis. Photophobia indicates **ocular sensitivity** to light and is commonly found in patients with uveitis.

**13. What rheumatic disorders, other than rheumatoid arthritis, may exhibit subcutaneous nodules?**

| | |
|---|---|
| Systemic lupus erythematosus | Multicentric reticulohistiocytosis |
| Rheumatic fever | Sarcoid |
| Tophaceous gout | Vasculitis |
| Juvenile chronic arthritis | Panniculitis |
| Limited scleroderma (calcinosis) | Type II hyperlipoproteinemia |
| Erythema nodosum | Lupus profundus |

**14. What historical or physical features are essential for the diagnosis of Raynaud's phenomenon?**

Raynaud's phenomenon is a reversible, vasospastic disorder characterized by transient, stress-induced (e.g., cold temperature) ischemia of the digits, nose-tip, and/or ears. As a result of vasospastic alterations in blood flow, a triphasic color response is usually observed. The initial color is **white** (ischemic pallor), then **blue** (congestive cyanosis), and finally **red** (reactive hyperemia). The diagnosis of Raynaud's phenomenon best correlates with the initial "dead-white" pallor of ischemia.

**15. Describe the examination of a patient with suspected median nerve entrapment of the wrist (carpal tunnel syndrome).**

Thenar atrophy is a reliable sign of carpal tunnel syndrome (CTS) but occurs only as a consequence of chronic disease with damage to the motor nerve. Acute or subacute CTS symptoms are typically sensory (the median nerve supplies sensory innervation to the palmar surface of the thumb, index finger, middle finger, and radial half of the ring finger). Its symptoms may be reproduced by the provocation tests of Tinel and Phalen. **Tinel's test** is best performed with the wrist in extension. The full width of the transverse carpal ligament is then percussed using a broad-headed, reflex hammer or the examiner's long finger. In contrast, **Phalen's test** is performed by gently positioning the wrist at full volar flexion for 60 seconds. Nerve conduction velocity studies are useful in confirming the clinical diagnosis of CTS.

**16. In the examination of an arthritic hand, what features enable you to differentiate rheumatoid arthritis from osteoarthritis?**

*Clinical Features of Rheumatoid Arthritis Versus Osteoarthritis*

| FEATURE | RHEUMATOID ARTHRITIS | OSTEOARTHRITIS* |
|---|---|---|
| Symmetry | Yes | Occasional |
| Synovitis | Yes | Rarely† |
| Nodules | Yes | No |
| Digital infarcts | Seldom | No |
| Bony hypertrophy | No | Yes |
| Joint involvement | | |
| DIP | No | Heberden's nodes |
| PIP | Yes | Bouchard's nodes |
| MCP | Yes | No‡ |
| CMC | No | Thumb |
| Wrist | Yes | No§ |
| Deformities | Swan neck<br>Boutonniere<br>Subluxation<br>Ulnar Drift | DIP or PIP angulation |

* Osteoarthritis may occur secondary to any inflammatory arthritis.
† Synovitis can occur in inflammatory erosive osteoarthritis.
‡ Osteoarthritis of the index and middle finger MCP joints may be a feature of hemochromatosis.
§ Osteoarthritis of the wrist may occur secondary to trauma or crystalline arthritis.

**17. What is Finkelstein's test?**

Finkelstein's test is a useful adjunct to direct palpation in the clinical diagnosis of wrist **tenosynovitis (deQuervain's)**. The test is initially performed by asking the patient to make a fist enclosing the thumb. While stabilizing the patient's forearm, the examiner gently bends the fist toward the ulnar styloid. If extreme discomfort occurs at the "anatomic snuffbox," deQuervain's tenosynovitis of the **abductor pollicis longus** and **extensor pollicis brevis** tendons is present. Occasionally crepitus may also be felt or heard with the stethoscope.

**18. How do you diagnose "tennis elbow" (lateral epicondylitis)?**

In addition to direct palpation, tennis elbow may be diagnosed by stressing the wrist extensor muscles at their origin, the lateral epicondyle. This provocation maneuver requires the patient to form a fist and maintain the wrist in extension. The examiner then flexes the wrist against resistance, while supporting the patient's forearm. Pain arising from the lateral epicondyle confirms the diagnosis. Patients also report grabbing and lifting a full milk carton reproduces the pain.

**19. When examining a swollen, inflamed elbow, how can you differentiate olecranon bursitis from true arthritis?**

Differentiation may be difficult as a result of swelling, pain, and limitation of range (extension and flexion). Rotation of the forearm, with the elbow flexed at 90°, is one maneuver that can help differentiate the two disorders. True arthritis of the elbow will inhibit pronation and supination of the radiohumeral joint, whereas in olecranon bursitis, the joint moves freely. Synovitis usually distends the normal sulcus of the ulnar groove not over the tip of the olecranon. Full extension of the elbow exacerbates true arthritis, while it doesn't affect olecranon bursitis.

**20. In the evaluation of shoulder pain, what single maneuver can best differentiate glenohumeral joint involvement from that of the periarticular tissues?**

Significant glenohumeral joint pathology can usually be excluded if **passive external rotation** of the shoulder is pain free.

**21. What does shoulder impingement mean?**

This multifactorial disorder represents a continuum of degenerative, inflammatory, and attrition of the structures in the subacromial space (SITS muscles, subdeltoid bursae, capsule, and bicipital tendon). Pain occurs during passive and active shoulder abduction between an arc of 70 and 120 degrees. Occasionally, the shoulder may be passively abducted beyond 120 degrees with relief of symptoms. Impingement commonly occurs following weakness or destruction of the rotator cuff muscles, which function to stabilize the humeral head against the shallow glenoid fossa. Active abduction by the large deltoid muscle would force the humeral head to migrate superiorly into the narrow subacromial space were it not for the counter force applied by intact rotator cuff muscles.

**22. Name the four shoulder muscles comprising the rotator cuff. How do you physically assess their integrity?**

The rotator cuff is comprised of the **SITS** muscles. Function of these muscles is tested by resistance maneuvers. Resistance is best performed with the patient's arm against the side and the elbow flexed to 90 degrees.

| MUSCLE | RESISTANCE MANEUVER |
|---|---|
| Supraspinatus | Abduction |
| Infraspinatus | External rotation |
| Teres Minor | External rotation |
| Subscapularis | Internal rotation |

**23. What are Speed's test and Yergason's maneuver?**

These are tests for bicipital tendinitis of the shoulder:

- **Speed's test**—pain in bicipital groove with resisted elevation of the humerus while elbow and forearm are fully extended forward.
- **Yergason's maneuver**—pain in bicipital groove with resisted supination of the forearm with elbow flexed to 90 degrees and held at patient's side.

Recurrent bicipital tendinitis (and/or rotator cuff tendinitis) should prompt an evaluation for impingement syndrome (see Chapter 66).

**24. How do you perform *Adson's test* to evaluate for vascular compromise in thoracic outlet syndrome?**

While the examiner palpates the radial pulse, the patient's arm is abducted, extended, and externally rotated. The patient is then asked to look *toward* the side being tested and inhale deeply. Diminution or loss of the radial pulse with development of a supraclavicular bruit is suggestive of significant subclavian artery compression.

**25. When a patient has true hip joint pathology, where is the pain usually reported and how is the hip joint examined?**

Despite misconceptions of the lay public, true hip pain is felt in the **groin** region in 90% of cases. In contrast, pain in the lateral hip region or buttock is usually referred from the lumbar spine or trochanteric bursa. Hip pain may occasionally radiate from the groin to the anteromedial thigh, greater trochanter, buttock, and knee. Assessment of hip mobility may help differentiate hip pathology from other causes of groin pain (e.g., adductor tendinitis). The origin of the hip joint as the source of pain can be confirmed by one of two maneuvers: Reproducing the pain during passive external or internal rotation of the hip in the seated position, or rotating the lower leg while the subject is supine with the knee in extension using the hip joint as a pivot (log roll). ROM of the hip can best be assessed while supine by hip flexion (with the knee flexed), whereas abduction and adduction should be assessed with the knee extended. Hip extension requires the patient to position the ipsilateral pelvis off the examining table so the lower leg can be extended posteriorly. In hip disease, the motion lost first is internal rotation.

The **Patrick** test (**Fabere** maneuver) is done with the patient lying supine and the examiner **f**lexes, **ab**ducts, and **e**xternally **r**otates the patient's leg so that the foot is on top of the opposite knee (forms a 4). The examiner lowers the leg toward the examining table. If there is a difference between the two legs, the test indicates hip disease or sacroiliitis.

**26. What does a positive Trendelenburg's test indicate?**

A positive Trendelenburg's test reveals weakness of the **gluteus medius** muscle, which may indicate hip joint pathology. The test is performed by observing the patient from behind as he or she stands on one leg. Normally, gluteus medius contraction of the ipsilateral, weight-bearing limb will elevate or allow the contralateral pelvis to remain level. In contrast, a weakened gluteus medius muscle cannot support the contralateral pelvis, and thus it will drop. Neurogenic causes (i.e., L5 nerve root compression) of gluteus medius weakness should also be excluded.

**27. Why examine a patient for leg-length inequality, and how is this measured?**

Leg-length discrepancy is associated with several "mechanical disorders," such as chronic back pain, trochanteric bursitis, and degenerative hip disease. **True** leg-length discrepancy reflects measurable differences (congenital or acquired) of both limbs using the anterior, superior iliac spines and lateral malleoli as landmarks. **Apparent** or functional leg-length discrepancy is primarily a measure of "pelvic tilt" typically induced by scoliosis or hip contractures. This apparent inequality is determined in the supine position by measuring the distance from the umbilicus to each medial malleoli. True leg-length measurement is usually *equal* in disorders of apparent leg-length discrepancy. Correction of significant inequality (≥ 1 cm) with a simple shoe lift can be therapeutic.

**28. Describe the physical findings of a patient with meralgia paresthetica.**

Meralgia paresthetica (lateral femoral cutaneous nerve syndrome) results from entrapment of the lateral femoral cutaneous nerve as it passes under the inguinal ligament medial to the anterior pelvic brim. Typical symptoms include burning dysesthesias and pain over the anterolateral thigh. In some patients, these symptoms may be elicited by performing **Tinel's test** at the site of entrapment.

**29. How do you diagnose trochanteric bursitis?**

The diagnosis of trochanteric bursitis is best made by direct palpation of the soft tissues overlying the greater trochanter of the femur. Trochanteric bursa pain may also be elicited by hip abduction, flexion, and external rotation.

**30. What is the Ober test?**

The Ober test evaluates the iliotibial band for contracture. The patient lies on the side with the lower leg flexed at the hip and knee. The examiner abducts and extends the upper leg with the knee flexed at 90 degrees. The examiner slowly lowers the limb with the muscles relaxed. A positive test result occurs if the leg does not fall back to the level of the table top. This indicates iliotibial band tightness, which can lead to altered gait causing low back pain, recurrent trochanteric bursitis, and lateral knee pain due to "snapping" of the iliotibial band over the lateral femoral condyle causing iliotibial bursitis.

**31. When examining a swollen knee, how can you tell if it is inflamed?**

In the absence of erythema, **warmth** may be the best indicator of inflammation in a swollen knee. Knee temperature is generally cooler than the quadriceps muscles or pretibial skin in normal individuals. Thus, if comparative palpation reveals the anterior knee skin to be warmer than these regions or the contralateral knee, inflammation is likely.

**32. When examining a swollen knee, how can you determine if an effusion is present?**

In addition to comparing the symmetry of the medial knee region to the unaffected knee, the patellar **bulge** test is most useful when evaluating minimal effusions. To perform this maneuver, the supine patient should relax the quadriceps muscle and have the supported knee flexed to 10 degrees. The examiner's palm is used to "milk" a potential effusion from the *medial* knee to the suprapatellar or lateral compartment. A reverse, similar maneuver is then performed on the lateral side. If rapid filling of the *medial* patellar fossa occurs, the bulge test is positive.

**33. What is the patellofemoral compression test?**

This test is used to evaluate damage (e.g., osteoarthritis) to the retropatellar surface. With the knee in flexion, the examiner compresses the patella against the femoral condyles. The patient is then asked to extend the knee forcefully, thus contracting the quadriceps muscle. With quadriceps contraction, the patella will be displaced proximally against the femur. If this maneuver produces pain, the test is positive. Patients usually report squatting or stair climbing reproduces their pain.

**34. How do you differentiate prepatellar bursitis from knee arthritis?**

A typical feature of acute inflammatory arthritis of the knee is loss of extension as a result of pain with an associated effusion. In prepatellar bursitis, the swelling tends to be localized anteriorly over the patella and pain is increased during knee flexion. Thus, if an inflamed knee demonstrates full extension without pain and a negative bulge sign, the disease is likely extra-articular.

**35. When evaluating an unstable knee, how do you perform Lachman's test?**

Lachman's test is a type of drawer test used to evaluate the integrity of the anterior cruciate ligament. It is best performed by holding the knee in 15–20 degrees of flexion. While stabilizing the thigh with one hand, the examiner uses the other hand to pull the tibia forward. A mild "give," or forward subluxation, is suggestive of anterior cruciate laxity or tear. Congenital laxity (hypermobility) must be excluded by comparison of both knees.

**36. Where is the pes anserine bursa?**

The pes anserine ("goose foot") bursa is on the medial side of the knee between the aponeurosis of the hamstring's insertion and the medial collateral ligament, approximately 5 cm below the anteromedial joint line. It is a common cause of medial knee pain and frequently mistaken for osteoarthritis of the knee.

**37. Describe the ankle joint examination.**

The ankle is a hinge joint. Palpation for synovitis is best done over the anterior (not lateral) aspect of the joint. When the ankle is at the normal position of rest (right angle between foot and leg), the ankle normally has 20 degrees of dorsiflexion and 45 degrees of plantar flexion. Subtalar (talocalcaneal) joint motion is tested by the examiner grasping the calcaneus with a hand and inverting (25 degrees) and everting (15 degrees) the foot while the ankle joint is held motionless. Muscular strength is assessed by the patient walking on his toes and heels.

**38. List some common causes of heel pain.**

- Achilles tendonitis—insertional or noninsertional. Usually due to overuse or overpronation of foot.
- Preadventitial Achilles bursitis—pump bump. Usually due to rubbing from shoe wear.
- Retrocalcaneal bursitis—inflammation of bursa between Achilles tendon and calcaneus.

- Calcaneal stress fracture.
- Plantar fasciitis—pain along medial plantar aspect of heel. Pain worse on first getting out of bed in morning with weight stretching plantar fascia. Not due to heel spurs.

**39. What type of patient usually gets posterior tibialis tendonitis (PTT)?**

PTT dysfunction occurs commonly in women ages 45–65 years old. It is associated with flatfoot deformity, obesity, and rheumatoid arthritis. Pain and swelling occur along medial aspect of ankle. Patients can't stand on their toes owing to pain and/or weakness.

**40. How should the foot be examined?**

With shoes and socks off! The foot is usually neglected in the physical examination but can be a source of lower extremity pain. Have the patient stand and put weight on his feet to see if there is excessive pronation (flat feet) or a high-arched cavus deformity. Check the range of motion of the MTP joints. The range of motion for functional ambulation is 65–75 degrees of dorsiflexion for first MTP joint and 60 degrees for lesser MTP joints. Have the patient ambulate in his bare feet. Foot deformity and lack of range of motion of toes can result in gait abnormalities that can contribute to ankle, knee, hip, and low back pain.

ACKNOWLEDGMENT

The editor and author wish to thank Dr. Danny Williams for his contributions to this chapter in the previous edition.

BIBLIOGRAPHY

1. American College of Rheumatology Ad Hoc Committee on Clinical Guidelines: Guidelines for the initial evaluation of the adult patient with acute musculoskeletal symptoms. Arthritis Rheum 39:1, 1996.
2. Buchanan WW, de Ceulaer K, Balint GP: Clinical Examination of the Musculoskeletal System: Assessing Rheumatic Conditions. Baltimore, Williams & Wilkins, 1997.
3. Hoppenfeld S: Physical Examination of the Spine and Extremities. New York, CT, Applelon-Century-Crofts, 1976.
4. Moder KG, Hunder GG: Examination of the joints. In Ruddy S, Harris ED, Sledge CB (eds): Kelley's Textbook of Rheumatology, 6th ed, Philadelphia, WB Saunders, 2001, pp 347–366.
5. Polley HF, Hunder GG: Rheumatologic Interviewing and Physical Examination of the Joints, 2nd ed. Philadelphia, WB Saunders, 1978.
6. Simms RW: Field Guide to Soft Tissue Pain: Diagnosis and Management. Lippincott, Williams & Wilkins, 2000.

# 9. LABORATORY EVALUATION

*Kathryn Hobbs, M.D.*

**1. Which laboratory tests are used most commonly in the clinical assessment of ongoing inflammation?**

Most clinicians follow the erythrocyte sedimentation rate (ESR) and/or C-reactive protein levels. These tests are nonspecific but may be useful for monitoring disease activity in rheumatoid arthritis, polymyalgia rheumatica, and the vasculitides.

**2. What is the erythrocyte sedimentation rate? How is it measured, and what influences its result?**

The ESR is a measurement of the distance in millimeters that red blood cells (RBCs) fall within a specified tube (Westergren or Wintrobe) over 1 hour. The ESR is an indirect measurement of alterations in acute-phase reactants and quantitative immunoglobulins. Acute-phase reactants are a heterogeneous group of proteins (fibrinogen, haptoglobin, C-reactive protein, alpha-1-antitrypsin, and others) that are synthesized in the liver in response to inflammation. Interleukin-6, an inflammatory cytokine, is an important mediator that stimulates the production of acute-phase reactants. Any condition that causes either a rise in the concentration of these asymmetrically charged acute-phase proteins or hypergammaglobulinemia (polyclonal or monoclonal) will cause an elevation of the ESR by increasing the dielectric constant of the plasma. This dissipates inter-RBC repulsive forces, and leads to closer aggregation of RBCs (i.e., rouleaux formation), which causes them to fall faster, increasing the result of the ESR. Aging, female sex, obesity, pregnancy, and possibly race are noninflammatory conditions that can elevate the sedimentation rate. Anemia and polycythemia may also affect the ESR, and alterations in size or shape of erythrocytes may physically interfere with rouleaux formation. Normal ranges of values therefore vary with patient characteristics as well as with technique. It costs about $10–12 to run.

**Pearl**: A rough rule of thumb is that the age-adjusted upper limit of normal for ESR is:

Male=age/2 Female = (age + 10)/2

**3. How do the Westergren and Wintrobe methods differ?**

The Westergren method uses a 200-mm tube, has a dilution step that corrects for the effect of anemia, and is the preferred method. The Wintrobe method uses a 100-mm tube and has no dilution step. Owing to its longer tube, only the Westergren method can detect an ESR > 50–60 mm/hr.

**4. What causes an extremely high or extremely low ESR?**

Markedly elevated ESR (> 100 mm/hr)
- Infection, bacterial (35%)
- Connective tissue disease: giant cell arteritis, polymyalgia rheumatica, SLE, other vasculitides (25%)
- Malignancy: lymphomas, myeloma, others (15%)
- Other causes (25%)

Markedly low ESR (0 mm/hr)
- Afibrinogenemia/dysfibrinogenemia
- Agammaglobulinemia
- Extreme polycythemia (hematocrit > 65%)
- Increased plasma viscosity

**5. Describe your approach to the evaluation of an elevated ESR.**

a. Complete history and physical examination and routine screening laboratories (complete blood count, chemistries, liver enzymes, urinalysis). Make sure that routine health care maintenance is up-to-date. Repeat ESR to ensure it is still elevated and there was no laboratory error.

b. If there is no clear association after step a, consider the following:
- Review medical record to compare with any previously obtained ESR.
- Check serum protein electrophoresis (SPEP) and CRP for evidence of acute-phase response, as well as to rule out myeloma or polyclonal gammopathy.

c. If still no obvious explanation, recheck ESR in 1–3 months. Up to 80% of patients will normalize. Follow patient for development of other symptoms or signs of disease if ESR remains elevated.

**6. What is the C-reactive protein (CRP)?**

CRP is a pentameric protein comprised of five identical, non-covalently linked 23-kD subunits arranged in cyclic symmetry in a single plane. It is present in trace concentrations in the plasma of all humans, and it has been highly conserved over hundreds of millions of years of evolution. Although its exact function is unknown, it shows important recognition and activation properties. Ligands recognized by CRP include phosphocholine as well as other phospholipids and some histone proteins. CRP is able to activate the classic complement pathway, and it can bind to and modulate the behavior of phagocytic cells in both pro- and anti-inflammatory ways. CRP is produced as an acute-phase reactant by the liver in response to interleukin-6 and other cytokines. Elevation occurs within 4 hours of tissue injury with peaks within 24–72 hours. In the absence of inflammatory stimuli, it falls rapidly, with a half-life of about 18 hours. CRP is measured by immunoassay or nephelometry, and testing costs around $25. A normal value is typically, < 1.0 mg/dL.

**Pearl**: Levels > 8–10 mg/dl should suggest bacterial infection, systemic vasculitis, or widely metastatic cancer.

**7. When should you order a CRP instead of an ESR?**

Both tests measure components of the acute-phase response and are useful in measuring generalized inflammation. The ESR is affected by multiple variables and, as such, is somewhat imprecise. Nevertheless, it is inexpensive and easy to perform. The CRP test measures a specific acute-phase reactant, and thus it is more specific. It rises more quickly and falls more quickly than the ESR, which tends to remain elevated for a longer time (decreases by 50% in 1 week) after inflammation subsides. The major drawback of the CRP is its increased cost relative to the ESR.

**8. What is the most sensitive test for detecting inflammatory change?**

The serum protein electrophoresis, while the most expensive, directly quantifies the acute-phase response. Inflammation is followed by characteristic protein alterations that are reflected on high-resolution electrophoresis. The typical pattern includes increases in immunoglobulins as well as increases in the α-1 and -2 zones (e.g., α-1 antitrypsin and haptoglobin) and the β-γ area (fibrinogen and CRP). Decreases are seen in pre-albumin, albumin, and the β zone (transferrin).

**9. When is it appropriate to order an antinuclear antibody (ANA) test?**

An ANA should be ordered when the clinical assessment of the patient suggests the presence of an autoimmune disease. An ANA should generally not be used as a screening test or as part of a "fishing expedition" to work-up a confusing case.

**10. How are antinuclear antibodies measured?**

The major method currently in use is fluorescence microscopy. Permeabilized cells are fixed to a microscope slide and incubated with the patient's serum, allowing ANAs to bind to the cell nuclei. After washing, a fluoresceinated second antibody is added, which binds to the patient's antibodies (which are bound to the nucleus). Cells are visualized through a fluorescence microscope to detect nuclear fluorescence. The amount of ANAs in a patient's serum is determined by diluting the patient's serum prior to adding the serum to the fixed cells—the greater the dilution (titer) at which nuclear fluorescence is detected, the greater the amount of ANAs present in the patient's serum.

Most laboratories now use HEp-2 cells (a proliferating cell line derived from a human epithelial tumor cell line) for the substrate to detect ANAs instead of frozen sections of rodent organ cells (mouse liver/rat kidney). This is because rapidly growing and dividing cells contain a larger array and higher concentration of nuclear antigens (such as SS-A and centromere antigens). Recently, enzyme-linked immunoassay methods (ELISA) have become available to detect ANAs. These assays vary among manufacturers and may not detect certain ANAs that are detected by the immunofluorescent method.

**11. What is an LE cell?**

The LE cell (lupus erythematosus cell) was the major method of measuring ANAs in the 1950s and 1960s. In this test, a bare nucleus stripped of cytoplasm is incubated with the patient's serum, allowing ANAs to bind to the nucleus. Normal polymorphonuclear leukocytes (PMNs) are then added, and if sufficient antibodies have been bound to the nucleus, the nucleus is opsonized and the PMNs engulf the nuclear material. A PMN containing phagocytosed nuclear material is known as an LE cell. This test is relatively insensitive in detecting ANAs and is difficult to interpret. The fluorescent ANA therefore has replaced it.

**12. At what point is an ANA test considered positive?**

A positive ANA is arbitrarily defined as that level of antinuclear antibodies that exceeds the level seen in 95% of the normal population. Each laboratory must determine the level that it considers positive, and this level may vary significantly among labs. In most laboratories, this level is a titer of 1:40 to 1:80. In laboratories where HEp-2 cells are used as substrate to detect an ANA, clinically significant titers are usually ≥ 1:160.

**13. What is the clinical significance of a positive ANA?**

That depends on the clinical context. A positive ANA in isolation never makes a specific diagnosis, and a negative ANA does not absolutely exclude autoimmune diseases. The ANA should be used primarily as a confirmatory test when the physician strongly suspects systemic lupus erythematosus (SLE) or other autoimmune disease.

**14. Can a positive ANA occur in a normal individual?**

Yes. The high level of sensitivity of the technique leads to the detection of ANA in patients with a wide variety of rheumatic and nonrheumatic diseases. A positive ANA is defined as the level (titer) of ANA that exceeds the level found in 95% of normal individuals. Thus, by definition, 5% of normals can be ANA-positive. In these individuals, titers are usually ≤ 1:320, and the nuclear staining pattern is most often speckled or homogenous. In addition, up to 20% of healthy relatives of patients with rheumatic disease, and up to 75% of elderly individuals without apparent disease, may have a positive ANA.

**15. Can a patient with SLE ever be ANA-negative?**

Yes. A very few patients (1–2%) with active, untreated SLE will have a negative ANA. These patients usually have antibodies to the nuclear antigen SS-A and are ANA-negative because the substrate used in the fluorescent ANA test did not contain sufficient SS-A antigen to allow detection of those antibodies. While such patients are ANA negative on rodent tissue substrates, they are almost always positive when HEp-2 substrate is used. Some cases of SLE may have antibodies restricted to cytoplasmic constituents (e.g., ribosomes, ribosomal P, and others). In addition, a larger number of SLE patients (10–15%) will become ANA-negative with treatment or as their disease becomes inactive. SLE patients with end-stage renal disease on dialysis frequently become ANA-negative (40–50%).

**16. What medical conditions are associated with a positive ANA?**

| CONDITION | % ANA-POSITIVE |
|---|---|
| SLE | 99 |
| Drug-induced lupus | 95–100 |
| Mixed connective tissue disease (MCTD) | 95–100 |
| Autoimmune liver disease (autoimmune hepatitis, primary biliary cirrhosis) | 60–100 |
| Progressive systemic sclerosis (PSS) | 80–95 |
| Polymyositis | 30–80 |
| Sjögren's syndrome | 75–90 |
| Rheumatoid arthritis | 30–50 |
| Multiple sclerosis | 25 |
| Patients with silicone breast implants | 15–25 |
| Healthy relatives of SLE patients | 15–25 |
| Neoplasia | 15–25 |
| Normal elderly (> 70 years) | 20 |

**17. Can the ANA titer be used to follow disease activity in patients with SLE or other autoimmune diseases?**

No. There is no evidence that variations in ANA titer (level) as measured by the screening ANA correlate with disease activity.

**18. What is the significance of the pattern of ANA?**

ANA patterns refer to the patterns of nuclear fluorescence observed under the fluorescence microscope. Certain patterns of fluorescence are associated with certain diseases, although these associations are not specific:

| | |
|---|---|
| Homogenous (diffuse) | SLE, drug-induced LE, other diseases |
| Rim (peripheral) | SLE, autoimmune hepatitis |
| Speckled | SLE, MCTD, Sjögren's, PSS, other diseases |
| Nucleolar | PSS, hepatocellular ca |
| Centromere | Limited scleroderma (CREST) |

Patterns of staining provide a clue to the category of nuclear antigens involved and are dependent upon the type of substrate used, and to a certain extent, the experience of the technician. Reliance on ANA patterns has largely been replaced by identification of specific antinuclear antibodies through the ANA profile (see Questions 21 and 22).

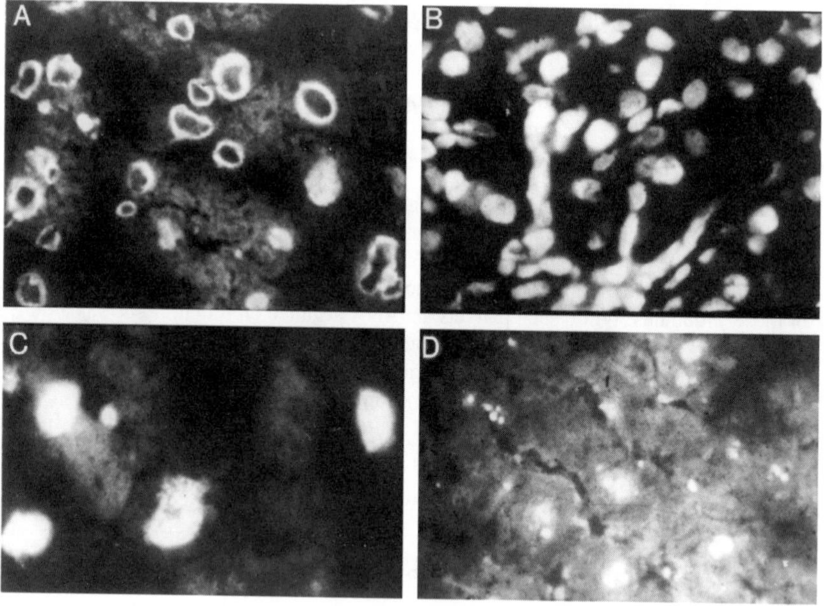


Patterns of ANA fluorescence: *A*, rim (peripheral); *B*, homogenous (diffuse); *C*, speckled; *D*, nucleolar. (From the Clinical Slide Collection on the Rheumatic Diseases. Atlanta, American College of Rheumatology, 1991; with permission.)

**19. Is the ANA a good screening test for SLE?**

No. Simple mathematics indicate that if 5% of the normal American population is ANA-positive, then 12.5 million normal individuals have a positive ANA. In contrast, even if 100% of SLE patients are ANA-positive, because the prevalence of SLE is only approximately 1/1000, there are only 250,000 individuals with SLE who are ANA-positive. Thus, if the entire population were screened for ANA, more normal individuals would be detected who are ANA-positive than SLE individuals (i.e., 50 to 1). The clinical value of an ANA test is tremendously enhanced by ordering an ANA when there is a reasonable pre-test probability (i.e., clinical suspicion) of an autoimmune disease.

**20. Which drugs can induce a positive ANA?**

| Common | Unusual |
|---|---|
| Procainamide | Up to 60 different drugs have been implicated as unusual causes of a positive ANA |
| Hydralazine | |
| Phenothiazines | |
| Diphenylhydantoin | |
| Isoniazid | |
| Quinidine | |

The clinical syndrome of drug-induced lupus occurs in only a small percentage of patients with drug-induced ANAs (see Chapter 21). ANA may remain positive months to years after discontinuing the drug. The ANA is usually directed against the epitope formed by the (H2A-H2B)–DNA complex, although hydralazine causes an ANA primarily against the H3–H4 histone dimer. The best test to order in patients with suspected drug-induced lupus and a homogenous ANA is antichromatin antibodies and not antihistone antibodies.

**21. What is meant by an "ANA profile"?**

An ANA profile consists of a battery of tests that measure ANAs specific for certain nuclear antigens. The standard profile includes tests to measure antibodies to double-stranded DNA, ribonuclear protein (RNP), Smith antigen (Sm), SS-A (Ro), SS-B (La), and centromere. Other disease-specific antinuclear antibodies [SCL-70 (topoisomerase I), PM-SCL (PM-1), histones, Th/To, Mi-2, and cytoplasmic antibodies (Jo-1, ribosomal P, mitochondrial)] have to be ordered individually.

**22. Which diseases are associated with the different antibodies measured in the ANA profile?**

| | dsDNA | RNP | SM | SS-A | SS-B | CENTROMERE |
|---|---|---|---|---|---|---|
| SLE | 60% | 30% | 30% | 30% | 15% | Rare |
| Rheumatoid arthritis | (-) | (-) | (-) | Rare | Rare | (-) |
| Mixed connective tissue disease | (-) | > 95% (high titer) | (-) | Rare | Rare | Rare |
| Scleroderma* | (-) | (low titer) | (-) | Rare | Rare | 10–15% |
| Limited scleroderma (CREST) | (-) | (-) | (-) | (-) | (-) | 60–90% |
| Sjögren's syndrome | (-) | Rare | (-) | 70% | 60% | (-) |

* Scleroderma = progressive systemic sclerosis (PSS).

**23. When is it appropriate to order an ANA profile?**

An ANA profile should be ordered when the screening ANA is positive and when additional information is desired regarding the type of autoimmune disease. Occasionally, antibodies to SS-A are detected on the ANA profile even in the face of a negative immunofluorescent ANA. Therefore, if the physician has a strong suspicion of SLE or another SS-A–associated disease, antibodies to SS-A should be ordered even despite a negative ANA.

**24. What syndromes are associated with antibodies to SS-A?**

SLE
Primary Sjögren's syndrome
Subacute cutaneous lupus (SCLE) (a variant of lupus characterized by prominent photosensitivity and rash)
Neonatal lupus
Congenital heart block
Secondary Sjögren's syndrome (rarely)

**25. In some diseases, antibodies against cytoplasmic antigens can be more helpful diagnostically than antibodies against nuclear antigens. Which diseases?**

*Autoimmune Diseases Associated with Anticytoplasmic Antibodies*

| DISEASE | CYTOPLASMIC ANTIGEN | FREQUENCY |
|---|---|---|
| Polymyositis | tRNA synthetase (anti-Jo-1, others) | 20–30% |
| SLE | Ribosomal P | 5–10% |
| Wegener's granulomatosis | Serine proteinase-3 (seen only in neutrophils) | 90% |
| Microscopic polyarteritis (+ other vasculitides) | Myeloperoxidase, others (seen only in neutrophils) | 70% |
| Primary biliary cirrhosis | Mitochondria | 80% |

Patients with these diseases frequently lack antibodies to nuclear antigens and hence are often ANA negative. Consequently, the specific anticytoplasmic antibody should be ordered when these diseases are suspected.

**26. Which of the ANAs measured in the ANA profile are useful to follow disease activity?**

Antibodies to dsDNA often parallel disease activity in SLE. High titers of antibody to dsDNA are associated with lupus nephritis, and increases in dsDNA antibody levels are frequently predictive of a flare of lupus activity. Other antibodies included in the ANA profile are markers of disease subsets but do not fluctuate with disease activity.

**27. Which antibodies are useful in a patient who is suspected of having progressive systemic sclerosis?**

Anticentromere (antikinetochore) antibodies are seen in up to 98% of patients with the limited form of scleroderma (CREST syndrome), and from 22–36% in patients with diffuse scleroderma. Antibodies to SCL-70 (anti-topoisomerase I) are seen in 22–40% of patients with diffuse systemic sclerosis, and generally predict diffuse cutaneous disease and proximal skin involvement, longer disease duration or association with cancer, pulmonary fibrosis, digital pitting scars, and cardiac involvement.

**28. What is the significance of antibodies to ribonuclear protein (RNP)?**

Antibodies to RNP produce a speckled pattern on immunofluorescent ANA, reflective of the focal distribution of their target; the spliceosomal snRNPs in the nucleoplasm. These antibodies are seen in a number of autoimmune diseases, including SLE, progressive systemic sclerosis, and mixed connective tissue disease (MCTD). The presence of very high levels of anti-RNP is highly suggestive of MCTD, a syndrome of overlapping disease manifestations with features of progressive systemic sclerosis, SLE, and polymyositis.

**29. Describe how the ANA pattern and antigen specificity are used in the diagnosis of the connective tissue diseases. (See Figure, top of next page.)**

**30. How would you evaluate an unexplained positive ANA in a patient with nonspecific arthralgias?**

- History and physical examination: Look for signs of a connective tissue disease and particularly occult Sjögren's syndrome.
- Obtain an ANA profile: ANA titers ≥ 1:160 or the presence of disease-specific autoantibodies usually indicates the ANA is significant.
- Obtain additional studies looking for evidence of immune hyperactivity:
  CBC: Look for anemia of chronic disease, neutropenia, and thrombocytopenia.
  Liver enzymes: If elevated, consider autoimmune hepatitis.

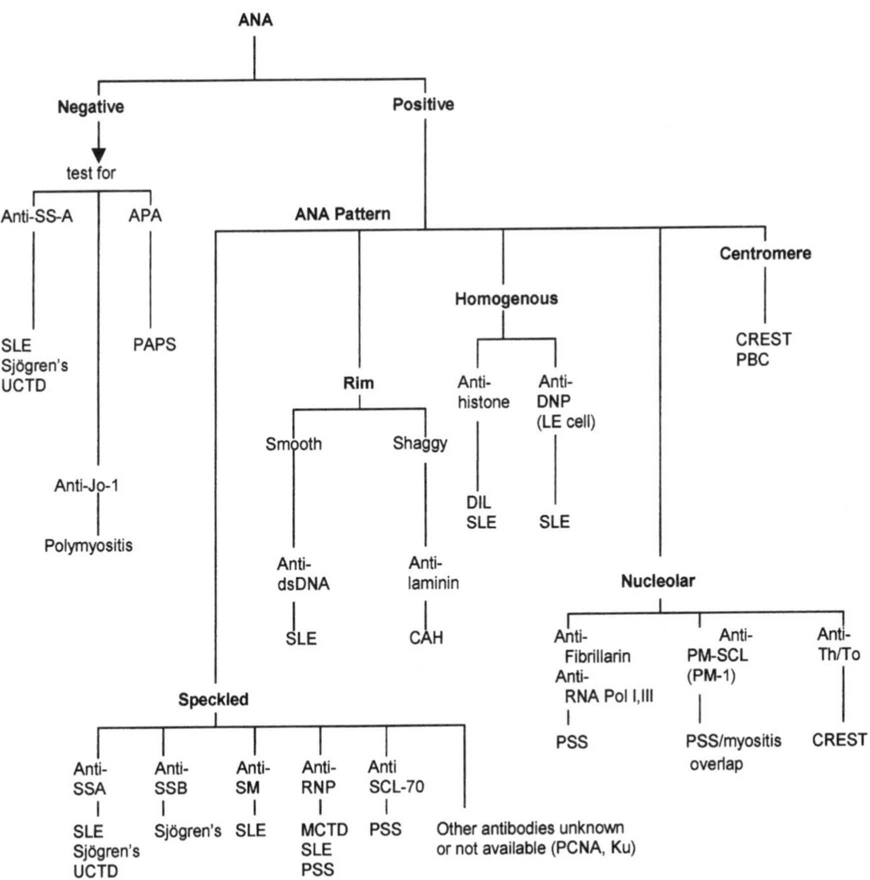


APA = antiphospholipid antibodies (lupus anticoagulant, anticardiolipin antibodies); CAH = chronic active hepatitis; DIL = drug-induced lupus; MCTD = mixed connective tissue disease; PAPS = primary antiphospholipid antibody syndrome; PSS = progressive systemic sclerosis (scleroderma); SCL-70 = topoisomerase I; UCTD = undifferentiated connective tissue disease; RNA Pol = RNA polymerase.

C3, C4: Look for hypocomplementemia.
SPEP: Look for polyclonal gammopathy.
RF, ESR, VDRL (false-positive), PTT (lupus anticoagulant).
Electrolytes, creatinine, urinalysis for completeness.

If any of the above are abnormal, the ANA may be indicative of an evolving autoimmune disease, and the patient will need to be followed closely.

**31. What are rheumatoid factors, and how are they measured?**

Rheumatoid factor (RF) is the general term used to describe an autoantibody directed against antigenic determinants on the Fc fragment of immunoglobulin G. RF may be of any isotype: IgM, IgG, IgA, or IgE. IgM RF is the only one routinely measured by clinical laboratories, using nephelometry, ELISA, and latex agglutination techniques.

**Pearl**: Formula to convert latex agglutination titer to nephelometry units:

$$\frac{\text{titer}}{10} \times 1.5.$$

Less than 24 is negative by this formula.

**32. What are the causes of a positive rheumatoid factor?**

The common denominator for the production of RF is chronic immune stimulation. The most common diseases associated with RF production are: CHRONIC, as the mnemonic indicates:

- **CH** *Ch*ronic disease, especially hepatic and pulmonary diseases
- **R** *R*heumatoid arthritis, 80–85% of patients
- **O** *O*ther rheumatic diseases, such as SLE (15–35%), PSS (20–30%), MCTD (50–60%), Sjögren's (75–95%), polymyositis (5–10%), sarcoid (15%)
- **N** *N*eoplasms, especially after radiation or chemotherapy
- **I** *I*nfections, e.g., AIDS, mononucleosis, parasitic infections, chronic viral infections, chronic bacterial infections (tuberculosis, subacute bacterial endocarditis, others)
- **C** *C*ryoglobulinemia, 40–100% of patients especially with hepatitis C

**33. In a patient with a known clinical diagnosis of rheumatoid arthritis (based on history and physical examination), what is the value of measuring rheumatoid factor?**

A positive RF does not make the diagnosis of rheumatoid arthritis. However, once rheumatoid arthritis has been diagnosed, patients who are RF-positive tend to have more aggressive disease, with more severe joint inflammation and destruction than in patients who are RF-negative. Patients with high-titer RF are also at increased risk to develop extra-articular manifestations of rheumatoid arthritis.

**34. Do changes in rheumatoid factor level reflect changes in rheumatoid arthritis disease activity?**

No. Disease activity of rheumatoid arthritis is best determined by clinical assessment.

**35. Rheumatoid factors are present in some normal people, especially the elderly. What are the false-positive rates?**

In normal individuals who are RF-positive, males and females are affected equally, and in only 20% of cases is the RF level significantly positive.

*Frequency of Positive RF in Normal Individuals of Different Ages*

| AGE | FREQUENCY OF RF |
|---|---|
| 20–60 yrs | 2–4% |
| 60–70 yrs | 5% |
| > 70 yrs | 10–25% |

**36. What are anti-neutrophil cytoplasmic antibodies (ANCA)?**

Antibodies directed against specific antigens present in the cytoplasm of neutrophils. There are two different types of ANCAs.

ANCAs reactive with myeloperoxidase (MPO), elastase, lactoferrin, and others give a perinuclear pattern of staining on immunofluorescence of ethanol-fixed neutrophils and are termed perinuclear, or P-ANCA. Antibodies to serine proteinase-3 (PR3) give diffuse cytoplasmic staining on immunofluorescence and are called cytoplasmic, or C-ANCA.. Patients who are ANCA positive should have specific antigen testing for MPO and PR3.

**37. Which diseases are associated with ANCAs?**

ANCAs are most strongly associated with necrotizing vasculitis. Disease associations differ for C-ANCA and P-ANCA:

| **C-ANCA** | **P-ANCA** |
|---|---|
| Wegener's granulomatosis | Microscopic polyarteritis (MPO positive) |
| Microscopic polyarteritis | Pauci-immune glomerulonephritis (MPO positive) |
| Churg-Strauss vasculitis (rare) | Churg-Strauss vasculitis (MPO positive) |
| | Drug-induced syndromes (hydralazine, PTU, penicillamine, minocycline) (MPO positive) |

| C-ANCA | P-ANCA |
|---|---|
| | Ulcerative colitis (MPO negative)<br>Autoimmune disease (liver, RA, SLE) (MPO negative)<br>HIV infection (MPO negative)<br>Certain other chronic infectious or neoplastic diseases (rare) (MPO negative) |

**Pearl**: If C-ANCA not against PR3 or P-ANCA not against MPO, look for causes other than vasculitis for the positive ANCA.

**38. Do ANCA titers fluctuate with disease activity?**

In Wegener's granulomatosis, the titer of C-ANCA can correlate with disease activity (in 60% of cases) and has been used to predict flares of disease. However, it remains controversial as to whether changes in C-ANCA titers should be used as the sole basis for changes in therapy. There is little evidence that P-ANCA titers fluctuate with disease activity.

**39. What are the causes of decreased circulating complement components?**

Serum complement may be decreased as a result of:

1. Decreased production, owing to either a hereditary deficiency or liver disease (complement components are synthesized in the liver).

2. Increased consumption (proteolysis), as a result of complement activation. A major cause of complement consumption is increased levels of circulating immune complexes, which activate the classic pathway.

**40. What clinical conditions are associated with hereditary complement deficiencies?**

| COMPLEMENT COMPONENTS | DISEASE |
|---|---|
| Early (C1, C2, C4) | SLE-like disease<br>Glomerulonephritis |
| Mid (C3, C4) | Recurrent pyogenic infections<br>SLE-like disease |
| Terminal (C5-C9) | Recurrent infections (especially gonococci and meningococci) |
| Regulatory (C1 INH) | Angioedema (hereditary or acquired) |

**41. Can a patient with active inflammation involving circulating immune complexes have a normal complement level?**

Yes. The serum level of complement components represents a balance between consumption and production. Complement components are acute-phase reactants, so their production by the liver increases with inflammatory states. If increased production keeps pace with consumption, the result will be a normal level of complement. Clinically, this means that while a decreasing level of complement is confirming evidence for complement consumption, normal complement levels cannot exclude complement consumption.

**42. What diseases are associated with decreased levels of complement (not deficiency)?**

**Rheumatic diseases**

SLE
Systemic vasculitis (especially polyarteritis nodosa, urticarial vasculitis)
Cryoglobulinemia
Rheumatoid arthritis with extra-articular manifestations (rare)

**Infectious diseases**

Subacute bacterial endocarditis
Bacterial sepsis (pneumococcal, gram-negative)
Viremias (especially hepatitis B)
Parasitemias

**Glomerulonephritis**
Post-streptococcal
Membranoproliferative

**43. What complement components should one order?**

Levels of C3 and C4, measured by nephelometry, are as a rule decreased with increased severity of disease in SLE, especially renal disease. Serial observations often reveal decreased levels preceding clinical exacerbations; reductions in C4 occur before reductions in C3. As attacks subside, levels return toward normal in the reverse order, with C4 remaining depressed longer. Some SLE patients have partial C4 deficiency and consequently will have persistently low C4 levels.

The total hemolytic complement assay, CH50, requires all components of the complement pathway to be present. It is a good screen for complement deficiency. A CH50 level of 0 or "unmeasurable" is suggestive of a hereditary (and homozygous) complement deficiency. It is not a good disease activity marker as, in active inflammation, its level can be either low, normal, or high, reflecting the end result of balance between production and consumption of the complement components.

**44. How do you separate iron deficiency anemia (IDA) from the anemia of chronic disease (ACD) in a patient with a chronic inflammatory disease like rheumatoid arthritis?**

In patients with uncomplicated IDA, measurement of iron status with serum level of iron (low), percent iron saturation (low), TIBC (high), and ferritin (low) are adequate. However, in patients with inflammatory disease, the TIBC and ferritin can be normal as a result of the acute phase reaction. Thus, to separate IDA from ACD, a bone marrow biopsy had to be done. Recently, studies have shown that a serum ferritin greater than 100 μg/liter excludes iron deficiency in patients with an active inflammatory disease as indicated by an elevated ESR/CRP. Likewise, a serum ferritin less than 50 μg/liter, particularly when associated with an elevated serum transferrin receptor level, is highly specific for IDA in patients with rheumatoid arthritis.

**45. Other than elevated ESR, CRP, and ACD, what additional tests suggest systemic inflammation?**

Patients with a systemic inflammatory disease such as vasculitis frequently have a reactive thrombocytosis, mild elevation of hepatic alkaline phosphatase, and low albumin. The low albumin is due to hepatic synthesis of acute-phase reactants (CRP, etc.) at the expense of albumin. Thus, the low albumin is not due to malnutrition, which is frequently postulated.

## Acknowledgment

The editor and author wish to thank Dr. J. Woodruff Emlen for his contribution to this chapter in the previous edition.

## BIBLIOGRAPHY

1. Bultink IEM, Lems WF, Vande Stadt RJ: Ferritin and serum transferrin receptor predict iron deficiency in anemic patients with rheumatoid arthritis. Arthritis Rheum 44:979–981, 2001.
2. Hoffman GS, Specks U: Antineutrophil cytoplasmic antibodies (ANCA). Arthritis Rheum 41:1521–1537, 1998.
3. Homburger HA: Cascade testing for autoantibodies in connective tissue diseases. Mayo Clin Proc 70:183–184, 1995.
4. Kavanaugh A, et al: Guidelines for clinical use of the antinuclear antibody test and tests for specific autoantibodies to nuclear antigens. Arch Pathol Lab Med 124:71–81, 2000.
5. Peng SL, Craft J: Antinuclear antibodies. In Ruddy S, Harris ED, Sledge CB (eds): Kelley's Textbook of Rheumatology, 6th ed. Philadelphia, W.B. Saunders, 2001, pp 161–174.
6. Ruddy S: Complement. In Ruddy S, Harris ED, Sledge CB (eds): Kelley's Textbook of Rheumatology, 6th ed. Philadelphia, W.B. Saunders, 2001, pp 185–194.
7. Shmerling RH, Delbanco TL: The rheumatoid factor: An analysis of clinical utility. Am J Med 91:528–534, 1991.

8. Slater CA, Davis RB, Shmerling RH: Antinuclear antibody testing: a study of clinical utility. Arch Int Med 156:1421–1425, 1996.
9. Sox HC, Liang MH: The erythrocyte sedimentation rate: Guidelines for rational use. Ann Intern Med 104:515–523, 1986.
10. Tighe H, Carson DA: Rheumatoid factor. In Ruddy S, Harris ED, Sledge CB (eds): Kelley's Textbook of Rheumatology, 6th ed. Philadelphia, W.B. Saunders, 2001, pp 151–160.

# 10. ARTHROCENTESIS AND SYNOVIAL FLUID ANALYSIS

*Robert T. Spencer, M.D.*

**1. When should arthrocentesis be performed?**

Without doubt, the single most important reason to perform arthrocentesis is to check for joint infection. Timely identification and treatment of a patient with septic arthritis are of paramount importance to a favorable clinical outcome. In addition, arthrocentesis is generally indicated to gain diagnostic information through synovial fluid (SF) analysis in the patient with a mono- or polyarticular arthropathy of unclear etiology characterized by joint pain and swelling.

**2. When is arthrocentesis contraindicated?**

When the clinical indication for obtaining SF is strong, such as in the patient with suspected septic arthritis, there is no absolute contraindication to joint aspiration. Relative contraindications include **bleeding diatheses**, such as hemophilia, anticoagulation therapy, or thrombocytopenia; however, these conditions frequently can be treated or reversed prior to arthrocentesis. **Cellulitis** overlying a swollen joint can make the approach to the joint space difficult, but this rarely precludes the ability to perform the procedure.

**3. How safe is arthrocentesis in patients on warfarin (Coumadin)?**

Although hemarthrosis has been reported following joint aspiration in anticoagulated patients, it appears to be uncommon. A recent study found no hemorrhagic complications in patients on Coumadin with INR < 4.5. Using the smallest needle necessary for the procedure and applying prolonged pressure following the arthrocentesis are recommended.

**4. What techniques should be used when performing arthrocentesis?**

The procedure should be performed using **aseptic technique**. A topical antiseptic, such as povidone-iodine, should be applied to the area. Nonsterile gloves should always be worn as part of universal precautions. Sterile gloves should be used if palpation of the area is foreseen subsequent to antiseptic prep and prior to placement of the needle. A 25-gauge needle should be used to administer a local anesthetic (e.g., 1% lidocaine). The aspiration itself should be performed using an 18-gauge, 1.5-inch needle, when possible, and a 10–30-ml syringe. Aspiration techniques for individual joints are described in other references.

**5. What precautions should be done if the patient is "allergic" to povidone-iodine, lidocaine, or latex?**

- Patients with topical iodine reactions can have their skin cleansed with Hibiclens or pHisoHex followed by an alcohol pad.
- True "caine" allergy is extremely rare. Many of the symptoms that occur during dental procedures are due to the epinephrine or preservatives (parabens) in the lidocaine (Xylocaine) and not an IgE-mediated reaction. To be absolutely sure, skin testing and subcutaneous incremental challenge would have to be done. This is usually not practical; therefore, options

include numbing the area with a skin refrigerant (ethyl chloride, Frigiderm) only or using a local anesthetic from the benzoic acid ester group that does not cross-react with lidocaine such as chloroprocaine (Nesacaine). Note that a patient with a procaine (Novocain) reaction can use lidocaine (Xylocaine).

- Most latex allergies are minor local reactions. However, some patients can have a severe latex allergy. In these patients, arthrocentesis must be performed using latex-free gloves and syringes. The rubber stopper on the top of the lidocaine must be removed because sticking a needle through this can result in latex protein being introduced into the lidocaine.

**6. What are the potential complications of arthrocentesis?**

- Infection (risk < 1 in 10,000)
- Bleeding/hemarthrosis
- Vasovagal syncope
- Pain
- Cartilage injury

**7. What studies should be performed for synovial fluid analysis?**

Because the single most important determination of SF analysis is for the presence of infection, **Gram stain** and **culture** should be performed on samples from joints with even relatively low suspicion for infection. Determining **total leukocyte count** and **differential** helps in differentiating between non-inflammatory and inflammatory joint conditions. Lastly, **polarized microscopy** should be done to evaluate for the presence of pathologic crystals. Chemistry determinations, such as glucose, total protein, and lactate dehydrogenase, are unlikely to yield helpful information beyond that obtained by the previous studies, and therefore they should not be routinely ordered.

**8. How should the SF sample be handled?**

Once fluid has been obtained, samples should be allocated into sterile vacuum tubes and sent for analysis. Fluid for culture and Gram stain may be sterilely transferred to a red-top tube. Fluid for crystal analysis may be place in a red- or green-top tube, depending on the lab's preference. Fluid for cell count and differential should be placed in a green- or purple-top tube.

**9. What if no SF is obtained (a "dry tap")?**

Even if no fluid is aspirated into the syringe, frequently one or two drops of fluid and/or blood can be found within the needle and its hub. This amount is sufficient for culture, in which case the syringe with capped needle should be submitted to the microbiology lab. If one extra drop can be spared, it can be placed on a microscope slide with a coverslip for polarized microscopy. When microscopy is completed, the coverslip can be removed and the specimen may then serve as a smear for Gram stain. The specimen remaining on the coverslip may be an adequate smear on which to perform a Wright stain, allowing determination of leukocyte differential. Thus, two drops of fluid can yield the same important diagnostic information as that obtained from a larger specimen, with the exception of a leukocyte count. The lesson to be learned from this is that when a "dry tap" is encountered, the needle and syringe should not be reflexively discarded!

**10. What are some causes of "dry taps"?**

Inability to obtain synovial fluid from a joint with an obvious effusion can be from:

- SF too thick to aspirate through the lumen of needle.
- Obstruction of the needle lumen with debris such as rice bodies (infarcted pieces of synovium in SF) or thick fibrin.
- Chronically inflamed synovium can undergo fat replacement and become markedly thickened (lipoma arborescens), so that the needle never makes it into the effusion.
- In the knee, a medial plica or medial fat pad (especially in obese patients) may block the needle. In this case, aspirate from lateral aspect of the knee.
- Poor technique and not getting into joint with needle.

**11. Within what time frame should SF analysis occur?**

SF should be analyzed as soon as possible after the fluid is drawn. If it is delayed more than 6 hours, results may be spuriously altered. Problems that can arise include:

- Decrease in leukocyte count (due to cell disruption)
- Decrease in number of crystals (primarily calcium pyrophosphate dihydrate)
- Appearance of artifactual crystals

**12. How may synovial fluid WBC count be estimated by "wet drop" examination?**

At the time polarized microscopy is performed, the synovial fluid WBC count can be easily estimated. The finding of 2 or fewer WBCs per high-power field (40X high dry objective) confidently suggests a noninflammatory fluid (< 2000 WBCs per mm$^3$). If greater than 2 WBCs per high-power field are seen, there is a significant chance the synovial fluid is inflammatory and formal determination of the WBC count should be ordered.

**13. Describe the classification based on SF analysis.**

*Synovial Fluid Classification*

| FLUID TYPE | APPEARANCE | TOTAL WBC COUNT/MM$^3$ | % PMNS |
|---|---|---|---|
| Normal | Clear, viscous, pale yellow | 0–200 | < 10% |
| Group 1 (noninflammatory) | Clear to slightly turbid | 200–2000 | < 20% |
| Group 2 (inflammatory) | Slightly turbid | 2000–50,000 | 20–70% |
| Group 3 (pyarthrosis) | Turbid to very turbid | > 50,000 | > 70% |

WBC, white blood cell (leukocyte); PMN, polymorphonuclear cell.

**14. Name some causes of noninflammatory (group 1) joint effusions.**

Osteoarthritis, joint trauma, mechanical derangement, pigmented villonodular synovitis, and avascular necrosis.

**15. Group 2 (inflammatory) synovial fluid is typical for which rheumatic disorders?**

Rheumatoid arthritis
Gout
Pseudogout
Psoriatic arthritis
Ankylosing spondylitis
Reiter's syndrome
Juvenile rheumatoid arthritis
Rheumatic fever
Systemic lupus erythematosus
Polymyalgia rheumatica
Giant cell arteritis
Wegener's granulomatosis
Hypersensitivity vasculitis
Polyarteritis nodosum
Familial Mediterranean fever
Sarcoidosis
Infectious arthritis
- Viral (hepatitis B, rubella, HIV, parvovirus, others)
- Bacterial (gonococci)
- Fungal
- Mycobacterial
- Spirochetal (Lyme disease, syphilis)

Subacute bacterial endocarditis
Palindromic rheumatism

**16. Other than joint sepsis, which conditions are associated with a group 3 fluid (pyarthrosis)?**

When a group 3 fluid is discovered, septic arthritis must be assumed until proved otherwise by SF culture. A few disorders may cause noninfectious pyarthrosis, sometimes referred to as joint **pseudosepsis**.

Gout
Reiter's syndrome
Rheumatoid arthritis

**17. List some causes of a hemarthrosis.**

- Trauma
- Bleeding diatheses
- Tumors
- Pigmented villonodular synovitis
- Hemangiomas
- Scurvy
- Iatrogenic (post-procedure)
- Arteriovenous fistula
- Intense inflammatory disease
- Charcot's joint

**18. Compare the polarized light microscopic findings of synovial fluid from a joint with gout and one with pseudogout.**

| | GOUT | PSEUDOGOUT |
|---|---|---|
| Crystal | Urate | Calcium pyrophosphate dihydrate (CPPD) |
| Shape | Needle | Rhomboid or rectangular |
| Birefringence | Negative | Positive |
| Color of crystals parallel to axis of red-plate compensator | Yellow | Blue |

**Pearl**: For the crystal color, use the mnemonic **ABC** (**A**lignment, **B**lue, **C**alcium). If the crystal aligned with the red-plate compensator is blue, it is calcium pyrophosphate dihydrate. Urate crystals are the opposite, being yellow when parallel to the compensator.

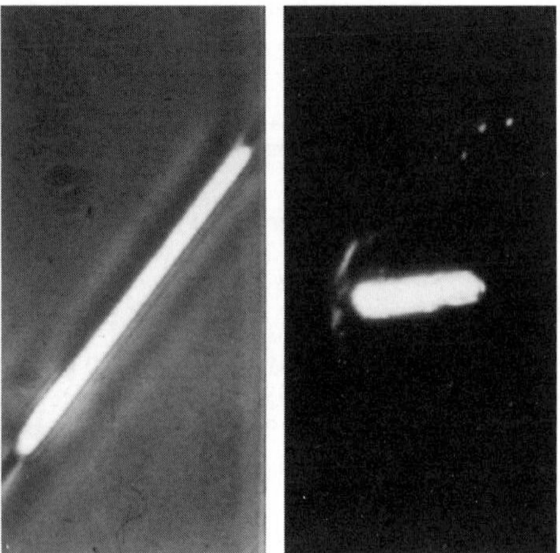

*Left*, Urate crystal of gout, showing needle shape. *Right*, CPPD crystal of pseudogout, showing rhomboid shape.

**18. Are there any "tricks" that can be done to increase the yield of finding uric acid crystals in a patient who clinically has gout?**

Rarely you may encounter a patient who clinically has gout but you can't find crystals on synovial fluid examination. Some "tricks" that have been tried are to spin the fluid and examine the centrifugate for crystals. Another is to cool the fluid in the refrigerator, although this usually doesn't work. Finally, putting fluid on a microscope slide and allowing it to dry for 2–3 hours may allow overhydrated uric acid crystals to dehydrate and be drawn toward each other to form spherules that are easier to see.

**19. What are the crystals shown below?**

Talc crystals that come from the examiner's gloves. To avoid this, it is best to wash hands after the aspiration procedure and before you prepare the slide with coverslip.

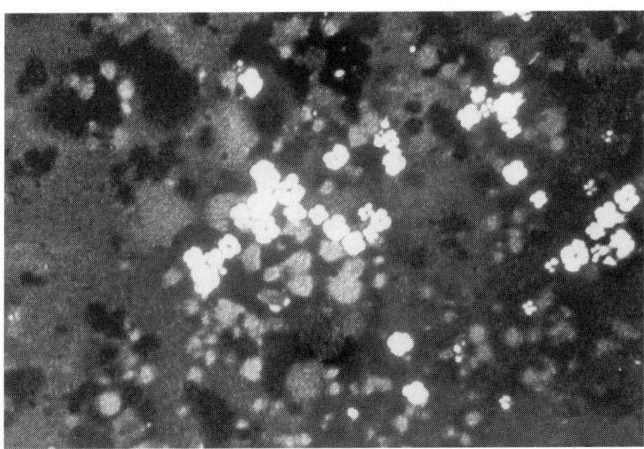

Talc crystals.

BIBLIOGRAPHY

1. Clayburne G, Daniel DG, Schumacher HR: Estimated synovial fluid leukocyte numbers on wet drop preparations as a potential substitute for actual leukocyte counts. J Rheumatol 19:60, 1992.
2. Doherty M, Hazelman BL, Hutton CW, et al (eds): Rheumatology Examination and Injection Techniques. Philadelphia, W.B. Saunders, 1992.
3. Fiechtner JJ, Simkin PA: Urate spherulites in gouty synovia. JAMA 245:1533–1536, 1981.
4. Hasselbacher P: Arthrocentesis, synovial fluid analysis, and synovial biopsy. In Schumacher HR, Klippel JH, Koopman WJ (eds): Primer on the Rheumatic Diseases, 10th ed. Atlanta, Arthritis Foundation, 1993.
5. Kerolus G, Clayburne G, Schumacher HR: Is it mandatory to examine synovial fluids promptly after arthrocentesis? Arthritis Rheum 32:271, 1989.
6. Roberts WN, Hayes CW, Breitbach SA, Owen DS: Dry taps and what to do about them: A pictorial essay on failed arthrocentesis of the knee. Am J Med 100:461, 1996.
7. Schumacher HR: Synovial fluid analysis and synovial biopsy. In Harris ED, Ruddy S, Sledge CB (eds): Kelley's Textbook of Rheumatology, 6th ed. Philadelphia, W.B. Saunders, 2001.
8. Shmerling RH, et al: Synovial fluid tests: What should be ordered? JAMA 264:1009, 1990.
9. Thumboo J, O'Duffy JD: A prospective study of the safety of joint and soft tissue aspirations and injections in patients taking warfarin sodium. Arthritis Rheum 41:736, 1998.

# 11. RADIOGRAPHIC AND IMAGING MODALITIES

*Kevin* M. *Rak*, M.D.

**1. Describe the radiographic modalities available in the assessment of arthritis.**

**Plain film radiographs** are the cornerstone of radiologic diagnosis in the arthritides. They typically define the character and distribution of bone erosions, abnormalities of the cartilaginous space, malalignment, soft tissue swelling, or calcifications. Conventional radiography is the least expensive modality available and readily depicts the extent of disease as well as progression of disease.

**Computed tomography** (CT) permits cross-sectional images to be displayed with excellent contrast resolution. CT is helpful in diagnosis of arthritides in complex joints (e.g., sacroiliac, subtalar, and sternoclavicular joints), in evaluation of bone tumors (e.g., osteoid osteoma), and in assessment of trauma, particularly in the spine and pelvis, as it defines and characterizes fractures better than plain radiographs.

**Arthrography** has been replaced somewhat by MRI in the assessment of intra-articular disorders. In the knee, arthrograms are rarely performed, except in cases of prior meniscectomy. Arthrography is still performed in other joints, such as the shoulder, wrist, ankle, and hip, particularly if MRI results are inconclusive. Aspiration arthrography is certainly indicated in a patient with a painful hip or knee prosthesis, to differentiate infection from aseptic loosening.

**Magnetic resonance imaging** (MRI) has no radiation, is noninvasive, and permits imaging in any plane or axis. It has outstanding sensitivity but, unfortunately, commonly lacks specificity. The excellent contrast resolution provided by MRI has made it the study of choice in evaluating internal disorders of the knee, rotator cuff tears, avascular necrosis, herniated nucleus pulposus, and spinal stenosis. In osteomyelitis, MRI is complementary to nuclear medicine scans, but its superior spatial resolution permits depiction of the full extent of marrow infection or edema. MRI also may be effective with contrast enhancement in determining the degree of synovial proliferation accompanying arthritides.

**Ultrasound** in the musculoskeletal system has a somewhat limited role. It is useful for evaluating superficial soft tissue structures. It is largely operator-dependent but, in experienced hands, can be effective in identifying and characterizing joint effusions and abnormalities of tendons, ligaments, and muscle.

**2. Does nuclear medicine have a role in musculoskeletal imaging?**

Bone scanning is routinely performed with $^{99m}$Tc-labeled diphosphonates, which are adsorbed onto the surface of bone proportional to the local osteoblastic activity and skeletal vascularity. Bone scans are therefore sensitive in detecting bone abnormalities but somewhat nonspecific, as tumor, trauma, infection, or other pathology can all cause increased tracer uptake. Bone scanning is the screening examination of choice for evaluating bony metastatic disease, as it images the entire skeleton. Bone scanning will commonly detect metastatic disease or osteomyelitis while plain radiographs are still normal, since up to 50% of bone must be decalcified for plain film detection of tumor or infection versus 1% for bone scanning. Bone scanning can also detect stress fractures earlier than plain radiographs and may detect avascular necrosis or bone infarcts not seen by MRI.

In arthritis, there is increased concentration of radionuclide in the bone adjacent to affected joints. This increased tracer uptake may be due to synovitis with increased vascularity, or the periarticular uptake may be due to direct bone involvement. Although the various forms of arthritis cannot be distinguished except by distribution of uptake, the bone scan is helpful in diagnosis and in documenting extent of disease. Other common indications for bone scanning are in the evaluation of Paget's disease or metabolic bone disease.

**3. What are the relative costs of the radiographic procedures used in musculoskeletal imaging of a specific joint (e.g., the shoulder)?**

| | | | |
|---|---|---|---|
| Plain radiograph | $120 | Bone scan | 600 |
| Ultrasound | 230 | CT scan | 700 |
| Arthrography | 450 | MRI scan | 700–1100 |

**4. Is there a pattern approach to interpreting a radiograph for arthritis?**

In assessing a skeletal radiograph, a pattern approach using **ABCDES** can be very helpful:

**A** —Alignment. Rheumatoid arthritis (RA) and systemic lupus erythematosus (SLE) are characterized by deformities such as ulnar deviation at metacarpophalangeal joints.
—Ankylosis. Seronegative spondyloarthropathies frequently cause ankylosis.

**B** —Bone mineralization. Periarticular osteoporosis is typical of RA or infection, and is rare in crystal diseases, seronegative spondyloarthropathies, and degenerative joint disease.
—Bone formation. Reactive bone formation (Periostitis) is the hallmark of seronegative spondyloarthropathies. Osteophytosis is seen in degenerative joint disease and calcium pyrophosphate disease and can be present in any end-stage arthritis.

**C** —Calcifications. Soft tissue calcifications may be seen in gouty tophi, SLE, or scleroderma. Cartilage calcification is typical of calcium pyrophosphate disease.
—Cartilage space. Symmetric and uniform cartilage or joint-space narrowing is typical of inflammatory disease. Focal or nonuniform joint-space loss in the area of maximal stress in weight-bearing joints is the hallmark of osteoarthritis.

**D** —Distribution of joints. For example, RA usually has symmetric distribution of affected joints, whereas seronegative spondyloarthropathies are asymmetric. Also, target sites of involvement may permit differentiation of arthritides.
—Deformities. Swan neck or boutonniere deformities of the hands are typical of RA.

**E** —Erosions. In addition to their presence or absence, the character of erosions may be diagnostic, such as overhanging edges and sclerotic margins in gout.

**S** —Soft tissue and nails. Look for distribution of soft tissue swelling, nail hypertrophy in psoriasis, and sclerodactyly in scleroderma.
—Speed of development of changes. Septic arthritis will rapidly destroy the affected joint.

**Pearl**: When obtaining radiographs on patients with arthritis, always order weight-bearing radiographs to evaluate joint-space narrowing in lower extremity joints (i.e., hip, knee, ankles).

**5. Describe the radiographic features of an inflammatory arthritis.**

1. Soft tissue swelling
2. Periarticular osteoporosis
3. Uniform loss of cartilage (i.e., diffuse joint-space narrowing)
4. Bony erosion in "bare" areas

Synovial inflammation causes soft tissue swelling. The inflammation also results in hyperemia, which, coupled with the inflammatory mediators released (such as prostaglandin $E_2$), causes periarticular (juxta-articular) osteoporosis. With chronicity, inflammatory arthritis may lead to more diffuse osteoporosis due to disuse (and other factors) of the joints due to pain. As the inflammation leads to synovial hypertrophy and pannus formation, the pannus erodes into the bone. These erosions occur first in the marginal "bare areas" where synovium abuts bone that does not possess protective cartilage (see figure). The pannus ultimately extends over the cartilaginous surface and/or erodes through the bone to the undersurface of the cartilage. Cartilage destruction results either by enzymatic action of the inflamed synovium and/or by interference with normal cartilage nutrition. Owing to its generalized nature, this cartilage destruction is radiographically seen as uniform or symmetric, diffuse joint-space narrowing observed best in weight-bearing joints.

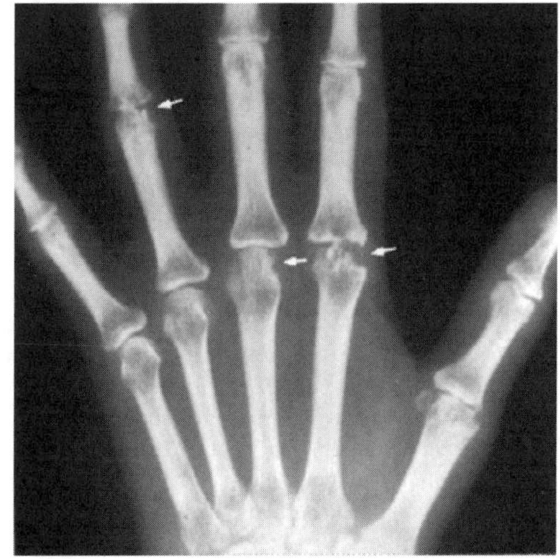

Radiograph of hand showing periarticular osteoporosis and bony erosions (arrows) compatible with an inflammatory arthritis. Patient had rheumatoid arthritis.

**6. What is the "bare area"? Why do the earliest erosions begin here?**

In synovial articulations, hyaline articular cartilage covers the ends of both bones. The articular capsule envelopes the joint cavity and is composed of an outer fibrous capsule and a thin inner synovial membrane. The synovial membrane typically does not extend over cartilaginous surfaces but lines the nonarticular portion of the synovial joint and also covers the intracapsular bone surfaces that are not covered by cartilage. These unprotected bony areas occur at the peripheral aspect of the joint and are referred to as "bare areas" (see figure).

In these areas, the bone does not have a protective cartilage covering. Consequently, the inflamed synovial pannus, which occurs in inflammatory arthritides such as rheumatoid arthritis, comes in direct contact with bone, resulting in marginal erosions. These "bare areas" are where you should look for the earliest evidence of erosions. With progression of disease, the pannus proliferates to cover the cartilage surfaces, resulting in cartilage destruction (joint-space narrowing) and more diffuse bony erosions.

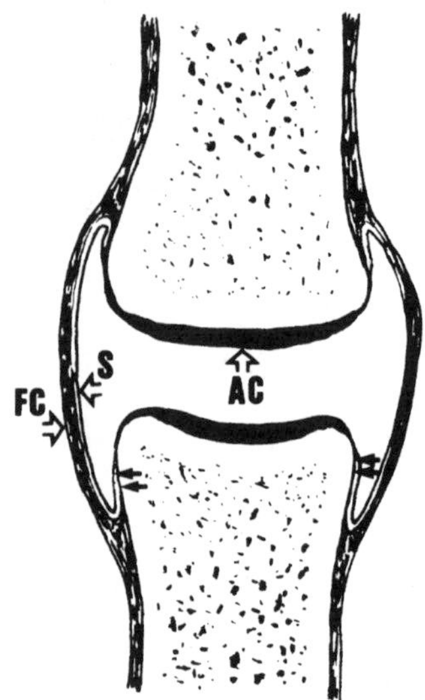


Diagram of typical synovial joint. Small black arrows point to "bare areas" where bone is exposed to synovium without protective cartilage covering. AC, articular cartilage; S, synovium; FC, fibrous capsule.

**7. List the rheumatic disease categories that typically cause radiographic features of an inflammatory arthritis.**

- Rheumatoid arthritis (adult and juvenile)
- Connective tissue diseases (SLE)
- Seronegative spondyloarthropathies
- Septic arthritis

**8. Describe the radiographic features of noninflammatory, degenerative arthritis.**

1. Sclerosis/osteophytes
2. Nonuniform loss of cartilage (focal joint-space narrowing in area of maximal stress in weight-bearing joints)
3. Cysts/geodes

The causes of degenerative arthritis are multifactorial. However, the primary problem and end result is cartilage degeneration. As the cartilage degenerates, the joint space narrows. However, in contrast to uniform, diffuse narrowing seen with inflammatory arthritides, the noninflammatory, degenerative arthritides tend to have nonuniform, focal joint-space narrowing, being most pronounced in the area of the joint where stresses are more concentrated (e.g., superolateral aspect of hip, medial compartment of the knee) (see figure).

Following cartilage loss, subchondral bone becomes sclerotic or eburnated, owing to trabecular compression and reactive bone deposition. With denudation of cartilage, synovial fluid can be forced into underlying bone, forming subchondral cysts or geodes with sclerotic margins. As an attempted reparative process, the remaining cartilage undergoes endochondral ossification to develop osteophytes. Such osteophytes commonly occur first at margins or nonstressed aspects of the joint (e.g., medial and lateral aspects of the distal femur and proximal tibia of the knee). Teleologically, osteophytes are believed to be the way the body attempts to restrict motion of a degenerating joint and a way to further spread forces across a joint.

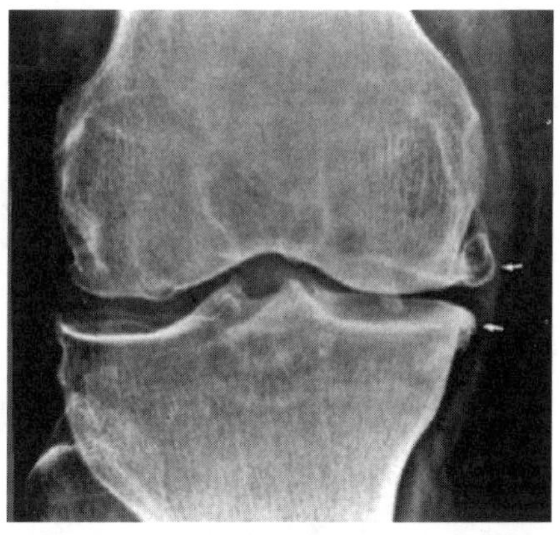

Knee radiograph demonstrating osteophytes (arrows) and medial joint-space narrowing consistent with degenerative arthritis.

**9. List the rheumatic disease categories that typically cause radiographic features of a noninflammatory arthritis.**

- Degenerative joint disease (e.g., primary osteoarthritis and secondary causes of osteoarthritis, such as traumatic arthritis, congenital bone diseases, others)
- Metabolic or endocrine disease (e.g., diseases associated with calcium pyrophosphate deposition, ochronosis, acromegaly)
- Miscellaneous (e.g., hemophilia, avascular necrosis)

**10. What are the typical sites of joint involvement in primary (idiopathic) osteoarthritis compared with secondary causes of noninflammatory, degenerative arthritis?**

**Primary** (idiopathic) osteoarthritis can cause noninflammatory, degenerative arthritic changes in the following joints:

Hands
- Distal interphalangeal joints (DIPs)
- Proximal interphalangeal joints (PIPs)
- First carpometacarpal joint (CMC) of thumb

Acromioclavicular joint of shoulder
Cervical, thoracic, and lumbosacral spine
Hips—subchondral cysts (Eggar's cysts) in superior acetabulum are characteristic
Knees
Feet
- First metatarsophalangeal joints (MTP)

**Secondary** causes of degenerative arthritis can result in noninflammatory, degenerative changes in any joint (not just those for primary disease). Consequently, if a patient has degenerative changes in any of the following joints, you must consider secondary causes of ortheoarthritis:

- Hands
  - MCPs (see figure)
- Wrist (see figure)
- Elbow
- Glenohumeral joint of shoulder
- Ankle
- Feet, other than first MTP

If the degenerative changes involve only one joint, consider traumatic arthritis. If multiple joints are involved, consider a metabolic or endocrine disorder that has caused the cartilage to degenerate in several joints. Note that the end stage of an underlying inflammatory arthritis that has destroyed the cartilage can result in degenerative changes superimposed on the inflammatory radiographic features.

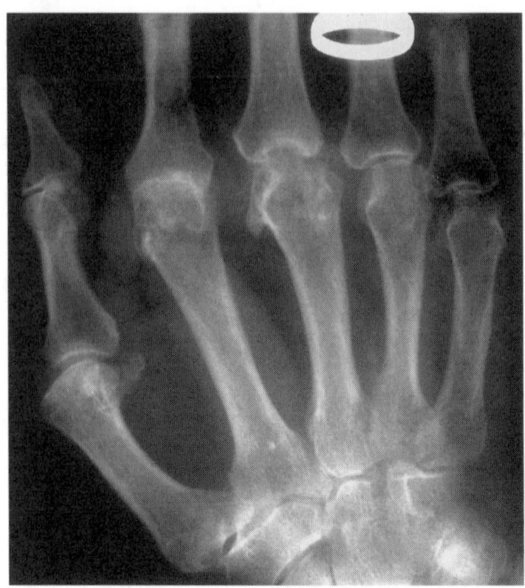

Hand radiograph with degenerative arthritis of MCPs and wrist. Patient had hemochromatosis.

**11. Describe the radiographic features of chronic gouty arthritis.**

- Erosions with sclerotic margins and an overhanging edge (see figure). These are caused by tophaceous deposits in the synovium slowly expanding into bone. The bone reacts and forms a sclerotic margin around the erosion.
- Relative preservation of joint space until late in disease
- Relative lack of periarticular osteoporosis for the degree of erosion seen
- Nodules in soft tissue (i.e., tophi). Unlike rheumatoid nodules, tophi can become calcified.

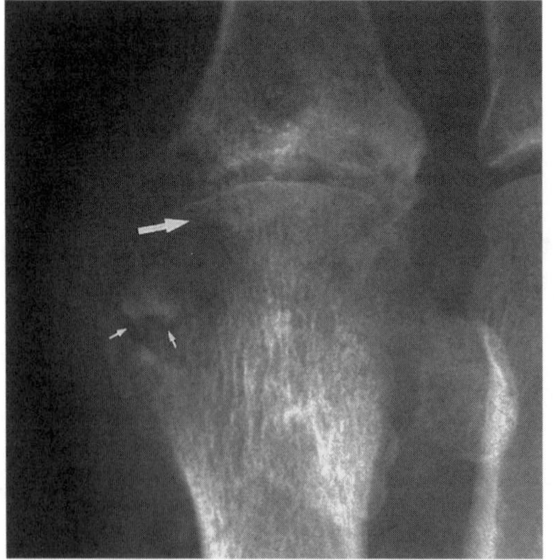

Radiograph of foot showing gouty erosions of first MTP with the characteristic overhanging edge (arrow). Note calcium in tophi (small arrows).

**12. What other diseases can give radiographic features similar to those of chronic gouty arthritis?**

*Mycobacterium tuberculosis* and some fungal infections
Pigmented villonodular synovitis
Amyloidosis
Multicentric reticulohistiocytosis
Synovial osteochondromatosis

**13. Compare the radiographic features of inflammatory and noninflammatory spinal arthritis.**

Inflammatory spinal arthritis is typically related to either infection or a seronegative spondyloarthropathy. Hematogenous spread of infection usually results in **osteomyelitis** originating near the endplate regions with subsequent spread to the intervertebral disc. The typical radiographic appearance of osteomyelitis is disc-space narrowing with poorly defined cortical endplates and destruction of the adjacent vertebrae (see figure). Although this appearance is very suggestive of infection, other inflammatory arthropathies, such as RA, seronegative spondyloarthropathies, and calcium pyrophosphate deposition disease, can rarely give a similar appearance.

**Ankylosing spondylitis** (AS) is associated with squared anterior vertebral bodies with sclerotic anterior corners, syndesmophytes (ossification of the annulus fibrosus), discovertebral erosions, and vertebral and apophyseal fusion (see figure). Psoriasis or Reiter's syndrome may cause spinal changes similar to AS; however, more typical is the presence of paravertebral ossifications or large, nonmarginal syndesmophytes near the thoracolumbar junction. Radiographic sacroiliitis will also be present in spondyloarthropathy patients who have inflammatory spinal disease (see Chapters 38–41).

**Noninflammatory lumbar arthritis** is characterized by disc-space narrowing and vacuum phenomenon, osteophytosis, and bony sclerosis in the absence of sacroiliitis (see figure). Degenerative diseases of the vertebral column can affect cartilaginous joints (discovertebral junction), synovial joints such as apophyses, or ligaments (enthesopathy). Typically, dehydration of the disc results in cartilage fissuring, with subsequent diminution in height and vacuum phenomenon (gas within the disc) and ultimately, bony sclerosis (intervertebral osteochondrosis). Osteophytosis (spondylosis deformans) is generally believed to be initiated by annulus fibrosus disruption. Ligamentous degeneration also occurs; ligamentum flavum hypertrophy may contribute to spinal stenosis, while ossification of the anterior longitudinal ligament is characteristic of diffuse idiopathic skeletal hyperostosis (DISH) (see Chapter 55).

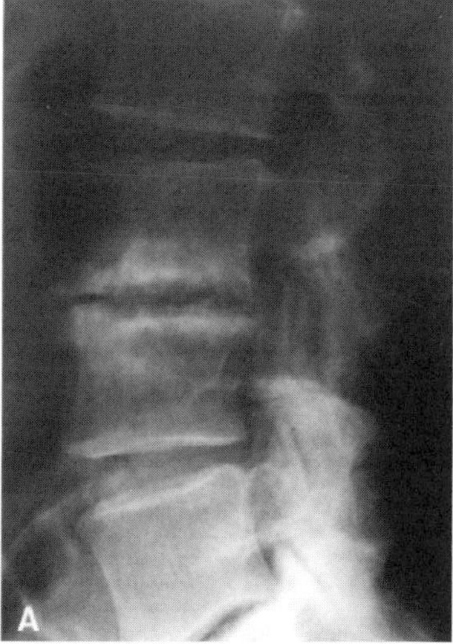


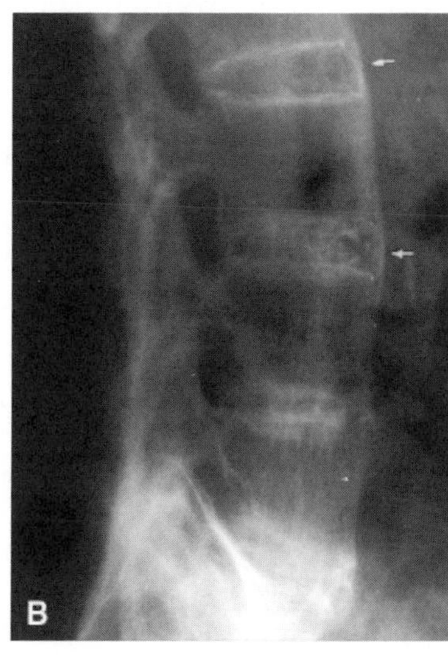

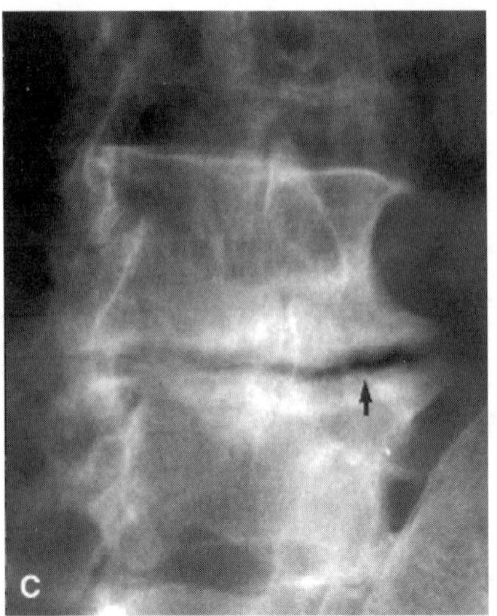


*A*, Lateral radiograph of lumbar spine demonstrating osteomyelitis at L3–4 with erosive/destructive changes of the adjoining cortical endplates. *B*, Lateral radiograph of lumbar spine demonstrating ankylosing spondylitis with anterior squaring of vertebrae and syndesmophytes (arrows). *C*, Oblique radiograph of lumbar spine showing degenerative disc disease, vacuum sign (arrow), and osteophytes.

*Radiographic Features of Inflammatory versus Noninflammatory Spinal Arthritis*

| | INFLAMMATORY | | NONINFLAMMATORY |
|---|---|---|---|
| | INFECTION | SPONDYLOARTHROPATHY | |
| Sacroiliac joints | Normal | Erosions | Normal |
| Vertebral bodies | Irregular, eroded endplates | Squaring± erosions | Sclerosis |
| Disc space | Narrowed | May be destroyed or convex | Narrowed, vacuum |
| | One site | Multiple sites | |
| Syndesmophytes | – | + | – |
| Osteophytes | – | – | + |
| Osteoporosis | + | + | – |
| Soft tissue mass | + | – | – |

### 14. What is the difference between an osteophyte and a syndesmophyte?

| FEATURE | OSTEOPHYTE | SYNDESMOPHYTE |
|---|---|---|
| Disorder | Osteoarthritis | Spondyloarthropathy* |
| Vertebral involvement | Lower cervical<br>Lumbar | Lower thoracic<br>Upper lumbar<br>Cervical |
| Vertebral orientation | Horizontal | Vertical |
| Pathogenesis | Endochondral ossification | Outer annulus fibrosus calcification |
| | "Bony spurs" | "Vertebral bridging" |
| Complications | Radiculopathy<br>Vertebrobasilar ischemia | Ankylosis<br>"Bamboo spine"<br>Fracture |

* Includes ankylosing spondylitis, psoriatic arthritis, Reiter's syndrome, inflammatory bowel disease arthritis.

**15. What rheumatic disease categories typically have unique radiographic features and are difficult to categorize using the inflammatory, noninflammatory, or gout-like patterns of radiographic changes?**

Collagen vascular disease (e.g., scleroderma, SLE)

Endocrine arthropathies (e.g., hyperparathyroidism, acromegaly, hyperthyroidism)

Miscellaneous (sickle cell disease, hemophilia, Paget's disease, avascular necrosis, Charcot joints, sarcoidosis, hypertrophic osteoarthropathy)

Tumors (e.g., synovial osteochondromatosis)

**16. List the most common diseases associated with the following radiographic changes seen in the hands.**

**Extensive arthritis of multiple DIP joints**
- Primary osteoarthritis
- Psoriatic arthritis
- Multicentric reticulohistiocytosis (MRH)

**First CMC joint arthritis**
- Primary osteoarthritis

**Second and third MCP joint arthritis**
- Hemochromatosis and acromegaly if degenerative arthritis with hook-like osteophytes
- Rheumatoid arthritis or psoriatic arthritis if erosive changes

**Arthritis mutilans of the hands (or feet)**
- Psoriatic arthritis
- Rheumatoid arthritis
- Chronic gouty arthritis
- Other less common diseases (multicentric reticulohistiocytosis)

Ulna impaction syndrome—ulna that is too long abuts on triquetrium causing DJD

**17. Outline the approach to the radiographic diagnosis of a patient with peripheral arthritis.**

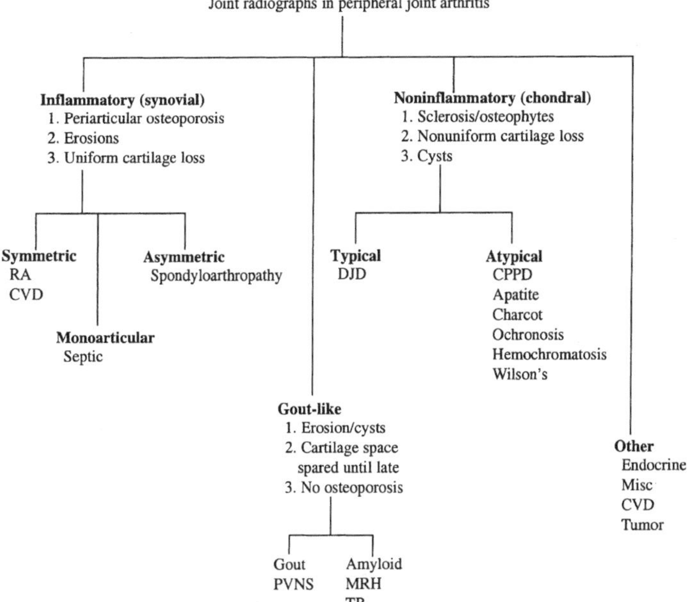


CVD, collagen vascular disease; DJD, degenerative joint disease; CPPD, calcium pyrophosphate deposition disease; PVNS, pigmented villonodular synovitis; MRH, multicentric reticulohistiocytosis; TB, tuberculosis.

**18. List the most common diseases associated with the following radiographic changes seen in the upper extremity and shoulder.**

**Radioulnar joint arthritis**
- Rheumatoid arthritis
- Juvenile rheumatoid arthritis
- Calcium pyrophosphate deposition disease (CPPD)

**Swan neck and/or ulnar deviation deformities**
- Rheumatoid arthritis if erosive changes and nonreversible deformities
- SLE if nonerosive and reversible deformities

**Elbow nodules in soft tissue**
- Rheumatoid arthritis
- Tophaceous gout (particularly if contains calcium deposits)
- Scleroderma-associated calcium deposits

**"Pencilling" of clavicle distal end**
- Rheumatoid arthritis
- Hyperparathyroidism

**19. Outline an approach to the radiographic diagnosis of a patient with arthritis of the back.**

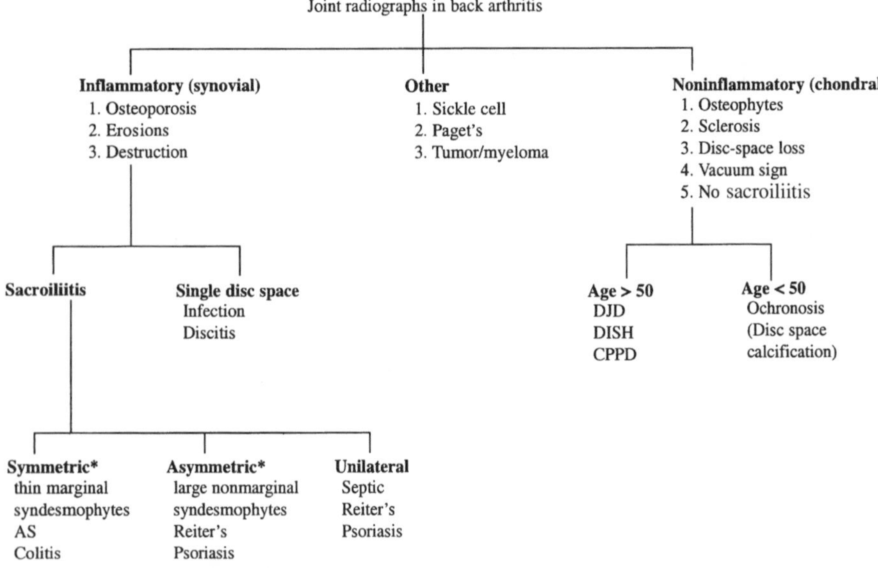


AS, ankylosing spondylitis; DISH, diffuse idiopathic skeletal hyperostosis.

**20. List the most common diseases associated with the following radiographic changes seen in the feet.**

**Destructive arthritis of great-toe interphalangeal joint**
- Reiter's syndrome
- Psoriatic arthritis
- Gout and rheumatoid arthritis, less commonly

**Destructive arthritis at great-toe MTP joint**
- Rheumatoid arthritis
- Chronic gouty arthritis
- Reiter's and psoriatic arthritis, less commonly
- Primary osteoarthritis if noninflammatory degenerative changes

**MTP joint erosive arthritis**
Reiter's or psoriatic if asymmetric distribution
Rheumatoid arthritis if symmetric distribution

**Calcaneal spurs**
Traction spurs (noninflammatory)—blunted spur with well-corticated margin
Seronegative spondyloarthropathies (inflammatory spurs)—pointed spur with poorly corticated margin

**21. In the spine?**

**Vacuum disc sign**
Degenerative disc disease (essentially this sign excludes infection at this disc level)

**Disc space calcification at multiple levels**
Ochronosis if patient young (< 30 yrs)
CPPD and others

**Sacroiliitis**
Ankylosing spondylitis (usually symmetric sacroiliitis)
Enteropathic arthritis (usually symmetric sacroiliitis)
Reiter's syndrome (frequently asymmetric sacroiliitis)
Psoriatic arthritis (frequently asymmetric sacroiliitis)
Infection (unilateral sacroiliitis)
[Don't get fooled by DISH. Can cause large osteophyte looking like sclerosis at junction of upper 1/3 and lower 2/3 of SI joint.]

**Syndesmophytes**
Ankylosing spondylitis and enteropathic arthritis (thin, marginal bilateral syndesmophytes)
Reiter's syndrome and psoriatic arthritis (large, nonmarginal, asymmetric syndesmophytes)
[Don't get fooled by DISH with its calcification of the anterior longitudinal ligament (sacroiliac joints will be normal).]

Ossification of posterior longitudinal ligament (OPLL)—usually C3–C4. Can cause spinal stenosis. Frequently in Asian patients.

**22. And other places (or everywhere)?**

**Chondrocalcinosis**
Idiopathic CPPD
Hyperparathyroidism
Hemochromatosis
Others, but they are rare diseases

**Erosions (hallmark of inflammatory synovial-based arthritis)**
Rheumatoid arthritis or juvenile rheumatoid arthritis
Seronegative spondyloarthropathies
Chronic gouty arthritis
Septic (infectious) arthritis
Others (SLE rarely, mixed connective tissue disease, multicentric reticulohistiocytosis, pigmented villonodular synovitis)

**Isolated patellofemoral degenerative arthritis**
CPPD

**23. Give the characteristic radiographic features of the different arthritides.**

**Rheumatoid arthritis—Symmetric, erosive arthritis**, uniform joint-space narrowing. Most common sites are small joints of hands and feet (MCPs, PIPs, wrists, MTPs) and cervical spine. Soft tissue nodules that do not calcify. Swan neck deformities and ulnar deviation.

**Juvenile chronic arthritis**—Osteoporosis, but joint-space narrowing and erosions typically absent until late. Periosteal reaction and **bony fusion** (carpus, facets in cervical spine) may distinguish it from RA. Whenever it looks as if someone has fused the wrist with a blowtorch, think juvenile rheumatoid arthritis.

**Ankylosing spondylitis—bilateral, symmetric sacroiliitis** with ankylosis. **Bilateral, thin, marginal** syndesmophytes in the spine may cause spinal fusion (bamboo spine). Peripheral arthropathy affects axial joints (shoulders, hips).

**Reiter's syndrome**—Can be bilateral or **unilateral, asymmetric sacroiliitis**. Peripherally, there is a predilection for **lower extremities** (especially the interphalangeal joint of great toe), with erosions and fluffy periostitis. Enthesopathy with erosions and calcifications at tendon insertions into calcaneus. Frequently, asymmetric joint involvement. Large, asymmetric, nonmarginal (jug-handle) syndesmophytes.

**Psoriatic arthritis**—Axial arthropathy similar to Reiter's. Peripherally, it has an **upper extremity predilection; DIP or PIP fusion. "Pencil-in-cup" deformity**. Enthesopathy and periostitis. **Erosions of several joints of a single digit** (MCP, PIP, and DIP of one finger). Frequently, asymmetric joint involvement. Acro-osteolysis. Jug-handle syndesmophytes.

**Gout—Erosions with overhanging edge and sclerotic margins**. Preserved joint space. Soft tissue tophi that can contain calcium.

**Calcium pyrophosphate dihydrate deposition** (CPPD)—Osteoarthritic changes at sites **atypical for degenerative joint disease (DJD)** (MCPs, elbow, radiocarpal, ankle, shoulder).

**Chondrocalcinosis**. Uniform joint-space narrowing despite being a cause of degenerative arthritis. **Isolated patellofemoral DJD**.

**Degenerative joint disease** (primary osteoarthritis)—Nonuniform joint-space narrowing, sclerosis, **osteophytosis**, cysts. Most common sites include the DIPs, PIPs, first CMC, knees, hips, and spine.

**Neuropathic joint (Charcot)**—Destruction, disorganization, density (i.e., sclerosis), debris, dislocation (**the 5 Ds**).

**Systemic lupus erythematosus** (SLE)—**Reversible swan neck and ulnar deviation deformity and subluxation**, but absence of erosions.

**Scleroderma**—Tapered, atrophic soft tissues (**sclerodactyly**) with soft tissue calcifications. Acro-osteolysis of terminal phalanges.

**Hemochromatosis**—Chondrocalcinosis. **Degenerative changes at MCPs** (especially second and third) with "hook-like" spurs. Cystic changes of radiocarpal joint of wrist.

**Ochronosis—Vertebral disc calcification**, chondrocalcinosis, osteoarthritis in multiple joints (especially spine) at young age.

**Acromegaly—widened joint and disc spaces**. Large spurs at bases of distal phalanges (**spade phalanges**).

**Hyperparathyroidism—subperiosteal resorption** at radial side of middle phalanges. Soft tissue calcifications, chondrocalcinosis, **"salt and pepper" skull**, ligament and tendon ruptures.

**Avascular necrosis—crescent sign, stepoff sign**. Hips and shoulders are most commonly affected

**Hypertrophic osteoarthropathy (periosteal reaction)**—pachydermoperiostitis (primary), lung cancer, and liver disease (secondary). Other causes of periosteal reaction include thyroid disease, tuberous sclerosis, stasis, infection.

**24. What is the difference between T1- and T2-weighted images on MRI?**

T1- or T2-weighting typically refers to the spin echo MR sequence. TR is the repetition time, or time between 90° radiofrequency pulses, whereas TE is the echo time, or time between the 90° pulse and the time the signal is received. **T1-weighted images** are short TR (300–1000 ms) and short TE (10–30 ms) and provide excellent anatomic detail. In contrast, **T2-weighted images** are long TR (1800–2500 ms) and long TE (40–90 ms), sensitive for detecting edema. A proton density sequence combines T1 and T2 weighting by having a long TR (> T1) and short TE (< T2). This technique can be used to separate cartilage from bone. The TR and TE numbers are printed in the corner of the MRI film so that you can tell if the image is T1- or T2-weighted.

Two other sequences commonly used are gradient echo and STIR (short tau [T1] inversion recovery). **Gradient echo** sequences can be either T1- or T2-weighted and permit very rapid acquisition with thin-section, high-quality images. **STIR** is effectively a fat-suppression technique, very sensitive in detection of fluid or edema. These images greatly aid in detection of marrow and soft tissue disease, and we routinely rely on these sequences for detecting pathology such as muscle tears, osteomyelitis, bone marrow edema, or tumor involvement

Gadolinium is a paramagnetic element used as a contrast agent in MRI. It is nonallergenic and nonradioactive, but it adds $100 to the cost of MRI. On T1-weighted images, gadolinium is distributed to areas of increased blood flow, so it is a good marker of vascularity of tumors or of inflammation.

**25. Describe the appearances of the various tissues on T1- and T2-weighted MR images.**

| STRUCTURE | T1 INTENSITY | T2 INTENSITY |
|---|---|---|
| Fat, fatty marrow | High | Lower |
| Hyaline cartilage | Intermediate | Intermediate |
| Muscle | Intermediate | Intermediate |
| Fluid, edema | Low | High |
| Neoplasm | Low | High |
| Cortical bone | Very low | Very low |
| Tendon, ligaments | Very low | Very low |

High appears white on MRI; low appears black on MRI. The brightness on MRI is compared with muscle.

**26. In which clinical situations is CT scan superior to MRI and vice versa?**

Plain radiographs should be obtained before a CT scan or MRI when evaluating musculoskeletal disorders. If the plain radiographs do not delineate the abnormality, CT scan and MRI may add further information.

**CT scan** is superior to MRI in:

| | |
|---|---|
| Acute trauma (fracture and dislocations) | Sacroiliac joint erosions |
| Tarsal coalition | Intra-articular osteocartilaginous loose bodies |
| Sternoclavicular joint arthritis | Crowned dens syndrome—CPPD at C2 dens |

**MRI scan** is superior to CT scan in:

| | |
|---|---|
| Cervical spine disease or instability | Osteomyelitis |
| Spinal stenosis or disc disease | Soft tissue tumors or skeletal muscle pathology |
| Internal derangement of knee | Pigmented villonodular synovitis (PVNS) |
| Rotator cuff tears and tendinitis | Inflammatory sacroiliitis |
| Avascular necrosis | Synovitis and tenosynovitis (rarely needed) |

MRI is complementary to CT scan and bone scintigraphy when evaluating bone tumors.

**27. What imaging features are typically seen in infections of bones or joint spaces?**

In acute osteomyelitis, the earliest radiographic abnormality is **soft tissue swelling** with obliteration of normal tissue planes. Hyperemia results in osteoporosis, and bone destruction or periostitis may not be visualized for 7–14 days. Thus, nuclear medicine scanning or MRI is much more sensitive for detection of early osteomyelitis. MRI is particularly helpful in defining the full extent of osteomyelitis, particularly when amputation is a therapeutic option (see figure, top of next page). Subacute osteomyelitis is frequently referred to as a Brodie's abscess, usually in the metaphysis of tubular bones. A well-marginated **lucent defect** (commonly elongated) is seen surrounded by a thick band of sclerosis. With chronic osteomyelitis, radiodense spicules of necrotic bone, referred to as **sequestra**, may be seen within the lucent defect.

**28. What are some of the potential uses for ultrasound in evaluation of musculoskeletal conditions?**

Ultrasound is good at detecting abnormalities of superficial structures. Its resolution is 1 mm, compared with 3 mm for MRI. It is also much less expensive than MRI. Some conditions it can be used in:

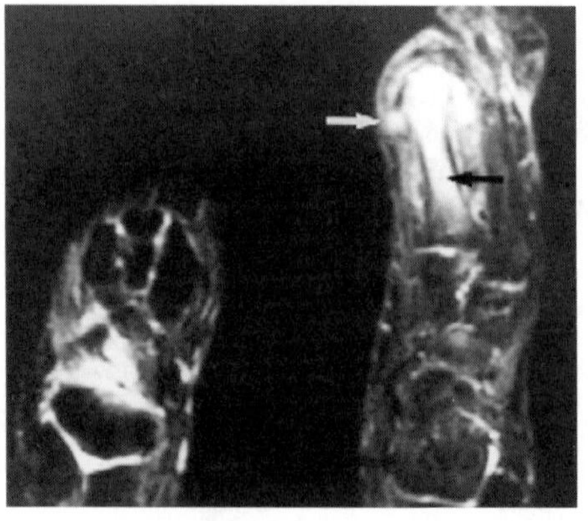

STIR MR image depicts the high-signal edema (black arrow) corresponding to osteomyelitis involving the entirety of the first metatarsal. Focus of high signal in the adjacent soft tissues represents an abscess (white arrow).

- Tendon pathology—tears and inflammation in posterior tibial tendon, Achilles tendon, or finger tendons. Accuracy of picking up rotator cuff tears is very operator dependent but can be > 90% in experienced operators.
- Soft tissue masses—can pick up foreign bodies better than MRI. Also good for Morton's neuromas > 5 mm in size and ganglions.
- Joint and bursal inflammation—synovitis and effusion of superficial joints. Picks up erosions of 2nd and 5th MCP joints before plain radiographs.

**29. What is a three phase bone scan?**

A three phase scan looks at blood flow to a particular area of the musculoskeletal system during the first two phases and then bony uptake in the delayed third phase. This is different from the standard bone scan that just looks at bony uptake in the delayed phase. The first phase is imaged within 2 minutes of $^{99m}$Tc diphosphonate injection and measures blood flow to an area. The second phase (blood pool phase) is imaged 20 minutes after injection, and the third phase 3–5 hours postinjection. Areas of inflammation or increased vascularity will have increased uptake in first two phases, while areas of bony injury will have uptake in third phase.

**30. Where can a three phase bone scan be useful?**

It is sometimes difficult separating cellulitis from joint pathology clinically. A three phase bone scan can help:

| | CELLULITIS | SYNOVITIS | OSTEOMYELITIS |
|---|---|---|---|
| First phase | + | + | + |
| Second phase | + | + | + |
| Third phase* | – | + | + |

* In the third phase, synovitis will have uptake on both sides of a joint while osteomyelitis will have bony uptake on one side.

Another place for these scans may be in patients with arthralgias but limited physical examination findings who are seeking disability. A negative three phase scan is good evidence of no significant underlying pathology, i.e., "a nuclear medicine sedimentation rate."

**31. What is the radiation exposure to an individual undergoing one of these techniques?**

The conversion for radiation units is as follows:

- 1 Sievert (Sv) = 1 Gray (Gy) = 100 Rem = 100 Rad
- Note that 1 Sv will suppress bone marrow. Chernobyl workers received 5 Sv.

The acceptable radiation exposure is:

- General public 5 m Sv/year = 5000 u Sv/year
- Occupational exposure 50 m Sv/year = 50,000 u Sv/year

The average background radiation exposure a person is exposed to is:

- Natural background = 5–8 u Sv/day
- Roundtrip flight from New York to Los Angeles = 60 u Sv
- Average annual dose = 3600 u Sv/year

The average radiation exposure for radiologic procedures is:

- Mammography—50 u Sv
- Chest x-ray—100 u Sv
- Lumbar spine x-ray—1300 u Sv
- Bone scan—4000 u Sv
- UGI—7500 u Sv
- Barium enema—11,000 u Sv (with fluroscopy)

DEXA—1–3 u Sv/site
Quantitative CT (bone density)—50 u Sv
Head CT scan—2000 u Sv
Ultrasound—0
MR—0

## BIBLIOGRAPHY


1. Battafarano DF, West SG, et al: Comparison of bone scan, computed tomography and magnetic resonance imaging in the diagnosis of sacroiliitis. Semin Arthritis Rheum 23:161–176, 1993.
2. Bloem JL, Sartoris DJ (eds): MRI and CT of the Musculoskeletal System. Baltimore, Williams & Wilkins, 1992.
3. Brower AC, Flaming DJ (eds): Arthritis in Black and White, 2nd ed. Philadelphia, W. B. Saunders, 1997.
4. Early PJ, Sodee DB: Principles and Practice of Nuclear Medicine. St. Louis, Mosby, 1995.
5. Rafii M (ed): The shoulder. Magn Reson Imag Clin North Am 1(1): 1993.
6. Resnick D: Bone and Joint Imaging. Philadelphia, W.B. Saunders, 1996.
7. van Holsbeeck MT (ed): Musculoskeletal ultrasound. Radiol Clinics North Amer 37:612–877, 1999.
8 Weissman BN, Resnick D, Kaushik S, et al: Imaging. In Ruddy S, Harris ED, Sledge CB (eds): Kelley's Textbook of Rheumatology, 6th ed. Philadelphia, W.B. Saunders, 2001, pp 621–684.


# 12. SYNOVIAL BIOPSIES

*Sterling* G. *West*, M.D.

**1. What are the indications to perform a synovial biopsy?**

The main indication for synovial biopsy is a chronic (> 6–8 weeks), nontraumatic, inflammatory (synovial fluid WBC count > 2000 cells/mm$^3$) arthritis limited to one or two joints in which the diagnosis has not been made by history, physical examination, laboratory studies, or synovial fluid analysis with culture (including both fungi and mycobacteria).

**2. What diseases can be diagnosed with a synovial biopsy?**

- Chronic infections
  - Fungal arthritis
  - Mycobacterial arthritis
  - Spirochetal arthritis (Lyme disease, syphilis)
  - Whipple's disease
  - Chlamydia
- Chronic sarcoidosis
- Infiltrative/deposition diseases*
  - Amyloidosis
  - Ochronosis
  - Hemochromatosis
  - Crystal-induced arthritis
- Tumors
  - Pigmented villonodular synovitis
  - Synovial osteochondromatosis
  - Synovial cell sarcoma
  - Leukemia/lymphoma
  - Metastatic disease to the joint
- Others
  - Multicentric reticulohistiocytosis
  - Plant thorn and other foreign-body synovitis

* Synovial biopsy is usually not necessary in these diseases.

**3. Does a synovial biopsy help in the diagnosis of a systemic connective tissue disease such as rheumatoid arthritis?**

No. Although biopsy of the synovium in a patient with rheumatoid arthritis may be compatible with the diagnosis, it is not pathognomonic. Clearly, spondyloarthropathy can produce synovial biopsies that look very much like those obtained from rheumatoid arthritis patients.

**4. How can synovial tissue be obtained?**

| METHOD | SIZE OF HOLE |
|---|---|
| Closed-needle biopsy (Parker-Pearson or other needle) | 14-gauge needle (1.6 mm) |
| Needle arthroscopy | 1.8 mm |
| Arthroscopy | 4–5 mm |
| Open surgical biopsy | Several inches |

**5. List the advantages and disadvantages of the different methods of synovial biopsy.**

*Comparison of Synovial Biopsy Techniques*

| | ADVANTAGES | DISADVANTAGES |
|---|---|---|
| Needle biopsy | Least expensive<br>Least traumatic<br>One skin incision | Small biopsy specimens |
| Needle arthroscopic biopsy | Minimally invasive<br>Direct visualization | Two skin incisions<br>Moderately expensive |
| Arthroscopic biopsy | Direct visualization<br>Large biopsy specimen | Expensive<br>Invasive |
| Open surgical biopsy | Direct visualization<br>Large biopsy specimen<br>Best if suspected tumor or foreign body<br>Can be done on any joint | Expensive<br>Most invasive<br>Longest postop recovery time |

**6. Which joints can be biopsied with a closed-biopsy needle?**

Usually large joints, most commonly the knee. Smaller joints can be biopsied also.

**7. How many specimens must be obtained by a closed-biopsy needle to minimize sampling error?**

Five to eight specimens from the joint being biopsied.

**8. Who invented arthroscopy?**

1918 Japanese physician, Dr. Takagi, performs first knee arthroscopy with a cystoscope.

1930s German rheumatologist, Dr. Vaupel, proposes use of arthroscopy to follow the course of arthritis.

1957 Dr. M. Watanabe performs first partial menisectomy through arthroscope.

1969 Dr. N. Matsui performs first arthroscopic synovectomy.

## BIBLIOGRAPHY

1. Arnold W: Arthroscopy in the diagnosis and therapy of arthritis. Hosp Pract 27:43–53, 1992.
2. Gibson T, Fagg N, Highton J, et al: The diagnostic value of synovial biopsy in patients with arthritis of unknown cause. Br J Rheumatol 24:232–241, 1985.

3. Saaibi DL, Schumacher HR: Percutaneous needle biospy and synovial histology. Baillieres Clin Rheumatol 10:535, 1996.
4. Schumacher HR: Needle biopsy of the synovial membrane: Experience with the Parker-Pearson technique. N Engl J Med 286:416–419, 1972.
5. Schumacher HR: Synovial fluid analysis and synovial biopsy. In Ruddy S, Harris ED, Sledge CB (eds): Kelley's Textbook of Rheumatology, 6th ed. Philadelphia, W.B. Saunders Co., 2001, pp 605–619.

# 13. ELECTROMYOGRAPHY AND NERVE CONDUCTION STUDIES

*Cliff A. Gronseth*, M.D.

**1. What is an EMG?**

It is a term used in two ways:

- As a global description of the entire spectrum of tests performed in electrodiagnostic medicine, such as nerve conduction studies (NCS) and electromyography (EMG).
- More specifically, to describe the type of procedure that uses a needle (needle EMG) or surface electrodes (surface EMG) to analyze the neural control mechanism of muscle (the motor unit).

**2. What is the motor unit?**

The anatomic unit of function for the motor portion of the peripheral nervous system. It includes the **motor neuron** found within the anterior horn of the spinal cord, its **axon**, the **neuromuscular junction**, and the **muscle fibers** supplied by the peripheral nerve. The electrodiagnostic physician can utilize a combination of EMG, nerve conduction studies (NCS), repetitive stimulation, and other electrophysiologic tests to assess individual components of the motor unit.

**3. What is an innervation ratio?**

For each efferent motor axon, there are a variable number of terminal axons and muscle fibers. Depending on the specific requirement of control, the ratio may be quite low or extremely high. The innervation ratio of the extraocular muscles is typically 1:3, owing to the fine control required for binocular vision. Conversely, the innervation ratio of the gastrocnemius can be as high as 1:2000, since most movements involving the plantar flexors of the ankle are relatively large motions requiring more force than accuracy.

**4. Name some other types of electrodiagnostic tests.**

- **Nerve conduction studies** (NCS), sometimes called nerve conduction velocities (NCVs), are used to assess the amplitude and velocity of electrical signals carried within the peripheral nerve.
- **Repetitive stimulation studies** are utilized for the evaluation of the neuromuscular junction (i.e., myasthenia gravis).
- **Somatosensory evoked potentials** are used to evaluate conduction within the spinal cord and brain.
- Other less frequently used tests include single-fiber EMG, motor-evoked potentials, and nerve root stimulation.

**5. What are the clinical indications for ordering an EMG? An NCS?**

An EMG is ordered to determine the localization and severity of neuropathic disorders and/or to document myopathic disorders. NCS are ordered to localize anatomic abnormalities of the peripheral motor and sensory nervous systems and to assess the severity of axonal or demyelinating pathology.

**6. Describe the components of a normal EMG.**

**Insertional/Spontaneous Activity**: An EMG needle inserted into normal muscle should evoke brief electrical discharges of muscle fibers. Increased or prolonged electrical activity may indicate abnormalities of the muscle fibers or the nerves supplying them. Fibrillations, positive sharp waves, and complex repetitive discharges (CRDs) are electrical signals that often represent abnormal spontaneous firing of muscle fibers, and possibly nerve and/or muscle damage. There should be no spontaneous activity when the muscle is at rest.

**Motor Unit Analysis**: The patient slightly contracts the muscle to allow analysis of the configuration and recruitment of isolated **motor unit action potentials** (MUAPs). Normal initial MUAPs have a duration of 5–15 msec, 2–4 phases (usually 3), an amplitude of 0.5–3 mV (depending on the muscle stimulated), and recruitment frequency of < 20 Hz. For the electromyographer, motor unit analysis is an important assessment tool that takes both visible and auditory training and skills.

**Interference Pattern**: The patient fully contracts the muscle. Normally, a sufficient number of motor units are recruited so that MUAPs overlap each other, resulting in "full interference pattern" or obliteration of the resting baseline. Sometimes pain prevents a patient from maximally contracting the muscle.

**7. What is an incremental response?**

Both the sensory and motor components of the nervous system function in an all-or-none fashion. For example, when the anterior horn cell of a single motor unit is activated, the entire motor unit depolarizes. Gradients or values of sensory or motor response are assessed or controlled by the CNS by the progressive addition of incremental responses. For example, when one motor unit is firing, a muscle may have little or no assessable change in tone. As additional motor units discharge, muscle tone increases to the point of visible contraction with progressively more force.

**8. How do fasciculations, fibrillations, and positive sharp waves differ on EMG?**

A **fasciculation** is an involuntary firing of an entire motor unit, i.e., single motor neuron and all its innervated muscle fibers. This is seen as a large electrical spike on EMG testing of a relaxed muscle. It is sometimes clinically visible in the patient as a brief, irregular undulation of muscle (worms under the skin). This can be a normal finding, but in excess is the hallmark of amyotrophic lateral sclerosis (Lou Gehrig's disease).

A **fibrillation** ("fib") is an involuntary contraction of a single muscle fiber that usually indicates denervation or muscle damage has occurred. Unlike a fasciculation, a fibrillation usually does not cause clinically visible muscle movement. Fibrillations occur as a result of spontaneous firing of muscle fibers that have developed an increased number of acetylcholine receptors on their surfaces following denervation (Cannon's law). Any extraneous acetylcholine in the area causes the muscle fiber to contract, generating electrical activity that is seen as a spontaneous fibrillation on the resting muscle EMG.

**Positive sharp waves** ("p-waves") are similar to fibrillation potentials in that they often represent abnormal muscle fiber firing from nerve or muscle damage. They are identified by their initial positive deflection from the baseline, as opposed the initial negative deflection of a fib.

**9. How do normal EMG findings compare with the findings seen in a denervated muscle (neuropathic process)?**

| EMG | NORMAL | DENERVATED MUSCLE | REINNERVATED MUSCLE |
|---|---|---|---|
| **Rest** | | | |
| Insertional activity | Normal | Increased | Normal to increased |
| Spontaneous activity | None | Fibrillations, positive sharp wave | None |
| **Mild contraction** MUAP | Normal | Normal, limited recruitment | Large, polyphasic, limited recruitment |
| **Maximal contraction** Interference pattern | Full | Reduced | Reduced |

Note that fibrillations and positive sharp waves are not seen in resting muscles until 7–14 days after the onset of axonal degeneration. Full reinnervation of the denervated muscle, resulting in large, polyphasic motor unit action potentials (MUAPs), may take 3–4 months.

**10. How do normal EMG findings compare with the findings seen in myopathic processes?**

| EMG | NORMAL | MYOPATHY | INFLAMMATORY MYOSITIS |
|---|---|---|---|
| **Rest** | | | |
| Insertional activity | Normal | Normal | Increased |
| Spontaneous activity | None | None | Fibrillations, positive sharp waves |
| **Mild contraction** | | | |
| MUAP | Normal | Small units, early recruitment | Small units, early recruitment |
| **Maximal contraction** | | | |
| Interference pattern | Full | Full, low amplitude | Full, low amplitude |

Up to 30% of patients with a noninflammatory (steroid) myopathy may have a normal EMG. Inflammatory myositis (i.e., polymyositis, dermatomyositis) has both neuropathic and myopathic EMG abnormalities. The spontaneous activity of fibrillations and positive sharp waves seen on EMG are due to inflammation affecting the nerve endings in the muscle, and represent denervation. The injured muscle fibers shrink, causing low-amplitude MUAPs, a key feature of EMG myopathic findings.

**11. Is the amplitude of a normal sensory nerve action potential (SNAP) higher or lower than a normal MUAP?**

The SNAP varies depending on the size and accessibility of distal nerves. It ranges from 10 to 100 microvolts, which is more than 1/20th the size of a normal MUAP, 2000–10,000 microvolts.

**12. Is the normal nerve conduction velocity (NCV) the same throughout the length of the nerve?**

NCVs vary among nerves and along their lengths. Normally, proximal nerve conduction is faster than distal nerve conduction as a result of the increased temperature and larger diameter of the proximal nerve segments. For example, median nerve conduction velocity from wrist to palm should be faster than from palm to finger. If not, carpal tunnel syndrome may be present.

**13. Why is temperature recorded during the course of an electrodiagnostic examination?**

NCVs change by 2.0–2.4 m/sec per degree Celsius reduction in both sensory and motor nerves. These changes can be significant, particularly in cooler climates. An astute question for a non-electromyographer to ask when results are borderline is, "What was the patient's temperature during the examination, or was the limb warmed before the NCV measurements were obtained?" Failure to warm the limb can result in false-positive studies, leading to a misdiagnosis of carpal tunnel syndrome or generalized sensory motor neuropathy.

**14. What are the H-reflex and F-wave? How are they clinically useful?**

The **H-reflex** is the electrical counterpart of the ankle jerk and gives information on the S1 afferent-efferent reflex arc. The H-reflex may be abnormal in neuropathies, S1 radiculopathies, or sciatic mononeuropathies.

The **F-wave** is a delayed motor potential following the normal MUAP and can give information about the proximal part of the nerve. An F-wave is obtained by powerfully stimulating a motor nerve in the distal limb and recording the delayed or late response of the muscle. The electrical stimulation travels proximally, bounces off the axon hillock, and returns down the nerve to contract the muscle slightly. Abnormal F-waves can indicate radiculopathy, plexopathy, or proximal nerve dysfunction such as in Guillain-Barré.

**15. How are sensory and motor portions of the peripheral nervous system tested?**

Sensory and motor nerve conduction studies are the primary means to test the peripheral nerves. The amplitude of the waveform, its point of onset, and its peak are compared with standardized normal values and with those from the opposite extremity. The waves created are summations of incremental depolarization of individual axonal fibers. Late responses (F-waves and H-reflexes) provide assessment of the more proximal, anatomically difficult-to-reach portions of the peripheral nervous system. These tests are also utilized to assess nerve conduction over a long segment of nerve fiber. F-waves, in particular, are an important screening test in the diagnosis of Guillain-Barré syndrome. Other less common techniques for assessing the peripheral nerves include somatosensory evoked potentials, dermatomal somatosensory evoked potentials, and selected nerve root stimulation.

**16. What disorders are characteristic of the peripheral nerve?**

Functionally, the peripheral nerve starts in the vicinity of the neural foramen, where sensory and motor fibers join. At its most proximal level, peripheral nerve injury in the form of **radiculopathy** is caused by compression of the nerve root by a herniated disc or bony fragment. **Plexus involvement** by disease or injury may occur in the upper (brachial plexus) or lower extremity (lumbar or lumbosacral plexopathy).

Peripheral nerve conditions can be acquired or congenital. Congenital anomalies include the hereditary sensory and motor neuropathies (e.g., Charcot-Marie-Tooth types I and II). Acquired conditions can include neuropathic disorders, such as diabetes, or those caused by toxins or metabolic insufficiencies.

**Focal neural entrapment** can be caused by carpal tunnel syndrome, ulnar neuropathy, or tarsal tunnel syndrome, to name just a few. It is very important for the electrodiagnostic physician to have taken a good history prior to commencing the examination.

**17. Describe the three main types of nerve injury.**

Nerves sustain a gradient of injury, which was originally defined by Seddon:

1. **Neurapraxia** is the functional loss of conduction without anatomic change of the axon. Demyelination may occur. However, with remyelination, NCV returns to normal.
2. In **axonotmesis**, the axonal continuity is lost. With its loss, wallerian degeneration occurs in the distal segment. Recovery, which is frequently not complete, occurs as a result of axonal regrowth at a rate of 1–3 mm/day (1 inch/month or 1 foot/year) in otherwise healthy individuals.
3. **Neurotmesis** results from separation of the entire nerve, including its supporting connective tissue. Regeneration frequently does not occur. Nerves with this degree of trauma frequently need surgical attention for any recovery to occur.

**18. Do the three types of nerve injuries ever occur together?**

Neurapraxia and axonotmesis commonly occur as a result of the same injury. When compression is relieved from the involved segment of nerve, two periods of healing typically occur. One is relatively immediate, from hours to weeks, as the neurapraxia resolves. A second period of healing, from weeks to months, may occur as a result of axonal regrowth.

**19. How can a demyelinating peripheral neuropathy and an axonal peripheral neuropathy be differentiated by EMG and NCS?**

**Demyelinating neuropathies** show moderate to severe slowing of motor conduction, with temporal dispersion of the MUAP, normal distal amplitudes, reduced proximal amplitudes, and delayed distal latencies. **Axonal neuropathies** show a milder slowing in NCV, with generally low MUAP amplitudes at all sites of stimulation. The EMG shows denervation abnormalities early in axonal neuropathies and only later in demyelinating neuropathies, when axons begin to degenerate.

**20. Which systemic diseases cause predominantly a demyelinating peripheral neuropathy? An axonal peripheral neuropathy?**

Peripheral polyneuropathies due to systemic disease can be classified (1) as acute, subacute, or chronic in onset; (2) as affecting predominantly sensory or motor nerves; and (3) as causing an axonal or demyelinating injury. Note that over time, most axonal neuropathies will develop myelin degeneration subsequently.

*Characteristic Polyneuropathies in Systemic Disease*

| | AXONAL | | DEMYLINATING | |
|---|---|---|---|---|
| | ACUTE | SUBACUTE/CHRONIC | ACUTE | SUBACUTE/CHRONIC |
| Diabetes mellitus | – | S, SM | – | S,SM |
| Uremia | – | SM | – | – |
| Porphyria | M | – | – | – |
| Vitamin deficiency | – | SM, S (B12 def.) | – | – |
| Amyloidosis | – | SM | – | – |
| Carcinoma | – | S (breast), SM (lung) | – | – |
| Lymphoma | – | SM | – | SM |
| Myeloma | – | SM | – | SM |
| Cryoglobulinemia and vasculitis | SM | SM | – | – |
| Diphtheria toxin | – | – | SM | – |

S = sensory; SM = sensorimotor; M = motor. In addition to these diseases, several drugs and environmental toxins can produce a polyneuropathy.

**21. How is EMG/NCS used in diagnosing carpal tunnel syndrome? Ulnar nerve entrapment at the elbow (cubital tunnel syndrome)?**

**Carpal tunnel syndrome** (CTS) or compressive median neuropathy at wrist is the most common entrapment neuropathy, affecting 1% of the population. CTS may show segmental nerve conduction slowing across the wrist. Sensory nerve action potential latencies of the median nerve (palmar latency) are delayed most often, but with increasing severity, motor latencies can be affected. Denervation of the thenar muscles seen on needle EMG indicates moderate to severe CTS. Clinical correlation is recommended for mild CTS as sometimes NCS/EMG studies are normal despite classic symptoms of hand pain/numbness in a median nerve distribution.

In **cubital tunnel syndrome**, the ulnar nerve is compressed at the elbow causing motor and/or sensory nerve conduction slowing. EMG assesses denervation in the ulnar-innervated muscles of the hand and forearm. The ulnar nerve can also be compressed at the wrist.

**22. What is a double crush syndrome?**

A double crush syndrome is controversial but may exist when carpal tunnel syndrome occurs in association with degenerative cervical spine disease. Proximal nerve entrapment may occur at the cervical root level, causing a disruption in axoplasmic flow in both afferent and efferent directions. A second point of entrapment distally, usually at the carpal tunnel, can result in a second physiologic insult along the course of the axon. While electromyographers speak of the syndrome, it is very difficult to quantify and document as a true clinical entity.

**23. Which other entities can be differentiated by EMG/NCS from the common peripheral nerve syndromes?**

| PERIPHERAL NERVE SYNDROME | DIFFERENTIAL DIAGNOSIS |
|---|---|
| CTS | Pronator teres syndrome<br>Other areas of median nerve entrapment |
| Ulnar entrapment at the elbow | C8 radiculopathy<br>Brachial plexus lesion |
| Radial nerve palsy | C7 radiculopathy |
| Suprascapular nerve lesion | C5–6 radiculopathy |
| Peroneal nerve palsy | L4–5 radiculopathy |
| Femoral nerve lesion | L3 radiculopathy |

**24. How is EMG used in the diagnosis and prognosis of myasthenia gravis, myotonic dystrophy, and Bell's palsy?**

**Myasthenia gravis**: Slow repetitive nerve stimulation of a motor nerve at 2–3 Hz will show a 10% or greater decremental motor response in 65–85% of patients. Single-fiber EMG, which measures the delay in transmission between terminal nerve fibers and their muscle fibers, is abnormal in 90–95% of patients.

**Myotonic dystrophy**: EMG shows MUAPs that vary in amplitude and frequency and are heard on the loud speaker as "dive bombers."

**Bell's palsy**: Facial NCS, done 5 days after the onset of palsy can indicate the prognosis for recovery. If NCV latencies and amplitudes are normal at this time, the prognosis for recovery is excellent.

ACKNOWLEDGMENT

The editor and author wish to thank Dr. Douglas Hemler for his contributions to this chapter in the previous edition.

BIBLIOGRAPHY

1. Aminoff MJ: Electrodiagnosis in Clinical Neurology, Churchill Livingstone, 1999.
2. Campbell WW: Essentials of Electrodiagnostic Medicine. Baltimore, Williams & Wilkins, 1999.
3. Dumitru D: Electrodiagnostic Medicine, 2nd ed. Philadelphia, Hanley & Belfus, 2001.
4. Kimura J: Electrodiagnosis in Diseases of Nerve and Muscle: Principles and Practice, 2nd ed. Philadelphia, F.A. Davis, 1989.
5. Liveson JA: Peripheral Neurology: Case Studies in Electrodiagnosis. Oxford, New York, Oxford University Press, 2000.
6. Johnson EW, Pease WS: Practical Electromyography. Baltimore, Williams & Wilkins, 1997.
7. Preston DC: Electromyography and Neuromuscular Disorders: Clinical-Electrophysiologic Correlations, Boston, Butterworth-Heinemann, 1998.

# 14. APPROACH TO THE PATIENT WITH MONOARTICULAR SYMTPOMS

*Robert A. Hawkins, M.D.*

**1. What conditions can be mistaken for a monoarticular process?**

Several common inflammatory processes occur in the soft tissues around, but not in, the joints. These conditions can be painful and may mimic arthritis. Examples include rotator cuff tendonitis of the shoulder, olecranon bursitis of the elbow, and prepatellar bursitis of the knee. It is important to distinguish these disorders from true joint disease because their management is often quite different from that of monoarticular arthritis. Careful history and physical examination usually allow correct identification of the affected region. (See also Chapter 66.)

**2. List the diseases that commonly present with monoarthritis.**

*Diseases Causing Monoarticular Symptoms*

| **Septic** | **Traumatic** |
|---|---|
| Bacterial | Fracture |
| Mycobacterial | Internal derangement |
| Lyme disease | Hemarthrosis |
| Fungal | |

(*Table continued on next page.*)

*Diseases Causing Monoarticular Symptoms (cont.)*

| Crystal deposition diseases | Other |
|---|---|
| Gout | Osteoarthritis |
| Calcium pyrophosphate dihydrate deposition disease (pseudogout) | Juvenile rheumatoid arthritis |
| Hydroxyapatite deposition disease | Coagulopathy |
| Calcium oxalate deposition disease | Avascular necrosis of bone |
| Palindromic rheumatism | Foreign-body synovitis |
| | Pigmented villonodular synovitis |
| | Synovioma |

**3. What polyarticular diseases occasionally present with a monoarticular onset?**

| | |
|---|---|
| Rheumatoid arthritis | Reiter's syndrome/reactive arthritis |
| Juvenile rheumatoid arthritis | Psoriatic arthritis |
| Viral arthritis | Enteropathic arthritis |
| Sarcoid arthritis | Whipple's disease |

**4. What is the most critical diagnosis to consider in the patient with monoarticular symptoms?**

Joint infection, one of the few rheumatologic emergencies! The septic joint must be diagnosed quickly and managed aggressively. Bacterial infections, especially those due to gram-positive organisms, can destroy the joint cartilage within a few days. Prompt and proper treatment of the septic joint will usually leave it without permanent structural damage. Additionally, as the septic joint is usually the result of hematogenous spread of infection from another body site, early recognition of the joint process allows more timely diagnosis and treatment of the primary infection. When evaluating a patient with acute monoarticular arthritis, a good rule of thumb is to assume that the joint is infected until proven otherwise.

**5. What nine questions should you ask when obtaining a history from a patient with monoarticular arthritis?**

1. Did the pain come on suddenly, in seconds or minutes? (Consider fracture and internal derangement.)
2. Did the pain come on over several hours or 1–2 days? (Consider infection, crystal deposition diseases, inflammatory arthritis syndromes, and palindromic rheumatism.)
3. Did the pain come on insidiously over days to weeks? (Consider indolent infections, such as mycobacteria and fungi, osteoarthritis, tumor, and infiltrative diseases.)
4. Has the joint been overused or damaged, either recently or in the past? (Consider traumatic causes.)
5. Is there a history of intravenous drug abuse? Has the patient had a recent infection of any kind? (Consider infection.)
6. Has the patient ever experienced previous acute attacks of joint pain and swelling that resolved spontaneously in any joint? (Consider crystal deposition diseases and other inflammatory joint syndromes.)
7. Has the patient recently been treated with a prolonged course of corticosteroids for any reason? (Consider infection or osteonecrosis of bone.)
8. Has the patient had symptoms, such as a skin rash, low-back pain, diarrhea, urethral discharge, conjunctivitis, or mouth sores? (Consider Reiter's syndrome, psoriatic arthritis, or enteropathic arthritis.)
9. Is there a history of a bleeding diathesis? Is the patient being treated with anticoagulants? (Consider hemarthrosis.)

**6. Is the age of the patient useful in the differential diagnosis?**

Yes! With the exception of infection (which occurs in all age groups), some joint diseases presenting as monoarthritis are more likely to occur at certain ages.

- In children, consider congenital dysplasia of the hip, slipped capital femoral epiphysis, or a monoarticular presentation of juvenile rheumatoid arthritis. Children are unlikely to have crystalline arthritis.
- In young adults, consider seronegative spondyloarthropathy, rheumatoid arthritis, or internal derangement of the joint. They are less likely to have crystalline arthritis. A septic joint in this age group is often due to gonococcal infection.
- Older adults are more likely to have crystalline arthritis, osteoarthritis, osteonecrosis, or internal derangement of the joint. A septic joint in these individuals is less likely due to gonococcal organisms.

**7. Is fever a useful sign?**

Yes, but it can be misleading. Fever is often present in infectious arthritis, but it may be absent. Fever, however, can also be a feature of acute attacks of gout and CPPD disease, rheumatoid arthritis, juvenile rheumatoid arthritis, sarcoidosis, and Reiter's syndrome. Many clinicians have been fooled by a gout attack masquerading as cellulitis or a septic joint.

**8. How does the presentation of gonococcal arthritis differ from that of nongonococcal bacterial arthritis?**

Gonococcal arthritis is often **polyarticular** and **migratory** in its earliest phase. It then progresses, in many instances, to a monoarticular joint phase. Two other characteristic features of disseminated gonococcal infection are tenosynovitis and skin involvement. **Tenosynovial inflammation** usually involves the dorsum of the hands and feet, wrists, and Achilles tendons. The **skin lesions** are unique to this septic arthritis and include tender vesicopustular lesions on an erythematous base and hemorrhagic papules.

**9. What are the most likely diagnoses in hospitalized patients who develop acute monoarticular arthritis following admission for another medical or surgical disease?**

Acute gout, pseudogout, and infection are by far the most common causes of acute attacks of such monoarthritis. These patients are often middle-aged or elderly, the primary age range for the crystalline arthropathies. In addition, they often have hospitalization-related risk factors known to provoke gout or pseudogout attacks: trauma, surgery, hemorrhage, infection, or medical stress such as renal failure, myocardial infarction, and stroke. One must be especially careful to exclude infection in these hospitalized patients.

**10. What is the single most useful diagnostic study in the initial evaluation of monoarthritis?**

Synovial fluid analysis.

**11. List the most common indications for arthrocentesis and synovial fluid analysis.**

1. **Suspicion of infection**. As little as 2 ml of fluid is sufficient for Gram stain, culture, and white blood cell (WBC) count and differential. A positive Gram stain will allow for rapid initiation of appropriate therapy. A positive culture will provide a definitive diagnosis. As previously stressed, failure to initiate timely and appropriate therapy can be disastrous for a septic joint.
2. **Suspicion of crystal-induced arthritis**. The sensitivity of polarizing microscopy in identifying birefringent crystals approaches 90% in acute gout and 70% in acute pseudogout. The benefits of joint aspiration in crystal-induced arthritis include exclusion of concomitant infection and the therapeutic effects of aspiration. Precise diagnosis of crystal deposition diseases also allows the most appropriate institution of both acute and chronic therapy in gout. It also prevents the use of inappropriate therapy (allopurinol, probenecid) in pseudogout.
3. **Suspicion of hemarthrosis**. Bloody joint fluid is characteristic of traumatic arthritis, clotting disorder, and pigmented villonodular synovitis.
4. **Differentiating inflammatory from noninflammatory arthritis**. The degree of elevation of synovial fluid WBC count can be useful in narrowing the list of possible causes of monoarthritis in a given patient. (See also Chapter 10.)

**12. If gonococcal arthritis is suspected, what special procedures should be performed?**

*Neisseria gonorrhoeae* and *N. meningitidis* are unusually fragile organisms outside the human host. Fewer than 25% of gonorrhea-infected joint aspirates grow in culture. This rate can be improved by plating the joint fluid at the bedside or by informing the laboratory that they should immediately inoculate the specimen on chocolate agar. Cervical, urethral, anal, and pharyngeal cultures for gonococci should also be obtained, as directed by the history of sexual contact.

**13. Does a crystal-proven diagnosis of gout or pseudogout rule out infection?**

No. Either gout or pseudogout can coexist with a septic joint.

**14. What other diagnostic studies are most useful in the initial evaluation of monoarthritis?**

**Almost always indicated**

1. *Radiograph of the joint*: Although frequently normal, the radiograph may disclose important information. It may diagnose unsuspected fracture, osteonecrosis, osteoarthritis, or juxtaarticular bone tumor. The presence of chondrocalcinosis, a radiologic feature of CPPD disease, increases suspicion for a pseudogout attack. Tumor, chronic fungal or mycobacterial infection, and other indolent destructive processes may be revealed. Contralateral joint radiograph for comparison may be useful, especially in children.
2. *Complete blood count*: Leukocytosis supports the possibility of infection.

**Indicated in selected patients**

1. *Cultures of blood, urine*, or other possible primary sites of infection: Mandatory when a septic joint is being considered.
2. *Serum prothrombin and partial thromboplastin time*: Useful if the patient is receiving anticoagulation or if a coagulation disorder is suspected.
3. *Erythrocyte sedimentation rate*: Although results are often nonspecific, significant elevation may suggest an inflammatory process.

**Rarely indicated**

1. *Serologic tests for antinuclear antibodies and rheumatoid factor*: However, the antinuclear antibody determination is frequently positive in the pauciarticular form of juvenile rheumatoid arthritis.
2. *Serum uric acid levels*: Notoriously unreliable in making or excluding the diagnosis of gout. These levels may be spuriously elevated in acute inflammatory conditions not related to gout and may be acutely diminished in a true gout attack. Also, by their uricosuric action, analgesics such as aspirin, which may have been taken by patients during the acute attack of arthritis, may lower serum uric acid levels into the normal range.

**15. If infection cannot be adequately ruled out by initial diagnostic studies, what should you do?**

The patient should be hospitalized and treated presumptively for a septic joint until culture results become available. This is usually indicated in the patient with synovial fluid findings suggesting a highly inflammatory process (synovial fluid WBC count > 50,000/mm$^3$) but with a negative synovial fluid Gram stain and no obvious primary source of infection. To lessen confusion regarding response to therapy, anti-inflammatory drugs should be withheld during this period.

**16. A diagnosis is always established by the end of the first week of onset of acute monoarticular arthritis. Right?**

No. Many patients defy initial attempts at diagnosis despite appropriate evaluation. A few achieve spontaneous remission, leaving the physician frustrated about the diagnosis, but relieved. Many patients, however, continue to have symptoms.

**17. The initial evaluation is unrevealing and the arthritis persists. What should be done?**

If the initial evaluation was carefully accomplished, a period of watchful waiting is often useful at this time. As noted previously, some processes will resolve spontaneously. Others become poly-articular, and the differential diagnosis will change to reflect the new joint involvement. New findings, such as the skin rash of psoriasis, occasionally emerge to aid in diagnosis. In a small number of patients, the monoarthritis persists.

**18. What is the definition of chronic monoarticular arthritis? Why is it useful to consider this as a category separate from acute monoarticular arthritis?**

Chronic monoarticular arthritis can be arbitrarily defined as **symptoms persisting within a single joint for > 6 weeks**. The differential diagnosis shifts away from some important and common causes of acute arthritis, such as pyogenic infection and acute crystal deposition diseases. In patients with an inflammatory synovial fluid, the likelihood of chronic inflammatory syndromes, such as mycobacterial or fungal septic arthritis, or a seronegative spondyloarthropathy increases. In patients with a noninflammatory process, a structural abnormality or internal derangement is a possibility.

**19. Name the most likely causes of chronic monoarticular arthritis.**

| INFLAMMATORY | NONINFLAMMATORY |
|---|---|
| Mycobacterial infection | Osteoarthritis |
| Fungal infection | Internal derangement of the knee |
| Lyme arthritis | Avascular necrosis of bone |
| Monoarticular presentation of rheumatoid arthritis | Pigmented villonodular synovitis |
| Seronegative spondyloarthropathies | Synovial chondromatosis |
| Sarcoid arthritis | Synovioma |
| Foreign-body synovitis | |

**20. What seven questions should you ask when obtaining a history from a patient with chronic monoarticular arthritis?**

1. Did the pain come on insidiously over days to weeks? (Consider indolent infections, such as mycobacteria and fungi, osteoarthritis, tumor, and infiltrative diseases.)
2. Is there a history of tuberculosis or a positive tuberculin skin test? (Consider mycobacterial disease.)
3. Is the patient a farmer, gardener, or floral worker, or does the patient have a similar exposure to soil or decaying vegetation? (Consider sporotrichosis.)
4. If the knee is involved, has the joint been damaged in the past? Does it ever "lock" in flexion? (Consider internal derangement and osteoarthritis.)
5. Has the patient ever experienced previous acute attacks of joint pain and swelling that resolved spontaneously in any joint? (Consider inflammatory joint syndromes.)
6. Has the patient recently been treated with a prolonged course of corticosteroids for any reason? (Consider osteonecrosis of bone.)
7. Has the patient had symptoms such as a skin rash, low-back pain, diarrhea, urethritis, conjunctivitis, or uveitis? (Consider the spondyloarthropathies.)

**21. What physical findings are useful in the differential diagnosis of a chronic monoarticular arthritis?**

1. Extra-articular features of the spondyloarthropathies, such as skin rashes (psoriasis, keratoderma blennorrhagicum), oral ulcers, urethral discharge, conjunctivitis, uveitis
2. Erythema nodosa, a feature of sarcoidosis and inflammatory bowel syndrome
3. A positive McMurray maneuver in the knee examination, suggesting internal derangement

**22. In evaluating chronic monoarthritis, what initial studies should be obtained?**

**Almost always indicated**

1. *Radiograph of the joint*: Although radiographs are frequently normal in acute arthritis, they are often revealing in chronic arthritis. Chronic infections by mycobacteria and fungi often

cause radiographically detectable abnormalities. Osteoarthritis, avascular necrosis of bone, and other causes of noninflammatory chronic arthritis also have characteristic radiographic appearances. Radiographs of the contralateral joint for comparison may be helpful, especially in children.

2. *Synovial fluid analysis*, if at all possible: This analysis is extremely useful in dividing possible causes of the joint process into the two broad diagnostic categories—inflammatory and noninflammatory arthritis. The presence of a bloody synovial effusion points to pigmented villonodular synovitis, synovial chondromatosis, or synovioma. Cultures of synovial fluid may demonstrate mycobacterial or fungal infection.

**Indicated in selected patients**

1. *Erythrocyte sedimentation rate*: Although results are often nonspecific, significant elevation may suggest an inflammatory process.
2. *Radiograph of sacroiliac joints*: This may demonstrate asymptomatic sacroiliitis in young males presenting with a chronic monoarticular arthritis as an initial manifestation of a spondyloarthropathy.
3. *Chest radiograph*: To detect evidence of a prior mycobacterial disease or to assess for pulmonary sarcoidosis.
4. *Skin test reaction to tuberculin*: A negative test is useful in excluding mycobacterial infection.
5. *Serologic tests for Lyme disease* (Borrelia burgdorferi), *rheumatoid factor*, *antinuclear antibody, and HLA B27.*

**23. Are other diagnostic studies useful in the evaluation of chronic monoarthritis?**

1. **Arthroscopy**: Arthroscopy allows direct visualization of many important articular structures and provides the opportunity for synovial biopsy in all large and some medium-sized joints. It is particularly useful for diagnosing internal derangement of the knee.
2. **Synovial biopsy**: Microscopic evaluation with culture of synovial tissue is useful in the diagnosis of:

| | |
|---|---|
| Tumors | Sarcoid arthritis |
| Pigmented villonodular synovitis | Foreign-body synovitis |
| Synovial chondromatosis | Fungal and mycobacterial infection |
| Synovioma | |

3. **Magnetic resonance imaging of the joint**

| | |
|---|---|
| Avascular necrosis | Internal derangement of the knee |
| Osteomyelitis | Destruction of periarticular bone |
| Pigmented villonodular synovitis | |

4. **Bone scan**

| | |
|---|---|
| Avascular necrosis | Osteomyelitis |
| Stress fracture | |

**24. How often is a specific diagnosis made in patients with chronic monoarthritis?**

Appropriate evaluation yields a diagnosis in approximately two-thirds of patients. Fortunately, the most serious and treatable diseases yield to diagnosis if a carefully reasoned clinical approach is taken.

## BIBLIOGRAPHY


1. American College of Rheumatology Ad Hoc Committee on Clinical Guidelines: Guidelines for the initial evaluation of the adult patient with acute musculoskeletal symptoms. Arthritis Rheum 39:1–8, 1996.
2. Baker DG, Schumacher HR: Acute monoarthritis. N Engl J Med 329:1013–1020, 1992.
3. Carias K, Panush RS: Acute arthritis. Bull Rheum Dis 43(7):1–4, 1994.
4. Cucurull E, Espinoza LR: Gonococcal arthritis. Rheum Dis Clin North Am 24:305–322, 1998.
5. El-Gabalawy WS, et al: Evaluating patients with arthritis of recent onset. JAMA 284(18):2368–2373, 2000.

6. Ho G, DeNuccio M: Gout and pseudogout in hospitalized patients. Arch Intern Med 153:2787–2790, 1993.
7. Hubscher O: Pattern recognition in arthritis. In Klippel JH, Dieppe PA (eds): Rheumatology. London, Mosby, 1998, pp 2-3.1–2-3.6.
8. McCarty DJ: Gout without hyperuricemia. JAMA 271:302–303, 1994.
9. McCune WJ, Golbus J: Monarticular arthritis. In Ruddy S, Harris ED, Sledge CB (eds): Kelley's textbook of rheumatology, 6th ed. Philadelphia, W.B. Saunders, 2001, pp 367–377.
10. Nissenbaum MA, Adamis MK: Magnetic resonance imaging in rheumatology: An overview. Rheum Dis Clin North Am 20:343–360, 1994.
11. Sack K: Monoarthritis: Differential diagnosis. Am J Med 102:30S–34S, 1997.
12. Shmerling RH: Synovial fluid analysis: A critical reappraisal. Rheum Dis Clin North Am 20:503–512, 1994.

# 15. APPROACH TO THE PATIENT WITH POLYARTICULAR SYMPTOMS

*Robert A. Hawkins, M.D.*

**1. What are the most important tools that the clinician can use on a patient with polyarticular symptoms?**

A careful history and physical examination. Laboratory testing and radiographic or other imaging studies provide definitive answers in only a few instances. Tests are often most useful in confirming the suspected diagnosis or in providing prognostic information. When confronted with a patient with polyarticular symptoms, an inexperienced clinician often will slight the most important, the history and physical examination, opting instead for "shotgun" laboratory testing. While tests such as rheumatoid factor, uric acid, ASO titers, and antinuclear antibodies may be indicated in many instances, the history and physical examination will reveal 75% of the information required for diagnosis.

**2. How are the many diseases causing polyarticular symptoms classified?**

No single classification scheme can be used to differentiate the wide variety of diseases presenting with polyarticular symptoms. A few diseases have a single descriptive finding that is essentially diagnostic, such as a positive synovial fluid culture in gonococcal polyarthritis, a high serum titer of anti-double-stranded DNA in systemic lupus erythematosus (SLE), or the rash of psoriasis in psoriatic arthritis. Most polyarticular diseases, however, are diagnosed by their characteristic clinical findings, such as the triad of urethritis, conjunctivitis, and oligoarticular arthritis in Reiter's syndrome, or the symmetrical synovitis and morning stiffness involving the small joints of the hands in rheumatoid arthritis.

In most instances, the clinician uses several variables in combination to reduce the number of diagnostic possibilities. These variables include:

Acuteness of onset of the process
Degree of inflammation of the joints
Temporal pattern of joint involvement
Distribution of joint involvement
Age and sex of the patient

Additionally, many systemic diseases with polyarticular involvement have characteristic extra-articular features that contribute substantially to the diagnosis. As previously stressed, these variables are often identified by the medical history and physical examination. The clinician can apply selected tests to the few remaining likely diseases to confirm the diagnosis.

**3. Which diseases commonly present with acute polyarticular symptoms?**

| **Infection** | **Other Inflammatory** |
|---|---|
| Gonococcal | Rheumatoid arthritis |
| Meningococcal | Polyarticular and systemic juvenile rheumatoid arthritis |
| Lyme | Systemic lupus erythematosus |
| Acute rheumatic fever | Reiter's syndrome |
| Bacterial endocarditis | Psoriatic arthritis |
| Viral (esp. rubella, hepatitis B and C, parvovirus, Epstein-Barr, HIV) | Polyarticular gout |
| | Sarcoid arthritis |
| | Serum sickness |

**4. Which diseases commonly present with chronic (persisting > 6 weeks) polyarticular symptoms?**

| **Inflammatory** | |
|---|---|
| Rheumatoid arthritis | Enteropathic arthritis |
| Polyarticular juvenile rheumatoid arthritis | Polyarticular gout |
| Systemic lupus erythematosus | Calcium pyrophosphate deposition (CPPD) disease |
| Progressive systemic sclerosis | Sarcoid arthritis |
| Polymyositis | Vasculitis |
| Reiter's syndrome | Polymyalgia rheumatica |
| Psoriatic arthritis | |
| Polyarticular gout | |
| **Noninflammatory** | |
| Osteoarthritis | Paget's disease |
| Calcium pyrophosphate deposition (CPPD) disease | Fibromyalgia |
| Polyarticular gout | Benign hypermobility syndrome |
| | Hemochromatosis |

**5. How do polyarthritis, polyarthralgias, and diffuse aches and pains differ?**

**Polyarthritis** is definite inflammation (swelling, tenderness, warmth) of > 4 joints demonstrated by physical examination. (A patient with 2–4 involved joints is said to have pauci- or oligoarticular arthritis.) The acute polyarticular diseases (see Question 3) and chronic inflammatory diseases (see Question 4) commonly present with polyarthritis. Most of the chronic noninflammatory diseases do not manifest significant joint inflammation. The exceptions are CPPD disease and polyarticular gout, which can present with either polyarthritis or polyarthralgia.

**Polyarthralgia** is defined as pain in > 4 joints without demonstrable inflammation by physical examination. SLE, systemic sclerosis, vasculitis, polymyalgia rheumatica, and the chronic noninflammatory arthritides commonly present with polyarthralgias.

**Diffuse aches and pains** are poorly localized symptoms originating in joints, bones, muscles, or other soft tissues. The joint examination does not reveal inflammation. Polymyalgia rheumatica, fibromyalgia, SLE, polymyositis, and hypothyroidism commonly present with these symptoms.

**6. Describe the three characteristic temporal patterns of joint involvement in polyarthritis.**

1. **Migratory pattern**: Symptoms are present in certain joints for a few days and then remit, only to reappear in other joints. Rheumatic fever, gonococcal arthritis, and the early phase of Lyme disease are famous examples.

2. **Additive pattern**: Symptoms begin in some joints and persist, with subsequent involvement of other joints. This pattern is nonspecific, being common in rheumatoid arthritis, SLE, and many other polyarticular syndromes.

3. **Intermittent pattern**: This pattern is typified by repetitive attacks of acute polyarthritis with complete remission between attacks. A prolonged observation may be necessary to establish

this phenomenon. Rheumatoid arthritis, polyarticular gout, sarcoid arthritis, Reiter's syndrome, and psoriatic arthritis may present in this manner.

**7. How is the distribution of joint involvement helpful in the differential diagnosis of polyarthritis?**

Different diseases characteristically affect different joints. Knowledge of the typical joints involved in each disease is a cornerstone of diagnosis in polyarthritis. In practice, knowledge of which joints are spared in each form of arthritis is also quite useful.

*Distribution of Joint Involvement in Polyarthritis*

| DISEASE | JOINTS COMMONLY INVOLVED | JOINTS COMMONLY SPARED |
|---|---|---|
| Gonococcal arthritis | Knee, wrist, ankle, hand IP | Axial |
| Lyme arthritis | Knee, shoulder, wrist, elbow | Axial |
| Rheumatoid arthritis | Wrist, MCP, PIP, elbow, glenohumeral, cervical spine, hip, knee, ankle, tarsal, MTP | DIP, thoracolumbar spine |
| Osteoarthritis | First CMC, DIP, PIP, cervical spine, thoracolumbar spine, hip, knee, first MTP, toe IP | MCP, wrist, elbow, glenohumeral, ankle, tarsal |
| Reiter's syndrome | Knee, ankle, tarsal, MTP, toe IP, elbow, axial | |
| Psoriatic arthritis | Knee, ankle, MTP, toe IP, wrist, MCP, hand IP, axial | |
| Enteropathic arthritis | Knee, ankle, elbow, shoulder, MCP, PIP, wrist, axial | |
| Polyarticular gout | First MTP, instep, heel, ankle, knee | Axial |
| CPPD disease | Knee, wrist, shoulder, ankle, MCP, hand IP, hip, elbow | Axial |
| Sarcoid arthritis | Ankle, knee | Axial |
| Hemochromatosis | MCP, wrist, knee, hip, feet, shoulder | |

Joints: IP, interphalangeal; MCP, metacarpophalangeal; PIP, proximal interphalangeal; CMC, carpometacarpal; DIP, distal interphalangeal; MTP, metatarsophalangeal.

**8. Name the two most common causes of chronic polyarthritis.**

1. **Osteoarthritis**: The prevalence of osteoarthritis rises steeply with age. Between 10–20% of people 40 years old have evidence of osteoarthritis, and 75% of women over age 65 have osteoarthritis. This very high prevalence makes osteoarthritis the single most likely diagnosis in older patients complaining of polyarticular pain who have noninflammatory signs and symptoms.

2. **Rheumatoid arthritis**: The prevalence in U.S. whites is approximately 1%, making it the most common chronic inflammatory joint disease.

**9. What are the most likely diagnoses in women aged 25–50 who present with chronic polyarticular symptoms?**

Osteoarthritis, rheumatoid arthritis, systemic lupus erythematosus, fibromyalgia, and benign hypermobility syndrome.

**10. What are the most likely diagnoses in men aged 25–50 who present with chronic oligoarticular or polyarticular symptoms?**

Gonococcal arthritis, Reiter's syndrome, ankylosing spondylitis, osteoarthritis, and hemochromatosis.

**11. And in patients over age 50 presenting with chronic polyarticular symptoms?**

Osteoarthritis, rheumatoid arthritis, CPPD disease, polymyalgia rheumatica, and paraneoplastic polyarthritis.

**12. What is morning stiffness? How is it useful in sorting out the causes of polyarticular symptoms?**

Morning stiffness refers to the amount of time it takes for patients with polyarthritis to "limber up" after arising in the morning. This rough measure is useful in differentiating inflammatory from noninflammatory arthritis. In inflammatory arthritis, morning stiffness lasts > 1 hour. In untreated rheumatoid arthritis, it averages 3.5 hours and tends to parallel the degree of joint inflammation. In contrast, noninflammatory processes, such as osteoarthritis, may produce transient morning stiffness that lasts < 15 minutes.

**13. List the differential diagnosis of fever and polyarthritis.**

**Infectious arthritis**: septic arthritis, bacterial endocarditis, Lyme disease, acid-fast bacterial or fungal arthritis, viral arthritis

**Reactive arthritis**: enteric infections, Reiter's syndrome, rheumatic fever, inflammatory bowel disease

**Systemic rheumatic diseases**: rheumatoid arthritis, SLE, Still's disease, systemic vasculitis

**Crystal-induced arthritis**: gout, pseudogout

**Miscellaneous disease**: malignancy, familial Mediterranean fever, sarcoidosis, dermatomyositis, Behçet's disease, Henoch-Schönlein purpura, Kawasaki's, erythema nodosum, erythema multiforme, pyoderma gangrenosum, pustular psoriasis

**14. Define tenosynovitis. How is its presence useful in the differential diagnosis of polyarticular symptoms?**

Tenosynovitis is inflammation of the synovial-lined sheaths surrounding tendons in the wrists, hands, ankles, and feet. Physical examination usually reveals tenderness and swelling along the track of the involved tendon *between* the joints. It is a characteristic feature of rheumatoid arthritis, gout, Reiter's syndrome, gonococcal arthritis, and tuberculous and fungal arthritis. It is distinctly uncommon in other causes of polyarticular disease.

**15. List skin lesions that can be useful in the diagnosis of acute or chronic polyarthritis.**

Erythema chronicum migrans (Lyme arthritis)
Erythema nodosum (sarcoid arthritis, enteric arthritis)
Psoriatic plaques (psoriatic arthritis)
Keratoderma blennorrhagicum (Reiter's syndrome)
Erythema marginatum (acute rheumatic fever)
Palpable purpura (vasculitis)
Livedo reticularis (vasculitis)
Vesicopustular lesions or hemorrhagic papules (gonococcal arthritis)
Butterfly rash, discoid lupus, or photosensitive rash (SLE)
Thickening of the skin (systemic sclerosis)
Heliotrope rash on eyelids, upper chest, and extensor aspects of joints (dermatomyositis)
Gottron's papules overlying the extensor aspects of the MCP and IP joints of the hands (dermatomyositis)
Gray/brown skin hyperpigmentation (hemochromatosis)

**16. Which rheumatic diseases should be considered in a patient with Raynaud's phenomenon and polyarticular symptoms?**

Progressive systemic sclerosis (prevalence of 90%)
Systemic lupus erythematosus (prevalence of 20%)
Polymyositis/dermatomyositis (prevalence of 20–40%)
Vasculitis (variable prevalence, depending on the particular syndrome)

**17. What other systemic features are seen in diseases causing polyarthritis?**

*Extra-articular Organ Involvement in Polyarticular Rheumatic Diseases*

| DISEASE | LUNG | PLEURA | PERI-CARDIUM | HEART MUSCLE | HEART VALVE | KIDNEY | GI TRACT | LIVER |
|---|---|---|---|---|---|---|---|---|
| Acute rheumatic fever | | • | • | • | • | | | |
| Viral arthritis | | | | | | | | • |
| Bacterial endocarditis | | | | | • | • | | |
| Rheumatoid arthritis | • | • | • | • | • | | | |
| SLE | • | • | • | • | • | • | | |
| Systemic sclerosis | • | • | • | • | | • | • | • |
| Polymyositis/ dermatomyositis | • | • | • | • | | | | |
| Reiter's syndrome | | | | | • | | • | |
| Enteropathic arthritis | | | | | | | • | • |
| Polyarticular gout | | | | | | • | | |
| Sarcoid arthritis | • | | | | | | | • |
| Vasculitis | • | | | | | • | | |
| Polymyalgia rheumatica | | | | | | | | • |
| Hemochromatosis | | | | • | | | | • |

JRA, juvenile rheumatoid arthritis.

**18. Which tests are most useful in evaluating a patient with chronic polyarticular symptoms?**

Complete blood count
Erythrocyte sedimentation rate
Antinuclear antibodies (ANA)
Rheumatoid factor
Liver enzymes
Serum creatinine
Urinalysis

Others to consider
- Serum uric acid
- Thyroid stimulating hormone
- Iron studies
- HLA-B27 antigen
- Radiographs
- Synovial fluid analysis

**19. What is the significance of a positive ANA in a patient with chronic polyarticular symptoms?**

A patient with polyarthralgia or polyarthritis who has a significantly elevated ANA titer often will have one of the following diseases: SLE (including drug-induced lupus), rheumatoid arthritis, Sjögren's syndrome, polymyositis, systemic sclerosis, or mixed connective tissue disease.

The history and physical examination should be directed toward the clinical findings in these diseases. A careful medication history may reveal that the patient has received procainamide or hydralazine, two common causes of drug-induced lupus (see Chapter 12 for other drugs known to induce positive ANA). Finally, it must be stressed that a positive ANA is a feature of several other chronic diseases and can also be found in normal healthy individuals, although usually in low titer. (See also Chapter 9.)

**20. Why should a rheumatoid factor not be ordered in the evaluation of patients with acute polyarticular symptoms?**

Rheumatoid factor (RF) has a low sensitivity and specificity for rheumatoid arthritis in patients with acute polyarticular symptoms. Serum RF is frequently positive in acute infectious syndromes caused by hepatitis B, Epstein-Barr, influenza, and other viruses but disappears as the viral syndrome resolves. Although RF will eventually become positive in 75–85% of patients with rheumatoid arthritis, it is positive in early rheumatoid arthritis in only 25–70% of patients.

**21. Which chronic polyarticular diseases are most likely to be associated with low serum complement levels?**

SLE and several of the vasculitis syndromes. Low serum complement levels (C3, C4, and total hemolytic complement) usually suggest the presence of immune complex disease. In SLE and in many diseases causing vasculitis, immune complexes often activate the complement cascade, resulting in consumption of individual complement components. In many instances, the liver is unable to produce these components as rapidly as they are consumed, resulting in a fall in serum levels.

**22. When should arthrocentesis for synovial fluid analysis be considered in the evaluation of polyarthritis?**

When the diagnosis has not been established *and* joint fluid can be obtained. Both of these requirements need to be met. For example, a patient with obvious osteoarthritis established by history and physical examination does *not* require a diagnostic aspiration in an uncomplicated knee effusion. If it can be obtained, synovial fluid analysis can be useful in the diagnosis of bacterial joint infection and crystal-induced arthritis. Even if a specific diagnosis is not forthcoming, synovial fluid analysis reduces the list of diagnostic possibilities by categorizing the process as either inflammatory or noninflammatory.

**23. Should radiographs of affected joints always be obtained?**

Not always. As a general rule, patients with acute polyarticular arthritis will not benefit from joint radiographs. Radiographs are most valuable in evaluating chronic arthritis that has been relatively long-standing and that has resulted in characteristic changes in joints. Osteoarthritis, chronic rheumatoid arthritis, psoriatic arthritis, gout, CPPD disease, systemic sclerosis, and sarcoidosis all have specific appearances on radiographs that are very useful in diagnosis. Remember, though, that osteoarthritis is so common that it may coexist with other arthritis syndromes, and that radiographic changes may be a mixture of both types of arthritis in a given patient.

**24. Why should the rheumatologist think in "geologic" time?**

Because many chronic polyarticular diseases require months or years to diagnose, tremendous and profound patience is often required. This prolonged period often seems like "geologic" time to many patients who may expect an accurate diagnosis in one or two visits. The characteristics of many chronic polyarticular diseases require this extraordinary degree of patience, in that:

- Many present insidiously with few objective findings for prolonged times.
- Many initially masquerade as other diseases before finally settling into their usual pattern. Rheumatoid arthritis, for example, can present as a monoarticular arthritis before assuming its more typical polyarticular course.
- Characteristic laboratory abnormalities may require months or years to develop. Patients with rheumatoid arthritis may have symptoms for a prolonged period before the development of RF in serum.
- The joint symptoms of many conditions precede the extra-articular features of the disease in some patients by months or years. The skin plaques of psoriasis and the bowel symptoms of inflammatory bowel disease may be the last and final diagnostic features of these arthritis syndromes.
- Joint radiographs may not show characteristic changes of the arthritis for months or years.

## BIBLIOGRAPHY

1. American College of Rheumatology Ad Hoc Committee on Clinical Guidelines: Guidelines for the initial evaluation of the adult patient with acute musculoskeletal symptoms. Arthritis Rheum 39:1–8, 1996.
2. Bomalaski JS: Acute rheumatologic disorders in the elderly. Emerg Med Clin North Am 8:341–359, 1990.
3. Carias K, Panush RS: Acute arthritis. Bull Rheum Dis 43(7):1–4, 1994.
4. Cucurull E, Espinoza LR: Gonococcal arthritis. Rheum Dis Clin North Am 24:305–322, 1998.

5. Liang MH, Sturrock RD: Evaluation of musculoskeletal symptoms. In Klippel JH, Dieppe PA (eds): Rheumatology. London, Mosby–Year Book Europe, 1994, pp 2,1.1–2,1.18.
6. Panush RS, Kisch A: Gonococcal arthritis. In Hurst W (ed): Medicine, 3rd ed. Boston, Butterworths, 1992, pp 215–217.
7. Pinals RS: Polyarthritis and fever. N Engl J Med 330:769–774, 1994.
8. Schumacher HR: Reactive arthritis. Rheum Dis Clin North Am 24:261–273, 1998.
9. Sergent JS: Polyarticular arthritis. In Ruddy S, Harris ED, Sledge CB (eds): Kelley's Textbook of Rheumatology, 6th ed. Philadelphia, W.B. Saunders, 2001, pp 379–385.

# 16. APPROACH TO THE PATIENT WITH NEUROMUSCULAR SYMPTOMS

Robert A. Hawkins, M.D.

**1. Discuss the relationship between rheumatic diseases and neuromuscular disease.**

Many primary rheumatic diseases, such as systemic lupus erythematosus, rheumatoid arthritis, and systemic vasculitis, are frequently complicated by neurologic or myopathic disease. Chronic synovitis, joint contractures, and deformities seen in rheumatoid arthritis lead to muscle atrophy and weakness. Other rheumatic diseases such as polymyositis are dominated by immune-mediated inflammation of muscle, and the differential diagnosis of myopathy is quite broad. Neuromuscular manifestations of rheumatic diseases may present as early and dominant findings, or as late complications of well-established diseases. They may also be complications of therapy for rheumatic diseases, as with the use of corticosteroids or D-penicillamine.

**2. What are the cardinal symptoms of neuromuscular lesions?**

**Weakness** and/or **pain** are the most common symptoms reported by patients. Weakness should be differentiated from fatigue and malaise. Fatigue differs from weakness in that fatigue is a loss of strength with activity that recovers with rest. Malaise is a subjective feeling of weakness without objective findings.

**3. Many patients complain of weakness. What is the best way to determine the cause of weakness in a given patient?**

The first step is to exclude **systemic causes** of fatigue or weakness, such as cardiopulmonary disease, anemia, hypothyroidism, malignancy, or depression. Many of these patients have malaise rather than weakness, and their examination usually fails to reveal true muscle weakness if they give their best effort. The carefully directed history and physical examination, combined with focused laboratory testing, are usually effective in eliminating these causes of weakness.

*Common Systemic Causes of Weakness or Fatigue*

| | | |
|---|---|---|
| Cardiopulmonary disease | Hypothyroidism | Malignancy |
| Anemia | Hyperthyroidism | Depression |
| Chronic infection | Poor physical conditioning | Chronic inflammatory disease |

**4. Once systemic causes of weakness have been excluded, what is the next step?**

The neuromuscular causes of weakness should be considered. A very useful method of categorizing neuromuscular diseases is by their customary level of anatomic involvement, beginning with the spinal cord and proceeding distally through nerve roots, peripheral nerves, neuromuscular junctions, and muscle.

*Diseases Affecting Neuromuscular Structures, by Level of Anatomic Involvement*

| SPINAL CORD | NERVE ROOT | PERIPHERAL NERVE | NEUROMUSCULAR JUNCTION | MUSCLE |
|---|---|---|---|---|
| Amyotrophic lateral sclerosis | Herniated nucleus pulposus | Vasculitis | Myasthenia gravis | Polymyositis |
| Transverse myelitis | Cervical spondylosis | Guillain-Barré syndrome | Eaton-Lambert syndrome | Hypothyroidism |
| Vasculitis | Lumbar spondylosis | Collagen vascular diseases | | Hyperthyroidism |
| Collagen vascular diseases | | Nerve compression | | Muscular dystrophy |
| | | Amyloidosis | | Corticosteroid use |
| | | | | Vasculitis |
| | | | | Collagen vascular diseases |

**5. Many patients complain of pain. What historical features are most useful in the differential diagnosis of pain?**

Neurologic lesions may or may not cause pain, depending on the level of involvement and the cause of the abnormality. Pure spinal cord lesions generally do not produce pain, although occasionally painful flexor muscle spasms will occur. Nerve root compression commonly produces pain in the affected nerve distribution. Peripheral nerve disease is often manifested by numbness, tingling, and paresthesias (pins and needles sensation). Some diseases such as Guillain-Barré syndrome, on the other hand, affect primarily the motor aspect of the peripheral nerve. Their predominant manifestation is weakness rather than pain. Diseases of the neuromuscular junction are not painful.

Myopathies may or may not be painful. In sorting them out, the following concepts are useful:
- Inflammatory myopathies are usually dominated by weakness, not pain. The exception to this rule is when the inflammatory myopathy has a fulminant onset, when pain may be as dominant a feature as weakness.
- Muscle pain on exertion is suggestive of claudication (vascular insufficiency) or rarer diseases of muscle metabolism.
- Myopathies do not produce numbness or paresthesias.

**6. How does the distribution of weakness or pain aid in differentiating neurologic from muscular lesions?**

**Myopathies** tend to cause *proximal* and *symmetrical* (bilateral) weakness or pain involving the shoulder girdle and hip girdle. Patients with proximal upper extremity weakness will note difficulty in combing hair or brushing their teeth. Patients with lower extremity weakness will complain of difficulty in rising from a chair or climbing stairs. If present, pain may be reported as aching or cramping.

**Peripheral neuropathies**, as a rule, cause *distal* (hands and feet) weakness and/or pain that is often *asymmetrical*. Typically, patients report their upper extremity weakness as clumsiness of the hands or a tendency to drop things. Lower extremity distal weakness is often manifested by foot dragging or tripping over rugs or rough surfaces. Asymmetrical peripheral weakness points toward a regional neurologic condition, such as median nerve compression in carpal tunnel syndrome.

**Nerve root compression** causes asymmetric weakness and pain that may be either proximal or distal, depending on the level of the involved nerve root.

**Spinal cord lesions** usually are associated with a distinct sensory level described as a tightness bilaterally around the trunk or abdomen. Distal spastic weakness, often with loss of bowel and bladder sphincter function, is also a feature of spinal cord disease.

**7. How does the temporal pattern of weakness or pain aid in diagnosis?**

1. **Abrupt onset** of weakness is characteristic of Guillain-Barré syndrome, poliomyelitis, and hypokalemic periodic paralysis.

2. **Intermittent** weakness may occur with myasthenia gravis, the rare causes of metabolic myopathy, and hypokalemic periodic paralysis.

3. **Gradual onset** of weakness or pain is typical of most muscle diseases, including inflammatory myopathies, the muscular dystrophies, and endocrine myopathies, as well as most neuropathies. It may also occur with myasthenia gravis.

**8. What is meant by fatigability? How is it useful in diagnosing neuromuscular disease?**

Fatigability is defined as progressive weakness of muscle with repetitive use, followed by recovery of strength after a brief period of rest. It is a classic finding in myasthenia gravis. Eaton-Lambert syndrome is often referred to as reverse myasthenia gravis, owing to the paradoxical increase in muscle strength observed with repetitive muscle contraction.

**9. How does the family history aid in diagnosis?**

Many of the muscular dystrophy syndromes have strong patterns of inheritance.

| | |
|---|---|
| Duchenne muscular dystrophy | X-linked |
| Limb-girdle muscular dystrophy | Autosomal recessive or dominant |
| Facioscapulohumeral muscular dystrophy | Autosomal dominant |
| Myotonic dystrophy | Autosomal dominant |
| Peroneal muscular atrophy (Charcot-Marie-Tooth disease) | Autosomal dominant |

**10. Name three hormones whose deficiency or excess is associated with myopathy.**

Thyroxine (hypothyroidism or hyperthyroidism)
Cortisol (Addison's disease or Cushing's disease)
Parathyroid hormone (hypoparathyroidism or hyperparathyroidism)

**11. Which drugs are most commonly responsible for neuromuscular symptoms?**

| | | | | |
|---|---|---|---|---|
| Corticosteroids | Chloroquine | Alcohol | D-Penicillamine | Clofibrate, |
| Emetine | Hydroxychloroquine | Colchicine | Cocaine | lovastin, other cholesterol lowering agents |
| Zidovudine | | | | |

**12. What toxins should be sought in the evaluation of neuromuscular symptoms?**

- **Organophosphates**: These esters are used in pesticides, petroleum additives, and modifiers of plastic. Their toxicity affects peripheral nerves. With progression of the neuropathy, pyramidal tract signs and spasticity may develop.
- **Lead**: Lead toxicity can result in encephalopathy and psychiatric problems (children), abdominal pain, and peripheral neuropathy appearing in the hands before the feet (adults).
- **Thallium**: This toxin is used in rodenticides and industrial processes. Patients present with a sensory and autonomic neuropathy. Alopecia usually develops at the onset of symptoms.
- **Arsenic, mercury** (electrical and chemical industry), and industrial solvents containing aliphatic compounds can also cause neuromuscular symptoms.

**13. What are the key elements of the physical examination in the evaluation of neuromuscular symptoms?**

| **System** | **Examine for** |
|---|---|
| General | Cardiopulmonary disease, infection, thyroid disease, malignancy |
| Joints | Synovitis, deformities, contractures |
| Muscles | Muscle bulk, tenderness, weakness, fasciculations |
| Neurologic | Sensory abnormalities, deep tendon reflexes, weakness |

**14. What is Gower's sign?**

A patient attempts to rise from a seated position by climbing up his legs with his hands. It is seen in patients with proximal lower extremity muscular weakness due to myopathy.

**15. How is muscle weakness graded by the physical examiner?**

The most commonly accepted scale is the Medical Research Council Grading System. Because there is a wide range of muscle strength between grades 5 and 4, it is common to assign intermediate values such as 5- or 4+ to many muscle groups in the examination.

| Grade | Degree of Strength |
|---|---|
| 5 | Normal strength |
| 4 | Muscle contraction possible against gravity plus some examiner resistance |
| 3 | Muscle contraction possible against gravity only |
| 2 | Muscle contraction possible only with gravity removed |
| 1 | Flicker of muscle contraction observed but without movement of extremity |
| 0 | No contraction |

**16. How are deep tendon reflexes graded by the physical examiner?**

| Grade | Strength of Contraction |
|---|---|
| 4 | Clonus |
| 3 | Exaggerated |
| 2 | Normal |
| 1 | Present but depressed |
| 0 | Absent |

**17. Can alterations in deep tendon reflexes aid in differentiation of neuromuscular diseases?**

The following generalizations are useful:

- Spinal cord lesions (above L2) and upper motor neuron disease usually produce exaggerated deep tendon reflexes and pathologic plantar reflexes.
- Nerve root and peripheral nerve lesions usually produce depressed or absent reflexes.
- Primary muscle diseases do not usually *present* with altered deep tendon reflexes. Late in the disease process, however, substantial muscle atrophy may cause reduction or loss of the reflex.
- Hyperthyroidism produces exaggerated tendon reflexes.
- Hypothyroidism produces depressed deep tendon reflexes with slow relaxation phase.
- Many people over age 60 experience a natural loss of their ankle reflexes.

**18. Which screening laboratory tests can evaluate for systemic causes of neuromuscular symptoms?**

Complete blood count
Serum electrolytes, calcium, magnesium, phosphorus
Serum muscle enzymes
Erythrocyte sedimentation rate
Serum liver enzyme tests
Serum renal function tests
Thyroid function tests
Chest radiograph
Electrocardiogram

**19. Which serum enzymes are elevated in muscle disease?**

| Serum Enzyme | Clinical Utility |
|---|---|
| Creatine kinase (CK) | Most sensitive and specific for muscle disease |
| Aldolase | Elevated in muscle, liver, and erythrocyte diseases |
| Lactic dehydrogenase | Elevated in muscle, liver, erythrocyte, and other diseases |
| Aspartate aminotransferase (AST) | Most specific for inflammatory muscle disease |

**20. What are other causes of elevation of serum creatine kinase besides myopathy?**

Intramuscular injections
Muscle crush injuries

Recent strenuous exercise
Myocardial infarction
Race of individual (healthy blacks may have significantly higher CK levels than the "normal" values derived from the entire population).

**21. Are additional specific tests useful in the evaluation of neuromuscular symptoms?**

| SPECIFIC TEST | SUSPECTED DISEASE PROCESSES |
|---|---|
| Serum antinuclear antibodies | Inflammatory myopathy, vasculitis |
| Serum rheumatoid factor | Inflammatory myopathy, vasculitis |
| Serum complement assay | Inflammatory myopathy, vasculitis |
| Serum cryoglobulins | Vasculitis |
| Hepatitis B surface antigen and hepatitis C antibody | Vasculitis |
| Anti-neutrophil cytoplasmic antibodies | Vasculitis |
| Acetylcholine receptor antibodies | Myasthenia gravis |
| Serum parathyroid hormone | Parathyroid disease |
| Electromyography and nerve conduction tests | Disease of nerve roots, peripheral nerves, or myopathies |
| Muscle biopsy | Inflammatory or metabolic myopathies, vasculitis |
| Nerve biopsy | Vasculitis |
| Magnetic resonance scan | Spinal cord, nerve root, and myopathic processes |

**22. What is mononeuritis multiplex?**

Mononeuritis multiplex is a pattern of motor and sensory involvement of multiple individual peripheral nerves that is a classic neurologic presentation of systemic vasculitis. First, one peripheral nerve becomes involved (usually with burning dysesthesias), followed by other individual nerves, often with motor dysfunction as well. The patchy nature of nerve involvement reflects the patchy vasculitis of the vasa nervorum, which is the underlying cause of the neuropathy.

**23. Is mononeuritis multiplex seen only in patients with vasculitis?**

No. The differential diagnosis of mononeuritis multiplex also includes:

Vasculitis
Diabetes mellitus
Lead neuropathy
Sarcoidosis
Wartenburg's relapsing sensory neuritis

**24. Is mononeuritis multiplex the only pattern of neuropathy seen in vasculitis?**

No. Two patterns of peripheral neuropathy are usually seen. Although mononeuritis multiplex is the most famous pattern, a **stocking-glove** pattern of neurologic involvement is seen more frequently. A stocking-glove pattern involves both feet, the calves, and hands. Most patients with vasculitic neuropathy will have a combination of mononeuritis multiplex and a stocking-glove neuropathy.

**25. What are the most common causes of proximal shoulder girdle and hip girdle aches, pains, and/or weakness? How are they differentiated?**

Six diseases are responsible for > 90% of diffuse, proximal aches or weakness. The first step is to decide which is the dominant clinical finding: pain or weakness. To determine if true weakness is present, the examiner should ask the patient to ignore any pain that may occur during muscle strength testing so that a true measure of muscle strength can be determined. Although patients with fibromyalgia syndrome and polymyalgia rheumatica may complain of weakness in addition to pain, they are not truly weak on physical examination.

| DISEASE | PAIN | WEAKNESS | ESR | SERUM CK | SERUM T4 |
|---|---|---|---|---|---|
| Fibromyalgia | Yes | No | Normal | Normal | Normal |
| Polymyalgia rheumatica | Yes | No | Marked elevation | Normal | Normal |
| Polymyositis | Usually none | Yes | Usually normal | Elevated | Normal |
| Corticosteroid myopathy | No | Yes | Normal | Normal | Normal |
| Hyperthyroidism | No | Yes | Normal | Normal | Elevated |
| Hypothyroidism | Yes | No | Normal | Elevated | Depressed |

ESR, erythrocyte sedimentation rate; T4, thyroxine.

**26. What is the diagnostic significance of "strokes in young folks"? What rheumatic syndromes should be considered in the differential diagnosis of cerebrovascular disease?**

Most cerebrovascular disease occurs in patients over age 50 as a result of long-standing hypertension, atherosclerosis, and cardiac emboli. When ischemic cerebrovascular disease occurs in patients under age 50, the possibility of several rheumatic syndromes should be especially considered:

| | |
|---|---|
| Systemic lupus erythematosus | Isolated angiitis of the CNS |
| Antiphospholipid antibody syndrome | Polyarteritis nodosa |
| Takayasu's arteritis | Wegener's granulomatosis |

## BIBLIOGRAPHY


1. Black HR, Quallich H, Gareleck CB: Racial differences in serum creatine kinase levels. Am J Med 81:479–481, 1986.
2. Bohlmeyer AHB, et al: Evaluation of laboratory tests as a guide to diagnosis and therapy of myositis. Rheum Dis Clin North Am 19:845–856, 1994.
3. Brick JE, Brick JF: Neurologic manifestations of rheumatic disease. Neurol Clin 7:629–639, 1989.
4. Kissel JT, Mendell JR: Vasculitic neuropathy. Neurol Clin 10:761–781, 1992.
5. Nissenbaum MA, Adamis MK: Magnetic resonance imaging in rheumatology: An overview. Rheum Dis Clin North Am 20:343–360, 1994.
6. Pascuzzi RM: Drugs and toxins associated with myopathies. Curr Opin Rheum 10:511–520, 1998.
7. Plotz PH: Not myositis: A series of chance encounters. JAMA 268:2074–2077, 1992.
8. Sergent JS: Weakness. In Ruddy S, Harris ED, Sledge CB (eds): Kelley's Textbook of Rheumatology, 6th ed. Philadelphia, WB Saunders, 2001, pp 387–391.
9. Tervaert JWC, Kallenberg C: Neurologic manifestations of systemic vasculitides. Rheum Dis Clin North Am 19:913–940, 1994.
10. Wolf PL: Abnormalities in serum enzymes in skeletal muscle diseases. Am J Clin Pathol 95:293–296, 1991.
11. Wortmann RL: Muscle disease symptoms: Evaluation and significance. Bull Rheum Dis 43(6):1–4, 1994.
12. Wortmann RL: Inflammatory disease of muscle and other myopathies. In Ruddy S, Harris ED, Sledge CB (eds): Kelley's Textbook of Rheumatology, 6th ed. Philadelphia, WB Saunders, 2001, pp 1273–1295.

# 17. HEALTH STATUS MEASUREMENTS

*Sterling G. West, M.D.*

**1. What are the most important concerns of a patient with a newly diagnosed chronic rheumatic disease?**

- Why did this happen to me?
- How well can my pain and other symptoms be controlled?
- Will I become disabled and lose the ability to be independent?

**2. What should be the primary goal of health care for a patient with a chronic rheumatic disease?**

The goal of health care for patients with any chronic disease is to maintain, or restore, the individual's ability to function successfully in personal, family, and community life.

**3. How do physicians traditionally assess rheumatic disease activity and/or response to therapy?**

**History**: How well is the patient doing compared with the last evaluation, including the amount of pain.

**Physical examination**: Number of tender and swollen joints; joint range of motion; document deformities; neuromuscular and other organ-specific examination.

**Laboratory** (sedimentation rate, other) and **radiographic** tests.

From this evaluation, the physician documents impairments (i.e., loss of range of motion, demonstrable deformities, others) and disease activity. This evaluation, however, does not necessarily tell the physician anything about the patient's functional disabilities.

**4. How do you determine the overall functional status of a patient with a chronic rheumatic disease (or any chronic disease for that matter)?**

In addition to a history, physical examination, and laboratory evaluation, other assessments that should be done include:

Physical function assessment
Psychological/cognitive function assessment
Social function assessment

**5. What "open-ended" questions can you ask a rheumatic disease patient to get an idea of his or her functioning?**

1. Are you able to do the things you want to?
2. What's the most difficult thing for you to do?
3. What do you need to do that you can't do or have difficulty doing?
4. What do you want to do that you can't do or have difficulty doing?
5. During a typical day, what limitations do you have to overcome?
6. How do you function in your family?
7. Do you have trouble sleeping and/or bathing?

**6. What is involved in the assessment of physical function?**

The assessment of physical function consists of evaluating the following areas:

- Ability to perform activities of daily living (ADLs)
- Recreational (avocational) or leisure-time activities
- Occupational (vocational) activities, including job, housework, and schoolwork
- Sexual activities
- Sleep

**7. What aspects are assessed when evaluating a patient's ability to perform activities of daily living?**

ADLs include the ability to do personal (self) care, which assesses upper-extremity function, as well as the ability to be mobile and ambulate, which assesses lower-extremity function.

**Personal care assessment**

Bed/bedroom—bed activities and dressing
Bathroom—toileting, bathing, grooming
Kitchen—eating, cooking
Other household activities—reaching, gripping

**Mobility and ambulation assessment**

Walking
Climbing stairs
Transfers/rising from a seated or supine position

**8. List the areas involved in the assessment of psychological function.**

Cognitive function, affective function (depression, anxiety, mood), coping skills, compliance with treatment plan, self-efficacy vs. helplessness.

**9. Which areas are evaluated in the assessment of social function?**

- Social support systems (with family, friends, and community)
- Interpersonal relationships (with family, friends, and community)
- Social integration (with family, friends, and community)
- Ability to fulfill social roles
- Family functioning
- Socioeconomic/financial
- Access to health care

**10. What methods can be used in clinical practice to assess a rheumatic disease patient's overall functioning?**

Several multidimensional health status questionnaires have been developed that can measure simultaneously multiple areas of functional status and disease activity at one point in time. Many of these questionnaires can be filled out by the patient or administered by trained personnel and take only a few minutes to complete. These questionnaires can be used to identify functional disabilities that are a problem for the patient and need to be further evaluated and treated. They also can be administered over time to detect changes in clinical and functional status and to help assess how well a patient is responding to a specific therapy.

**11. Name some multidimensional health status questionnaires commonly used to evaluate patients with chronic rheumatic diseases.**

**General health status questionnaires**

Sickness Impact Profile (SIP)
Medical Outcomes Study 36-Item Short-Form Health Survey (SF-36)

**Rheumatic disease–specific questionnaires**

Rheumatoid arthritis
Arthritis Impact Measurement Scales (AIMS 1 and 2)
Stanford Heath Assessment Questionnaire (HAQ)
Modified HAQ (MHAQ)
McMaster-Toronto Arthritis Questionnaire (MACTAR)
Spondyloarthropathy
Bath Anylosing Spondylitis Indices
Childhood rheumatic disorders
Juvenile HAQ

Systemic lupus erythematosus (SLE)
British Isles Lupus Assessment Group (BILAG) Index
SLE Disease Activity Index (SLE-DAI)
SLE Activity Measure (SLAM)
SLE (ACR/SLICC) Damage Index
Osteoarthritis
Western Ontario and McMaster WOMAC)
Osteoarthritis Index
Low back pain
Oswestry Low Back
Pain Disability Questionnaire
Fibromyalgia
Fibromyalgia Impact Questionnaire (FIQ)
**Pain**
Visual analogue pain scale (VAPS)
McGill Pain Questionnaire
**Fatigue**
Multidimensional Assessment of Fatigue
**Depression**
PRIME—MD
Center for Epidemiology Studies—Depression (CES-D) instrument

The AIMS and HAQ have also been adapted for use in many rheumatic diseases other than rheumatoid arthritis. Some of these multidimensional health status questionnaires are available in foreign languages. Note that these questionnaires can identify functional limitations but cannot determine the *etiology* of that disability.

**12. What are some problems with the use of multidimensional health status questionnaires in clinical practice?**

- Intrapatient variability in filling out self-reported forms.
- Inter-rater variability in filling out forms administered to the same patient.
- Ability of questionnaires to detect change over time and agreement on what degree of change in score is significant clinically
- Length of time to administer

**13. Describe the American College of Rheumatology criteria for classification of global functional status.**

**Class I**: Able to perform usual ADLs (self-care, vocational, and avocational).

**Class II**: Able to perform usual self-care and vocational activities but limited in avocational activities.

**Class III**: Able to perform usual self-care activities but limited in vocational and avocational activities.

**Class IV**: Limited in ability to perform usual self-care, vocational, and avocational activities.

In this classification, a patient is assigned to a specific functional class by a physician depending on an evaluation.

**14. Discuss the HAQ, SLE-DAI, and WOMAC.**

- HAQ—most widely used instrument. It addresses eight domains of activities of daily living in 24 questions and yields a score between 0 (complete ability) and 3 (complete inability). It takes less than 5 minutes to complete. Scores greater than 1.5 reflect significant impairment in ADLs. The minimally significant change in response to therapy is .21.
- SLE-DAI—a disease activity index for SLE, which is a weighted index of 9 organ systems. Maximum score theoretically is 105, but most patients are under 45. Patients with scores greater than 20 usually have severely active disease. The minimally significant change in response to therapy is 4. It takes only a few minutes to fill out.

- WOMAC—a multidimensional instrument that emphasizes pain, stiffness, and impairment of physical activities related to osteoarthritis of hip or knee. It takes less than 10 minutes to fill out.

## BIBLIOGRAPHY

1. American College of Rheumatology Glossary Committee: Dictionary of the Rheumatic Diseases: Vol III. Health Status Measurement. Atlanta, American College of Rheumatology, 1988.
2. Bellamy N, Carr AJ: Health outcome assessment. In Ruddy S, Harris ED, Sledge CB (eds): Kelley's Textbook of Rheumatology, 6th ed. Philadelphia, W.B. Saunders, 2001, pp 777–787.
3. Calkins DR, Rubenstein LV, Cleary PD, et al: Failure of physicians to recognize functional disability in ambulatory patients. Ann Intern Med 114:451–454, 1991.
4. Hochberg MC, et al: The American College of Rheumatology 1991 revised criteria for classification of global functional status in rheumatoid arthritis. Arthritis Rheum 35:498–502, 1992.
5. Meenan RF: Health status assessment. In Schumacher HR Jr (ed): Primer on the Rheumatic Diseases, 10th ed. Atlanta, Arthritis Foundation, 1993, pp 81–82.
6. Wolfe F: Health status questionnaires. Rheum Dis Clin North Am 21:445–464, 1995.
7. Wolfe F, Pincus T: Listening to the patient: A practical guide to self-report questionnaires in clinical care. Arthritis Rheum 42:1797–1808, 1999.

# 18. PREOPERATIVE ASSESSMENT OF PATIENTS WITH RHEUMATIC DISEASE

*Kimberly P. May, M.D.*

**1. Why is it important for rheumatic disease patients to be evaluated preoperatively?**

In general, rheumatic disease patients who go to surgery do not have postoperative complications related to the procedure performed or the anesthetic used, but to exacerbations of antecedent medical conditions. Patients with rheumatic diseases can have unique problems because of advanced disease, complications of medical therapy, and limitations in functional status. The preoperative evaluation can identify those factors that may contribute to surgical risk so that appropriate action can be taken to avoid complications.

**2. List the essential items to review in the preoperative evaluation of a patient with a rheumatic disease.**

A comprehensive evaluation should include the "ABCDE'S":

**A**—adjust medications
**B**—bacterial prophylaxis
**C**—cervical spine disease
**D**—deep vein thrombosis prophylaxis
**E**—evaluate extent and activity of disease
**S**—stress-dose steroid coverage

**3. How are patients "cleared" for surgery?**

The term "clearance" was formerly used at a time when the goal of the preoperative assessment was to crudely divide patients into those able to tolerate surgery ("cleared") and those unable to tolerate surgery. The term is archaic since today patients are rarely excluded from being considered for an operative procedure on the basis of their underlying medical conditions, but they may be at increased risk for a complication. A more appropriate goal of the preoperative assessment is risk stratification, with identification of potential perioperative problems whose risk can be reduced by preoperative management.

**4. What laboratory tests are routinely required for patients with rheumatic diseases scheduled for elective surgery?**

There is no consensus on preoperative screening, however, a complete blood count, blood urea nitrogen, creatinine, glucose, coagulation studies, urinalysis, chest radiograph, and electrocardiogram are commonly obtained on all patients. Other tests in asymptomatic patients may include:

| TEST | ORDER IN A PATIENT WITH |
|---|---|
| Liver function tests | NSAID, gold, methotrexate, leflunomide use |
| Prothrombin time/partial thromboplastin time | Liver disease or bleeding disorder<br>Antiphospholipid antibody syndrome |
| Electrocardiogram | Age > 40<br>Coronary disease or risk factors |
| Bleeding time | Controversial; possibly in recent NSAID users |
| Chest x-ray | Long-standing arthritis<br>Pulmonary or cardiovascular disease<br>Thoracic surgery<br>Age > 60 |
| Pulmonary function tests/arterial blood gases | Same as chest x-ray |
| Cervical spine x-ray | Rheumatoid arthritis, juvenile rhuematoid arthritis |

**5. Are patients with rheumatic diseases at increased risk for perioperative complications compared with other patients?**

Patients with rheumatic diseases may have a higher incidence of postoperative wound infections and impaired wound healing than nonrheumatic patients, usually owing to the medications used to treat their diseases. Accelerated coronary artery disease (CAD) may be seen in patients with chronic steroid use, and CAD may be silent if severe joint disease limits activity. A low threshold for CAD evaluation is appropriate in this patient population.

**6. Should rheumatoid patients with active synovitis be taken to elective surgery?**

No. Postoperatively, patients with active synovitis will have significant pain from their arthritis, which can impair functional status, impede progress with rehabilitation, and prolong hospitalization. Patients with active synovial disease and its consequent disability should have the inflammation controlled as much as possible prior to elective surgical procedures.

**7. Why is it important to evaluate patients with rheumatoid arthritis (RA) for cervical spine disease prior to surgery?**

Instability of the cervical spine may be found in up to 30–40% of patients with RA awaiting elective surgical procedures. Proliferative synovitis along the articular surfaces of the cervical vertebrae can lead to erosion of surrounding bone and destruction or laxity of the supporting ligaments. In particular, **atlanto-axial subluxation** can occur owing to weakening of the transverse ligament, which holds the odontoid process of C2 against the anterior arch of C1. Manipulation of the neck during intubation and transport of the patient, especially extreme flexion or extension, can cause compression of the spinal cord by the odontoid process.

**8. What factors increase the risk for cervical spine disease in patients with rheumatoid arthritis?**

**C**—corticosteroid use
**S**—seropositive RA
**P**—peripheral joint destruction
**I**—involvement of cervical nerves (paresthesias, neck pain, weakness)
**N**—nodules (rheumatoid)
**E**—established disease (present > 10 yrs)

Most anesthesiologists advocate preoperative radiographs for all RA patients, because significant disease may be present but asymptomatic.

**9. How is atlanto-axial instability diagnosed?**

Instability of C1–C2 is diagnosed when the odontoid process is found to be displaced > 3 mm from its normal position against the anterior arch of the atlas in the lateral flexion and extension radiographs.

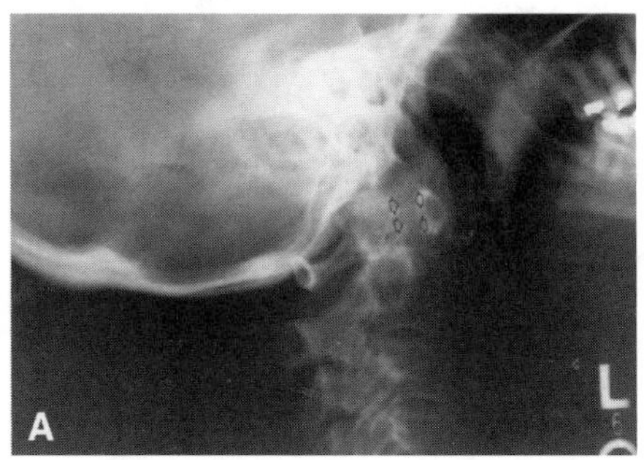


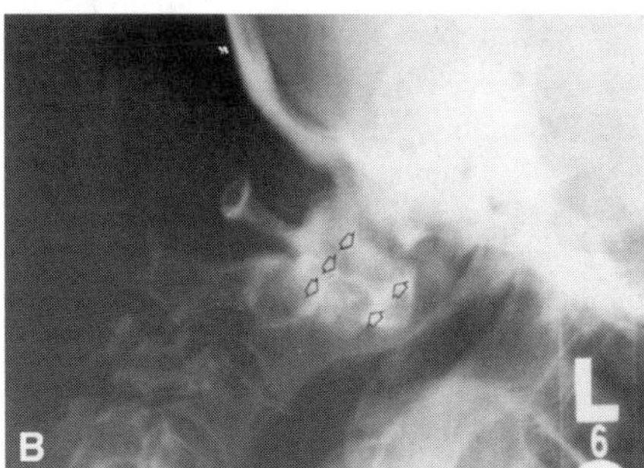


Atlanto-axial instability. Arrows show wide separation of the odontoid process of C2 from the anterior arch of C1 in extension (*panel A*) and flexion (*panel B*) in a patient with severe RA.

**10. How are patients with cervical spine disease managed?**

Symptomatic patients should have surgical stabilization performed before the planned procedure. Patients with asymptomatic or mild disease may be considered for intubation with fiberoptic assistance to minimize the extremes of motion associated with routine intubation. A soft cervical collar worn throughout the perioperative period will serve as a visual reminder that these patients should be handled with care, but it does not offer support to an unstable spine.

**11. What is cricoarytenoid disease? How can it impact on anesthetic complications?**

The cricoarytenoid (CA) joint is a true diarthrodial articulation and is subject to the same destructive changes that occur in other small joints in patients with RA. Proliferative synovium can spread across the articular surface of the CA joint during episodes of disease activity and impair the mobility of the vocal cords, giving symptoms of tracheal pain, dysphonia, stridor, dyspnea, and dysarthria. Other patients can have minor symptoms related to synovitis but over time develop fibrous replacement of the normal cartilage and ankylosis across the joint space. In the latter group, the diagnosis of CA disease may be clinically silent until attempts at endotracheal intubation by standard techniques result in trauma to the adducted vocal cords, with subsequent edema, inflammation, and airway obstruction.

**12. Who is at risk for developing cricoarytenoid disease?**

The degree of involvement correlates with the extent and activity of the peripheral joint disease. The prevalence of laryngeal abnormality noted by laryngoscopy is as high as 25%, though clinically significant disease is rare.

**13. How is cricoarytenoid disease managed?**

Preoperative fiberoptic laryngoscopy is recommended for all patients with symptoms of CA disease. Mild cases may be treated preoperatively with systemic steroids (prednisone, 20 mg orally three times daily) or injection of the CA joint with triamcinolone acetonide. Intubation under fiberscopic guidance is also recommended at the time of surgery. Patients with severe disease should be considered for elective tracheostomy if the vocal cords are found to be chronically adducted.

**14. Should aspirin be discontinued preoperatively in rheumatic disease patients?**

Patients treated with aspirin and acetylsalicylate-containing medications may be at risk for increased surgical bleeding, because these drugs impair platelet aggregation for the life of the platelet (7–10 days). However, the clinical significance of the excess blood loss and the ability of a preoperative bleeding time (BT) to predict it have been questioned. Regardless, it is the practice of most surgeons to recommend discontinuation of acetylsalicylate-containing medications 7–10 days prior to a planned surgical procedure. In the perioperative period, acetaminophen (up to 4 gm daily), prednisone (5–10 mg daily), and selective COX-2 inhibiting NSAIDs may be used. Aspirin may be restarted 3–4 days postoperatively.

**15. What about other nonsteroidal anti-inflammatory drugs (NSAIDs)?**

COX-1 inhibiting NSAIDs affect platelet aggregation in the same way as aspirin, but their effects are reversible with discontinuation of the medicine. These drugs have also been associated with more frequent episodes of gastrointestinal bleeding when given perioperatively. All COX-1 inhibiting NSAIDs should be held preoperatively for a time equal to four to five half-lives of the drug to allow return of normal platelet function, and they may be restarted 2–3 days postoperatively. COX-2 selective NSAIDs may be given safely perioperatively because they do not affect platelet function or BT (See also Chapter 84).

**16. How does the normal adrenal gland respond to surgery?**

In a baseline state, the adrenal gland secretes the equivalent of 30 mg of hydrocortisone (7.5 mg of prednisone) per day, but with stress, it may produce the equivalent of 200–400 mg of hydrocortisone (50–100 mg of prednisone) per day. With surgery, typical secretion is on the order of 50–100 mg hydrocortisone-equivalent per day. Cortisol levels typically peak within 24 hours of the time of surgical incision and return to normal after 72 hours if no other factors contribute to perioperative stress.

**17. What causes perioperative adrenal insufficiency?**

The administration of exogenous corticosteroids can interfere with the normal dynamics of the hypothalamic-pituitary-adrenal axis and blunt endogenous cortisol excretion. With stress, the adrenal output may become inadequate to support physiologic demands, leading to hemodynamic instability, fever, nausea, and other signs of adrenal insufficiency. A routine part of the preoperative evaluation should be to consider whether the patient is at risk for adrenal insufficiency.

**18. Who is at risk for adrenal insufficiency?**

1. Patients treated with daily administration of supraphysiologic doses of prednisone (> 10 mg) for > 1 week during the 12 months preceding surgery.
2. Patients who overuse steroid inhalers to treat inflammatory lung disease.
3. Rarely, patients who receive intra-articular steroid injections.
4. Patients on chronic steroids, even low-dose prednisone (< 10 mg daily).

**19. How can patients at risk for adrenal insufficiency be tested preoperatively?**

The Cortrosyn (cosyntropin) stimulation test is a simple and reliable method to evaluate the adrenal gland's ability to respond to stress. After a baseline cortisol level is obtained, 25 units of Cortrosyn (an ACTH analogue) is injected intravenously, and a cortisol level is collected after 60 minutes. Patients with a normal hypothalamic-pituitary-adrenal axis should demonstrate a stimulated value of > 20 mg/dL.

**20. How are stress-dose steroids given?**

Guidelines for steroid dosing in patients at risk for adrenal insufficiency are given below. Because the risks of coverage are minimal, and the complications avoided can be life-threatening, it is best to err on the side of safety when considering steroid administration.

**Major surgery**
100 mg hydrocortisone IV on call to the OR, *then*
100 mg hydrocortisone IV q 6–8 hrs × 3 doses, *then*
50 mg hydrocortisone IV q 6–8 hrs × 3 doses, *then*
25 mg hydrocortisone IV q 6–8 hrs × 3 doses, *then* Stop.
**Minor surgery**
100 mg hydrocortisone IV on call to the OR, *then*
100 mg hydrocortisone IV q 6–8 hrs for 24 hrs, *then* Stop.

Elaborate tapering schedules are not required unless postoperative complications prolong stress after surgery. Patients on oral steroids preoperatively may resume their normal dose after this protocol is complete. The oral prednisone equivalent can be given once the patient can take oral medications (1 mg prednisone = 4 mg hydrocortisone).

**21. Name the two most common organisms to infect a prosthetic joint at the time of surgery.**

*Staphylococcus aureus*
*Staphylococcus epidermidis*

**22. What is standard antibiotic prophylaxis for prosthetic joint surgery?**

- Cefazolin, 1 gm IV within 60 min of incision, then every 8 hrs
- Vancomycin, 1 gm IV every 12 hrs, in penicillin-allergic patients

Prophylactic antibiotics should not be continued for > 24 hours postoperatively.

**23. Should patients who have prosthetic joints have antibiotic prophylaxis prescribed before undergoing dental procedures?**

There is not yet a consensus among orthopedic surgeons, dentists, and primary care providers as to the utility of antibiotic prophylaxis during dental procedures in patients with prosthetic joints.

**For**

1. The risk of prosthetic joint infections is similar to that for prosthetic heart valves, in which prophylactic antibiotics have significantly reduced morbidity following dental procedures.
2. Animal models confirm the occurrence of hematogenous seeding of prosthetic joints.
3. Numerous case reports of prosthetic joint infections following dental procedures have been documented.
4. Consequences of infection are severe, including removal of the prosthesis, prolonged sepsis, and death.
5. Routine antibiotic administration would be cost-effective, even allowing for the cost of adverse drug reactions.

**Against**

1. Prosthetic joints are not similar to prosthetic heart valves in terms of their likelihood of being infected following dental manipulation, and there is no evidence to support routine prophylaxis.
2. The inoculum used during animal studies was large (half the animals died of septicemia or shock) and was not representative of the transient bacteremia induced by dental procedures.
3. Episodes of adverse reactions to antibiotics, including fatal anaphylaxis, would impose a risk of administration that would far outweigh the benefits of reduced numbers of infections.
4. Routine antibiotic administration to an unselected population would not be cost-effective.

The latter argument against the routine use of prophylaxis has some merit. However, it has been recognized that several clinical factors, including a history of RA, corticosteroid use, diabetes, and operations for prosthesis replacement, may increase the risk of prosthetic joint infection. Antibiotics prescribed for these select patients would probably provide benefit without excess risk. In the absence of good data, amoxicillin (2 grams), cephradine (2 grams), cephalexin (2 grams), or clindamycin (600 mg) for the penicillin allergic patient, dosed 1 hour prior to the procedure, appears to be a rational choice.

**24. What are the options for deep vein thrombosis prophylaxis in patients undergoing joint replacement procedures?**

- Coumadin, 10 mg the day before surgery, then 5 mg the evening of surgery, then dose by sliding scale to a target prothrombin time of 16–18 sec (INR 2–3) until time of discharge
- Heparin, 3500 units subcutaneously prior to surgery, then 3500 units every 8 hours after surgery, adjusted by sliding scale every day to maintain the adjusted partial thromboplastin time within 4 seconds of the upper limit of normal.
- Pneumatic compression devices, worn on the lower extremities at all times starting the morning of surgery, until the patient is ambulatory or discharged.
- Low molecular weight heparins may be used for prophylaxis (check product recommendations for prophylactic dosage). Best efficacy achieved by giving half the high-risk dose between 2 hours preoperatively and 6–8 hours postoperatively.

**25. Should cytotoxic/remittive agents be stopped prior to elective surgery?**

Most drugs are safe to continue perioperatively. No data support the discontinuation of hydroxychloroquine, oral or parenteral gold, sulfasalazine, azathioprine, or cyclophosphamide preoperatively. Several studies suggest that methotrexate should be discontinued 1–4 weeks prior to a planned procedure, because of concern for increased risk of infection and decreased wound healing. This is a reasonable strategy if the patient's disease can be controlled with the addition of NSAIDs or low-dose prednisone. Practically, many rheumatologists recommend discontinuation of methotrexate the week of and the week after surgery. Because of concern for diminished wound healing in patients taking d-penicillamine, it may also be held for 1–2 weeks prior to and following surgery.

**26. A patient with RA is found to have a swollen, warm, and tender knee on postoperative day 4 after a cholecystectomy. Should the patient have an arthrocentesis performed?**

Yes. An acutely inflamed joint postoperatively should always be aspirated to exclude a septic joint. Do not assume that the symptoms are due to a flare of RA, especially if the involved joint seems "out of synch" with the rest of the patient's disease activity.

**27. A patient with chronic tophaceous gout has the acute onset of left knee pain and swelling postoperatively. Aspiration reveals negatively birefringent needle-shaped crystals. Can you be certain of the diagnosis of acute gouty arthritis?**

Not yet. Patients with chronic gout can have uric acid crystals seen on synovial fluid aspirated from an asymptomatic joint, and so in this case their presence is not diagnostic. Sepsis and gout can also occur simultaneously, so Gram stain and culture of the fluid are mandatory.

**28. What predisposes patients to postoperative gout attacks?**

Dehydration
Increased uric acid production due to adenosine triphosphate breakdown (energy utilization) during surgery
Medicines (diuretics, heparin, cyclosporine)
Minor trauma to the joint during surgery and transport
Infections
Hyperalimentation
Surgical stress

**29. What are the options for treating patients with acute gouty arthritis postoperatively when they are NPO?**

- Indomethacin, 50 mg three times daily per nasogastric tube or suppositories per rectum.
- Colchicine, 2 mg in 20 ml of normal saline, infused over 20 min. May repeat with 1 mg every 6 hrs for two additional doses. (No oral colchicine for 7 days after intravenous use.) Reduce the colchicine dose if renal or liver disease is present.

- ACTH, 20 units intravenous slowly, or 40 units intramuscularly.
- Triamcinolone acetonide, 40 mg intramuscularly. This is the safest option in most cases.
- Triamcinolone preparation injected into the joint if you are sure it is not infected.

ACKNOWLEDGMENT

The author and editor would like to thank Dr. Richard Shea for his contribution to the previous edition of this chapter.

## BIBLIOGRAPHY

1. American Dental Association and American Academy of Orthopaedic Surgeons: Antibiotic prophylaxis for dental patients with total joint replacements. J Am Dent Assoc 128:1–6, 1997.
2. Antimicrobial prophylaxis in surgery. Med Lett Drugs Ther 41:75–80, 1999.
3. Dockery KM, Sismanis A, Abedi E: Rheumatoid arthritis of the larynx: The importance of early diagnosis and corticosteroid therapy. South Med J 84:95–96, 1991.
4. Goldman DR: Surgery in patients with endocrine dysfunction. Med Clin North Am 71:499–509, 1987.
5. Hull RD, Pineo GF, Stein PD, et al: Timing of initial administration of low-molecular-weight heparin prophylaxis against deep vein thrombosis in patients following elective hip arthroplasty. Arch Intern Med 161:1952–1960, 2001.
6. MacKenzie CR, Sharrock NE: Perioperative medical considerations in patients with rheumatoid arthritis. Rheum Dis Clin North Am 24:1–17, 1998.
7. Merli GJ: Deep vein thrombosis and pulmonary embolism prophylaxis in joint replacement surgery. Rheum Dis Clin North Am 25:639–656,1999.
8. Nierman E, Zakrzewski K: Recognition and management of preoperative risk. Rheum Dis Clin North Am 25:585–622,1999.
9. Shaw M, Mandell BF: Perioperative management of selected problems in patients with rheumatic diseases. Rheum Dis Clin North Am 25:623–638, 1999.

# IV. *Systemic Connective Tissue Diseases*

*The wolf, I'm afraid, is inside tearing up the place.*
Letter to Sister Mariella Gable from Flannery O'Connor, a sufferer of systemic lupus erythematosus, July 5, 1964

*[P.S.] Prayers requested. I am sick of being sick.*
Letter to Louise Abbot from Flannery O'Connor, May 28, 1964

## 19. RHEUMATOID ARTHRITIS

*Jennifer* R. Elliott, M.D., *and James* O'Dell, M.D.

**1. What is rheumatoid arthritis?**

Rheumatoid arthritis (RA) is a chronic, systemic, inflammatory disorder of unknown etiology that is characterized by its pattern of diarthrodial joint involvement. Its primary site of pathology is the synovium of the joints. The synovial tissues become inflamed and proliferate, forming **pannus** that invades bone, cartilage, and ligament and leads to damage and deformities. Rheumatoid factor positivity and extra-articular manifestations commonly accompany the joint disease, but arthritis represents the major manifestation.

**2. What is the etiology and pathogenesis of RA?**

Despite extensive research, the cause of RA remains unknown. It is thought to be multifactorial, with genetic factors and environmental factors playing important roles. RA is strongly associated with HLA-DR4 and, to a lesser extent, HLA-DR1 and DR14 positivity, with the susceptibility gene or "shared epitope" postulated on the third hypervariable region of HLA-DRB1. HLA-DR4 positivity also occurs in 20–30% of the general population; therefore, other factors must be present for the disease to develop. A variety of bacteria and viruses have been thought to trigger RA in a genetically susceptible host, but none have been consistently implicated. These and other factors are the subject of active research and debate.

Most research in RA has been on its pathogenesis. RA is thought to be initiated by T-lymphocytes recognizing antigens in the synovial tissue. Activated T-cells, macrophages, and fibroblasts produce pro-inflammatory cytokines that play a key role in synovitis and tissue destruction in RA. TNF alpha and Il-1 are two main pro-inflammatory cytokines that enhance synovial proliferation and stimulate secretion of matrix degrading metalloproteinases, other inflammatory cytokines, adhesion molecules, and prostaglandin E2.

Current treatment strategies with monoclonal anti-TNF antibodies (infliximab) and TNF receptor blockers (etanercept) have shown clinically significant responses. Also, minocycline, an inhibitor of matrix metalloproteinases, has reduced the need for other antirheumatic medication in some patients when used in early RA.

**3. Does the HLA associations ("shared epitope hypothesis") with RA explain the genetic risk for this disease?**

No. Familial aggregation studies show the concordance rate for RA for monozygotic twins is 30–50% and for dizygotic twins and siblings is the same at 2–3%. Overall, the risk to unaffected siblings for developing RA (if one sibling has RA) is 5–10 times that of the general population. Genetic analysis suggests that only 30% of this increased risk can be ascribed to HLA, indicating a substantial role for non-HLA genes (30,000 to choose from).

**4. List the criteria for the classification of RA.**

*The 1987 Revised Criteria for the Classification of Rheumatoid Arthritis*

1. Morning stiffness in and around joints lasting at least 1 hour before maximal improvement*
2. Soft-tissue swelling (arthritis) of 3 or more joint areas observed by a physician*
3. Swelling (arthritis) of the proximal interphalangeal (PIP), metacarpophalangeal (MCP), or wrist joints*
4. Symmetric arthritis*
5. Subcutaneous nodules
6. Positive test for rheumatoid factor (RF)
7. Radiographic erosions or periarticular osteopenia in hand or wrist joints

* Present for at least 6 weeks.

From Arnett FC, Edworthy SM, Bloch DA, et al: The American Rheumatism Association 1987 revised criteria for the classification of rheumatoid arthritis. Arthritis Rheum 31:315–324, 1988; with permission.

To be classified as having RA, a patient must meet four or more criteria. The criteria demonstrate 92% sensitivity and 89% specificity for RA when compared with control subjects with non-RA rheumatic disease. These new criteria also have been used to diagnose RA (controversial).

It is important to point out that the first five criteria are all obtained by history or physical examination. Thus, the diagnosis of RA is an extremely clinical one. Most patients with RA have a **symmetric polyarthritis** involving the small joints of the hands (MCPs, PIPs), wrists, and frequently the feet [metatarsophalangeals (MTPs)]. Up to 85% of patients are RF-positive, and most develop periarticular erosions of the small joints within the first 2 years of disease.

**5. What other diseases should be excluded before making the diagnosis of RA?**

**Common Diseases**

Seronegative spondyloarthropathies
Connective tissue diseases (SLE, scleroderma, polymyositis, vasculitis, MCTD, polymyalgia rheumatica)
Polyarticular gout
Behçet's syndrome
Parkinson's disease
Calcium pyrophosphate deposition disease
Osteoarthritis
Viral infection (EBV, HIV, hepatitis B, parvovirus, rubella, hepatitis C)
Fibromyalgia
Reactive arthritis

**Uncommon Diseases**

Hypothyroidism
Subacute bacterial endocarditis
Hemochromatosis
Hypertrophic pulmonary osteoarthropathy
Hyperlipoproteinemias (types II, IV)
Hemoglobinopathies (sickle cell disease)
Relapsing polychondritis
Rheumatic fever
Sarcoidosis
Lyme disease
Amyloid arthropathy
Malignancy and paraneoplastic syndrome

**Rare Diseases**

Familial Mediterranean fever
Multicentric reticulohistiocytosis
Remitting seronegative symmetrical synovitis with pitting edema (RS3PE)
Whipple's disease
Angioimmunoblastic lymphadenopathy

A clinician should consider a diagnosis *other than* RA particularly in patients who have an asymmetric arthritis, migrating pattern, predominantly large-joint arthritis, DIP joint involvement, rash, back disease, renal disease, RF-negative status, leukopenia, hypocomplementemia, or no erosions on radiographs after many months of disease.

**6. Discuss the epidemiologic characteristics of RA.**

- Race—worldwide, all races
- Sex distribution—females > males 3:1

- Age—women 40–60 years, men later
- Occurs in about 1% of adults in the United States. The prevalence increases with age.

**7. How does RA usually have its onset?**

It usually has a subacute (20%) or insidious (70%) onset with arthritic symptoms of pain, swelling, and stiffness, with the number of joints involved increasing over weeks to months. About 10% of patients have an acutely severe onset, and a few start with episodic symptoms that progress to persistent disease.

**8. Which joints are commonly affected in RA?**

*Most Common Joints Involved During the Course of RA*

| | | | |
|---|---|---|---|
| MCP | 90–95% | Ankle/subtalar | 50–80% |
| Wrist | 80–90% | Cervical spine (esp. C1–2) | 40–50% |
| PIP | 65–90% | Hip | 40–50% |
| Knee | 60–80% | Elbow | 40–50% |
| MTP | 50–90% | Temporomandibular | 20–30% |
| Shoulder | 50–60% | | |

The joints most commonly involved *first* are the MCPs, PIPs, wrists, and MTPs. Larger joints generally become symptomatic after small joints. Patients may start out with only a few joints involved (oligoarticular onset) but progress to involvement of multiple joints (polyarticular) in a **symmetric distribution** within a few weeks to months.

Involvement of the thoracolumbar, sacroiliac, or hand distal interphalangeal (DIP) joints is very rare in RA and should suggest another diagnosis, such as a seronegative spondyloarthropathy (sacroiliac joints), psoriatic arthritis (DIP joints), or osteoarthritis (lumbar spine, DIP joints).

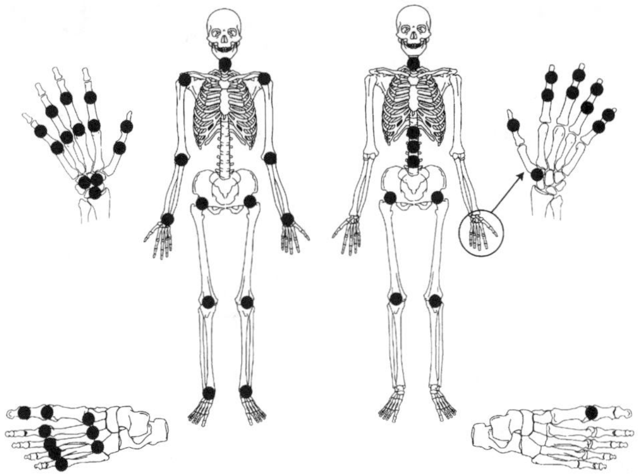

Joint distribution of RA (left) and osteoarthritis (OA) (right).

**9. What is meant by symmetrical involvement of joints?**

The most obvious meaning is that both sides of the body are involved similarly. Additionally, in RA, the whole joint surface is involved, as compared with osteoarthritis, which usually involves only the weight-bearing areas of the joint.

**10. What is pannus?**

The synovium is the primary site for the inflammatory process in RA. The inflammatory infiltrate consists of mononuclear cells, primarily CD4$^{+}$ (helper) T lymphocytes, as well as activated macrophages and plasma cells (some making RF). The synovial cells proliferate, and the inflamed synovium becomes boggy and edematous and develops villous projections. This proliferative synovium is called **pannus**, and it is capable of invading bone and cartilage, causing destruction of the joint.

Few if any polymorphonuclear leukocytes (PMNs) are found in the synovium, whereas it is the predominant cell in the inflammatory synovial fluid of RA patients. Degradative enzymes from these synovial fluid PMNs also contribute to destruction of the joint cartilage.

**11. What are the common deformities of the hand in RA?**

**Fusiform swelling**—Synovitis of PIP joints, causing them to appear spindle-shaped.

**Boutonniere deformity**—Flexion of the PIP and hyperextension of the DIP joint, caused by weakening of the central slip of the extrinsic extensor tendon and a palmar displacement of the lateral bands. This deformity resembles a knuckle being pushed through a buttonhole.

**Swan-neck deformity**—Results from contraction of the flexors of the MCPs, resulting in flexion contracture of the MCP joint, hyperextension of PIP, and flexion of the DIP joint.

**Ulnar deviation of fingers** with subluxation of MCP joints.

**"Piano key" ulnar head** secondary to destruction of ulnar collateral ligament.

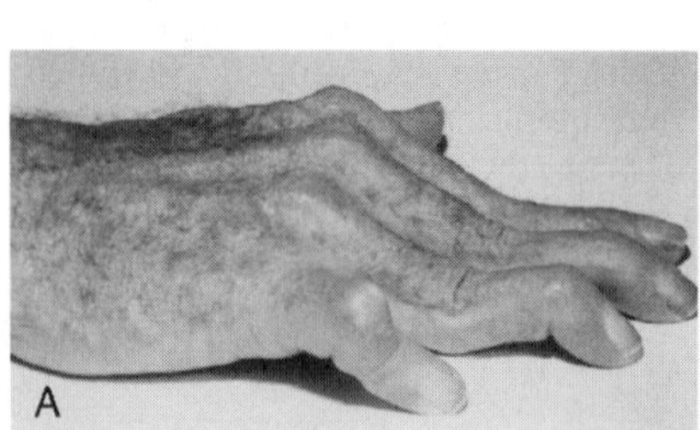


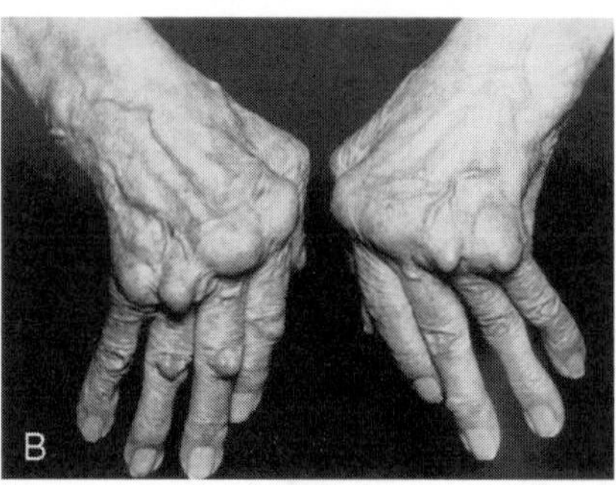


*A*, Swan neck (2nd to 4th fingers) and boutonniere (5th finger) deformities. *B*, Ulnar deviation of fingers (note rheumatoid nodules). (From the Revised Clinical Slide Collection on the Rheumatic Diseases. Atlanta, American College of Rheumatology, 1991; with permission.)

**12. Does RA affect the feet?**

Yes, the most common deformity in the foot of RA patients is the **claw toe**, or **hammer toe**. This is due to inflammation of the MTP joints leading to subluxation of the metatarsal heads. When this problem occurs, the patient has problems fitting his or her toes into the shoe as the tops of the toes rub on the shoe box, resulting in callous or ulcer formation. Additionally, because the soft tissue pad that normally sits underneath the metatarsal heads is displaced, the heads of the metatarsal bones are no longer cushioned and become very painful to walk on, frequently resulting in calluses on the inferior surface of the foot. Patients commonly complain that it feels as though they are walking on pebbles or stones. Arthritic involvement of the tarsal joint and subtalar joint can result in flattening of the arch of the foot and hindfoot valgus deformity.

**13. Describe the radiographic features of RA.**

The mnemonic **ABCDE'S** is a convenient way to remember these:

**A**—*Alignment*, abnormal; no ankylosis

**B**—*Bones*—periarticular (juxta-articular) osteoporosis; no periostitis or osteophytes

**C**—*Cartilage*—uniform (symmetric) joint-space loss in weight-bearing joints; no cartilage or soft tissue calcification

**D**—*Deformities* (swan neck, ulnar deviation, boutonniere) with symmetrical *distribution*

**E**—*Erosions*, marginal

**S**—*Soft-tissue swelling*; nodules without calcification

The radiographic changes in RA take months to develop. Juxta-articular osteopenia is seen early in the course of the disease, followed later by more diffuse osteopenia. Joint erosions typically occur at the margins of small joints. Later, joint-space narrowing and deformities develop. The earliest erosions occur in the hands (2,3,5 MCPs) before feet in 1/3 of patients, the feet (1,5 MTPs) before the hands in 1/3, and in both hands and feet at the same time in 1/3 of patients.

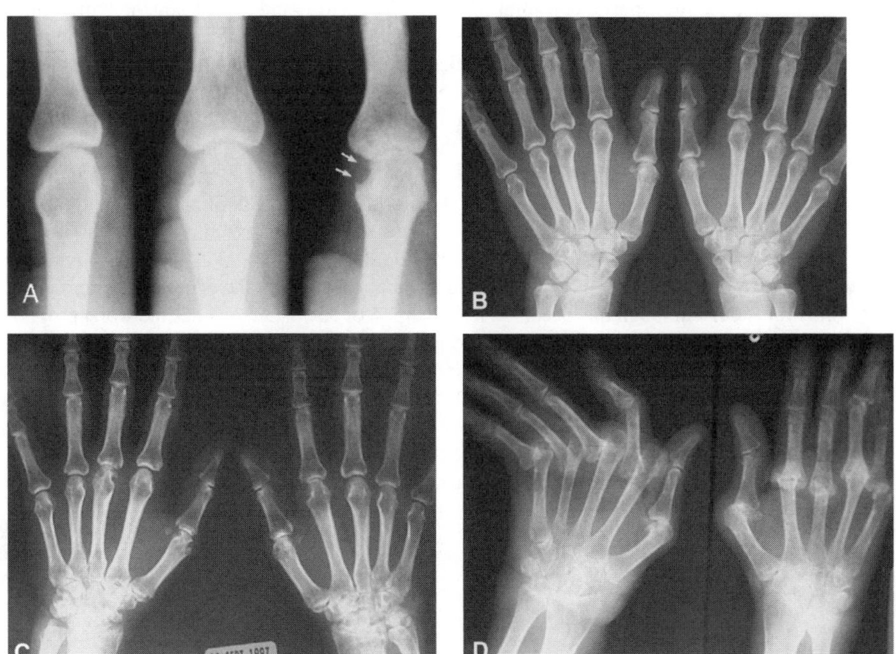


*A*, Progressive marginal erosions (arrows) of an MCP joint. (From the Revised Clinical Slide Collection on the Rheumatic Diseases. Atlanta, American College of Rheumatology, 1991; with permission.) *B*, Early RA with symmetrical joint space narrowing and juxta-articular osteoporosis. *C*, Same patient, 5 years later, with significant marginal erosions and severe wrist involvement. *D*, Severe RA with destruction of MCP joints, subluxation of MCP joints (left) leading to ulnar deviation, and marked wrist involvement.

**14. Compare the radiographic features of RA with those of OA.**

| | RA | OA |
|---|---|---|
| Sclerosis | ± | ++++ |
| Osteophytes | ± | ++++ |
| Osteopenia | +++ | 0 |
| Symmetry | +++ | + |
| Erosions | +++ | 0 |
| Cysts | ++ | ++ |
| Narrowing | +++ | +++ |

**15. What are the typical features of the synovial fluid in RA?**

The synovial fluid is inflammatory, with WBC counts typically between 5000 and 50,000/mm$^3$. Rarely, synovial fluid WBC count can exceed 100,000/mm$^3$ (pseudoseptic) but infection must always be ruled out. Generally the differential shows a predominance (> 50%) of PMNs. The protein level is elevated, and the glucose level may be low compared with serum values (40–60% of serum glucose). There are no crystals in the fluid, and cultures are negative. Unfortunately, there are no specific findings in the synovial fluid that allow a definitive diagnosis of RA.

**16. How is the cervical spine involved in RA?**

The cervical spine is involved in 30–50% of RA patients, with C1–2 the most commonly involved level. Arthritic involvement of the cervical spine can lead to instability with potential impingement of the spinal cord; thus it is important for the clinician to obtain radiographs of the cervical spine prior to surgical procedures requiring intubation. It is important to note that cervical spine disease parallels peripheral joint disease. The earliest and most frequent symptom of subluxation is pain radiating to the occiput. Pain, neurologic involvement, and death are the main concerns with subluxation. The patterns of cervical spine involvement include:

- **C1–2 Subluxation** (50% of patients)—The most common C1–2 (atlantoaxial) subluxation is **anterior**, resulting in > 3mm between the arch of C1 and the odontoid of C2. This is caused by synovial proliferation around the articulation of the odontoid process with the anterior arch of C1, leading to stretching and rupture of the transverse and alar ligaments, which keep the odontoid in contact with the arch of C1. The risk of spinal cord compression is greatest when the anterior atlanto-odontoid interval is ≥ 9 mm or the posterior atlanto-odontoid interval is ≤ 14 mm. **Vertical** atlantoaxial subluxation occurs as a result of collapse of the lateral articulations between C1 and C2, causing the odontoid to impinge on the brainstem. Although this occurs in less than 5% of RA patients, it has the worst prognosis neurologically, especially when the odontoid is ≥ 5 mm above Ranawat's line. **Lateral** (rotary) and **posterior** atlantoaxial subluxations also occur.
- **C1–2 Impaction** (35% of patients)—Destruction between the occipitoatlantal and atlantoaxial joints.
- **Subaxial involvement** (10–20% of patients)—Involvement of typically C2–3 and C3–4 facets and intervertebral disks. This can lead to "stair-stepping" with one vertebrae subluxing forward on the lower vertebrae.

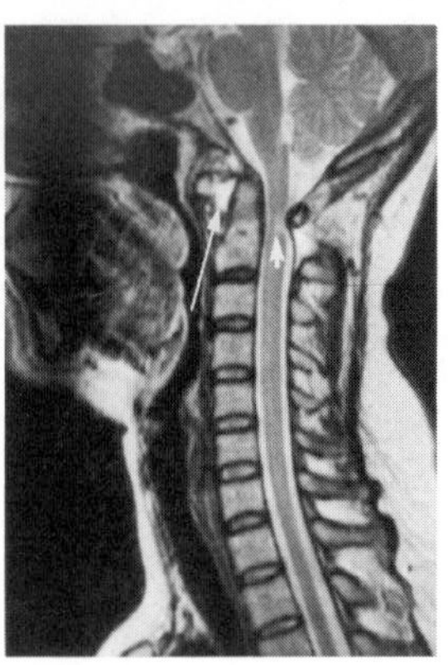

MRI of the cervical spine demonstrating pannus formation of the C1–2 articulation (long arrow) and impingement of the odontoid on the spinal cord (arrow).

**17. What are the typical laboratory findings in RA patients?**

Most patients with active RA have an anemia of chronic disease and elevated platelet counts, which both correlate with the activity of the disease. WBC counts are generally normal but may be low in patients with Felty's syndrome. Erythrocyte sedimentation rate (ESR) and C-reactive protein (CRP) values are elevated. Rheumatoid factor is positive. ANAs are positive in about 30% of patients. Urinalysis, renal function, liver function, metabolic function, and uric acid are normal. C3, C4, and CH50 levels are usually normal or elevated. Hypocomplementemia is rare and seen only in patients with severe vasculitis associated with RA.

**18. Which laboratory tests correlate with activity of disease?**

Clearly, the degree of **anemia** and the degree of **thrombocytosis** may correlate with the activity of the disease. However, the best correlation is found with the **ESR** and **CRP**. When choosing a laboratory test to follow in patients with RA, you would probably select one of these indicators, keeping in mind that both are very nonspecific. Serum albumin is frequently low because it acts as a negative acute phase reactant during active disease. RF titer does not correlate with disease activity.

**19. What is rheumatoid factor? How commonly is it found in RA patients?**

RF is a series of antibodies that recognize the Fc portion of an IgG molecule as their antigen. RFs can be of any isotype (IgM, IgG, IgA, IgE), but their distinguishing feature is the recognition of IgG as their antigen. Most of the RFs that are measured clinically are, in fact, IgM RFs. Teleologically, RFs probably developed in humans as a mechanism to help remove immune complexes from the circulation. Therefore, many conditions associated with chronic inflammation are also associated with RF positivity (discussed in Chapter 9). In RA patients, approximately 70% are RF-positive at disease onset, and an additional 10–15% (overall 85%) become RF-positive over the first 2 years after onset. It is important to note that a positive RF without clinical evidence of RA does not suggest RA. Also, diseases with arthritis other than RA can have a positive RF such as hepatitis C (40%), SLE (20%), Sjögren's (70%), and others like subacute bacterial endocarditis.

**20. What is the significance of RF in RA patients?**

RF positivity is associated with more severe disease, with extra-articular manifestations including subcutaneous nodules, and with increased mortality.

**21. Are antinuclear antibodies (ANAs) found in patients with RA?**

About 30% of RA patients have ANA, but these ANAs are not directed against any of the antigens typically tested for in the ANA profile (SS-A, SS-B, Sm, RNP, DNA). ANA-positive patients tend to have more severe disease and a poorer prognosis than RA patients who are ANA-negative.

**22. What is the significance of the anti-cyclic citrullinated peptide antibody?**

- This antibody reacts with the common epitope, which has been identified in the past by anti-filaggrin, anti-perinuclear, and anti-keratin antibodies.
- Highly specific (98%) for rheumatoid arthritis.
- Seen in up to 70% of patients with seropositive RA and 33% of patients with seronegative RA. Can be present for years before articular manifestations.
- May be useful in differentiating RA from disorders with articular symptoms plus RF positivity (hepatitis C, others) and in the early diagnosis of RA in patients who are seronegative.

**23. List some of the extra-articular manifestations of RA.**

**General**
Fever
Lymphadenopathy
Weight loss
Fatigue
**Dermatologic**
Palmar erythema
Subcutaneous nodules
Vasculitis
**Ocular**
Episcleritis
Scleritis
Choroid and retinal nodules
**Pulmonary**
Pleuritis
Nodules
Interstitial lung disease
Bronchiolitis obliterans
Arteritis

**Cardiac**
Pericarditis
Myocarditis
Coronary vasculitis
Nodules on valves
**Neuromuscular**
Entrapment neuropathy
Peripheral neuropathy
Mononeuritis multiplex
**Hematologic**
Felty's syndrome
Large granular lymphocyte syndrome
Lymphomas
**Others**
Sjögren's syndrome
Amyloidosis

**24. Which patients with RA are most likely to get extra-articular manifestations?**

Patients who are RF-positive, HLA-DR4-positive, and males are more likely to have extra-articular manifestations. It is important for clinicians to rule out other causes (infection, malignancy, medications, etc.) for an extra-articular manifestation before ascribing it to RA, especially if the patient is RF-negative.

**25. How commonly do fever and lymphadenopathy occur in RA patients?**

They are uncommon and generally seen only in those patients with severely active disease. Infection and lymphoreticular malignancy should always be considered in an RA patient with these symptoms.

**26. What are rheumatoid nodules? Where are they found?**

Rheumatoid nodules are subcutaneous nodules that have the characteristic histology of a central area of fibrinoid necrosis surrounded by a zone of palisades of elongated histiocytes and a peripheral layer of cellular connective tissue. They occur in about 20–35% of RA patients, who typically are RF-positive and have severe disease. They tend to occur on the extensor surface of the forearms, in the olecranon bursa, over joints, and over pressure points, like sacrum and occiput. They frequently develop and enlarge when the patient's RA is active and may resolve when disease activity is controlled. Methotrexate therapy has caused increased nodulosis in some RA patients, even when the disease is well-controlled.

**27. Which diseases should be considered in a patient with subcutaneous nodules and arthritis?**

| | |
|---|---|
| Rheumatoid arthritis | Xanthoma |
| Gout (tophi) | SLE (rare) |
| Amyloidosis | Rheumatic fever (rare) |
| Sarcoidosis | |

**28. Which cutaneous disorder can cause lesions that pathologically are similar to rheumatoid nodules?**

**Granuloma annulare** lesions have been called "benign" rheumatoid nodules. Patients with granuloma annulare do not have arthritis and are RF-negative. These lesions are more common in childhood.

**29. What are the ocular manifestations of RA?**

Both episcleritis and scleritis can occur as extra-articular manifestations of RA. If scleral inflammation persists, scleral thinning and scleromalacia perforans can occur. Sicca symptoms of dry eyes frequently accompany coexistent Sjögren's syndrome.

**30. Discuss the pulmonary manifestations of RA.**

**Pleural disease**: Pleurisy and pleural effusions can occasionally be the first manifestations of RA. Pleural effusions are characterized as cellular exudates with high protein and lactate dehydrogenase levels, a low glucose level (due to a defect in the transport of glucose across the pleura), and frequently a low pH (suggesting an infection).

**Nodules**: Rheumatoid nodules in the lung may be solitary or multiple and can cavitate or resolve spontaneously. Caplan's syndrome involves multiple rheumatoid nodules occurring in the lungs of RA patients who are coal miners.

**Interstitial pulmonary fibrosis (IPF)**: Fibrosing alveolitis occurs commonly in RA patients but is symptomatic and progressive in < 10%. Patients can have progressive dyspnea, Velcro rales, and fibrosis primarily in the lower lobes on chest radiography. Rapidly progressive IPF is called Hamman-Rich syndrome.

**Bronchiolitis obliterans (BO)**: Patients have dyspnea, hyperinflated chest x-ray, and small airways obstruction on pulmonary function tests. This condition can be rapidly fatal. Penicillamine therapy has occasionally been associated with causing this disease.

**Bronchiolitis obliterans with organizing pneumonia (BOOP)** and **nonspecific interstitial pneumonitis (NSIP)** can also occur and are more responsive to corticosteroid therapy than IPF or BO.

**31. What are the clinical consequences of the cardiac manifestations of RA?**

| | |
|---|---|
| **Pericarditis** | Pain (1% of RA patients) |
| | Tamponade (rare) |
| | Constriction (uncommon) |
| **Nodules** | Conduction abnormalities |
| | Valvular problems |
| **Coronary arteritis** | Myocardial infarction |
| **Myocarditis** | Congestive heart failure |

Pericarditis is the most common cardiac manifestation of RA and is present in up to 50% of patients at autopsy. It usually manifests as asymptomatic pericardial effusions, which may be found by echocardiography in about 30% of patients. These effusions are rarely large enough to cause tamponade but may result in constrictive pericarditis late in the course of the disease. RA may also cause nodules to form in and around the heart, leading to conduction defects and occasionally valvular insufficiency.

**32. Which types of vasculitis occur in RA patients?**

Vasculitis most commonly occurs in RA patients with long-standing disease, significant joint involvement, high-titer RF, and nodules. The types of vasculitis are:

- **Leukocytoclastic vasculitis**—Usually presents as palpable purpura and results from inflammation of postcapillary venules.
- **Small arteriolar vasculitis**—Presents as small infarcts of digital pulp and frequently is associated with a mild distal sensory neuropathy caused by vasculitis of vasa nervorum.
- **Medium-vessel vasculitis**—Can resemble polyarteritis nodosa with visceral arteritis, mononeuritis multiplex, and livedo reticularis.
- **Pyoderma gangrenosum**

**33. What three findings make up the classic triad of Felty's syndrome?**

Felty's syndrome is **RA** in combination with **splenomegaly** and **leukopenia**. Felty's syndrome is seen in 1% of RA patients who have RF, subcutaneous nodules, and other extra-articular manifestations. 95% of patients are HLA-DR4 and RF positive. Articular disease parallels those of RF-positive patients, but Felty's syndrome patients have more extra-articular manifestations. The leukopenia is generally a neutropenia (< 2000/mm$^3$); thrombocytopenia may occur. The major complications of Felty's syndrome include bacterial infections (20-fold increase compared with other RA patients) and chronic non-healing ulcers. Severe bacterial infections correlate with the neutrophil counts of < 1000/mm$^3$. Also, patients with Felty's syndrome have a 13-fold increased risk of developing non-Hodgkin's lymphoma. Some patients develop nodular regenerative hyperplasia of the liver with portal hypertension and varices that can bleed.

Treatment is the same as for RA patients with joint disease. Splenectomy has been used in the past for severe, recurrent bacterial infections or chronic non-healing leg ulcers in patients who were not responsive to drug therapy. However, splenectomy and other therapies such as lithium are now out of favor. Granulocyte colony stimulating factor (G-CSF) has been used and shown effective at increasing WBC counts and decreasing infections in some patients (neutrophils < 1000/mm$^3$). G-CSF [filgrastim (Neupogen)] is given in doses of 2–5 μg/kg/day to RA patients with recurrent infections until neutrophils > 1500/mm$^3$ and then weekly to maintain this level. However, G-CSF can cause increased arthritis and vasculitis in some Felty's patients when the WBC count is raised.

**34. What other clinical problems occur with increased frequency in RA patients?**

**Sjögren's syndrome**—Up to 20–30% of RA patients develop secondary Sjögren's syndrome with dry eyes and dry mouth. They are frequently ANA positive but typically do not have the anti-SS-A or SS-B antibodies commonly seen in primary Sjögren's syndrome.

**Amyloidosis**—Up to 5% of RA patients develop secondary or AA-associated amyloidosis. This occurs in long-standing, poorly controlled RA and usually presents as nephrotic syndrome.

**Osteoporosis**—Seen in the majority of RA patients and related to disease activity, immobility, and medications. Insufficiency fractures of the spine, sacrum, and other areas are common in long-standing disease.

**Entrapment neuropathy**—Median nerve (carpal tunnel), posterior tibial nerve (tarsal tunnel), ulnar nerve (cubital tunnel), and posterior interosseous branch of the radial nerve are most commonly involved.

**Laryngeal manifestations**—Cricoarytenoid arthritis can present as pain, dysphagia, hoarseness, and rarely, stridor.

**Ossicles of ear**—Tinnitus and decreased hearing.

**Renal and gastrointestinal involvement**—Rare. Usually abnormalities are due to NSAIDs causing renal insufficiency or gastric ulcers with hemorrhage. Other medications, such as gold and penicillamine, can cause a membranous nephropathy with significant proteinuria.

**Large granular lymphocyte (LGL) syndrome**—A syndrome of neutropenia, splenomegaly, susceptibility to infections, and large granular lymphocytes bearing CD2, 3, 8, 16, and 57 surface phenotypes in the peripheral blood smear. These cells have natural killer and antibody-dependent cell-mediated cytotoxicity activity. It is now recognized that when this syndrome occurs in RA patients, it is a subset of Felty's syndrome. About 1/3 of Felty's patients have significant clonal expansions of these cells on their peripheral smear, and these patients are HLA-DR4 positive similar to Felty's patients without LGL expansion.

**35. Are patients with RA at increased risk for joint infections?**

Unfortunately, yes. Joint infections tend to occur in abnormal joints, and RA patients have lots of these. Patients are also at increased risk secondary to immunosuppressive medication. Any time an RA patient presents with one or two joints that are swollen, red, and hot, out of proportion to the other joints, the clinician should suspect infection. In addition, following joint replacement surgeries, an infected artificial joint is a constant concern. The most common infecting organism is *Staphylococcus aureus*.

**36. Do any markers help predict if an RA patient will have severe disease and a poor prognosis?**

RF positivity and poor functional status [high health assessment questionnaire (HAQ) score > 1] at presentation are the best predictors of subsequent disability and joint damage. Other factors include:

1. Generalized polyarthritis involving both small and large joints (>20 total joints)
2. Extra-articular disease, especially nodules and vasculitis
3. Persistently elevated ESR or C-reactive protein
4. Radiographic erosions within 2 years of disease onset
5. HLA-DR4 genetic marker
6. Education level < 11th grade (frequently have manual labor job contributing to joint damage)

**37. Discuss the management principles for the initial treatment of RA.**

Traditionally, RA patients were initially started on NSAIDs, then disease-modifying antirheumatics (DMARDs) were added when joint damage was seen. Patients unfortunately experienced poor long-term outcomes, as 70% of RA patients have radiographic damage within 2 years. Over the last decade, treatment strategies have changed as RA has become known as a severe, progressive disease with poor long-term consequences.

Current strategies include early aggressive treatment with one or more DMARDs in addition to symptomatic therapy with NSAIDs, low-dose prednisone, physical therapy, occupational therapy, rest, patient education, and calcium supplementation to prevent osteoporosis (for rehabilitation techniques, see Chapter 91).

Methotrexate has been the most effective antirheumatic drug used, but alone seldom leads to remission. New biological response modifiers, including etanercept and infliximab, have shown good clinical responses. Minocycline, an inhibitor of matrix metalloproteinases, has induced remissions and reduced the need for antirheumatic medications when used early in RA. Combinations of DMARDs have been studied, and to date six clinical trials have shown advantages to using combination therapy in the treatment of RA. Combinations of methotrexate, sulfasalazine, and hydroxychloroquine, and methotrexate with infliximab or etanercept, have shown significant clinical improvement when compared with single therapy or placebo. Interestingly, no increased toxicity was seen with combination therapy. Thus, the side effects of DMARDs do not outweigh the benefits of controlling the consequences of RA. (More information about medications used in the treatment of RA are found in Chapters 86 and 87.)

**38. What is the long-term prognosis for RA patients?**

RA is clearly a disease that shortens survival and produces significant disability. Approximately 50% of patients will be functional class III or IV within 10 years of disease onset. Over 33% of RA patients who were working at the time of onset of their disease will leave the workforce within 5 years. In addition, the standardized mortality ratio is 2–2.5 to 1 compared with people of same sex and age without RA. Overall, RA shortens the lifespan of patients by 5–10 years. Patients with the poorest functional status and multiple joint involvement had a 5-year survival rate of 50% or less, which is similar to survival of stage IV Hodgkin's disease or three-vessel coronary artery disease in the 1970s. The patients with a poorer long-term outcome can be identified by prognostic markers (see Question 36). Aggressive DMARD therapy can reduce disability by 30% over 10–20 years.

**39. What causes the increased mortality in RA patients?**

- **Cardiovascular**—42%. Frequency, however, is not increased over the general population.
- **Infections** (especially pneumonias)—9%. Increased five times over that in the general population.
- **Cancer and lymphoproliferative malignancies**—14% Increased five to eight times over the rate in the general population. It is unclear whether malignancy is associated with RA and chronic immunostimulation or whether it is from immunosuppressive therapy with methotrexate, cyclosporine, and cyclophosphamide.
- **Others**, including renal disease due to amyloidosis, gastrointestinal hemorrhage due to NSAIDs (4%), and RA complications (5%).

Ten percent of deaths are due to RA itself, primarily vasculitis, atlanto-axial dislocation, rheumatoid involvement of lungs and heart, and medication induced. Excess mortality has not changed in four decades, although the general population's survival has increased.

**40. What is "seronegative" RA?**

It is one term to identify patients who are thought to have RA but are RF-negative. In general, RA patients who are RF-negative have a better prognosis, fewer extra-articular manifestations, and better survival. Additionally, a number of these patients over time will, in fact, be found to have some other disease. Thus, when dealing with seronegative RA patients, the clinician should always look for the possibility of psoriatic arthritis, lupus arthritis, calcium pyrophosphate crystal deposition disease, gout, hemochromatosis, or another form of arthritis other than RA. Testing for anti-cyclic citrullinated peptide may be helpful if it returns positive.

**41. What is the RS3PE syndrome?**

A syndrome characterized by the acute severe onset of symmetrical synovitis of the small joints of the hands, wrists, and flexor tendon sheaths accompanied by pitting edema of the dorsum of the hand (''boxing-glove" hand). Other joints may be involved. This syndrome affects mostly elderly (mean age 70) white men (M/F ratio 4:1). All patients are RF-negative. Symptoms do not respond to NSAIDs but are very sensitive to low-dose prednisone and hydroxychloroquine. Bony erosions do not occur. The disease predictably remits in < 36 months and, unlike RA, does not recur after withdrawal of medications. Severe hand pitting edema has also been reported in polymyalgia rheumatica and as a paraneoplastic syndrome.

## BIBLIOGRAPHY


1. Felson DT, Anderson JJ, Boers M, et al: American College of Rheumatology preliminary definition of improvement in rheumatoid arthritis. Arthritis Rheum 38:727–735, 1995.
2. Firestein GS: Etiology and pathogenesis of rheumatoid arthritis. In Ruddy S, Harris ED, Sledge CB (eds): Kelley's Textbook of Rheumatology, 6th ed. Philadelphia, W.B. Saunders, 2001, pp 921–966.
3. Fries JF, Williams CA, Morfeld D, et al: Reduction in long-term disability in patients with rheumatoid arthritis by disease-modifying antirheumatic drug-based treatment strategies. Arthritis Rheum 39:616–622, 1996.
4. Gabriel SE, Crowson CS, and O'Fallon WM: Mortality in rheumatoid arthritis: Have we made an impact in four decades? J Rheum 26:2529–2533, 1999.
5. Guedes C, et al: Mortality in rheumatoid arthritis. Rev Rheum 66:492–498, 1999.
6. Guidelines for the management of rheumatoid arthritis: 2002 update. Arthritis Rheum 46:328–346, 2002.
7. Harris ED: Clinical features of rheumatoid arthritis. In Ruddy S, Harris ED, Sledge CB (eds): Kelley's Textbook of Rheumatology, 6th ed. Philadelphia, W.B. Saunders, 2001, pp 967–1000.
8. Hochberg MC, Chang RW, Dwosh I, et al: The American College of Rheumatology 1991 revised criteria for the classification of global functional status in rheumatoid arthritis. Arthritis Rheum 35:498–502, 1992.
9. Kirwan JR: The effect of glucocorticoids on joint destruction in rheumatoid arthritis. N Engl J Med 333:142–146, 1995.
10. Kroot EJ, de Jong BAW, van Leeuwen MA, et al: The prognostic value of the antiperinuclear factor, anti-citrullinated peptide antibodies and rheumatoid factor in early rheumatoid arthritis. Clin Exp Rheumatol 17:689–697, 1999.
11. Landewé RBM, Boers M, Verhoeven AC, et al: COBRA combination therapy in patients with early rheumatoid arthritis: Long-term structural benefits of a brief intervention. Arthritis Rheum 46:347–356, 2002.
12. Luthra HS: Extra-articular rheumatoid arthritis. In Koopman WJ (ed): Arthritis and Allied Conditions, 14th ed. Philadelphia, Lea & Febiger, 2001, pp 1187–1201.
13. McCarty DJ, O'Duffy JD, Pearson L, Hunter JB: Remitting seronegative symmetrical synovitis with pitting edema ($RS_3PE$) syndrome. JAMA 254:2763–2767, 1985.
14. O'Dell JR, Haire CE, Erikson N, et al: Treatment of rheumatoid arthritis with methotrexate alone, sulfasalazine and hydroxychloroquine, or a combination of all three medications. N Engl J Med 334: 1287–1291, 1996.
15. O'Dell JR, Paulsen G, Haire CE, et al: Treatment of early seropositive rheumatoid arthritis with minocycline. Arch Intern Med 160:437–444, 2000.
16. Pinals RS: Felty's syndrome. In Ruddy S, Harris ED, Sledge CB (eds): Kelley's Textbook of Rheumatology, 6th ed. Philadelphia, W.B. Saunders, 2001, pp. 1023–1026.
17. Pincus T, Brooks RH, Callahan LF: Prediction of long-term mortality in patients with rheumatoid arthritis according to simple questionnaire and joint count measures. Ann Intern Med 120:26–34, 1994.
18. Pincus, T, O'Dell JR, Kremer JM: Combination treatment with multiple disease-modifying antirheumatic drugs in rheumatoid arthritis: A preventive strategy. Ann Intern Med 131:768–774, 1999.
19. Scott DL: Prognostic factors in early rheumatoid arthritis. Rheum 39(Suppl):24–29, 2000.
20. van Everdingen AA, Jacobs JWG, van Reesema DRS, Bijlsma JWJ: Low dose prednisone therapy for patients with early active rheumatoid arthritis: Clinical efficacy, disease-modifying properties and side effects. Ann Int Med 136:1–12, 2002.


# 20. SYSTEMIC LUPUS ERYTHEMATOSUS

*Brian* L. *Kotzin*, M.D.

**1. Who is the typical patient with systemic lupus erythematosus (SLE)?**

The typical patient is a female between the ages of 15 and 45 years. Although SLE can occur at nearly any age, the incidence of disease clearly increases in women of child-bearing age. The female-to-male ratio during these ages may be > 8:1, but during childhood or after the menopause, the ratio is closer to 2:1. This pattern strongly suggests that sex hormones influence the probability of developing or expressing SLE, a conclusion that is supported by studies in animal models of lupus. It should be emphasized that although males develop disease less frequently, their illness is not milder than in females. Also, the incidence of SLE is about 2 to 4 times greater in blacks and Hispanics than in whites in the United States.

**2. Describe the criteria used in the classification of SLE.**

Any person having 4 or more of the following 11 criteria, serially or simultaneously, during any interval of observation is considered to have SLE for the purposes of clinical studies (> 90% sensitivity and specificity).

| CRITERION | DEFINITION |
|---|---|
| 1. Malar rash | Fixed erythema, flat or raised over the malar eminences, tending to spare the nasolabial folds |
| 2. Discoid rash | Erythematous raised patches with adherent keratotic scaling and follicular plugging; atrophic scarring may occur in older lesions |
| 3. Photosensitivity | Skin rash as a result of unusual reaction to sunlight, by patient history or physician observation |
| 4. Oral ulcers | Oral or nasopharyngeal ulceration, usually painless, observed by a physician |
| 5. Arthritis | Nonerosive arthritis involving two or more peripheral joints, characterized by tenderness, swelling, or effusion |
| 6. Serositis | Pleuritis: convincing history of pleuritic pain or rub heard by physician or evidence of pleural effusion, *or*<br>Pericarditis documented by EKG or rub or evidence of pericardial effusion |
| 7. Renal disorder | Persistent proteinuria >0.5 gm/day or >3+ if quantitation not performed, *or*<br>Cellular casts (red cell, hemoglobin, granular, tubular, or mixed) |
| 8. Neurologic disorder | Seizures in the absence of offending drugs or known metabolic derangements, e.g., uremia, ketoacidosis, or electrolyte imbalance, *or*<br>Psychosis in the absence of offending drugs or known metabolic derangements, e.g., uremia, ketoacidosis, or electrolyte imbalance |
| 9. Hematologic disorder | Hemolytic anemia with reticulocytosis, *or*<br>Leukopenia < 4000/mm$^3$ total on two or more occasions, *or*<br>Lymphopenia < 1500/mm$^3$ on two or more occasions, *or*<br>Thrombocytopenia < 100,000/mm$^3$ in the absence of offending drugs |
| 10. Immunologic disorders | Positive LE cell preparation, *or*<br>Anti-DNA (antibody to native DNA in abnormal titer) *or*<br>Anti-Sm (presence of antibody to Sm nuclear antigen) *or*<br>* False-positive serologic test for syphilis known to be positive for at least 6 months and confirmed by TPI or FTA-ABS+ |
| 11. Antinuclear antibody(ANA) | An abnormal titer of ANA by immunofluorescence or an equivalent assay at any point in time and in the absence of drugs known to be associated with drug-induced lupus |

Adapted from Tan EM, et al: The 1982 revised criteria for the classification of systemic lupus erythematosus. Arthritis Rheum 25:1271, 1982.

* The Diagnostic and Therapeutic Criteria Committee of the American College of Rheumatology (ACR) has recommended that this criterion be replaced with a positive test for antiphospholipid antibodies (elevated serum level of anticardiolipin antibodies or positive test for lupus anticoagulant using a standard method).

+ TPI, *Treponema pallidum* immobilization test; FTA-ABS, fluorescent treponemal antibody absorption test.

**3. How do the criteria for the classification of SLE relate to making a diagnosis of SLE?**

Although these criteria are extremely helpful when considering the diagnosis of SLE for an individual patient, it should be emphasized that these criteria were designed for classification and not diagnosis. Especially for mild cases and patients with early disease, the classification criteria may not be sensitive for making the diagnosis. For example, a patient with a classic malar rash and a high positive test for ANA almost certainly has SLE, and yet would not satisfy the classification criteria. Similarly, a patient with glomerulonephritis, elevated anti-DNA antibodies, and a positive ANA almost certainly has SLE.

**4. What is the evidence that heredity is important in the development of SLE?**

The best evidence that SLE is genetically determined is from studies of familial aggregation (i.e., an increased frequency of persons with SLE in the same family). For example, an identical twin of a patient with SLE may have a 1 in 4 chance of developing the disease, but this risk is much less if the affected twin was nonidentical (risk~2 to 5%). Still, this latter risk is much greater than that in the general population (~1 in 1000 for white females). Population-based studies have also shown that susceptibility to SLE, like other autoimmune diseases in humans, is linked to particular class II genes of the major histocompatibility complex (HLA) in humans. Additional evidence comes from animal models of lupus in which mice can be bred to develop lupus-like autoantibody production and disease.

**5. What is the laboratory hallmark of SLE?**

ANA. Greater than 98% of patients with SLE demonstrate elevated serum levels of ANA, which is considered to be the laboratory hallmark of this disease. This test, however, is not specific for SLE.

**6. How is a screening test for ANA usually performed in a clinical laboratory?**

An indirect immunofluorescence test is the most common assay used to detect ANA. The patient's serum is diluted and then layered onto a slide on which either tissue or cells have been fixed. After any unbound antibodies are washed off, a fluorescein-tagged antibody reagent directed to human immunoglobulin is added as a secondary reagent. Any antibodies (from the patient) bound to the nucleus will be stained, and the nucleus will fluoresce when viewed under a fluorescence microscope. The results are registered as positive or negative and the strength of a positive reaction at particular serum dilutions. In many laboratories, the highest dilution of serum giving a positive reaction is commonly recorded as the test result. Frequently, serum dilutions begin at about 1:40, and a dilution of at least 1:80 may be required to consider a test significantly positive.

The ANA test is not specific for the diagnosis of SLE or rheumatic disease. In a recent study of 15 international laboratories, the frequency of a positive ANA in healthy individuals was 32% at a 1:40 serum dilution and 13% at 1:80. Less than 1 in 40 people with a positive test at 1:80 will have SLE. False-positive reactions also increase with age. It is emphasized that SLE is a clinical diagnosis supported by a positive ANA test. Since almost all patients with SLE have a positive ANA test, a negative ANA at 1:40 or 1:80 is an excellent screening test result to strongly suggest that the diagnosis is not SLE. A positive test at titers above 1:160 and tests for specific types of ANA (see below) provide the best laboratory support for the diagnosis of SLE.

The laboratory also reports a pattern of nuclear staining (rim, diffuse, speckled, or nucleolar). The peripheral or rim pattern (corresponding to autoantibodies to deoxynucleoproteins) is the most specific pattern for SLE, whereas a speckled pattern, which is the most common pattern in both SLE and other diseases, is the least specific. Patterns have less significance today because a positive test is usually followed up with an ANA profile, which tests for specific types of autoantibodies including those highly specific for SLE. (See figure, top of next page.)

**7. Which ANAs are most specific for the diagnosis of SLE?**

The screening ANA test is fairly nonspecific in that patients with other rheumatic diseases (Sjögren's, MCTD, scleroderma, RA, polymyositis) or other types of inflammatory disorders (autoimmune hepatitis, hepatitis C, lymphoma, IPF) may also be positive. Certain ANA are more specific for the diagnosis of SLE, especially antibodies to double-stranded (ds) DNA and to the Sm antigen. The higher the levels of antibodies to these nuclear antigens, the greater the specificity for SLE.

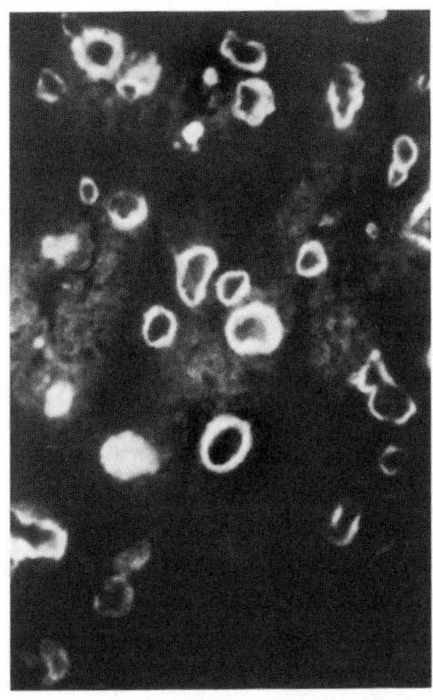

Indirect immunofluorescence test demonstrating a positive rim pattern.

**8. List the most common autoantibodies found in SLE and some of their major clinical associations.**

*Autoantibodies in SLE and Some of Their Clinical Associations*

| TARGET | CLINICAL ASSOCIATIONS |
|---|---|
| dsDNA | High diagnostic specificity for SLE<br>Correlation with disease activity (esp. activity of lupus nephritis) |
| ssDNA | Low diagnostic specificity |
| Histones<br>(H1, H2A, H2B, H3, H4) | SLE and drug-induced lupus |
| Sm (SnRNP core proteins<br>B, B', D, E) | High diagnostic specificity for SLE<br>No correlation with disease activity |
| U1-RNP (SnRNP specific proteins<br>A, C, 70-kDa) | Mixed connective tissue disease /related overlap syndrome<br>(when not accompanied by anti-Sm antibodies) |
| Ro/SS-A<br>(60-kDa and 52-kDa proteins) | Neonatal lupus (with anti-SS-B/La)<br>Photosensitivity<br>Subacute cutaneous lupus |
| La/SS-B (48-kDa protein) | Neonatal lupus (with anti-SS-A/Ro)<br>Associated Sjögren's syndrome |
| Ku | Diagnostic specificity for SLE |
| Proliferating cell nuclear antigen<br>(PCNA)/cyclin) | High diagnostic specificity for SLE |
| Ribosomal P proteins | High diagnostic specificity for SLE<br>Cytoplasmic staining<br>Psychiatric disease |
| Phospholipids<br>(β2-glycoprotein 1) | Inhibition of in vitro coagulation tests (lupus anticoagulant)<br>Thrombosis<br>Recurrent abortions/fetal wasting<br>Neurologic disease (focal presentations)<br>Thrombocytopenia |

(*Table continued on next page.*)

*Autoantibodies in SLE and Some of Their Clinical Associations (cont.)*

| TARGET | CLINICAL ASSOCIATIONS |
|---|---|
| Cell surface antigens | |
| Red blood cells | Hemolytic anemia |
| Platelets | Thrombocytopenia |
| Lymphocytes | Lymphopenia |
| Neuronal cells | Neurologic disease (diffuse presentations) |

RNP, ribonucleoprotein.

**9. Describe four different types of rash associated with SLE.**

1. **Malar or butterfly rash**. The malar rash typifies acute photosensitive rashes in SLE and indicates that the patient has active systemic disease. The rash extends from the cheeks over the bridge of the nose and spares the nasolabial folds. It can be macular but is usually erythematous and raised with papules and/or plaques. These lesions heal without scarring. Other causes of red face must be excluded, including rosacea, seborrhea, contact dermatitis, atopic dermatitis, and actinic dermatitis.

2. **Acute photosensitive rashes elsewhere**. Many of the acute rashes in SLE are related to photosensitivity and therefore are more likely to occur in sun-exposed areas. These rashes have similar characteristics to the malar rash, including healing without scarring. UV-B (290–320 nm) > UV-A (320–400 nm) light is a problem for SLE patients. Sunscreens block UV-B and short wave UV-A light. Only clothing blocks long wave UV-A light. Glass blocks UV-B but not UV-A.

3. **Subacute LE**. These raised erythematous lesions are also commonly related to sun exposure and are frequently associated with antibodies to Ro/SS-A. Rash occurs on chest, back, and outer arms but tends to spare midfacial areas. The lesions are symmetric, nonfixed, and can be annular or serpiginous, sometimes with central areas of scaling. These lesions usually heal without scarring but can leave areas of depigmentation, which can be especially prominent in dark-skinned individuals. May have negative lupus band test on biopsy.

4. **Discoid LE**. These lesions may begin as erythematous papules or plaques and evolve into larger, coin-shaped (discoid), chronic lesions with central areas of epithelial thinning and atrophy and with follicular plugging and damage. Lesions can expand with active erythematous inflammation at the periphery, leaving depressed central scarring, depigmentation, and patches of alopecia. Discoid lesions frequently leave scars after healing. The most affected skin areas include the face (85%), scalp (50%), ears (50%), neck, and extensor surfaces of the arms. Some patients can have prolonged discoid disease and not develop systemic disease. However, about 15 to 30% of patients with SLE demonstrate discoid disease at some time in their disease course. On biopsy, discoid lesions typically have inflammation around skin appendages (hair follicles, etc.) and vacuolization at the dermal-epidermal junction. A positive lupus band test with immune reactants (IgG, IgM, C3 > IgA, fibrin) at the dermal-epidermal junction is also characteristic.

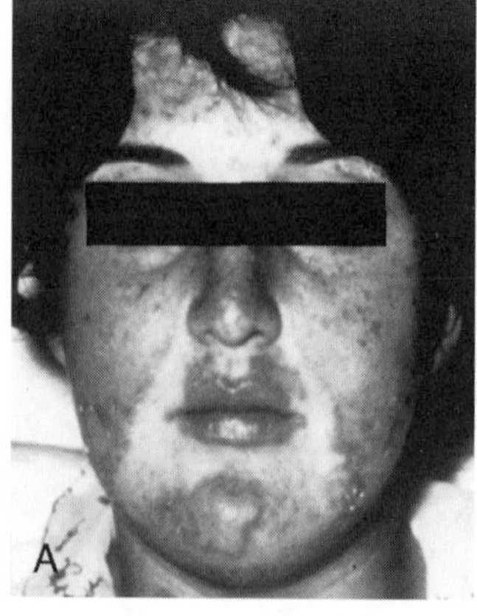


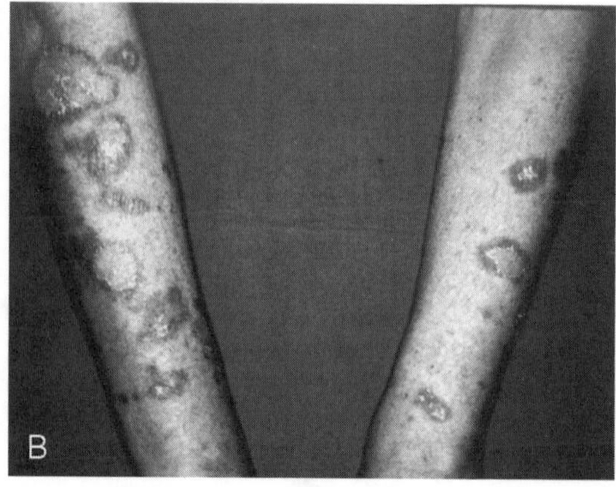

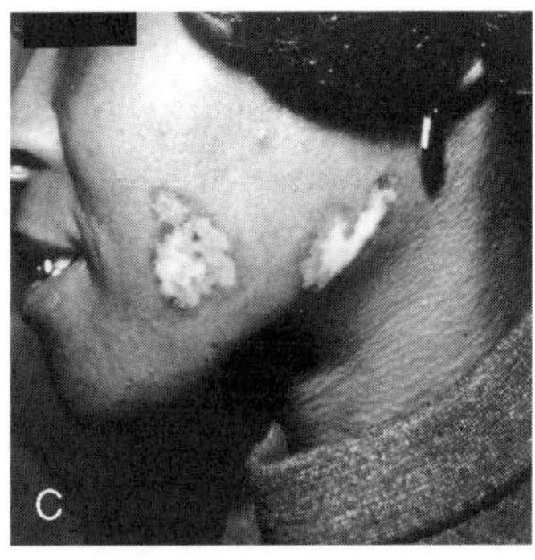


Rashes associated with SLE. *A*, Malar rash. *B*, Subacute cutaneous. *C*, Discoid. (From the Revised Clinical Slide Collection on the Rheumatic Diseases. Atlanta. American College of Rheumatology. 1991; with permission.)

Less common rashes include bullous lesions, palpable purpura secondary to small vessel vasculitis, urticaria that may also be related to small vessel vasculitis, panniculitis with subcutaneous nodules, and livedo reticularis frequently associated with anti-phospholipid antibodies.

**10. Which type of hand rash strongly suggests the diagnosis of SLE?**

The rash on the left is almost pathognomonic for SLE. There are erythematous lesions over the dorsum of the hands and fingers, affecting the skin *between* the joints. In contrast, the right panel shows lesions *over* the MCP and PIP joints, and this rash (Gottron's papules) is characteristic of dermatomyositis.

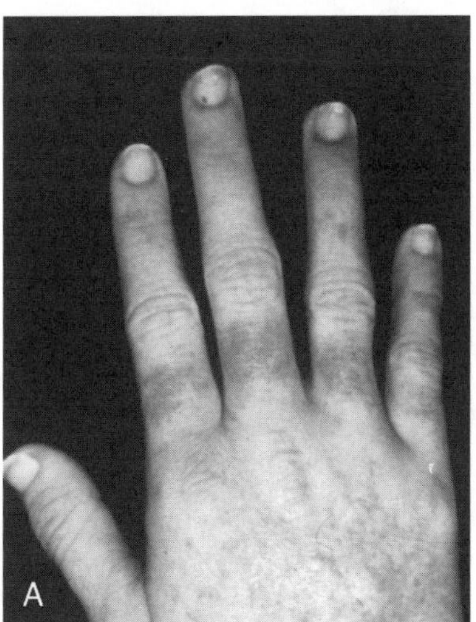


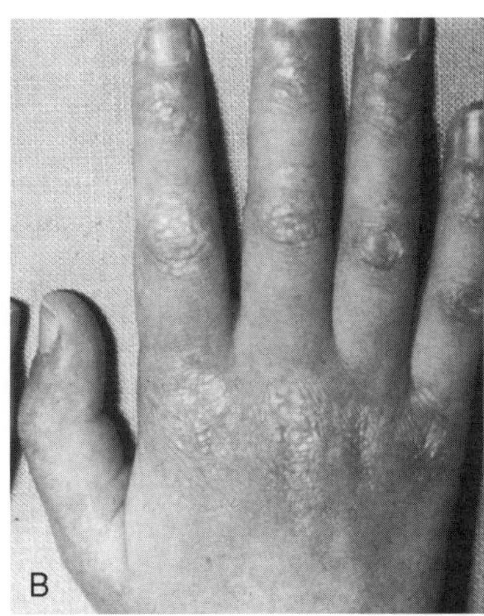


Hand rash. (From the Revised Clinical Slide Collection on the Rheumatic Diseases. Atlanta. American College of Rheumatology. 1991: with permission.)

**11. Name three causes of alopecia in the setting of SLE.**

1. Active systemic disease can result in diffuse alopecia, which is reversible once disease activity is controlled.
2. Discoid disease results in patchy hair loss corresponding to the distribution of discoid skin lesions. This hair loss is permanent because the hair follicles are damaged by the inflammation.
3. Drugs such as cyclophosphamide can result in diffuse hair loss, which is reversible after therapy is discontinued and disease activity decreases.

**12. What therapies are recommended for the skin lesions occurring in SLE patients?**

**General**

- Avoid sun: clothing, sunscreens (Shade Gel SPF 30 or equivalent, no PABA), avoid hot part of day with most UV-B light (10:00 a.m.–4:00 p.m.), camouflage cosmetics
- Stop smoking so antimalarials work better
- Thiazides and sulfonylureals may exacerbate skin disease

**Routine therapy**

- Topical steroids, intralesional steroids
- Hydroxychloroquine
- Oral corticosteroids
- Dapsone for bullous lesions

**Advanced therapy for resistant causes**

- Subacute cutaneous lupus—mycophenylate mofetil, retinoids, or cyclosporine
- Discoid lesions—chloroquine ± quinacrine, clofazimine (Lamprene), thalidomide, or cyclosporine
- Lupus profundus—dapsone
- Chronic lesions over > 50% of body—topical nitrogen mustard, BCNU, or tacrolimus
- Vasculitis—may need immunosuppressives

**13. You are caring for a patient with SLE who has arthritis and complains of severe joint pains. What is the likelihood that this patient will develop severe deformities of her hands?**

The arthritis associated with SLE is rarely erosive or destructive of bone and therefore is quite different from rheumatoid arthritis. Joint deformities are unusual and, when they occur, are secondary to ligament loosening rather than cartilage and bone destruction. Occasionally, SLE patients demonstrate ulnar deviation and swan-neck deformities of the hands (called Jaccoud's arthritis).

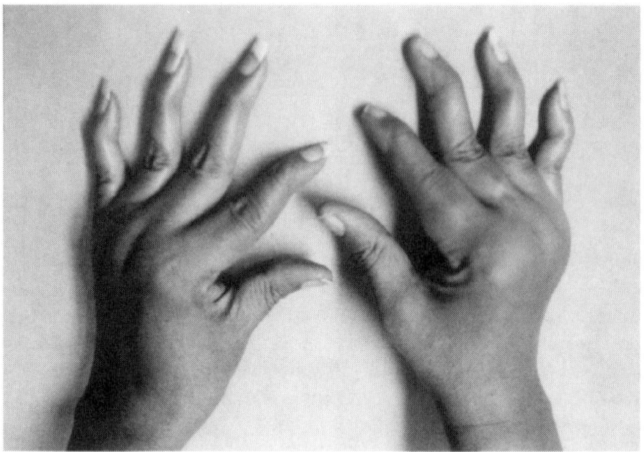

Swan-neck deformities in SLE, which are reversible.

**14. What are the best approaches for therapy in an SLE patient with arthritis who has no evidence of internal organ involvement?**

The first line of therapy is NSAIDs. Cycloxoygenase-2 specific inhibitors may be used but may contribute to thrombotic risk in patients with antiphospholipid antibodies. Patients can also benefit remarkably from antimalarial drugs, usually given in the form of low doses of daily oral hydroxychloroquine (200 mg twice a day).

**15. Identify five manifestations of lupus that warrant high-dose corticosteroid therapy.**

The most common problems that warrant this therapy include:

1. Severe lupus nephritis

2. CNS lupus with severe manifestations
3. Autoimmune thrombocytopenia with extremely low platelet counts (e.g., < 30,000/mm$^3$)
4. Autoimmune hemolytic anemia
5. Acute pneumonitis caused by SLE

Additional problems that may warrant aggressive corticosteroid therapy (with doses ≥ 60 mg/day in an adult) include severe vasculitis with visceral organ involvement, serious complications that result from serositis (pleuritis, pericarditis, or peritonitis), and sometimes severe systemic disease. It is important to emphasize that several problems in SLE should not be treated with high doses of corticosteroids (i.e., lupus arthritis, skin rashes, etc.).

**16. How does WHO classify the different pathologic forms of lupus nephritis?**

| CLASS | DESCRIPTION |
|---|---|
| I | Normal |
| II | Mesangial nephritis |
| III | Focal proliferative glomerulonephritis |
| IV | Diffuse proliferative glomerulonephritis |
| V | Membranous nephropathy |
| VI | Advanced sclerosing glomerulonephritis |

Overall, the World Health Organization (WHO) histological scheme correlates with clinical severity and prognosis in patients with lupus nephritis. However, it has been emphasized that knowledge of the WHO histological type of renal disease may add little clinically useful information over and above what is already known from clinical laboratory studies (urinalysis, protein excretion, and especially renal function studies).

When interpreting histological findings in lupus nephritis, keep in mind that the renal biopsy is only a reflection of what is going on currently in the kidney and that changes from one pathologic stage to another over time are well documented in patients with lupus nephritis. In patients biopsied a second time, up to 40% have undergone a change to another WHO class.

**17. Describe the key histologic findings of the various pathologic forms of lupus nephritis and their clinical implications.**

**Mesangial nephritis** (WHO class II) is characterized by immune deposits in the mesangium that are best seen by immunofluorescence and electron microscopy. Biopsies that are normal on light microscopy are designated as WHO class IIA. Class IIB designates biopsies that show mesangial hypercellularity and/or increased matrix on light microscopy. Deposits in the capillary loops are not apparent in this class of disease. Patients with mesangial nephritis usually demonstrate little clinical evidence of renal involvement, with normal or near-normal urinalysis and renal function, and rarely require any treatment for their renal disease.

**Focal proliferative glomerulonephritis** (WHO class III) is characterized histologically by hypercellularity due to increases in mesangial, endocapillary, and/or infiltrating cells. These changes result in encroachment of the glomerular capillary space. Active inflammatory lesions are present, often in a segmental pattern (i.e., involving only one area of a glomerulus) and involving < 50% of the glomeruli. Immune complex deposits are present in the capillary loops. Patients with this pattern usually demonstrate proteinuria and hematuria, but severe (nephrotic range) proteinuria or progressive loss of renal function is less common than with diffuse disease. Focal proliferative nephritis should be viewed on a continuum with diffuse disease because the lesions are qualitatively similar but less extensive. Up to one third of patients with focal proliferative nephritis will progress to diffuse proliferative disease.

**Diffuse proliferative glomerulonephritis (DPGN)** (WHO class IV) is seen in most SLE patients who progress to renal failure. DPGN is characterized by involvement of > 50% of the glomeruli, with generalized hypercellularity of mesangial and endothelial cells. Inflammatory cellular infiltrates and areas of necrosis are common. These changes may ultimately lead to obliteration of the capillary loops and sclerosis. Regions of basement membrane thickening are also present. Immunofluorescence microscopy demonstrates extensive deposition (full house pattern) of immunoglobulin (IgG, IgM, IgA) and complement (C3, C1q) in the mesangium and capillary loops, and electron microscopy frequently shows immune complex deposits in both subendothelial and subepithelial distributions. Clinically, patients almost always have proteinuria (frequently nephrotic) and hematuria and, not infrequently, decreases in renal function. Hypertension is common.

**Membranous nephropathy** (WHO class V) is characterized histologically by diffuse thickening of the basement membrane. Glomeruli usually have normal cellularity. Deposits containing immunoglobulin and complement are apparent along the basement membrane on electron microscopy and immunofluorescence microscopy. Clinically, patients who have pure membranous disease frequently have extensive proteinuria but only minimal hematuria or renal functional abnormalities. A subset of patients (10 to 30%) slowly progress to chronic renal failure within a 10-year period. Membranous disease can also be observed as a transition stage after treatment for proliferative glomerulonephritis.

**18. In the analysis of a renal biopsy from a patient with SLE, what criteria are used in the *activity* and *chronicity* indices?**

*Pathologic Indices of Activity and Chronicity*

| CHRONICITY INDEX | ACTIVITY INDEX |
|---|---|
| Glomerular sclerosis | Cellular proliferation |
| Fibrous crescents | Fibrinoid necrosis |
| Tubular atrophy | Cellular crescents |
| Interstitial fibrosis | Hyaline thrombi |
| | Leukocyte infiltration in glomerulus |
| | Mononuclear cell infiltration in interstitium |

To obtain a **chronicity score**, each parameter is graded 0 to 3 depending on severity of involvement, and the grades are added. Glomerular sclerosis and fibrous crescents are graded as follows: 0, absent; 1+, < 25% of glomeruli involved; 2+, 25 to 50% of glomeruli involved; 3+, > 75% of glomeruli involved. Tubular atrophy and interstitial fibrosis are graded as follows: 0, absent; 1+, mild; 2+, moderate; 3+, severe. The maximal chronicity score is 12.

To obtain an **activity score**, each parameter is graded 0 to 3 depending on the severity of involvement, and the individual grades are added. Fibrinoid necrosis and cellular crescents have been given a "weighting" factor of 2. The maximal activity score is 24.

**19. What is the importance of evaluating biopsies for the extent of chronic damage?**

The histologic scoring systems for lupus nephritis using chronicity and activity indexes have been developed in an effort to more accurately predict renal outcome and to help determine which patients are most likely to benefit from aggressive therapy. The **chronicity index** measures four histologic components of chronic *irreversible* renal damage, and the **activity index** measures six histologic components of activity of lupus nephritis.

In the last several years, these systems have come into major use, as a number of studies have reported on their predictive associations and usefulness. Most, but not all, studies have found that a higher chronicity index is associated with greater risk for progression to renal failure. Based on its apparent validity as a prognostic indicator as well as the fact that the presence of chronic damage identifies disease with destructive potential, several investigators have recommended the use of the chronicity index as a guide to the aggressiveness of therapy. In particular, treatment with agents such as cyclophosphamide was predicted to be most beneficial for patients with intermediate chronicity index scores.

In contrast to the chronicity index, the validity of the activity index as a predictor of renal outcome is less clear; approximately half of these studies have shown that a higher score correlates with increased risk of renal failure. This may relate to the caveat that active lesions are amenable to therapy, whereas chronic lesions represent irreversible destruction. It seems likely that the activity index also identifies patients most likely to respond to aggressive treatment.

**20. Which serologic tests are most useful when following a patient with lupus nephritis?**

Only one ANA has been shown to correlate with the activity of lupus nephritis, antibodies to dsDNA. Therefore, serial monitoring should be limited to tests that specifically quantitate anti-dsDNA antibodies. In addition, patients with active lupus nephritis have decreased levels of complement components (e.g., C3 and C4) as well as total hemolytic complement ($CH_{50}$), which also correlate with the activity of renal disease. Remember that many SLE patients have partial C4 deficiency and may always have a low C4 level.

**21. What is the evidence that anti-dsDNA antibodies are important in the pathogenesis of lupus nephritis?**

IgG antibodies directed to dsDNA appear to play a prominent role in lupus nephritis. The evidence for this includes:

1. Detection of anti-dsDNA antibodies in the glomeruli of patients and animals with active disease
2. Studies showing enrichment of IgG anti-dsDNA antibodies in glomerular tissues relative to serum and other organs
3. Longitudinal studies in a subset of SLE patients demonstrating that high levels of circulating anti-dsDNA antibodies frequently precede or coincide with active glomerulonephritis
4. Demonstration in animals that injection of certain monoclonal IgG anti-dsDNA antibodies or expression of genes that encode pathogenic IgG anti-dsDNA activity can lead to glomerular pathology

It should be emphasized that the correlation of anti-dsDNA autoantibody levels with the extent of renal damage is a general one. For example, numerous studies have shown that glomerulonephritis in SLE can occur in the absence of elevated serum levels of anti-DNA antibodies. Although these cases may represent a failure of the sensitivity of currently available techniques to detect anti-DNA antibodies, it also suggests that in some cases, autoantibodies directed to non-DNA antigens may participate in renal damage in lupus nephritis.

**22. What are the proposed mechanisms by which anti-dsDNA antibodies cause glomerulonephritis in SLE?**

Anti-DNA antibodies do not appear to mediate renal damage in SLE through the deposition of circulating immune complexes. Even in patients with active glomerulonephritis or animal models with actively increasing amounts of anti-DNA antibodies in the glomerulus, DNA-anti-DNA complexes have been difficult to demonstrate in the circulation. Thus, two alternative theories have been proposed to explain the pathogenic mechanisms of these antibodies.

In the first, DNA-anti-DNA complexes are proposed to form in the glomerulus (in-situ complex formation) rather than being deposited from the blood. Evidence supports a model in which DNA or chromatin first binds to the glomerulus and is then recognized and bound by anti-DNA antibodies. It is of interest that increased amounts of circulating DNA have been detected in the blood of patients with SLE. The circulating nuclear material, resembling nucleosomes, could thus become the planted renal target for a subset of pathogenic anti-DNA antibodies.

In an alternative model, the subset of pathogenic anti-DNA antibodies have been hypothesized to cross-react with glomerular antigens that are not DNA in origin. This model is supported by data showing that anti-DNA antibodies do contain other specificities and can bind to different glomerular structures.

The activation of complement components through the classical pathway, with amplification by the alternative pathway, appears to be involved in the pathogenesis of glomerular damage.

Complement activation may cause direct damage as well as recruit inflammatory cells to the sites of immune complexes. Based on this scheme, IgG anti-DNA antibodies that are complement-fixing are likely to be more pathogenic.

**23. What are some of the prognostic indicators of a good or poor prognosis in a SLE patients with DPGN?**

| GOOD INDICATORS | POOR INDICATORS |
|---|---|
| White race | Black race |
| Baseline Cr < 1.4 mg/dl | Hypertension |
| Activity index < 12 | Increase in Cr of 0.3 mg/dl or doubling of proteinuria over baseline after 4 weeks of therapy |
| Chronicity index < 4 | Doubling of baseline creatinine at any time |
| Normalization of creatinine and decrease in proteinuria to less than 1 gram/day by 6 months of therapy. | Persistent nephrotic range proteinuria |
| Stabilize creatinine and decrease proteinuria to less than 2 grams/day | Crescents > 50% of glomeruli |
| | High chronicity index |

**24. What is the first-line of therapy for patients with severe lupus nephritis?**

Previously untreated patients with active lupus nephritis and severe clinical manifestations (i.e., decreasing renal function and/or high-grade proteinuria) first receive high doses of corticosteroids. An attempt should be made to control disease activity quickly. The initial dose of the most commonly used drug, **prednisone**, should be approximately 1 mg/kg/day (~60 to 80 mg/day) in three divided doses. It may take several weeks to achieve control of active nephritis.

**25. When are cytotoxic drugs indicated in the treatment of lupus nephritis?**

The toxicity of continuous high-dose corticosteroid therapy is cumulative and severe. If a 6- to 8-week course of high-dose prednisone has not restored serum creatinine levels to normal or the proteinuria continues at > 1 gm/day, a renal biopsy can be done to determine whether glomerular sclerosis, fibrous crescents, and irreversible tubulointerstitial changes are present. If these poor prognostic indicators are observed, especially with evidence of continued activity, the addition of cytotoxic drugs or other immunosuppressive modalities should be considered.

The use of cytotoxic drugs in the treatment of lupus nephritis should be reserved for the subgroup of patients with severe, refractory disease. These include (1) patients with evidence of active and severe glomerulonephritis despite treatment with high-dose prednisone; (2) patients who have responded to corticosteroids but who require an unacceptably high dose to maintain a response; and (3) patients with unacceptable side effects from corticosteroids. In addition, as discussed in an earlier question, evidence of chronic damage on a renal biopsy and other indicators of a poor prognosis may suggest the need for early introduction of cytotoxic drug therapy.

**26. Which cytotoxic agents are most frequently used?**

Oral azathioprine (or 6-mercaptopurine if nausea on azathioprine), oral cyclophosphamide, or intermittent intravenous cyclophosphamide. Daily oral chlorambucil has been used occasionally as an alternative to cyclophosphamide. Mycophenylate mofetil or cyclosporine has also been used, especially in membranous glomerulonephritis. Each of these drugs are given in association with a dose of prednisone (usually 0.5 mg/kg/day) required to control extrarenal manifestations. Cytotoxic drugs in combination with prednisone have been shown to prevent progression to renal failure in some patients more effectively than prednisone alone. However, because of potentially severe toxicity, overall improvements in mortality have been more difficult to demonstrate.

**27. Are there any advantages of intermittent intravenous cyclophosphamide compared with daily oral cyclophosphamide therapy in the treatment of lupus nephritis?**

There are two major ways to use cyclophosphamide (Cytoxan) in the treatment of SLE patients with severe manifestations such as severe lupus nephritis:

1. Daily oral therapy with doses of ~1.0 to 2.0 mg/kg/day
2. Monthly boluses of 0.5 to 1.0 gm/m$^2$ given intravenously (iv) with vigorous hydration

The major advantage of intermittent IV cyclophosphamide relates to a markedly decreased incidence of bladder damage and hemorrhagic cystitis. Theoretically, IV therapy also appears to work more rapidly than continuous oral treatment. There is not much evidence to suggest that the IV regimen is actually more efficacious than oral cyclophosphamide, although trends have been seen in some controlled trials.

**28. Describe a protocol for using monthly IV cyclophosphamide.**

There are many different protocols that can be used. The following is one example:

**Prior to cyclophosphamide**

- Premedication 15–30 minutes prior to cyclophosphamide—dexamethasone 10 mg, lorazepam 1 mg, and ondansetron (Zofran) 8 mg or ganisetron (Kytril) 1 mg in 100 cc normal saline intravenously
- Mesna (25% of cyclophosphamide dose in milligrams) in 500 cc normal saline.

**Cyclophosphamide infusion**

- Cyclophosphamide 0.75 grams/m$^2$ of body surface area in 1000 cc normal saline for initial dose. If creatinine clearance less than 35–40 cc/min, then decrease initial dose to 0.50 grams/m$^2$ of BSA.
- Subsequent monthly doses depend on white blood cell (WBC) counts at 10 to 14 days post cyclophosphamide.
  - If nadir < 3000/mm$^3$, reduce dose by 0.25 gm/m$^2$.
  - If nadir > 4000/mm$^3$ dose can be increased if necessary to maximum of 1 gm/m$^2$.

**Post cyclophosphamide infusion**

- Mesna (25% of cyclophosphamide dose in mg) in 500 cc normal saline
- Compazine SR 15 mg BID for 2–3 days

**Dose interval for cyclophosphamide**

- Monthly for 6 doses, *then*
- Every 2 months for 3 doses, *then*
- Every 3 months for 4 doses, *then*
- Maintenance with azathioprine or mycophenylate mofetil.

**29. A 30-year-old woman with severe nephritis and end-stage renal failure is referred for further evaluation and treatment. The patient, who has been on dialysis for nearly 5 years, is being considered for transplantation but is afraid that her lupus will just destroy the donor kidney. She asks for your opinion.**

Approximately 20 to 30% of patients with severe lupus nephritis will progress over a 10-year follow-up period to end-stage renal disease, and lupus nephritis accounts for up to 3% of cases of end-stage renal failure requiring dialysis or transplantation. For unclear reasons, SLE patients with progressive renal failure and those on dialysis frequently demonstrate a decrease in nonrenal clinical manifestations of active SLE as well as a decrease in serologic markers of active disease. In SLE patients with absent or minimal disease activity, the clinical course and survival on dialysis compare favorably with those of other patient groups. Although controversial, it has been recommended that SLE patients should wait 6 to 12 months on dialysis prior to transplantation. With time, SLE patients appear to be excellent candidates for transplantation, and the recurrence of active lupus nephritis in the transplant is unusual (< 10%). However, recent follow-up studies have suggested that renal allograft survival in SLE patients is lower compared with most other patient groups.

**30. List the manifestations of CNS involvement in SLE.**

CNS involvement can be either diffuse or focal. Manifestations of diffuse disease include intractable headaches, generalized seizures, aseptic meningitis, organic brain syndrome, psychiatric disease (especially psychosis and severe depression), and coma. Manifestations of focal disease include stroke syndromes such as hemiparesis, focal seizures, movement disorders such as chorea, and transverse myelitis.

**31. Name three types of autoantibodies that have been associated with CNS involvement in SLE.**

1. Serum anti-phospholipid antibodies associated with focal neurologic manifestations in CNS lupus.
2. Cerebrospinal fluid anti-neuronal antibodies associated with diffuse manifestations of CNS lupus.
3. Serum antibodies to ribosomal P proteins (anti-P antibodies) associated with psychiatric problems (severe depression and psychosis) in SLE.

**32. How does SLE cause CNS involvement?**

CNS lupus (also referred to as neuropsychiatric lupus erythematosus) with **diffuse** manifestations appears to be primarily caused by autoantibodies directed to neuronal cells or their products. These autoantibodies are hypothesized to affect neuronal function in a generalized manner. Studies suggest that increased levels of inflammatory cytokines, induction of nitric oxide production, oxidative stress, and excitatory amino acid toxicity also may contribute to diffuse CNS dysfunction in SLE. Patients with organic brain syndrome frequently demonstrate elevated levels of anti-neuronal antibodies or other evidence of autoantibody production in the cerebrospinal fluid. As in multiple sclerosis, elevated levels of IgG and oligoclonal bands are markers of abnormal autoantibody production within the CNS and are frequently present in CNS lupus with diffuse manifestations. In patients with diffuse CNS lupus who present with primarily psychiatric disease, serum anti-P antibodies appear to be a helpful diagnostic marker.

CNS lupus with **focal** manifestations is most likely to be related to intravascular occlusion. MRI, which is much more sensitive than CT or brain scanning, almost always shows abnormalities characteristic of ischemic damage in these patients. Furthermore, these patients frequently demonstrate significantly elevated serum levels of anti-phospholipid antibodies (APAs), which are associated with intravascular occlusion. Less commonly, evidence of vasculitis is apparent. Cardiac emboli should always be ruled out with an echocardiogram.

**33. A 40-year-old woman with severe lupus nephritis has been treated with 60 mg of prednisone for the last 2 weeks but now seems disoriented and demonstrates bizarre behavior with delusional thinking. Describe the appropriate evaluation and treatment.**

The differential diagnosis for the change in behavior in this patient should include CNS lupus, prednisone-induced psychosis, and a separate problem such as infection or metabolic disturbance. First, the patient should be examined carefully, especially for evidence of active lupus, an organic brain syndrome (i.e., decreased intellectual function), and any additional neurologic (especially focal) deficits. Any positive neurologic findings would strongly suggest that the change in behavior was not directly caused by the high doses of prednisone.

Laboratory tests should exclude the possibility of a new metabolic problem and determine the activity of nephritis and/or other organ involvement. Studies directed at the CNS should include MRI, electroencephalogram (which should be normal in steroid-induced psychosis), and lumbar puncture (for standard tests such as cell count, protein level, and culture). In a patient on high doses of steroids, the possibility of infection must be considered and excluded. In addition, analysis of the cerebrospinal fluid should include tests for increased CNS IgG production, oligoclonal bands, and anti-neuronal antibodies. Serologic tests should include anti-P antibodies (which have been associated with psychosis caused by CNS lupus) as well as studies for the systemic activity of disease.

If the evaluation is negative, the most likely cause for the change in behavior is steroid-induced psychosis, and the appropriate treatment would be to decrease its dose. In contrast, evidence for CNS lupus would warrant therapy directed at the pathogenic process. This might include increasing the dose of steroids and/or adding a cytotoxic drug.

**34. In what ways can the heart be involved in SLE?**

Pericarditis
Myocarditis
Vasculitis
Secondary atherosclerotic coronary artery disease and myocardial infarction
Secondary hypertensive disease
Valvular disease—more frequent in patients with antiphospholipid antibodies

**35. In what ways can the lung be involved in SLE?**

Pleuritis
Acute lupus pneumonitis with or without pulmonary hemorrhage
Chronic interstitial lung disease and pulmonary fibrosis
Pulmonary hypertension
Pulmonary embolism, especially in patients with antiphospholipid antibodies
"Shrinking lung syndrome" (decreased lung volumes without parenchymal disease)
Secondary infection

**36. The hematocrit in a patient with SLE has been dropping over the last several months to a steady level of 31%. RBC indices are otherwise normal, as is the rest of the CBC. Recent medications have included prednisone (5 mg/day) and intermittent low doses of NSAIDs. What is the most likely cause for the anemia in this patient?**

The most likely cause is the so-called **anemia of chronic disease**, secondary to the persistent inflammation that occurs in SLE. The mechanisms of this type of anemia mostly relate to decreased production of red blood cells (RBCs) as well as slightly decreased RBC survival. There is an inability for iron to be handled normally by the reticuloendothelial system, and blood tests frequently disclose a low serum iron concentration as well as a low total iron-binding capacity. Ferritin is normal or elevated.

The evaluation in this patient should rule out the possibility of an autoimmune hemolytic anemia. This should include a reticulocyte count to determine (in conjunction with a stable hematocrit) whether there is active destruction of RBCs and possibly tests for autoantibodies to RBCs (direct Coombs tests). Remember, however, that many more SLE patients will have a positive Coombs test than a hemolytic anemia. The patient should also be evaluated for the possibility of gastrointestinal blood loss and iron deficiency related to the continued use of NSAIDs.

It is important to determine that the patient has the anemia of chronic disease because it implies ongoing inflammation, prompting careful follow-up of the patient. Patients demonstrating this form of anemia are more likely to demonstrate flares of lupus activity in the near future.

**37. A patient with SLE has a low WBC count of 2500/mm$^3$ (70% neutrophils, 20% lymphocytes, 8% monocytes, 2% eosinophils). Her prednisone has been tapered to 5 mg/day, and there are no clinical manifestations of active disease. A review of systems and the physical exam are negative, except for a mild malar rash. Laboratory tests show no evidence for lupus nephritis or other internal organ involvement. How do you evaluate and treat this leukopenia?**

This degree of leukopenia, which includes both a neutropenia and lymphopenia, is not uncommon in SLE and warrants no further evaluation or treatment. It is not associated with an increased risk of infection. It does imply continued disease activity, so the patient needs to be followed carefully.

**38. A 25-year-old woman with SLE has had difficulty with severe thrombocytopenia. Previous bone marrow biopsies showed increased numbers of megakaryocytes and no other abnormalities. Past therapy with high doses of corticosteroids has been successful in raising the platelet count to normal levels, but tapering to 20 mg/day has resulted in a progressive decline in platelet counts to < 20,000/mm$^3$. The patient is taking no other medications, and her physical examination is normal. Discuss the options for therapy in this patient.**

There are several therapeutic options to consider in this patient with autoimmune thrombocytopenia. One consideration would be **splenectomy**. If the patient had idiopathic thrombocytopenic purpura (ITP) without SLE, this would probably be recommended. However, the value of splenectomy in lupus-related thrombocytopenia has been debated, and its use is controversial. Some studies (retrospective and anecdotal) have suggested a high rate of failure in maintaining adequate platelet counts long-term. Other reports (equally anecdotal) maintain that splenectomy is as valuable a long-term therapy in SLE as it is in ITP. Considering that the patient has no other severe problems from SLE and is a young woman, splenectomy would be a reasonable option.

Another option is **danazol**, an androgen that increases platelet counts and allows the steroid dose to be decreased. Doses of 800 mg/day may be necessary, and the androgenic side effects in a young female may be troubling.

A separate option is the addition of an **immunosuppressive** or **cytotoxic drug** such as azathioprine. This addition will decrease platelet destruction and allow the prednisone dose to be tapered. Azathioprine is less toxic than cyclophosphamide, especially in terms of causing hemorrhagic cystitis, ovarian failure, and probably secondary lymphoma/leukemia, and would certainly be preferred in this setting.

On a separate note, high doses of **intravenous immunoglobulin** (IVIG) have been a very effective therapy to raise platelet counts acutely. For example, this treatment could be used in preparation for splenectomy or if the patient showed signs of bleeding. Because of its cost, however, repeated treatments with IVIG are not a reasonable long-term therapeutic option.

**39. A 25-year-old woman with SLE presents with fever, altered mental status, worsening renal function, hemolytic anemia, and thrombocytopenia. What is your next step?**

This patient has the five major manifestations of acute thrombotic thrombocytopenic purpura (TTP). Patients with SLE can develop TTP, which can be misdiagnosed as a flare of SLE. Making the correct diagnosis is essential so appropriate therapy can be instituted. The quickest way is to examine the peripheral blood smear for schistocytes, which will confirm a microangiopathic hemolytic anemia (Coombs negative) seen in TTP and rule out the Coombs positive autoimmune hemolytic anemia seen in SLE.

The etiology of TTP occurring in SLE may be similar to idiopathic TTP. Acute TTP recently has been found to be from IgG autoantibody against the metalloprotease responsible for cleavage of the monomeric subunits of von Willebrand factor. This allows for the accumulation of unusually large multimers of von Willebrand factors secreted by endothelial cells into the plasma. These multimers bind to platelet glycoprotein receptors, causing platelet adhesion and microthrombi. The treatment of acute TPP in SLE patients includes plasmapheresis to remove the autoantibody and large multimers of von Willebrand factor, followed by fresh frozen plasma to replace the metalloprotease. Antiplatelet agents, corticosteroids, and/or immunosuppressive drugs have been used, but are not as effective as plasmapheresis and plasma replacement. However, corticosteroids and immunosuppressives may be needed to prevent recurrence by suppressing autoantibody formation.

**40. What is the lupus anticoagulant? What are its clinical associations?**

Lupus anticoagulant refers to a subset of autoantibodies to phospholipids that interfere with certain clotting tests. It is usually picked up by an abnormally elevated partial thromboplastin time (PTT) and can be further demonstrated by specific clotting studies, such as the Russell viper venom test. Anti-phospholipid antibodies (APAs) can also be detected by a test for anti-cardiolipin antibodies, which have been shown to be mostly directed to β2-glycoprotein I (usually with bound phospholipid).

The term lupus anticoagulant is truly a misnomer, since the major clinical association of anti-phospholipid antibodies (APAs) is thrombosis (not bleeding), and these autoantibodies can occur (and are even more common) in the absence of SLE. Disease from these autoantibodies is referred to as the **primary anti-phospholipid antibody syndrome** (see Chapter 27). Complications associated with APAs include arterial and venous thrombosis, miscarriage and fetal wastage, thrombocytopenia, livedo reticularis, and autoimmune hemolytic anemia. APAs and their complications are a major issue in the care of patients with SLE. The mechanism by which these antibodies cause these complications is unknown.

**41. A 25-year-old woman with severe SLE on prednisone and azathioprine complains of progressive right hip pain located in the groin for the past month. She denies fever and chills. She has good range of motion of the hip with some pain. What is your next step?**

Although septic arthritis is always a concern, this presentation is worrisome for osteonecrosis of the hip (see Chapter 58). Patients with SLE are more prone to develop osteonecrosis than patients with other disease states treated with corticosteroids. Patients who become cushingoid on steroids, who have antiphospholipid antibodies, and those treated with greater than 20 mg of prednisone are at increased risk. The femoral head and knee are involved more than other joint areas. Evaluation should start with a radiograph followed by a magnetic resonance imaging (MRI). Both hips should be done even if only one is symptomatic, since the contralateral femoral head is involved in 50% of cases. In patients with greater than 25% of the femoral head involved, without bony collapse, core decompression should be considered. All patients put on corticosteroids should be warned about this complication and documented in the chart, since this is a major cause of malpractice claims.

**42. In a SLE patient who is pregnant, which lupus-related autoantibodies can cause problems for the fetus?**

Antibodies to **Ro/SSA**, especially when in conjunction with antibodies to **La/SS-B** (25–70%), have been associated with the neonatal lupus syndrome. The major manifestation of this complication is congenital heart block, which is frequently severe and abrupt and may require a cardiac pacemaker. A neonatal rash may also be part of this syndrome. Anti-Ro/SSA antibodies inhibit inward L-type calcium currents of cardiocytes, which may explain damage to the atrioventricular node leading to complete heart block. The sinoatrial node can also be involved.

**Anti-phospholipid antibodies** have been associated with recurrent spontaneous abortion and stillbirths (fetal wastage). One hypothesis for this complication is intravascular thrombosis and placental insufficiency.

**Anti-platelet antibodies** can occasionally cause autoimmune thrombocytopenia in the fetus with associated hemorrhage, especially at the time of delivery. The management of this complication can be difficult.

**43. How often will a SLE patient who has antibodies to Ro/SSA deliver a baby with neonatal lupus syndrome?**

SLE patients with anti-Ro/SSA antibodies (especially directed against the 52-kD component, which is more common in those with associated Sjögren's) may have up to a 4 to 5% overall risk of having a baby with the neonatal lupus syndrome. Of these babies, 40% have only rash, 40% have complete heart block (CHB), and 10–20% will have both rash and CHB. Of the babies with CHB, approximately 50% will require a permanent pacemaker, and 10% will die despite the pacemaker. Once a SLE patient with anti-Ro/SSA antibodies has had one child with CHB, there is a 15% overall risk of her next baby having CHB. Patients at risk for having babies with CHB should have weekly fetal echocardiograms from the 18th to 24th weeks of gestation to measure the mechanical PR interval. If the fetus demonstrates development of heart block, treatment of the mother with dexamethasone (not prednisone, since it is metabolized by placental 11-B hydroxygenase) and plasmapheresis may occasionally reverse the heart block. All infants born to mothers with anti-Ro/SSA antibodies should have an EKG to evaluate for first degree AV block because postnatal progression to CHB has been reported.

**44. A 25-year-old patient with SLE, currently on 5 mg of prednisone per day, and quiescent disease for the last few years wants to become pregnant. What advice can you offer her about potential problems for her or the fetus?**

Pregnancy in SLE can be difficult and warrants special consideration. The optimal time for the patient to consider becoming pregnant is when disease activity is quiescent and medications are minimal. Thus, for this patient, this would be a relatively good time to become pregnant. Careful follow-up is essential during pregnancy. Although controversial, some experienced physicians believe that pregnancy increases the risk for disease flares, especially during the third trimester and the immediate post-partum period. Patients need to be followed carefully for blood pressure elevations and evidence of glomerulonephritis. Useful laboratory tests to follow patients include anti-dsDNA antibodies and complement levels. The mainstay of therapy for serious lupus flares during pregnancy is prednisone.

**45. A patient with SLE and active lupus nephritis wants to become pregnant. Current medications include prednisone, 20 mg/day. What do you recommend?**

In contrast to a SLE patient with quiescent disease, this patient should be counseled against becoming pregnant at this time. There is an increased chance of worsening disease activity that could result in renal functional deterioration and increased problems related to hypertension and pre-eclampsia. It has been estimated that patients with active lupus nephritis have a 50 to 60% chance of nephritis exacerbation during pregnancy or immediately post-partum. In contrast, for patients with quiescent disease, the risk of nephritis exacerbation is < 10%.

Flares of lupus nephritis during pregnancy can be very severe. In patients with active lupus, there is also a high chance for problems in the fetus. For example, the risk of prematurity may be as high as 60%. Furthermore, if the renal disease should worsen, certain therapies such as cyclophosphamide are contraindicated. This would limit therapeutic options, although azathioprine has been used successfully because it is metabolized by the placenta and little gets into the fetal circulation.

**46. What are the four most common causes of death in patients with SLE?**

1. Infection
2. Lupus nephritis, renal failure, and its complications
3. Cardiovascular disease
4. CNS lupus

Outcome in SLE has been steadily improving over the last 30 years. A large fraction of the deaths are now secondary to infection and atherosclerotic disease. Some have emphasized the bimodal pattern of mortality in SLE. Death early in the disease is generally a reflection of active lupus or its treatment. Infection in SLE appears to be mostly related to the complications of immunosuppressive therapy, especially to prolonged use of high-dose corticosteroids. Coronary artery disease is the leading cause of death late in the course of SLE. The risk of coronary artery disease is increased 10-fold in SLE patients (50-fold in SLE patients 35–44 years old). Factors playing a role in the coronary artery disease of SLE patients include corticosteroid therapy, hyperlipidemia, hypertension, smoking, coagulation abnormalities, homocystinemia, obesity, and vasculopathy from immune injury. The presence and extent of renal disease are probably the most important prognostic factors in SLE. This relates not only to the possibility of developing renal failure but also to the probability of receiving potentially toxic therapy (high-dose prednisone and cytotoxic drugs) required to treat this manifestation of disease.

**47. Discuss some of the management principles other than immunosuppression used in the treatment of SLE patients.**

- Avoid possible disease triggers—sulfa antibiotics, sun, high estrogen–containing birth control pills, alfalfa sprouts, echinacea.

- Prevent atherosclerosis—control blood pressure (target 130/80), hyperlipidemia (target LDL cholesterol < 130), stop smoking, treat hyperhomocystinemia (folate 1–5 mg/d, pyridoxine 25 mg/d, vitamin $B_{12}$ 500 μg/d or combination pill), one baby aspirin per day taken prior to other NSAIDs.
- Prevent osteoporosis—calcium (1500 mg), vitamin D (800 IU), lower corticosteroid dosage, bisphosphonates if on ≥ 10–20 mg of prednisone a day for ≥ 3 months. Rule out low testosterone in males with SLE.
- Prevent infections—pneumococcal vaccine because SLE patients have hyposplenism, influenza vaccine. Patients on immunosuppressive agents and/or prednisone ≥ 20 mg/d may not mount a satisfactory immune response and should not be given live attenuated vaccines (measles, mumps, rubella, polio, BCG, and yellow fever). Immunization does not flare SLE. *Pneumocystis carinii* prophylaxis if on cyclophosphamide and glucocorticoids.
- Prevent progression of renal disease in patients with nephritis—avoid NSAIDs, control BP (target 120/80), limit proteinuria (use ACE inhibitors).
- Prevent clots in patients with antiphospholipid antibodies (not on warfarin)—low-dose aspirin, use of hydroxychloroquine, avoid unnecessary surgeries and vascular catheterizations, treat infections promptly, avoid Cox-2 specific inhibitors, avoid exogenous estrogen.
- Treat fatigue—rule out hypothyroidism, metabolic disturbances, myopathy, anemia, depression, and sleep apnea. Eliminate drugs that can cause fatigue. Antimalarials and DHEA (200 mg/day) can help fatigue.

**48. Can patients with SLE receive exogenous estrogens? (Controversial)**

Since SLE is primarily a disease of premenopausal females, there is concern that exogenous estrogens may cause an exacerbation of SLE. Furthermore, venous thromboembolism and precipitation of coronary thrombosis or stroke in patients with underlying atherosclerosis are potential complications. However, exogenous estrogens in birth control pills (BCPs) can help prevent pregnancy and hormone replacement therapy (HRT) in post menopausal women can help vasomotor symptoms, atrophic vaginitis, and osteoporosis. Until the results of the SELENA trial are available, the following are suggested guidelines:

- Avoid BCPs and HRT in patients with active SLE, history of clot, active lupus nephritis with or without nephrotic syndrome, and high-titer antiphospholipid antibodies.
- Avoid selective estrogen receptor modulators (SERMs) such as raloxifene in patients with history of clot or significant risk factors for clot.
- Preferred methods of contraception in SLE patients are barriers, tubal ligation, or progesterone-only contraceptives. The intrauterine device is an option if not on immunosuppressive drugs. If patient demands BCP, use low estrogen–containing BCP.
- In postmenopausal patients without history of clot or risk factors for clot, HRT has been safe and not associated with disease exacerbations.
- In postmenopausal patients with risk factors for clot but no previous history of clot, use estrogen patch that does not stimulate liver to make coagulation factors.

**49. How does the erythrocyte sedimentation rate (ESR), C-reactive protein (CRP), and white blood cell count help in following disease activity in SLE? Help distinguish infection?**

Unlike rheumatoid arthritis, the ESR and CRP are not helpful in following disease activity in SLE. The ESR remains elevated even when the disease is controlled, usually owing to a persistent polyclonal gammopathy. On the other hand, CRP usually does not rise much even during disease flare unless there is a systemic vasculitis or associated infection. A SLE patient with fever and an elevated C-reactive protein should have an infection aggressively ruled out and treated. Remember when an SLE patient "flares," the WBC count frequently goes down. When a SLE patient gets infected, the WBC count may rise to the "normal" range if the patient is usually leukopenic. Any febrile SLE patients with a high WBC count should be investigated for an infection and empirically treated with antibiotics until cultures return.

**50. Discuss the experimental therapies that are being evaluated for the treatment of SLE.**

A variety of experimental therapies have been tested and are being evaluated for the treatment of SLE, especially in patients with severe lupus nephritis. Studies have shown that plasmapheresis does not have long-term benefit in the treatment of lupus nephritis, and it cannot be recommended as a routine adjunct to drug treatment. Therapies utilized in the setting of transplantation, such as cyclosporine, tacrolimus (FK506), mycophenolate mofetil, and total lymphoid irradiation, have been reported in the treatment of lupus nephritis as an alternative to cyclophosphamide therapy with at least anecdotal efficacy. However, none have been shown to be an acceptable alternative to cyclophosphamide in patients with severe disease. Animal studies and anecdotal case series initially suggested that mycophenylate mofetil may be efficacious in lupus nephritis. A recent controlled study in patients with relatively mild DPGN showed that initial remission rates with this drug and prednisolone were comparable with responses with oral cyclophosphamide and prednisolone (followed by azathioprine and prednisolone). However, the study design did not allow conclusions regarding whether mycophenylate mofetil will be able to prevent progression to renal failure similar to cyclophosphamide, especially in patients with more severe disease. Because of the potential toxicity of prolonged cyclophosphamide therapy, there has also been consideration to replace maintenance therapy with less toxic regimens such as azathioprine or mycophenylate mofetil. It remains unclear whether these approaches to reduce toxicity will be successful at maintaining remission and preventing long-term progression. Recent work has suggested that very high dose (immunoablative) cyclophosphamide, with or without bone marrow transplantation, may provide long-term benefit for patients with very severe disease, and trials are in progress to test this idea.

There is also great excitement about several new biologic inhibitors being developed for therapy of patients with SLE. For example, inhibitors of the CD40-CD40 ligand interaction with monoclonal antibodies to CD40 ligand and the CD28-B7 interaction with CTLA4-Ig, especially in combination, have demonstrated potent suppression of lupus nephritis in murine models. These agents are based on the well-demonstrated importance of T helper cells for IgG autoantibody production in SLE. Based on the demonstrated importance of certain molecular pathways in SLE and initial results in murine lupus, clinical trials are also being started with biologic agents that inhibit the production or signaling of interferon-$\gamma$, the activity of cytokines that stimulate B cells such as BLys-1, and the activation of complement component C5. Finally, trials are underway investigating if antibodies against B cells (anti CD20, rituximab) can be useful in treating SLE patients.

## BIBLIOGRAPHY

1. ACR Ad Hoc Committee on Neuropsychiatric Lupus Nomenclature: The American College of Rheumatology nomenclature and case definitions for neuropsychiatric lupus syndromes. Arthritis Rheum 42:599, 1999.
2. Austin HA, Boumpas DT, Vaughan EM, Balow JE: Predicting renal outcomes in severe lupus nephritis: Contributions of clinical and histologic data. Kidney Int 45:544–550, 1994.
3. Balow JE, Boumpas DT, Austin HA: Systemic lupus erythematosus and the kidney. In Lahita RG (ed): Systemic Lupus Erythematosus, 3rd ed. San Diego, Academic Press, 1999, pp 657–685.
4. Brooks E, Liang MH: Evaluation of recent clinical trials in lupus. Curr Opin Rheum 11:341–347, 1999.
5. Buyon JP, Kim MY, Copel JA, Friedman DM: Anti-Ro/SSA antibodies and congential heart block: Necessary but not sufficient. Arthritis Rheum 44:1723–1727, 2001.
6. Chan TM, Li FK, Tang CSO, et al: Efficacy of mycophenylate mofetil in patients with diffuse proliferative lupus nephritis. N Engl J Med 343:1156–1162, 2000.
7. Gourley MF, Austin HA 3rd, Scott D, et al: Methylprednisolone and cyclophosphamide, alone or in combination, in patients with lupus nephritis. A randomized, controlled trial. Ann Intern Med 125:549–557, 1996.
8. Karrar A, Sequeira W, Block JA: Coronary artery disease in systemic lupus erythematosus: A review of the literature. Semin Arthritis Rheum 30:436–443, 2001.
9. Kelley VR, Wuthrich RP: Cytokines in the pathogenesis of systemic lupus erythematosus. Semin Nephrol 19:57–66. 1999.

10. Kotzin BL, West SG: Systemic lupus erythematosus. In Rich RR, Fleisher TA, Shearer WT, et al (eds): Clinical Immunology: Principles and Practice, 2nd ed., London, Mosby, 2001.
11. Kotzin BL, Achenbach GA, West SG: Renal involvement in systemic lupus erythematosus. In Schrier RW, Gottschalk CW (eds): Diseases of the Kidney, 7th ed. Philadelphia, Lippincott, Williams & Wilkins, 2001.
12. McMurray RW: Nonstandard and adjunctive medical therapies for systemic lupus erythematosus. Arthritis Care Res 45:86–100, 2001.
13. Mok CC, Lau CS, Wong RWS: Use of exogenous estrogens in systemic lupus erythematosus. Semin Arthritis Rheum 30:426–435, 2001.
14. Roubey RA: Update on antiphospholipid antibodies. Curr Opin Rheumatol 12:374–378, 2000.
15. Rus V, Hochberg, MC: The epidemiology of systemic lupus erythematosus. In Wallace DJ, Hahn BH (eds): Dubois' Lupus Erythematosus, 6th ed. Baltimore, Williams & Wilkins, 2002, pp 65–86.
16. Stone JH, Amend WC, Criswell LA: Outcome of renal transplantation in ninety-seven cyclosporine-era patients with systemic lupus erythematosus and matched controls. Arthritis Rheum 41:1438–1445, 1998.
17. Tan EM, Feltkamp TE, Smolen JS: Range of antinuclear antibodies in healthy individuals. Arthritis Rheum 40:1601–1611, 1997.
18. Vyse TJ, Kotzin BL: Genetic susceptibility to systemic lupus erythematosus. Annu Rev Immunol 16:261–292, 1998.
19. Wallace DJ, Hahn BH (eds): Dubois' Lupus Erythematosus, 6th ed. Baltimore, Williams & Wilkins, 2002.
20. West SG, Emlen W, Wener MH, Kotzin BL: Neuropsychiatric lupus erythematosus: A 10-year prospective study on the value of diagnostic tests. Am J Med 99:153–163, 1995.

# 21. DRUG-INDUCED LUPUS

*Brian* L. *Kotzin*, M.D.

**1. Name seven drugs definitely associated with antinuclear antibodies and manifestations of lupus-like disease.**

Procainamide, hydralazine, quinidine, isoniazid, methyldopa, chlorpromazine, and minocycline

**2. For these drugs, provide an estimate of the risk of developing drug-induced lupus (DIL) (from high to low).**

Procainamide (high)
Hydralazine (high)
Quinidine (moderate)
Isoniazid (low)
Methyldopa (low)
Chlorpromazine (low)
Minocycline (low)

**3. List any other drugs for which there is more than anecdotal evidence for lupus-inducing potential.**

Mephenytoin, phenytoin, beta-adrenergic blocking agents, carbamazepine, sulfasalazine, and D-penicillamine.

**4. How do the clinical manifestations occurring most commonly in procainamide-induced lupus compare with the manifestations of idiopathic systemic lupus erythematosus (SLE)?**

Patients with DIL have a different distribution of clinical manifestations than those with idiopathic SLE. In procainamide-induced lupus, severe nephritis or manifestations of CNS involvement (e.g., organic brain syndrome, seizures, or psychosis) are very rare. In contrast, nearly 50%

of patients with SLE will demonstrate clinical evidence of nephritis during their disease course, and neurologic and/or psychiatric manifestations occur in up to two-thirds of SLE patients. Furthermore, rashes such as a malar rash or discoid lesions are unusual in drug-induced disease but are common in patients with SLE. Frequent problems seen in drug-induced disease include fever, myalgias, arthralgia/arthritis, and pleuritis, with 30 to 40% of patients having acute pulmonary infiltrates. Although pleuritis is also relatively common in SLE, acute infiltrates not related to infection are uncommon and are usually seen only in patients who are acutely ill.

**5. How do the clinical manifestations of hydralazine-induced lupus differ from those of procainamide-induced disease?**

Like those with procainamide-induced lupus, patients with hydralazine-induced lupus are also likely to have fever, myalgias, and arthritis/arthralgias and rarely manifest either severe lupus nephritis or CNS involvement. Compared with procainamide-induced disease, serositis and pulmonary parenchymal involvement are much less common, and rashes are more likely to be seen, although the classic malar rash and discoid lesions are unusual.

**6. Will patients with either DIL or SLE usually have a positive test for antinuclear antibodies (ANA)?**

Yes. By definition, essentially all patients with DIL will demonstrate a positive ANA test.

**7. Which autoantibodies are most commonly seen in DIL? How do these compare with the autoantibodies seen in idiopathic SLE?**

The spectrum of ANAs in DIL is much more limited than that seen in SLE. **Anti-histone antibodies** are the most common autoantibody specificity in DIL, and most patients with symptomatic drug-induced disease demonstrate elevated levels of IgG anti-histone antibodies. Antibodies to histones are also frequent in SLE, detectable in 50 to 80% of patients, depending on disease activity. Antibodies to single-stranded DNA are also common in both DIL and SLE, but antibodies to double-stranded DNA are highly specific for SLE and rarely found in DIL. Antibodies to Sm (~30% of SLE), Ro/SS-A (~60% of SLE), and La/SS-B (~15 to 20% of SLE) are also rarely if ever seen in DIL. Antiphospholipid antibodies can be seen in both DIL and idiopathic SLE. Hypocomplementemia is uncommon in DIL but not SLE.

**8. Is testing for anti-histone antibodies clinically useful to distinguish drug-induced disease from idiopathic SLE in a patient taking either procainamide or hydralazine?**

Testing for anti-histone antibodies can occasionally be useful in situations in which the diagnosis of DIL is being considered. As discussed, nearly all patients with symptomatic procainamide- or hydralazine-induced lupus demonstrate elevated serum levels of IgG anti-histone antibodies. Thus, a negative test would make this diagnosis unlikely. However, a positive test for anti-histone antibodies has much less diagnostic value because 50 to 80% of patients with active SLE also have a positive test. Furthermore, some patients taking either procainamide or hydralazine will have a positive test but not symptoms of lupus-like disease. Remember that in most cases in which drug-induced disease is being considered, performing an ANA test and (if positive) taking the patient off the offending agent may be the most cost-effective approach to the situation.

**9. Contrast the type of anti-histone antibodies found in drug-induced lupus versus idiopathic SLE.**

In certain specialized research laboratories, the specificity of anti-histone antibodies for individual histones (i.e., H1, H2A, H2B, H3, and H4), histone complexes, or intra-histone epitopes can be distinguished. Overall, anti-histone antibodies in DIL tend to be much more focused on certain histone complexes compared with SLE. For example, in procainamide-induced lupus (and most other causes of DIL), the onset of symptomatic disease has been associated with the production of IgG antibodies to the H2A-H2B-DNA complex. Although this complex is also a target in about 15% of patients with SLE, autoantibodies in the idiopathic disease are frequently also directed to other individual histones and other histone complexes. In hydralazine-induced disease, one study has suggested that the major targets are histones H3 and H4 and the H3-H4 complex. In contrast to procainamide-induced lupus and SLE, the autoantibodies induced by hydralazine appear to be directed more to determinants hidden within chromatin rather than exposed on the surface.

**10. What percentage of patients taking procainamide or hydralazine develop a positive test for ANA even without symptoms of DIL?**

Nearly 75% of patients receiving procainamide therapy will develop a positive ANA test within the first year of treatment, and over 90% develop a positive ANA by 2 years. Thirty to 50% of patients taking hydralazine will demonstrate a positive test after a year of drug therapy. For both drugs, the probability of developing a positive ANA test depends on the dose and duration of drug therapy. With long-term drug use, perhaps 10 to 30% of ANA-positive patients go on to develop symptoms of lupus. It is important to note that many more patients will demonstrate a positive ANA test than develop DIL, and the presence of a positive test is not a valid reason for stopping the medication. In DIL, the onset of symptoms can be insidious or acute, and an interval of 1 to 2 months frequently passes before the diagnosis is made and the drug is withdrawn.

**11. Do similar genetic factors predispose patients to develop DIL and SLE?**

The genetic risk factors in DIL and idiopathic SLE appear to be quite separate. The major risk for procainamide- or hydralazine-induced lupus appears to be **acetylator phenotype**. Metabolism of these drugs involves the hepatic enzyme *N*-acetyltransferase, which catalyzes the acetylation of amine or hydrazine groups. The rate at which this reaction takes place is under genetic control. Approximately 50% of the U.S. white population are fast acetylators, and the rest are slow acetylators. The slow acetylators, when treated with procainamide or hydralazine, develop ANA earlier and at higher titers and are more likely to develop symptomatic disease compared with fast acetylators. In one study, hydralazine-induced disease developed only in slow acetylators. It should also be noted that *N*-acetylprocainamide, despite its chemical similarity to procainamide and its similar drug action, has not been associated with drug-induced ANA production or DIL.

In SLE, acetylator phenotype does not appear to be involved in genetic susceptibility. Instead, HLA class II genes, complement deficiencies, and multiple other genes are important in the complex genetic basis of SLE (see Chapter 20).

**12. What age, sex, and racial groups are most at risk for DIL? For idiopathic SLE?**

The incidence of SLE increases greatly in women of childbearing age, and the female-to-male ratio overall is about 8:1. In contrast, the usual age of patients with DIL is 50 years old, reflecting the age of the population being treated with drugs such as procainamide and hydralazine. The female-to-male ratio in DIL is also much closer to unity (procainamide-induced disease may be slightly more frequent in females). The frequency of SLE may be two to four times increased in blacks and Hispanics compared with whites. In contrast, the frequency of DIL may be 6-fold lower in blacks than whites.

**13. Will the severity of clinical manifestations of DIL frequently progress after the offending drug is discontinued?**

No. In nearly all cases, disease manifestations begin to improve within a few days to weeks after the drug is discontinued. If this does not occur, question the diagnosis.

**14. Is the use of procainamide or other drugs associated with DIL contraindicated in patients with SLE? Can they exacerbate disease activity?**

No. The population at risk for developing DIL is very different compared with that developing SLE. There is no evidence that drugs capable of causing DIL will change or worsen disease activity in a patient with SLE. However, if an alternative drug is available, it may be prudent to use it so that there won't be any confusion if the SLE patient has a disease flare in the future.

**15. What is the mainstay of therapy for DIL?**

The first and most important aspect of treatment is to *discontinue the offending medication.*

**16. Describe the management of a patient with procainamide-induced lupus who has fevers, arthritis, and pleuritis as the major manifestations of disease.**

First, discontinue procainamide. Many patients with these symptoms can be controlled with NSAIDs, while the symptoms of drug-induced disease gradually resolve after discontinuing the offending drug. A small percentage of patients with severe symptoms may require a short course of prednisone, especially if complications of pleuritis or pericarditis or if pulmonary infiltrates are apparent. If necessary, steroids are usually very effective in reversing the features of DIL. More toxic medications, such as azathioprine or cyclophosphamide, are almost never required in the treatment of DIL.

**17. A patient returns to your clinic 8 months after being treated for procainamide-induced lupus. Her symptoms resolved about 4 weeks after stopping procainamide and required a short course of prednisone. She has been off prednisone for over 6 months and remains asymptomatic, but a repeat ANA test is still positive in a high titer. What changes in your therapeutic plan are required at this time?**

No therapy is required at this time. It is not unusual for the ANA to remain positive for months to years after an episode of DIL, despite the rapid resolution of all symptoms of lupus-like disease. As long as the patient is not rechallenged with the offending drug, symptoms should not recur.

**18. How do medications such as procainamide and hydralazine induce lupus-like autoantibody production and disease? Is there evidence from animal models of DIL?**

The failure to metabolize these drugs via *N*-acetyltransferase to an inactive metabolite is likely involved in the induction of disease. Thus, persons who are slow acetylators are more likely to produce ANA and develop symptoms. One study showed that activated neutrophils can convert lupus-inducing drugs to products that are cytotoxic for lymphocytes and other cells. This conversion required the enzymatic action of myeloperoxidase. It was hypothesized that exposure of the immune system to these cytotoxic metabolites is important in the induction of lupus-like disease, perhaps by generating the release of autoantigens or by causing an immune dysregulation. In other animal studies, the injection of procainamide-hydroxylamine (an active metabolite of procainamide) into the thymus of mice was shown to induce anti-chromatin autoantibodies and chromatin-reactive T cells. Studies suggested that the drug disrupted central T cell tolerance during intrathymic T cell development. Still other studies have suggested that lupus-inducing drugs inhibit DNA methylation, which causes peripheral T cells to alter gene expression and become autoreactive.

Despite these interesting clues and the importance of the question in terms of gaining insight into the mechanisms of autoimmunity, nobody truly understands the pathogenesis of DIL. There is also no established or reproducible animal model that resembles human DIL.

**19. What are the characteristic clinical features of minocycline-induced lupus?**

Minocycline is a semisynthetic tetracycline frequently used to treat acne. There have been multiple cases of DIL affecting young individuals (females > males, ages 14–31) after an average of 30 months (range 6–72) of use in doses of 50 to 200 mg a day. All patients have arthritis/arthralgias and a positive ANA. Fever (33%), rash (20%), pleuritis (10%), hepatitis, and anticardiolipin antibodies (33%) can be seen. Interestingly, only 10–15% have antihistone antibodies but 75–80% have a positive pANCA. Treatment is discontinuing minocycline, which should result in rapid resolution of symptoms.

## BIBLIOGRAPHY

1. Jiang X, Khursigara G, Rubin RL: Transformation of lupus-inducing drugs to cytotoxic products by activated neutrophils. Science 266:810–813, 1994.

2. Kretz-Rommel A, Rubin RL: Disruption of positive selection of thymocytes causes autoimmunity. Nat Med 6:298–305, 2000.
3. Lawson TM, Amos N, Bulgen D, Williams BD: Minocycline-induced lupus: Clinical features and response to rechallenge. Rheumatology 40:329–335, 2001.
4. Monestier M, Kotzin BL: Antibodies to histones in systemic lupus erythematosus and drug-induced lupus syndromes. Rheum Dis Clin North Am 18:415–436, 1992.
5. Portanova JP, Arndt RE, Tan EM, Kotzin BL: Anti-histone antibodies in idiopathic and drug-induced lupus recognize distinct intrahistone regions. J Immunol 138:446–451, 1987.
6. Rao T, Richardson B: Environmentally induced autoimmune diseases: Potential mechanisms. Environ Health Perspect 107(Suppl 5):737–742, 1999.
7. Rubin RL: Etiology and mechanisms of drug-induced lupus. Curr Opin Rheumatol 11:357–363, 1999.
8. Rubin RL: Drug-induced lupus. In Wallace DJ, Hahn BH (eds): Dubois' Lupus Erythematosus, 6th ed. Baltimore, Williams & Wilkins, 2002, pp 885–916.

# 22. SYSTEMIC SCLEROSIS

*David* H. *Collier,* M.D.

**1. Define systemic sclerosis.**

Systemic sclerosis is an uncommon connective tissue disease with the most prominent feature being thickening or fibrosis of the skin. It is a heterogeneous disorder, both in the involvement of internal organs and joints and in the pace and severity of its clinical course. It is a subcategory of scleroderma (*sclero* = thickened, *derma* = skin).

The American College of Rheumatology (ACR) has proposed preliminary criteria for the diagnosis of this condition:

Major criteria
- Scleroderma proximal to the metacarpophalangeal or metatarsophalangeal joints

Minor criteria
- Sclerodactyly
- Digital pitting scars
- Bibasilar pulmonary fibrosis

One major and two minor criteria are needed for diagnosis of definite systemic sclerosis. However, these criteria will not define a significant minority of patients with limited systemic sclerosis. It has recently been suggested that the ACR criteria be expanded to include abnormal capillary microscopy, dilated capillaries and avascular areas at the nailbeds, and anti-centromere antibodies to the preliminary criteria to more adequately incorporate patients with limited systemic sclerosis.

**2. How is scleroderma classified?**

1. **Localized scleroderma**: cutaneous changes consisting of dermal fibrosis without internal organ involvement
   a. **Morphea**: single or multiple (generalized) plaques commonly on the trunk
   b. **Linear scleroderma**: bands of skin thickening commonly on the legs or arms but sometimes on the face (*en coup de sabre*) that typically follow a linear path
2. **Systemic sclerosis**
   a. **Diffuse systemic sclerosis**: fibrotic skin proximal to the elbows or knees excluding the face and neck. This category of patients may have the onset of Raynaud's phenomenon within a year of developing systemic sclerosis and are more likely to have pulmonary, renal, or cardiac involvement. They are more likely to have autoantibodies to topoisomerase-1 (anti-Scl-70) and much less likely to have an anti-centromere antibody.

b. **Limited systemic sclerosis**: fibrotic skin limited to the hands and forearms, feet, neck, and face. This category of patients usually has Raynaud's phenomenon for years and may have telangiectasias, skin calcifications, and a late incidence of pulmonary hypertension. These patients have a high incidence of anti-centromere antibody.

3. **Overlap syndromes**: scleroderma associated with other autoimmune diseases

**3. What is the CREST syndrome?**

This term describes a subgroup of patients with limited systemic sclerosis having:

**C** — **C**alcinosis
**R** — **R**aynaud's phenomenon
**E** — **E**sophageal dysmotility
**S** — **S**clerodactyly
**T** — **T**elangiectasias

The term **limited systemic sclerosis** is preferable because the term CREST describes only a narrow part of the spectrum of limited systemic sclerosis.

**4. Who gets systemic sclerosis?**

Systemic sclerosis is most commonly seen in women (F:M = 3:1) between the ages of 35 to 64. Systemic sclerosis is rare in children and men under age 30. It is slightly more common in black women during child-bearing years, but over all ages, there is probably no significant predominance among blacks.

**5. Describe the cutaneous abnormalities in systemic sclerosis.**

The hallmark of systemic sclerosis is **thickened skin**, thought to be due to the abnormal production by a subset of fibroblasts of normal type I collagen along with the accumulation of glycosaminoglycan and fibronectin in the extracellular matrix. There is loss of sweat glands and hair loss in areas of tight skin. Although patients seem to have areas of involved and uninvolved skin, as based on the presence of procollagen-1 and adherence molecules, all skin is abnormal. Skin thickening begins on the fingers and hands in virtually *all* cases of systemic sclerosis. When it begins elsewhere, other localized forms of scleroderma or eosinophilic fascitis should be considered.

**Calcinosis** consists of cutaneous deposits of basic calcium phosphate that characteristically occur in the hands (especially over the proximal interphalangeal joints and fingertips), periarticular tissue, and over bony prominences (especially the extensor surface of the elbows and knees) but can occur virtually anywhere on the body. The deposits of calcium are firm, irregular, and generally nontender, ranging in diameter from 1 mm to several centimeters. They can become inflamed, infected, or ulcerated or may discharge a chalky white material.

**Telangiectases** are dilated venules, capillaries, and arterioles. In systemic sclerosis, they tend to be *matte* telangiectases, which are oval or polygonal macules 2–7 mm in diameter found on the hands, face, lips, and oral mucosa. They are seen more commonly in limited systemic sclerosis. When they occur in GI mucosa, they can bleed, leading to iron deficiency anemia.

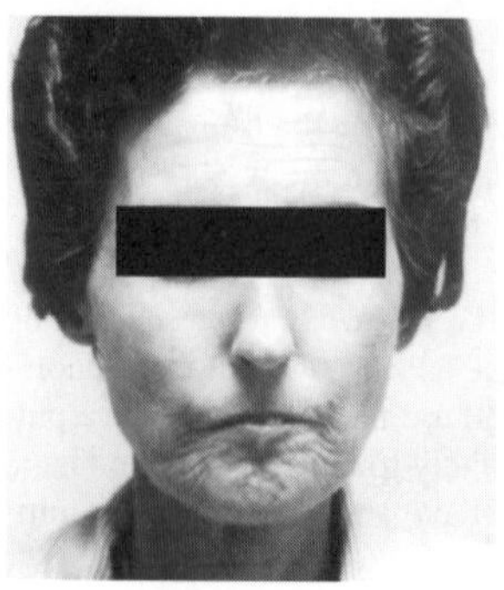

Scleroderma patient demonstrating tightened facial skin. Note exaggerated radial furrowing about the lips (tobacco pouch sign).

**6. Discuss the natural history of these cutaneous abnormalities.**

The progression of **skin tightening** is quite variable. However, most patients' skin, with no therapy, softens or atrophies over 3–10 years. Internal organ involvement does not mimic the skin improvement and may worsen over time.

**Calcinosis** can be persistent for years. It is extremely difficult to treat, and no therapy is consistently successful. Therapies used have included warfarin (1–2.5 mg/day, in an attempt to inhibit the vitamin K–dependent Gla matrix protein), aluminum hydroxide, diltiazem, probenecid, and high doses of bisphosphonates.

**Telangiectases** are usually harmless and a cosmetic problem. They may disappear spontaneously over time. Laser therapy has been used to remove them with some success, but commonly they will return.

**7. What is Raynaud's phenomenon?**

Raynaud's phenomenon is an episodic self-limited and reversible vasomotor disturbance manifested as color changes bilaterally in the fingers, toes, and sometimes ears, nose, and lips. The color changes are **pallor**, **cyanosis**, and then **erythema** (white, blue, and then red) that occur in response to environmental cold and/or emotional stress. There does not need to be a three-color change to diagnose Raynaud's phenomenon; episodic pallor or cyanosis that reverses to erythema or normal skin color may be all that is seen. Patients may describe symptoms of numbness, tingling, or pain on recovery. (See also Chapter 78.)

**8. In a patient with new-onset Raynaud's phenomenon, what findings would suggest early systemic sclerosis?**

- Positive antinuclear antibodies, anti-centromere antibodies, or anti-topoisomerase 1 (Scl-70) antibodies
- Nailfold capillary abnormalities of capillary drop-out and/or dilatation (see Chapter 78)
- Tendon friction rubs
- Puffy, swollen fingers or legs
- Associated esophageal reflux

**9. At the onset of systemic sclerosis, how might the timing of the onset of Raynaud's phenomenon and skin thickening help suggest if the patient will develop the diffuse form of systemic sclerosis versus the limited form of systemic sclerosis?**

If the Raynaud's phenomenon precedes any skin changes by a year or longer, the patient most likely will develop the limited form of systemic sclerosis. If the Raynaud's phenomenon occurs simultaneously with the skin changes, the patient will most likely develop the diffuse form of systemic sclerosis.

**10. How is Raynaud's phenomenon treated?**

First, keep hands *and* body warm. Many patients carry gloves at all times. When going to cold places, patients may bring exothermic reaction bags (chemical heat packs), which can be obtained at sporting goods, hardware, and other stores. Repeated soaking in warm water sometimes helps.

The patient should stop smoking. For primary Raynaud's, biofeedback can be very successful if the patient is committed to learning and practicing this technique. Systemic sclerosis patients rarely benefit from biofeedback.

Various prescription vasodilators can be used. Calcium channel blockers are the first choice. The most studied is nifedipine, but diltiazem works well and the newer calcium channel blockers are used if the patient is having side effects from the nifedipine. Verapamil does not work. The dose of these drugs is increased until the desired effect is obtained or the patient cannot tolerate the side effects. Antiadrenergic agents such as prazosin, doxazosin, methyldopa, and reserpine and the angiotensin-converting enzyme inhibitors are also used as vasodilators but appear to be less effective than the calcium channel blockers. More recently, good results have been obtained with angiotensin II receptor antagonists such as losartan, valsartan, or irbesartan. Topical nitroglycerin ointment applied sparingly over the affected area for 20 minutes three times a day can be helpful, but commonly the patient has an accompanying headache. One-half aspirin a day to inhibit platelet activation is also recommended. Niacin is also used starting at 50 mg twice a day and working up to 500 mg BID to TID. The limiting factor is the flushing that niacin can cause. In severe cases of Raynaud's associated with scleroderma, full anticoagulation with warfarin can be used. The use of intravenous prostacyclin and its analogue (iloprost) appears promising in severe cases of Raynaud's. Intravenous *N*-acetylcysteine has shown promise in one pilot study.

**11. Compare and contrast the organ system involvement in diffuse and limited systemic sclerosis.**

| ORGAN SYSTEM INVOLVEMENT | DIFFUSE | LIMITED |
|---|---|---|
| Skin thickening | 100% | 95% |
| Telangiectasias | 30 | 80 |
| Calcinosis | 5 | 45 |
| Raynaud's phenomenon | 85 | 95 |
| Arthralgias or arthritis | 80 | 60 |
| Tendon friction rubs | 65 | 5 |
| Myopathy | 20 | 10 |
| Esophageal hypomotility | 75 | 75 |
| Pulmonary fibrosis | 35–59 | 35 |
| Pulmonary hypertension | < 1 | 12 |
| Congestive heart failure | 10 | 1 |
| Renal crisis | 15 | 1 |

**12. Discuss the pathophysiologic progression of gastrointestinal involvement in systemic sclerosis.**

Although no longitudinal studies have been done to document the anatomic progression in the GI system, there is good circumstantial evidence to suggest an orderly series of steps leading to progressive dysfunction. First, there is neural dysfunction thought to be due to arteriolar changes of the vasa nervorum leading to dysmotility. Second, there is smooth muscle atrophy. Third, there is fibrosis of the muscle.

**13. How is esophageal dysmotility assessed in patients with systemic sclerosis?**

Esophageal dysmotility is documented by manometry, cine-esophagraphy, or by a routine upper GI series with barium swallow. Practically speaking, manometry, although the most sensitive, is so uncomfortable that it is rarely performed. Endoscopy is used to assess reflux esophagitis, candidiasis, Barrett's esophagus, and strictures of the lower esophageal area.

**14. How is esophageal dysmotility treated in patients with systemic sclerosis?**

Treatment is designed to decrease complications of acid reflux, such as esophagitis, stricture, or nocturnal aspiration of stomach contents. The head of the bed should be elevated 4 inches; adding more pillows to sleep on may only make matters worse by decreasing stomach area. The patient should not eat for 2–3 hours before bedtime. The acid content in the stomach should be decreased in the evening with antacids, $H_2$ blockers, or, for progressive problems, proton pump inhibitors such as omeprazole, esomeprazole, lansoprazole, pantoprazole, and rabeprazole. Motility agents such as metoclopramide before meals are sometimes helpful early in the disease, but as the GI smooth muscles fibrose, these agents become ineffective.

**15. What is a "watermelon stomach"?**

Watermelon stomach is a descriptive term for gastric antral venous ectasia. This can be a cause of upper gastrointestinal bleeding in scleroderma patients.

**16. Patients with systemic sclerosis may have small and large bowel involvement. What symptoms and signs do these patients have?**

The major manifestations are due to diminished peristalsis with resulting stasis and dilatation. The diminished peristalsis can lead to bacterial overgrowth (hydrogen breath test, high folate). Later, malabsorption can be a major problem (low albumin, low $B_6$/$B_{12}$/folate/25OH vit D, high fecal fat, low D-xylose absorption test, low carotene). Patients may complain of abdominal distention and pain due to dilated bowel, obstructive symptoms from intestinal pseudo-obstruction, or diarrhea from bacterial overgrowth or malabsorption. If the malabsorption becomes severe, the patient may have signs of vitamin deficiencies or electrolyte abnormalities.

Patients with large bowel involvement may demonstrate wide mouth diverticulae on barium enema. It should be emphasized that barium studies are relatively contraindicated in systemic sclerosis patients with poor GI motility, owing to the risk of barium impaction.

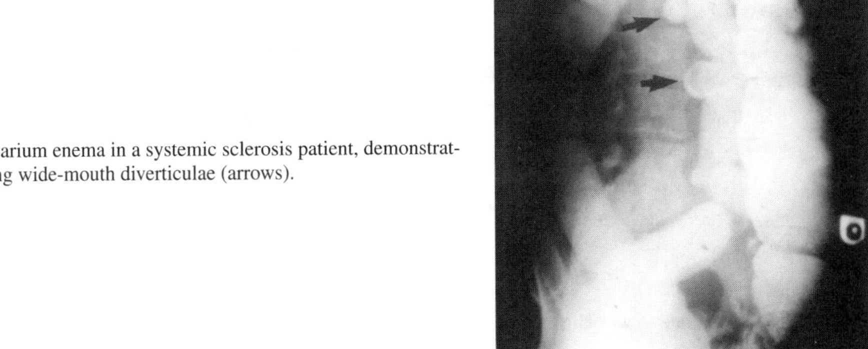

Barium enema in a systemic sclerosis patient, demonstrating wide-mouth diverticulae (arrows).

**17. How are small and large bowel problems managed in these patients?**

Stimulation of gut motility with metoclopramide is tried initially. Erythromycin, a motilin agonist, can be given one-half hour before meals to stimulate gut motility. There is limited evidence that daily injectable octreotide (50 µg qhs subq) may help in severe cases. Fiber may help colonic dysmotility but may make small bowel problems worse. Fiber is worth an empiric trial.

Diarrhea is treated initially as if it were due to bacterial overgrowth. An antibiotic is given that can partially decrease gut flora, such as metronidazole (250 mg TID), tetracycline (250 mg QID), amoxicillin or ciprofloxacin (250 mg BID) for 10 days. In most cases, this stops the diarrhea. Agents that slow intestinal motility, such as paregoric or loperamide, should be avoided. If the diarrhea persists, a malabsorption work-up should be pursued. Most patients with malabsorption can be treated with supplemental vitamins, minerals, and predigested liquid food supplements. A rare patient will need total parenteral nutrition.

**18. Which scleroderma patients get interstitial lung disease? Which get pulmonary hypertension?**

| CLASSIFICATION | INTERSTITIAL LUNG DISEASE | PULMONARY HYPERTENSION |
|---|---|---|
| Localized | None | None |
| Limited systemic sclerosis (LSSc) | Typically bibasilar (20%) and usually nonprogressive | 8–28%<br>Poor prognosis |

(*Table continued on next page.*)

| CLASSIFICATION | INTERSTITIAL LUNG DISEASE | PULMONARY HYPERTENSION |
|---|---|---|
| Diffuse systemic sclerosis | More common than LSSc (31–59%) and can be progressive, leading to death | Very rare |
| Overlap | Common (19–85%, average 38%) can progress | 21–29% |

**19. Describe the clinical characteristics of lung disease associated with systemic sclerosis.**

Many patients with laboratory evidence of **interstitial lung disease** are asymptomatic. Clinical symptoms can be insidious and include exertional dyspnea, easy fatigability, and exertional nonproductive cough, but later may progress to dyspnea at rest. Clinical signs are typically early inspiratory fine or Velcro crackles. Pleuritic chest pains are rare in systemic sclerosis.

Patients with **pulmonary hypertension** usually have an insidious onset of exertional dyspnea, which can rapidly become dyspnea at rest with pedal edema. Physical exam can reveal an increased pulmonic component of the second heart sound ($P_2$), right ventricular gallops, pulmonic or tricuspid insufficiency murmur, jugular venous distention, and pedal edema. Chest radiographs and CT scans demonstrate interstitial fibrosis predominantly of the lower lobes.

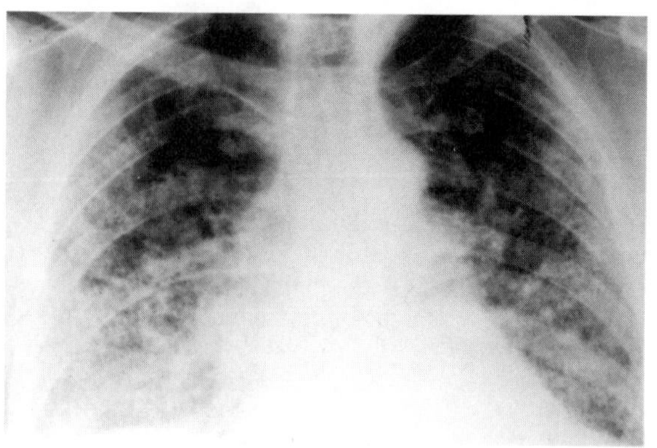

Interstitial lung disease in a systemic sclerosis patient.

**20. What is the treatment for interstitial lung disease (ILD) associated with systemic sclerosis?**

Many patients with systemic sclerosis have basilar ILD that never spreads to the middle or upper lung fields. This does not have to be treated. However, many patients will have progression of their lung disease to the middle and upper lobes. Patients who are most likely to respond to immunosuppressive therapy have evidence of active alveolitis on bronchoalveolar lavage [elevated percentage of neutrophils and/or eosinophils (> 5% of BAL fluid cellularity)] and/or nonspecific interstitial pneumonitis (NSIP) on high resolution CT scan (ground glass, no honey combing) or lung biopsy (VATS or open). These patients may respond to prednisone and cyclophosphamide. Other immunosuppressive medications have also been used. Patients with progression of lung disease without active alveolitis and/or usual interstitial pneumonia (UIP) on HRCT scan (honey combing, subpleural fibrosis) or lung biopsy usually do not respond to therapy similar to patients with idiopathic pulmonary fibrosis (IPF). This is because these patients most likely develop fibrosis due to fibroblastic foci and not due to inflammation. In these patients, antifibrotic therapy would be beneficial, but none is available. Experimentally, gamma interferon has been effective in treating IPF and has been suggested for treatment of UIP associated with systemic sclerosis.

**21. What is the treatment for pulmonary hypertension?**

Initially, patients are placed on nasal oxygen. Calcium channel blockers such as nifedipine and diltiazem can be tried for their vasodilator effect. Full anticoagulation with warfarin is often administered. For severe pulmonary hypertension, patients may go on to continuous intravenous infusion of epoprostenol ($PGI_2$). A new oral nonspecific endothelin antagonist, bosentan (Tracleer, 125 mg BID), is now available for severe pulmonary hypertension. Contraindications to bosentan are pregnancy, cyclosporine, and glyburide. Hepatotoxicity and interaction with other medications are possible. If the patient progresses on the above regimen, lung transplantation is then recommended.

**22. Describe the cardiac involvement in systemic sclerosis.**

Autopsy studies find cardiac involvement unrelated to lung or renal disease relatively common (50%). However, clinically significant heart problems are rare. Pericardial effusion is common at autopsy, but symptomatic pericarditis is rarely seen. Similarly, endocardial involvement is described but clinically insignificant. The most common manifestation of scleroderma heart disease is myocardial fibrosis, usually focal but equally distributed throughout the right and left heart myocardium. This can lead to an uncommon cause of cardiomyopathy. Premature coronary artery disease has also been noted in many patients, probably as part of the diffuse vasculopathy occurring in these patients. The use of high-dose corticosteroids is also thought to enhance coronary artery disease. Patients may present with conduction defects and congestive heart failure. The conduction defects, unless showing significant ventricular arrhythmia, are usually not treated. Congestive heart failure is treated in standard ways.

**23. Renal failure is one of the most feared complications of systemic sclerosis. What is the presentation of this complication?**

Renal failure may present as acute renal crisis, after prolonged hypertension, and less commonly as normotensive renal failure.

**Renal crisis** is the abrupt onset of arterial hypertension, appearance of grade III (flame-shaped hemorrhages and/or cotton-wool exudates) or grade IV (papilledema) retinopathy, and the rapid deterioration of renal function (within a month). Abnormal laboratory tests include elevated renal function tests, consumptive thrombocytopenia, microangiopathic hemolysis, and elevated renin levels (twice the ULN or greater). Renal crisis usually occurs in the patient with **diffuse** systemic sclerosis. Generally, renal crisis occurs early in the course of the disease, with a mean onset of 3.2 years, and more often in the fall and winter months. Prognosis for recovery is poor.

**Prolonged hypertension** seems to predispose to renal failure. There is a minority of patients who develop normotensive renal failure with no evidence of renal crisis. The use of high-dose corticosteroids probably increases the risk for renal failure in systemic sclerosis.

**24. Which therapeutic intervention has helped avoid renal failure in patients with systemic sclerosis?**

The use of **angiotensin converting enzyme (ACE) inhibitors** has dramatically changed the incidence and outcome of renal involvement in systemic sclerosis. The diastolic blood pressure should be kept below 90 mm Hg in all patients with systemic sclerosis. Captopril and enalapril are the most studied ACE inhibitors in scleroderma, but probably any of the ACE inhibitors are effective. In a small series of scleroderma patients who went into renal crisis, the angiotensin II receptor antagonists did not seem to reverse the renal crisis but when switched to an ACE inhibitor, their renal function improved.

**25. Describe the bone and articular involvement in systemic sclerosis.**

Bone involvement is usually demonstrated by resorption of bone. Acrosclerosis with osteolysis is common. Resorption of ribs, mandible, acromion, radius, and ulna have been reported. Arthralgias and morning stiffness are relatively common, but erosive arthritis is rare. Hand deformities and ankylosis are seen, but these are attributed to the tethering effects of skin thickening instead of joint involvement. Tendon sheaths can become inflamed and fibrinous, mimicking arthritis. Tendon friction rubs can be palpated typically over the wrists, ankles, and knees. Mainly, the diffuse systemic sclerosis patients develop tendon friction rubs.

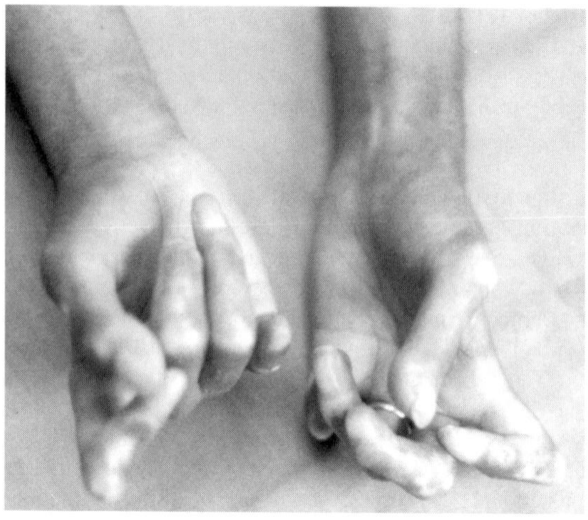

Articular and cutaneous involvement in systemic sclerosis. The skin is taut and thickened, leading to deformity and limited motility of the fingers. Note sclerodactyly and digital ulcerations.

**26. Discuss the three types of muscle abnormalities seen in systemic sclerosis.**

1. Mild proximal weakness due to a noninflammatory benign myopathy. On histology, this myopathy looks normal or shows muscle fiber type 2 atrophy. This pattern of fiber loss is seen with inactivity and corticosteroid use. The muscle enzymes are typically normal.

2. Mild elevation of muscles enzymes with waxing and waning of symptoms. Muscle biopsy reveals interstitial fibrosis and fiber atrophy. Minimal inflammatory cell infiltration is noted.

3. Inflammatory type of myopathy with elevated muscle enzymes (as seen with polymyositis). These patients are considered to have an overlap syndrome, and many fit the definition of mixed connective tissue disease.

**27. Which autoantibodies are seen in diffuse and limited systemic sclerosis?**

| ANTIBODIES | DIFFUSE SYSTEMIC SCLEROSIS | LIMITED SYSTEMIC SCLEROSIS |
|---|---|---|
| Antinuclear antibody* | 90–95% | 90–95% |
| Anti-topoisomerase I (Scl-70) | 20–30 | 10–15 |
| Anti-centromere antibody | 5 | 50–90 |
| Anti-RNA polymerase III | 25 | 6 |
| Anti U3 RNP (fibrillarin) | 7 | — |
| Anti Th/To+ | — | 4–16 |

* Patients with systemic sclerosis frequently have ANA with nucleolar pattern. ANA against topoisomerase 1, RNA polymerase III, fibrillarin, Th/To, PM-Scl (PM-1) all give nucleolar staining.

+ A patient with limited systemic sclerosis, nucleolar ANA, and negative anticentromere antibody frequently has anti Th/To.

**28. Which chemicals have been implicated in inducing a scleroderma-like condition?**

Vinyl chloride—a number of reports
Silica dust—noted first in gold miners
Rapeseed oil contaminated with aniline dye—toxic oil syndrome noted in Spain in 1981
Contaminated L-tryptophan—implicated in an epidemic of eosinophilia myalgia syndrome

Organic solvents
  Aromatic hydrocarbons—toluene, benzene
  Aliphatic hydrocarbons
    Chlorinated—trichloroethylene, perchlorethylene
    Nonchlorinated—naphtha-n-hexane, hexachloroethane
Epoxy resins
Drugs
  Bleomycin
Appetite suppressants
Silicone—breast implants (controversial)

**29. What traditional medicines have been used to treat the skin involvement in systemic sclerosis?**

No treatment has been shown definitively to be successful in treating scleroderma. The following treatments have been tried in small studies:

- Colchicine (0.6 mg bid)—relatively safe but usually ineffective
- *p*-Aminobenzoic acid (3 gm qid)—safe; used to treat keloid formation; all studies in systemic sclerosis are uncontrolled
- D-Penicillamine (increase slowly to 1000 mg/day)—the most studied drug in systemic sclerosis; a number of retrospective and uncontrolled studies have demonstrated help with tight skin and possibly interstitial lung disease; a relatively toxic drug. A recent large, randomized, multicenter, double-blind study in early diffuse systemic sclerosis patients comparing low dose (62.5 mg daily) with high dose (750 mg daily) D-penicillamine found no difference in skin scores, mortality, or the incidence of renal crisis.
- Chlorambucil—showed no help in a prospective study in patients with disease an average of 7.9 years.
- Corticosteroids—thought to increase the incidence of renal crisis and probably should be avoided. Used for comfort in patients with very actively inflamed and tight skin. Also used for inflammatory myositis.

**30. What experimental drugs or therapies have been proposed recently?**

- Relaxin—a natural hormone made during pregnancy. Although an initial phase I/II study showed promise, a larger, multicenter, double-blind controlled study demonstrated no difference from placebo.
- Methotrexate—small studies suggested this drug might help the skin. A large, multicenter, placebo-controlled, blinded study out of Canada demonstrated a trend in favor of methotrexate but no statistical difference in skin scores in early diffuse patients.
- Extracorporeal photochemotherapy (photophoresis)—an initial study in 1992 showed a modest but statistical benefit. A more recent study in 1999 showed no difference in skin scores.
- 5-Fluorouracil—in small uncontrolled series has shown some benefit in skin scores.
- Cyclosporine—has shown modest benefit in uncontrolled series but had unacceptable renal toxicity.
- Gamma-interferon—in small series has shown benefit in skin scores, although some patients went into renal crisis. It has been proposed to treat interstitial lung disease.
- Plasmapheresis.
- Immunosuppression has been proposed as the best direction to treat rapidly progressive diffuse patients. In this regard, oral and intravenous cyclophosphamide, mycophenolate mofetil, and autologous hematopoietic stem cell transplantation are being studied as interventions in early diffuse systemic sclerosis.
- Transforming growth factor–beta (TGF-beta) is a pivotal cytokine involved in fibrosis. Strategies to neutralize this cytokine with decorin (a small TGF-beta binding proteoglycan), latency-associated peptide (a potent inhibitor of TGF-beta isoforms), soluble receptors, and chimeric antibodies are all being pursued.

**31. Is there an association between cancer and systemic sclerosis (SS)?**

Breast cancer has been described to develop in close proximity prior to or at the onset of SS. Lung cancer is increased 1.8-fold in patients with lung fibrosis ("scar carcinoma"). Despite chronic reflux, esophageal cancer is not increased unless the patient has Barrett's esophagus.

**32. What is the cause of systemic sclerosis (SS)?**

Unknown. What does appear to be important is endothelial disruption and fibroblast proliferation. The fibroblasts produce an excess of collagen (type I and III). The collagen is normal, and the ability to break down the collagen is normal. However, it is made in excessive amounts for the normal breakdown mechanisms to control, so it accumulates. Cytokines such as TGF-β are believed to play a role. Platelet activation due to endothelial disruption is also important to the intimal proliferative process.

The trigger is unknown. Environmental factors have been implicated (see Question 28). Recently, individuals with SS have been shown to have persistence of fetal cells in higher numbers in their peripheral circulation, skin, and lung. This fetal microchimerism suggests that mechanisms similar to graft-versus-host disease (scleroderma-like skin, sicca, ILD following bone marrow transplant) may play a role in systemic sclerosis.

## BIBLIOGRAPHY

1. Althan RD, Medsger TA, Bloch DA, Michel BA: Predictors of survival in systemic sclerosis (scleroderma). Arthritis Rheum 34:403–413, 1991.
2. Badesch DB, Tapson VF, McGoon MD, et al: Continuous intravenous epoprostenol for pulmonary hypertension due to the scleroderma spectrum of diseases: A randomized clinical trial. Ann Int Med 132:425–434, 2000.
3. Borg EJT, Piersma-Wichers G, Smit AJ, et al: Serial nailfold capillary microscopy in primary Raynaud's phenomenon and scleroderma. Semin Arthritis Rheum 24:40–47, 1994.
4. Claman HN, Giorno RC, Seibold JR: Endothelial and fibroblastic activation in scleroderma: The myth of the "uninvolved skin." Arthritis Rheum 34:1495–1501, 1991.
5. Clements PJ, Furst DE (eds): Systemic Sclerosis. Baltimore, Williams & Wilkins, 1996.
6. Clements PJ, Furst DE, Wong WK, et al.: High-dose versus low dose D-penicillamine in early diffuse systemic sclerosis: Analysis of a two-year, double blind, randomized, controlled clinical trial. Arthritis Rheum 42:1194–1203, 1999
7. Donohoe JF: Scleroderma and the kidney. Kidney Int 41:462–477, 1992.
8. Furst DE: Rational therapy in the treatment of systemic sclerosis. Curr Opin Rheumatol 12:540–544, 2000.
9. Geirsson AJ, Wollheim FA, Akesson A: Disease severity of 100 patients with systemic sclerosis over a period of 14 years: Using a modified Medsger scale. Ann Rheum Dis 60:1117–1122, 2001.
10. Janosik DL, Osborn TG, Moore TL, et al: Heart disease in systemic sclerosis. Semin Arthritis Rheum 19:191–200, 1989.
11. Leighton C: Drug treatment of scleroderma. Drugs 61:419–427, 2001.
12. LeRoy EC, Black C, Fleischmajer R, et al: Scleroderma (systemic sclerosis): Classification, subsets and pathogenesis. J Rheumatol 15:202–205, 1988.
13. Nelson JL: Pregnancy and microchimerism in autoimmune disease: Protector or insurgent? Arthritis Rheum 46:291–297, 2002.
14. Pope JE, Bellamy N, Seibold JR, et al: A randomized, controlled trial of methotrexate versus placebo in early diffuse scleroderma. Arthritis Rheum 44:1351–1358, 2001.
15. Rosas I, Conte J, Yang S, et al: Lung transplantation and systemic sclerosis. Ann Transplantation 5:38–43, 2000.
16. Sjogren RW: Gastrointestinal motility disorders in scleroderma. Arthritis Rheum 37:1265–1282, 1994.
17. Soudah HC, Hasler WL, Owyang C: Effect of octreotide on intestinal motility and bacterial overgrowth in scleroderma. N Engl J Med 325:1461–1467, 1991.
18. Steen VD, Costantino JP, Shapiro AP, et al: Outcome of renal crisis in systemic sclerosis: Relation to availability of angiotensin converting enzyme (ACE) inhibitors. Ann Intern Med 113:352–357, 1990.
19. Steen VD, Medsger TA: Epidemiology and natural history of systemic sclerosis. Rheum Dis Clin North Am 16:641–654, 1990.
20. Steen VD: Treatment of systemic sclerosis. Am J Clin Dermatol 2:315–25, 2001.
21. Varga J: Progress in systemic sclerosis: Novel therapeutic paradigms. Curr Rheumatol Rep 2:481–485, 2000.

22. Weiner ES, Hildebrandt S, Senecal JL, et al: Prognostic significance of anti-centromere antibodies and anti-topoisomerase 1 antibodies in Raynaud's disease: A prospective study. Arthritis Rheum 34: 68–77, 1991.
23. White B, Moore WC, Wigley FM, et al: Cyclophosphamide is associated with pulmonary function and survival benefit in patients with scleroderma and alveolitis. Ann Int Med 132:947–954, 2000.

# 23. EOSINOPHILIA-MYALGIA SYNDROME, DIFFUSE FASCIITIS WITH EOSINOPHILIA, AND RHEUMATIC DISEASE ASSOCIATED WITH SILICONE BREAST IMPLANTS

*Gregory J. Dennis, M.D.*

## EOSINOPHILIA-MYALGIA SYNDROME

**1. List characteristic clinical features of the eosinophilia-myalgia syndrome (EMS) seen at onset of the disease.**

Myalgias (severe)
Maculopapular erythematous skin rashes
Peripheral edema
Fever
Fatigue
Weight loss
Cough
Skin induration (especially trunk, lower extremities)

This acute phase is abrupt in onset and lasts weeks to months.

**2. What are some typical findings that occur later in the disease process in EMS?**

Scleroderma-like skin thickening
Xerostomia
Alopecia
Proximal myopathy
Peripheral neuropathy
Cognitive dysfunction

This chronic phase can last for years.

**3. Is EMS recognized as a New or Old World disease?**

EMS was recognized during 1989 as an epidemic. Although the initial cases were recognized in Los Alamos, New Mexico, the outbreak was nationwide. Relatively few cases have occurred outside of the United States, where the highest prevalence rates occurred in the western states. Cases reported from California represented 19% of the U.S. total.

**4. Which chemical product was implicated with EMS?**

L-tryptophan. Numerous trace level impurities have been identified in cases of EMS suggesting the possibility that impurities ingested in combination with L-tryptophan results in the characteristic pathological features. Whether the syndrome derives from the L-tryptophan content, an impurity, a combination of the two, or some as yet undetermined external factor remains unknown.

**5. What three essential features of the disease were established by the Centers for Disease Control and Prevention (CDC) as the surveillance case definition?**

1. Blood eosinophil count greater than $10^9$/liter (> 1000 cells/mm$^3$)
2. Generalized myalgia of sufficient severity to limit activity
3. Exclusion of neoplasm or infection to account for symptoms

**6. Approximately how many cases of EMS were reported in the United States that fulfilled the CDC criteria?**

More than 1500 cases, with 38 deaths, were reported that fulfilled the CDC criteria. Many more were probably affected that did not fulfill the criteria.

**7. List some clinical problems that could potentially lead to disability in patients with EMS.**

| | |
|---|---|
| Sclerodermatous skin thickening | Neuropathy |
| Hyperpigmentation | Myopathy |
| Myalgia | Dyspnea |
| Muscle cramping | Subjective cognitive impairment |
| Arthralgia | Fatigue |

**8. Describe the cutaneous findings in EMS.**

The cutaneous findings are similar to those seen in eosinophilic fasciitis and systemic sclerosis. During the acute phase, alopecia, erythematous macules, papular eruptions, and subcutaneous edema occurred in many patients. Edema at times had a *peau d'orange* quality. In contrast to scleroderma, the face and the acral portions of the body were usually spared.

**9. When in relation to the onset of disease did the cutaneous manifestations of EMS appear?**

The cutaneous findings in EMS had onset during the initial 3–6 months of disease. Preexisting edema was not uniformly present, but skin changes often were associated with the presence of papular mucinosis. The distribution of sclerodermatous thickening is similar to that of the subclasses of skin involvement in idiopathic systemic sclerosis—i.e., diffuse, limited, or localized. There is a wide range of sclerodermatous involvement, increasing from 44% to 82% after 14 to 36 months from disease onset in several series. Hyperpigmentation is also seen in EMS patients.

**10. What features of idiopathic systemic sclerosis are not characteristic of patients with EMS?**

Patients with EMS generally lack Raynaud's phenomenon, digital ischemic lesions, tendon friction rubs, and acral sclerosis.

**11. List four features that distinguishes EMS from eosinophilic fasciitis (EF).**

- EMS patients were more likely to require hospitalization, develop fever, and have systemic involvement.
- Inflammation in EMS characteristically occurred in cutaneous and subcutaneous areas, whereas the inflammation in EF is primarily subcutaneous.
- Perineural inflammatory infiltrates are more common in EMS.
- More immunoglobulin and complement deposition in EF biopsies.

**12. Briefly discuss the manifestations of muscle involvement in EMS.**

The abrupt onset of myalgia is considered one of the hallmarks of EMS and persists in greater than 50% of individuals after 1 year of disease. Severe muscle cramps occur in 43–90% of patients with chronic EMS. Myopathy may be present in early or late disease, most commonly as a result of perimyositis. Rarely, myonecrosis or microangiopathy may be responsible for the myopathic process.

**13. What types of peripheral neurologic abnormalities have been reported in patients with EMS?**

An axonal sensorimotor polyneuropathy has been the most common peripheral neuropathy reported. Others include mononeuritis multiplex, demyelinating neuropathy, and postural tremor.

**14. Do clinical manifestations of neuropathy in EMS correlate with findings on electrodiagnostic testing?**

Clinical findings of a sensory neuropathy are common, but there may be discordant findings when the patient undergoes electrodiagnostic tests. This discrepancy may be related to the inability of standard nerve conduction velocities to detect involvement of small dermal nerves.

**15. How significant is fatigue in patients with EMS?**

Fatigue is a significant problem in most patients from the onset. It is one of the principal disabling aspects of chronic EMS, being present in as many as 95% of afflicted individuals.

**16. Describe pathognomonic signs in EMS.**

There are no pathognomonic signs. Initially, patients show few abnormal findings. Palpable muscle tenderness and skin rash may be all that is present. A flu-like prodrome is often present, including muscle aches, cough, shortness of breath, and fatigue. Nonspecific symptoms and constitutional symptoms may also be present.

**17. Which manifestation was considered to be the hallmark of EMS?**

A high eosinophil count is considered to be the hallmark of the disease. The eosinophil count, however, is often transient and is found only early in the disease process. The absence of eosinophilia should not preclude a diagnosis of EMS. Eosinophil degranulation in tissue samples has been shown to occur.

**18. How is EMS treated?**

Discontinuation of L-tryptophan–containing products was a necessity, but did not always lead to improvement. Variable responsiveness to glucocorticoid medications was observed; however, long-term efficacy was not demonstrated. Other immunomodulating therapies resulted in inconsistent responses. The myalgias frequently required narcotics for pain relief during the acute phase.

**19. What long-term complications have been noted in EMS?**

Although many patients improved after elimination of L-tryptophan, many others persisted with chronic problems. Myalgias, muscle cramps, fatigue, paresthesias, and scleroderma-like skin changes were reported in greater than 50% of patients after 18–24 months. Only 26% reported being able to perform normal daily activities.

**20. Is there currently any marketing restriction of dietary supplements containing L-tryptophan and related compounds?**

At the present time, an import alert exists limiting the importation of L-tryptophan into the United States except for an exempted use. The FDA permits the use of L-tryptophan in accordance with the provisions of Title 21 of the Code of Federal Regulations in foods that are intended for use under medical supervision to meet nutritional requirements in specific medical conditions, i.e., infant formulas, enteral and approved parenteral products.

**21. What other disease epidemic resembled EMS?**

In the summer of 1981, 20,000 people in Spain developed an epidemic of acute pneumonitis followed by a chronic stage of scleroderma-like skin thickening, neuromyopathy, and sicca syndrome. This was called toxic oil syndrome and was traced to ingestion of tainted rapeseed oil used for cooking.

## EOSINOPHILIC FASCIITIS (DIFFUSE FASCIITIS WITH EOSINOPHILIA)

**22. Is eosinophilic fasciitis (EF) associated with ingestion of chemicals?**

To date, EF is considered to be an idiopathic connective tissue disorder of uncertain etiology. First described in 1974, no association with the ingestion of chemicals has been convincingly demonstrated. Two cases have been reported in association with prolonged exposure to the solvent trichloroethylene. It is often classified in a category with scleroderma and scleroderma-like syndromes, but in contrast to scleroderma, individuals with EF generally do not have Raynaud's phenomenon and have normal nailfold capillaries. Strenuous physical exertion may precede its onset in some patients.

**23. List three common early clinical manifestations of EF.**

Diffuse swelling
Stiffness
Tenderness of the involved areas

**24. Is there a characteristic distribution of involvement in EF?**

There is usually simultaneous involvement in all affected areas. The most frequent pattern includes involvement of both the arms and legs in a symmetrical fashion with sparing of the fingers and toes. The proximal areas of the extremities are generally more affected than the distal.

**25. Describe a characteristic feature of the cutaneous involvement.**

The initial manifestations of EF are often followed by the development of severe induration of the skin and subcutaneous tissues of the affected areas. The skin becomes taut and woody with a coarse orange-peel appearance (*peau d'orange*). Although the induration often remains confined to the extremities, it may variably affect extensive areas of the trunk and face.

**26. Are there any common musculoskeletal problems that individuals with EF develop?**

Because of involvement of the fascia, carpal tunnel syndrome is an early feature in many patients. Flexion contractures of the digits and extremities may occur as a consequence of the fascial involvement.

**27. Is eosinophilia uniformly present throughout the course of an EF patient's illness?**

No. Eosinophilia is often present only during the early stages of the patient's illness and tends to decline later in the illness. The degree of eosinophilia does not closely parallel disease activity.

**28. Is there any reason to expect hematologic abnormalities to be associated with EF?**

The pathogenesis of these conditions is thought to involve autoimmune mechanisms. Hematologic problems have been significantly appreciated. Those described in a small number of patients include thrombocytopenia, aplastic anemia, and myelodysplasia. These complications may occur at any time in the course of EF and do not correlate with the severity of disease.

**29. How is the diagnosis of EF confirmed histologically?**

Histologically, the diagnosis is best confirmed by performing a deep wedge en-bloc full thickness biopsy of an involved area. The biopsy should be deep enough to acquire skin, subcutis, fascia, and muscle for study. Although inflammation and fibrosis are generally found in all layers, they are usually most intense in the fascia. The inflammatory infiltrate consists of abundant lymphocytes, plasma cells, and histiocytes. Eosinophilic infiltration may be particularly striking, especially early in the disease process.

**30. What laboratory abnormality other than eosinophilia is commonly found in patients with EF?**

Other than eosinophilia, the only other commonly reported laboratory abnormality that is generally present is **hypergammaglobulinemia**. The IgG fraction appears to be primarily responsible for the elevation in the total gammaglobulin pool.

**31. Describe the course of illness in patients with EF.**

In many patients, the illness is self-limited with spontaneous improvement. Occasionally complete remission occurs after 2 or more years. Some patients, unfortunately, have persistent or recurrent disease. Fixed joint contractures may be responsible for permanent disability in some patients.

**32. Are any therapies effective in patients with EF?**

Corticosteroids often result in marked and rapid improvement in both the eosinophilia and the presence of fasciitis. Other medications, such as cimetidine, hydroxychloroquine, penicillamine, and immunosuppressive agents, have been used with variable success.

**33. Without therapy, what percentage of individuals will develop progressive disease?**

If untreated, fascial inflammation will lead to joint contractures in 85%. In addition, the skin that is initially indurated frequently may become bound down and develop a *peau d'orange* appearance.

**34. Does the inflammatory process in EF ever extend beyond the fascia?**

Deeper layers of the dermis have been involved with cellular infiltration in over 30% of cases. The inflammatory infiltrate has been noted to extend to the epi- and perimysial connective tissue. However, muscle fiber neurosis and phagocytosis are rare.

**35. When should the diagnosis of EF be considered?**

The diagnosis should be considered in an individual with the following:

Scleroderma-like skin tightening
Peripheral eosinophilia
Skin thickening that spares the digits
No Raynaud's phenomenon

## RHEUMATIC DISEASE ASSOCIATED WITH SILICONE BREAST IMPLANTS

**36. List the commonly recognized complications of breast implant augmentation.**

- Infection
- Hemorrhage
- Local skin necrosis
- Capsule formation
- Implant rupture

**37. When were the first reports of connective tissue diseases in patients with breast implants?**

The first report of a connective tissue disease after breast augmentation appeared in the Japanese literature in 1964. One of these patients had dramatic improvement after removal of the foreign substance. The first report in the English literature was in 1979. These early reports were mostly in women receiving breast augmentation with injections of non–medical-grade silicone or paraffin rather than breast implants. The connective tissue diseases reported in patients with breast implants have included systemic sclerosis, mixed connective tissue disease, rheumatoid arthritis, SLE, sicca syndrome (Sjögren's) and atypical connective tissue disease. Many patients have had complaints of chronic fatigue, arthralgias, and myalgias that defy classification into a specific category of connective tissue disease.

**38. Which types of medical-grade polymers are under consideration in the association of silicone with connective tissue disease?**

**Polydimethylsiloxane** (PDMS) polymers are widely used in applications ranging from the manufacture of food-processing materials to the production of cosmetics and medical devices. Gels used in breast implants that have been implicated with connective tissue disease are generally produced by the addition of vinyl to PDMS.

**39. Which connective tissue disease has the greatest likelihood of being associated with breast implants?**

While a number of connective tissue disease syndromes were thought to be significantly associated with silicone breast implants, except for possibly Sjögren's syndrome, no convincing evidence is available at this time.

**40. Do patients' symptoms resolve or improve when the silicone breast implants are removed?**

Improvement and resolution of the patient's problems on removal of the implants have been reported in multiple cases, but this occurs in only a minority of patients. These patients have usually been classified as having rheumatoid arthritis or SLE. The reversibility of illnesses after removal of the implants has perpetuated the notion that there may be a link between silicone implants and connective tissue disease.

**41. Can laboratory variables be used to identify connective tissue disease in patients who have had silicone breast implants?**

To date, there are no laboratory markers that exist to distinguish those who have problems with implants from those without. Likewise, those with problems cannot be distinguished serologically or otherwise from those having idiopathic connective tissue disease. Antinuclear antibodies have been commonly detected in those with silicone breast implants, but acute-phase reactants primarily correlate with objective evidence of inflammatory disease.

**42. Are imaging studies helpful in the evaluation of patients with possible connective tissue disease?**

Imaging studies such as mammography or breast MRI may be helpful in detecting implant rupture prior to operative intervention. However, breast implant imaging studies are not helpful in predicting which individuals are at risk for developing a connective tissue disease.

**43. Does breast implant rupture increase the risk of connective tissue disease occurrence?**

The presence of objective implant rupture thus far has not been shown to correlate with the risk of developing connective tissue disease. Fragmentation of the surface of most breast implants occurs over time, resulting in leakage, migration, or transport of implant contents into surrounding tissue. In the absence of rupture, it is hypothesized that silicone gel may migrate through the elastomeric envelope.

**44. What specific recommendations have been made regarding silicone breast implants in the United States?**

Silicone gel-filled breast implants are currently not authorized for use in the United States. A committee of the Institute of Medicine convened during 2000 and concluded that there is insufficient evidence to support an association of silicone breast implants with defined connective tissue disease and no rigorous convincing scientific support for atypical connective tissue or any new disease in women that is associated with silicone breast implants.

## BIBLIOGRAPHY

1. Angell M: Do breast implants cause systemic disease? Science in the courtroom. N Engl J Med 330:1748–1749, 1994.
2. Clauw DJ, Pincus T (eds): Eosinophilia-myalgia syndrome: Review and reappraisal of clinical, epidemiologic and animal studies symposium, December 7–8, 1994, Georgetown University, Washington, DC. J Rheumatol Suppl 46, 1996.
3. Committee of the Institute of Medicine: Safety of silicone breast implants, epidemiological studies of connective tissue or rheumatic diseases and breast implants. The National Academy Press, copyright 2000.
4. Fock KM, Feng PH, Tey BH: Autoimmune disease developing after augmentation mammoplasty: Report of 3 cases. J Rheumatol 11:98–100, 1984.
5. Haseler LJ, Sibbitt WL Jr, Sibbitt RR, Hart BL: Neurologic, MR imaging, and MR spectroscopic findings in eosinophilia myalgia syndrome.Am J Neuroradiol 19(9):1687–1694, 1998.
6. Janowsky EC, Kupper LL, Hulka BS: Meta-analyses of the relation between silicone breast implants and the risk of connective-tissue diseases. N Engl J Med 342:781–790, 2000.
7. Martin RW, Duffy J, Engel AG, et al: The clinical spectrum of the eosinophilia-myalgia syndrome associated with L-tryptophan ingestion. Ann Intern Med 113:124–134, 1990.
8. Naschitz JE, Boss JH, Misselevich I, et al: The fasciitis-panniculitis syndromes. Medicine 75:6–16, 1996.

9. Philen RM, Posada M: Toxic oil and eosinophilia-myalgia syndrome: May 8–10, 1991, World Health Organization meeting report. Semin Arthritis Rheum 23:104–124, 1993.
10. Rodnan GP, Di Bartolomeo AG, Medsger TA: Eosinophilic fasciitis: Report of seven cases of a newly recognized scleroderma-like syndrome. Arthritis Rheum 18:422–423, 1975.
11. Shulman LE: Diffuse fasciitis with eosinophilia: A new syndrome. Arthritis Rheum 20:133, 1977.
12. Sullivan EA, Kamb ML, Jones JL, et al: The natural history of eosinophilia-myalgia syndrome in a tryptophan-exposed cohort in South Carolina. 156:973–979, 1996.
13. Varga J, Kahari VM: Eosinophilia-myalgia syndrome, eosinophilic fasciitis, and related fibrosing disorders. Curr Opin Rheumatol 9(6):562–570, 1997.
14. Varga J, Schumacher HR, Jimenez SA: Systemic sclerosis after augmentation mammoplasty with silicone implants. Ann Intern Med 111:377–383, 1989.
15. Tugwell P, Wells G, Peterson J, et al: Do silicone breast implants cause rheumatologic disorders? Arthritis Rheum 44:2477–2484, 2001.
16. U.S. Food and Drug Administration Center for Food Safety and Applied Nutrition, Office of Nutritional Products, Labeling, and Dietary Supplements: Information paper on L-tryptophan and 5-hydroxy-L-tryptophan. Feb 2001.

# 24. INFLAMMATORY MUSCLE DISEASE

*Robert* T. *Spencer*, M.D.

**1. Idiopathic inflammatory myopathies comprise which disorders?**

**Polymyositis** (PM) and **dermatomyositis** (DM) are the most common of these uncommon disorders, which cause nonsuppurative muscle inflammation. Other disorders in this classification include inclusion body myositis, eosinophilic myositis, giant cell myositis, and focal or localized myositis. Other inflammatory myopathies include those caused by infections, drugs, and toxins.

**2. How are PM and DM classified?**

Although several classification schemes have been devised, the system proposed by Bohan and Peter in 1975 remains the one most commonly referred to:

1. Adult polymyositis
2. Adult dermatomyositis
3. PM/DM associated with malignancy
4. Childhood DM (less often PM)
5. PM/DM associated with other connective tissue disorders

**3. What are some of the epidemiologic features of these disorders?**

- Annual incidence of 2–10 cases/million
- Peak age of onset is bimodal in distribution: one peak at 10–15 years of age, and the other at 45–55 years
- Female to male ratio is 2–3:1 overall. Female to male ratio in childhood DM is close to 1:1, and in PM/DM associated with other connective tissue disorders it is 8–10:1.
- In the United States, African-Americans are affected more commonly than whites at a ratio of 3–4:1

**4. What are the major diagnostic criteria for PM/DM?**

- **Proximal motor weakness**: Weakness occurs earliest and insidiously over 3–6 months. It occurs most severely around the shoulder/pelvic girdles and neck flexors. Ocular and facial motor weakness is strikingly unusual. Pain is typically absent or minimal.
- **Elevated serum muscle enzymes**: Creatine kinase (CK) is elevated in almost all patients at some time during the course of active disease. Other markers of muscle damage include

elevated levels of aldolase, myoglobin, aspartate and alanine aminotransferase (AST and ALT), and lactate dehydrogenase (LDH). Myoglobinuria can be seen in active disease.

- **Abnormal neurodiagnostic studies**: The electromyogram (EMG) in PM/DM reveals polyphasic motor unit action potentials (MUAPs) with short duration and low amplitude. This pattern is in contrast to those seen in neuropathic disorders, which are characterized by large-amplitude, long-duration, polyphasic MUAPs (see Chapter 13). Nerve conduction velocity (NCV) studies are abnormal in neuropathic diseases. They are normal in the idiopathic inflammatory myopathies, with the exception of inclusion-body myositis in which neuropathic disease can develop along with the myopathy.
- **Muscle biopsy**: Muscle biopsy should be performed in all cases to confirm the suspected diagnosis. Typical findings are perivascular and endomysial inflammation with accompanying muscle fiber necrosis and muscle fiber regeneration. In PM, endomysial infiltration by chronic inflammatory cells is seen; most of these cells are cytotoxic CD8+ T cells. In DM, a somewhat different picture is seen in that the chronic inflammatory cell infiltration develops in perivascular as well as perifascicular regions and consists of a higher proportion of CD4+ T cells in addition to B cells. Perifascicular atrophy is diagnostic of DM.
- **Characteristic rash of dermatomyositis (see below)**.

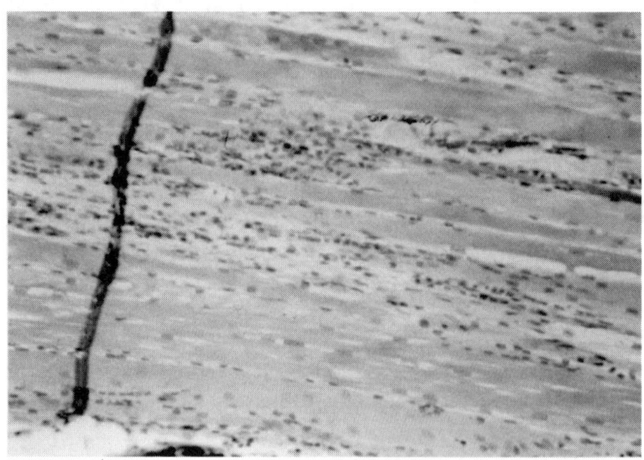

Muscle biopsy demonstrating inflammatory infiltrate and muscle fiber necrosis in a patient with polymyositis.

5. **Describe the dermatologic manifestations of dermatomyositis.**

**Heliotrope** (lilac-colored) **rash**: Purple to erythematous rash affecting the eyelids, malar region, forehead, and nasolabial folds. (Eyelids and nasolabial folds are typically spared in the rash of SLE).

**Gottron's papules**: Purple to erythematous flat or raised lesions over the interphalangeal regions of the fingers (i.e., knuckles). (See Chapter 20.)

**V-sign rash**: Confluent erythematous rash over the anterior chest and neck.

**Shawl-sign rash**: Erythematous rash over the shoulders and proximal arms.

**Mechanic's hands**: Characterized by cracking and fissuring of the skin of the finger pads.

**Nailfold abnormalities**: Periungual erythema, cuticular overgrowth, dilated capillary loops. (See Chapter 78.)

**Subcutaneous calcification**: Seen nearly exclusively in the juvenile form of DM; can be very extensive.

**Dermatomyositis mimics**: These can include cutaneous manifestations of trichinosis, allergic contact dermatitiis, and drug reactions (hydroxyurea, penicillamine, diclofenac).

6. **What measures can be taken to maximize muscle biopsy yield?**

- Biopsy a muscle that is clearly weak, but not severely so.

- Biopsy the muscle contralateral to one that is abnormal by EMG (i.e., perform neurodiagnostic studies unilaterally, and biopsy the contralateral side based on EMG results). Do not biopsy a muscle that has undergone recent EMG evaluation to avoid spurious results (i.e., EMG artifact).
- MRI scanning can be helpful to direct muscle biopsy in difficult cases. Areas of inflamed muscle demonstrate increased signal on T2-weighted and STIR images but not T1-weighted images, denoting areas of edema/inflammation.

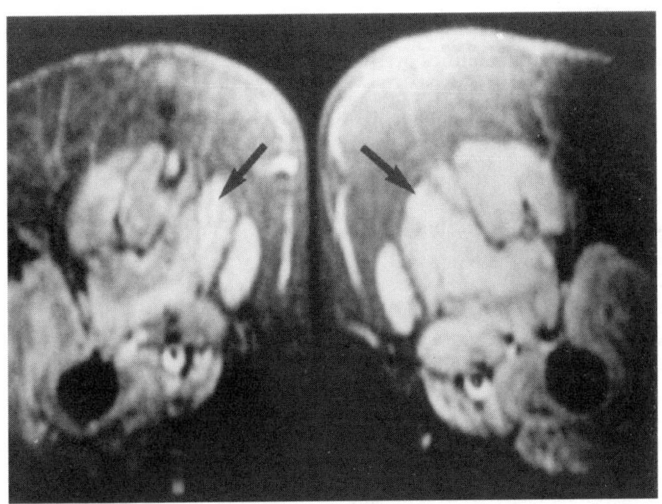

MRI scan of a patient with polymyositis. T2-weighted images demonstrate increased signal intensity of affected muscle tissue (arrows).

**7. What is amyotrophic dermatomyositis?**

Occasionally, the cutaneous manifestations of DM occur in the absence of clinically apparent muscle involvement. Such is referred to as **amyotrophic dermatomyositis**. Perhaps half or more of such patients will develop muscle disease over time, but a significant proportion will manifest skin-limited disease only.

**8. List some of the extramuscular or extradermatologic manifestations of PM/DM.**

**Constitutional symptoms**: fatigue, low-grade fever, weight loss

**Musculoskeletal**: arthralgias/arthritis (20–70%)

**Pulmonary**: interstitial lung disease (5–10%); aspiration pneumonia; respiratory muscle weakness; pulmonary hypertension

**Gastrointestinal**: esophageal dysmotility (10–30%); intestinal perforation due to vasculitis (primarily in juvenile DM)

**Cardiac**: ECG abnormalities (dysrhythmias, conduction blocks); myocarditis

**Vascular**: vasculitis causing livedo reticularis, skin ulcerations (juvenile DM); Raynaud's phenomenon (20–40%)

**Other**: manifestations of other connective tissue diseases when PM/DM occurs in "overlap" syndromes or in association with mixed connective tissue disease (MCTD)

**9. Is there an association between PM/DM and underlying neoplastic disease?**

Associated cancers are present at diagnosis, or at some point during follow-up (usually within first 3 years), in about 10% of adult patients with PM and in about 15% of adult patients with DM. Cancers reported in association with PM/DM include, among others, lung, stomach, ovary, breast, pancreas, and Hodgkin's lymphoma. This association has long been controversial, but recent studies have shown a 3–6 times increased risk for malignancy in DM and a 1.4–2 times increased risk for PM. Therefore, it is generally advised that patients with PM, and especially those with adult DM, be screened for underlying neoplastic disease. This screen should be age appropriate and include a complete history and exam (including breast, pelvis, prostate), stool occult blood testing, chest x-ray, mammogram, and routine laboratory tests. Some clinicians recommend an abdominal/pelvic CT scan owing to the high incidence of lymphoma and ovarian cancer. If initial cancer screen is negative, the physician should be alert for future development of cancer over the next 3–5 years.

**10. Which laboratory abnormalities are seen in PM/DM?**

- **Nonspecific abnormalities**
  Elevated muscle enzymes: Some patients have elevated aldolase and normal CPK. The combination of elevated CPK, aldolase, AST, and CPK MB > 2% is highly characteristic of an inflammatory myopathy.
  Erythrocyte sedimentation rate (elevated in 50%)
- **Myositis-associated autoantibodies**
  ANA (50–80%)
  Anti-RNP antibody (MCTD and "overlap" syndromes)
  Anti-PM-Scl antibody (PM-scleroderma overlap)
  Anti-Ku antibody (PM-scleroderma overlap)
- **Myositis-specific autoantibodies**

**11. Does an elevated serum CPK MB band indicate myocardial involvement?**

Elevations in CPK MB do not correlate with the presence or extent of myocardial disease, as regenerating skeletal muscle fibers release this isoform of the enzyme. Troponin is elevated in PM/DM patients with myocardial involvement.

**12. What are some of the more common myositis-specific autoantibodies?**

| AUTOANTIBODY | ANTIGEN | PREVALENCE PM/DM | IN CLINICAL ASSOCIATION | HLA ASSOCIATION |
|---|---|---|---|---|
| Antisynthetase* (e.g., anti-Jo-1) | Aminoacyl-tRNA synthetase | 20–50% | Antisynthetase syndrome | DRw52, DR3 |
| Anti-SRP | Signal recognition particle | < 5% | Severe, resistant PM | DRw52, DR5 |
| Anti-Mi-2 | Helicase components of histone acetylase complexes | 5–10% | Classic DM | DRw53, DR7 |

* Include anti Jo-1 (histidyl), PL-7 (threonyl), PL-12 (alanyl), EJ (glycyl), OJ (isoleucyl), KS (asparaginyl).

**13. What is the clinical significance of myositis-specific autoantibodies?**

Presence of these autoantibodies helps to predict clinical manifestations and prognosis. For example, the presence of anti-Jo-1 antibody is associated with an increased risk for interstitial lung disease (ILD), among other somewhat unique problems.

| | ANTI-SYNTHETASE | ANTI-SRP | ANTI-MI-2 |
|---|---|---|---|
| Onset | Acute; spring | Very acute; winter | Acute |
| Clinical manifestations | PM>>DM<br>ILD (40–60%)<br>Arthritis (deforming, nonerosive)<br>Mechanic's hands<br>Raynaud's phenomenon | Severe PM<br>Cardiac involvement | Classic DM<br>V-sign and shawl-sign rashes<br>Periungual erythema<br>Cuticular overgrowth |
| Steroid response | Moderate | Poor | Good |

**14. Which conditions should be considered in the differential diagnosis of inflammatory myopathies?**

**Drug and toxin induced myopathies** (especially statins, colchicine, antimalarials, AZT, alcohol)

**Neuromuscular disorders**
Muscular dystrophies (e.g., Duchenne's)
Neuromuscular junction disorders (e.g., myasthenia gravis, Eaton-Lambert syndrome)
Denervating conditions (e.g., amyotrophic lateral sclerosis)

**Endocrine disorders**
Hypothyroidism (may see CK as high as 3000)
Hyperthyroidism
Acromegaly
Cushing's disease
Addison's disease

**Miscellaneous**
Other rheumatic disorders (e.g., polymyalgia rheumatica, fibromyalgia syndrome, inflammatory arthritides, systemic vasculitis)
Carcinomatous neuromyopathy
Acute rhabdomyolysis
Organ failure (uremia, liver failure)

**Infectious myositis**
Bacterial (*Staphylococcus*, *Streptococcus*, *Borrelia burgdorferi*)
Viral (e.g., HIV, adenovirus, influenza)
Parasitic (e.g., *Toxoplasma*, *Trichinella*, *Taenia*)

**Metabolic myopathies**
Glycogen storage diseases (e.g., McArdle's or myophosphorylase deficiency, acid maltase deficiency)
Abnormalities of lipid metabolism (e.g., carnitine deficiency, carnitine palmitoyl transferase deficiency)
Mitochondrial myopathies
Nutritional disorders (malabsorption, vitamin D and E deficiencies)
Electrolyte disorders (hypo- and hypercalcemia, hypokalemia, hypophosphatemia)
Sarcoidosis

**15. What is the approach to treatment of PM/DM?**

**Corticosteroids** are the mainstay of therapy for PM/DM. Commonly, prednisone is started at a dose of 1–1.5 mg/kg/day in divided doses, and the dose is maintained until remission is achieved (improved strength and normalization of muscle enzymes). Subsequently, the dose is slowly tapered while monitoring for recurrence of disease activity.

**Immunosuppressive agents** are used in life-threatening disease and in disease resistant to corticosteroids alone. Methotrexate and azathioprine are used most often. Cyclophosphamide, Cellcept, chlorambucil, and cyclosporine are used rarely but have been reported to be of potential benefit in refractory disease. Hydroxychloroquine can be a helpful adjunct in treating the cutaneous manifestations of DM.

Of **experimental therapies**, intravenous immunoglobulin (IVIG) has been reported to be effective in severe, refractory DM/PM. Plasmapheresis has been tried in small numbers of patients and is of questionable benefit.

In the initial stages of disease, when muscle inflammation is most severe and when the patient is most weak, **rehabilitation** is recommended to involve only passive/active assisted range of motion exercises. Later, as strength returns and muscle inflammation subsides, exercise for strengthening can slowly be added to the physical therapy regimen.

**16. What is the overall prognosis for these disorders?**

**Clinical subgroups**: Similar 5-year survivals are seen in idiopathic PM/DM and in those cases with associated connective tissue diseases (≥ 85%). In patients with associated neoplastic disease, a much poorer survival rate is observed.

**Serologic subgroups**: Patients with the anti-Mi-2 antibody appear to have a very favorable prognosis, with a 5-year survival of > 90%. Patients who are myositis-specific antibody negative and those with anti-synthetase antibodies have a less favorable prognosis, but still have 5-year survivals > 65%. The worst prognosis is seen in patients with an associated anti-SRP antibody, in whom 5-year survival is approximately 30%.

**17. What is inclusion body myositis?**

Inclusion body myositis (IBM) predominantly affects white males over age 50. Onset of weakness is slow and insidious. Proximal muscles are involved, but distal muscles are also affected early in the disease course. Weakness is usually bilateral, but asymmetry is common. The legs, especially the anterior thigh, are typically affected more than the arms, and muscle atrophy can be prominent. At presentation, CPK may be normal (20–30%) and if elevated is less than 600–800 mg/dL.

Some patients have a mild peripheral neuropathy with loss of deep tendon reflexes. EMG usually shows both myopathic and neuropathic changes. Extraskeletal muscle involvement of the lungs, joints, and heart rarely occurs in these patients. Antinuclear antibodies can be present, but myositis-specific autoantibodies (e.g., anti-Jo-1) do not occur. Muscle biopsy shows foci of chronic inflammatory cells without perifascicular atrophy. The inflammatory infiltrate is predominantly CD8+ T cells. The characteristic findings in IBM on muscle biopsy are red-rimmed vacuoles containing beta-amyloid. Patients respond poorly to immunosuppressive therapy, and the course is typically progressive. Rarely a patient will respond to prednisone alone or in combination with methotrexate or azathioprine.

**18. How does inclusion body myositis differ from polymyositis?**

Despite IBM and polymyositis both being inflammatory myopathies, there are several clinical and immunologic differences that distinguish between them.

| | IBM | POLYMYOSITIS |
|---|---|---|
| Demographics | M > F<br>Age > 50 | F > M<br>All ages |
| Muscle involvement | Proximal and distal<br>Asymmetric | Proximal<br>Symmetric |
| Other organ involvement | Neuropathy | Interstitial lung disease, arthritis, heart involvement |
| Antinuclear antibodies | Sometimes | Frequent |
| Myositis-specific antibodies | No | Yes |
| EMG | Myopathic and neuropathic | Myopathic |
| Muscle biopsy | CD8+ T-cell infiltrate<br>Red-rimmed vacuoles with beta-amyloid | CD8+ T-cell infiltrate |
| Response to immunosuppressive therapy | No | Frequent |

**Pearl**: A patient with PM who fails to respond to prednisone should be reexamined for IBM.

**19. How do you separate steroid myopathy from polymyositis exacerbation?**

Polymyositis patients initially responding to prednisone may later complain of weakness while maintained on prednisone, especially when greater than 20 mg a day. Keep in mind that this may represent development of a steroid myopathy. To separate the two look, at the CPK. Steroid myopathy does not cause elevated CPK or aldolase because it causes type IIb muscle fiber atrophy, whereas polymyositis causes inflammation with CPK elevations. If still not certain, a muscle MRI with STIR images will identify if active inflammation is still present.

## BIBLIOGRAPHY

1. Adams EM, Plotz PH: The treatment of myositis. How to approach resistant disease. Rheum Dis Clin North Am 21:179, 1995.
2. Amato A, Barohn RJ: Idiopathic inflammatory myopathies. Neurol Clinics 15:615–648, 1997.
3. Askanas V, Engel WK: Inclusion-body myositis: Newest concepts of pathogenesis and relation to aging and Alzheimer's disease. J Neuropathol Exp Neurol 60:1–14, 2001.

4. Buchbinder R, Forbes A, Hall S, et al: Incidence of malignant disease in biopsy-proven inflammatory myopathy. Ann Int Med 134:1087–1095, 2001.
5. Callen JP: Dermatomyositis. Lancet 355:53–57, 2000.
6. Dalakas MC: Medical progress: Polymyositis, dermatomyositis, and inclusion-body myositis. N Engl J Med 325:1487, 1991.
7. Dalakas MC: Molecular immunology and genetics of inflammatory muscle diseases. Arch Neurol 55:1509–1512, 1998.
8. Dalakas MC, Illa I, Dambrosia JM, et al: A controlled trial of high-dose intravenous immune globulin infusions as treatment for dermatomyositis. N Engl J Med 329:1993, 1993.
9. Hill CL, Zang Y, Sigurgeirsson B, et al: Frequency of specific cancer types in dermatomyositis and polymyositis: A population-based study. Lancet 357:96–100, 2001.
10. Joffe MM, Love LA, Leff RL, et al: Drug therapy of the idiopathic inflammatory myopathies: Predictors of response to prednisone, azathioprine, and methotrexate and a comparison of their efficacy. Am J Med 94:379, 1993.
11. Park JH, Olsen NJ: Imaging of skeletal muscle. In Wortmann RL (ed): Diseases of Skeletal Muscle. Philadelphia, Lippincott, Williams & Wilkins, 2000, pp 293–312.
12. Plotz PH, Rider LG, Targoff IN, et al: Myositis: Immunologic contributions to understanding cause, pathogenesis, and therapy. Ann Intern Med 122:715, 1995.
13. Rendt K: Inflammatory myopathies: Narrowing the differential diagnosis. Cleve Clinic J Med 68:505–519, 2001.
14. Wortmann RL: Idiopathic inflammatory diseases of muscles. In Weisman MH, Weinblatt ME (eds): Treatment of the Rheumatic Diseases. Companion to the Textbook of Rheumatology. Philadelphia, WB Saunders, 1995, pp 201–216.
15. Wortmann RL: Inflammatory diseases of muscle. In Ruddy S, Harris ED, Sledge CB (eds): Kelley's Textbook of Rheumatology, 6th ed. Philadelphia, WB Saunders, 2001, pp 1273–1296.

# 25. MIXED CONNECTIVE TISSUE DISEASE, OVERLAP SYNDROMES, AND UNDIFFERENTIATED CONNECTIVE TISSUE DISEASE

*Vance J. Bray, M.D.*

**1. What is the difference between mixed connective tissue disease (MCTD), undifferentiated connective tissue disease (UCTD), and overlap syndromes?**

Mixed connective tissue disease, first described by Sharp et al. in 1972, is characterized by a combination of manifestations similar to those seen in systemic lupus erythematosus (SLE), scleroderma (PSS), rheumatoid arthritis (RA), and myositis (PM); the diagnosis requires the presence of high-titer anti-U1-RNP antibodies. These patients lack other autoantibodies such as anti-Sm, anti–SS-A, anti–SS-B, and anti–double-stranded DNA. UCTD typically describes a syndrome in which a patient develops clinical features of an autoimmune disease and nonspecific autoantibodies without developing enough manifestations to meet criteria for a more specific diagnosis (e.g., a patient with inflammatory arthritis and a positive antinuclear antibody but no other manifestations suggestive of lupus). Overlap syndromes occur when patients meet criteria for the diagnosis of more than one connective tissue disease (e.g., patients with SLE may develop a positive rheumatoid factor and an erosive arthritis in a distribution similar to RA; the overlap of SLE and RA is known as RUPUS). It is estimated that up to 25% of patients with one connective tissue disease will develop an overlap syndrome. Although the features of both diseases may occur concurrently, usually one syndrome gradually takes on the features of another. Recently, the existence of MCTD as a distinct clinical entity has become controversial. Some patients initially believed to have MCTD eventually develop clinical manifestations typical of another defined rheumatic disease. Opponents of MCTD feel that UCTD should be applied to these patients until their disease develops and fits established criteria. However, proponents note that genetic, serologic and clinical data provide enough evidence to allow designation of MCTD as a specific disease entity. It is suggested that development of additional CTD manifestations should be regarded as "clinical spreading" rather than as differentiation from an undifferentiated state.

**2. Describe the typical MCTD patient.**

MCTD is 15 times more common in women than men. The mean age at diagnosis is 37 years, with a range of 4–80 years. There are no apparent racial or ethnic predispositions. Although the exact prevalence is not known, MCTD is thought to be more common than PM-DM, not as common as SLE, and about as common as scleroderma.

**3. What are the early clinical manifestations of MCTD, and how do they change over time?**

The onset of MCTD is characterized by features of scleroderma, SLE, RA, and myositis that occur in concert or sequentially (see following table). The most common lupus-like manifestation at onset is arthralgia or nondeforming arthritis. Skin changes seen in the early stages of scleroderma are usually limited to edematous hands; only a minority of patients have more widespread skin changes. Raynaud's phenomenon occurs in over 90% of patients. Esophageal dysmotility is common. Myositis is present in up to 75% of the patients early in the disease course. It is unusual to have renal disease. These patients generally respond to therapy with corticosteroids. Over time, the manifestations of MCTD tend to become less severe and less frequent. Inflammatory symptoms become much less common. Persistent problems are most often those associated with scleroderma, such as sclerodactyly, Raynaud's phenomenon, and esophageal dysmotility. These patients have fewer problems with arthralgias, arthritis, serositis, fever, hepatomegaly, and splenomegaly. Lymphadenopathy and symptomatic muscle disease also become less frequent with time. Renal disease continues to be unusual. Pulmonary hypertension is the primary disease-associated cause of death.

*Clinical Features of Patients with Mixed Connective Tissue Disease at Onset and at Follow-up (Average Follow-up Duration of 12 Years)*

| CLINICAL MANIFESTATION | PRESENCE % | |
|---|---|---|
| | AT ONSET | AT FOLLOW-UP |
| Joint symptoms | 93 | 64 |
| Swelling or sclerodermatous changes of the hands | 71 | 43 |
| Raynaud's phenomenon | 93 | 71 |
| Esophageal dysmotility | 57 | 43 |
| Muscle involvement | 50 | 29 |
| Lymphadenopathy | 71 | 21 |
| Fever | 36 | 0 |
| Hepatomegaly | 21 | 0 |
| Serositis | 29 | 0 |
| Splenomegaly | 21 | 0 |
| Renal disease | 7 | 7 |
| Anemia | 64 | 14 |
| Leukopenia | 57 | 57 |
| Hypergammaglobulinemia | 79 | 64 |

**4. What are the common gastrointestinal manifestations of MCTD?**

Gastrointestinal (GI) symptoms and their frequencies were recorded in 61 patients with MCTD and are listed in the following table. The most common manifestations are similar to those of scleroderma: upper and lower esophageal sphincter hypotension, esophageal dysmotility, gastroesophageal reflux disease with its complications, and pulmonary aspiration. Esophageal function is abnormal in up to 85% of patients, although it may be asymptomatic. In some patients, esophageal pressures improve with corticosteroid therapy. Small bowel and colonic disease is less common in MCTD than in scleroderma. Other less common GI complications include intestinal vasculitis, acute pancreatitis, and chronic active hepatitis.

*Gastrointestinal Symptoms in Patients with Mixed Connective Tissue Disease*

| SYMPTOM | FREQUENCY (%) |
|---|---|
| Heartburn or acid reflux | 48 |
| Dysphagia | 38 |
| Dyspepsia | 20 |
| Diarrhea | 8 |
| Constipation | 5 |
| Vomiting | 3 |

**5. What are the pulmonary manifestations of MCTD, and how are they managed?**

Involvement of the lungs is common in MCTD, although most patients are asymptomatic; two-thirds to three-fourths of patients evaluated have some abnormality. The typical manifestations and their frequencies are detailed below.

*Pulmonary Manifestations of Mixed Connective Tissue Disease*

| | |
|---|---|
| Symptoms | |
| Dyspnea | 16% |
| Chest pain and tightness | 7% |
| Cough | 5% |
| Chest x-ray findings | |
| Interstitial changes | 19% |
| Small pleural effusions | 6% |
| Nonspecific pneumonitis | 4% |
| Pleural thickening | 2% |
| Segmental atelectasis | 1% |
| Pulmonary function studies | |
| Restrictive pattern | 69% |
| Decreased carbon monoxide diffusion | 66% |
| Pulmonary hypertension | 23% |

Management involves identifying the specific abnormalities and directing therapy appropriately. Active inflammation, such as interstitial inflammation or pleuritis, may respond to nonsteroidal anti-inflammatory drugs or corticosteroids. Other medications such as azathioprine or cyclophosphamide may be used to treat interstitial lung disease, although the data are not adequate to assess their efficacy. Pulmonary hypertension is a major cause of mortality and morbidity in patients with MCTD. It may result from vasoconstriction associated with hyperreactivity of the muscular arteries, hypoxemnia associated with progressive pulmonary fibrosis, recurrent thromboemboli, pulmonary vasculitis, or plexogenic arteriopathy. Pulmonary hypertension may respond to antihypertensive therapy, particularly calcium channel blockers or ACE inhibitors. Recently, prostacyclin infusion has been used successfully. Aspiration secondary to esophageal disease may also contribute to pulmonary compromise, so treatment with antacids, even in the absence of reflux symptoms, is indicated.

**6. What are the common nervous system manifestations of MCTD?**

Severe central nervous system involvement is unusual with MCTD. Trigeminal neuralgia is the most common problem, as it is in PSS. Headaches are also relatively common, but convulsions and psychosis rarely occur.

**7. What are the typical laboratory findings in a patient with MCTD?**

The typical findings are detailed below.

*Laboratory Findings in Patients with MCTD*

| ABNORMALITY | FREQUENCY (%) |
|---|---|
| Anemia | 75 |
| Leukopenia | 75 |
| False-positive VDRL | 10 |
| Rheumatoid factor | 50 |
| Antinuclear antibody | 100 |
| Anti-U1-RNP | 100 |
| Hypocomplementemia | 25 |

Anemia is usually that of chronic disease. Coombs' positivity is detected in 60% of patients, although overt hemolytic anemia is uncommon. Thrombocytopenia is uncommon. The sedimentation rate is usually elevated and can be related to disease activity. Hypocomplementemia is not associated with any particular clinical manifestation. Antibodies against other common nuclear antigens are rarely seen.

**8. What is U1-RNP?**

U1-RNP is a uridine rich (hence U) small nuclear ribonucleoprotein (snRNP) that consists of U1-RNA and U1-specific polypeptides 70 kD, A, and C. U1-RNP is one of the spliceosomal snRNPs (U1, U2, U4/U6, U5, U7, U11, U12) complexes whose function is to assist in splicing premessenger RNA to mature RNA. Patients with MCTD form high titers of antibodies against U1-RNP, particularly U1-70kD and U1-RNA, but also polypeptides A and C, which results in a high-titer ANA with a speckled pattern. This antibody can be present in other autoimmune diseases such as SLE and scleroderma but in low titer. Patients with MCTD appear to mount an antigen-driven immune response directed against U1-RNP. One hypothesis is that a genetically predisposed (i.e. HLA-DR4) individual mounts a specific immune response against a microbial antigen (cytomegalovirus glycoprotein) that cross-reacts with U1-70kD peptide that has been modified during cellular apoptosis.

**9. What is the course and prognosis of MCTD?**

There is a low incidence of life-threatening renal disease and neurologic disease in MCTD. The major mortality results from progressive pulmonary hypertension and its cardiac sequelae. Patients with abnormal nailfold capillaries and/or anticardiolipin antibodies are predisposed to developing pulmonary hypertension. The general consensus is that patients with MCTD have a better prognosis than those with SLE, but because there is tremendous variability in disease severity and manifestations, it is misleading to tell an individual that he or she has an excellent prognosis. The development of end-organ involvement dictates the morbidity and mortality.

As a general rule, the SLE-like features of arthritis and pleurisy are treated with NSAIDs, antimalarials, low-dose prednisone (< 20 mg/day), and occasionally methotrexate. Inflammatory myositis is treated with high doses of prednisone (60 mg/day) and rarely methotrexate or azathioprine. PSS-like features of Raynaud's phenomenon, dysphagia, and reflux esophagitis are treated as described in Chapter 22. Vigorous therapy of myocarditis and/or early pulmonary hypertension with corticosteroids and cyclophosphamide can be beneficial. Symptomatic and progressive pulmonary hypertension is treated with trials of intravenous prostacyclin, bosentan (endothelin antagonist), ACE inhibitors, and/or calcium channel blockers, usually with limited success. Lung transplantation may be the only option in severe cases, although experience with this procedure in MCTD is limited.

**10. What is the most common disease in overlap syndromes, and with which other diseases is it associated?**

Sjögren's syndrome is the most common overlap and is seen with RA, SLE, PSS, PM, MCTD, primary biliary cirrhosis (PBC), necrotizing vasculitis, autoimmune thyroiditis, chronic active hepatitis, mixed cryoglobulinemia, and hypergammaglobulinemic purpura.

**11. What other overlap syndromes are seen?**

Other overlap syndromes not associated with high titer anti-U1-RNP antibodies are:

- SLE is associated with polymyositis in 4–16% of cases.
- SLE can be associated with RA (RUPUS) with positive rheumatoid factor, nodules, and erosive polyarthritis.
- Scleroderma can be associated with myositis. Antibodies to PM-Scl are found in 40–50% of patients. The PM-Scl antigen is a complex of 16 polypeptides located at the site of ribosomal assembly in the nucleolus. Thus, patients will have a nucleolar ANA. Anti-PM-Scl antibodies are strongly associated with HLA-DR3. In Japanese patients, who rarely are HLA-DR3 positive, anti-Ku antibodies are more commonly found in patients with this overlap.
- Limited scleroderma (CREST) can be associated with primary biliary cirrhosis (PBC). CREST antedates PBC by an average of 14 years. Antimitochrondrial antibody can be seen in 18–27% of CREST patients. Many also have Sjögren's.
- RA can overlap with scleroderma, SLE, or Sjögren's syndrome.

**12. How common is undifferentiated connective tissue disease (UCTD)?**

Up to 50% of patients with early connective tissue disease symptoms may not fulfill criteria for a defined connective tissue disease at time of presentation. However, over time (1–3 years) 30–50% of these cases will evolve into a defined connective tissue disease, leaving about 15–20% of all connective tissue diseases being UCTD.

**13. What are the clinical and serologic characteristics of UCTD? Do any predict the future development of a defined CTD?**

The most frequent manifestations of UCTD are arthralgias/arthritis, Raynaud's phenomenon, mucocutaneous manifestations, and sicca symptoms. Major organ involvement is rare. Most patients are ANA positive but lack specific autoantibodies against Sm, dsDNA, and centromere. Some patients have anti-SSA antibodies, which correlates with sicca symptoms and mucocutaneous lesions; others have low titer anti-RNP antibodies, which correlates with Raynaud's and arthritis.

UCTD patients with fever and anti-dsDNA antibodies are more likely to develop SLE; patients with Raynaud's and nucleolar ANA developed scleroderma; and patients with xerostomia and anti-SSA antibodies developed Sjögren's.

**14. What are suggested classification criteria for UCTD?**

- Signs and symptoms of a connective tissue disease, but not fulfilling the criteria for any of the defined CTDs for at least 3 years,

*and*

- Presence of antinuclear antibodies on two different occasions.

## BIBLIOGRAPHY

1. Burdt MA, Hoffman RW, Deutsher SL, et al: Long-term outcome in mixed connective tissue disease. Arthritis Rheum 42:899–909, 1999.

2. Jury EC, D'Cruz D, Morrow WJW: Autoantibodies and overlap syndromes in autoimmune rheumatic disease. J Clin Pathol 54:340–347, 2001.
3. Lundberg I, Hedfors E: Clinical course of patients with anti-RNP antibodies: A prospective study of 32 patients. J Rheumatol 18:1511–1519, 1991.
4. Mosca M, Neri R, Bombardieri S: Undifferentiated connective tissue disease (UCTD). Clin Exp Rheumatol 17:615–620, 1999.
5. Prakash UBS: Respiratory complications in mixed connective tissue disease. Clin Chest Med 19:733–746, 1998.
6. Sharp GC, Irvin WS, Tan EM, et al: Mixed connective tissue disease—an apparently distinct rheumatic disease syndrome associated with a specific antibody to an extractable nuclear antigen (ENA). Am J Med 52:148–159, 1972.
7. Smolen JS, Steiner G: Mixed connective tissue disease, to be or not to be? Arthritis Rheum 41:768–777, 1998.

# 26. SJÖGREN'S SYNDROME

*Vance* J. *Bray*, M.D.

**1. Who was Sjögren, and what is his syndrome?**

Henrich Sjögren was born in 1899 in Stockholm and received his M.D. from the Karolinska Institut in 1927. In 1933, he published a monograph associating dry eyes with arthritis. He also introduced Rose Bengal staining to identify corneal lesions and introduced the term **keratoconjunctivitis sicca (KCS)** to describe the ocular manifestations. Sjögren's syndrome (SS) refers to a systemic disease most frequently manifested by dry eyes, dry mouth, and arthritis.

**2. What are the alternative names for SS?**

Sjögren's syndrome has also been known as Mikulicz's disease, Gougerot's syndrome, sicca syndrome, and autoimmune exocrinopathy. Hadden, Leber, and Mikulicz initially described the association of dry eyes, dry mouth, and glandular enlargement in the late 1800s. Gougerot in 1925 and Sjögren in 1933 associated these findings with polyarthritis and systemic disease.

**3. Who typically develops SS?**

The typical patient is a middle-aged female. The female to male ratio is 9:1, and the mean age at diagnosis is 50 years. Sjögren's has rarely been reported in children.

**4. What is the difference between primary and secondary SS?**

The clinical manifestations of primary and secondary SS are the same. **Primary** Sjögren's is diagnosed in the absence of another underlying rheumatic disease, is immunogenetically associated with HLA-B8-DR3, and is associated with antinuclear antibodies to Ro/SS-A and La/SS-B. **Secondary** Sjögren's is diagnosed when there is accompanying evidence of another connective tissue disease, most frequently rheumatoid arthritis (RA). The immunogenetic and serologic findings are usually those of the accompanying disease (e.g., HLA-DR4-positive if associated with RA).

**5. How common is SS?**

An estimated 1–2 million people in the United States have Sjögren's, and most are undiagnosed. Primary Sjögren's occurs at a rate of 1/1000 individuals, which is equal to the frequency of systemic lupus erythematosus. Secondary Sjögren's accounts for the remainder of cases. Approximately 30% of patients with RA have secondary Sjögren's syndrome. It takes about 9 years for Sjögren's patients to be diagnosed appropriately, even after they develop sicca symptoms. The average duration of SS symptoms is estimated at 7 years for dyspareunia, 1–5 years for dry mouth, and 1 year for dry eyes. Many patients may be too embarrassed to mention painful intercourse unless directly asked about the problem.

**6. What are the common initial manifestations of primary SS?**

| | |
|---|---|
| Xerophthalmia | 47% |
| Xerostomia | 42% |
| Arthralgias/arthritis | 28% |
| Parotid gland enlargement | 24% |
| Raynaud's phenomenon | 21% |
| Fever/fatigue | 10% |
| Dyspareunia | 5% |

**7. What is the underlying pathology of SS?**

The manifestations of SS result from lymphocytic infiltration of glandular and nonglandular organs. Lymphocytic infiltration of the lacrimal glands and salivary glands interferes with the production of tears and saliva, respectively. Lymphocytic infiltration of other organs, such as the lungs and GI tract, results in a variety of major organ manifestations. The lymphocytes are predominantly CD4+ helper T cells. B cells account for 20% of the lymphocytes and are responsible for increased immunoglobulin production.

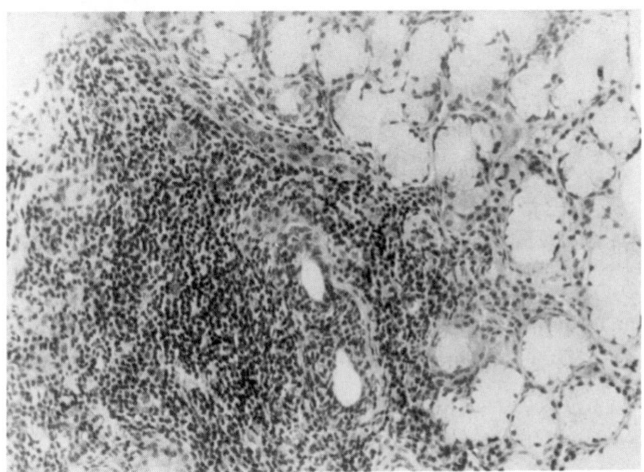

Minor salivary gland biopsy demonstrating mononuclear cell infiltration and salivary gland destruction. (From the Clinical Slide Collection on the Rheumatic Diseases. Atlanta, American College of Rheumatology, 1991; with permission.)

**8. What are the most common ocular symptoms of SS?**

Patients most often complain of dry eyes or painful eyes, also known as **KCS** or **xerophthalmia**. These symptoms result from a deficient aqueous middle layer of precorneal tear film, which normally comprises 90% of tear volume. These patients may experience a foreign-body or gritty sensation, a burning sensation, itchiness, blurred vision, redness, and/or photophobia. Symptoms worsen as the day progresses, owing to evaporation of ocular moisture during the time that the eyes are open. This pattern contrasts with blepharitis, a low-grade infection of the meibomian glands, in which there is crusting and discomfort most pronounced in the morning on awakening. KCS can lead to infections, corneal ulceration, and visual loss.

**9. What are other causes of dry eyes besides Sjögren's?**

Blepharitis, viral infections, contact lens irritation, and medications such as antihistamines, diuretics, tricyclic antidepressants, and benzodiazepines.

**10. What tests are used to document dry eyes in a patient with suspected Sjögren's?**

The most common tests of tear production and adequacy are the **Schirmer's test** and tests using vital dyes that detect disturbances in the normal mucin coating of the conjunctival surface. The **Schirmer's I test** involves placing a piece of filter paper under the inferior eyelid and measuring the amount of wetness over a specified time. Wetting of < 5 mm in 5 minutes is a strong indication of diminished tear production. **Schirmer's II test** involves putting a Q-tip into the nose, which will maximally stimulate output of major and minor lacrimal glands through the nasolacrimal gland reflex. There is a 15% false-positive and false-negative rate with Schirmer's testing.

**Rose Bengal** or lissamine green dyes can be applied topically and are taken up by devitalized or damaged epithelium of the cornea and conjunctiva, thus documenting dryness of enough severity to injure corneal tissue. The area of maximum uptake is along the palpebral fissure, where the maximum exposure to the environment and evaporation of tears occur. There is a 5% false-positive and false-negative rate with Rose Bengal staining. Tests for ocular osmolarity and for tear proteins are under development.

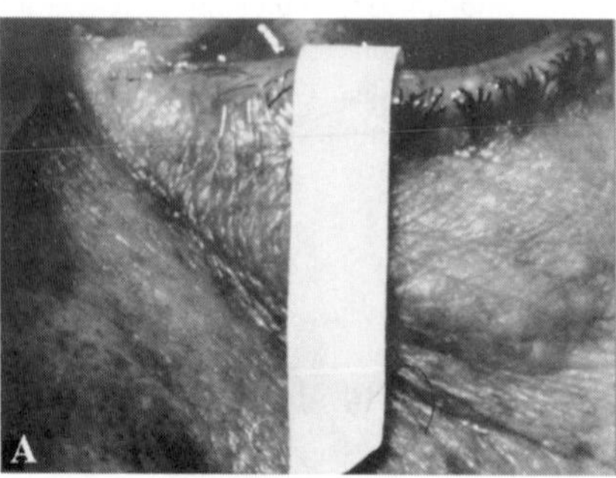


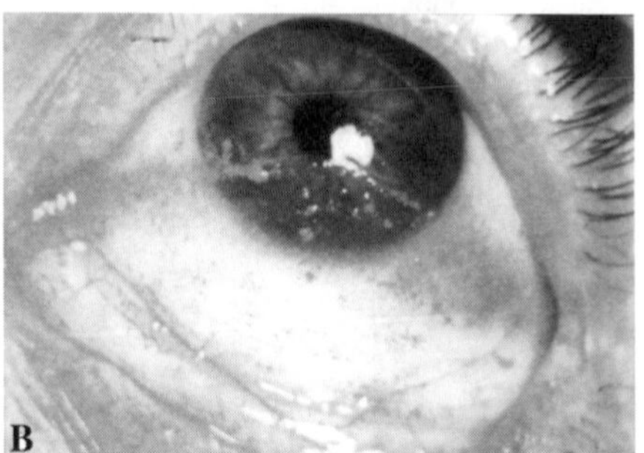


*A*, Schirmer's test demonstrating decreased tear production. *B*, Rose Bengal test with increased dye uptake in areas of devitalized epithelium. (From the Clinical Slide Collection on the Rheumatic Diseases. Atlanta, American College of Rheumatology, 1991; with permission.)

**11. What are the common symptoms of decreased production of saliva?**

Decreased saliva production is known as **xerostomia**. It may result in a variety of problems, including:

Difficulty swallowing dry food (17%)
Inability to speak continuously
Change in taste (33%)
Burning sensation (30–40%)
Increase in dental caries
Problems wearing dentures
Gastroesophageal reflux symptoms (due to lack of salivary buffering)
Disturbed sleep (due to dry mouth and/or nocturia)
Predisposition to oral candidiasis

**12. How can salivary gland involvement be determined?**

A variety of methods are used to determine salivary function. **Lashley cups** can be used to quantitate saliva production. Alternatively, a patient can place a dry **sponge** in his or her mouth; the difference between dry and wet weights indicates the amount of saliva produced. **Sialography** will outline the salivary duct anatomy but may be painful, predispose to infections, or cause obstruction. **Scintigraphy** utilizes the uptake and secretion of $^{99m}$Tc pertechnetate during a 60-minute period following intravenous injection to quantitate salivary flow rates.

Finally, **minor salivary gland** involvement will demonstrate lymphocytic infiltration. An incisional **biopsy** through the lower labial mucosa yielding 5–10 minor glands is adequate for assessment. An area of > 50 lymphocytes around salivary gland acini or ducts is defined as a focus, with > 1 focus/4 $mm^2$ supporting the diagnosis of the salivary component of Sjögren's. The findings in the minor salivary glands generally parallel involvement of other organs, so biopsy of the parotid glands or major salivary glands is generally not necessary. The minor salivary gland biopsy also may be abnormal before decreased salivary flow can be documented with scintigraphy, because it takes time for the infiltrate to destroy enough salivary gland tissue to cause decreased saliva production.

**13. What are the common causes of decreased salivary secretion?**

**Temporary**

Short-term drug use (e.g., antihistamines)
Viral and bacterial infections (especially mumps)
Dehydration (thermal, trauma, diabetes)
Psychogenic causes (fear, depression)

**Chronic**

Chronically administered drugs (antidepressants, anticholinergics, neuroleptics, clonidine, diuretics)
Systemic diseases
- Sjögren's syndrome
- Granulomatous diseases (sarcoid, tuberculosis, leprosy)
- Amyloidosis
- HIV infection
- Hepatitis C infection
- Graft-versus-host disease
- Cystic fibrosis
- Diabetes mellitus (uncontrolled)

**Other**

Therapeutic radiation to the head and neck
Trauma or surgery to the head and neck
Absent or malformed glands (rare)
Type V hyperlipidemia
Multiple sclerosis

**14. What is the differential diagnosis of salivary gland enlargement?**

**Usually unilateral**

Primary salivary gland neoplasms
Bacterial infection
Chronic sialadenitis
Obstruction

**Usually bilateral** (asymmetric, with hypofunction)

Viral infection (mumps, cytomegalovirus, influenza, coxsackie A)
Sjögren's syndrome
Granulomatous diseases (sarcoid, tuberculosis, leprosy)
Recurrent parotitis of childhood
HIV infection (DILS)

**Bilateral, symmetric** (soft, nontender)

| | | |
|---|---|---|
| Idiopathic | Hepatic cirrhosis | Acromegaly |
| Diabetes mellitus | Anorexia/bulimia | Gonadal hypofunction |
| Hyperlipoproteinemia | Chronic pancreatitis | Phenylbutazone ingestion |

**15. What is DILS?**

**Diffuse infiltrative lymphocytosis syndrome** (DILS) is a disorder that mimics Sjögren's and is seen in patients infected with the human immunodeficiency virus (HIV). Common clinical features include fever, lymphadenopathy, weight loss, and bilateral parotid gland enlargement. In contrast to most patients with primary Sjögren's, patients with DILS experience more xerostomia than xerophthalmia and keratoconjunctivitis sicca. DILS patients may also experience recurrent sinus and middle ear infections, lymphocytic interstitial pneumonitis, lymphocytic hepatitis, infiltration of the gastric mucosa (which can mimic linitus plastica), lymphocytic interstitial nephritis, aseptic meningitis, sensorimotor neuropathies, uveitis, and cranial nerve palsies.

DILS differs from SS in that the infiltrating lymphocytes in DILS are CD8+ cells, not CD4+ as seen in Sjögren's. DILS patients also lack antibodies to Ro/SS-A and La/SS-B. In contrast to other patients infected with HIV, DILS patients maintain their CD4 counts in the range of asymptomatic HIV-infected individuals and tend not to develop opportunistic infections or Kaposi's sarcoma. However, they are four times more likely to develop a high-grade non-Hodgkin's B-cell lymphoma in the salivary or lacrimal glands and elsewhere.

**16. List the common extraglandular manifestations of primary Sjögren's syndrome.**

| | |
|---|---|
| Arthralgias/arthritis | 60–70% |
| Raynaud's phenomenon | 35–40% |
| Esophageal dysfunction | 30–35% |
| Lymphadenopathy | 15–20% |
| Vasculitis | 5–10% |
| Lung involvement | 10–20% |
| Kidney involvement | 10–15% |
| Liver involvement | 5–10% |
| Peripheral neuropathy | 2–5% |
| Myositis | 1–2% |
| Lymphoma | 5–8% |

**17. Describe the arthritis of primary Sjögren's.**

The distribution of Sjögrens' arthritis is similar to that of rheumatoid arthritis. The patient experiences symmetric arthralgias and/or arthritis of the wrists, metacarpophalageal and proximal interphalangeal joints, frequently associated with morning stiffness and fatigue. In contrast to rheumatoid arthritis, Sjögren's arthritis is nonerosive and tends to be mild. It usually responds to medications such as NSAIDs, antimalarials (hydroxychloroquine), and/or low doses of prednisone (≤5 mg).

**18. Are there typical laboratory and autoantibody findings in patients with primary Sjögren's syndrome?**

| | |
|---|---|
| Erythrocyte sedimentation rate | 80–90% |
| Hypergammaglobulinemia | 80% |
| Anemia of chronic disease | 25% |
| Leukopenia | 10% |
| Thrombocytopenia | Rare |
| Autoantibodies | |
| Rheumatoid factor | 80–95% |
| Antinuclear antibody (ANA) | 90% |
| anti-SS-A antibody | 50–90% |
| anti-SS-B antibody | 50–90% |

**Pearl**: It is difficult to make a diagnosis of Sjögren's without serologic evidence of autoimmunity (i.e., positive RF or ANA).

**19. What is the risk of cancer in Sjögren's syndrome patients?**

Sjögren's patients are at a 44-fold greater risk of developing lymphoma than age-matched controls, with an overall frequency of lymphoma of 5–8%. Lymphomas are usually non-Hodgkin's B cell lymphomas. The onset of lymphoma may be preceded by the development of a monoclonal gammopathy. Alternatively, concern for lymphoma is raised by the loss of a previously positive rheumatoid factor, the loss of the monoclonal gammopathy, or the development of hypogammaglobulinemia. Other clues of excessive lymphoproliferation include regional or generalized lymphadenopathy, hepatosplenomegaly, pulmonary infiltrates, renal insufficiency, purpura, and leukopenia.

**20. Which criteria have been proposed to diagnose Sjögren's syndrome?**

**Primary Sjögren's**

Dry eyes with keratoconjunctivitis sicca documented by an abnormal Schirmer's and positive Rose Bengal test

Dry mouth documented by abnormal salivary scintigraphy or positive minor salivary gland biopsy

Abnormal serologies manifested by a positive rheumatoid factor, positive ANA, and/or positive anti-SSA or anti-SSB (or both)

**Secondary Sjögren's**

Dry eyes (as documented above)

Dry mouth (as documented above)

Associated autoimmune disease (usually rheumatoid arthritis)

**21. How is the xerophthalmia of SS treated?**

Dry eyes are treated with eye drops, with preservative-free artificial tears generally being less irritating. Many preparations with differing degrees of viscosity are available. Those with a watery consistency may require frequent applications; more viscous preparations (Refresh, Celluvisc) may provide longer benefit but may blur vision in some patients. Lubricant ointments (Refresh PM, Lacrilube) are available and may be especially useful during the night. Slow-release artificial tears (Lacriserts) are also available but require a small amount of residual tear production to be effective. Humidifiers are useful in arid climates and at high altitudes. Evaporation of tears may be slowed by the use of glasses with side shields; swim goggles are an inexpensive means of obtaining occlusive eyewear. Punctal occlusion, performed by the ophthalmologist, will obstruct the normal lacrimal drainage system, allowing tears to last longer. Temporary plugs are generally inserted before permanent obstruction is considered. Severe ocular surface disease (scleritis, inflammatory nodules, corneal ulcers) may respond to autologous serum, topical steroids, or topical cyclosporine.

**22. Describe the management for other mucosal dryness in Sjögren's.**

The complications of xerostomia are best prevented by good dental care, with frequent use of fluoridated toothpaste and mouthwash as well as regular professional dental attention. Sugar-free (not just sugarless) mints or candies may stimulate salivary flow without increasing the risk of dental caries. Saliva substitutes (MouthKote, Salivart) and systemically administered cholinergic drugs (pilocarpine, cevimeline) are also available. Oral candidiasis is best treated with oral application of nystatin vaginal tablets. Nystatin is preferred because other available oral preparations contain glucose or sucrose, which would promote dental caries. Topical drugs may be necessary because with significant salivary hypofunction systemically administered antifungal drugs do not reach the mouth in therapeutically adequate amounts. Dentures must be removed while the mouth is being treated and may also need to be treated in order to cure and prevent recurrence of oral candidiasis. Oral fluconazole for 2 weeks can be used in resistant cases. Avoidance of alcohol, frequent water ingestion, and removal of nasal polyps to limit mouth breathing will help oral dryness. Vaginal dryness is treated with topical lubricants. Dry skin usually improves with lotions and creams.

**23. How do the cholinergic drugs help dryness?**

Patients with significant oral and ocular dryness have been noted to have only 30% of their salivary/lacrimal glands infiltrated with lymphocytes and only 30–50% of the glands destroyed. Consequently, the remaining functioning glands can be stimulated to produce more tears and saliva.

Pilocarpine (Salagen 5 mg QID) and cevimeline (Evoxac 30 mg TID) stimulate the M3 muscarinic receptors on lacrimal and salivary acinar glands. This results in stimulation of ATPase needed for secretion. Cevimeline has longer half-life (4 hrs vs 1.5 hrs) and higher specificity of the M3 receptor, thereby lessening cardiac and pulmonary toxicity (heart and lungs have M2 receptors). Patients with some tear production on Schirmer's II testing are more likely to respond to these drugs. Patients with narrow-angle glaucoma, asthma, or on beta blockers should avoid these drugs or be monitored closely. Common side effects are sweating and gastrointestinal disturbances.

**24. How are the other manifestations of Sjögren's managed?**

Fatigue is a common symptom that may be difficult to alleviate (rule out hypothyroidism). If associated with poor sleep, treatment similar to that recommended for fibromyalgia may be of benefit, although tricyclic antidepressants are likely to aggravate dryness of the mucous membranes. The best TCA is desipramine, owing to low anticholinergic effects. If there are associated inflammatory parameters, such as an elevated sedimentation rate and/or hypergammaglobulinemia, the patient may benefit from treatment with an antimalarial or a low dose of prednisone (controversial).

Arthritis generally responds to NSAIDs, antimalarials, and low doses of prednisone. Severe extraglandular disease may require higher doses of systemic corticosteroids, azathioprine, or cyclophosphamide. Lymphoma should be treated in consultation with an oncologist and based on the type and stage of disease.

## BIBLIOGRAPHY


1. Alexander E: Central nervous system disease in Sjögren's syndrome. Rheum Dis Clin 18:637–672, 1992.
2. Bell M, Askari A, Bookman A, et al: Sjögren's syndrome: A critical review of clinical management. J Rheumatol 26:2051–2061, 1999.
3. Chan EKL, Andrade LEC: Antinuclear antibodies in Sjögren's syndrome. Rheum Dis Clin 18:551–570, 1992.
4. Constantopoulous SH, Tsianos EV, Moutsopoulos HM: Pulmonary and gastrointestinal manifestations of Sjögren's syndrome. Rheum Dis Clin 18:617–635, 1992.
5. Daniels TE: Evaluation, differential diagnosis, and treatment of xerostomia. J Rheumatol 61:6–10, 2000.
6. Fox RI, Michelson P: Approaches to the treatment of Sjögren's syndrome. J Rheumatol 61:15–21, 2000.
7. Fox RI: Treatment of the patient with Sjögren's syndrome. Rheum Dis Clin 18:699–709, 1992.
8. Fox RI, Kang H: Pathogenesis of Sjögren's syndrome. Rheum Dis Clin 18:517–538, 1992.
9. Itescu S, Winchester R: Diffuse infiltrative lymphocytosis syndrome: A disorder occurring in human immunodeficiency virus-1 infection that may present as sicca syndrome. Rheum Dis Clin 18:683–697, 1992.
10. Lemp MA: Evaluation and differential diagnosis of keratoconjunctivitis sicca. J Rheumatol 61:11–14, 2000.
11. Moutsopoulos HM, Tzioufas AG: Sjögren's syndrome. In Klippel JH, Dieppe PA (eds): Rheumatology. London, Mosby–Year Book Europe Ltd, 1994.
12. Provost TT, Watson R: Cutaneous manifestations of Sjögren's syndrome. Rheum Dis Clin 18:609–616, 1992.
13. Ramos-Casals M, Garcia-Carrasco M, Cervera R, et al: Hepatitis C virus infection mimicking Sjögren's syndrome. Medicine 80:1–7, 2001.
14. Reveille JD, Arnett FC: The immunogenetics of Sjögren's syndrome. Rheum Dis Clin 18:539–550, 1992.


# 27. ANTIPHOSPHOLIPID ANTIBODY SYNDROME

*Karen E. Hansen, M.D.*

**1. What are antiphospholipid antibodies?**

Antiphospholipid antibodies (**aPL**) are a heterogeneous group of antibodies that bind to plasma proteins with an affinity for phospholipid surfaces. Most of the antigens (for example, prothrombin and β2-glycoprotein I) are involved in blood coagulation. These antibodies include the **anticardiolipin antibodies, lupus anticoagulant**, β2-glycoprotein I, and anti-prothrombin antibodies. In a given patient, one or more of these antibodies may be present.

**2. How are aPL measured?**

a. Anticardiolipin antibodies are measured by an ELISA assay for IgG, IgM, and IgA isotypes, and the results are reported in quartiles.
b. To test for the lupus anticoagulant, a phospholipid-dependent screening assay is performed and if prolonged, normal plasma is added in a 1:1 mix. If the lupus anticoagulant is present, addition of normal plasma does not correct the prolonged assay but addition of excess phospholipid does. If a factor deficiency is present, the assay does correct with addition of normal plasma.
c. The β2-glycoprotein I antibody is measured by ELISA.
d. Anti-prothrombin antibodies are also measured by an ELISA test.

**3. What is the value of a false-positive VDRL?**

The VDRL measures agglutination (flocculation) of lipid particles that contain cholesterol and the negatively charged phospholipid cardiolipin. Antiphospholipid antibodies bind to the cardiolipin in these particles and cause flocculation, indistinguishable from that seen in patients with syphilis. A false-positive VDRL may be a clue to the presence of an antiphospholipid antibody, but in and of itself, is not a good way to test for the presence of aPL. A false-positive VDRL or RPR is seen in, at most, 50% of subjects with anticardiolipin antibodies and as such, is not recommended as an additional laboratory test in assessing an individual with suspected aPL.. Patients with only a false-positive VDRL and no other aPL are not at increased risk for clot or fetal loss.

**4. What is the clinical significance of a positive aPL result?**

Positive aPL are seen in up to 8% of the normal population, and are associated with a variety of chronic infections including HIV and hepatitis C. They are present in about 20% of patients with systemic vasculitis but do not correlate statistically with the development of thrombosis.

Primary antiphospholipid antibody syndrome (referred to as PAPS) is the presence of aPL in the setting of thrombosis. Thrombocytopenia, recurrent miscarriage, and/or livedo reticularis may be present. Virtually any venous or arterial site has been affected by thrombosis from these antibodies. In a large group of subjects with thrombosis related to aPL, about 2/3 of thrombotic events are venous, while 1/3 are arterial. The site of initial thrombosis often predicts the site of recurrent thrombosis in a given individual. Typical thrombotic events include deep vein thrombosis, pulmonary embolus, transient ischemic attack, stroke, and myocardial infarction. Antiphospholipid antibodies account for about 15% of women who experience recurrent miscarriage.

About half of subjects with systemic lupus erythematosus have aPL, and the presence of aPL has now been added to the list of criteria for diagnosis of systemic lupus erythematosus (under the "Immunologic" criterion). In the group with both lupus and aPL, up to one-half will subsequently develop a thrombotic event. Prospectively, 3–7% of patients per year who have aPL will experience a new thrombotic event. A field of ongoing research involves developing a model that predicts which subjects are most likely to sustain a thrombotic event, so that intervention trials may be designed to prevent potentially life-threatening or disabling events.

Overall, the positive predictive value of an aPL predicting a future stroke, venous thrombosis, or recurrent fetal loss is between 10 and 25%.

**5. How does the lupus anticoagulant affect the prothrombin time (PT) and activated partial thromboplastin time (aPTT)?**

In about half of subjects with the lupus anticoagulant, the aPTT is prolonged. Therefore, a normal aPTT does not exclude the presence of the lupus anticoagulant. Up until recently, it was thought that the PT was unaffected by the lupus anticoagulant. Moll and Ortel took blood samples from 22 subjects with the lupus anticoagulant, and measured the PT in each patient using 9 different assays from companies across the United States. What they found was that the lupus anticoagulant does affect the PT! In one subject, the INR was less than 2 with one reagent and greater than 8 with another. As you can imagine, this is crucial in a subject with the lupus anticoagulant who is taking Coumadin to prevent further thrombosis. With one result, the doctor would ask the patient to increase the dose of Coumadin, while with the other result, the doctor would ask the patient to hold Coumadin! Therefore, in a patient with the lupus anticoagulant initiating Coumadin therapy, it is important to check an assay *insensitive* to this antiphospholipid antibody at the same time as an INR is drawn. That will reveal whether the lupus anticoagulant is interfering with the reliability of the INR result. Two tests that are not affected by the lupus anticoagulant are **chromogenic factor X** and the **prothrombin-proconvertin time**.

**6. What is the Russell viper venom time (RVVT)?**

The RVVT is a confirmatory test for the lupus anticoagulant. Russell viper venom directly activates factor X and thereby bypasses the factors required in the intrinsic pathway of coagulation. RVVT is performed like the aPTT, except intrinsic coagulation factors proximal to factor X are not required and less phospholipids are present in the reaction. Therefore, the RVVT is not affected by factor deficiencies and is more sensitive in the detection of lupus anticoagulant than prolongation of the aPTT.

**7. What is the significance of a prolonged PT in a patient with the lupus anticoagulant?**

A prolonged PT might indicate an extremely high level of lupus anticoagulant, but could also indicate the presence of a prothrombin (factor II) deficiency. This condition can be caused by liver disease, vitamin K deficiency, or anticoagulation with warfarin. In addition, isolated factor II deficiency is rarely associated with autoimmune disorders, including systemic lupus erythematosus. It is extremely important to detect factor II deficiency, since it is associated with excessive bleeding rather than hypercoagulability. If both the aPTT and PT are prolonged, a prothrombin level should be measured directly to exclude a deficiency.

**8. In a patient with thrombosis due to aPL, how frequently are the lupus anticoagulant (LA) and anticardiolipin antibodies (aCL) both positive?**

- aCL positive and LA positive 70%
- aCL positive and LA negative 15%
- aCL negative and LA positive 15%
- aCL negative and LA negative < 1%

**9. Can a patient with thrombosis due to aPL ever have both a negative LA and negative aCL antibodies?**

Yes. Rarely, patients with large clots will presumably consume the aPL in the clot, leading to false-negative results. Consequently, repeating the tests for aPL 6 weeks after the thrombotic event may show they are positive.

Another possibility is that the pathogenic aPL are directed against other targets not detected by the LA and aCL assays. Such candidate antigens include prothrombin, phosphatidylserine, thrombomodulin, annexin V, protein C, and protein S. Furthermore, antibodies directed specifically against β2-glycoprotein I and not picked up by the aCL ELISA assay have been reported to be associated with clots in some individuals.

Other causes for thrombosis should always be assessed in patients with negative LA and aCL tests. The concept of "seronegative" antiphospholipid antibody syndrome is not recognized.

**10. What is the antigenic determinant for anti-β2-glycoprotein I antibodies? What is the clinical significance of anti-β2-glycoprotein I antibodies?**

β2-Glycoprotein I (apolipoprotein H) is a lipid-binding anticoagulant protein. It becomes antigenic on binding to a negatively charged surface, at which time it undergoes a conformational change, exposing a cryptic antigen and leading to clustering of molecules to provide a high antigen density. The anti-β2-glycoprotein I antibody binds to an octapeptide in the fifth domain of β2-glycoprotein I. In vivo, β2-glycoprotein I binds to phosphatidylserine on activated or apoptotic cell membranes.

Notably, a positive anticardiolipin antibody ELISA test is usually due to binding by anti-β2-glycoprotein I antibodies. Patients (usually those with infections) who have positive anticardiolipin antibody by ELISA but negative anti-$\beta_2$-glycoprotein I tests are not at increased risk for clotting.

**11. What is the clinical significance of anti-prothrombin antibodies?**

Antibodies to prothrombin may be responsible for a positive lupus anticoagulant test increasing the risk for thrombosis. Conversely, antibodies to prothrombin may deplete prothrombin leading to hemorrhage.

**12. Is the level of aPL stable over time?**

No. aPL levels may fluctuate widely over time spontaneously or in response to clinical events such as a flare of lupus, change in pregnancy status, or thrombosis. aPL levels may or may not change with immunosuppressive therapy or anticoagulation for thrombosis.

**13. List the main types of diseases associated with increased aPL production.**

Increased aPL production is frequently associated with chronic immune stimulation. The primary conditions can be remembered by the mnemonic **MAIN**:

**M** — Medications
**A** — Autoimmune diseases
**I** — Infectious diseases
**N** — Neoplasms

**14. What medications are associated with elevated levels of aPL?**

Although many drugs have been associated with elevated aPL, the most common are the phenothiazines and other drugs associated with drug-induced lupus: chlorpromazine (a phenothiazine), hydralazine, phenytoin, procainamide, and quinidine.

**15. Which infectious diseases are associated with elevated levels of aPL, and what is the clinical significance?**

Many acute infections, both bacterial and viral, have been associated with transiently or persistently elevated levels of aPL. Chronic infections, such as HIV and hepatitis C, are also associated with increased aPL; 60–80% of patients who are HIV-positive have elevated levels of aPL. aPL induced by infections are in general not associated with increased thrombotic risk because they are not directed against β2-glycoprotein I.

**16. Which neoplasms are associated with aPL?**

Many neoplasms have been reported, but the most common is lymphoma.

**17. Which clinical syndromes are associated with elevated levels of aPL?**

aPL are associated with a hypercoagulable state characterized by:

**C** — Clot: recurrent arterial and/or venous thromboses (clots)
**L** — Livedo reticularis: lace-like rash over the extremities and trunk exaggerated by cold
**O** — Obstetrical loss: recurrent fetal loss
**T** — Thrombocytopenia

**18. How is the primary antiphospholipid antibody syndrome (PAPS) defined? What is the catastrophic vascular occlusion syndrome?**

PAPS includes the presence of aPL and one of the following: thrombosis, recurrent fetal loss, or thrombocytopenia. There can be no underlying disorder as the cause of aPL, such as SLE, HIV infection, or vasculitis. However, up to 10% of PAPS patients will evolve into SLE within 10 years. The catastrophic antiphospholipid antibody syndrome is a life-threatening complication of PAPS where multiple thromboses of medium and small arteries in three or more organs occur over a few days.

**19. What is the risk of thrombosis in a subject with aPL?**

This depends on the clinical setting and the type of aPL present. Listed below are the odds ratios of thrombosis in SLE patients with aPL.

| APL | ODDS RATIO |
|---|---|
| Anti-β2-glycoprotein I | 3.02 |
| Anticardiolipin antibody | 2.2 |
| Lupus anticoagulant | 5.6 |

**20. In a patient with their first deep vein thrombosis, how often are aPL responsible?**

In two separate papers evaluating subjects admitted for suspected deep vein thrombosis, the incidence of aPL in those with thrombosis was 15%. Factor V Leiden can account for about 20–30% of first deep vein thrombosis, while the prothrombin gene polymorphism (20210 G) accounts for about 6% of first deep vein thrombosis.

**21. What central nervous system (CNS) thrombotic manifestations can occur in patients with aPL?**

Stroke is the most common CNS manifestation. aPL have been found in 5–10% of unselected patients with stroke and 45–50% of patients less than 50 years old with stroke. This gives a relative risk of 2.3 for aPL and stroke for all patients and 8.3 for young stroke patients. Notably, multiple strokes can lead to dementia.

Thromboses can occur in other areas leading to ischemic optic neuropathy, retinal artery or vein occlusion, sensorineural hearing loss, chorea, and cavernous or sagittal sinus thrombosis causing pseudotumor cerebri. Some patients with neurologic symptoms have been misdiagnosed as having multiple sclerosis, based on brain MRI results. However, patients with aPL and neurologic symptoms usually have a normal IgG index and negative oligoclonal bands.

**22. What other thrombotic manifestations can occur in patients with aPL?**

Virtually any organ can be involved. Skin thrombosis can cause cutaneous ulceration. Digital gangrene can result from arterial occlusion. Renal artery or vein thrombosis and a thrombotic microangiopathy can cause renal insufficiency. Pulmonary emboli occur in 30% of patients with PAPS and can lead to pulmonary hypertension in 5%. Budd-Chiari syndrome due to venous thrombosis of the liver has been reported. Avascular necrosis is increased in SLE patients with aPL.

**23. How do elevated levels of aPL cause thrombosis in vivo?**

Because many of the antigens involved in the production of aPL are components of the clotting cascade, it is believed that the antibodies directly interfere with normal anticoagulation. For example, it was shown that aPL target β2-glycoprotein I, which is an anticoagulant. However, this does not explain why some subjects with aPL never develop a thrombotic event. The two-hit hypothesis is that aPL *plus* another prothrombotic factor are both necessary to "tip" the clotting cascade toward thrombosis. The prothrombotic factors that coexist in aPL subjects with and without thrombosis is an area of ongoing research.

**24. Does the level or type of aPL affect the risk of developing thrombosis?**

This issue is controversial and unresolved. However, research suggests that high levels of aPL are associated with a higher thrombotic risk and that IgG antibodies are more thrombogenic than IgM or IgA antibodies. The presence of a lupus anticoagulant is associated with a higher risk of thrombosis than aCL. However, these generalizations are not strong enough to alter therapy; in a patient with clinical thrombosis and elevated aPL, treatment should not be altered based on the isotype of aPL.

**25. What factors may increase the risk of thrombosis in a patient with aPL?**

- **Antibody characteristics**
  - IgG with anti-β2-glycoprotein I reactivity
  - High titers of antibody
  - Lupus anticoagulant
- **Increased tissue factor release**
  - Infection
  - Surgery
- **Abnormal endothelium**
  - Active vasculitis/inflammatory disease
  - Atherosclerosis and risk factors (diabetes, etc.)
  - Catheterization for arteriography/IV access
- **Prothrombotic risk factors**
  - Smoking
  - Oral contraceptives
  - Pregnancy
  - Homocystinemia
  - Hereditary hypercoagulable disorders
    - Factor V Leiden (APC resistance)
    - Protein C or S deficiency
    - Prothrombin gene mutation (20210 G)
    - Antithrombotin III deficiency
- **History of previous thrombosis or fetal loss**
- **Use of cycloxygenase-2 specific inhibitors** (controversial)

**26. How should heparinization be monitored in patients who already have a prolonged aPTT from the lupus anticoagulant?**

In patients who are heparinized, heparin levels can be monitored directly to give an indication of anticoagulant effect. In addition, the thrombin time, which measures the clotting system distal to the effects of aPL, can be used as a good indicator of heparinization. In a patient on warfarin, the PT is primarily affected and, as discussed, is not usually profoundly affected by the lupus anticoagulant.

**27. What is the treatment for a patient who has had venous or arterial thrombosis and elevated levels of aPL?**

Because the risk of recurrent thrombosis is between 44 and 69%, most individuals will require lifelong anticoagulation (unless a mitigating factor is present). The intensity of anticoagulation has been hotly debated, with some authors recommending INRs of 2–3, and others recommending an INR over 3. It is certainly possible that the discrepancies in the literature are because in some patients in the studies, recurrent thrombosis occurred with a high INR because the lupus anticoagulant was interfering with the INR result. In general, standard intensity anticoagulation is first given, and if the lupus anticoagulant is present, *an assay insensitive to this antibody* (chromogenic factor X or prothrombin-proconvertin time) should be measured to ensure that the INR is reliable. If recurrent thrombosis occurs with an INR between 2–3, then higher intensity anticoagulation is needed. Adequate anticoagulation is felt to be achieved when the factor X level is less than 15% of normal.

**28. When do fetal losses typically occur in patients with aPL?**

Up to 2% of normal pregnant women have aPL, while 15% of women with recurrent pregnancy losses have these antibodies. The pregnancy is usually lost before the tenth week. Patients with aPL are at risk for preeclampsia, intrauterine growth retardation, and pre-term labor.

**29. What is the best treatment for the pregnant patient with elevated aPL who has had prior fetal loss?**

An aspirin daily is prescribed prior to conception. Once conception has occurred, subcutaneous heparin 5000 units every 8 hours is added. With this combination, the rate of live births increases dramatically, with some clinicians reporting a 100% success rate (average 80%). Heparin is stopped prior to delivery and then continued 6–12 weeks post delivery. Coumadin is contraindicated during pregnancy owing to fetal malformations. All patients with aPL should have the placenta examined for evidence of infarction even if no problems occurred during pregnancy.

**30. What other clinical manifestations are associated with aPL?**

- Migraine headaches (controversial).
- Seizures (even with normal brain MRI).
- Valve disease—mitral > aortic valve. Occurs in up to 50% of patients with aPL and SLE. Can cause embolic strokes, and 5% need valve replacement.
- Accelerated atherosclerosis (controversial).
- Hemolytic anemia.

**31. When should tests for aPL be ordered?**

Measurement should be considered as part of the standard hypercoagulation work-up, especially in patients with deep venous thrombosis, pulmonary emboli, or early onset stroke or myocardial infarction. Since aPL has recently been added as one of the criteria to diagnose SLE, it should be routinely measured in patients who have SLE, or can be measured to provide an additional criteria for diagnosing this disease. In addition, women with recurrent spontaneous abortions should be examined for aPL.

**32. How can aPL be detected in a patient who is already anticoagulated?**

Measurement of anticardiolipin antibodies is not affected by anticoagulation and can therefore be used to determine aPL levels in a patient on heparin or warfarin. However, coagulation tests to detect the lupus anticoagulant are affected by heparin and warfarin, and care must be taken in determining lupus anticoagulants in these situations. In the patient on heparin, plasma can be treated with heparinase to remove the heparin prior to the coagulation tests. In a patient on warfarin, it is the PT that is primarily affected, and the aPTT is usually not prolonged. Thus, prolongation of aPTT in a patient on warfarin is still suggestive of the presence of a lupus anticoagulant. Because warfarin depletes vitamin K–dependent factors, a 1:1 mix of the patient's plasma with normal plasma should correct the factor deficiencies induced by warfarin. Thus, if the alterations of clotting parameters are due to warfarin, the PT as well as aPTT will correct. However, as discussed earlier, a prolonged aPTT that does not correct in this situation is indicative of a lupus anticoagulant.

**33. How should you treat an individual with elevated levels of aPL but with no history of thrombosis or recurrent fetal loss?**

There are no prospective trials to date, guiding our treatment of asymptomatic subjects. Retrospective trials disagree on whether an aspirin daily is protective against future thrombosis. An aspirin daily probably protects a subject with aPL from future thrombosis and has low risk of harm; therefore, most clinicians prescribe an aspirin daily.

**34. Can low molecular weight heparin (LMWH) be used in patients with thrombosis and aPL?**

There have been no controlled trials of the use of LMWH in patients with antiphospholipid antibody syndrome. However, there have been several cases of failure to prevent extension of clots in patients with a new episode of thrombosis. Therefore, in patients presenting with an active clot, it is best to control their initial clot with unfractionated heparin and switch them to warfarin. If patients get subtherapeutic on warfarin, they can use LMWH until their INR is back to ≥ 3. Use LMWH cautiously if CrCl < 20–30 cc/min, since they are cleared by the kidney.

| | Cost |
|---|---|
| • Enoxaparin (Lovenox) 1 mg/kg bid | $85/d |
| • Dalteparin (Fragmin) 100 IU/kg bid | $63/d |
| • Tinzaparin (Innohep) 175 IU/kg qd | $51/d |

**35. If patients with aPL develop heparin-induced thrombocytopenia (HIT) and need anticoagulation until warfarin is therapeutic, what can be done?**

There are thrombin inhibiting medications that can be substituted for heparin in such a situation and will not cause HIT:

- Argatroban—given IV, cleared by liver, monitor with PTT
- Lepirudin—given IV, cleared by kidney, monitor with PTT
- Danaparoid—given subcutaneously, cleared by kidney, monitor with heparin levels

**Note**: You cannot use LMWH as a substitute in patients with HIT.

**36. A patient with aPL antibody syndrome on warfarin comes in with a dangerously high INR. What can be done?**

Most patients will not have bleeding risk unless INR is 5 or greater. Most of the time you can instruct the patient to hold warfarin until the INR decreases to the desired range. If you must decrease it more quickly, the patient can be given 1 mg of vitamin K orally or intravenously (not subcutaneously). This will decrease the excessive anticoagulation within 12 hours without making them resistant to warfarin for several days, which happens if vitamin K is given subcutaneously. If the patient has high INR and is severely bleeding, they need to receive fresh frozen plasma to replace coagulation factors acutely.

**37. What other therapies have been found to be clinically effective in patients with antiphospholipid antibody syndrome?**

- Aspirin
- Antiplatelet agents—ticlopidine, etc.
- Hydroxychloroquine

ACKNOWLEDGMENT

The editor and author wish to thank Dr. Woodruff Emlen for his contributions to this chapter in the previous edition.

## BIBLIOGRAPHY

1. Asherson RA, Cervera R, Piette JC, et al: Catastrophic antiphospholipid syndrome. Medicine 77:195–207, 1998.
2. Cuadrado MJ, Khamashta MA, Ballesteros A, et al: Can neurologic manifestations of Hughes syndrome be distinguished from multiple sclerosis? Medicine 79:57–68, 2000.
3. Galli M, Finazzi G, Barbui T: Antiphospholipid antibodies: Predictive value of laboratory tests. Thromb Haemost 78:75–78, 1997.
4. Ginsberg JS, Wells PS, Brill-Edwards P, et al: Antiphospholipid antibodies and venous thromboembolism. Blood 86:3685–3691, 1995.
5. Horbach DA, Oort EV, Donders RCJM, et al: Lupus anticoagulant is the strongest risk factor for both venous and arterial thrombosis in patients with systemic lupus erythematosus. Thrombosis Haemost 76:916–924, 1996.

6. Khamashta MA (ed): Antiphospholipid (Hughes) syndrome. Rheumatic Disease Clinics North America 27:499–671, 2001.
7. Khamashta MA, Cuadrado MJ, Mujie F, et al: The management of thrombosis in the antiphospholipid-antibody syndrome. N Engl J Med 332:993–997, 1995.
8. Krnic-Barrie S, O'Connor CR, et al: A retrospective review of 61 patients with antiphospholipid syndrome. Arch Intern Med 157:2101–2108, 1997.
9. Levine SR, Brey RL, Joseph CLM, Havstad S: Risk of recurrent thromboembolic events in patients with focal cerebral ischemia and antiphospholipid antibodies. Stroke 23(suppl I):I-29–I-32, 1992.
10. Lockshin MD: Antiphospholipid antibody syndrome. In Ruddy S, Harris ED, Sledge CB (eds): Kelley's Textbook of Rheumatology, 6th ed. Philadelphia, W.B. Saunders, 2001, pp 1145–1152.
11. Love PE, Santoro SA: Antiphospholipid antibodies: Anticardiolipin antibodies and the lupus anticoagulant in systemic lupus erythematosus (SLE) and in non-SLE disorders. Ann Intern Med 112:682–698, 1990.
12. Moll S, Ortel TL: Monitoring warfarin therapy in patients with lupus anticoagulants. Ann Intern Med 127:177–185, 1997.
13. Rai R, Cohen H, Dave M, Regan L: Randomised controlled trial of aspirin and aspirin plus heparin in pregnant women with recurrent miscarriage associated with phospholipid antibodies (or antiphospholipid antibodies). Brit J Med 314:253–257, 1997.
14. Rosove MH, Brewer PMC: Antiphospholipid thrombosis: Clinical course after the first thrombotic event in 70 patients. Ann Intern Med 117:303–308, 1992.
15. Wahl DG, Guillemin F, de Maistre E, et al: Risk for venous thrombosis related to antiphospholipid antibodies in systemic lupus erythematosus—a meta-analysis. Lupus 6(5):467–473, 1997.

# 28. ADULT-ONSET STILL'S DISEASE

*Vance* J. *Bray*, M.D.

**1. What is Still's disease?**

Still's disease is a variant of juvenile rheumatoid arthritis that is characterized by seronegative chronic polyarthritis in association with a systemic inflammatory illness. It was initially described in 1897 by George F. Still, a pathologist. The characteristic features of this illness have subsequently been reported in adults, as detailed by Eric Bywaters in 1971.

**2. How do adults with Still's disease generally present?**

Patients are usually young adults (75% before age 35) who present with a prolonged course of nonspecific signs and symptoms. The most striking manifestations are severe arthralgias, myalgias, malaise, weight loss, and fever. A prodromal sore throat occurring days to weeks before other symptoms occurs in 70%. These patients appear severely ill and have often received numerous courses of antibiotics for presumed sepsis, although cultures are negative. As many as 5% of patients being evaluated for "fever of unknown origin" may be diagnosed eventually with Still's disease. A few patients may have had similar episodes of illness as children.

**3. Describe the characteristic fever of Still's disease.**

The fever in Still's disease generally occurs only once or twice a day, usually in the early morning and/or late afternoon and lasts 2–4 hours. The temperature elevation is marked (66% fever > 40°C), although between fever spikes the patient's temperature is normal or below normal. This pattern is known as either **quotidian** or **diquotidian**. Patients with Still's disease generally feel very ill when febrile but feel well when their body temperature is normal. This poses a dilemma for physicians, because hospital rounds and clinic visits may not occur during the times when the patient is febrile. The fever pattern in Still's disease contrasts with the pattern seen in the setting of infection; infections generally cause a baseline elevation in body temperature in addition to episodic fever spikes.

**4. What are the common signs and symptoms seen in Still's disease?**

*Signs and Symptoms of Adult-Onset Still's Disease*

| MANIFESTATION | FREQUENCY |
|---|---|
| Arthralgias | 98–100% |
| Fever (>39°C) | 83–100% |
| Myalgias | 84–98% |
| Arthritis | 88–94% |
| Sore throat | 50–92% |
| Rash | 87–90% |
| Weight loss | 19–76% |
| Lymphadenopathy | 48–74% |
| Splenomegaly | 45–55% |
| Pleuritis | 23–53% |
| Abdominal pain | 9–48% |
| Hepatomegaly | 29–44% |
| Pericarditis | 24–37% |
| Pneumonitis | 9–31% |

Unusual manifestations include alopecia, Sjögren's syndrome, subcutaneous nodules, necrotizing lymphadenitis (Kikuchi's), amyotrophy, acute liver failure, pulmonary fibrosis, cardiac tamponade, aseptic meningitis, peripheral neuropathy, proteinuria, microscopic hematuria, amyloidosis, hemolytic anemia, disseminated intravascular coagulation, thrombotic thrombocytopenic purpura, orbital pseudotumor, cataracts, sensorineural hearing loss, and hemophagocytic syndrome.

**5. Describe the rash associated with Still's disease.**

Although the rash is said to occur in the vast majority of patients with Still's disease, it is often unappreciated unless specifically sought. The characteristic appearance is that of an evanescent, salmon-colored, macular or maculopapular lesion that is nonpruritic. It is usually seen on the trunk, arms, legs, or areas of mechanical irritation. Often, it is only seen when the patient is febrile. The rash can sometimes be elicited with heat, such as that produced by applying a hot towel or taking a hot bath or shower. Koebner phenomenon (i.e., the rash can be induced by rubbing the skin) is reported in approximately 40% of patients. Skin biopsies and immunofluorescent studies are nondiagnostic, showing a perivascular mononuclear cell infiltrate.

**6. Describe the arthritis associated with Still's disease.**

The arthritis associated with Still's disease may be overshadowed by the systemic features of the illness. It may not be present at the time of disease onset, may involve only one or a few joints, or be fleeting. With time, the arthritis frequently becomes polyarticular affecting both small and large joints. The joints involved are those typical for other forms of rheumatoid arthritis: knees, wrists (very common), ankles, proximal interphalangeals (PIPs), elbows, shoulders, metacarpophalangeals (MCPs), metatarsophalangeals (MTPs), hips, distal interphalangeals (DIPs), and temporomandibular joints (TMJ). Neck pain is seen in 50%. Arthrocentesis generally yields class II inflammatory synovial fluid, and radiographs usually reveal soft-tissue swelling, effusions, and occasionally periarticular osteoporosis. Joint erosions and/or fusion of the carpal bones (50%), tarsal bones (20%) and cervical spine (10%) may be seen. A destructive arthritis occurs in up to 20–25%.

**7. What are the characteristic laboratory features of Still's disease?**

*Laboratory Findings in Adult-onset Still's Disease*

| FREQUENCY | | |
|---|---|---|
| Elevated erythrocyte sedimentation rate (> 50) | 96–100% | |
| Leukocytosis (range 12–40,000/mm$^3$) | 71–97% | |
| Anemia | 59–92% | |
| Neutrophils (≥ 80%) | 55–88% | |
| Hypoalbuminemia | 44–85% | |
| Elevated hepatic enzymes | 35–85% | |
| Thrombocytosis | 52–62% | |
| Positive antinuclear antibodies | 0–11% | Should be |
| Positive rheumatoid factor | 2–8% | negative |

There are no diagnostic tests for Still's disease. Rather, the diagnosis is one of exclusion, made in the setting of the proper clinical features and laboratory abnormalities and the absence of another explanation (such as infection or malignancy).

An extremely elevated serum ferritin level is suggestive of Still's disease, with a value of ≥ 1000 mg/dl in the proper clinical setting being confirmatory of the diagnosis, especially if associated with a low glycosylated ferritin level. Values > 4000 are seen in less than 50%. The reason for this elevation is not known, although ferritin is an acute-phase reactant and reflects inflammation. C-reactive protein is frequently greater than 10 times upper limit of normal.

**8. How is Still's disease treated?**

In 20–60% of cases, nonsteroidal anti-inflammatory drugs (especially indomethacin 150 mg/d) adequately control Still's disease. However, most patients require corticosteroid therapy. Approximately one-third of patients require at least 60 mg of prednisone daily. When prednisone cannot be tapered to a low dose without disease recurrence, one of the slow-acting antirheumatic drugs or immunosuppressive agents (methotrexate) may be used. Anti-tumor necrosis factor therapy (etanercept, infliximab) may be beneficial, although some reports suggest it is more helpful for articular than systemic manifestations. Intravenous gammaglobulin, azathioprine, mycophenolate mofetil, leflunomide, and cyclosporine have been used for resistant cases.

**9. What is the clinical course and prognosis of Still's disease?**

The median time to achieve clinical and laboratory remission while receiving therapy is 10 months. The median time to enter remission requiring no therapy is 32 months.

The course of illness generally follows one of three patterns, with approximately one-third of patients pursuing each: self-limited illness, intermittent flares of disease activity, or chronic Still's disease. The patients who experience a self-limited course undergo remission within 6–9 months. Of those with intermittent flares, two-thirds will only have one recurrence, occurring from 10 to 136 months after the original illness. The minority of patients in this group will experience multiple flares, with up to 10 flares being reported at intervals of 3–48 months. The recurrent episodes are generally milder than the original illness and respond to lower doses of medications. In the group that experiences a chronic course, arthritis and loss of joint range of motion become the most problematic manifestations and may result in the need for joint arthroplasty, especially of the hip. The systemic manifestations tend to become less severe.

The presence of polyarthritis or large-joint (shoulder, hip) involvement at onset is a poor prognostic sign and is associated with the development of chronic disease. The 5-year survival rate in adult-onset Still's disease is 90–95%, which is similar to the survival rate for lupus. Deaths occurring in Still's disease have been attributed to infections, liver failure, amyloidosis, adult respiratory distress syndrome, heart failure, carcinoma of the lung, status epilepticus, and hematologic manifestations including disseminated intravascular coagulation and thrombotic thrombocytopenic purpura.

**10. What is the cause of Still's disease?**

Unknown, although an infectious trigger is suspected. The circadian release of proinflammatory cytokines such as interleukin-6 appears to account for many clinical features. Interleukin-18 is also elevated and can stimulate ferritin synthesis in monocytes/macrophages.

## BIBLIOGRAPHY


1. Bray VJ, Singleton JD: Disseminated intravascular coagulation in Still's disease. Semin Arthritis Rheum 24:222–229, 1994.
2. Bywaters EGL: Still's disease in the adult. Ann Rheum Dis 30:121–133, 1971.
3. Cush JJ, Medsger TA, Christy WC, et al: Adult-onset Still's disease: Clinical course and outcome. Arthritis Rheum 30:186–194, 1987.
4. Elkon KB, Hughes GRV, Bywaters EGL, et al: Adult-onset Still's disease: Twenty-year follow-up and further studies of patients with active disease. Arthritis Rheum 25:647–654, 1982.
5. Elliott MJ, Woo P, Charles P, et al: Suppression of fever and the acute-phase response in a patient with chronic arthritis treated with monoclonal antibody to tumour necrosis factor–alpha (cA2). Br J Rheumatol 36:589–593, 1997.
6. Esdaile JM, Tannenbaum H, Hawkins D: Adult Still's disease. Am J Med 68:825–830, 1980.
7. Fautrel B, LeMoël G, Saint-Marcoux B, et al: Diagnostic value of ferritin and glycosylated ferritin in adult onset Still's disease. J Rheumatol 28:322–329, 2001.
8. Kietz DA, Pepmueller PH, Moore TL: Clinical response to etanercept in polyarticular course juvenile arthritis. J Rheumatol 28:360–362, 2001.
9. Ohta A, Yamaguchi M, Tsunematsu T, et al: Adult Still's disease: A multicenter survey of Japanese patients. J Rheumatol 17:1058–1063, 1990.
10. Ota T, Higashi S, Suzuki H, et al: Increased serum ferritin levels in adult Still's disease. Lancet 1:562–563, 1987.
11. Pouchot J, Sampalis JS, Beaudet F, et al: Adult Still's disease: Manifestations, disease course, and outcome in 62 patients. Medicine 70:118–136, 1991.
12. Reginato AJ, Schumacher HR, Baker DG, et al: Adult onset Still's disease: Experience in 23 patients and literature review with emphasis on organ failure. Semin Arthritis Rheum 17:39–57, 1987.
13. Schmeling H, Mathony K, John V, et al: A combination of etanercept and methotrexate for the treatment of refractory juvenile idiopathic arthritis: a pilot study. Ann Rheum Dis 60:410–412, 2001.
14. Still GF: On a form of chronic joint disease in children. Med Chir Trans 80:47–49, 1987. [Reprinted in Arch Dis Child 16:156–65, 1941.]


# 29. POLYMYALGIA RHEUMATICA

*James D. Singleton, M.D.*

**1. How does "SECRET" describe the clinical features of polymyalgia rheumatica?**

**S** = Stiffness and pain
**E** = Elderly individuals
**C** = Constitutional symptoms, caucasians
**R** = Arthritis (rheumatism)
**E** = Elevated erythrocyte sedimentation rate (ESR)
**T** = Temporal arteritis

**2. Where did the term polymyalgia rheumatica originate?**

Reports of this syndrome appeared in the medical literature for years under a variety of designations. The name polymyalgia rheumatica (PMR) was introduced by Barber in 1957 in a report of 12 cases.

**3. Define polymyalgia rheumatica.**

PMR is an inflammatory syndrome of older individuals that is characterized by pain and stiffness in the shoulder and/or pelvic girdles. Formal criteria have included:

- Patient age > 50 years
- Bilateral symptoms involving two of three areas (neck, shoulder girdle, or hip girdle) for at least 1 month
- ESR > 40 mm/hr
- Exclusion of other diagnoses except temporal arteritis

Constitutional symptoms and arthritis are common. Some definitions have included a rapid response to glucocorticoid therapy (prednisone equivalent of 10–15 mg daily).

**4. Who is affected by PMR?**

PMR is a relatively common syndrome that rarely affects those under age 50 and becomes more common with increasing age. Most patients are > 60 years of age, with the mean age of onset being approximately 70 years. Women are affected twice as often as men. PMR, like temporal arteritis, largely affects whites and is uncommon in black, Hispanic, Asian, and Native American individuals. Whites in the southern United States appear to be less frequently affected than those in northern areas.

**5. Describe the typical stiffness and pain of PMR.**

- Stiffness and pain are usually insidious in onset, symmetric, and profound, and they involve more than one area (neck, shoulders, pelvic girdle). However, at times, the onset is abrupt or the initial symptoms are unilateral and then progress to symmetric involvement.
- The shoulder is often the first area to be affected, and a single area may be the predominant source of pain.
- The magnitude of the pain limits mobility; stiffness and gelling phenomena are dramatic. Pain at night is common and may awaken the patient.
- Patients may complain of a sensation of muscle weakness due to the pain and stiffness.

**6. Describe the arthritis of PMR.**

Synovitis has been reported by many authors. In one series of patients followed over 16 years, 31% had clinical manifestations of synovitis. Effusions of the knees, wrist synovitis (often with carpal tunnel syndrome), and sternoclavicular synovitis are detected most frequently. Knee effusions can be large (30–150 ml). Peripheral arthritis, at times with pitting edema, has been reported in up to 38% of patients. It may be present initially or occur later during the course and is most often polyarticular.

**7. What are the findings on physical examination in patients with PMR?**

Physical findings are less striking than the history would lead one to believe. Patients may appear chronically ill as a result of the presence of weight loss, fatigue, depression, and low-grade fever. High, spiking fevers are unusual unless temporal arteritis is present. The neck and shoulders are often tender, and active shoulder motion may be limited by pain. With longer duration of illness, capsular contracture of the shoulder (limiting passive motion) and muscle atrophy may occur. Joint movement increases the pain, which is often felt in the proximal extremities, not the joints. Clinical synovitis is most frequently noted in the knees, wrists, and sternoclavicular joints. Carpal tunnel syndrome may be present. Muscle strength testing is often confounded by the presence of pain. However, strength is normal unless disuse atrophy has occurred.

**8. What is the etiology of PMR?**

The cause of PMR is unknown, but there is no evidence of an infectious agent or toxin. Clues are presumably provided by the epidemiology of the disease, yet the association of PMR with aging is without clear explanation. The preponderance of whites has suggested a genetic predisposition, and an association with HLA-DR4 has been reported. The immune system is implicated in the pathogenesis, but no persistent immune defects or characteristic antibodies have been identified.

**9. Explain the source of the symptoms of PMR.**

PMR is a systemic inflammatory syndrome, accounting for the frequent constitutional symptoms. Synovitis of the hips and shoulders is difficult to detect clinically but is believed by many authors to be the cause of the proximal stiffness and pain. This is supported by scintigraphic evidence of axial synovitis, documentation of synovitis by clinical observation, synovial fluid analysis, and synovial biopsy. Some authors have proposed tenosynovitis and bursitis and not synovitis as the source of symptoms. MRI of the shoulders has demonstrated this in some patients. Other authors contend that PMR is an expression of underlying arteritis and that synovitis has little to do with the clinical symptoms. Muscle biopsies are usually normal and, when abnormal, have shown nonspecific changes and no inflammation.

**10. What is the most characteristic laboratory finding? Is it always present?**

An elevated erythrocyte sedimentation rate (ESR), often > 100 mm/hr, is the characteristic lab finding. PMR may occasionally occur with a normal or only mildly elevated ESR.

**11. Are there other commonly encountered laboratory abnormalities?**

Findings reflecting the systemic inflammatory process (normochromic normocytic anemia, thrombocytosis, increased gamma globulins, elevated acute phase reactants) are common. Liver-associated enzyme abnormalities may be seen in up to one-third of patients; an increased alkaline phosphatase level is most common. Renal function, urinalysis, and serum creatine kinase level are normal. Tests for antinuclear antibodies and rheumatoid factor are negative.

**12. Describe the results of synovial fluid analysis.**

Synovial fluid is typically inflammatory with a poor mucin clot. However, leukocyte counts have varied from 1000–20,000 cell/mm$^3$ with 40–50% polymorphonuclear leukocytes. Culture and crystal examinations are negative.

**13. How are PMR and temporal arteritis (TA) related?**

These two disorders frequently occur synchronously or sequentially in individual patients. PMR has been noted in 40–60% of patients with TA and may be the initial symptom complex in 20–40%. Conversely, TA may occur in patients with PMR. In 1963, Alestig and Barr reported the presence of histologic TA in patients with PMR who had no clinical evidence of arteritis. Although studies from Scandinavia have shown TA to occur in almost 50% of PMR patients, only 15–20% of PMR patients in North America have coexistent TA. Interestingly, PET scans have shown increased uptake in the aorta of PMR patients suggesting subclinical arteritis can occur.

**14. When should a temporal artery biopsy be performed on a patient with PMR? (Controversial)**

Temporal artery biopsy is not necessary unless symptoms or signs suggest the presence of TA. The patient should be queried regarding current or recent headache, jaw claudication, visual disturbance, scalp tenderness, and other features of TA. The arteries of the head, neck, torso, and extremities should be examined for tenderness, enlargement, bruits, and decreased pulsation. Constitutional symptoms and laboratory values in PMR and TA are similar and therefore are not of discriminatory value. However, the failure of prednisone (15–20 mg/d) to significantly improve symptoms or to normalize the ESR/CRP within 1 month should suggest the presence of TA and prompt temporal artery biopsy.

**15. How is the diagnosis of PMR established?**

The diagnosis of PMR is a clinical one, relying on the features in the clinical definition.

**16. Should other diagnoses be considered? How are they differentiated?**

*Differential Diagnoses in Polymyalgia Rheumatica/Temporal Arteritis*

| DIAGNOSIS | DISTINGUISHING FEATURES |
|---|---|
| Fibromyalgia syndrome | Tender points, normal ESR |
| Hypothyroidism | Elevated thyroid-stimulating hormone, normal ESR |
| Depression | Normal ESR |
| Polymyositis | Weakness predominates; elevated creatine kinase; abnormal electromyography |
| Malignancy | Clinical evidence of neoplasm (there is no association of cancer with PMR) |
| Infection | Clinical suspicion of infection; cultures |
| Rheumatoid arthritis | Positive rheumatoid factor, small joint involvement, especially MTPs |

**17. How is PMR distinguished from rheumatoid arthritis?**

It is often difficult to distinguish PMR from the onset of rheumatoid arthritis in older patients, in whom constitutional symptoms and morning stiffness often surpass joint manifestations. Features that support the diagnosis of PMR are:

Absence of rheumatoid factor
Lack of involvement of small joints of hands and feet
Lack of development of joint damage
Absence of erosive disease during follow-up

The response to glucocorticoids is not a reliable distinguishing feature.

**18. How are NSAIDs used in the treatment of PMR?**

NSAIDs are an effective therapy in only 10–20% of patients and are best used in those with mild symptoms. As with other diseases, no individual NSAID is necessarily more effective than another, and selection is based on perception of tolerability and safety for the patient. NSAIDs may be added to glucocorticoid therapy to facilitate steroid tapering. However, the toxicities of NSAIDs need to be kept in mind, particularly given the age of these patients and the duration of therapy.

**19. Describe the initial use of glucocorticoids in PMR.**

Prednisone in a dose of 15–20 mg/day usually evokes a dramatic and rapid response. Most patients are significantly better within 1–2 days, though others may take longer to respond completely. A single daily dose is more effective than alternate-day dosing, and initial dosage selection is determined largely by the severity of symptoms (doses > 20 mg/day are unnecessary). The dose is reduced every 2–4 weeks, using the patient's response (symptoms and ESR/CRP) as the most reliable parameter to follow. The ESR should steadily decline, although normalization may take several weeks. Dosage is decreased by 2.5-mg increments until a dose of 10 mg/day is attained. Further tapering is by 1-mg increments as the patient and ESR are monitored.

**20. What is the course of PMR?**

The course of PMR is longer and recurrences more frequent than once believed. In one study, 70% of 246 patients were still taking prednisone after 2 years of treatment; some patients required glucocorticoids for up to 10 years. Relapses of PMR after therapy has been stopped are seen in about 20% and may occur months or years later. The ESR may not be as high as with the original presentation.

**21. Given the course of PMR, how long should prednisone be continued?**

Optimally, prednisone should be tapered and discontinued as quickly as possible. However, since too rapid a taper results in relapse, observe the patient for about 1 year after a prednisone dose of about 5 mg/day is attained. Side effects and toxicities are usually minimal at this dose and relapses unusual. If there is then no evidence of disease recurrence, prednisone is tapered by 1 mg every 1–2 months until discontinued.

If relapse occurs, control is often regained by only a small increase in dosage. A slow taper can again be done, halting at a dose just above that at which relapse occurred. Further tapering is attempted again after a period of 6 months to a year. Because of the often significant side effects and toxicities of prolonged steroid therapy, use of methotrexate or other steroid-sparing agents may be helpful.

**22. Other than medication, what should be included in the treatment plan of PMR?**

Reassurance
Patient education
Regular physician monitoring
Range of motion exercises, especially where muscle atrophy and/or contracture have occurred
Attention to glucocorticoid side effects, especially osteoporosis

## BIBLIOGRAPHY

1. Barber HS: Myalgic syndrome with constitutional effects: Polymyalgia rheumatica. Ann Rheum Dis 16: 230–237, 1957
2. Blockmans D, Stroobants S, Maes A, Mortelmans L: Positron emission tomography in giant cell arteritis and polymyalgia rheumatica: Evidence for inflammation of the aortic arch. Am J Med 108:246–249, 2000.
3. Evans JM, Hunder GG: Polymyalgia rheumatica and giant cell arteritis. Rheum Dis Clin North Am 26:493–515, 2000.
4. Gabriel SE, Sunku J, Salvarani C, et al: Adverse outcomes of antiinflammatory therapy among patients with polymyalgia rheumatica. Arthritis Rheum 40:1873–1878, 1997.
5. Gonzalez-Gay MA, Garcia-Porrua C, Salvarani C, Hunder GG: Diagnostic approach in a patient presenting with polymyalgia rheumatica. Clinical and Experimental Rheumatology 17:276–278, 1999.
6. Gran JT: Current therapy of polymyalgia rheumatica. Scand J Rheumatol 28:269–272, 1999.
7. Gran JT, Myklebust G: The incidence and clinical characteristics of peripheral arthritis in polymyalgia rheumatica and temporal arteritis: A prospective study of 231 cases. Rheumatology 39:283–287, 2000.
8. Hunder GG: Giant cell arteritis and polymyalgia rheumatica. In Ruddy S, Harris ED, Sledge CB (eds): Kelley's Textbook of Rheumatology, 6th ed. Philadelphia, WB Saunders, 2001, pp 1155–1164.
9. Proven A, Gabriel SE, O'Fallon WM, Hunder GG: Polymyalgia rheumatica with low erythrocyte sedimentation rate at diagnosis. J Rheumatol 26:1333–1337, 1999.
10. Salvarani C, Cantini F, Olivieri I, et al: Proximal bursitis in active polymyalgia rheumatica. Ann Int Med 127:27–31, 1997.
11. Salvarani C, Gabriel S, Hunder GG: Distal extremity swelling with pitting edema in polymyalgia rheumatica. Report on nineteen cases. Arthritis Rheum 39:73–80, 1996.
12. Salvarani C, Macchioni P, Boiardi L: Polymyalgia rheumatica. Lancet 350:43–47, 1997.
13. Weyand CM, Fulbright JW, Evans JM, et al: Corticosteroid requirements in polymyalgia rheumatica. Arch Int Med 159:577–584, 1999.

# V. The Vasculitides and Related Disorders

*We are too much accustomed to attribute to a single cause that which is the product of several, and the majority of our controversies come from that.*

Baron Justus Von Liegig (1803–1873)
German chemist

# 30. APPROACH TO THE PATIENT WITH SUSPECTED VASCULITIS

Marc D. Cohen, M.D.

**1. In simple terms, what is the definition of vasculitis?**

Vasculitis is inflammation and necrosis of a blood vessel with subsequent impairment of flow.

**2. What two vascular consequences of vasculitis result in clinical signs and symptoms?**

- Vessel wall destruction leading to perforation and hemorrhage into adjacent tissues
- Endothelial injury leading to thrombosis and ischemia/infarction of dependent tissues

**3. What are the characteristic histologic features of vasculitis?**

- Infiltration of the vessel wall by neutrophils, mononuclear cells, and/or giant cells
- Fibrinoid necrosis (panmural destruction of the vessel wall)
- Leukocytoclasis (dissolution of leukocytes, yielding "nuclear dust")

Perivascular infiltration is a nonspecific histologic finding observed in a variety of disease processes and is not considered diagnostic of vasculitis, even though it may coexist in vasculitic tissues.

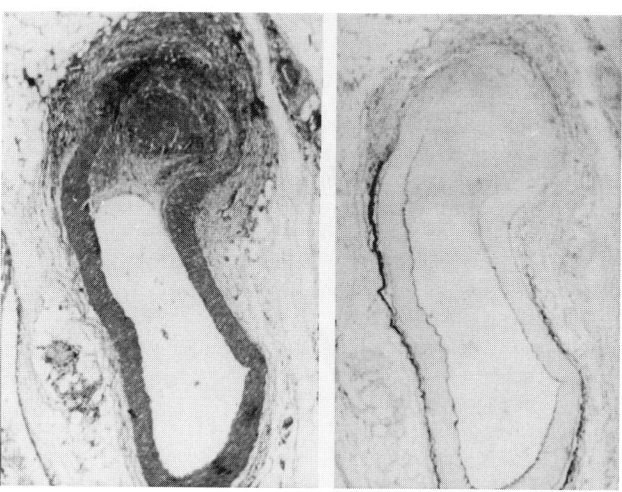

Necrotizing vasculitis in a bowel specimen from a patient with polyarteritis nodosa. The arterial lumen is partially occluded by thrombus. Adjacent arterial wall is necrotic, resulting in destruction of the elastic laminae (*Left*, hematoxylin-eosin; *right*, elastic tissue stain; lower power).

**4. Through which immune mechanisms does vasculitis occur?**

Depending on the type of vasculitis, either **cell-mediated** (granulomatous) or **humoral** (immune complex) mechanisms are involved. Examples of granulomatous vasculitis include giant cell arteritis, Takayasu's arteritis, Wegener's granulomatosis, Churg-Strauss syndrome, and isolated CNS vasculitis. Examples of immune complex vasculitis include polyarteritis nodosa, hypersensitivity vasculitis, cryoglobulinemic vasculitis, and perhaps Henoch-Schönlein purpura. The immune mechanisms of the other types of vasculitis are mixed or less certain.

**5. How is primary systemic vasculitis categorized when classified according to the size of the vessel involved (pathologic classification)?**

| VESSEL SIZE | VASCULITIS |
|---|---|
| Large | Takayasu's arteritis<br>Giant cell (temporal) arteritis (GCA) |
| Medium | Polyarteritis nodosa (PAN)<br>Kawasaki's disease |
| Small | Immune-complex associated<br>  Hypersensitivity vasculitis<br>  Cryoglobulinemic vasculitis<br>  Henoch-Schönlein purpura<br>Antineutrophil cytoplasmic antibody associated (pauci immune)<br>  Wegener's granulomatosis<br>  Microscopic polyangiitis (MPA)<br>  Churg-Strauss vasculitis |

**6. In general, how does one approach the diagnosis of vasculitis?**

1. Suspect the disease
2. Define the extent of disease
3. Rule out the vasculitis mimickers
4. Confirm the diagnosis

**7. How does vasculitis typically present? When should you suspect vasculitis mimickers?**

There is no single presentation typical of vasculitis. Vasculitis may present as a rash, headache, foot-drop, vague constitutional symptoms, or a major visceral event such as stroke, bowel infarction, or alveolar hemorrhage. Because of its protean manifestations, vasculitis can easily be confused with other diseases. "Mimickers" of vasculitis must be excluded early in the evaluation, since treatment varies dramatically, and misdiagnosis may result in morbidity and/or mortality. Vasculitis mimics should be suspected when there is:

1. New heart murmur [subacute bacterial endocarditis (SBE)]
2. Necrosis of lower extremity digits (cholesterol emboli)
3. Splinter hemorrhages (SBE)
4. Prominent liver dysfunction (hepatitis C)
5. Drug abuse (HIV, hepatitis C, cocaine, etc.)
6. Prior diagnosis of neoplastic disease
7. Unusually high fever (SBE)
8. History of high-risk sexual activity (HIV)

**8. What disorders can mimic vasculitis?**

**Large arteries**: Fibromuscular dysplasia, radiation fibrosis, neurofibromatosis, congenital coarctation of aorta

**Medium arteries**: *Cholesterol emboli syndrome, atrial myxoma*, lymphomatoid granulomatosis, thromboembolic disease, ergotism, type IV Ehlers-Danlos

**Small arteries**: *Infectious endocarditis, mycotic aneurysm with emboli, cholesterol microemboli syndrome, anti-phospholipid antibody syndrome, sepsis (gonococcal, meningococcal)*, ecthyma gangrenosum (pseudomonas), thrombocytopenia with hemorrhage, cocaine, amphetamines, HIV, hepatitis C

**Note**: Common clinical entities are in italics. To rule out vasculitis mimics, consider blood cultures, viral hepatitis studies, HIV test, urine toxicology screen, echocardiogram, antiphospholipid antibodies, and/or angiography/MRA depending on clinical situation.

**9. What clinical situations should provoke the consideration of vasculitis as a primary diagnosis?**

Multisystem inflammatory disease; fever of unknown origin and/or unexplained constitutional symptoms; ischemic signs and symptoms, especially in a young person; mononeuritis multiplex; suspicious skin lesions; and rapidly progressive organ dysfunction such as pulmonary-renal syndromes, strokes, or other organ infarctions.

**10. What localizing clinical features suggest the different types of vasculitis?**

- Jaw claudication, visual loss, and a palpable, thickened, tender temporal artery or a diminished temporal artery pulsation may be in seen in giant cell arteritis.
- Absent radial pulses or difficulty obtaining a blood pressure in one arm may indicate Takayasu's arteritis or large artery involvement in giant cell arteritis.
- Mononeuritis multiplex occurs in polyarteritis nodosa, Wegener's granulomatosus, and Churg-Strauss vasculitis. Sinus involvement suggests Wegener's granulomatosus or Churg-Strauss syndrome.
- Hypertension in a clinical context suggesting vasculitis may indicate renal vascular involvement from polyarteritis nodosa or Takayasu's arteritis. Alternatively, the hypertension may result from glomerular disease as seen in Wegener's granulomatosus and microscopic polyangiitis.
- The presence or history of asthma may help categorize a patient as having Churg-Strauss syndrome. Pulmonary involvement other than asthma is seen in Wegener's granulomatosus and is often seen in microscopic polyangiitis. Lung manifestations are rare in polyarteritis nodosa.
- Testicular tenderness may be seen in polyarteritis nodosa. The bloody diarrhea and crampy abdominal pain seen in Henoch-Schönlein may mimic inflammatory bowel disease, but biopsies from involved tissue demonstrate predominantly IgA deposition, which is diagnostic.
- Wegener's granulomatosus and microscopic polyangiitis may cause pulmonary-renal syndromes mimicking SLE and Goodpasture's syndrome.
- These features occur either before, during, or after the constitutional features. They may suggest a type of vasculitis, but are also relatively nonspecific with considerable overlap. Patients with systemic vasculitis feel sick.

**11. Which skin lesions are suggestive of vasculitis?**

Palpable purpura, livedo reticularis, subcutaneous nodules, "punched-out" ulcers, digital infarction, splinter hemorrhages, hemorrhagic macules, and urticaria lasting > 24 hours. (See figure, top of next page.)

**12. Which laboratory tests are useful in the evaluation of suspected vasculitis?**

- **Tests suggesting systemic inflammation**

  CBC—look for anemia of chronic disease and thrombocytosis. WBC and differential to look for neutrophilia or eosinophilia.

  Westergren ESR and C-reactive protein. An ESR > 100 mm/hr and a CRP > 10mg/dl in the absence of bacterial infection and widespread cancer should suggest vasculitis.

  Low albumin—this is a negative acute-phase reactant and goes down with systemic inflammation.

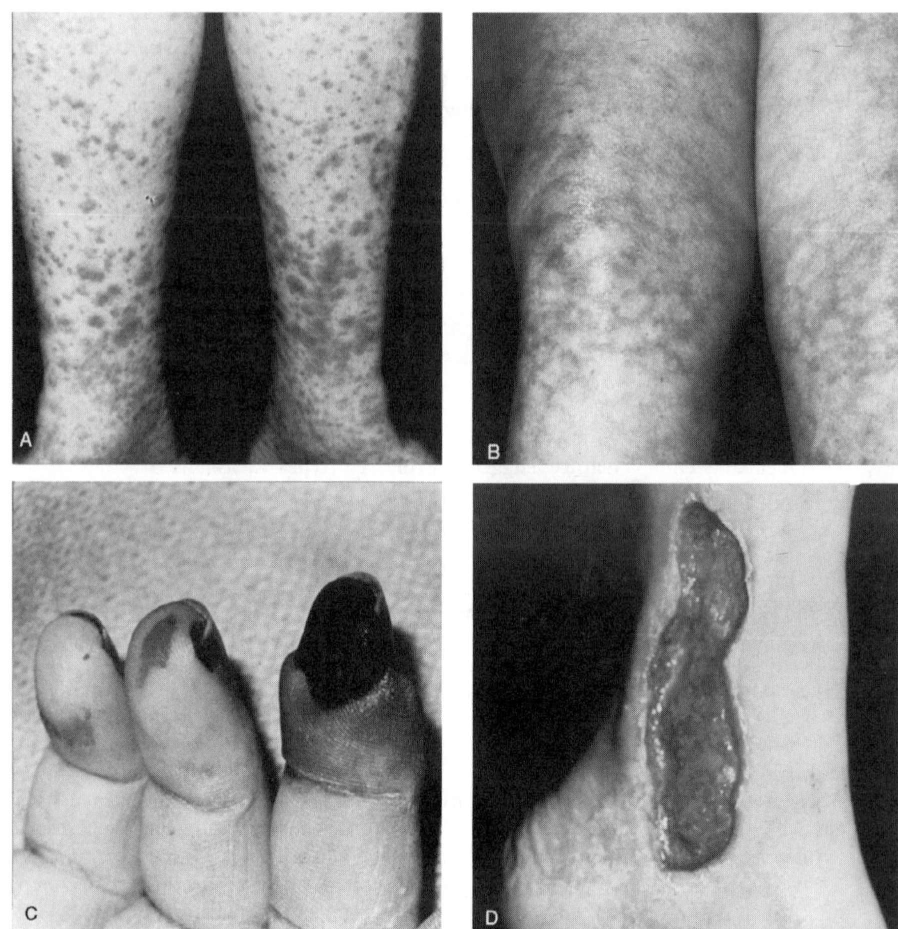


*A*, Palpable purpura; *B*, livedo reticularis; *C*, digital infarction; *D*, "punched out" ulcer. (From the Revised Clinical Slide Collection on the Rheumatic Diseases. Atlanta, American College of Rheumatology, 1991; with permission.)

- **Tests suggesting organ involvement**
  Creatinine and urinalysis
  Liver-associated enzymes—if extremely elevated, consider hepatitis B/C
  Creatine kinase
  Stool for occult blood
  Chest radiograph
  Brain MRI or abdominal CT scan if symptoms suggest involvement.
- **Tests suggesting immune complex formation and/or deposition**
  Rheumatoid factor (RF) and ANA. Should not be positive in primary vasculitis. If RF positive, consider cryoglobulinemia, and subacute bacterial endocarditis. If ANA positive, consider SLE or Sjögren's.
  Cryoglobulins—if positive, rule out hepatitis C.
  Complement levels—C3/C4 are low in cryoglobulinemia. Other vasculitides usually have normal values except polyarteritis nodosa, where they are low in 25% of cases, and some cases of hypersensitivity vasculitides.

- **Tests suggesting ANCA-related vasculitis**
  c-ANCA—if against serine proteinase 3, usually Wegener's granulomatosis. Sometimes MPA.
  p-ANCA—if against myeloperoxidase, consider MPA and Churg-Strauss vasculitis.
- **Tests suggesting etiology**
  Blood cultures—rule out SBE
  Infectious serologies—Hep BsAg (PAN), hepatitis C (cryoglobulinemia), parvovirus IgM (Wegener's, PAN), herpes (IgM), CMV (IgM), HIV (any vasculitis).
  SPEP—rule out myeloma
  CSF studies—herpes, varicella-zoster (VZV)

**Note**: All these tests are not ordered for all patients. Must choose based on clinical situation.

**13. How might ANCAs be helpful in differentiating vasculitis?**

The c-ANCA directed against serine proteinase 3 is highly specific for Wegener's granulomatosus with widespread systemic involvement (> 90%). Less specific is p-ANCA (antibody to myeloperoxidase), which may be found in microscopic polyangiitis and Churg-Strauss vasculitis. If p-ANCA is not against myeloperoxidase, inflammatory diseases other than vasculitis should be considered (inflammatory bowel disease, infections).

**14. When are hepatitis serologies helpful in vasculitis suspects?**

The presence of hepatitis B surface antigen may be found in some patients (25%) with polyarteritis nodosa. Hepatitis C antibody is often found in patients with essential mixed cryoglobulinemic vasculitis and more rarely in polyarteritis nodosa.

**15. Which other diagnostic studies are commonly used in the evaluation of suspected vasculitis?**

| | |
|---|---|
| Chest x-ray | Echocardiography |
| Sinus x-rays or CT scan | Angiography |
| Electromyography and nerve conduction studies | Tissue biopsy |

**16. Tissue biopsy is unquestionably the procedure of choice in the diagnosis of vasculitis. List some of the frequently approached biopsy sites.**

| **Common** | **Less Common** |
|---|---|
| Skin | Testicle (PAN) |
| Sural nerve (PAN, CSS) | Rectum/gut |
| Only biopsy if abnormal EMG/NCV | Liver |
| Temporal artery (GCA) | Heart |
| Muscle (PAN) | Brain (isolated angiitis of CNS) |
| Kidney (Wegener's, MPA) | Sinus (Wegener's) |
| Rare to see vasculitis, usually see focal necrotizing glomerulonephritis ± crescents. | |
| Lung (Wegener's, MPA) | |

**17. If tissue biopsy is not feasible, which alternative procedure can yield a diagnosis?**

Angiography may be helpful in certain types of vasculitis:

| **Site** | **Diagnosis** |
|---|---|
| Abdomen (celiac trunk, superior mesenteric, and renal arteries) | Polyarteritis nodosa |
| Aortic arch | Takayasu' arteritis<br>Giant cell arteritis with large vessel involvement |
| Extremity | Buerger's disease |
| Cerebral | Isolated angiitis of CNS |

**18. List two characteristic (but not diagnostic) angiographic features of vasculitis.**

- Irregular tapering and narrowing
- Aneurysms ("beading")

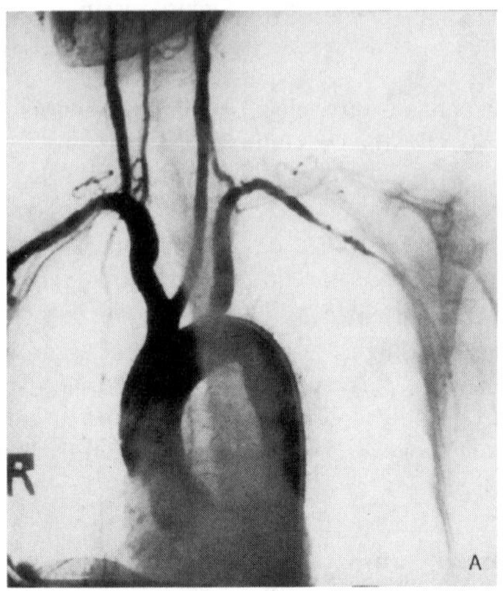


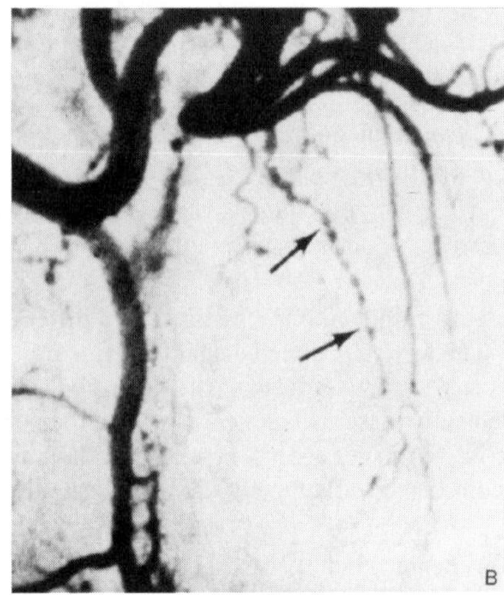


Angiography in vasculitis. *A*, Irregular tapering and narrowing of the left subclavian artery in Takayasu's arteritis; *B*, typical "rosary beading" aneurysm formation in a patients with isolated CNS vasculitis.

**19. What noninvasive tests can be used to determine vessel involvement in patients with vasculitis?**

- Doppler ultrasound of temporal arteries—localize area of narrowing in GCA. Help determine site of biopsy.
- MR angiogram of aorta—look for aortic wall thickening, enhancement with gadolinium indicating inflammation, and areas of stenosis in patients with Takayasu's arteritis or GCA with large artery involvement.
- PET scan—can see enhancement of aortic and subclavian vessel wall if active inflammation in patients with Takayasu's and GCA.

**20. Describe the general approach to the treatment of a vasculitis.**

- Identify and remove inciting agents (i.e., medications, etc.)
- Treat the primary underlying disease associated with the vasculitis (i.e., antibiotics for endocarditis; interferon-$\alpha$ for hepatitis B or C)
- Initiate anti-inflammatory and/or immunosuppressive therapy commensurate with the extent of vasculitis. Small-vessel vasculitis confined to the skin usually needs less aggressive treatment than systemic vasculitis involving large and/or medium-sized arteries
- Prevent complications—infection (PPD, Pneumovax, Septra prophylaxis if on cyclophosphamide), osteoporosis, and atherosclerosis (control blood pressure and lipids)

## BIBLIOGRAPHY

1. Atalay MK, Bluemke DA: Magnetic resonance imaging of large vessel vasculitis. Curr Opin Rheumatol 13:41–47, 2001.
2. Cohen MD, Conn DL: Approach to the patient with suspected vasculitis. Bull Rheum Dis 48:1–4, 1999
3. Gay RM, Ball GV: Vasculitis. In Koopman WJ (ed): Arthritis and Allied Conditions: A Textbook of Rheumatology, 13th ed. Baltimore, Williams & Wilkins, 1997, pp 1491–1525.
4. Hara M, Goodman PC, Leder RA: FDG-PET findings in early-phase Takayasu's arteritis. J Comput Assist Tomogr 23:16–18, 1999.
5. Hoffman GS, Specks U: Antineutrophil cytoplasmic antibodies. Bull Rheum Dis 47:5–8, 1998.

6. Jennette JC, Falk RJ: Disease associations and pathogenic role of antineutrophil cytoplasmic autoantibodies in vasculitis. Curr Opin Rheumatol 4:9–15, 1992.
7. Jennette JC, Falk RJ: Small-vessel vasculitis. N Engl J Med 337:1512–1523, 1997.
8. Jennette JC, Falk RJ, Andrassy K, et al.: Nomenclature of systemic vasculitides. Proposal of an international consensus conference. Arthritis Rheum 37:187–192, 1994.
9. Jennette CJ, Milling DM, Falk RJ: Vasculitis affecting the skin. A review [editorial]. Arch Dermatol 130:899–906, 1994.
10. Lie JT: Diagnostic histopathology of major systemic and pulmonary vasculitic syndromes. Rheum Dis Clin North Am 16:269–292, 1990.
11. Lie JT: Vasculitis simulators and vasculitis look-alikes. Curr Opin Rheumatol 4:47–55, 1992.
12. Mandell BF, Hoffman GS: Differentiating the vasculitides. Rheum Dis Clin North Am 20:409–442, 1994.
13. Schmidt WA, Kraft HE, Vorpahl K, et al: Color duplex ultrasonography in the diagnosis of temporal arteritis. N Engl J Med 337:1336–1342, 1997.
14. Stone JH, Taylor M, Stebbing J, et al: Test characteristics of immunofluorescence and ELISA tests in 856 consecutive patients with possible ANCA-associated conditions. Arthritis Care Res 13:424–434, 2000.

# 31. LARGE-VESSEL VASCULITIS: GIANT CELL ARTERITIS AND TAKAYASU'S ARTERITIS

*Gregory J. Dennis, M.D.*

**1. List the primary large-vessel vasculitides and the rheumatic diseases associated with large vessel vasculitis.**

Giant cell arteritis, Takayasu's arteritis, and other rheumatic diseases associated with aortitis such as the seronegative spondyloarthropathies, relapsing polychondritis, and Behçet's disease.

## GIANT CELL ARTERITIS

**2. What are other names for giant cell arteritis (GCA)?**

Cranial arteritis, temporal arteritis, and Horton's headache.

**3. Discuss the usual demographic characteristics of a patient with GCA.**

GCA occurs primarily in patients over age 50 years. The incidence increases with age, with GCA being almost 10 times more common among patients in their 80s than in patients aged 50–60 years. GCA is twice as common among women than men. Siblings of a patient with GCA are at increased risk (10-fold) of getting the disease. GCA has been most commonly reported in whites of Northern European descent. Epidemiological studies suggest that the incidence of GCA in blacks, Hispanics, and Asians is not as rare as once thought.

**4. How do patients with GCA present clinically?**

Most patients will present with one of four presentations:

- 20% Cranial symptoms with superficial headache, scalp tenderness, jaw and tongue claudication, and rarely scalp necrosis, diplopia, or blindness.
- 40% Polymyalgia rheumatica (PMR) with pain and stiffness of proximal muscle groups, such as neck, shoulders, hips, and thighs. Muscle symptoms are usually symmetric.
- 20% Both cranial and PMR symptoms. About 20–50% of patients with GCA have PMR symptoms.
- 15% Fever and systemic symptoms without any localized symptoms. Patients can present with a fever of unknown origin.
- 5% Other—cough, claudication (upper > lower extremity), or synovitis.

Onset of symptoms may be acute or insidious. Most patients have fever (40%), weight loss (50%), fatigue, and malaise (40%) as nonspecific symptoms.

**5. Are there any physical findings that may be helpful in suggesting a diagnosis of GCA?**

Several physical abnormalities are highly specific for temporal arteritis, but unfortunately, most have a low or only moderate degree of sensitivity for the diagnosis. **Scalp tenderness** and **temporal artery abnormalities**, such as a reduction in the pulse in conjunction with palpable tenderness, yield the greatest sensitivity for diagnosis. The presence of a visual abnormality (diplopia, amaurosis fugax, unilateral loss of vision, optic neuritis, and optic atrophy) may lend additional support for the diagnosis but is relatively less sensitive.

**6. Which are the five most common presenting clinical manifestations in GCA?**

| CLINICAL | FREQUENCY |
|---|---|
| Headache | 32 |
| PMR | 20 |
| Fever | 15 |
| Visual symptoms (without visual loss) | 7 |
| Fatigue/malaise | 5 |

**7. When should GCA be suspected?**

There are no pathognomonic clinical features. GCA should be suspected in individuals over age 50 who develop a new type of headache, jaw claudication, unexplained fever, or polymyalgia rheumatica.

**8. What is the most dreaded complication of GCA? How commonly does it occur?**

**Visual loss** occurs in 15% of patients, can be an early symptom, and is most commonly due to ischemic optic neuritis. Anatomic lesions that produce anterior ischemic optic neuritis result from arteritis involving the posterior ciliary branches of the ophthalmic arteries. The blindness is abrupt and painless. Retinal and ophthalmic artery thromboses are relatively less common causes of blindness. Blindness occurs in less than 1% of patients after corticosteroids are begun.

**9. The clinical manifestations of GCA might also include what other ocular problems?**

Blurring of vision, transient visual loss (amaurosis fugax), iritis, conjunctivitis, scintillating scotomata, photophobia, glaucoma, and ophthalmoplegia from ischemia of extraocular muscles may also occur. Visual blurring and/or amaurosis fugax are usually warning signs for months before sudden blindness occurs.

**10. Does GCA only involve the cranial circulation?**

Although cranial involvement is the most frequently recognized and characteristic anatomic location for GCA, the process is a generalized vascular disease not limited to the cranial vessels. Extracranial GCA usually involves the aorta and its major branches and is clinically detectable in 10–15% of patients. Positron emission tomography (PET) scans suggest that the aorta is involved even if not detectable clinically.

**11. Are neurologic complications common in patients with GCA?**

Neurologic complications are relatively rare in GCA. The internal carotid and vertebral arteries may be involved, leading to strokes, seizures, acute hearing loss, vertigo, cerebral dysfunction, and depression. Involvement of the intracranial arteries is unusual because these vessels lack an internal elastic lamina.

**12. List the resulting manifestation when GCA involves a particular vascular distribution.**

| VASCULATURE | COMPLICATION |
|---|---|
| Ophthalmic | Blindness |
| Subclavian | Absent pulses |

| VASCULATURE | COMPLICATION |
|---|---|
| Renal | Hypertension |
| Coronary | Angina pectoris |
| Carotid | Stroke |
| Vertebral | Dizziness, stroke |
| Iliac | Claudication |
| Mesenteric | Abdominal pain |

Note that GCA can involve both large- and medium-sized arteries. Pulmonary artery involvement is unusual. Small-artery involvement is much less common, so skin manifestations are rare.

**13. Which tests are most helpful in the diagnosis of GCA?**

The ESR is the most useful laboratory test and tends to be higher in GCA than in other vasculitides. It is almost always > 50 mm/hr, averaging 80–100 mm/hr by the Westergren method. Rarely, it may be normal when other acute phase reactants are not. Although in the appropriate clinical setting, the ESR is a sensitive indicator of GCA, its specificity is < 50%. Other laboratory abnormalities include anemia, thrombocytosis, abnormal liver function tests (especially alkaline phosphatase), and increased C-reactive protein (frequently to very high levels, > 10 mg/dl).

**14. Is it possible for patients with GCA to present with a normal ESR?**

Yes. Although the vast majority of patients present with ESRs > 50 mm/hr, there have been case reports and small series describing the association of biopsy-proven GCA with rates < 40 mm/hr. One series consisting of five such individuals emphasized an increased frequency of polymyalgia rheumatica or prior treatment with corticosteroid medications for other conditions as an explanation for this occurrence. When the ESR is normal, an elevated C-reactive protein might be helpful in detecting evidence in support of an acute phase response.

**15. Which test, if any, is used for confirmation of the clinical diagnosis of GCA?**

While color duplex ultrasound and positive emission tomography have been utilized for confirmation of the diagnosis, **biopsy** of the most abnormal segment of the temporal artery remains the technique of choice. In the presence of extracranial involvement, **angiography** may provide sufficient support of the diagnosis in the absence of a confirmatory biopsy.

**16. What characteristic of the disease process may hamper the ability to demonstrate vasculitis on biopsy?**

GCA is characterized by patchy or segmental arterial involvement. Consequently, a 3–6 cm segment should be obtained when the physical findings are indeterminate. The arterial biopsy specimen should be sliced like salami at 1–2 mm intervals and examined histologically at multiple levels.

**17. How often does a properly performed temporal artery biopsy define the need for therapy?**

A properly performed biopsy will define the need for therapy in approximately 80–85% of cases. However, if the biopsy is negative and the clinical suspicion for disease remains high, consideration should be given toward biopsy of the opposite side, which will be positive in an additional 10–15% of cases. Patients with posterior headaches may have a positive superficial occipital artery biopsy.

**18. Describe the characteristic histologic findings on temporal artery biopsy in GCA.**

Histologically, two patterns are seen. More commonly, there is granulomatous inflammation of the inner half of the media centered on the internal elastic membrane marked by a mononuclear infiltrate, multinucleate giant cells, and fragmentation of the internal elastic lamina. Less commonly, granulomas are rare or absent, and there is only a nonspecific panarteritis with a mixed inflammatory infiltrate composed largely of lymphocytes and macrophages admixed with some neutrophils and eosinophils without giant cells. Giant cells (multinucleated and Langerhans) occur in two thirds of cases.

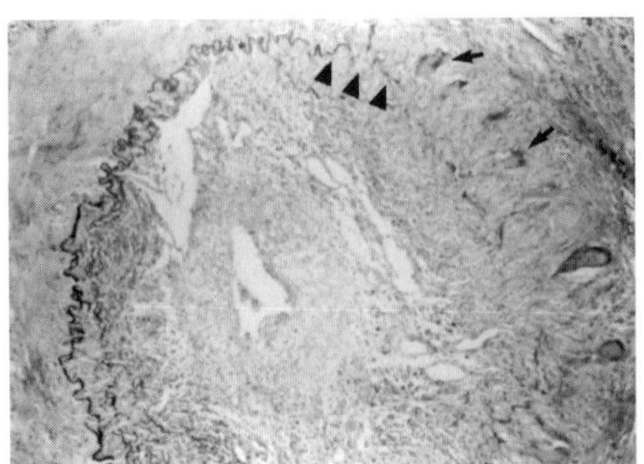

Temporal artery biopsy in a patient with GCA, showing the disrupted internal elastic lamina (arrowheads) and Langerhans' giant cells (arrows).

**19. What pitfalls can confuse a pathologist from correctly diagnosing giant cell arteritis from a temporal artery biopsy?**

- Up to 40% of positive biopsies show diffuse lymphocytic infiltrate without evidence of granulomatous inflammation or giant cells.
- Fragmentation and fraying of the internal elastic lamina is a constant feature of all aging arteries. It alone is not indicative of active or healed arteritis. There must be an inflammatory cell infiltrate to diagnose temporal arteritis.
- Healed temporal arteritis (because patient on long-term corticosteroids) can still be diagnosed, since it is characterized by intimal fibrosis, medial scarring, and eccentric destruction of internal elastic lamina. Corticosteroid therapy does not "normalize" the affected artery; it just gets rid of the inflammatory infiltrate.

**20. Is GCA a genetic disease? How does heredity relate to its pathogenesis?**

The cause of GCA is unknown, and its pathogenesis is poorly understood. The localization of the inflammatory reaction around the fragmented internal elastic lamina suggests that GCA may result from an autoimmune reaction to elastin or other macromolecules, although this is unproven. The inflammatory infiltrate is primarily macrophages and $CD4^+$ T lymphocytes of Th1 type, with approximately 25% being activated T cells. Recently, it has been discovered that the majority of GCA and PMR patients express the HLA-DR4 allele (60–70%). Interestingly, the association of GCA with the HLA-DRB1 genotype appears to confer increased susceptibility to the disease, but do not appear to be indicators of disease activity.

**21. Is there a standard treatment for the management of GCA?**

Currently, high-dose corticosteroids (prednisone, 20 mg three times a day) remain the cornerstone of therapy. Alternate-day corticosteroid regimens are not effective. Recent investigations to assess the efficacy of methotrexate as a steroid sparing medication have supported a promising role for it and perhaps others in the management of this disease. Other steroid-sparing agents such as anti-TNF$\alpha$ inhibitors are being investigated.

**22. Should one implement therapy before obtaining a temporal artery biopsy?**

It depends on the assessed risk for a serious complication and how soon the biopsy can be obtained. Symptoms for which corticosteroid therapy might be instituted sooner include the risk for visual loss, stroke, and angina. In general, there should be a low threshold for starting corticosteroids early in patients who have a clinical syndrome compatible with GCA.

**23. Does treatment with corticosteroids influence the biopsy findings?**

While it is possible that corticosteroid therapy may influence temporal artery biopsy findings, recent studies have shown that biopsies may show arteritis after greater than 14 days of corticosteroid therapy. In general, the biopsy should be obtained within 7 days of starting corticosteroid therapy whenever possible.

**24. Do patients respond rapidly to the initiation of appropriate therapy?**

Corticosteroids usually are dramatically effective in suppressing the systemic symptoms of GCA within 72 hours after initiation of therapy. Localized manifestations of arteritis, such as headaches, scalp tenderness, and jaw or tongue claudication, steadily improve over a longer period of time.

**25. Does the initiation of corticosteroid therapy prevent catastrophic events such as blindness and strokes?**

There have been many instances that support the prevention of catastrophic events by corticosteroids in patients with temporal arteritis. Sudden blindness and other stroke-like events have occasionally been reversed in patients by the institution of high-dose corticosteroid therapy (1 gram of intravenous methylprednisolone daily for 3 days) if started within 24 hours of the event.

**26. When should the level of corticosteroid medications be reduced?**

Patients should receive close periodic observation to identify potential harbingers of complications and the gradual discontinuation of corticosteroid therapy. When clinical evidence of the inflammatory process, including symptoms and laboratory evidence of inflammation, have subsided, the corticosteroid dosage can be lowered safely. A good rule of thumb is to begin tapering after clinical and laboratory parameters, particularly the ESR, have normalized. If patients do not achieve complete remission or are not able to be tapered to low doses of corticosteroids (< 10–20 mg prednisone a day), additional immunosuppressive medications should be considered. Some start low-dose weekly pulse methotrexate simultaneously with the institution of corticosteroids to allow tapering off corticosteroids more quickly. While there are studies that support this approach, additional studies are needed to demonstrate greater benefit than harm in using this approach long-term.

**27. How long do patients with GCA usually receive corticosteroid therapy?**

Treatment usually continues for at least 6 months, and often low-dose prednisone is needed for years. It has been well documented that discontinuation of corticosteroid medications too early is associated with worsening of disease activity. Moreover, recurrences are known to occur several years after the completion of an appropriate therapeutic regimen. Every effort should be made to limit side effects of corticosteroids such as osteoporosis (calcium and vitamin D therapy, bisphosphonates).

**28. Can you recommend a corticosteroid tapering schedule for a patient with GCA?**

After normalization of symptoms, ESR, and CRP (usually takes 1 month) on prednisone 30 mg twice a day, the following taper can be tried:

- Taper by 5 mg every 1–2 weeks to 30 mg once a day.
- Taper by 2.5 mg every 1–2 weeks to 15 mg once a day.
- Taper by 2.5 mg every 4 weeks to 7.5 mg daily.
- Taper by 2.5 mg every 12 weeks until off.

Spontaneous recurrences occur in up to 50%. Up to 40% (especially women) need corticosteroids for years.

**29. Is mortality increased in GCA patients compared with the general elderly population?**

The risk of death from GCA appears to be increased (3×) within the first 4 months of starting therapy. Patients typically die of vascular complications, such as stroke or myocardial infarction. After 4 months, the mortality is similar to that of an aged-matched general population except there is an increased prevalence (17×) of thoracic aortic aneurysm and aortic dissection. Patients with a history of GCA should be followed for the development of a new aortic insufficiency murmur. If one develops, further investigation for an aneurysm should be undertaken. Surgery is considered when the aneurysm enlarges to greater than 5 cm or dissects.

## TAKAYASU'S ARTERITIS

**30. List other names for Takayasu's arteritis (TA).**

Pulseless disease
Aortic arch syndrome
Occlusive thromboaortopathy

**31. Discuss the typical demographic characteristics of a patient with TA.**

TA occurs most commonly in young women. The average age is 10–30 years, but it can occur in younger and much older individuals. TA is eight times more common among women then men. TA occurs most commonly in Asian females but has been reported worldwide in all racial groups.

**32. What are the major clinical presentations of TA?**

A triphasic pattern of progression of disease has been described:

- **Phase I**—Pre-pulseless, inflammatory period characterized by nonspecific systemic complaints such as fever, arthralgias, and weight loss. These patients are often diagnosed as having a prolonged viral syndrome. Patients under age 20 frequently present with disease in this phase.
- **Phase II**—Vessel inflammation dominated by vessel pain and tenderness.
- **Phase III**—Fibrotic stage when bruits and ischemia predominate.

Patients can present in any phase or combination of phases because TA is a chronic, recurrent disease. Up to 10% present with no symptoms, and the incidental finding of unequal pulses/blood pressures, bruits, or hypertension prompts further evaluation.

**33. List some of the more common clinical features occurring in TA.**

| | | | |
|---|---|---|---|
| Bruits | 80% | Headache | 40% |
| Claudication | 70% | Hypertension | 30% |
| Decreased pulses | 60% | Dizziness | 30% |
| Arthralgias | 50% | Pulmonary | 25% |
| Asymmetric blood pressure | 50% | Cardiac | 10% |
| Constitutional symptoms | 40% | Erythema nodosum | 8% |

Symptoms occur primarily as a result of stenoses of the aorta and its branches. The aortic arch and abdominal aorta are most commonly affected. Upper-extremity and thoracic vessels (subclavian, carotid, vertebral) are more commonly involved than iliac arteries. Pulmonary artery involvement can occur in up to 70% of patients, with < 25% having symptoms of pulmonary hypertension. Cardiac involvement with angina, myocardial infarction, heart failure, sudden death, and aortic valvular regurgitation occurs in up to 15% of patients.

**34. Are there any specific laboratory tests useful for the diagnosis of TA?**

No. Nonspecific laboratory studies indicate active inflammation such as anemia of chronic disease, thrombocytosis, and an elevated ESR and C-reactive protein. The ESR does not always follow the degree of active, ongoing inflammation and may be normal in up to 33% of patients with active disease on biopsy.

**35. How is the diagnosis of TA made?**

Angiography is the gold standard for detecting arterial involvement in TA. Full aortography should be performed. The lesions of TA are most often long-segment stenoses or arterial occlusions of aorta and visceral vessels at their aortic origins. Aneurysms can occur but are uncommon (see Chapter 30).

Noninvasive imaging studies such as MRI are gaining popularity. With MRI, there is no radiation risk, and it is useful in detecting vessel wall thickness and inflammation as well as mural thrombus. It can also detect pulmonary artery involvement. Overall, MRI will miss some lesions, particularly in the proximal aortic arch or distal aortic branches, which are best detected by angiography.

**36. Is the histopathologic description of TA the same as that for GCA?**

The histologic appearance of TA is a focal panarteritis that can be very similar to GCA. Like GCA, focal "skip lesions" are common. One point that helps separate TA from GCA is that the cellular infiltrate in TA tends to localize in the adventitia and outer parts of the media including vasa vasorum, whereas the inflammation of GCA concentrates around the inner half of the media. Biopsy of a vessel is not necessary to establish the diagnosis of TA if the angiogram and clinical symptoms are characteristic.

**37. Is TA genetic disease?**

The etiology and pathogenesis of TA are unknown. Studies linking RA to HLA class I and II genes have provided conflicting results. There is no link to HLA-DR4 as is seen in GCA.

**38. What is the treatment of TA?**

High-dose corticosteroids (prednisone, 20 mg three times a day) are the initial therapy for active inflammatory TA. Alternate-day regimens are not successful. Corticosteroids are maintained at high doses until symptoms and laboratory evidence (ESR, CRP) of inflammation normalize. Unfortunately, the ESR does not always reflect the degree of inflammation observed if a blood vessel is biopsied. With control of inflammation, corticosteroids are tapered.

Relapses do occur, and up to 40% of TA patients will require cytotoxic therapy. Methotrexate is preferred, owing to its limited toxicity and its ability to induce remission in 80% of patients. However, up to 20% of TA patients never achieve remission. These patients require cyclophosphamide, mycophenylate mofetil, or another immunosuppressive medication.

Other medical therapy includes antihypertensive therapy (vasodilators should be avoided unless the patient has heart failure), antiplatelet therapy to prevent thrombosis, calcium therapy to prevent osteoporosis, and control of hyperlipidemia. Surgery is used to bypass stenotic lesions that fail to improve with medical management. Percutaneous transluminal angioplasty has been used in some patients to treat stenotic vessels once inflammation is controlled.

**39. If a normal ESR does not reflect the degree of ongoing inflammation of the great vessels in TA, are there any other ways to assess disease control?**

- MRI with gadolinium. Increased gadolinium uptake in the aortic wall suggests ongoing inflammation.
- PET scan—Increased uptake of fluorodeoxyglucose (FDG) suggests ongoing inflammation.
- Vessel wall biopsy—Practical only if patient having a vessel bypass as a result of stenosis.

**40. What is the prognosis for patients with TA?**

Sudden death may occur as a result of myocardial infarction, stroke, or aneurysmal rupture or dissection. Cardiac and renal failure can occur. Long-term survival rates are 80–90%.

## BIBLIOGRAPHY


1. Achkar AA, Lie JT, Hunder GG, et al: How does previous corticosteroid treatment affect the biopsy findings in giant cell (temporal) arteritis? Ann Intern Med 120:987–992, 1994.
2. Cantini F, Niccoli L, Salvarani C, et al: Treatment of longstanding active giant cell arteritis with inflix-imab: Report of four cases. Arthritis Rheum 44:2933–2935, 2001.
3. Diana E, Schieppati A, Remizzi G: Mycophenylate mofetil for the treatment of Takayasu arteritis. Ann Int Med 130:422, 1999.
4. Evans MR, O'Fallon WM, Hunder GG: Increased incidence of aortic aneurysm and dissection in giant cell (temporal) arteritis: A population based study. Ann Int Med 122:502, 1995.
5. Gonzalez-Gay MA, et al: Biopsy negative giant cell arteritis: Clinical spectrum and predictive factors for positive temporal artery biopsy. Semin Arthritis Rheum 30:249, 2001.
6. Hara M, Goodman PC, Leder RA: FDG-PET finding in early-phase Takayasu arteritis. J Computer Assisted Tomog 23:16–18, 1999.
7. Hoffman GS, Leavitt RY, Kerr GS: Treatment of glucocorticoid-resistant or relapsing Takayasu arteritis with methotrexate. Arthritis Rheum 37:578–582, 1994.

8. Jover JA, et al: Combined treatment of giant cell arteritis with methotrexate and prednisone: A randomized, double-blind, placebo-controlled trial. Ann Int Med 134:106, 2001.
9. Kerr GS, Hallahan CW, Giordano J, et al: Takayasu's arteritis. Ann Intern Med 120:919–929, 1994.
10. Lie JT, Brown AL, Carter ET: Spectrum of aging changes in temporal arteries. Arch Pathol Lab Med 90:278, 1970.
11. Mitomo T, et al: Giant cell arteritis and magnetic resonance angiography. Arthritis Rheum 41:1702, 1998.
12. Nesher G, Sonnenblick M, Friendlander Y: Analysis of steroid related complications and mortality in temporal arteritis: A 15 year survey of 43 patients. J Rheumatol 21:1283–1286, 1994.
13. Ninet JP, Bachet P, Dumontet CM, et al: Subclavian and axillary involvement in temporal arteritis and polymyalgia rheumatica. Am J Med 88:13–20, 1990.
14. Nordborg E, Nordborg C, Malmvall BE, et al: Giant cell arteritis. Rheumatic Dis Clin North Am 21:1013–1026, 1995.
15. Salvarani C, Hunder G: Giant cell arteritis with low erythrocyte sedimentation rate: Frequency of occurrence in a population-based study. Arthritis Care Res 45:140–145, 2001.
16. Schmidt WA, et al: Color duplex ultrasonography in the diagnosis of temporal arteritis. N Engl J Med 337:1336, 1997.
17. Tanigawa K, Eguchi K, Kitamura Y, et al: Magnetic resonance imaging detection of aortic and pulmonary artery wall thickening in the acute stage of Takayasu's arteritis. Arthritis Rheum 35:476, 1992.
18. Turlakow, et al: Fludeoxyglucose positron emission tomography in the diagnosis of giant cell arteritis. Archives Int Med 161:1003, 2001.

# 32. MEDIUM-VESSEL VASCULITIDES: POLYARTERITIS NODOSA, THROMBOANGIITIS OBLITERANS, AND PRIMARY ANGIITIS OF CNS

*Ramon A. Arroyo*, M.D.

**1. What are the medium vessel vasculitides?**

- Polyarteritis nodosa (PAN)
- Kawasaki's disease (see Chapter 75)
- Thromboangiitis obliterans (TO) (Buerger's disease)
- Primary angiitis of the CNS (PACNS)

**2. Are there other size vessels involved in the medium-vessel vasculitides?**

Yes, pathologic changes are not restricted to medium-size vessels alone. Large- and, more frequently, small-vessel changes are often found.

## POLYARTERITIS NODOSA

**3. What is polyarteritis nodosa (PAN)?**

PAN is a multisystem condition characterized by inflammation of small and medium-sized arteries. It most commonly involves vessels of the skin, kidney, peripheral nerves, muscle, and gut. Involvement of other organs is rare.

**4. How common is PAN?**

It's uncommon. PAN has an annual incidence of 5–10 cases per 1,000,000. It is more common in males by a ratio of 2:1. It affects all racial groups, with an average age at diagnosis ranging from the mid-40s to mid-60s.

**5. What are the clinical features of this condition?**

The disease presents in a variety of ways. Typically, the patient experiences constitutional features of fever, malaise, and weight loss along with the following manifestations of multisystem involvement.

| ORGAN | MANIFESTATION | ESTIMATED PREVALENCE | COMMENTS |
|---|---|---|---|
| Peripheral nerves | Mononeuritis multiplex | 50–70% | Motor and sensory deficits |
| Kidney | Focal necrotizing glomerulonephritis | 70% | Hypertension, occasionally severe |
| Skin | Palpable purpura, infarction, livedo | 50% | Mainly over the lower extremities |
| Joint | Arthralgias<br>Arthritis | 50%<br>20% | |
| Muscle | Myalgias | 50–60% | |
| Gut | Abdominal pain, liver function abnormalities | 30% | Due to mesenteric arteritis |
| Heart | Congestive heart failure, myocardial infarction | Low | |
| CNS | Seizures, stroke | Low | |
| Lung | Interstitial pneumonitis | Low | |
| Temporal artery | Jaw claudication | Low | |
| Testis | Pain | 20% | More common with hepatitis B |
| Eye | Retinal hemorrhage | Low | |

However, PAN can be limited to one organ without detectable systemic involvement. This usually is seen as cutaneous PAN, which may represent 10% of cases.

**6. Are any specific laboratory tests helpful in the diagnosis of PAN?**

No, most tests are nonspecific and reflect the systemic inflammatory nature of this condition. Elevated ESR/C-reactive protein, normocytic normochromic anemia, thrombocytosis, and diminished levels of albumin are usually present. Decreased complement occurs in about 25% of cases during active disease. Hepatitis B surface antigen is present in 10–50%, depending on the series. Patients with hepatitis B associated PAN will also be HBeAg and HBV DNA positive. By definition, antineutrophil cytoplasmic (ANCA) antibodies are absent in this condition.

**7. How do you make the diagnosis of PAN?**

It's often difficult. You should suspect PAN in any patient who presents with constitutional symptoms and multisystem involvement. Key **clinical features** suggestive of PAN include skin lesions (e.g., palpable purpura, livedo, necrotic lesions, infarct of the fingertips), peripheral neuropathy (most frequently mononeuritis multiplex), and renal sediment abnormalities. Once you suspect PAN, **biopsying** accessible tissues should determine the diagnosis. If clinically involved tissues are not amenable to biopsy, a visceral **angiogram** should be considered.

**8. Which tissue should be sampled to diagnose PAN?**

The likelihood of finding arteritis is greatest when symptomatic sites are examined. The most accessible tissues are skin, sural nerve, skeletal muscle, liver, rectum, and testicle. Biopsy of asymptomatic sites is not recommended.

**9. Can a kidney biopsy be diagnostic of PAN?**

No. In cases with abnormalities of urinary sediment or proteinuria, renal biopsy will usually reveal a focal necrotizing glomerulonephritis. This can be seen in almost all the vasculitides, so renal biopsy is not helpful in differentiating between medium-vessel vasculitides, but it could be useful if no other tissues are involved or available for diagnosis.

**10. Describe the histologic features in PAN.**

The pathologic lesion defining classic PAN is a **focal segmental necrotizing vasculitis** of medium-sized and small arteries (see figure), less commonly arterioles, and rarely, venules. Involvement of large vessels such as the aorta is virtually unknown.

The lesions occur in all parts of the body, but usually less so in the pulmonary and splenic arteries. The inflammation is characterized by fibrinoid necrosis and pleomorphic cellular infiltration of the vessel wall, predominantly PMNs and variable numbers of lymphocytes and eosinophils. The normal architecture of the vessel wall, including the elastic laminae, is disrupted. Thrombosis or aneurysmal dilation may occur at the site of the lesion. Healed areas of arteritis show proliferation of fibrous tissue and endothelial cells, which may lead to vessel occlusion. Remember, the lesions are focal and sectorial, involving only parts of the arterial circumference.

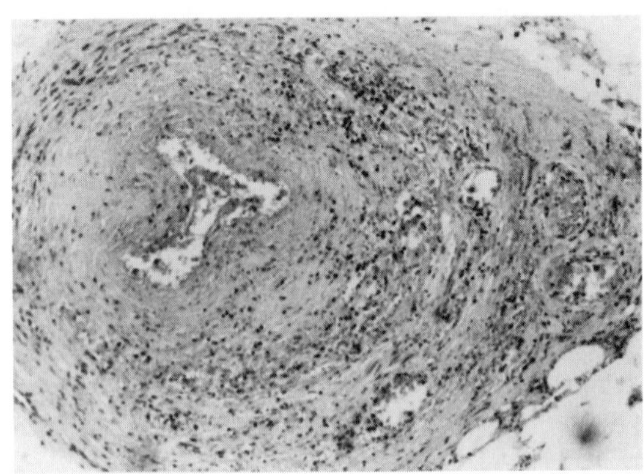

PAN involving a medium-sized artery.

**11. When do you perform an angiogram for the diagnosis of PAN?**

When clinically involved tissue is not available for biopsy (i.e., a patient who presents with constitutional symptoms and digital ischemia). Angiographic evaluation for PAN usually requires study of the abdominal viscera. The best plan is to study the kidney, liver, spleen, stomach, and small bowel. In rare cases, hand or foot arteriography is necessary.

**12. Describe the angiographic findings in PAN.**

Small aneurysms (microaneurysm), occlusion, and stenoses of the small and medium-sized vessels of the viscera (see figure, top of next page).

**13. What are some other diseases which can give aneurysms on abdominal visceral angiography?**

- Segmental mediolytic arteriopathy—noninflammatory arterial disease seen at any age that can give angiogram that mimics PAN. Probably a variant of fibromuscular dysplasia, affects hepatic, splenic, and celiac arteries most commonly. Can cause thrombosis, hemorrhage, and dissection. Diagnosis made by biopsy.
- Ehlers Danlos, type IV—aneurysms due to vessel wall weakening caused by defect in production of type III collagen.
- Fibromuscular dysplasia.

* Others—pseudoxanthoma elasticum, neurofibromatosis, atrial myxoma, others.

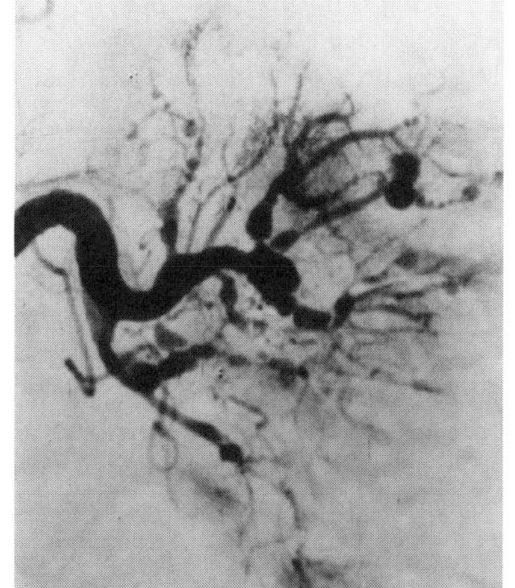

Angiogram of the kidney in a patient with PAN demonstrating multiple aneurysmal dilatations.

**14. What causes PAN?**

Unknown. An immune complex–mediated mechanism is frequently considered, but immune complex deposits or complement components are seldom found in involved vessels. Direct endothelial injury with subsequent release of cytokines and mediators of inflammation is another theory, but the triggering factor or antigen has not been found. Several conditions have been associated with PAN or PAN-like vasculitis, including:

Viral infections [e.g., hepatitis B, CMV, HTLV-1, HIV, parvovirus, EBV, hepatitis C (rare)]
Autoimmune disorders (e.g., SLE, rheumatoid arthritis, dermatomyositis, Cogan's syndrome)
Medications (e.g., allopurinol, sulfa)
Hairy cell leukemia

**15. How is PAN treated?**

Decisions regarding the initial management of PAN without HBV infection depends on the extent of disease, rate of disease progression, and organs involved. Treatment of this systemic vasculitis should include high doses of corticosteroids. If severe, intravenous pulse methylprednisolone 1 gm/day for 3 days is frequently used followed by prednisone at a dose of 1–2 mg/kg/day in divided doses. Gradually corticosteroids are changed to a single daily dose and slowly tapered. Cytotoxic medications such as cyclophosphamide (2 mg/kg daily oral or 500–1000 mg/m$^2$ IV each month) are added to the corticosteroids in cases with major organ involvement or inability to taper steroids.

**16. How does the therapy for hepatitis B virus (HBV) associated with PAN differ from that for PAN not associated with hepatitis B?**

Owing to hepatitis B vaccination, hepatitis B associated PAN now only accounts for < 10% of cases of PAN. PAN usually occurs within 6 months of acquisition of hepatitis B. Hepatitis B associated PAN has more orchitis, HBP, and renal infarcts. In HBV-associated PAN, the traditional treatment with corticosteroids and cyclophosphamide jeopardizes the patient's outcome by allowing the virus to persist and cause further liver damage and ongoing antigenemia. Consequently, patients who are HBeAg-positive are treated with a combination of prednisone (30 mg/day with rapid taper) to control systemic symptoms, plasmapheresis to remove circulating immune complexes (60 ml/kg exchanges, 9–12 plasma exchanges over 3 weeks), and antiviral agents (interferon$\alpha$-2b or lamivudine) to eliminate the virus. Successful therapy will be accompanied by seroconversion from HBeAg to anti-HBe antibodies. Patients who are negative for hepatitis C, HIV, and delta virus do best.

**17. What is the prognosis of PAN?**

The outcome of PAN depends on the presence and extent of visceral and CNS involvement. Most deaths occur within the first year, usually as a result of uncontrolled vasculitis, delay in diagnosis, or complications of treatment. Deaths occurring after the first year are usually due to complications of treatment, infections, or a vascular event such as myocardial infarction or stroke. The overall 5-year survival rate is 65–75% with aggressive treatment.

**18. Can PAN affect only one organ?**

Yes. Localized PAN is uncommon but has been reported as an isolated finding in the skin, gallbladder, uterus, appendix, and peripheral nerves. Cutaneous PAN is the most common presentation. Patients present with multiple, tender nodular skin lesions (.5–2 cm diameter) usually located on the legs and feet but can occur on arms and trunk. Livedo is found in 60%, and a mild polyneuropathy can be seen. Internal organ involvement is absent, but fever and arthralgias can be seen in the acute phase. Only 10% progress to systemic PAN in follow-up. Owing to the benign prognosis, patients can be treated with prednisone 20–40 mg a day with subsequent taper. Low-dose methotrexate, azathioprine, dapsone, and colchicine have been used successfully as steroid-sparing agents. Cyclophosphamide is not needed, unlike in systemic PAN. In patients who develop cutaneous PAN after a streptococcal infection, antibiotic therapy is effective.

## THROMBOANGIITIS OBLITERANS

**19. Is thromboangiitis obliterans (TO) a true vasculitis?**

TO, also known as Buerger's disease, is an inflammatory, obliterative, nonatheromatous vascular disease that most commonly affects the small- and medium-sized arteries, veins, and nerves. In the acute phase of this condition, a highly inflammatory thrombus will form, and although there is some inflammation in the blood vessel wall itself, the inflammatory changes are not nearly as prominent as in other forms of vasculitis. However, because of the associated mild inflammatory changes within the blood vessel, TO is pathologically considered as a vasculitis.

**20. What is the etiology of TO?**

Although it is clear that tobacco use plays a major role in the initiation and continuation of this disease, the pathogenesis remains unknown. Other etiologic factors may be important as well, such as genetic predisposition and possibly autoimmune mechanisms.

**21. Who is affected by TO?**

Typically young smokers aged 18–50 years, and rarely beyond. The average age at diagnosis is the mid-30s. Most reports describe heavy smokers, but TO have been reported in smokers using 3–6 cigarettes a day for a few years. The disease has also been reported in pipe smokers and tobacco chewers.

TO is predominantly a disease of males but is seen in women as well. The disease is more prevalent in the Middle East and Far East than in North America and Western Europe.

**22. What are the clinical features of this condition?**

Usually TO's initial manifestation is ischemia or claudication of both legs, and sometimes hands, which begins distally and progresses cephalad. Two or more limbs are commonly involved. Superficial thrombophlebitis, and Raynaud's phenomenon are described in 40% of cases.

**23. What are some of the presenting symptoms that prompt the patient to seek medical attention?**

1. Claudication, pain at rest, and digital ulceration are the primary manifestations. Because the disease starts distally, dysesthesias, sensitivity to cold, rubor, or cyanosis prompts the patient to seek medical attention in one-third of cases.

2. Pedal (instep) claudication is characteristic of TO, and patients often seek special shoes or orthopedic or podiatry care before the process is fully appreciated.

3. Gangrene and ulceration or rest pain is the presenting complaint in one-third of the patients. This occurs predominantly in the toes and fingers. It may occur spontaneously but more often follows trauma, such as nail trimming or pressure from tight shoes.

4. Superficial migratory thrombophlebitis.

**24. How is TO diagnosed?**

To confirm your clinical diagnosis, you need to exclude conditions that mimic TO. The most important and common of these are atherosclerosis, emboli, autoimmune diseases, hypercoagulable state, and diabetes. There are no specific tests to aid in the diagnosis. Complete blood count, liver function tests, urinalysis, fasting blood glucose, acute phase reactants, and serologic tests (ANA, RF) are usually normal or negative. All patients suspected of having TO should undergo an echocardiogram to rule out cardiac thrombi and an arteriogram to rule out atherosclerosis. The arteriogram will also help confirm your clinical diagnosis of TO, as arteriographic findings are suggestive (though not pathognomonic) of the disease.

**25. Describe the arteriographic findings in TO.**

Although no single arteriographic feature is specific for TO, the radiographic constellation in conjunction with the clinical picture *is* diagnostic. On arteriograms, there is involvement of the small- and medium-sized blood vessels, most commonly the digital arteries of the fingers and toes as well as the palmar, plantar, tibial, peroneal, radial, and ulnar arteries (see figure). The angiographic appearance is bilateral focal segments of stenosis or occlusion with normal proximal or intervening vessels. An increase in collateral vessels often occurs around areas of occlusion, giving a tree root, spider web, or corkscrew appearance. Note that in the arteriographic description, the affected arteries may have normal segments, but most important is that the proximal arteries are normal without evidence of atherosclerosis or emboli.

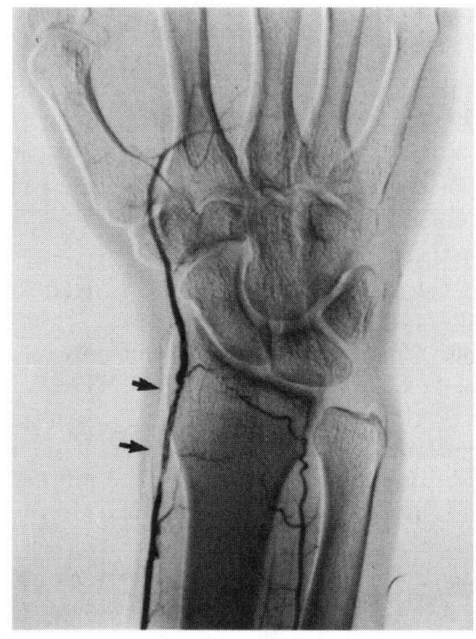

Angiogram of hand in TO. Note irregularity of radial artery (arrows) and cutoff of palmar arch vessels with no digital vessels.

**26. Is a biopsy needed to make the diagnosis?**

Pathologic specimens are not commonly obtained during the acute phase of TO. Reluctance to obtain biopsy specimens of these vessels is because the distal extremity is usually ischemic and biopsy may lead to new ulceration. Therefore, most pathologic specimens come from amputated limbs. In the acute phase, a panvasculitis with a highly cellular thrombus with microabscesses in the thrombus is seen. In the sub-acute phase, the thrombus is less cellular and recanalization of the thrombus is apparent. There may be perivascular fibrosis during this phase. In the late phase, there is often organized and recanalized thrombus and perivascular fibrosis. Unlike other medium-vessel vasculitides, the internal elastic membrane is preserved and venulitis is frequently found.

**27. What conditions should be included in the differential diagnosis of TO?**

Systemic lupus erythematosus
Rheumatoid arthritis
Scleroderma
PAN
Anti-phospholipid antibody syndrome
Giant cell or Takayasu's arteritis
Small-vessel vasculitides
Various blood dyscrasias (hyperviscosity syndrome)
Occupational hazards
Hypothenar hammer syndrome and thoracic outlet syndrome
Embolic disease (cholesterol emboli and atrial myxoma)
Premature atherosclerosis

**28. How do you treat TO?**

1. **Complete discontinuation** of smoking or tobacco use in any form including nicotine replacements. (Many patients continue to smoke despite disease severe enough to result in amputation.) Stop smoking!
2. Treatment of local ischemic ulceration.
   Foot care (lubricate skin with lanolin-based cream, place lamb's wool between toes, avoid trauma)
   Trial of calcium channel blockers and/or pentoxifylline
   Iloprost (helps patients with critical limb ischemia get through the period when they first discontinue smoking)
   Sympathectomy
3. Treat cellulitis with antibiotics.
4. Treat superficial phlebitis with NSAIDs.
5. Amputate limb when all else fails.

**29. Is surgical recanalization an option in the treatment of TO?**

Usually not. Because vascular involvement is distal, appropriate sites for bypass graft insertion are generally not present. In the few patients who have undergone arterial bypass, long-term results are poor.

## PRIMARY ANGIITIS OF THE CNS (PACNS)

**30. What other names are commonly used to describe PACNS?**

- Granulomatous angiitis of CNS (GACNS)
- Isolated angiitis of CNS

**31. How common is PACNS, and who get it?**

Rare. Can affect any age or sex. Most common in adults 30–50 years old.

**32. What are the presenting manifestations?**

The onset can be acute or insidious (over 1–3 months). Patients almost always have a headache. Common presentations are:

- Chronic meningitis (headaches)
- Recurrent focal neurologic symptoms
- Unexplained diffuse neurologic dysfunction (encephalopathy, behavioral changes, seizures)
- Unexplained spinal cord dysfunction (myelopathy, radiculopathy)

**33. How is the clinical diagnosis of PACNS confirmed?**

- Cerebrospinal fluid—pleocytosis and elevated protein. High IgG index and oligoclonal bands can occasionally be seen.
- Angiogram—alternating areas of stenosis and ectasia in multiple vessels in more than a single vascular bed. Sensitivity is 56–90% and predictive value 30–50%.
- Brain MRI—almost always abnormal but nonspecific with predictive value of 40–70%.
- Brain biopsy (gold standard)—granulomatous vasculitis more diagnostic than lymphocytic vasculitis. Highest yield is from a lesion. Can't be obtained from needle biopsy. If no lesion, then biopsy leptomeninges and cortex from nondominant temporal lobe. Sensitivity is 75% and specificity 90–100%.

**34. What are the three clinical subsets of PACNS?**

- Benign angiopathy of CNS—usually women who present with acute headache or focal neurologic dysfunction. Frequently seen during pregnancy or with use of vasoconstricting medications such as diet pills. They will have an abnormal MRI and cerebral angiogram but normal CSF. Treatment with corticosteroids, verapamil, and aspirin.
- GACNS—focal or diffuse symptoms present or recurring for more than 3 months. Abnormal MRI, angiogram, and CSF. Biopsy demonstrates granulomatous vasculitis. Treatment with corticosteroids, cyclophosphamide, verapamil, and aspirin. Poor prognosis.
- PACNS—similar to GACNS, but cerebral biopsy does not show granulomatous vasculitis. Treat same as GACNS.

**35. What other diseases can give CNS vasculitis and must be excluded prior to giving a patient the diagnosis of PACNS?**

- Infections—herpes, HIV, varicella zoster, syphilis, others
- Malignancy-associated vasculitis—lymphoma, lymphomatoid granulomatosis
- Drugs°amphetamines, cocaine, heroin, ephedrine, phenylpropanolamine. May cause vasospasm and not vasculitis.
- Connective tissue diseases—SLE, Sjögren's, Behcet's, PAN, Churg-Strauss, Wegener's.

**36. Is the cerebral angiogram specific for PACNS?**

No. Several other diseases can give angiographic features similar to PACNS, including severe hypertension, amyloid angiopathy, drug-induced vasospasm, syphilis, CNS lymphoma, and thrombotic disorders.

## BIBLIOGRAPHY


1. Abgrall S, Mouthon L, Cohen P, et al: Localized neurological necrotizing vasculitides. Three cases with isolated mononeuritis multiplex. J Rheumatol 28:631–633, 2001.
2. Calabrese LH, Duna GF, Lie JT: Vasculitis in the central nervous system. Arthritis Rheum 40:1189, 1997.
3. Chan RJ, Goodman TA, Lie JT: Segmental mediolytic arteriopathy of the splenic and hepatic arteries mimicking systemic necrotizing vasculitis. Arthritis Rheum 41:935–938, 1998.
4. Chu CT, Gray L, Goldstein LB, et al: Diagnosis of intracranial vasculitis: A multi-disciplinary approach. J Neuropathol Exper Neurol 57:30, 1998.
5. Daod MS, Hutton KP, Gibson LE: Cutaneous polyarteritis nodosa: A clinicopathologic study of 79 cases. Br J Dermatol 136:706–713, 1997.
6. Erhardt A, Sagir A, Guillevin L, et al: Successful treatment of hepatitis B virus associated polyarteritis nodosa with a combination of prednisolone, alpha-interferon, and lamivudine. J Hepatology 33: 677–683, 2000.
7. Gayraud M, Guillevin L, le Toumelin P, et al: Long-term follow-up of polyarteritis nodosa, microscopic polyangiitis, and Churg-Strauss syndrome: Analysis of four prospective trials including 278 patients. Arthritis Rheum 44:666–675, 2001.
8. Guillevin L, Lhote F: Treatment of polyarteritis nodosa and microscopic polyangiitis. Arthritis Rheum 41:2100–2105, 1998.
9. Guillevin L, Lhote F, Cohen P, et al: Polyarteritis nodosa related to hepatitis B virus. A prospective study with long-term observation of 41 patients. Medicine 74:238–253, 1995.

10. Olin JW: Thromboangiitis obliterans (Burger's disease). N Engl J Med 343:8864–8869, 2000.
11. Rose BD, Appel GB, Hunder GG: Polyarteritis nodosa. In 2000 Up To Date, Vol. 8, No.2, Jan 2000.
12. Sergent JS: Polyarteritis and related disorders. In Ruddy S, Harris ED, Sledge CB (eds): Kelley's Textbook of Rheumatology, 6th ed. Philadelphia, .B Saunders, 2001, pp 1185–1196.
13. Sigal LH: Cerebral vasculitis. In Koopman W (ed): Arthritis and Allied Conditions, 14th ed. Baltimore, Williams & Wilkins, 2001, pp 1696–1710.
14. Trepo C, Guillevin L: Polyarteritis nodosa and extra hepatic manifestations of HBV infection: The case against autoimmune intervention in pathogenesis. J Autoimmun 16:269–274, 2001.

# 33. WEGENER'S GRANULOMATOSIS AND OTHER ANCA-ASSOCIATED DISEASES

*Mark Malyak*, M.D.

**1. Define Wegener's granulomatosis.**

Wegener's granulomatosis (WG) is a clinicopathologic syndrome of unknown etiology. Its generalized form is characterized by:

- Extravascular granulomatous inflammation, granulomatous vasculitis of predominantly small-sized vessels, and necrosis of the **upper and lower respiratory tracts**
- **Glomerulonephritis**, usually pauci-immune, focal and segmental, and necrotizing
- Variable involvement of **other organ systems** with granulomatous vasculitis of mostly small-sized vessels, extravascular granulomatous inflammation, and necrosis
- Strong association with cytoplasmic anti-neutrophil cytoplasmic antibodies (C-ANCA) and anti-proteinase 3 antibodies

Though WG is considered a primary vasculitis syndrome, the inflammatory changes, including granulomas, often occur in parenchymal sites outside vessel walls. Indeed, extravascular granulomatous infiltration may be the predominant lesion in WG. Limited WG is defined as absence of renal involvement. Generalized WG implies involvement of all three major end-organs.

**2. How does the American College of Rheumatology define WG?**

The College has proposed the following criteria for WG. Patients meeting two or more of these four criteria can be classified (? diagnosed) as having WG with a sensitivity of 88% and a specificity of 92%. Of note, these criteria were formulated prior to general availability of ANCA testing.

- Nasal or oral inflammation characterized as oral ulcers or purulent or bloody nasal discharge
- Abnormal chest radiograph showing nodules, fixed infiltrates, or cavities
- Abnormal urinary sediment showing microhematuria or RBC casts
- Characteristic granulomatous inflammation in the wall of an artery or in perivascular/extravascular areas

**3. How is the upper respiratory tract affected clinically by WG?**

Chronic inflammation of the mucosa of the upper respiratory tract characterized by granulomatous inflammation, vasculitis, and necrosis may lead to clinical manifestations in the following locations:

**Paranasal sinuses**—Chronic sinusitis is a common presenting manifestation (50%) that ultimately affects 80% of patients with WG.

**Nasal mucosa**—Chronic inflammation occurs in approximately 70% of patients, resulting in chronic purulent nasal discharge, epistaxis, mucosal ulcerations, and, less commonly, perforation of the nasal septum and disruption of the supporting cartilage of the nose (saddle-nose deformity).

**Oral mucosa**—Chronic inflammation may lead to oral ulcers that may or may not be painful.

**Pharyngeal mucosa**—Chronic inflammation may lead to obstruction of the auditory canal, resulting in acute suppurative otitis media or chronic serous otitis media.

**Pearl**: New onset otitis media in an adult, think WG.

**Laryngeal and tracheal mucosa**—Chronic inflammation may lead to subglottic stenosis, which, in severe cases, may result in stridor and respiratory insufficiency.

**4. Describe the pathologic findings in the lower respiratory tract in WG.**

*Lower Respiratory Tract Pathology in WG*

Extravascular inflammation
- Chronic: granulomatous
- Acute: neutrophilic infiltration

Vasculitis
- Chronic: granulomatous
- Acute: capillaritis, characterized by neutrophilic infiltration and fibrinoid necrosis

Fibrosis

Pulmonary disease in WG is characterized by variable degrees of chronic (granulomatous) and acute (neutrophilic) inflammation and necrosis of the alveolar septa and small blood vessels. Airways and larger blood vessels are involved less commonly.

**Chronic inflammation** results in the characteristic lesion of WG, the granuloma, typically occurring in the extravascular interstitium of the alveolar septa, but also within vessel and airway walls. **Acute inflammation** results in infiltration of neutrophils and other inflammatory cells in vessel walls, extravascular interstitium, and alveolar spaces.

If acute or chronic inflammation resolves, it may be characterized by resolution (healing) or organization (collagen deposition and scar formation). Also, acute inflammation may evolve into a chronic inflammatory process with granulomatous infiltration. Many patients with WG have variable degrees of both acute and chronic inflammation on pathologic examination, often with one type predominating. When inflammation occurs adjacent to the serosal surface of the lung, chronic fibrinous pleuritis may result.

**5. How does lower respiratory tract involvement manifest clinically in WG?**

*Lower Respiratory Tract Involvement in WG*

| CLINICAL SYNDROME | PATHOLOGY | RADIOGRAPHIC FINDINGS |
|---|---|---|
| Asymptomatic (common) | Predominantly chronic inflammation | Fixed, focal infiltrates and/or nodules |
| Chronic cough, without other symptoms of pulmonary involvement (common) | Predominantly chronic inflammation | Fixed, focal infiltrates and/or nodules |
| Alveolar hemorrhage syndrome (uncommon) | Capillaritis within alveolar septa | Fleeting, focal alveolar infiltrates |
| Acute/subacute pneumonitis with acute respiratory failure (uncommon) | Predominantly acute inflammation | Transient focal or diffuse interstitial/alveolar infiltrates |
| Chronic respiratory insufficiency (uncommon) | Chronic inflammation and/or fibrosis | Fixed diffuse infiltrates |
| Pleuritis (uncommon) | Chronic fibrinous pleuritis | ± Pleural effusion |

Clinical evidence of pulmonary disease is common on presentation (50%) in WG, ultimately affecting 85% of patients. Approximately one-third of these patients, despite having radiographically evident pulmonary disease, do not have lower respiratory tract symptoms. The clinical manifestations of pulmonary involvement are highly variable, but can be explained by the underlying pathologic process.

**Chronic** inflammation with granuloma infiltration of the alveolar septa and small blood vessels may lead to the formation of nodules and/or fixed infiltrates on chest radiographs (see figure). If this process is extensive, subacute or chronic respiratory insufficiency may result. Chronic respiratory insufficiency may also be caused by diffuse fibrosis resulting from organization of previous chronic or acute inflammation.

**Acute** inflammation with necrotizing vasculitis of small blood vessels and neutrophilic infiltration of extravascular sites (alveolar septa and intra-alveolar spaces) may lead to a diffuse acute pneumonitis and consequent acute respiratory insufficiency/failure. It may also lead to capillaritis of alveolar septa, which may result in an alveolar hemorrhage syndrome with hemoptysis and variable degrees of acute respiratory insufficiency/failure.

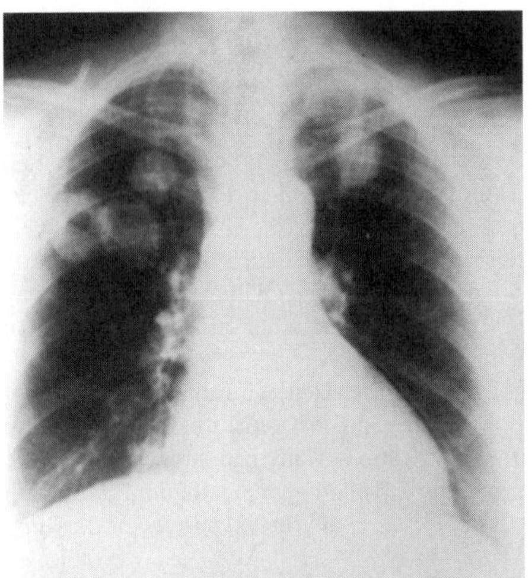

Chest radiograph demonstrating nodules (some cavitating) in a patient with WG. (From the Clinical Slide Collection on the Rheumatic Diseases. Atlanta, American College of Rheumatology, 1991; with permission.)

**6. Besides direct involvement, how else may the upper and lower respiratory tracts be affected in WG?**

Bacterial sinusitis, most often due to *Staphylococcus aureus*, is common in patients with upper respiratory tract involvement in WG. Obstruction of the paranasal sinus ostia by the inflammatory process is the usual cause. Similarly, obstruction of bronchi by nodules or intrabronchial lesions may lead to postobstructive suppurative bacterial pneumonia.

Infections may also result as a complication of treatment-induced immunosuppression. The two agents most commonly used, glucocorticoids and cyclophosphamide, can suppress both humoral and cellular immunity. Thus, patients are predisposed to pulmonary infections with opportunistic organisms such as *Pneumocystis carinii*, herpesviruses, mycobacteria, fungi, and *Legionella*, as well as the common suppurative bacteria such as *Streptococcus pneumoniae*.

Finally, medications may have direct toxic effects on the lungs. Cyclophosphamide, even in the relatively low doses used to treat WG, may rarely lead to pulmonary fibrosis. Methotrexate is also associated with pneumotoxicity.

**7. How does involvement of the kidney by WG manifest clinically and pathologically?**

Clinical evidence of renal disease occurs in approximately 15% of patients with WG on presentation, ultimately affecting 50%.

The typical renal lesion is a pauci-immune, focal and segmental, necrotizing **glomerulonephritis**. In more severe cases, crescentic glomerulonephritis may occur. Immunofluorescent studies often reveal little or no deposition of immunoglobulin, immune complexes, or complement;

thus the designation pauci-immune. Renal vasculitis is less common and may be characterized as necrotizing vasculitis with or without granulomatous infiltration.

Most patients with glomerulonephritis have asymptomatic renal disease, manifesting as an "active" urinary sediment (hematuria, pyuria, proteinuria, and cellular casts) with variable degrees of disturbance of renal function (characterized by an elevated serum creatinine). Patients with more severe renal involvement may develop progressive renal disease leading to acute or chronic renal failure.

**8. Besides the upper and lower respiratory tracts and kidney, what other organ systems may be affected?**

All organ systems may be affected to variable degrees by WG. Additionally, "constitutional symptoms," such as anorexia, weight loss, fatigue, malaise, and fever, are common and likely result from circulating cytokines, particularly interleukin-1 (IL-1), interleukin-6 (IL-6), and tumor necrosis factor-α (TNF-α), elaborated by the inflammatory process.

The **eye** is commonly involved, eventually affecting 50% of patients. Proptosis due to inflammatory and fibrotic infiltration of the retro-orbital space (retro-orbital pseudotumor) eventually affects 15% of patients with WG. This process may result in loss of visual acuity as a result of impingement upon the optic nerve and loss of conjugate gaze due to infiltration of the extraocular muscles. Other less-specific ocular abnormalities include scleritis, episcleritis, uveitis, conjunctivitis, optic neuritis, and retinal artery thrombosis. Eye involvement may be the initial presentation of WG before other manifestations occur.

The **skin** is eventually involved in 50% of patients with WG. Lesions include palpable purpura, ulcers, subcutaneous nodules, and vesicles. Pathologic examination may reveal necrotizing vasculitis with or without granulomatous infiltration of the vessel walls, in addition to extravascular granulomatous infiltration and necrosis. Children with WG may present with palpable purpura and be misdiagnosed as having Henoch-Schönlein purpura.

Involvement of the **musculoskeletal system** commonly manifests as arthralgia and myalgia, eventually affecting 67% of patients. Synovitis is less common and, when present, does not result in erosive disease, articular destruction, or joint deformity.

Involvement of the peripheral and central **nervous systems** occurs in 15% and 8% of patients, respectively. The most common peripheral neuropathy is mononeuritis multiplex. CNS syndromes include cranial neuropathy, cerebrovascular events, seizures, and diffuse white matter disease presumably due to vasculitis.

Approximately 5% of patients develop **pericarditis**, which rarely results in interference with ventricular filling. Involvement of the myocardium, endocardium, and coronary vasculature is unusual, but may result in significant morbidity and, rarely, mortality.

Involvement of other organ systems, including the gastrointestinal and genitourinary tracts, occurs less frequently but may occasionally result in life-threatening complications.

**9. Discuss the epidemiology of WG.**

The true prevalence and incidence of WG are unknown, but it is a rare disorder. It is much less common than other rheumatologic disorders such as rheumatoid arthritis, systemic lupus erythematosus (SLE), polymyalgia rheumatica, and giant cell arteritis. The mean age at diagnosis is 41 years. Although the age range is 5–78 years, only 16% of patients are < 18 years old. The male:female ratio is 1:1. Approximately 97% of patients are white; only 2% are African-American.

**10. Define ANCA.**

ANCA (anti-neutrophil cytoplasmic antibodies) are antibodies directed against specific proteins in the cytoplasm of neutrophils and are present in the sera of patients having several underlying diseases. When alcohol-fixed neutrophils are used as a source of antigen in the indirect immunofluorescence test, three categories of ANCA may be detected by their resulting pattern: C-ANCA, P-ANCA, and atypical patterns (see figure). The **cytoplasmic**, or C-ANCA, is characterized by diffuse staining of the neutrophil cytoplasm; the **perinuclear**, or P-ANCA, results in perinuclear cytoplasmic staining; patterns not clearly C-ANCA or P-ANCA are labeled **atypical**. The protein actually recognized by C-ANCA is nearly always proteinase-3, a serine proteinase present in the primary granules of the neutrophil. The protein recognized by P-ANCA is often myeloperoxidase and, less commonly, elastase and other proteins within the granules of neutrophils. The protein target of the atypical ANCA is usually unclear, but in some cases it is common to P-ANCA.

In addition to the indirect immunofluorescence ANCA, specific ELISA for proteinase-3 and myeloperoxidase antibodies are now universally available. All three of these tests should be requested when evaluating a patient for suspected ANCA-associated vasculitis, in an attempt to better understand the underlying process.

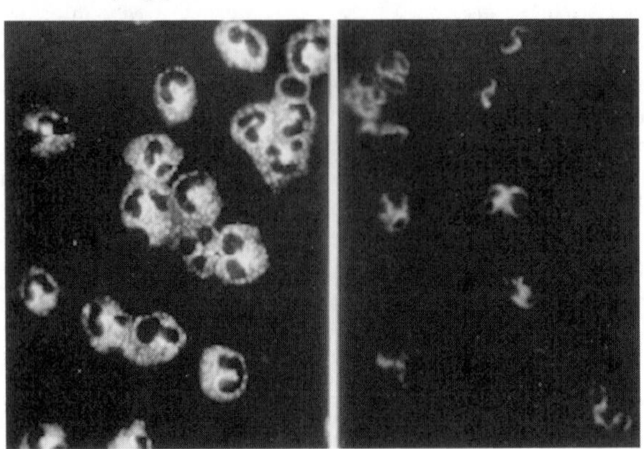

C-ANCA (*left*) and P-ANCA (*right*) immunofluorescence pattern using alcohol-fixed neutrophils as antigen source.

**11. What is the clinical association of ANCA and WG?**

C-ANCA, due to the presence of anti-proteinase 3 antibodies, is strongly associated with WG. The sensitivity and specificity of C-ANCA for WG are 30–90% and 98%, respectively. The wide range of sensitivity is due to the fact that the presence and titer of C-ANCA depend upon the extent of the disease and disease activity. Thus, patients with active WG clinically limited to the upper and lower respiratory tracts have lower C-ANCA titers and more false-negative tests than patients with clinical involvement of the upper and lower respiratory tracts and kidneys. Regardless of the extent of disease, disease activity as assessed clinically is an important factor determining the presence and titer of C-ANCA. Overall, C-ANCA titers correlate with WG disease activity in 60% of cases. Furthermore, some studies suggest that a rise in the C-ANCA titer of patients with clinically inactive WG heralds an exacerbation of disease. Additionally, since the ANCA titers tend to rise in exacerbations of WG whereas they usually do not in acute infection, the ANCA may aid in distinguishing an exacerbation of WG from an infectious process in patients with previously quiescent disease. Some patients with WG also have detectable P-ANCA.

**12. What other disorders are associated with C-ANCA?**

| DISEASE ENTITY | SENSITIVITY OF | |
|---|---|---|
| | ANTI-PROTEINASE 3 | ANTI-MYELOPEROXIDASE |
| WG | 85% | 10% |
| Microscopic polyangiitis | 15–45% | 45–80% |
| Idiopathic crescentic glomerulonephritis | 25% | 65% |
| Churg-Strauss syndrome | 10% | 60% |
| Polyarteritis nodosa | 5% | 15% |

Adapted from Kallenberg CGM, et al: Anti-neutrophil cytoplasmic antibodies: Current diagnostic and pathophysiological potential. Kidney Int 46:1–15, 1994.

Although the presence of C-ANCA, and thus anti-proteinase 3 antibodies, is quite specific (98%) for WG, there are a number of other disease associations, particularly microscopic polyangiitis and idiopathic crescentic glomerulonephritis. Interestingly, the glomerular lesions of these three disorders are indistinguishable and are characterized by scant or no deposition of immunoglobulin (pauci-immune). Thus, these C-ANCA-associated pauci-immune disorders are a distinct category of autoimmune disease and can be distinguished from immune complex disease (e.g., SLE) and anti-basement membrane antibody disease (Goodpasture's disease), which can also affect the kidneys (and lungs).

**13. Which disorders are associated with P-ANCA and atypical ANCA?**

Whereas C-ANCA represents the presence of anti-proteinase 3 antibodies and is associated with a small number of diseases, P-ANCA and atypical ANCA may be due to a variety of different antibodies and may be present in a wide range of diseases. Specific antibodies that may result in a positive P-ANCA or atypical ANCA include antibodies directed against myeloperoxidase, elastase, cathepsin G, lactoferrin, and β-glucuronidase. P-ANCA in the setting of idiopathic crescentic glomerulonephritis, Churg-Strauss syndrome, microscopic polyangiitis, polyarteritis nodosa, or WG is usually due to anti-myeloperoxidase antibodies. P-ANCA present in other disorders is less well characterized but is usually not due to antibodies directed against myeloperoxidase. Finally, a number of medications are associated with induction of ANCA, with or without associated clinical manifestations.

**Pearl**: P-ANCA should be against myeloperoxidase if it is due to a vasculitis.

*Disease Associations of P-ANCA and Atypical ANCA*

| DISEASE CATEGORY/EXAMPLE | CHARACTERISTICS |
|---|---|
| Primary vasculitis syndrome | |
| WG | P-ANCA due to anti-MPO (10%)<br>C-ANCA due to anti-P3 (85%) |
| Microscopic polyangiitis | P-ANCA due to anti-MPO (45-80%)<br>C-ANCA due to anti-P3 (15-45%) |
| Idiopathic crescentic glomerulonephritis | P-ANCA due to anti-MPO (65%)<br>C-ANCA due to anti-P3 (25%) |
| Churg-Strauss syndrome | P-ANCA due to anti-MPO (60%)<br>C-ANCA due to anti-P3 (10%) |
| Polyarteritis nodosa | P-ANCA due to anti-MPO (15%)<br>C-ANCA due to anti-P3 (5%) |
| Diffuse connective tissue disease | |
| SLE | P-ANCA and atypical ANCA (20%) due to anti-elastase, lactoferrin, MPO, other |
| Rheumatoid arthritis | P-ANCA and atypical ANCA (25%) due to anti-elastase, lactoferrin, MPO, other |
| Inflammatory bowel disease | |
| Ulcerative colitis | P-ANCA and atypical ANCA (70%) due to anti-lactoferrin, cathepsin G, other |
| Crohn's disease | P-ANCA and atypical ANCA (30%) due to anti-lactoferrin, cathepsin G, other |
| Autoimmune liver disease | |
| Primary sclerosing cholangitis | P-ANCA and atypical ANCA (70%) due to anti-lactoferrin, cathepsin G, other |
| Chronic active hepatitis | P-ANCA and atypical ANCA not characterized |
| Primary biliary cirrhosis | P-ANCA and atypical ANCA not characterized |
| Infection | |
| HIV | ANCA not characterized |
| Cystic fibrosis with infection | ANCA not characterized |
| Bacterial endocarditis | ANCA not characterized |

(*Table continued on next page.*)

*Disease Associations of P-ANCA and Atypical ANCA (cont.)*

| DISEASE CATEGORY/EXAMPLE | CHARACTERISTICS |
|---|---|
| Medications | |
| Hydralazine | P-ANCA due to anti-MPO |
| Propylthiouracil | P-ANCA due to anti-MPO |
| D-penicillamine | P-ANCA due to anti-MPO |
| Minocycline | P-ANCA due to anti-MPO |

MPO, myeloperoxidase; P3, proteinase 3. Adapted from Kallenberg et al: Anti-neutrophil cytoplasmic antibodies: Current diagnostic and pathophysiological potential. Kidney Int 46:1–15, 1994; and Savige et al: Anti-neutrophil cytoplasmic antibodies (ANCA): Their detection and significance: Report from workshops. Pathology 26:186–193, 1994.

**14. Besides the ANCA, what other laboratory tests may be abnormal in WG?**

C-ANCA and anti-proteinase 3 antibodies are the only specific laboratory tests abnormal in WG. Other abnormal laboratory tests in WG reflect the presence of systemic inflammation and end-organ involvement.

The systemic inflammatory nature of WG often results in anemia of chronic inflammation, leukocytosis, thrombocytosis, and elevation of the ESR. Low serum albumin and elevated globulin levels may also be present. These abnormalities are likely due to circulating cytokines, such as IL-1, IL-6, and TNF-α, elaborated by the inflammatory process. Importantly, leukopenia and thrombocytopenia are unusual, often helping to distinguish WG from other autoimmune disorders.

Evidence of glomerulonephritis is suggested by the presence of hematuria, pyuria, cellular casts, and proteinuria. If renal function is compromised by the inflammatory process, elevated serum creatinine is expected. Other laboratory tests may be helpful in the investigation of specific end-organ damage, such as electrocardiography and echocardiography for pericarditis, nerve conduction velocity for mononeuritis multiplex, and MRI for retro-orbital infiltration.

**15. The prototypic pulmonary-renal syndromes are WG, Goodpasture's disease, and SLE. Since routine hematoxylin and eosin staining of these kidney biopsies is nonspecific, what other studies performed on renal tissue may aid in distinguishing these three disorders?**

Immunofluorescence studies. **Goodpasture's disease** results from the presence of circulating anti-basement membrane antibodies, which bind to epitopes in the basement membranes of glomeruli and alveoli. The resultant antibody-antigen interaction leads to fixation of complement and initiation of the inflammatory process, causing glomerulonephritis and alveolar hemorrhage. Immunofluorescence staining with antibodies against immunoglobulin (Ig) detects the **linear** deposition of Ig in the glomerular basement membranes.

Glomerulonephritis due to **SLE** results from immune complex deposition in the glomerulus. Immunofluorescence studies detect **granular** (lumpy) deposition of Ig, characteristic of immune complex deposition, within the glomerulus.

The pathophysiology of glomerulonephritis in **WG** is unclear, but the disease does not appear to be due to immune complexes or detectable direct antibody binding to epitopes within the glomerular tissue. Thus, immunofluorescence studies usually are negative or reveal only scant Ig deposition, usually in areas of necrosis.

**16. Discuss the differential diagnosis of WG.**

*Differential Diagnosis of WG*

| SYNDROME | EXAMPLE | DISTINGUISHING FEATURES |
|---|---|---|
| Primary vasculitis syndromes | Churg-Strauss syndrome | Atopic history<br>Marked eosinophilia |
| | Microscopic polyangiitis | Destructive upper airway disease unusual |

(*Table continued on next page.*)

*Differential Diagnosis of WG (cont.)*

| SYNDROME | EXAMPLE | DISTINGUISHING FEATURES |
|---|---|---|
| | | Cavitary pulmonary nodules unusual<br>Absence of granuloma |
| Angiocentric immuno-proliferative lesions | Lymphomatoid granulomatosis | Glomerulonephritis unusual |
| Pulmonary renal syndromes | Goodpasture's disease | Anti-basement membrane antibodies<br>Immunofluorescence: linear deposition |
| | Immune complex disease (e.g., SLE) | ANA<br>Anti-dsDNA, Sm antibodies<br>Immunofluorescence: granular deposition |
| Granulomatous infections | Mycobacterium<br>Fungi<br>Actinomycosis<br>Syphilis | Proper stains and cultures |
| Intranasal drug abuse | Cocaine | History<br>Predominantly nasal septal pathology |
| Pseudovasculitis syndromes | Atrial myxoma | Echocardiography |
| | Subacute bacterial endocarditis | Blood cultures<br>Echocardiography |
| | Cholesterol emboli syndrome | Transesophageal echocardiography<br>Angiography<br>Biopsy |

**17. What causes WG?**

The etiology is unknown. The clinical disease frequently begins within the upper respiratory tract, followed by the lower respiratory tract and later the kidneys, which suggests that the etiologic agent may be airborne and inhaled. Despite vigorous study of various tissues from affected patients, no infectious or noninfectious agent has been identified. Specifically, agents demonstrated to cause granulomatous disease have not been found.

**18. Describe its pathophysiology.**

The pathophysiology of WG is also unknown. Because of the absence of significant Ig deposition in affected tissue, WG does not appear to be due to typical immune complex disease, such as SLE, or to autoantibodies against structural components, such as Goodpasture's disease. The presence of granulomata and numerous $CD4^+$ T cells suggests the possibility of cell-mediated immunopathology. Additionally, anti-proteinase 3 antibodies conceivably may play a pathologic role. Under certain conditions, such as a typical viral or bacterial infection, neutrophils and endothelial cells produce and express proteinase 3 on their surfaces. Anti-proteinase 3 antibodies may bind to surface proteinase 3 on endothelial cells, fix complement, and initiate an inflammatory event within vessel walls, resulting in vasculitis. Anti-proteinase 3 antibody binding to surface proteinase 3 on neutrophils and monocytes may activate these cells, amplifying the inflammatory response. These possibilities are being studied and remain controversial.

**19. What is the natural history of WG?**

The presentation and natural history of WG are highly variable. The spectrum of clinical presentation may range from relatively mild disease limited to the upper respiratory tract to fulminant life-threatening involvement of the upper and lower respiratory tract, kidneys, and other end-organs. The disease progression is also variable and protean, including protracted mild disease remaining in the upper respiratory tract despite absence of treatment, wide-spread but relatively mild and slowly progressive disease, and rapidly progressive pulmonary and renal disease manifesting as alveolar hemorrhage syndrome and rapidly progressive renal failure upon presentation. A further caveat is the observation that relatively mild and limited disease may rapidly progress to more diffuse and active disease at any time during the course of disease. At present, it is unknown if upper respiratory tract–limited disease may remain limited indefinitely. These considerations obviously have implications regarding treatment.

The natural history of untreated generalized WG is well understood. It is a uniformly fatal disorder with a mean survival time of < 1 year. Death may result from respiratory failure, renal failure, infection, other end-organ involvement, or as a complication of treatment.

**20. How do you treat WG?**

Standard treatment for generalized WG, or limited WG with severe involvement of the lower respiratory tract or other end-organ, is oral cyclophosphamide (2 mg/kg/day) and oral prednisone (1 mg/kg/day). After 4 weeks and if a substantial clinical response has occurred, prednisone may be converted to an alternate-day regimen over a period of 1–2 months, followed by gradual and complete tapering as tolerated. Cyclophosphamide should be continued for approximately 1 year after complete clinical response, followed by tapering by 25-mg amounts every 2–3 months as tolerated. A major acute complication of this regimen is leukopenia; often the cyclophosphamide dose must be adjusted in order to maintain the total WBC level above 3000–3500/ml and the neutrophil level above 1000–1500/ml. This regimen has resulted in complete remission in 75% of patients, with marked improvement in an additional 16%. In patients attaining complete remission, approximately half will experience a relapse of WG up to 16 years later.

In patients who present with fulminant life-threatening WG, initially more aggressive therapy may be warranted. Cyclophosphamide may be started at 3–5 mg/kg/day as tolerated. Glucocorticoids may be administered parenterally at prednisone-equivalent doses of 2–15 mg/kg/day.

Oral trimethoprim/sulfamethoxazole (one double-strength tablet three times a week) provides prophylaxis against *Pneumocystis carinii* in patients with vasculitis who are receiving high-dose glucocorticoid therapy and cyclophosphamide. This antibiotic therapy also limits recurrent sinus infections, which can cause exacerbations of WG. Therapy to prevent osteoporosis should also be instituted.

**21. What other therapeutic approaches are being tried in WG?**

Because daily oral cyclophosphamide therapy is associated with significant morbidity (40% of patients) including infection, hemorrhagic cystitis, and infertility as well as occasionally mortality, less rigorous regimens are being studied for patients who have limited or less active WG or can't tolerate cyclophosphamide. These include:

- Intermittent pulse intravenous cyclophosphamide—can induce remission, but relapses are more common than with daily oral therapy.
- Methotrexate—consider in milder disease with little renal compromise. More severe disease should be brought under control with 3 months of cyclophosphamide and then switched over to weekly methotrexate (20–25 mg a week).
- Cyclosporin—has been used alone and in combination with cyclophosphamide. Not to be used if significant kidney disease. Does not cause leukopenia.
- Anti-tumor necrosis factor α therapy—owing to high TNF levels in WG patients' lesions, anti-TNF therapy is being investigated in combination with cyclophosphamide or methotrexate. Anti-TNFα therapy is not effective alone in inducing remissions.
- Mycophenylate mofetil, leflunomide, and azathioprine are being studied.
- Intravenous gammaglobulin has been added to other regimens in patients in whom standard therapy is failing.

**Pearl**: Daily oral cyclophosphamide and high-dose prednisone are best to induce remission in patients with severe disease. They then can be switched to less toxic medication to maintain remission.

**22. How can relapses be prevented in WG patients?**

Patients who have been in complete remission for 12–18 months on standard therapy have a 50% risk of relapse once that therapy is stopped. Studies have demonstrated that one double-strength

Bactrim or Septra daily or weekly methotrexate can help prevent relapses. Methotrexate is probably more effective. Patients with WG who have persistent C-ANCA positivity even if in clinical remission should probably be maintained on weekly methotrexate to prevent relapses.

**23. Can WG patients who go into renal failure receive a kidney transplant?**

Yes. However, the WG should be under control and the C-ANCA titer low or absent before transplant. The use of mycophenylate and cyclosporine post-transplant to prevent rejection should help prevent recurrence of WG.

## BIBLIOGRAPHY


1. de Groot K, Reinhold-Keller E, Tatsis E, et al: Therapy for the maintenance of remission in sixty-five patients with generalized Wegener's granulomatosis. Methotrexate versus trimethoprim/sulfamethoxazole. Arthritis Rheum 39:2052–2061, 1996.
2. Duna GF, Galperin C, Hoffman GS: Wegener's granulomatosis. Rheumatic Dis Clinics North America 21:949–986, 1995.
3. Guillevin L, Cordier J-F, Lhote F, et al: A prospective, multicenter, randomized trial comparing steroids and pulse cyclophosphamide versus steroids and oral cyclophosphamide in the treatment of generalized Wegener's granulomatosis. Arthritis Rheum 40:2187–2198, 1997.
4. Hoffman GS, Kerr GS, Leavitt RY, et al: Wegener granulomatosis: An analysis of 158 patients. Ann Intern Med 116:488–498, 1992.
5. Kallenberg CGM, Brouwer E, Weening JJ, Tervaert JWC: Anti-neutrophil cytoplasmic antibodies: Current diagnostic and pathophysiological potential. Kidney Int 46:1–15, 1994.
6. Langford CA, Talar-Williams C, Barron KS, Sneller MC: A staged approach to the treatment of Wegener's granulomatosis. Arthritis Rheum 42:2666–2673, 1999.
7. Savige JA, Davies DJ, Gatenby PA: Anti-neutrophil cytoplasmic antibodies (ANCA): Their detection and significance: Report from workshops. Pathology 26:186–193, 1994.
8. Stone J, Tun W, Hellmann D: Treatment of non-life threatening Wegener's granulomatosis with methotrexate and daily prednisone as the initial therapy of choice. J Rheumatol 26:1134–1139, 1999.
9. Stone JH, Uhlfelder ML, Hellmann DB, et al: Etanercept combined with conventional treatment in Wegener's granulomatosis. Arthritis Rheum 44:1149–1154, 2001.


# 34. SMALL-VESSEL VASCULITIDES

*Ramon A. Arroyo, M.D.*

## IMMUNE COMPLEX–MEDIATED SMALL VESSEL VASCULITIS

**1. What are the small vessel vasculitides due to immune complex deposition?**

Small-vessel vasculitis includes a variety of conditions that are grouped together because of involvement of small blood vessels of the skin, especially arterioles and postcapillary venules. **Leukocytoclastic vasculitis** (LCV) and **necrotizing vasculitis** are terms used to describe the usual histopathology, in which small blood vessels are infiltrated with polymorphonuclear neutrophils (PMNs) and/or mononuclear cells. As the process evolves, fibrinoid necrosis of the vessel wall with leukocyte fragments (leukocytoclasis) and destruction of the blood vessel wall is seen. The conditions associated with small-vessel cutaneous vasculitis due to immune complex deposition include:

| CONDITIONS | COMMENTS |
|---|---|
| 1. Hypersensitivity vasculitis | Drugs reactions or idiopathic |
| 2. Urticarial vasculitis | If hypocomplementemic, possibly a subset of SLE |

(*Table continued on next page.*)

| CONDITIONS | COMMENTS |
| --- | --- |
| 3. Henoch-Schönlein purpura | Renal and GI involvement, IgA in lesion |
| 4. Mixed cryoglobulinemia | Hepatitis B and C; rarely HIV, and cancer |
| 5. Rheumatic disorders | RA, SLE, Sjogren's syndrome |
| 6. Infections | SBE, *Neisseria*, influenza, mononucleosis, HIV, hepatitis B and C |
| 7. Malignancy | Leukemia, lymphoma, myeloma, solid tumors, myelodysplastic syndromes |
| 8. Erythema elevatum diutinum | Over extensor surfaces of joints (hands, knees) and buttocks. Responds to dapsone. |

**2. What causes this group of small-vessel vasculitides?**

The cause of cutaneous vasculitis is not a single factor and is dependent on the underlying associated condition(s). The vascular injury is believed to be triggered by the deposition of immune complexes in the vessel wall with activation of complement, leading to migration of PMNs to the area, release of lysosomal enzymes, and damage to the vessel wall.

**3. What is the major clinical manifestation in small-vessel vasculitis?**

**Palpable purpura** is the most common primary lesion in cutaneous vasculitis. Typically, hundreds of discrete, subtly palpable, purpuric spots suddenly appear on the feet and lower extremities (see figure). The hands, arms, and other body sites also may be affected. In addition to the palpability, the presence of a central necrotic punctum is helpful in distinguishing a purpura of vasculitis from purpuras of other causes. These lesions are dynamic, often beginning as asymptomatic, nonpalpable, purpuric macules and eventually becoming palpable. Some may become nodular, bullous, infarctive, and ulcerative.

Urticarial lesions are the second most common cutaneous presentation. Other cutaneous manifestations include livedo reticularis and erythema multiforme–like lesions.

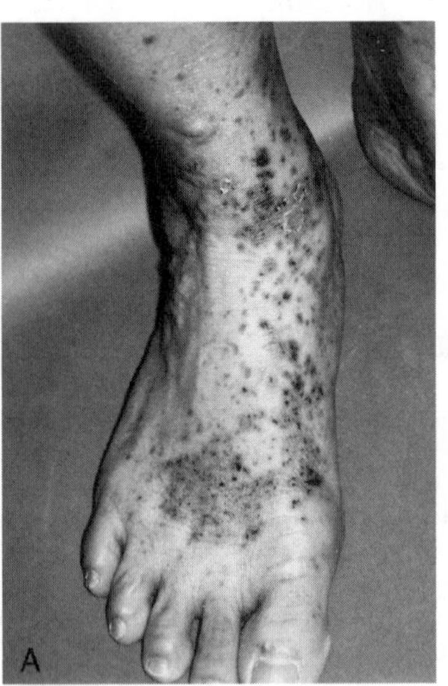


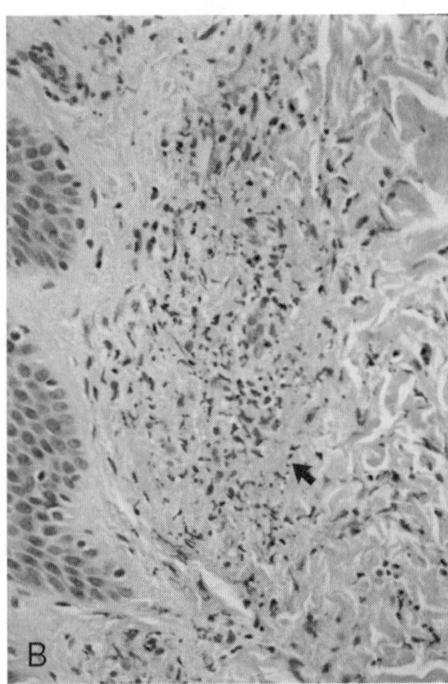


Small-vessel vasculitis. *A*, Palpable purpura. *B*, Histopathology of cutaneous blood vessel, demonstrating leukocytoclastic vasculitis with nuclear dust (arrow).

**4. Can patients with small vessel vasculitis have systemic manifestations??**

Yes. Constitutional symptoms, including fever, arthralgias and malaise, frequently accompany the appearance of the skin lesions. Arthritis is uncommon. Proteinuria, hematuria, and occasional renal insufficiency can occur. Gastrointestinal manifestations include abdominal pain and GI bleeding, which can be severe and life-threatening. Other organ involvement is less common.

5. **Are any laboratory findings specific for small-vessel vasculitis?**
The laboratory abnormalities are usually nonspecific. Normocytic, normochromic anemia, elevated ESR, or eosinophilia is seen in approximately two-thirds of the patients. In those patients with renal involvement, hematuria and proteinuria may be present, as well as an increase in serum creatinine. The ANA is positive in 10%, and rheumatoid factor is present in 20%. The clinical significance of these serologic findings is uncertain. Hypocomplementemia (low C3 and C4) is infrequent. Hepatitis B surface antigenemia and hepatitis C antigenemia with cryoglobulinemia have been associated with LCV in some patients. ANCA positivity in combination with the lack of immune deposits on skin biopsy may be helpful in identifying systemic vasculitides such as Wegener's, Churg-Strauss, PAN, and microscopic polyangiitis that occasionally present with cutaneous involvement (palpable purpura).

6. **How does one make the diagnosis of small-vessel vasculitis?**
The evaluation of these patients requires a full medical evaluation and appropriate lab tests depending on the clinical situation. Diagnosis is made by **skin biopsy**, identifying the presence of cutaneous vasculitis. Immunofluorescent study of the skin is helpful in differentiating systemic diseases like microscopic polyangiitis and HSP. The lack of immune deposits distinguishes microscopic polyangiitis from HSP and mixed cryoglobulinemia, in which immunoglobulins are deposited in vascular walls. However, skin biopsy cannot discern the etiology of cutaneous vasculitis (infections, drugs, cryoglobulinemia, malignancy etc.). Therefore, a complete evaluation must be undertaken with history, physical exam, and selected laboratory tests.

7. **How is small-vessel vasculitis treated?**
Treatment has to be determined individually. If the associated disorder can be identified, treating this problem may suffice. Any potential drug or antigen should be discontinued or removed. An underlying infection should be properly treated. Mild cases without internal organ involvement may be self-limited, requiring no specific treatment. If systemic symptoms are present and skin lesions are diffuse, or if internal organ involvement is present, glucocorticoids are usually the treatment of choice.

8. **What are the histopathologic features of Henoch-Schönlein purpura (HSP)?**
The histopathologic features of HSP are leukocytoclastic vasculitis or necrotizing small-vessel vasculitis. The characteristic direct immunofluorescence finding is predominantly **IgA deposition** in affected blood vessels. IgA can also be found in the glomerular mesangium. The skin biopsy finding of IgA deposition is what makes this syndrome pathologically different from the other forms of small-vessel vasculitis.

9. **What is the role of IgA in the pathogenesis of HSP?**
Immunoglobulin A (IgA) plays a pivotal role in the pathogenesis of HSP. There are two subclasses of IgA, IgA1 and IgA2. IgA1 accounts for 80–90% of serum IgA, whereas only 50% of secretory IgA. HSP is associated only with deposition of IgA1 and not IgA2. Notably, IgA nephropathy (Berger's disease) involves IgA1 exclusively also. For both HSP and Berger's disease, investigators have found that the hinge region O-linked glycans of IgA1 are deficient in galactose and/or sialic acid content. IgA1 molecules with these deficiencies have a tendency to form macromolecular complexes and have the ability to activate the alternative complement pathway. In addition, IgA can bind to mesangial cells in the kidney leading to proliferation and release of proinflammatory cytokines. This kidney receptor binds IgA1 at its hinge region more readily when the IgA1 is deficient in sialic acid or galactose.

10. **Describe the clinical manifestations of the HSP syndrome.**
The classic tetrad of palpable purpura, arthritis, abdominal pain, and renal disease occurs in up to 80% of cases. The rash may begin as a macular erythema and urticarial lesions, but may

progress rapidly to purpura. The lower extremities and buttocks are the most common sites for the rash. Scrotal and scalp edema can be seen, particularly in children. The joints are involved in 60–84% of patients. The involvement is symmetrical and most commonly involves the ankles and knees; usually they are swollen, warm, and tender. Gastrointestinal lesions may cause severe cramping, abdominal pain, intussusception, hemorrhage, and, rarely, ileal perforation. Renal involvement is seen in 50% of patients and is usually manifested by asymptomatic proteinuria and hematuria. However, more marked findings may occur including nephrotic syndrome and acute renal failure.

HSP is often acute in onset, and resolution is rapid and complete in 97% of cases, except in a minority of patients (3–5%) with chronic renal disease. Persons of any age can be affected, but it occurs primarily in children between ages 2 and 10 years old. Adults have a more severe disease with higher frequency of renal involvement. Patients of any age suspected to have HSP but have no IgA on skin biopsy should be evaluated for Wegener's granulomatosis.

**11. How is HSP treated?**

The disease is generally self-limited, lasting from 6–16 weeks. For mild cases, supportive treatment alone may be adequate. Arthritis responds to NSAID. Systemic glucocorticoids may be used in patients with GI involvement or bleeding. Progressive renal disease is difficult to treat and usually does not respond to glucocorticoids. Aggressive treatment with high-dose pulse glucocorticoids and cytotoxics should be considered in patients with poor prognostic factors: proteinuria > 1 gm/day, nephrotic syndrome, and crescentic glomerulonephritis > 50% crescents. Remember to rule out Wegener's.

**12. What is urticarial vasculitis?**

Urticarial vasculitis (UV) is a small-vessel vasculitis presenting with urticarial lesions instead of the more typical palpable purpura. Because of this unusual presentation, urticarial vasculitis was separated from the other types of necrotizing small-vessel vasculitis. Most patients with UV have and an associated underlying disease (secondary UV). In a minority of patients, UV is a local process not associated with a specific disorder (primary or idiopathic UV).

**13. How is urticarial vasculitis differentiated from typical urticaria?**

- UV lesions typically last for more than 24 hours and often resolve with residual hyperpigmentation. True urticaria/hives lesions last for 2 to 8 hours and leave no trace.
- UV lesions are often characterized by pain and burning rather than pruritus, the sensory hallmark of true urticaria/hives.
- UV lesions are typically 0.5–5 cm in diameter, while true urticaria may coalesce into large lesions > 10 cm.
- Symptoms or signs of systemic disease, such as fever, arthralgias, abdominal pain, lymphadenopathy, or abnormal urine sediment, tend to occur in UV and rarely in allergic true urticaria.
- The histology of UV is LCV, while for true urticaria is edema of the upper dermis.

**14. Is there other organ involvement in urticarial vasculitis?**

Other clinical features include arthralgias and arthritis. There appears to be an increased incidence of obstructive pulmonary disease (50%) in UV patients who also are cigarette smokers. Other less common associations include uveitis (30%), episcleritis, fever, angioedema (50%), peripheral neuropathy, and seizures.

**15. What are the major laboratory abnormalities in urticarial vasculitis?**

Patients with UV can be classified into two different subsets according to their serum complement levels: those with hypocomplementemia (38%), and those with normal complements. Those patients with low complements are more likely to have SLE. An increased ESR is present in two-thirds of patients. ANA and rheumatoid factor are usually negative unless the vasculitis is associated with another connective tissue disease such as SLE.

**16. What are some of the conditions associated with urticarial vasculitis?**

Urticarial vasculitis has been described in association with SLE, Sjögren's syndrome, hepatitis B and C antigenemia, drug reactions, and sun exposure. The etiology is thought to be related to immune complex deposition. Some patients have serum IgG antibodies that react with C1q, leading to deposition and activation of complement in vasculitic lesions.

**17. How is urticarial vasculitis treated?**

Therapy consists of supportive measures and treatment of any associated or underlying disorder. Assuming that there is no internal organ involvement, conservative treatment is reasonable. Both $H_1$ (fexofenadine) and $H_2$ (ranitidine) antihistamines are used. NSAIDs (typically indomethacin) help with arthralgias and arthritis. In addition, prednisone in doses from 10–60 mg may be required. Dapsone and hydroxychloroquine have been reported to benefit some patients. For those patients with severe disease, use of azathioprine and cyclophosphamide has been reported in individual case reports. Cyclosporine may be beneficial for patients with UV who develop progressive airway obstruction.

## ANCA-ASSOCIATED SMALL VESSEL VASCULITIS

**18. What are the antineutrophil cytoplasmic antibody (ANCA)–associated small vessel vasculitides? (See Chapter 33, Question 10 for discussion of ANCA.)**

- Wegener's granulomatosis (see Chapter 33)
- Allergic angiitis and granulomatosis of Churg-Strauss (Churg-Strauss syndrome)
- Microscopic polyangiitis

**19. How does antineutrophil cytoplasmic antibody (ANCA) contribute to the development of these diseases? (Controversial.)**

Unknown. Under certain conditions such as infections, the release of cytokines (IL-1, TNFα) can cause neutrophils to transport serine proteinase 3 (PR-3) or myeloperoxidase (MPO) to their surfaces. Patients with C-ANCA can react with PR-3, while patients with P-ANCA react with MPO causing activation of neutrophils. Cytokines (IL-1, TNFα) also upregulate adhesion molecules on endothelial cells, which the activated neutrophils can bind to and transmigrate into the vessel wall causing vasculitis.

## CHURG-STRAUSS SYNDROME

**20. What is Churg-Strauss syndrome (CSS)?**

CSS, also known as allergic angiitis and granulomatosis of Churg-Strauss, is a granulomatous inflammation of small- and medium-sized vessels, frequently involving the skin, peripheral nerves, and lungs, which is associated with peripheral eosinophilia. It occurs primarily in patients with a previous history of allergic manifestations, such as rhinitis (often with nasal polyps) (70%) and adult-onset asthma (> 95%). Cytokines that affect the eosinophil (IL-5) and eosinophil granule proteins (major basic protein, cationic protein) appear to be important in the pathogenesis of this disease.

**21. Describe the three clinical phases of CSS.**

These phases may appear simultaneously and do not have to follow one another in the order presented here.

1. **Prodromal phase**. This phase may persist for years (3–7 years) and consists of allergic manifestations of rhinitis, polyposis, and asthma.

2. **Peripheral blood and tissue eosinophilia**, frequently causing a picture resembling Löffler's syndrome (shifting pulmonary infiltrates and eosinophilia), chronic eosinophilic pneumonia, or eosinophilic gastroenteritis. This second phase may remit or recur over years before the third phase.

3. **Life-threatening systemic vasculitis**. The asthma can abruptly abate as the patient moves into this phase.

**22. What are the major clinical features of Churg-Strauss syndrome?**

| ORGAN | CLINICAL MANIFESTATIONS |
|---|---|
| Paranasal sinus | Acute or chronic paranasal sinus pain or tenderness, rhinitis (70%), polyposis, opacifications of paranasal sinus on radiographs |
| Lungs | Asthma (usually adult onset), patchy and shifting pulmonary infiltrates, nodular infiltrates without cavitations, pleural effusions and diffuse interstitial lung disease seen on chest radiograph. Pulmonary hemorrhage can occur. |
| Nervous system (60%) | Mononeuritis multiplex or symmetric polyneuropathy; rarely CNS involvement |
| Skin (50%) | Subcutaneous nodules, petechiae, purpura, skin infarction, (they occur mainly during the vasculitic phase) |
| Joints | Arthralgias and arthritis (rare) |
| Gastrointestinal | Abdominal pain, bloody diarrhea, abdominal masses |
| Miscellaneous | Renal failure, congestive heart failure, corneal ulcerations, panuveitis, prostatitis |

**23. What laboratory abnormalities are seen in CSS?**

The characteristic laboratory abnormality is **eosinophilia**. Anemia, elevated ESR, and elevated IgE may be found. Antineutrophil cytoplasmic antibodies (ANCA) are present in 67% of patients. These are directed primarily against myeloperoxidase and give a P-ANCA pattern. There is no direct correlation between degree of eosinophilia and disease activity.

**24. How do you diagnose CSS?**

On the basis of its clinical and pathologic features. The diagnosis should be suspected in a patient with a previous history of allergy or asthma who presents with eosinophilia (> 1500/mm$^3$), and systemic vasculitis involving two or more organs. The diagnosis is corroborated by biopsy of involved tissue.

**25. Describe the histopathologic findings in CSS.**

The characteristic pathologic changes in CSS include **small necrotizing granulomas** as well as **necrotizing vasculitis of small arteries and veins**. Granulomas are usually extravascular near small arteries and veins. They are highly specific and composed of a central eosinophilic core surrounded radially by macrophages and giant cells (in contrast to a granuloma with basophilic core seen in other diseases). Inflammatory cells are also present, with eosinophils predominating with smaller numbers of PMNs and lymphocytes.

**26. What drugs have been reported to cause Churg-Strauss syndrome?**

The cysteinyl leukotriene type I receptor antagonists, zafirlukast (Accolate), montelukast (Singulair), and pranlukast, have been associated with CSS. Whether there is a direct cause is controversial. Some clinicians believe that CSS is unmasked when the patient uses these drugs because the patient is able to taper their glucocorticoids. Others feel it directly contributes to the development of CSS. Consequently, leukotriene inhibitors should not be used in patients with CSS.

**27. How is CSS differentiated from Wegener's granulomatosis?**

| | CSS | WEGENER'S GRANULOMATOSIS |
|---|---|---|
| ENT | Rhinitis, polyposis | Necrotizing lesions |
| Allergy, bronchial asthma | Frequent | No more frequent than in general population |
| Renal involvement | Uncommon | Common |
| Eosinophilia | 10% of peripheral leukocytes | Minimally elevated |
| Histology | Eosinophilic necrotizing granuloma | Necrotizing epithelioid granuloma |
| Prognosis (major cause of death) | Cardiac | Pulmonary and renal |
| ANCA | P-ANCA 67% | C-ANCA 90% |

**28. How do you treat CSS? What is its prognosis?**

The treatment of choice is glucocorticoids. Prednisone at high doses (60 mg/day) is usually sufficient to control the disease. In severe cases with life-threatening organ involvement, cyclophosphamide should be considered. In patients who fail cytotoxic therapy, interferon-( may be beneficial.

The 5-year survival rate for CSS is 78%. The major cause of death is cardiac involvement (50%) with myocardial infarction and congestive heart failure.

## MICROSCOPIC POLYANGIITIS (MPA)

**29. What is microscopic polyangiitis? How does it differ from classic PAN?**

MPA is defined as a systemic necrotizing vasculitis that clinically and histologically affects small vessels (i.e., capillaries, venules, or arterioles) with few or no immune deposits. Frequently associated with focal segmental necrotizing glomerulonephritis and pulmonary capillaritis. It can be separated from classic PAN primarily because it does not cause microaneurysm formation of abdominal or renal vessels. It can be differentiated from Wegener's granulomatosis in that it does not cause granuloma formation or a granulomatous vasculitis. The treatment of MPA is based on the same principles as those outlined for Wegener's granulomatosis.

| CLINICAL FEATURES | PAN | MPA |
|---|---|---|
| Kidney involvement | | |
| Renal vasculitis with infarcts and microaneurysms | Yes | No |
| Rapidly progressive glomerulonephritis with crescents | No | Yes |
| Lung involvement | | |
| Alveolar hemorrhage | No | Yes |
| Laboratory data | | |
| HBV-infection | Yes (10%) | No |
| P-ANCA | < 10% | 50–80% |
| Abnormal angiogram with microaneurysms | Yes | No |
| Histology | Necrotizing vasculitis | Necrotizing vasculitis (no granulomas) |
| Relapses | Rare | Common |

In the past, MPA was lumped with PAN or Wegener's, which is no longer done owing to the differences between these diseases.

**30. Who gets MPA?**

The disease affects males and females with peak age 30 to 50 years old. However, it can occur at any age.

**31. What is the usual presentation of MPA?**

Patients typically present with acute onset of rapidly progressive glomerulonephritis (100%) with up to 50% having pulmonary infiltrates and/or effusions. Up to 30% have diffuse alveolar hemorrhage with hemoptysis. Other manifestations include fever (50–70%), arthralgias (30–65%), purpura (40%), and peripheral or central nervous system involvement (25–30%). Although uncommon, some patients present with the insidious onset of these symptoms.

**32. What is the characteristic histopathology of MPA?**

The renal pathology is a focal, segmental necrotizing glomerulonephritis frequently with crescents. Immunofluorescence and electron microscopy show no immune deposits (i.e., pauci-immune glomerulonephritis). Lung biopsy shows pulmonary capillaritis with negative immunofluorescence. Skin biopsy shows leukocytoclastic vasculitis.

**33. How is the diagnosis of MPA made?**

The diagnosis is made on the basis of a characteristic clinical presentation and a renal biopsy showing necrotizing glomerulonephritis without immune deposits. A P-ANCA directed against myeloperoxidase is found in up ot 80% of patients and is supportive of the diagnosis. Notably, some patients may have C-ANCA (directed against serine proteinase 3) but will not have upper respiratory tract involvement (i.e., sinusitis) separating it from Wegener's.

**34. What other pulmonary-renal syndromes must MPA be separated from?**

SLE and Goodpasture's syndrome can present with rapidly progressive renal dysfunction and pulmonary hemorrhage. SLE patients will have diffuse proliferative glomerulonephritis with immune complex deposits on kidney biopsy as well as other clinical and serologic manifestations of SLE. Goodpasture's syndrome patients have a linear pattern of immunofluorescence on kidney and lung biopsy and a positive anti-glomerular basement membrane antibody in their serum.

**35. Described the recommended therapy for MPA and its prognosis.**

Owing to the serious presentation of this disease, most investigators recommend combined therapy with high-dose glucocorticoids and cyclophosphamide. Plasmapharesis and intravenous gammaglobulins have been used in a few patients with progressive renal failure or pulmonary hemorrhage.

Prognosis is guarded. Relapses are common (33%). Between 25% and 45% end up on dialysis. Pulmonary hemorrhage can be life-threatening. Overall, the 5-year survival is 65%.

## BIBLIOGRAPHY

1. Eustace JA, Nadasdy T, Choi M: Disease of the month: the Churg-Strauss syndrome. J Am Soc Nephrol 10:2048–2055, 1999.
2. Gonzales BG, Conn DL: Hypersensitivity vasculitis (small-vessel cutaneous vasculitis). In Ruddy S, Harris ED, Sledge CB (eds): Kelley's Textbook of Rheumatology, 6th ed. Philadelphia, W.B. Saunders, 2001, pp 1997–1204.
3. Guillevin L, Durand-Gasselin B, Cevallos, R, et al: Microscopic polyangiitis: Clinical and laboratory findings in eighty-five patients. Arthritis Rheum 42:421–430, 1999.
4. Harper L, Savage COS: Pathogenesis of ANCA-associated systemic vasculitis. J Pathol 190:349–359, 2000.
5. Hunder GG, Calabrese LH: Hypersensitivity vasculitis. In 2000 Up To Date, Vol. 8, No. 2, Jan 2000.
6. Jennings CA, King TE, Tuder R: Diffuse alveolar hemorrhage with underlying pauci-immune pulmonary capillaritis. Am J Respir Crit Care Med 155:1101, 1997.
7. Lhote F, Cohen P, Guillevin L: Polyarteritis nodosa, microscopic polyangiitis and Churg-Strauss syndrome. Lupus 7:238–258, 1998.

8. Saulsbury FT: Henoch-Schönlein purpura in children: report of 100 patients and review of literature. Medicine 78:395–409, 1999.
9. Wechsler ME, Garpestad E, Flier SR, et al: Pulmonary infiltrates, eosinophilia, and cardiomyopathy following corticosteroid withdrawal in patients with asthma receiving zafirlukast. JAMA 279:455, 1998.
10. Wisnieski J: Urticarial vasculitis. Curr Opin Rheumatol 12:24–31, 2000.

# 35. CRYOGLOBULINEMIA

*Raymond J. Enzenauer, M.D.*

**1. Define cryoglobulins.**

Cryoglobulins are immunoglobulins or immunoglobulin-containing complexes that spontaneously precipitate and form a gel at low temperatures. They become soluble again when the temperature rises.

**2. What are the three major types of cryoglobulins?**

Brouet et al. studied 86 patients with cryoglobulinemia and, from them, identified three groups of cryoglobulins:

**Type I** is a single homogeneous monoclonal immunoglobulin with only one class or subclass of heavy or light chain. In type I cryoglobulinemia, serum levels are usually high (5–30 mg/ml), and the immunoglobulin readily precipitates in the cold.

**Type II** comprises mixed cryoglobulins with a monoclonal component that acts as an antibody against polyclonal IgG (i.e., rheumatoid factor activity). Most are IgM-IgG, although IgG-IgG and IgA-IgG can also occur. Serum levels of type II cryoglobulins are usually high, with 40% at a level of 1–5 mg/ml and 40% with levels > 5 mg/ml.

**Type III** includes mixed polyclonal cryoglobulins that are consistently heterogeneous; they are composed of one or more classes of polyclonal immunoglobulins and sometimes nonimmunoglobulin molecules, such as complement proteins or lipoproteins. Most are also immunoglobulin-anti-immunoglobulin cryoglobulins. Type III cryoglobulins are usually more difficult to detect because they precipitate slowly and tend to be present in small quantities (0.1–1 mg/dl).

**3. Describe the requirements for collection of cryoglobulin specimens.**

1. Specimens must be collected at body temperature; otherwise, significant quantities of cryoglobulins may be lost.
2. Blood is drawn into a warmed syringe and immediately allowed to clot for 1–2 hours at 37°C.
3. After clotting, the serum is harvested at the warm temperature and then incubated at 4°C for 5–7 days.
4. Quantitation is accomplished by direct measurement of packed volume of precipitate after centrifugation (cryocrit) or spectrophotometric determination of protein concentration.

**4. What is the overall incidence of each cryoglobulin type?**

25% of patients have type I, 25% type II, and 50% type III.

**5. Which infection(s) is most commonly associated with mixed cryoglobulinemia?**

**Hepatitis C virus** (HCV). A possible causative role of hepatotrophic viruses in mixed cryoglobulinemia has been hypothesized, suggested by the presence of chronic hepatitis in almost two-thirds of patients. Although mixed cryoglobulinemia was first reported in 1977 as an extrahepatic manifestation of hepatitis B virus (HBV) infection, HBV represents a causative factor of mixed cryoglobulinemia in < 5% of individuals. In 1989, hepatitis C (HCV) was recognized as the major etiologic agent of post-transfusion and sporadic parenterally transmitted non-A, non-B hepatitis. Antibodies against hepatitis C were initially reported in up to 50% of mixed cryoglobulinemia patients, and with the introduction of second generation enzyme-linked immunosorbent assay (ELISA) and recombinant-based immunoblot assay (RIBA), the presence of serum anti-HCV in mixed cryoglobulinemia patients ranges from 70 to 100% of cases. A prevalence of cryoglobulinemia of 36% has been reported with chronic hepatitis C.

Various other infections have been reported in association with cryoglobulinemia, including that with other viruses (Epstein-Barr virus, cytomegalovirus, adenovirus, HIV), bacteria (subacute bacterial endocarditis, leprosy, post-streptococcal syndrome, syphilis, Q fever), fungi (coccidioidomycosis), and parasites (kala-azar, toxoplasmosis, echinococcosis, schistosomiasis, malaria).

**6. List the reported causes of cryoglobulinemia.**

Infection

| | |
|---|---|
| Viral | Bacterial |
| Fungal | Parasitic |

Autoimmune disease

| | |
|---|---|
| Systemic lupus erythematosus | Sarcoidosis |
| Rheumatoid arthritis | Henoch-Schönlein purpura |
| Polyarteritis nodosa | Behçet's disease |
| Sjögren's syndrome | Polymyositis |
| Scleroderma | Thyroiditis |

Lymphoproliferative disease

| | |
|---|---|
| Macroglobulinemia | Chronic lymphocytic leukemia |
| Lymphoma | Angioimmunoblastic lymphadenopathy |

Renal disease (proliferative glomerulonephritis)
Liver disease
Familial
Essential (most of these are due to HCV)
Experimental (post-vaccination)

**7. Which type of cryoglobulins are most commonly seen in association with autoimmune disease?**

Mixed cryoglobulins are a frequent finding in patients with connective tissue diseases, with two-thirds of cases having type III mixed cryoglobulinemia. Systemic lupus erythematosus and rheumatoid arthritis are the most common connective tissue diseases associated, with cryoglobulins seen in 50% and 25% of cases, respectively. Rheumatoid arthritis patients with cryoglobulins more often have rheumatoid vasculitis or Felty's syndrome. Other autoimmune diseases associated with cryoglobulinemia include polyarteritis nodosa, Sjögren's syndrome, scleroderma, sarcoidosis, thyroiditis, Henoch-Schönlein purpura, Behçet's disease, polymyositis, celiac disease, pulmonary fibrosis, and pemphigus vulgaris.

**8. What is the most common presenting symptoms of cryoglobulinemia?**

**Cutaneous manifestations** are the most common complaint of patients with cryoglobulinemia. Palpable purpura may be seen in 60–70% of patients with mixed cryoglobulinemia (types II and III), although this condition is seen in only 15% of patients with type I monoclonal cryoglobulins. Patients with monoclonal cryoglobulins more often present with distal ulceration/necrosis (40%). Other symptoms include Raynaud's phenomenon in 40–60% and arthralgias/arthritis in 35% (especially in low-level mixed cryoglobulinemias). Renal disease is seen in 20–25% of patients and peripheral neuropathy in 25%.

**9. What two main mechanisms are responsible for the clinical findings in cryoglobulinemia (Controversial)?**

1. **Intravascular deposits of cryoglobulin** were first suggested on clinical (cold-induced symptoms of vascular insufficiency) as well as histologic (occlusion of various sized

vessels) grounds. These symptoms are more commonly seen in patients with type I or type II cryoglobulins.

2. **Immunoglobulins** found in the cryoprecipitate have been demonstrated in blood vessel walls of patients with cryoglobulinemia. In addition, circulating immune complexes have been demonstrated in the serum of patients with mixed cryoglobulinemia. The cutaneous vasculitis and glomerulonephritis are consistent with an immune-complex–mediated disease, most frequently in patients with type II and type III mixed cryoglobulinemia.

**10. Summarize the major clinical and laboratory features of cryoglobulinemia.**

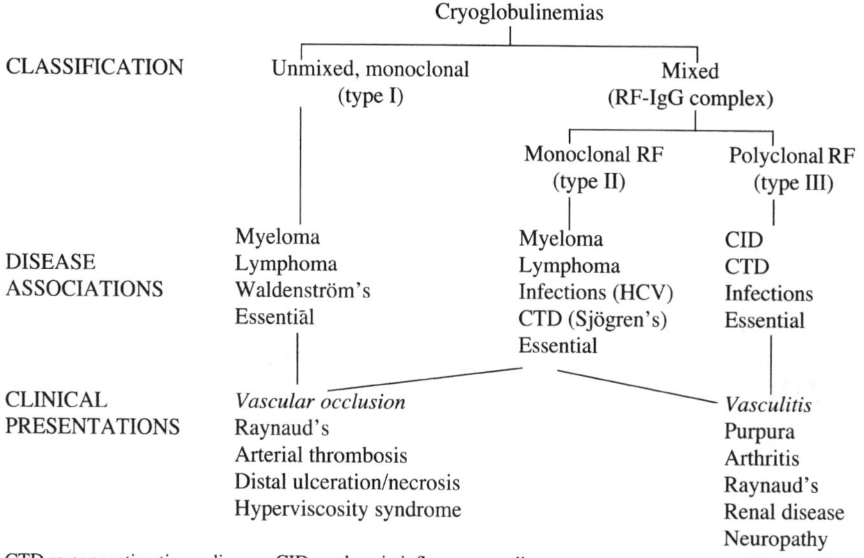


CTD = connective tissue disease; CID = chronic inflammatory disease.

**11. Renal complications are more common with which cryoglobulin type?**

Renal complications are more common in type II than in type III mixed cryoglobulinemia and range from isolated proteinuria with microscopic hematuria to an acute nephritic syndrome. Nephrotic syndrome and a more insidious progression to chronic renal failure also occur.

**12. Does any clinical parameter correlate with prognosis in mixed cryoglobulinemia?**

Prognosis is very much influenced by the presence of **renal disease**. In a 7-year follow-up period, 70% of patients with renal disease will die compared with 31% without renal involvement. Cryoglobulin levels, complement values, and titers of rheumatoid factor are not prognostic indicators of disease.

**13. What are the three leading causes of death in patients with mixed cryoglobulinemia?**

Renal disease, systemic vasculitis, and infection.

**14. Explain the pathogenesis of articular disease in cryoglobulinemia.**

The pathogenesis of the articular lesions is unknown. Their occurrence as a prominent feature during the early phase of disease, as well as the lack of frank arthritis or deforming disease even after years of symptoms, suggests that symptoms are related to circulating immune complex deposition.

**15. Cutaneous manifestations are virtually universal in patients with cryoglobulinemia and are a frequent presenting complaint. List the various cutaneous manifestations of cryoglobulinemia.**

| | |
|---|---|
| Palpable purpura | 60–97% |
| Pigmentary changes | 40% |
| Petechiae | 31% |
| Distal necrosis | 14% |
| Telangiectasias | 11% |
| Urticaria | 4–10% |
| Livedo | 10–19% |
| Leg ulcers | 10–25% |

**16. List the common signs and symptoms of cryoglobulinemia.**

| | |
|---|---|
| Cutaneous | 80% |
| Liver disease (due to HCV) | 70% |
| Arthralgia/arthritis | 35–50% |
| Renal disease | 55% |
| Raynaud's phenomenon | 10–50% |
| Neurologic | 7–17% |
| Acrocyanosis | 10% |
| Hemorrhage | 7% |
| Abdominal pain | 2% |
| Arterial thrombosis | 1% |

**17. What laboratory abnormalities are commonly seen in mixed cryoglobulinemia?**

| | |
|---|---|
| Serum protein electrophoresis | |
| Hypergammaglobulinemia | 60% |
| Hypogammaglobulinemia | 5% |
| Monoclonal gammopathy | 5% |
| Rheumatoid factor positive | 92% |
| > 1:640 | 45% |
| > 1:160 < 1:640 | 24% |
| < 1:160 | 32% |
| Elevated ESR | 70% |
| Hypocomplementemia | |
| Low $CH_{50}$ | 82% |
| Low C3 | 58% |
| Low C4 | 63–80% |
| Abnormal urinalysis | |
| Hematuria | 64% |
| Pyuria | 64% |
| Proteinuria | 73% |
| Anemia (hematocrit 35%) | 70% |
| Azotemia | 46% |
| Elevated transaminases | 50% |

**18. Pulmonary involvement is a frequent, often overlooked finding in mixed cryoglobulinemia. Describe the pulmonary abnormalities seen.**

Dyspnea is the most frequent pulmonary complaint, seen in 39% of patients. Less frequent complaints include cough (13%), asthma (9%), pleurisy (4%), and hemoptysis (4%). Roentgenographic findings show moderate interstitial involvement in 74% of patients. Pulmonary function testing is frequently abnormal and indicative of small airways disease.

**19. Is there liver involvement in mixed cryoglobulinemia?**

Clinical or biochemical evidence of liver dysfunction is seen in 84% of patients with mixed cryoglobulinemia. Hepatomegaly is detected in 77%, with splenomegaly detected in 54%.

Abnormalities in bilirubin, alkaline phosphatase, or serum aspartate aminotransferase (AST, SGOT) are seen in 77%. Only a minority of patients (11%) have overt liver disease. Up to 70% of patients will have serologic evidence of HBV and/or HCV infection.

**20. What is the major hypothesis of the cause of essential mixed cryoglobulinemia?**

Based on indirect evidence, it is thought that the rheumatoid factors that are responsible for the cryoglobulins result from an antigen driven process related to the HCV infection.

**21. Describe the treatment approach to patients with cryoglobulinemia.**

At present, the drug of choice for treating patients with mixed cryoglobulinemia is interferon-alfa 2-b. Although the optimal treatment regimen has not as yet been defined, typical regimens use 3 million units (MU) subcutaneously three times a week (tiw) for 6–12 months. Recent kinetic studies of HCV infection after interferon-alpha therapy indicate that daily and longer periods of treatment are required for eradication of the virus. Recently, a pegylated interferon alfa-2b has become available, which can be given once weekly with better efficacy. However, HCV typically relapses within 12 months following discontinuation of therapy. Side effects are relatively mild and only occasionally require withdrawal of therapy. The main side effects include a flu-like syndrome in 40%, effectively aborted with acetaminophen, and cytopenia or thrombocytopenia in 10% that usually does not require alteration of therapy. The addition of antiviral therapy (ribavirin [Rebetol] 1000 mg to 1200 mg daily) increases the biochemical and virological response in patients with chronic hepatitis C. The end point of therapy should be clearance of both serum HCV and cryoglobulins.

It is now clear that neither glucocorticoids nor immunosuppressives can be used as primary drugs in the therapy of cryoglobulinemia because of their potential for enhancing viral proliferation; however, these drugs may still have a role combined with antiviral drugs in patients with organ-threatening cryoglobulinemic vasculitis.

In patients with cryoglobulinemia not associated with hepatitis C, the patient's clinical condition is the main factor affecting treatment decisions. Patients without major organ involvement but who have complaints of arthralgia, mild purpura, and fatigue should be treated with protective measures against cold, bedrest, and NSAIDs. Antimalarial drugs may be of some benefit. Patients with severe vasculitis involving the kidneys, CNS, skin, or liver require more aggressive immunosuppressive therapy. Corticosteroids have been the most widely used drugs in the treatment of severe cryoglobulinemia. They may also be used in combination with other immunosuppressive/cytotoxic therapy, such as cyclophosphamide, azathioprine, and chlorambucil.

**22. What are the indications for plasmapheresis in cryoglobulinemia?**

Plasmapheresis should be saved for patients with acute, life-threatening forms of disease, including vasculitis, nephritis, malignant hypertension, severe CNS involvement, vascular insufficiency (distal necrosis), and hyperviscosity syndrome. Concomitant immunosuppressive therapy must be instituted to prevent rebound antibody production after pheresis.

## BIBLIOGRAPHY


1. Agnello V, Romain PL: Mixed cryoglobulinemia secondary to hepatitis C virus infection. Rheum Dis Clin North Am 22:1–21, 1996.
2. Agnello V: Therapy for cryoglobulinemia secondary to hepatitis C virus: The need for tailored protocols and multicentric studies. J Rheumatol 27:2065–2077, 2000.
3. Brouet J-C, Clauvel J-P, Danon F, et al: Biologic and clinical significance of cryoglobulins: A report of 86 cases. Am J Med 57:775–788, 1984.
4. Cohen SJ, Pittelkow MR, Su WPD: Cutaneous manifestations of cryoglobulinemia: Clinical and histopathologic study of seventy-two patients. J Am Acad Dermatol 25:21–27, 1991.
5. Ferri C, Greco F, Longombardo G, et al: Antibodies to hepatitis C virus in patients with mixed cryoglobulinemia. Arthritis Rheum 34:1606–1610, 1991.
6. Ferri C, Zignego AL: Relation between infection and autoimmunity in mixed cryoglobulinemia. Curr Opin Rheumatol 12:53–60, 2000.

7. Frankel AH, Singer DRJ, Winearls CG, et al: Type II essential mixed cryoglobulinemia: Presentation, treatment and outcome in 13 patients. Q J Med 82:101–124, 1992.
8. Lamprecht P, Gause A, Gross WL: Review: Cryoglobulinemic vasculitis. Arthritis Rheum 42:2507–2516, 1999.
9. Zuckerman E, Keren D, Slobodin G, et al: Treatment of refractory, symptomatic, hepatitis C virus related mixed cryoglobulinemia with ribavirin and interferon-alpha. J Rheumatol 27:2172–2178, 2000.

# 36. BEHÇET'S SYNDROME

*Raymond J. Enzenauer, M.D.*

**1. What are the criteria for Behçet's disease?**

**Recurrent oral ulceration**: Minor aphthous, major aphthous, or herpetiform ulceration observed by a physician or patient, which occurred at least 3 times in one 12-month period

*Plus 2 of the following*:

**Recurrent genital ulceration**: Aphthous ulceration or scarring observed by a physician or patient

**Eye lesions**: Anterior uveitis, posterior uveitis, or cells in vitreous on slit lamp examination; or retinal vasculitis observed by an ophthalmologist

**Skin lesions**: Erythema nodosum observed by physician or patient, pseudofolliculitis, or papulopustular lesions; or acneiform nodules observed by physician in postadolescent patients not on corticosteroid treatment

**Positive pathergy test**: 2 mm erythema 24–48 hrs after #25 needleprick to depth of 5 mm

Prior to publication in 1990 of the criteria of the International Study Group (ISG) for Behçet's Disease, five sets of criteria for the diagnosis of Behçet's disease had been in use, which hindered interpretation of different studies and collaborative research. Sensitivity and specificity of the ISG criteria are 95% and 98%, respectively, with more specificity and little loss of sensitivity compared with the other five sets of previously used criteria.

**2. Behçet's disease is a clinical diagnosis. What other diseases must be considered and ruled out in a patient presenting with possible Behçet's disease?**

Virtually all the features of Behçet's disease can be seen in Crohn's colitis. Inflammatory bowel disease must be considered particularly in patients with iron deficiency, markedly elevated ESR (> 100 mm/hr), or even minor bowel complaints. Other collagen vascular diseases with oral ulcers, ocular disease, and arthritis need to be considered, including systemic lupus erythematosus, Reiter's syndrome, and systemic vasculitis.

**3. Describe "pathergy."**

Pathergy is the hyperreactivity of the skin to any intracutaneous injection or needlestick (pathergy test). Originally described in 1935, this reaction is believed by some to be pathognomonic for Behçet's disease. The mechanism of pathergy in Behçet's is unknown, but it is thought to be related to increased neutrophil chemotaxis. The rate of a positive reactions varies in different populations, being more common in Japan and Turkey and less common in England and the United States.

**4. Who gets Behçet's disease?**

The disease occurs in both males and females equally, with the mean age of patients being about 40 years. 1–2% of cases occur in childhood.

**5. What is the relationship between this disease and the old Silk Route of Marco Polo?**

Although Behçet's disease occurs worldwide, it is much more prevalent in individuals living along the old Silk Route (trade trail of Marco Polo), extending from the Orient (Japan) through

Turkey and into the Mediterranean basin. The Japanese and eastern Mediterranean peoples have a 3–6 times increased incidence of HLA-B5, and subtype B51, in Behçet's disease patients compared with controls. The presence of HLA-B51 appears to be associated with a more complete expression of manifestations and a more severe clinical course of disease. HLA-B5 and B51 are not increased in frequency in Behçet's patients in the United States. Although first described 25 years ago, we still do not know whether the HLA-B51 or a gene in linkage disequilibrium with HLA-B51 is the predisposing locus for Behçet's disease.

**6. Describe the aphthous ulcers associated with Behçet's disease.**

Aphthous-like stomatitis is the initial manifestation in 25–75% of patients with Behçet's disease. Preferential sites of ulceration are the mucous membranes of the lips, gingiva, cheeks (buccal mucosa), and tongue. The palate, tonsils, and pharynx are rarely involved (unlike Reiter's or Stevens-Johnson syndrome). Most oral ulcers occur in crops and heal without scarring within 10 days.

**7. List a differential diagnosis of aphthous stomatitis.**

Underlying conditions may be identified in as many as 30% of patients with severe aphthous stomatitis. Most cases remain idiopathic, however.

| CONDITION | % OF AFFECTED POPULATION |
|---|---|
| Idiopathic | 70% |
| $B_{12}$/folate/iron deficiency | 22% |
| Gluten-sensitive enteropathy | 2% |
| Menstrually related | 2% |
| Severe aphthosis | 2% |
| Inflammatory bowel disease | 1% |
| Behçet's disease | 1% |

**8. What is complex aphthosis?**

This recently described entity describes patients without systemic manifestations of Behçet's disease who have recurrent oral and genital aphthous ulcers or almost constant multiple (> 3) oral aphthae. Differentiation from complex aphthosis may be difficult because the initial clinical presentation or Behçet's disease is often confined to oral and genital ulceration.

**9. How frequently do the various clinical symptoms of Behçet's disease occur?**

| | |
|---|---|
| Oral aphthous ulcers | 97–100% |
| Genital ulcers | 80–100% |
| Ocular symptoms | 50–79% |
| Arthritis | 30–50% |
| Skin lesions | 35–65% |
| CNS disease | 10–30% |
| Major vessel occlusion/aneurysm | 10–37% |
| Gastrointestinal involvement | 0–25% |

**10. Describe the genital ulcers of Behcet's disease.**

Aphthous ulcers similar to those in the mouth also occur on the genitalia, most frequently the scrotum and vulva. The penis and the perianal and vaginal mucosa may also be involved. Lesions in men tend to be more painful than those in women. The genital ulcers are usually deeper than oral lesions and may leave scars after healing. Vulvar ulcers often develop during the premenstrual stage of the cycle.

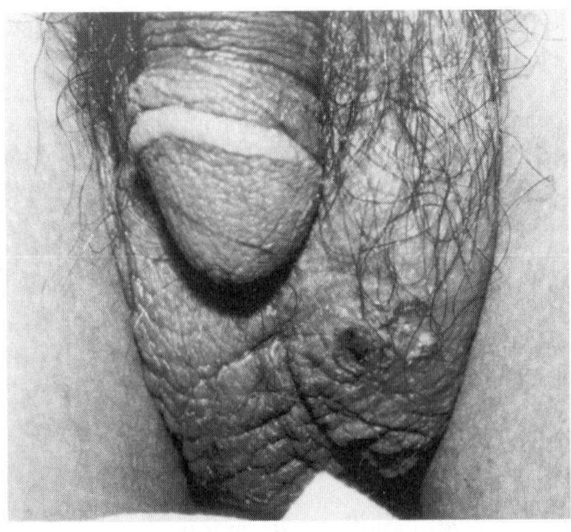

Scrotal ulcer in a patient with Behçet's disease. Oral aphthous ulcers have a similar appearance.

**11. Are nonvenereal genital ulcers commonly due to Behçet's?**

No. Although genital ulcers are virtually universal in Behçet's disease, Behçet's is a rare cause of genital ulceration. Venereal ulcers are the most common type of genital ulceration and include herpes simplex, syphilis, chancroid, lymphogranuloma venereum (LGV), and granuloma inguinale (donovanosis). Nonvenereal causes of genital ulceration include trauma (mechanical, chemical), adverse drug reactions, nonvenereal infections (nonsyphylitic spirochetes, pyogenic, yeast), vesiculobullous skin diseases, and various neoplasms such as precarcinoma (Bowen's disease) and carcinoma (basal cell carcinoma and squamous cell carcinoma). More common rheumatic causes of genital ulceration include Reiter's syndrome and Crohn's disease.

**12. What are the ophthalmologic manifestations of Behçet's disease?**

Anterior/posterior uveitis, conjunctivitis, corneal ulceration, papillitis, and arteritis. Blindness is limited mostly to patients with posterior uveitis, and occurs on average 4 years after onset of Behçet's disease.

**13. What is a hypopyon?**

The presence of inflammatory cells in the anterior chamber of the eye. While initially believed to be pathognomonic of ocular Behçet's disease, hypopyon is more commonly seen with severe B27-associated uveitis (see Chapter 79).

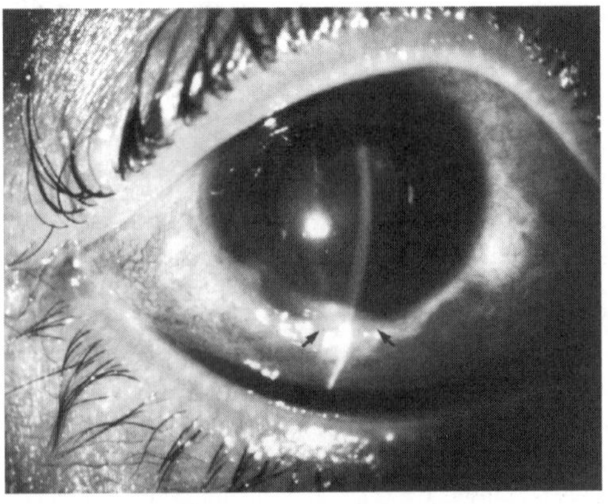

Hypopyon iritis (arrows).

**14. Behçet's disease is a leading cause of acquired blindness in Japan. True or false?**

True. Between 11 and 12% of all acquired blindness in or before middle age in Japan develops as a result of ocular involvement of Behçet's syndrome.

**15. Describe the arthritis associated with Behçet's disease.**

Slightly more than one-half of patients will develop signs or symptoms of joint involvement. The arthritis is usually migratory, mono- or oligoarticular, and asymmetric, principally affecting the knees, ankles, elbows, and wrists. Shoulders, spine, hips, and small joints of the hands and feet are infrequently involved. The arthritis may be polyarticular and occasionally resemble rheumatoid arthritis. Erosive changes are rare. Synovial fluid cell counts average 5000–10,000/mm$^3$, and neutrophils predominate. Note that **arthralgia** is more common but lacks diagnostic value.

**16. What are the cutaneous manifestations of Behçet's disease?**

Erythema nodosum
Thrombophlebitis
Acneiform skin eruption
Hyperirritability of skin (pathergy)

**17. A thrombotic tendency is a feature of Behçet's disease. Describe the vascular involvement in Behçet's disease.**

Thrombosis of the large veins and arteries may occur, as can arterial aneurysms. Vascular thrombosis may be seen in one-fourth of all patients and include thrombosis of the superior or inferior vena cava or the portal or hepatic veins. Up to a third of Behçet's patients with thrombosis may have the factor V Leiden mutation. Behçet's disease is virtually alone among the vasculitides as a frequent cause of fatal aneurysms of the pulmonary arterial tree.

**18. How often do neurologic manifestations occur in Behçet's disease?**

| | |
|---|---|
| Headaches (52%) | Cerebellar ataxia |
| Meningoencephalitis (28%) | Hemiplegia/paraparesis |
| Cranial nerve palsies (16%) | Pseudobulbar palsy |
| Seizures (13%) | Extrapyramidal signs |

Neurologic symptoms tend to recur during flares of oral, genital, and joint lesions. CNS involvement, which may be life-threatening, is usually a late manifestation occurring from 1–7 years after the initial onset of disease. The most commonly involved region is the brainstem. Intracranial hypertension, mostly resulting from dural sinus thrombosis, is seen in 25% of patients with neurologic disease. Mortality of CNS Behçet's disease may be 41%.

**19. Describe cardiac involvement in Behçet's disease.**

Apart from sporadic reports of valvular lesions, myocarditis, and pericarditis, cardiac involvement in Behçet's disease is uncommon. There is no significant difference in the prevalence of cardiac abnormalities among Behçet's disease patients and controls.

**20. What are the common laboratory findings in Behçet's disease?**

Laboratory parameters are nonspecific in Behçet's. Some of the common findings include increased serum levels of IgG, IgA, and IgM; increased C-reactive protein and $\alpha_2$-globulin; elevated CSF protein and cell count (in patients with neurologic involvement); leukocytosis; and an elevated ESR. These findings most often occur during disease exacerbation and often return to normal during remission.

**21. What are the major causes of mortality in Behçet's disease?**

| | |
|---|---|
| CNS involvement | Pulmonary disease (hemoptysis) |
| Vascular disease | Serious cardiac disease |
| Bowel disease (perforation) | |

Mortality may be 16% in 5 years.

**22. What is the drug-of-choice for severe meningoencephalitis or uveitis associated with Behçet's disease?**

**Chlorambucil** is the drug-of-choice for severe ocular or CNS disease. Cyclophosphamide has also been used. With proper management, loss of useful vision has been reduced from 75 to 20%.

**23. Which drugs are reported to be successful in treating the mucocutaneous lesions of Behçet's syndrome?**

Oral colchicine, 0.5–0.6 mg 2–3 times a day
Dapsone, 100 mg/day
Thalidomide, 100–400 mg/day
Levamisole, 150 mg/day for 3 days every 2 wks
Interferon alfa, $9 \times 10^6$ units 3 times a week for 3 months followed by $3 \times 10^6$ units 3 times a week

**24. Describe the use of antibiotics in the treatment of Behçet's disease.**

Based on the rationale that streptococci might play a possible role in the pathogenesis of Behçet's disease, several studies have evaluated the effectiveness of antibiotics in the treatment of Behçet's disease. Benzathine penicillin may be useful for treatment of mucocutaneous lesions and for prevention of arthritis in Behçet's disease. Minocycline may be useful for mucocutaneous lesions.

**25. Which immunosuppressive agents are reported to be successful in treating severe ocular/CNS Behçet's disease?**

Systemic corticosteroids
- Oral, 1–2 mg/kg/day
- IV, 1 gm/day for 3 days

Chlorambucil, 0.1–0.2 mg/kg/day
Azathioprine, 2.5 mg/kg/day orally
Cyclophosphamide
- IV, 0.5–1.0 gm/m$^2$ per month
- Oral, 1–2 mg/kg/day

Cyclosporine, 5–10 mg/kg/day
Levamisole, 150 mg po 2–3 times weekly
Methotrexate, 7.5–15 mg/wk po
Tacrolimus (FK506), 0.1 mg/kg/day

**26. Who was Behçet?**

Hulusi Behçet, a Turkish dermatologist, in 1937 described a chronic relapsing syndrome of oral ulceration, genital ulceration, and uveitis that now bears his name.

**27. Describe the MAGIC syndrome.**

Although chondritis has been noted in association with many other rheumatic diseases, the relationship between idiopathic relapsing polychondritis and Behçet's disease is particularly close. In 1985, Firestein and colleagues proposed the name "**M**outh **A**nd **G**enital ulceration with **I**nflamed **C**artilage" (MAGIC) syndrome in an attempt to encompass both clinical entities.

**28. Describe the pathogenesis of Behçet's disease**

The pathogenesis of Behçet's disease remains unclear. It might not have a primary autoimmune basis. No specific antibodies or clear-cut abnormalities in B cells have been demonstrated. T-cell hyperactivity has been reported in patients with Behçet's disease. Elevated levels of interleukin-12 have been reported in Behçet's disease, suggesting a Th1 pattern. Neutrophil hyperactivity has been reported in Behçet's disease with increased migration of neutrophils during attacks but not during remissions in Behçet's disease.

BIBLIOGRAPHY

1. Calguneri M, Kiraz S, Ertenli I, et al: The effect of prophylactic penicillin treatment on the course of arthritis episodes in patients with Behçet's disease: A randomized clinical trial. Arthritis Rheum 39:2062, 1996.
2. Friedman-Birnbaum R, Bergman R, Aizen E: Sensitivity and specificity of pathergy test results in Israeli patients with Behçet's disease. Cutis 45:261–264, 1990.
3. Hamuryudan V, Mat C, Saip S, et al: Thalidomide in the treatment of the mucocutaneous lesions of the Behçet's syndrome. Ann Intern Med 128:443, 1998.
4. Hutton KP, Rogers RS: Recurrent aphthous stomatitis. Dermatol Clin 5:761–768, 1987.
5. Imai H, Motegi M, Mizuki N, et al: Mouth and genital ulcers with inflamed cartilage (MAGIC syndrome): A case report and literature review. Am J Med Sci 314:330, 1997.
6. International Study Group for Behçet's Disease: Criteria for diagnosis of Behçet's disease. Lancet 335:1078–1080, 1990.
7. Kaklamani V, Vaiopoulos G, Kaklamanis PG: Behçet's disease. Semin Arthritis Rheum 27:197, 1998.
8. Kaklamani VG, Kaklamanis PG: Treatment of Behçet's disease—an update. Semin Arthritis Rheum 30:299–312, 2001.
9. Nussenblatt RB: Uveitis in Behçet's disease. Int Rev Immunol 14:67, 1997.
10. O'Duffy JD, Robertson DM, Goldstein NP: Chlorambucil in the treatment of uveitis and menigoencephalitis of Behçet's disease. Am J Med 76:75–84, 1984.
11. Sakane T, Suzuki N, Nagafuchi H: Etiopathology of Behçet's disease: Immunological aspects. Yonsei Med J 38:350, 1997.
12. Schreiner DT, Jorizzo JL: Behçet's disease and complex aphthosis. Dermatol Clin 5:769–778, 1987.
13. West SG, Ball GV: Uncommon rheumatic diseases. In Weisman MH, Weinblatt ME, Louie JS (eds): Treatment of Rheumatic Diseases. Companion to the Textbook of Rheumatology. Philadelphia, W.B. Saunders, 2001, pp 487–502.
14. Yazici H, Yurdakul S, Hamuryudan V: Behçet's syndrome. Curr Opin Rheumatol 11:53–57, 1999.
15. Zouboulis CC, Orfanos CE: Treatment of Adamantiades-Behçet's disease with systemic interferon alfa. Arch Dermatol 1334:1010, 1998.

# 37. RELAPSING POLYCHONDRITIS

*Marc D. Cohen, M.D.*

**1. Define relapsing polychondritis (RPC).**

Relapsing polychondritis is an uncommon episodic systemic disease characterized by recurrent inflammation and destruction of cartilaginous tissues.

**2. Who gets RPC?**

Patients are predominantly Caucasian with a slight female predominance and a range of 20–60 years with a peak in the fifth decade. There may be an association with HLA-DR4.

**3. Briefly discuss the etiopathogenetic hypothesis of RPC.**

The etiology of RPC is unknown. It is thought to be an autoimmune process for the following reasons: (1) lymphocytes of RPC patients, when confronted with cartilage mucopolysaccharide, induce lymphoblast transformation and macrophage migration responses indicative of cell-mediated immunity; and (2) antibodies to native type 2 collagen and circulating immune complexes have been identified in RPC patients, suggestive of humoral immunity. The degree of immune response correlates with clinical disease activity.

An inciting agent (infectious, toxic, immunologic) has not yet been identified. However, once stimulated, activated lymphocytes and macrophages are thought to secrete mediators that induce the release of lysosomal enzymes, especially proteases. The resulting inflammatory destruction of cartilage generates an attempt at repair by local fibroblasts and chondrocytes, leading to the formation of granulation tissue and fibrosis.

**4. Describe the histopathology of RPC.**

The histopathology of involved cartilage, regardless of location, is similar and highly characteristic. The cartilage matrix, which is normally basophilic (blue), becomes acidophilic (pink) when examined by routine hematoxylin and eosin staining. Inflammatory cell infiltrates (initially polymorphonuclear cells and later lymphocytes and plasma cells) are seen invading the cartilage from the periphery inward. Granulation tissue and fibrosis develop adjacent to inflammatory infiltrates, occasionally resulting in sequestration of cartilage segments. Increased lipids and lysosomes in chondrocytes are demonstrated by electron microscopy.

**5. Define the diagnostic criteria for RPC (set forth by McAdam in 1976).**

- Recurrent chondritis of both auricles
- Nonerosive inflammatory polyarthritis
- Chondritis of nasal cartilages
- Inflammation of ocular structures, including conjunctivitis, keratitis, scleritis/episcleritis, and/or uveitis
- Chondritis of the respiratory tract involving laryngeal and/or tracheal cartilages
- Cochlear and/or vestibular damage manifested by neurosensory hearing loss, tinnitus, and/or vertigo

The presence of three or more clinical features is considered diagnostic of RPC.

**6. Which target organs are most commonly involved in the clinical presentation and eventual course of RPC?**

*Clinical Manifestations of Relapsing Polychondritis**

| MANIFESTATION | PRESENTING SYMPTOM % | EVENTUAL INVOLVEMENT % |
|---|---|---|
| Auricular chondritis | 26 | 89 |
| Arthritis | 23 | 81 |
| Nasal chondritis | 13 | 72 |
| Ocular inflammation | 14 | 65 |
| Respiratory tract | 15 | 56 |
| Audiovestibular | 6 | 46 |
| Cardiovascular | — | 24 |
| Skin | — | 17 |

* Data from Michet CJ, Jr., McKenna CH, Luthra HS, O'Fallon WM: Relapsing polychondritis. Survival and predictive role of early disease manifestations. Ann Intern Med 104:74–78, 1986.

**7. Discuss the clinical features and potential complications of the auricular and nasal chondritis of RPC.**

**Auricular chondritis** is the most frequent and characteristic clinical feature of RPC. It typically presents as the sudden onset of burning pain, warmth, swelling, and purplish-red discoloration of the pinnas of both ears (see Figure *A*, top of next page). Because only the cartilaginous portion is affected, the inferior soft lobules are always spared, separating it from cellulitis. Attacks may last from a few days to several weeks. After one or more attacks, the external ear may lose its structural integrity owing to inflammatory dissolution of cartilage. This results in a dropping, floppy ear that has been termed "cauliflower ear" (see Figure *B*, top of next page).

**Nasal chondritis** develops suddenly as a painful fullness of the nasal bridge. Epistaxis occasionally accompanies the inflammation. It is less recurrent than auricular chondritis; however, even in the absence of clinical inflammation, cartilage collapse may occur, resulting in a "saddle nose" deformity (see figure, middle of next page).

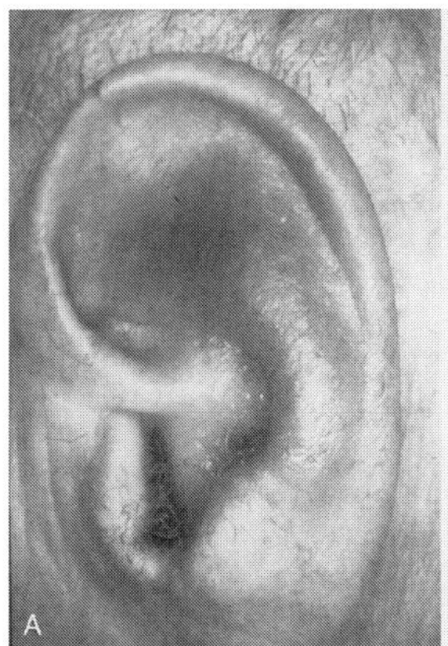


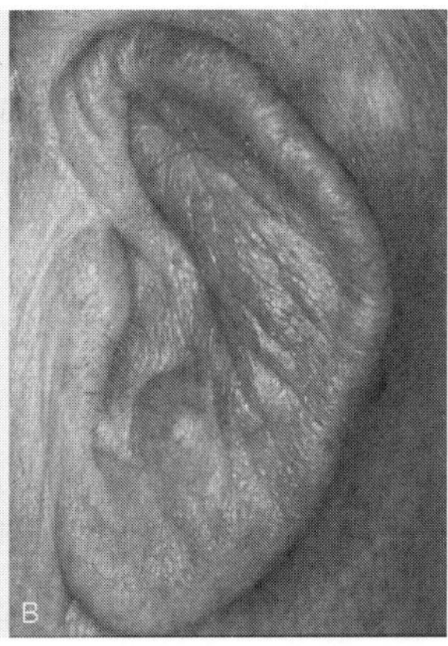


*A*, The ear in early inflammatory RPC. *B*, Chronic collapse of the cartilaginous pinna in a patient with RPC. (Reprinted from the Revised Clinical Slide Collection on the Rheumatic Diseases, copyright 1991. Used by permission of the American College of Rheumatology.)

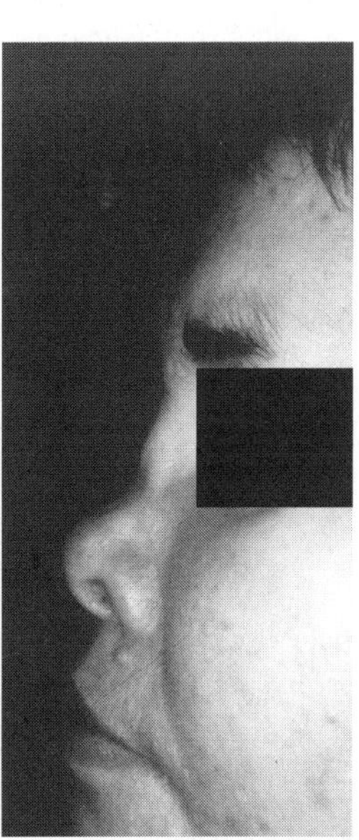

Saddle nose deformity due to nasal septal collapse. (Reprinted from the Revised Clinical Slide Collection on the Rheumatic Diseases, copyright 1991. Used by permission of the American College of Rheumatology.)

**8. Describe the arthritis of RPC.**

The arthritis of RPC is usually an oligo- or polyarticular asymmetric nonerosive inflammatory arthritis with a predilection for the large joints of the extremities and the sternoclavicular, costochondral, and sternomanubrial joints. When the small joints of the hands and feet are affected, the disease may mimic seronegative rheumatoid arthritis. Flail chest has been described secondary to inflammatory lysis of the costosternal cartilage.

**9. Describe the ocular involvement of RPC.**

Virtually every structure of the eye and surrounding tissues may be affected. Episcleritis, conjunctivitis, and uveitis are most common. Complications may include cataracts, optic neuritis, keratitis, proptosis, corneal ulcerations and thinning, and extraocular muscle palsies. Losses of visual acuity and even blindness have been reported.

**10. Discuss the distribution of disease, clinical symptoms, and potential complications of the respiratory tract in RPC.**

Cartilage inflammation may occur early in the larynx and trachea, and later in the first- and second-order bronchi. In mild cases, symptoms might consist of throat tenderness, hoarseness, and a nonproductive cough. In severe cases, laryngeal and epiglottal edema may cause choking, stridor, dyspnea, or respiratory failure requiring emergency tracheostomy. Repeated or persistent inflammation of the airways can lead to either tracheal stenosis or dynamic airway collapse caused by dissolution of the tracheal and bronchial cartilaginous rings. Flail chest can interfere with ventilatory efforts. In addition, respiratory tract infections may complicate the clinical course of these patients.

**11. Discuss audiovestibular damage in RPC.**

Audiovestibular involvement presents as hearing loss, tinnitus, vertigo, and fullness in the ear (due to serous otitis media). Conductive hearing loss results form inflammatory edema or cartilage collapse of the auricle, external auditory canal, and/or eustachian tubes. Sensorineural hearing loss can be caused by inflammation of the internal auditory artery.

**12. Describe the cardiac manifestations of RPC.**

Aortic insufficiency is the most common cardiac manifestation and, after respiratory involvement, is the most serious complication of RPC. It is usually due to progressive dilatation of the aortic root, which usually distinguishes it from the aortic insufficiency of other common rheumatic diseases (see following table). Less frequent cardiac complications include pericarditis, arrhythmias, and conduction defects.

*Aortic Insufficiency: Patterns of Disease Association*

| PATHOLOGY | UNDERLYING CONDITION |
|---|---|
| Valvulitis | Rheumatic fever<br>Rheumatoid arthritis<br>Ankylosing spondylitis*<br>Endocarditis<br>Reiter's syndrome*<br>Behçet's syndrome* |
| Congenital | Bicuspid aortic valve |
| Dilatation of valve ring | Marfan's syndrome<br>Syphilis<br>Relapsing polychondritis<br>Dissecting aneurysm<br>Idiopathic |

* Also dilation of valve ring.
From Trenham DE, Le CH: Relapsing polychondritis. In McCarty DJ, Koopman WJ (eds): Arthritis and Allied Conditions, 12th ed. Philadelphia. Lea & Febiger, 1993; with permission.

**13. What other clinical manifestations occur in RPC?**

**Vasculitis** may occur in up to 30% of cases. Involved vessels range in size from capillaries (leukocytoclastic vasculitis) to large arteries (aortitis).

**Neurologic manifestations** may include cranial neuropathies (second, sixth, seventh, eighth), headaches, and more rarely seizures, encephalopathy, hemiplegia, and ataxia.

**Renal disease**, although rare, does occur, usually focal glomerulonephritis, but a wide variety of renal lesions have been reported. Renal disease usually indicates a worse prognosis.

**Dermatologic features** range from alopecia, abnormal nail growth, and postinflammatory hyperpigmentary changes to leukocytoclastic vasculitis.

**14. What laboratory data support the diagnosis of RPC?**

Laboratory abnormalities in RPC are nonspecific and generally reflective of an inflammatory state: elevated erythrocyte sedimentation rate, leukocytosis, thrombocytosis, chronic anemia, and increased alpha and gamma globulins. Low titers of rheumatoid factor, antinuclear antibody, and antinuclear cytoplasmic antibodies may be seen. Antibodies to type II collagen have been found in approximately 20% of patients but are not prognostic of disease activity.

**15. Describe the radiographic abnormalities of RPC.**

Soft-tissue radiographs of the neck may demonstrate narrowing of the tracheal air column, suggestive of tracheal stenosis. Tomography or computerized axial tomography can more accurately define the degree of tracheal narrowing (see figure). Repeated inflammation may lead to cartilaginous calcification of the pinnas, which may be seen in other conditions, such as frostbite. Radiographs of the joints may occasionally demonstrate periarticular osteopenia, joint space narrowing, and erosions suggestive of rheumatoid arthritis.

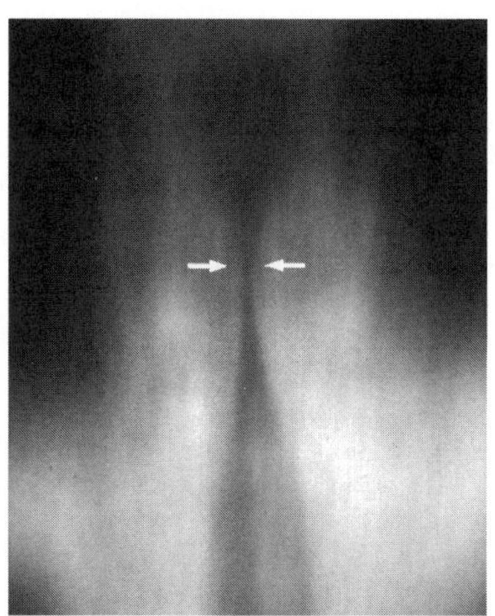

Tracheal tomogram demonstrating subglottic edema and tracheal narrowing (arrows) in a patient with RPC. This "steeple sign" is also seen in children with croup. (Reprinted from the Revised Clinical Slide Collection on the Rheumatic Diseases, copyright 1991. Used by permission of the American College of Rheumatology.)

**16. What is the differential diagnosis of RPC?**

Like RPC, syphilis and Wegener's granulomatosis also cause saddle nose deformities. Other disorders that destroy cartilage, such as infectious perichondritis, frostbite, and midline granuloma, do not present as multifocal chondritis. Inherited degenerative chondropathy is a recently described autosomal dominant disease caused by myxoid degeneration of thyroid and cricoid cartilage and characterized by saddle nose deformity at birth and laryngeal stenosis at 9–12 years of age.

**17. Which diseases commonly coexist in patients with RPC?**

Several rheumatologic diseases are seen in association with RPC, including systemic lupus erythematosus, rheumatoid arthritis, Sjögren's syndrome, spondyloarthropathy, and systemic vasculitis (most common). Usually the inflammatory rheumatologic disease precedes the onset of RPC. Hypothyroidism has also been associated with RPC. Myelodysplastic syndromes have also been reported, occurring before or simultaneously with the RPC.

**18. Which diagnostic modalities are useful in detecting and following disease activity and cartilage damage in patients with RPC?**

The erythrocyte sedimentation rate is an accurate predictor of disease activity in most patients. Functional complications may be demonstrated by radiographic imaging as outlined previously and by the use of pulmonary function testing with flow volume loops. Echocardiography is useful in the diagnosis and follow-up of valvular heart disease.

**19. What medications are used in the treatment of RPC?**

Glucocorticoids are the pharmacologic mainstay of therapy in RPC. During active disease, doses of 20–60 mg/day are used until control is attained. Continued inflammation or an inability to taper glucocorticoids to safe maintenance doses warrants the addition of a steroid-sparing agent. Dapsone (50–200 mg/d) has been useful in this regard in patients without major organ involvement. In patients with ocular, pulmonary, cardiovascular involvement, or systemic vasculitis, other immunosuppressives such as methotrexate, azathioprine, cyclophosphamide, and cyclosporine are used. A recommended approach in patients with severe disease is to control manifestations with corticosteroids and cyclophosphamide and later switch to less toxic medication like methotrexate.

**20. When does surgery play a role in the management of RPC?**

Tracheostomy may be required in patients with airway collapse. Airway obstruction caused by tracheal stenosis or tracheomalacia may require surgical resection. Intrabronchial stent placement has been reported as a potential remedy for dynamic airway collapse. Aortic insufficiency may require valve replacement, and aortic aneurysm formation may necessitate surgical grafting.

Surgical reconstruction of nasal septal collapse is ***not*** recommended because further collapse and deformity frequently occur postoperatively.

**21. What is the prognosis in patients with RPC?**

In 1976, McAdam et al. reported that the 5- and 10-year survival of 112 patients with RPC was 74% and 55%, respectively. Infection and systemic vasculitis were the major causes of death. Fifteen percent died as a direct consequence of cardiovascular or respiratory tract RPC. Poor prognostic indicators included coexistent vasculitis and early saddle nose deformity in younger patients, and the presence of anemia in older patients. In the 1998 study by Trentham et al., the average disease duration was 8 years and the survival rate was significantly improved at 94%.

ACKNOWLEDGMENT

The editor and author wish to thank Dr. Steven Older for his contributions to this chapter in the previous edition.

## BIBLIOGRAPHY

1. Balsa A, Expinosa A, Cuesta M, et al: Joint symptoms in relapsing polychondritis. Clin Exp Rheumatol 13:425–430, 1995.
2. Del Rosso A, Petix NR, Pratesi M, Bini A: Cardiovascular involvement in relapsing polychondritis. Semin Arthritis Rheum 26:840–844, 1997.
3. Diebold L, Rauh G, Jager K, Lohrs U: Bone marrow pathology in relapsing polychondritis: High frequency of myelodysplastic syndromes. Br J Haematol 89:820–830, 1995.
4. Hanslik T, Wechsler B, Piette JC, et al: Central nervous system involvement in relapsing polychondritis. Clin Exp Rheumatol 12:539–541, 1994.
5. Hochberg MC: Relapsing polychondritis. In Ruddy S, Harris ED, Sledge CB (eds): Kelley's Textbook of Rheumatology, 6th ed. Philadelphia, WB Saunders, 2001, pp 1463–1467.
6. McAdam LP, O'Hanlan MA, Bluestone R, Pearson CM: Relapsing polychondritis: Prospective study of 23 patients and a review of the literature. Medicine (Baltimore) 55:193–215, 1976.
7. Michet CJ: Vasculitis and relapsing polychondritis. Rheum Dis Clin North Am 16:441–444, 1990.
8. Michet CJ Jr, McKenna CH, Luthra HS, O'Fallon WM: Relapsing polychondritis. Survival and predictive role of early disease manifestations. Ann Intern Med 104:74–78, 1986.
9. Molina JF, Espinoza LR: Relapsing polychondritis. Baillieres Best Pract Res Clin Rheumatol 14:97–109, 2000.
10. Port JL, Khan A, Barbu RR: Computed tomography of relapsing polychondritis. Comput Med Imaging Graph 17:119–123, 1993.
11. Sarodia BD, Dasgupta A, Mehta AC: Management of airway manifestations of relapsing polychondritis: Case reports and review of literature. Chest 116:1669–1675, 1999.
12. Spraggs PD, Tostevin PM, Howard DJ: Management of laryngotracheobronchial sequelae and complications of relapsing polychondritis. Laryngoscope 107:936–941, 1997.
13. Tillie-Leblond I, Wallaert B, Leblond D, et al: Respiratory involvement in relapsing polychondritis. Clinical, functional, endoscopic, and radiographic evaluations. Medicine (Baltimore) 77:168–176, 1998.
14. Trentham DE, Le CH: Relapsing polychondritis. Ann Intern Med 129:114–122, 1998.
15. Zeuner M, Straub RH, Rauh G, et al: Relapsing polychondritis: Clinical and immunogenetic analysis of 62 patients. J Rheumatol 24:96–101, 1997.

# VI. Seronegative Spondyloarthropathies

*Which of your hips has the most profound sciatica?*
William Shakespeare (1564–1616)
*Measure for Measure*, I

## 38. ANKYLOSING SPONDYLITIS

Robert W. Janson, M.D.

**1. What is ankylosing spondylitis? How was the term derived?**

Ankylosing spondylitis (AS) is a chronic systemic inflammatory disease affecting the sacroiliac joints, spine, and, not infrequently, peripheral joints. Sacroiliitis is its hallmark. The name is derived from the Greek roots *ankylos*, meaning "bent" (*ankylosis* means joint fusion), and *spondylos*, meaning spinal vertebra. If AS occurs in association with reactive arthritis, psoriasis, ulcerative colitis, or Crohn's disease, it is called "secondary" AS.

**2. Ankylosing spondylitis is also known by what eponyms?**

Marie-Strümpell's or von Bechterew's disease, after physicians who contributed to the clinical description of the disease in the late 19th century.

**3. Describe the clinical characteristics of AS.**

The clinical manifestations of AS usually begin in late adolescence or early adulthood, with onset after age 40 being uncommon. It occurs more commonly in males than females (3:1), but AS is often more difficult to diagnose in females as a result of less-pronounced clinical features and possibly slower development of radiographic changes. Patients complain of back pain with prolonged morning and, often, nocturnal stiffness. This stiffness improves with movement and exercise. Physical examination reveals sacroiliac joint tenderness, decreased spinal mobility, and sometimes reduced chest expansion due to costovertebral joint involvement.

**4. What features in the history and physical examination are helpful in differentiating inflammatory low back pain (LBP) in AS from mechanical low back pain?**

*Differentiation of Low Back Pain*

| | INFLAMMATORY LBP | MECHANICAL LBP |
|---|---|---|
| Age of onset | < 40 yrs of age | Any age |
| Type of onset | Insidious | Acute |
| Symptom duration | > 3 mos | < 4 wks |
| Morning stiffness | > 60 min | < 30 min |
| Nocturnal pain | Frequent | Absent |
| Effect of exercise | Improvement | Exacerbation |
| Sacroiliac joint tenderness | Frequent | Absent |
| Back mobility | Loss in all planes | Abnormal flexion |
| Chest expansion | Often decreased | Normal |
| Neurologic deficits | Unusual | Possible |

**5. Describe six physical examination tests used to assess sacroiliac joint tenderness or progression of spinal disease in AS.**

- **Occiput-to-wall test**. Assesses loss of cervical range of motion. Normally with the heels and scapulae touching the wall, the occiput should also touch the wall. Any distance from the occiput to the wall represents a forward stoop of the neck secondary to cervical spine involvement with AS. The tragus-to-wall test could also be used.
- **Chest expansion**. Measured at the fourth intercostal space, normal chest expansion is approximately 5 cm.
- **Schober test**. Detects limitation of forward flexion of the lumbar spine. Place a mark at the level of the posterior superior iliac spine and another 10 cm above in the midline. With maximal forward spinal flexion with locked knees, the measured distance should increase from 10 cm to at least 15 cm (see figure).

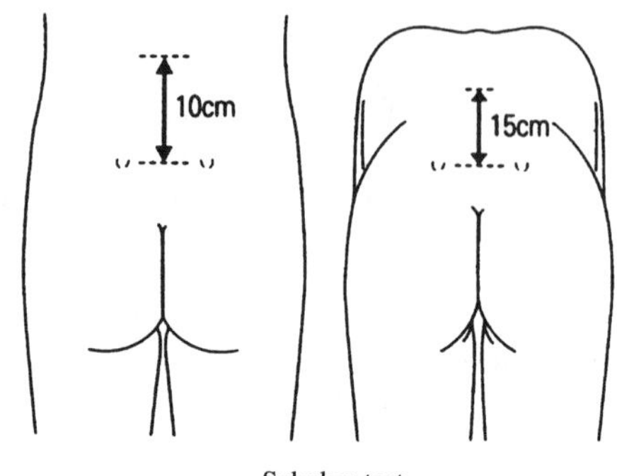


Schober test.

- **Pelvic compression**. With the patient lying on one side, compression of the pelvis should elicit sacroiliac joint pain.
- **Gaenslen's test**. With the patient supine, a leg is allowed to drop over the side of the exam table while the patient draws the other leg toward the chest. This test should elicit sacroiliac joint pain on the side of the dropped leg (see figure).
- **Patrick's test**. With the patient's heel placed on the opposite knee, downward pressure on the flexed knee with the hip now in *f*lexion, *ab*duction, and *e*xternal *r*otation (FABER) should elicit contralateral sacroiliac joint tenderness (see figure).

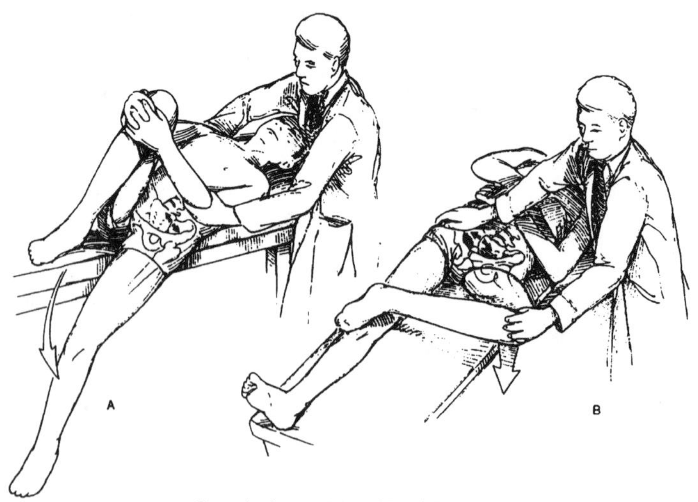


Gaenslen's test (*A*) and Patrick's test (*B*).

**6. What is an enthesis? How does it relate to the disease process in AS?**

An enthesis is a site of insertion of a ligament, tendon, or articular capsule into bone. In AS, the initial inflammatory process involves the enthesis, followed by a process that results in new bone formation or fibrosis. Sites of enthesopathy in AS include the sacroiliac joints; ligamentous structures of the intervertebral discs, manubriosternal joints, and symphysis pubis; ligamentous attachments in the spinous processes, the iliac crests (whiskering), trochanters, patellae, clavicles, and calcanei (Achilles enthesitis or plantar fasciitis); and capsules and intracapsular ligaments of large synovial joints.

**7. Which peripheral joints are most commonly involved in AS?**

The hips and shoulders. Rarely, arthritis of the sternoclavicular, temporomandibular, cricoarytenoid, or symphysis pubis occurs. Approximately 30% of patients with AS develop a peripheral arthritis.

**8. What are the extraskeletal manifestations of AS?**

Remembering the first few letters of the disease's name will help in recalling these.

**A** Aortic insufficiency, ascending aortitis, and other cardiac manifestations, such as conduction abnormalities, diastolic dysfunction, and pericarditis (10% of patients)
**N** Neurologic: atlantoaxial subluxations and cauda equina syndrome
**K** Kidney: secondary amyloidosis and chronic prostatitis

**S** Spine: cervical fracture, spinal stenosis, significant spinal osteoporosis
**P** Pulmonary: upper lobe fibrosis, restrictive changes
**O** Ocular: anterior uveitis (25–30% of patients)
**N** Nephropathy (IgA)
**D** Discitis or spondylodiscitis (Andersson lesions)

In addition, 30–60% of patients have asymptomatic microscopic colitis in their terminal ileum and colon.

**9. Which human leukocyte antigen (HLA) shows a strong association with AS? Does this association vary among different racial groups?**

HLA-B27 is present in over 90% of white AS patients and 50–80% of nonwhite patients with AS. Since the prevalence of the HLA-B27 allele is 8% in healthy whites and 3% in healthy North American blacks, an HLA-B27 positive individual has a 50 to 100 times increased relative risk of developing AS. Currently, there are over 20 subtypes (B*2701 to B*2723) known. B*2705 is the most prevalent subtype. No one subtype predisposes to AS, although B*2706 and B*2709 appear to lack an association with AS.

Twin studies show that there is a 60% disease concordance for AS in monozygotic twins and a 20–25% disease concordance in HLA-B27 dizygotic twins. This suggests that other genetic factors must be contributing to the risk of AS in addition to environmental factors.

**10. How prevalent is AS among individuals who are HLA-B27-positive? Among individuals who are HLA-B27-positive with a relative with AS? Among different ethnic groups?**

Two percent of HLA-B27-positive persons develop AS. Among those HLA-B27-positive persons with an affected first-degree relative, the rate rises to 15–20%. AS is associated with HLA-B27 in all ethnic groups. Since the prevalence of HLA-B27 in northern latitudes is high (up to 15% of Scandinavians) and low (< 1% of African blacks and Asians) in ethnic populations near the equator, there is an apparent decrease in the prevalence of AS going from north to south.

**11. When should an HLA-B27 test be ordered?**

Most patients with AS can be diagnosed on the basis of history, physical examination, and the finding of sacroiliitis on radiographs, obviating the need for HLA testing. Knowing the HLA-B27 status of a patient with back pain of an inflammatory nature with negative radiographic findings might be helpful, particularly in nonwhite individuals.

**12. How is HLA-B27 hypothesized to play a role in the pathogenesis of AS?**

Infection with an unknown organism or exposure to an unknown antigen in a genetically susceptible individual (HLA-B27+) is hypothesized to result in the clinical expression of AS.

- The arthritogenic response might involve specific microbial peptides that bind to HLA-B27 and then are presented to $CD8^+$ (cytotoxic) T cells.
- Abnormal cellular processing, transport, and folding of HLA-B27 could predispose certain HLA-B27+ individuals to AS.
- The induction of autoreactivity to self-antigens might develop as a result of "molecular mimicry" between sequences or epitopes on the infecting organism or antigen and a portion of the HLA-B27 molecule.
- The repertoire of "arthritogenic peptides" presented by HLA-B27 could change during bacterial infection.
- Endogenous HLA-B27 itself could be the source of the antigenic peptide resulting in the induction of an autoimmune response.
- HLA-B27 could function at the level of the thymus to select a repertoire of specific $CD8^+$ T cells that are involved in an arthrogenic response when exposed to certain microbial antigens.
- HLA-B27 might only be a marker for a disease susceptibility gene in linkage disequilibrium with HLA-B27.

The potential role of HLA-B27 in the pathogenesis of AS is further supported by the finding that transgenic rats expressing the HLA-B27 gene develop an inflammatory disease that resembles a spondyloarthropathy with axial and peripheral arthritis. Transgenic animals kept in a germ-free environment remain healthy, suggesting that an environmental trigger is also needed.

**13. Describe the typical radiographic features of AS.**

The radiographic changes of AS are predominantly seen in the axial skeleton (sacroiliac, apophyseal, discovertebral, and costovertebral) as well as at sites of enthesopathy ("whiskering" of the iliac crest, ischial tuberosities, femoral trochanters, calcaneus, and vertebral spinous processes). Sacroiliitis is usually bilateral and symmetric, and initially it involves the synovial-lined lower two-thirds of the sacroiliac joint (see figure). The earliest radiographic change is erosion of the iliac side of the sacroiliac joint, where the cartilage is thinner. Progression of the erosive process results in an initial "pseudo-widening" of the sacroiliac joint space with bony sclerosis eventually followed by complete bony ankylosis or fusion of the joint. In cases of early sacroiliitis where plain radiographs may be normal, magnetic resonance imaging (MRI) will demonstrate inflammation and edema.

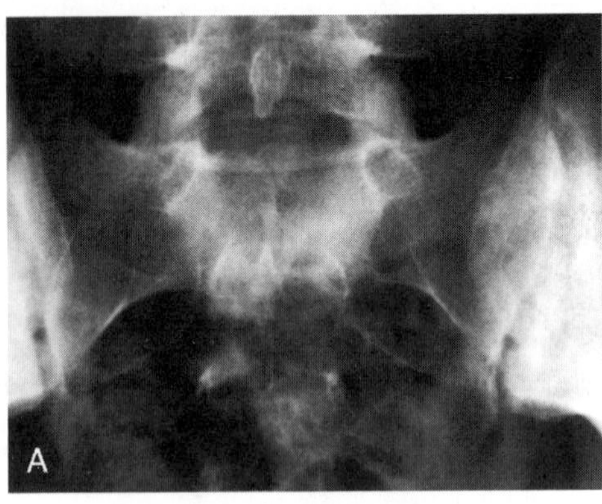


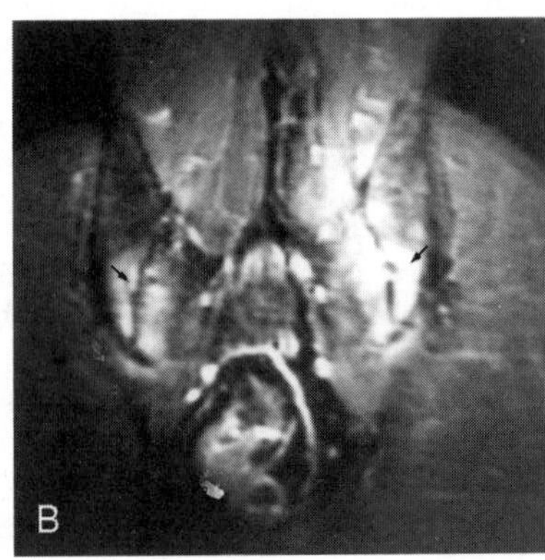


*A*, Radiograph of the pelvis demonstrating bilateral sacroiliitis. *B*, MRI of the sacroiliac joints demonstrating edema (arrows) due to inflammation of these joints.

Inflammatory disease of the spine involves the insertion of the annulus fibrosis to the corners of the vertebral bodies, resulting in initial "shiny corners" (Romanus lesion) followed by "squaring" of the vertebral bodies (see figure). Gradual ossification of the outer layers of the annulus fibrosis (Sharpey's fibers) forms intervertebral bony bridges called **syndesmophytes**. Fusion of the apophyseal joints and calcification of the spinal ligaments along with bilateral syndesmophyte formation can result in complete fusion of the vertebral column, giving the appearance of a "bamboo" spine.

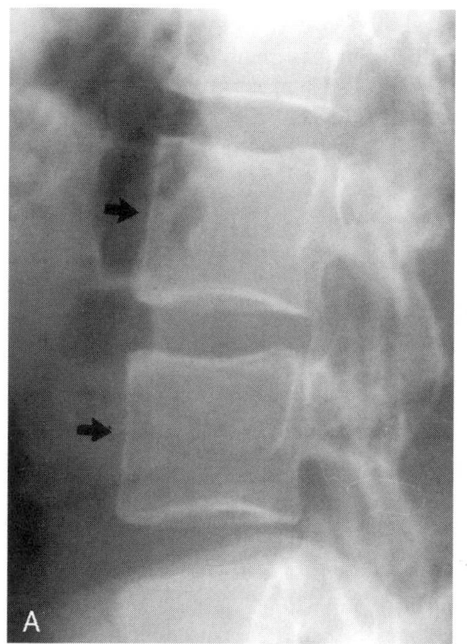


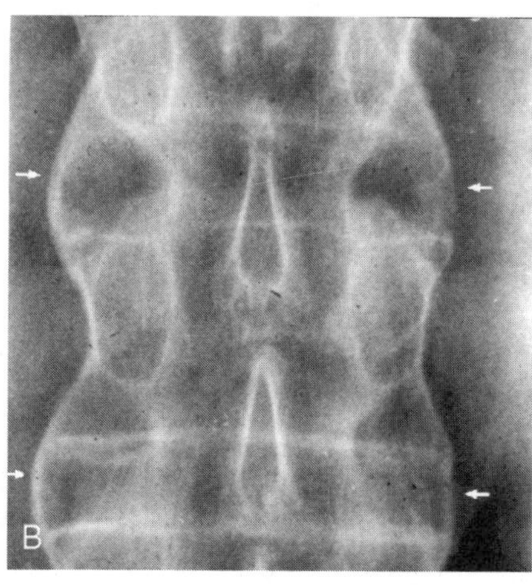


*A*, Lateral radiograph of the lumbar spine demonstrating anterior squaring of vertebrae (arrows). *B*, Anteroposterior radiograph of the spine demonstrating bilateral, thin, marginal syndesmophytes (arrows).

**14. What is osteitis condensans ilii (OCI)?**

An asymptomatic disorder of multiparous young women, OCI is characterized by radiographic findings of a triangular area of dense sclerotic bone only on the iliac side and adjacent to the lower half of the sacroiliac joints. This benign condition is not a form of AS and is not associated with HLA-B27 status.

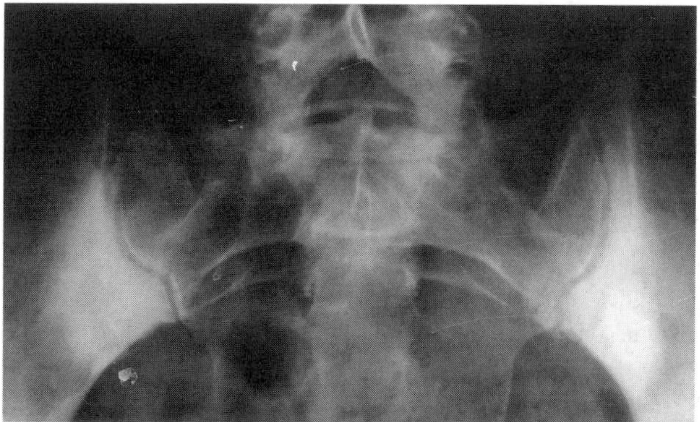

Radiograph of pelvis demonstrating osteitis condensans ilii.

**15. How are AS and diffuse idiopathic skeletal hyperostosis different?**

Diffuse idiopathic skeletal hyperostosis (DISH, Forestier's disease) is a noninflammatory disease occurring in males aged > 50 years. It is characterized by flowing hyperostosis (bone formation), calcification of the anterior longitudinal ligament of at least four contiguous vertebral bodies, and nonerosive enthesopathies (whiskerings). The disease is not associated with sacroiliitis, apophyseal joint ankylosis, or HLA-B27. The flowing osteophytes in DISH typically occur on the right side of the spine, contralateral to the heart. On a lateral spine radiograph, a linear area of radiolucency exists between the calcified anterior longitudinal ligament and the anterior surface of the vertebra. (See chapter 55.)

**16. What are other causes of radiographic sacroiliac joint abnormalities?**

**Inflammatory**: spondyloarthropathies, infection (bacterial, fungal, mycobacterial)

**Traumatic**: fracture, osteoarthritis, osteitis condensans ilii

**Generalized disease**: gout, hyperparathyroidism, Paget's disease, paraplegia, neoplastic metastases

**17. Name the radiographic view used to specifically visualize the sacroiliac joints.**

An **anteroposterior** projection of the pelvis (AP pelvis) is often sufficient to evaluate the inferior aspects of the sacroiliac joints. The **Ferguson** view (AP with the tube angled 25–30° cephalad) counteracts the overlap of the sacrum with the ilium, enabling a full view of the sacroiliac joint. This view is recognized because the symphysis pubis overlaps the sacrum.

**18. Describe the natural course of AS.**

Although the course is variable, most patients have a satisfactory functional outcome and maintain the ability to work. Factors that may influence overall prognosis include cervical spine ankylosis, hip joint involvement, uveitis, cardiovascular involvement, pulmonary fibrosis, and a persistent elevation of the sedimentation rate. It is likely that patients with mild AS have a normal life expectancy.

**19. Which medications are helpful in the management of AS?**

Although there is no cure for AS, most patients can be managed by controlling inflammatory symptoms and participating in an exercise program to minimize deformity and disability. The following modalities are helpful:

**NSAIDs**. Indomethacin is the most widely used NSAID for AS. Other NSAIDs may also be beneficial, and the choice is balanced by tolerance and effectiveness. Simple analgesics can be added for additional pain relief but should not be used as primary therapy.

**Second-line treatment**. Sulfasalazine (1500 mg bid) may be beneficial in patients with early progressive disease with peripheral arthritis. Although not well studied, low-dose weekly methotrexate therapy may benefit patients with prominent peripheral joint involvement.

**Corticosteroids**. Oral corticosteroids have *no* value in the treatment of the musculoskeletal aspects of AS. Local corticosteroid injections are useful in the treatment of enthesopathies and recalcitrant peripheral synovitis.

**Other treatments**. Preliminary studies suggest that anti-TNF-α therapy is effective in AS. It remains to be determined if this therapy prevents ankylosis. Bisphosphonates should be considered in AS patients with osteoporosis secondary to their inflammatory disease. Anterior uveitis can usually be managed with dilation of the pupil and corticosteriod eye drops.

**20. How is physiotherapy used in AS?**

Daily exercises need to be performed to maintain good posture and chest expansion and to minimize deformities. Hydrotherapy (swimming) provides the best environment to maximize the exercise program. Patients should sleep on a firm mattress on their back or in the prone position without a pillow in order to prevent progressive deformity. Cigarette smoking should be avoided in light of potential diminished chest expansion and apical lobe fibrosis.

**21. When is surgery indicated in AS?**

Total hip replacement is indicated in the setting of severe pain and limitation of motion. Bisphosphonates may be used for 3 months after surgery to prevent postoperative calcifications around the prosthesis. Vertebral wedge osteotomy to correct severe kyphotic deformities in some patients may be warranted, but it carries the risk of operative neurologic damage. Cardiac manifestations of AS may require aortic valve replacement or pacemaker insertion.

## BIBLIOGRAPHY


1. Boushea DK, Sundstrom WR: The pleuropulmonary manifestations of ankylosing spondylitis. Semin Arthritis Rheum 18:277–281, 1989.
2. Braun J, Haibel H, Cronely D, et al: Successful treatment of active ankylosing spondylitis with the anti-tumor necrosis factor α monoclonal antibody infliximab. Arthritis Rheum 43:1346–1352, 2000.
3. Brown M, Wordsworth P: Predisposing factors to spondyloarthropathies. Curr Opin Rheumatol 9:308–314, 1997.
4. Brown MA, Kennedy LG, MacGregor AJ, et al: Susceptibility to ankylosing spondylitis in twins: The role of genes, HLA, and the environment. Arthritis Rheum 40:1823–1828, 1997.
5. González S, Martinez-Bora J, Lopez-Larrea C: Immunogenetics. HLA-B27 and spondyloarthropathies. Curr Opin Rheumatol 11:257–264, 1999.
6. Gran JT, Husby G: Ankylosing spondylitis in women. Semin Arthritis Rheum 19:303–312, 1990.
7. Gran JT, Husby G: The epidemiology of ankylosing spondylitis. Semin Arthritis Rheum 22:319–334, 1993.
8. Haslock I: Spondyloarthropathies: Ankylosing spondylitis: Management. In Klippel JH, Dieppe PA (eds): Rheumatology, 2nd ed. London, Mosby, 1998, pp 6.19.1–6.19.10.
9. Hunter T: The spinal complications of ankylosing spondylitis. Semin Arthritis Rheum 19:172–182, 1989.
10. Inman RD: Seronegative spondyloarthropathies: D. Treatment. In Klippel JH (ed): Primer on the Rheumatic Diseases, 11th ed. Atlanta, Arthritis Foundation, 1997, pp 193–195.
11. Khan MA: Seronegative spondyloarthropathies: C. Ankylosing spondylitis. In Klippel JH (ed): Primer on the Rheumatic Diseases, 11th ed. Atlanta, Arthritis Foundation, 1997, pp 189–195.
12. Khan MA: Spondyloarthropathies: Ankylosing spondylitis: Clinical features. In Klippel JH, Dieppe PA (eds): Rheumatology, 2nd ed. London, Mosby, 1998, pp 6.16.1–6.16.10.
13. O'Neill TW, Breshnihan B: The heart in ankylosing spondylitis. Ann Rheum Dis 51:705–706, 1992.
14. Oostveen J, Prevo R, den Boer J, van de Laar M: Early detection of sacroiliitis on magnetic resonance imaging and subsequent development of sacroiliitis on plain radiography: A prospective, longitudinal study. J Rheumatol 26:1953–1958, 1999.
15. van der Linden S, van der Heijde D: Spondyloarthopathies: Ankylosing spondylitis. In Ruddy S, Harris ED Jr, Sledge CB (eds): Kelley's Textbook of Rheumatology, 6th ed. Philadelphia, W.B. Saunders, 2001, pp 1039–1053.


# 39. RHEUMATIC MANIFESTATIONS OF GASTROINTESTINAL AND HEPATOBILIARY DISEASES

*Sterling* G. *West*, M.D.

## ENTEROPATHIC ARTHRITIDES

**1. What bowel diseases are associated with inflammatory arthritis?**

- Idiopathic, inflammatory bowel disease (ulcerative colitis, Crohn's disease) and pouchitis
- Microscopic colitis and collagenous colitis
- Infectious gastroenteritis
- Whipple's disease
- Gluten-sensitive enteropathy (celiac disease)
- Intestinal bypass arthritis

**2. How often does an inflammatory peripheral and/or spinal arthritis occur in patients with idiopathic inflammatory bowel disease?**

| | ULCERATIVE COLITIS | CROHN'S DISEASE |
|---|---|---|
| Peripheral arthritis | 10% | 20% |
| Sacroiliitis | 15% | 15% |
| Sacroiliitis/spondylitis | 5% | 5% |

**3. What are the most common joints involved in ulcerative colitis (UC) and Crohn's disease?**

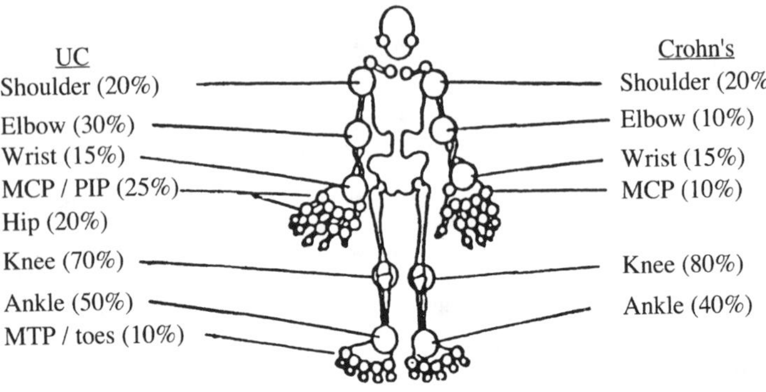


Upper extremity and small joint involvement are more common in UC than in Crohn's disease. Both UC and Crohn's-related arthritis affect the knee and ankle predominantly.

**4. Describe the clinical characteristics of the inflammatory peripheral arthritis associated with idiopathic inflammatory bowel disease (IBD).**

The arthritis occurs equally in males and females, and children are affected as commonly as adults. The arthritis is typically acute in onset, migratory, asymmetric, and pauciarticular (usually involves < 5 joints). Synovial fluid analysis reveals an inflammatory fluid with up to 50,000 white blood cells/mm$^3$ (predominantly neutrophils) and negative crystal examination and cultures. Most arthritic episodes resolve in 1–2 months and do not result in radiographic changes or deformities.

**5. What other extraintestinal manifestations commonly occur with idiopathic IBD and inflammatory peripheral arthritis?**

**P** Pyoderma gangrenosum (< 5%)
**A** Aphthous stomatitis (< 10%)
**I** Inflammatory eye disease (acute anterior uveitis) (5–15%)
**N** Nodosum (erythema) (< 10%)

**6. Do the extent and activity of the IBD and the activity of the peripheral inflammatory arthritis show any correlation?**

Ulcerative colitis and Crohn's disease patients are more likely to develop a peripheral arthritis if the colon is extensively involved. Most arthritic attacks occur during the first few years following onset of the bowel disease. The episodes coincide with flares of bowel disease in 60–70% of patients. Occasionally, the arthritis may precede symptoms of IBD, especially in children with Crohn's disease. Consequently, lack of gastrointestinal symptoms or even a negative stool guaiac test does not exclude the possibility of occult Crohn's disease in a patient who presents with a characteristic arthritis!

**7. What are the clinical characteristics of the inflammatory spinal arthritis occurring in idiopathic IBD?**

The clinical characteristics and course of spinal arthritis in IBD are similar to those for ankylosing spondylitis.

- Inflammatory spinal arthritis occurs more commonly in males than females (3:1).
- Patients complain of back pain and prolonged stiffness, particularly at night and upon awakening. This improves with exercise and movement.
- Physical examination reveals sacroiliac joint tenderness, global loss of spinal motion, and sometimes reduced chest expansion.

**8. Does the activity of inflammatory spinal arthritis correlate with the activity of the IBD?**

No. The onset of sacroiliitis/spondylitis can precede by years, occur concurrently, or follow by years the onset of IBD. Furthermore, the course of the spinal arthritis is completely independent of the course of the IBD.

**9. What human leukocyte antigen (HLA) occurs more commonly than expected with inflammatory arthritis secondary to IBD?**

HLA-B27. Eight percent of a normal healthy Caucasian population has the HLA-B27 gene, but a patient with IBD who possesses the HLA-B27 gene has a 7–10 times increased risk of developing an inflammatory sacroiliitis/spondylitis compared with IBD patients who are HLA-B27 negative.

*Frequency of HLA-B27 in IBD*

| | CROHN'S | UC |
|---|---|---|
| Sacroiliitis/spondylitis | 55% | 70% |
| Peripheral arthritis | Same as normal healthy control population | |

**10. What are the typical radiographic features of inflammatory sacroiliitis and spondylitis in IBD patients?**

They are similar to those of ankylosing spondylitis. (See Chapter 38.)

**11. What other rheumatic problems occur with increased frequency in IBD patients?**

- Achilles tendinitis/plantar fasciitis
- Clubbing (5%)
- Hypertrophic osteoarthropathy
- Psoas abscess or septic hip from fistula formation (Crohn's disease)
- Osteoporosis secondary to medications (i.e., prednisone)
- Vasculitis
- Amyloidosis

**12. What serologic abnormalities are seen in patients with inflammatory bowel disease?**

- Erythrocyte sedimentation rate (ESR) is elevated, while rheumatoid factor and ANA are negative.
- Antineutrophil cytoplasmic antibody (ANCA)—up to 50–60% of ulcerative colitis patients can have pANCA, which is directed against bactericidal permeability increasing protein (BPI), cathepsin G, lactoferrin, lysozyme, or elastase but not myeloperoxidase (MPO).
- Up to 50% of Crohn's disease patients can have antibodies against *Saccharomyces cerevisiae*.

**13. Which treatments are effective for alleviating symptoms of inflammatory peripheral arthritis and/or sacroiliitis/spondylitis in IBD patients?**

*Treatment of IBD-Related Inflammatory Peripheral or Spinal Arthritis*

| | PERIPHERAL ARTHRITIS | SACROILIITIS/SPONDYLITIS |
|---|---|---|
| NSAIDs* | Yes | Yes |
| Intra-articular corticosteroids | Yes | Yes (sacroiliitis) |
| Sulfasalazine | Yes | Maybe |
| Immunosuppressive medication | Yes | No |
| Antitumor necrosis factor α | Yes | Yes |
| Bowel resection | | |
| UC | Yes | No |
| Crohn's | No | No |

* Nonsteroidal anti-inflammatory drugs (NSAIDs) may exacerbate IBD.

**14. What rheumatic disorders have been associated with pouchitis, microscopic (lymphocytic) colitis (MC), and collagenous colitis (CC)?**

| | POUCHITIS | MC | CC |
|---|---|---|---|
| IBD-like peripheral inflammatory arthritis | Yes | Yes | Yes (10%) |
| Rheumatoid arthritis | No | Yes | Yes |
| Ankylosing spondylitis | No | Yes* | No |
| Thyroiditis/other autoimmune disease | No | Yes | Yes |

* Up to 50% of ankylosing spondylitis patients have asymptomatic microscopic colitis/Crohn's like lesions on right-sided colon biopsies.

**15. Why are patients with IBD prone to develop an inflammatory arthritis?**

One theory is that environmental antigens capable of inciting rheumatic disorders gain entry to the body's circulation by traversing the respiratory mucosa, skin, or gastrointestinal (GI) mucosa. The human GI tract has an estimated surface area of 1000 $m^2$ and functions not only to absorb nutrients but also to exclude potentially harmful antigens. The gut-associated lymphoid tissue (GALT), which includes Peyer's patches, the lamina propria, and intraepithelial T cells, constitutes 25% of the GI mucosa and helps to prevent entry of bacteria and other foreign antigens. Although the upper GI tract is normally not exposed to microbes, the lower GI tract is constantly in contact with millions of bacteria (up to $10^{12}$/g of feces). Inflammation, whether from idiopathic IBD or infection with pathogenic microorganisms, can disrupt the normal integrity and function of the bowel, leading to increased gut permeability. This increased permeability may allow **nonviable** bacterial antigens in the gut lumen to enter the circulation more easily. These microbial antigens could then either deposit directly in the joint synovia, leading to a local inflammatory reaction, or cause a systemic immune response, resulting in immune complexes that could then deposit in joints and other tissues.

**16. What rheumatic manifestations have been described in patients with celiac disease (gluten-sensitive enteropathy)?**

- Arthritis—symmetric polyarthritis involving predominantly large joints (knees and ankles > hips and shoulders). May precede enteropathic symptoms in 50% of cases.
- Osteomalacia due to steatorrhea from severe enteropathy
- Dermatitis herpetiformis

**17. What human leukocyte antigen (HLA) is more common in celiac disease patients than in normal healthy controls?**

HLA-DR3/DQ2, frequently in association with HLA-B8, is seen in 95% of celiac disease patients compared with 12% of the normal population.

**18. How is the diagnosis of celiac disease made?**

The gold standard is jejunal biopsy showing villous atrophy. However, autoantibody testing is very helpful in screening individuals prior to biopsy. During the acute phase, IgA antibodies against endomysium/tissue transglutaminase have a greater than 90% sensitivity and specificity for celiac disease. IgG antigliadin antibodies are 90% sensitive but seen in 10–15% of patients without celiac disease. IgA antigliadin antibodies are less sensitive (70%) but more specific (80–85%).

**19. How is the arthritis occurring in celiac disease treated?**

The arthritis responds to a **gluten-free diet** in 40% of cases.

**20. What is the intestinal bypass arthritis-dermatitis syndrome?**

This syndrome occurs in 20–80% of patients who have undergone intestinal bypass (jejunoileal or jejunocolic) surgery for morbid obesity. The arthritis is inflammatory, polyarticular, symmetric, and frequently migratory, and it affects both upper and lower extremity joints. Radiographs usually remain normal despite 25% of patients having chronic recurring episodes of arthritis. Up to 80% develop dermatologic abnormalities, the most characteristic of which is a maculopapular or vesiculopustular rash. The pathogenesis involves bacterial overgrowth in the blind loop, resulting in antigenic stimulation causing immune complex formation (frequently cryoprecipitates containing bacterial antigens), which may deposit in the joints and skin. Treatment includes NSAIDs and oral antibiotics, which usually improve symptoms. Only surgical reanastomosis of the blind loop can result in complete elimination of symptoms.

**21. What types of arthritis can be associated with carcinomas of the esophagus and colon?**

Carcinomatous polyarthritis can be the presenting feature of an occult malignancy of the GI tract. The arthritis is typically acute in onset, asymmetric, and predominantly involves lower extremity joints while sparing the small joints of the hands and wrists. Patients have an elevated ESR and a negative rheumatoid factor. Another type of arthritis associated with colorectal malignancy is septic arthritis due to *Streptococcus bovis*.

## RHEUMATIC SYNDROMES AND PANCREATIC DISEASE

**22. What pancreatic diseases have been associated with rheumatic syndromes?**

Pancreatitis, pancreatic carcinoma, and pancreatic insufficiency.

**23. What are the clinical features of the pancreatic panniculitis syndrome?**

Pancreatic panniculitis is a systemic syndrome occurring in some patients with pancreatitis or pancreatic acinar cell carcinoma. Its clinical manifestations include:

- Tender, red nodules, usually on the extremities, which are frequently misdiagnosed as erythema nodosum but really are areas of panniculitis with fat necrosis.
- Arthritis (60%) and arthralgias, usually of the ankles and knees. Synovial fluid is typically noninflammatory and creamy in color, and it contains lipid droplets that stain with Sudan black or oil red O.
- Eosinophilia
- Osteolytic bone lesions from bone marrow necrosis (10%), pleuropericarditis, fever

A good way to remember the manifestations is the mnemonic PANCREAS:

**P**ancreatitis
**A**rthritis

**N**odules secondary to fat necrosis
**C**ancer of the pancreas
**R**adiographic abnormalities (osteolytic lesions of bone)
**E**osinophilia
**A**mylase, lipase, and trypsin elevations
**S**erositis, including pleuropericarditis

**24. What causes the pancreatic panniculitis syndrome?**

Skin and synovial biopsies show fat necrosis, which is caused by release of trypsin, amylase, and lipase from the diseased pancreas.

**25. What other musculoskeletal problem can occur with pancreatic insufficiency?**

Osteomalacia due to fat-soluble vitamin D malabsorption.

## RHEUMATIC SYNDROMES AND HEPATOBILIARY DISEASE

**26. What is lupoid hepatitis?**

Lupoid hepatitis is now called type I autoimmune hepatitis (AIH). Patients are young (< age 40), predominantly female (70%), and have clinical (arthralgias) and laboratory manifestations that resemble systemic lupus erythematosus (SLE). Patients commonly have positive antinuclear antibodies (ANA), antibodies against smooth muscle antigen (F1 actin), and occasionally LE cells.

**27. To what degree is lupoid hepatitis (type I AIH) similar to SLE?**

*Comparison of Lupoid Hepatitis and SLE*

| | SLE | LUPOID HEPATITIS (TYPE I AIH) |
|---|---|---|
| Young women | + | + |
| Polyarthritis | + | + |
| Fever | + | + |
| Nephritis | + | – |
| Central nervous system disease | + | – |
| Photosensitivity | + | – |
| Oral ulcers | + | – |
| ANA | 99% | 70–90% |
| LE cells | 70% | 40–50% |
| Polyclonal gammopathy | + | + |
| Anti-Smith antibodies | 25% | 0 |
| + anti-ds DNA | 70% | Rare—40% |
| + anti-FI actin | Rare | 60–95% |

**28. What is the difference between anti-Sm and anti-SM antibodies?**

Anti-Sm antibodies are antibodies against the Smith antigen, which is an epitope on small nuclear ribonuclear proteins. It is highly diagnositc of SLE. Anti-SM antibody is an antibody against the smooth muscle antigen (FI actin). It is highly diagnostic of auotimmune hepatitis.

*Anti-Sm vs. Anti-SM Antibodies*

| | SLE | AUTOIMMUNE HEPATITIS |
|---|---|---|
| Anti-Smith (Sm) antibodies | Yes | No |
| Anti-Smooth muscle (SM) antibodies | No | Yes |

**29. List the common autoimmune diseases associated with primary biliary cirrhosis (PBC).**

Up to 80% of patients with PBC have one or more of the following disorders:

- Keratoconjunctivitis sicca (Sjögren's syndrome) 66%
- Autoimmune thyroiditis (Hashimoto's disease) 20%
- Scleroderma/Raynaud's disease* 20%
- Rheumatoid arthritis 10%

* CREST occurs in 4% of PBC patients and antedates PBC by 14 years.

**30. Compare and contrast the arthritis that may occur with PBC and rheumatoid arthritis.**

*PBC Arthritis vs. Rheumatoid Arthritis*

| | PBC ARTHRITIS | RHEUMATOID ARTHRITIS |
|---|---|---|
| Frequency in patients with PBC | 10% | 10% |
| Number of joints | Polyarticular | Polyarticular |
| Symmetry | Symmetric | Symmetric |
| Inflammatory | Yes | Yes |
| Rheumatoid factor | Sometimes | Yes (85%) |
| Erosions on radiograph | Rare | Common |

**31. What other musculoskeletal manifestations may occur in patients with PBC?**

- Osteomalacia due to fat-soluble vitamin D malabsorption
- Osteoporosis due to renal tubular acidosis
- Hypertrophic osteoarthropathy

**32. What autoantibodies commonly occur in patients with PBC?**

- Antimitochondrial antibodies 80%*
- Anticentromere antibodies 20%**

* The most specific antimitochondrial antibody for PBC is the M2 antibody directed against the E2 subunit of the pyruvate dehydrogenase complex on the inner mitochondrial membrane.

** Most patients also have manifestations of the CREST variant of scleroderma. (CREST = calcinosis, Raynaud's phenomenon, esophageal disease, sclerodactyly, and telangiectasia.)

**33. What dose adjustments need to be made for antirheumatic medications in patients with severe hepatobiliary disease?**

Severe liver disease can be defined as a combination of one or more of the following factors: elevated bilirubin > 3 mg/dl, albumin < 3 gm/dl with ascites, elevated protime not fully corrected by vitamin K, and/or cirrhosis on liver biopsy. Elevated transaminases greater than 3 times upper limit of normal should also be a concern. Also note that since creatine is synthesized in the liver, serum creatinine may be an overestimate of renal function.

Hepatobiliary disease may substantially impair the elimination or activation of drugs that the liver metabolizes or excretes. Although glucuronidation is spared, oxidation and acetylation are slowed. In addition, decreased synthesis of albumin may lead to increased free fraction of the active drug. Decreased synthesis of vitamin K–dependent clotting factors may lead to increased risk of bleeding if a medication affects platelet function or number.

The following are guidelines for antirheumatic drug therapy in severe liver disease:

- **Pro drug metabolism**—azathioprine, leflunomide, cyclophosphamide, prednisone, and sulindac need to be converted to active moiety by the liver. This is impaired in patients with severe hepatic insufficiency. Consequently, these drugs should be avoided or replaced with active form (i.e., 6-mercaptopurine, prednisolone).
- **Biliary excretion**—methotrexate, cyclosporine, colchicine, leflunomide, indocin, and sulindac are excreted in the bile and undergo enterohepatic circulation. These should be avoided in patients with impaired biliary function.

- **Change in drug dosage for severe liver disease**
  Antimalarials: Use with caution at lower doses.
  Anti-TNFα: Probably safe.
  Allopurinol: Little data. Use with caution. Can cause severe hepatitis.
  Azathioprine: Use 6-mercaptopurine instead.
  Bisphosphonates: Probably safe.
  Colchicine: Avoid.
  Cyclophosphamide: May not be converted to active form.
  Cyclosporine: Eliminated by liver, so avoid.
  Intramuscular gold: Use with some caution.
  Leflunomide: Avoid.
  Methotrexate: Avoid.
  Mycophenylate mofetil: No dosage change, but don't exceed 2 grams a day.
  Narcotics: Most metabolized by liver. Need to lower dose or extend interval. Avoid meperidine.
  NSAIDs: Lower dose 50%. Avoid diclofenac, sulindac, and indomethacin.
  Penicillamine: Probably safe.
  Prednisone: Use prednisolone instead.
  Sulfasalazine: Probably safe, but can cause hepatic failure rarely.
  Tramadol: Double dosing interval from 6 to 12 hours.

## BIBLIOGRAPHY

1. Balbir-Gurman A, Schapira D, Nahir M: Arthritis related to ileal pouchitis following total proctocolectomy for ulcerative colitis. Semin Arthritis Rheum 30:242–248, 2001.
2. Culp KS, Fleming CR, Duffy J, et al: Autoimmune associations and primary biliary cirrhosis. Mayo Clin Proc 57:365–370, 1982.
3. Dahl PR, Su WPD, Cullimore KC, Dicken CH: Pancreatic panniculitis. J Am Acad Dermatol 33:413–417, 1995.
4. Duffy J: Arthritis and liver disease. In Koopman W (ed): Arthritis and Allied Conditions, 14th ed. Philadelphia, Lea & Febiger, 2001, pp 1383–1399
5. Fomberstein B, Yerra N, Pitchumoni CS: Rheumatological complications of GI disorders. Amer J Gastroenterology 91:1090–1103, 1996.
6. Hall S, Czaja AJ, Kaufman DK, et al: How lupoid is lupoid hepatitis? J Rheumatol 13:95–98, 1986.
7. Keyser FD, Elewaut D, Devos M, et al: Bowel inflammation and the spondyloarthropathies. Rheumatic Dis Clinics North Amer 24:785–814, 1998.
8. Lubrano E, Cicacci C, Amers PR, et al: The arthritis of coeliac disease: Prevalence and pattern in 200 adult patients. Br J Rheumatol 35:1314–1318, 1996.
9. Makinen D, Fritzler M, Davis P, Sherlock S: Anticentromere antibodies in primary biliary cirrhosis. Arthritis Rheum 26:914–917, 1983.
10. Marx WJ, O'Connell DJ: Arthritis of primary biliary cirrhosis. Arch Intern Med 139:213–216, 1979.
11. Naschitz JE, Rosner I, Rozenbaum M, et al: Cancer associated rheumatoid disorders: Clues to occult neoplasia. Semin Arthritis Rheum 24:231–241, 1995.
12. Roubenoff R, Ratain J, Giardiello I, et al: Collagenous colitis, enteropathic arthritis, and autoimmune diseases: Results of a patient survey. J Rheumatol 16:1229–1232, 1989.
13. Schnabel A, Csernok E, Schultz H, et al: Bactericidal permeability increasing protein (BPI)-ANCA marked chronic inflammatory bowel diseases and hepatobiliary diseases. Med Klin 92:389–393, 1997.
14. Veloso FT, Carvalho J, Magro F: Immune-related systemic manifestations of inflammatory bowel disease: A prospective study of 792 patients. J Clin Gastroenterol 23:29–34, 1996.
15. Wands JR, LaMont TJ, Mann BS, et al: Arthritis associated with intestinal bypass procedure for morbid obesity: Complement activation and characterization of circulatory cryoproteins. N Engl J Med 294:121–124, 1976.

# 40. REITER'S SYNDROME AND REACTIVE ARTHRITIDES

Richard T. Meehan, M.D.

**1. What is Reiter's syndrome?**

As originally described in 1916, Reiter's syndrome is the clinical triad of urethritis, conjunctivitis, and arthritis following an infectious dysentery. Reiter's syndrome is now considered to be a form of reactive arthritis because two-thirds of patients do not have all three features of this triad.

**2. Define "reactive" arthritis.**

Reactive arthritis (ReA) is a sterile inflammatory synovitis following an infection by organisms that infect mucosal surfaces, especially urogenital or enteric infections. The clinical features of reactive arthritis among HLA-B27 positive patients are similar to those found in other seronegative spondyloarthropathies, whereas HLA-B27 negative patients usually resemble patients presenting with an undifferentiated oligoarthritis. ReA patients commonly exhibit systemic symptoms with unique extra-articular manifestations including skin, eye, and enthesopathy features.

**3. How is reactive arthritis acquired?**

Susceptibility to reactive arthritis may be conferred by specific class I major histocompatibility antigens (e.g., HLA-B27). However, its acquisition is strictly dependent on infection with certain gastrointestinal (enterogenic) or genitourinary (urogenital) pathogens. The most common organisms associated with disease among HLA-B27 patients include *Salmonella*, *Shigella*, *Yersinia*, *Chlamydia*, *Campylobacter* and *Clostridium*. Many studies using electron microscopy, molecular amplification and immunofluorescence techniques have identified microbacterial products including nucleic acids within the synovium of these patients.

**4. What infectious agents "cause" ReA?**

| | |
|---|---|
| Urogenital | ***Chlamydia*** trachomatis, *Ureaplasma urealyticum* |
| Enterogenic | ***Salmonella*** *typhimurium, S. enteritidis, S. heidelberg, S. cholerae-suis* |
| | ***Shigella*** *flexneri, S. sonnei* |
| | ***Yersinia*** *enterocolitica, Y. pseudotuberculosis* |
| | ***Campylobacter*** *jejuni* |
| Others | *Clostridium difficile* |
| | *Chlamydia pneumoniae* |
| | *Vibrio parahaemolyticus* |
| | *Borrelia burgdorferi* |
| | *Neisseria gonorrhoeae* |
| | *Streptococcus* (post-Streptococcal reactive arthritis) |
| | Hepatitis C |
| | *Giardia lamblia* |
| | *Mycoplasma* |

**5. Who gets reactive arthritis?**

Primarily young adults, ages 20–40 years. Patients with enterogenic reactive arthritis exhibit equal sex distribution, while those with the urogenital form are predominantly male. Reactive arthritis is rare in children and uncommon in blacks. Reiter's syndrome is the most common type of inflammatory arthritis affecting young adult males.

**6. After the initial infection, when do symptoms of reactive arthritis first appear?**

Though the initial infection may be mild or inapparent (10%), most patients will develop systemic symptoms within 1–4 weeks.

**7. List the extra-articular features associated with reactive arthritis.**

**Constitutional**
Low-grade fever
Weight loss (rare)

**Ocular**
Sterile conjunctivitis (60%)
Anterior uveitis (20%) (usually unilateral, HLA-B27+)

**Gastrointestinal**
Infectious ileitis/colitis
Sterile ileitis/colitis (60%)

**Cardiac** (rare in acute disease)
Heart block (1%)
Aortic regurgitation
Aortitis (1%)
Pericarditis

**Genitourinary**
Infectious urethritis
Sterile urethritis
Prostatitis (80%)
Hemorrhagic cystitis
Salpingitis, vulvovaginitis

**Mucocutaneous**
Circinate balanitis (30%)
Keratoderma blennorrhagicum (15%)
Hyperkeratotic nails (10%)
Painless oral ulcers (25%)

**Other**
Neuropathy (cranial or peripheral nerve)
IgA nephropathy
Renal amyloidosis
Thrombophlebitis, livedo reticularis
Erythema nodosum (*Yersinia*)

**8. What two cutaneous lesions are characteristic of Reiter's syndrome?**

**Circinate balanitis** and **keratoderma blennorrhagicum** are relatively specific for Reiter's syndrome. Circinate balanitis is a **painless**, serpiginous ulceration of the glans penis. Similarly, keratoderma blennorrhagicum refers to psoriasiform lesions occurring primarily on the plantar surface of the heel and metatarsal heads. Both lesions are predominantly associated with urogenital reactive arthritis and resolve spontaneously.

**9. Describe the musculoskeletal manifestations of reactive arthritis.**

**Arthritis**. In reactive arthritis, the joints tend to be moderately inflamed and characterized by prolonged stiffness. Joint involvement is typically asymmetric, oligoarticular (< 5 joints), and confined to the knees, ankles, and/or feet. Upper limb arthritis (e.g., wrist and digits) may also occur. Joint erosions may result from chronic disease.

**Enthesitis** is an inflammation of the ligament, tendon, joint capsule, or fascia insertion site into bone (enthesis). In reactive arthritis, enthesitis commonly causes heel pain (Achilles tendon and plantar fascia), metatarsalgia (plantar fascia), and "sausage" digits (dactylitis).

**Spondylitis**. Forty percent of patients with reactive arthritis may have axial skeleton symptoms, and 25% get radiographic changes. The risk of developing sacroiliitis and/or spondylitis is related to disease chronicity and HLA-B27.

**10. What is the differential diagnosis for reactive arthritis?**

| MOST LIKELY | LESS LIKELY |
|---|---|
| Gonococcal arthritis | Ankylosing spondylitis |
| Acute septic arthritis | Rheumatic fever |
| Psoriatic arthritis | Gout/pseudogout |
| Inflammatory bowel disease arthritis | Lyme disease |
| Rheumatoid arthritis | Behçet's syndrome |

In addition, reactive arthritis must always be considered as a possible complication of hepatitis C and HIV infection.

**11. Compare the clinical features of Reiter's syndrome with gonococcal arthritis.**

| FEATURE | REITER'S | GONOCOCCAL |
|---|---|---|
| Sex ratio | Male > female | Female > male |
| Age | 20–40 yrs | All ages, most 20–40 yrs |
| Migratory arthralgias | No | Yes |
| Arthritis | Lower limbs | Upper limbs, knees |
| Enthesitis | Yes | No |
| Spondylitis | Yes | No |
| Tenosynovitis | Yes | Yes |
| Dactylitis | Yes | No |
| Urethritis | Yes | Yes |
| Uveitis | Yes | No |
| Oral ulcers | Yes | No |
| Cutaneous lesions | Keratoderma, balanitis | Pustules |
| Culture positive | No | Yes (< 50%) |
| HLA-B27 positive | Yes (80%) | Same as rest of population (7%) |
| Penicillin responsive | No | Yes |

**12. Compare the clinical features of Reiter's syndrome with rheumatoid arthritis.**

| FEATURE | REITER'S SYNDROME | RA |
|---|---|---|
| Sex ratio | Male > female | Female > male |
| Age | 20–40 yrs | All ages |
| Arthritis | Oligoarticular<br>Large joints (asymmetric) | Polyarticular<br>MCP, PIP wrists, MTP (symmetric) |
| Enthesitis | Yes | No |
| Spondylitis | Yes | No |
| Ocular disease | Conjunctivitis, uveitis | Keratitis, scleromalacia |
| Lung disease | No | Yes |
| Urethritis | Yes | No |
| Cutaneous lesions | Keratoderma, balanitis | subcutaneous nodules, vasculitis |
| Rheumatoid factor positive | No | Yes (85%) |
| HLA association | HLA-B27 (80% of Caucasian males) | HLA-DR4 (70%) |

**13. Which laboratory investigations are useful in confirming the diagnosis of reactive arthritis?**

The diagnosis of reactive arthritis is clinical, and no laboratory investigation can substitute for a proper history and physical exam. However, they can be used in confirming the clinical diagnosis. Arthrocentesis is the most valuable test, since it excludes septic and crystalline arthritis.

| | *Expected Result* |
|---|---|
| **Primary (essential)** | |
| ESR and or CRP | Elevation |
| Complete blood count and differential | Polymorphonuclear leukocytosis<br>Thrombocytosis and anemia |
| Rheumatoid factor | Negative |
| Urinalysis | Pyuria, +/- bacteria |
| Synovial fluid analysis | Moderate leukocytosis<br>Neg Gram stain and no crystals |
| Cultures | |
| Throat | (+/-) culture |
| Urine | (+/-) culture |
| Stool | (+/-) culture |
| Synovial fluid | Neg culture |
| Urethra/cervix | (+/-) culture |
| **Secondary (optional)** | |
| Antinuclear antibody | Negative |
| Antibody serology | Positive (e.g., *Yersinia* and *Chlamydia*) |
| Blood cultures | Negative, unless septic |
| Radiographs | |
| Peripheral joints | Arthritis, enthesitis |
| Axial joints | Spondylitis, enthesitis |
| Anteroposterior pelvis | Sacroiliitis |
| Electrocardiogram | Heart block |
| Colonoscopy | Ileitis/colitis |

**14. What are the usual synovial fluid findings from a patient with reactive arthritis?**

The synovial fluid typically reveals a predominance of leukocytes, ranging from 5000–50,000 cells/mm$^3$. In acute reactive arthritis, most of these cells are neutrophils, but in chronic disease, either lymphocytes or monocytes may be prevalent.

Other synovial fluid characteristics include decreased viscosity, normal glucose level, and increased protein. Large, vacuolar macrophages (Reiter's cells), containing intact lymphocytes or fragmented nuclei, are occasionally seen but are not specific for reactive arthritis.

**15. Describe the radiographic features seen in patients with reactive arthritis.**

Remember your **ABCDE'S**. These radiographic features are typical of all seronegative spondyloarthropathies.

**A—Ankylosis** of the spine occurs in up to 20% of patients. There are large, nonmarginal syndesmophytes, called "jug-handle" syndesmophytes, which usually occur in an asymmetric distribution. These syndesmophytes can also occur in psoriatic spondylitis but differ from the thin, marginal, bilateral syndesmophytes seen in ankylosing spondylitis.

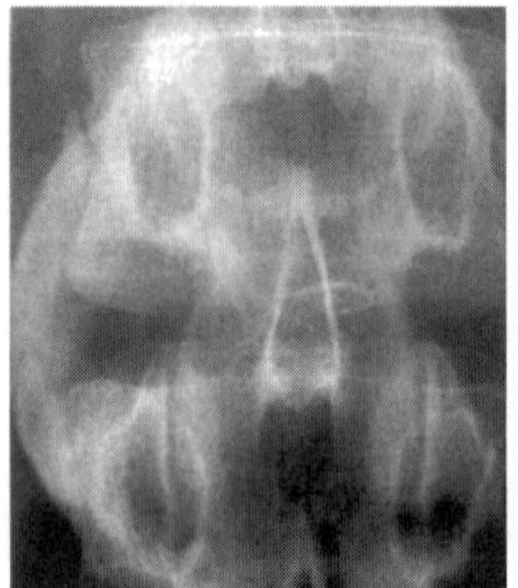

Radiograph of spine showing a large "jug-handle" syndesmophyte.

B—**Bony reactivity** and proliferation at enthesis sites (Achilles tendon and plantar fascia insertions) and periostitis are common. Ossification of tendons may occur. **Bone demineralization (osteopenia)** may be observed in a periarticular distribution compatible with an inflammatory arthritis.

C—**Cartilage**-space narrowing occurs uniformly across the joint space of weight-bearing joints compatible with an inflammatory arthritis. No abnormal cartilage or soft tissue **calcifications** are seen.

D—**Distribution** of arthritis is primarily in the lower extremity, whereas psoriatic arthritis usually affects the upper extremity. The sentinel joint involved may be the interphalangeal joint of the great toe.

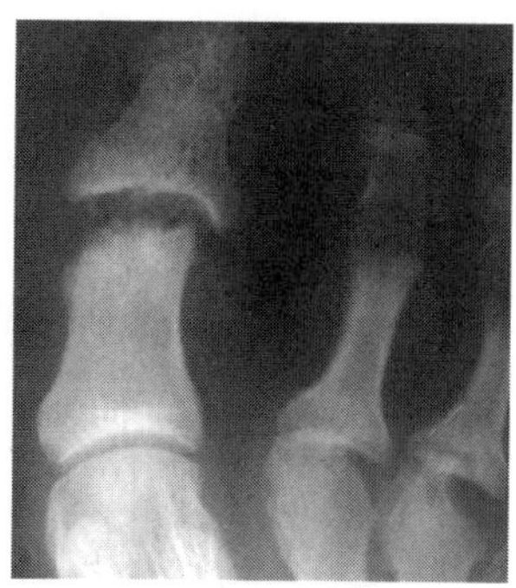

Radiograph of foot in a patient with Reiter' s syndrome showing erosions of the interphalangeal joint of the great toe and second and third MTP joints.

E—**Erosions** are common in the metatarsophalangeal joints (MTPs). Sacroiliac joint erosions tend to involve one sacroiliac joint more than the other (asymmetric), which contrasts to the symmetric involvement of ankylosing spondylitis.

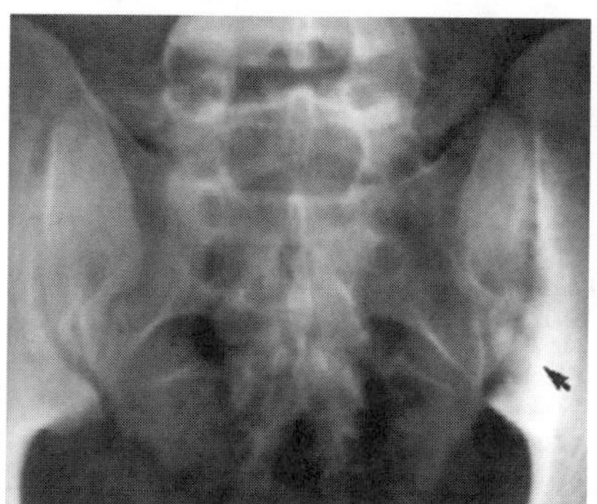

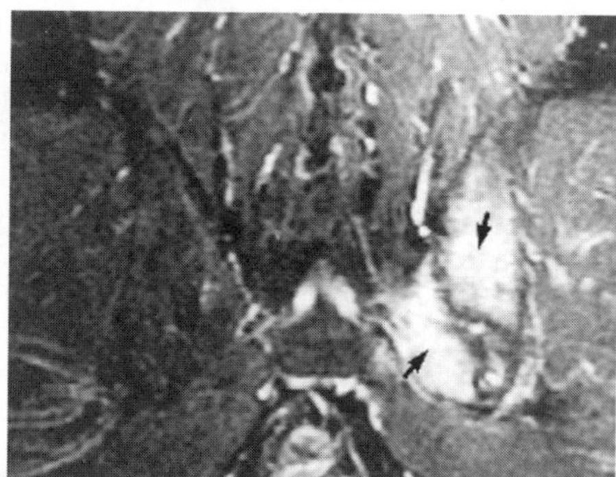

Radiograph (*left*) and MRI (*right*) of pelvis showing left sacroiliitis (arrows)

S—**Soft tissue** swelling and dactylitis (diffuse swelling of toes). Psoriatic arthritis causes dactylitis of the fingers more than toes.

**16. How do the radiographic features of sacroiliac and spine involvement in reactive arthritis compare with those in ankylosing spondylitis?**

| | ANKYLOSING SPONDYLITIS | REACTIVE ARTHRITIS |
|---|---|---|
| Sacroiliitis | Bilateral, symmetric | Unilateral or asymmetric |
| Spondylitis | Bilateral, thin, marginal syndesmophytes | Asymmetric, nonmarginal, "jug-handle" syndesmophytes |

Note that 100% of patients with ankylosing spondylitis develop radiographic changes in the sacroiliac joints, compared with only 25% of reactive arthritis patients. Patients with inflammatory bowel disease also develop radiographic changes of their spine similar in appearance to those of ankylosing spondylitis, whereas psoriatic arthritis produces changes similar to reactive arthritis.

**17. Is HLA-B27 determination useful?**

A sufficient number of patients with reactive arthritis will not be HLA-B27 positive, thus rendering HLA-B27 determination a poor diagnostic test in screening patients with low back pain, especially since 7% of the normal Caucasian population will be positive. Patients with reactive arthritis can usually be successfully diagnosed and managed without HLA-B27 determination. However, this test may be of value if the clinical picture is incomplete, such as in the absence of an antecedent infection or lack of extra-articular features. Many rheumatologists find it useful, however, to classify patients as having either "HLA-B27 associated" or "non-associated" forms of ReA. HLA-B27 status may have prognostic value, as positivity correlates with an increase in disease severity, chronicity, and frequency of exacerbations, as well as development of aortitis, uveitis, and spondylitis.

**18. Describe the nonpharmacologic management of reactive arthritis.**

Initial management begins with bed rest and splinting of the affected joints. Transient relief of joint inflammation may be obtained by use of ice packs and/or warm compresses. Once inflammation subsides (1–2 weeks), **passive** strengthening and range of motion exercises should be initiated. Progression to **active** exercises reduces the likelihood of muscle atrophy. Avoidance of behavior promoting reinfection is critical.

**19. Describe the pharmacologic management of reactive arthritis.**

**Infectious disease**. Elimination of the "triggering" infection with appropriate antibiotics is the first therapeutic goal in reactive arthritis. This is especially true for *Chlamydia* infections.

**Extra-articular disease**. The mucocutaneous features of reactive arthritis are usually self-limited and may require no specific therapy. Topical corticosteroids and keratolytic agents may help keratoderma blennorrhagicum. Symptoms of uveitis should be referred for ophthalmologic evaluation.

**Articular disease**. In most patients, reduction of inflammation and restoration of function can be achieved with NSAIDs alone. Indomethacin (150 mg/day) is the prototypic NSAID for treatment of reactive arthritis. Alternative NSAIDs (e.g., diclofenac) or cyclooxygenase 2 inhibitors may be necessary, owing to patient intolerance. Aspirin and propionic acid derivatives (e.g., ibuprofen) seem less effective and are not recommended for initial therapy.

Some patients with recurrent or chronic symptoms may require additional therapeutic measures for disease control. Intra-articular corticosteroids may be used judiciously to alleviate NSAID-resistant synovitis and sacroiliitis. Obviously, joint sepsis must be excluded prior to corticosteroid injection. Systemic corticosteroids are usually ineffective in reactive arthritis, but a therapeutic trial may be warranted in patients having resistant disease and disorders (e.g., AIDS) in which cytotoxic therapy is contraindicated. There is no cure for reactive arthritis.

**20. How do you treat refractory reactive arthritis?**

In most patients, remission of symptoms usually occurs within 2–6 months after disease onset. Patients experiencing symptom recurrence, persistence, and/or flare, despite adequate NSAID therapy, may require a disease-modifying agent. Sulfasalazine (2–3 gm/day) is the drug of choice for refractory reactive arthritis and may also be safely used in patients with HIV infection. Other disease-modifying agents, such as methotrexate, azathioprine, and cyclophosphamide, also have been used with variable success. TNF alpha blocking agents have been reported to be successful in some patients. In contrast, intra-muscular gold, antimalarials, and D-penicillamine seem ineffective.

**21. Should antibiotics be used in reactive arthritis? If so, for how long? (Controversial)**

Once an antecedent infection has triggered reactive arthritis, it is unlikely that antibiotics will affect the course of illness with the possible exception of *Chlamydia*-triggered ReA. Some rheumatologists advocate a 3-month trial of doxycycline or minocycline 100 mg bid for 3 months for *Chlamydia*-confirmed or suspected ReA. Antibiotic therapy for post-enteric associated ReA has not been demonstrated in trials to reduce severity of arthritis. The demonstration of bacterial cell wall antigens in synovial tissue suggests that bacterial antigens alone, *not* viable microorganisms, may perpetuate reactive arthritis. The beneficial effect of doxycycline or its analogues in some cases may also be due to the anti-inflammatory effects of this agent rather than exclusively any antibacterial activity.

**22. When should you suspect that reactive arthritis may be a complication of HIV infection?**

Reactive arthritis may be the first manifestation of HIV infection. Therefore, HIV antibody status and hepatitis serology should be determined when the appropriate risk factors and/or clinical features are present. Furthermore, patients with refractory reactive arthritis and risk factors for HIV should have antibody determination prior to the use of immunosuppressive agents.

**23. What is the prognosis for patients with reactive arthritis?**

Though the prognosis of reactive arthritis is variable, most patients fully recover from their initial illness. However, a significant number (15–50%) will have one or more recurrences of ocular disease, mucocutaneous lesions, and/or arthritis. Twenty percent of patients will manifest some form of chronic peripheral arthritis and/or axial skeleton disease. The spondylitis of reactive arthritis is common (15–30%) but typically mild. Factors such as reinfection, hip arthritis, ESR > 30 mm/hr, sausage digits, poor response to NSAIDs, genetic susceptibility (HLA-B27), and heel pain are associated with a poorer prognosis. In general, disability due to articular disease is related to responsiveness to medication in the absence of spontaneous remission. Overall, the long-term prognosis for post-dysenteric ReA is better than post-*Chlamydia* ReA.

ACKNOWLEDGMENT

The editor and author wish to thank Dr. Danny Williams for his contributions to this chapter in the previous edition.

## BIBLIOGRAPHY

1. Amor B: Reiter's syndrome diagnosis and clinical features. Rheum Dis Clin North Am 24:677, 1998.
2. Butler MDI, Russell AS, Percy JS, Lentil BC: A follow-up study of 48 patients with Reiter's syndrome. Am J Med 67:808, 1979.
3. Clegg DO, Redo DJ, Abdellatif M: Comparison of sulfasalazine and placebo for the treatment of axial and peripheral articular manifestations of the seronegative spondyloarthropathies. Arthritis Rheum 42:2325, 1999.
4. Dougados M, van der Linden S, Juhlin R, et al: The European Spondyloarthropathy Study Group preliminary criteria for the classification of spondyloarthropathy. Arthritis Rheum 34:1218, 1991.
5. Fox R, Calin A, Gerber RC, Gibson D: The chronicity of symptoms and disability in Reiter' s syndrome. Ann Intern Med 91:190, 1979.
6. Inman RD, Scofield RH: Etiopathogenesis of ankylosing spondylitis and reactive arthritis. Curr Opin Rheumatol 6:360, 1994.
7. Leirisalo-Repo M: Prognosis, course of disease, and treatment of the spondyloarthropathies. Rheum Dis Clin North Am 24:737, 1998.
8. Schumacher HR: Reactive arthritis. Rheum Dis Clin North Am 24:261,1998.
9. Sieper J, Fendler C, Laitko S, et al: No benefit of long-term ciprofloxacin treatment in patients with reactive arthritis and undifferentiated oligoarthritis. Arthritis Rheum 42:1386, 1999.
10. Toivanen A, Toivanen D: Reactive arthritis. Curr Opin Rheumatol 12:300–305,2000.
11. Yu DTY, Fan PT: Reiter' s syndrome and undifferentiated spondyloarthropathy. In Ruddy S, Harris EB, Sledge CB (eds): Kelley's Textbook of Rheumatology, 6th ed. Philadelphia, WB Saunders, 2001, p 1055.

# 41. ARTHRITIS ASSOCIATED WITH PSORIASIS AND OTHER SKIN DISEASES

*William* R. *Gilliland*, M.D.

**1. How prevalent is psoriasis and psoriatic arthritis in the general population?**

Epidemiologic studies suggest the prevalence of psoriasis is approximately 1.2%. While estimates of polyarthritis accompanying psoriasis range from 5–50%, major textbooks estimate the prevalence to be 5–7%. The prevalence of axial involvement is 2%.

**2. Do genetic factors play a role in psoriatic arthritis?**

Yes. Both family studies and HLA typing suggest a genetic predisposition to psoriatic arthritis. Moll and Wright found that first-degree relatives of psoriatic arthritis patients may be 50 times more likely to develop arthritis.

Certain HLA haplotypes are associated with various subsets of psoriatic arthritis. B38 and B39 are associated with peripheral arthritis, DR4 is associated with polyarthritis (rheumatoid-like), and B27 is associated with sacroiliitis and spondylitis.

**3. Does gender play a role in its prevalence?**

Unlike the classic connective tissue disorders such as systemic lupus erythematosus or rheumatoid arthritis, the overall prevalence of arthritis is relatively equal between the sexes. However, in patients with spinal involvement, the male to female ratio is almost 3:1. Men also tend to have a higher prevalence of DIP only involvement, while women tend to have a higher prevalence of symmetric polyarthritis.

**4. How old is the typical patient?**

Most patients present between the ages of 35 and 50. However, juvenile psoriatic arthritis is also well recognized and usually presents between ages 9 and 12.

**5. Is there a relationship between the onset of psoriasis and the onset of arthritis?**

| | |
|---|---|
| Psoriasis precedes arthritis | 67% |
| Arthritis precedes psoriasis or occurs simultaneously | 33% |

**6. If psoriasis is not obvious, what areas should be closely examined?**

Umbilicus, scalp, anus, and ears.

**7. Is there a relationship between the extent of skin involvement and arthritis?**

No particular pattern or extent of psoriasis is associated with arthritis. However, some suggest that arthritis is more deforming and widespread with extensive skin involvement.

**8. What are the characteristic patterns of joint involvement in psoriatic arthritis?**

Approximately 95% of patients with psoriatic arthritis have peripheral joint disease. Another 5% have axial spine involvement exclusively. In 1973, Moll and Wright divided psoriatic arthritis into five broad categories. In reality, they overlap, creating a heterogeneous combination of joint disease. (Even though several authors have advocated adding new subsets to Moll and Wright's classification, this early classification scheme remains the most useful.)

*Classification of Joint Involvement in Psoriatic Arthritis*

| SUBTYPE | PERCENTAGE | TYPICAL JOINTS |
|---|---|---|
| 1. Asymmetric oligoarticular disease | > 50% | DIPs and PIPs of hands and feet, MCPs, MTPs, knees, hips, and ankles |
| 2. Predominant DIP involvement | 5–10% | DIPs |
| 3. Arthritis mutilans | 5% | DIPs, PIPs |
| 4. Polyarthritis "rheumatoid-like" | 15–25% | MCPs, PIPs, and wrists |
| 5. Axial involvement | 20–40% | Sacroiliac, vertebral |

**9. What other features are associated with certain subtypes?**

Asymmetric oligoarthritis—Dactylitis
Predominant DIP involvement—Nail changes
Arthritis mutilans—Osteolysis of involved joints, "telescoping" of digits
"Rheumatoid-like" disease—Fusion of wrists
Axial involvement—Asymmetric sacroiliitis and syndesmophytes

**10. Which is the most "classic" pattern of psoriatic arthritis?**

Predominant DIP involvement, but note it is one of the least common patterns.

**11. How does the axial involvement in psoriatic arthritis differ from that in other seronegative spondyloarthropathies?**

Asymmetric sacroiliac involvement is typical of psoriatic arthritis and Reiter's syndrome. The other major seronegative spondyloarthropathies, ankylosing spondylitis and inflammatory bowel disease, tend to be more **symmetric**. Additionally, syndesmophytes are characteristically large, non-marginal ("jug handle"-like), as opposed to the thin, marginal, symmetric syndesmophytes that occur in ankylosing spondylitis.

**12. What clinical features suggest psoriatic arthritis rather than other polyarticular arthritic diseases such as rheumatoid arthritis?**

Asymmetric joint involvement
Absence of rheumatoid factor
Significant nail pits
Involvement of the DIPs in the absence of osteoarthritis
"Sausage digits"
Family history of psoriasis or psoriatic arthritis
Axial radiographic evidence of sacroiliitis, paravertebral ossification, and syndesmophytes
Peripheral radiographic evidence of erosive arthritis with relative lack of osteopenia

**13. Are there any extra-articular features associated with psoriatic arthritis?**

Unlike rheumatoid arthritis, psoriatic arthritis has only two major extra-articular features: nail changes and eye disease. **Nail changes** are seen in 80% of patients with arthritis, as opposed to only 30% with psoriasis only. These changes include pitting, transverse ridging, onycholysis, hyperkeratosis, and yellowing. **Eye disease** includes conjunctivitis in 20% and iritis in 7%. Iritis is more commonly associated with axial involvement.

**14. Are there additional concerns when someone presents acutely with severe psoriasis or psoriatic arthritis?**

Especially in young or middle-aged men, one needs to consider concurrent HIV infection. Clinically, psoriasis or psoriatic arthritis associated with HIV infection is more aggressive and difficult to control with traditional medical therapy. As you might suspect, the detection of HIV is also important therapeutically, because drugs such as methotrexate have been associated with worsening immunodeficiency and death. While it was initially thought that immunosuppressive drugs such as methotrexate were contraindicated in HIV-positive patients, with close monitoring many patients have been successfully treated with agents such as methotrexate.

**15. Can laboratory tests help in diagnosing psoriatic arthritis?**

By definition, psoriatic arthritis is classified as a "seronegative" arthritis, meaning that the rheumatoid factor is typically negative. When psoriatic patients have erosive disease and a positive rheumatoid factor, it most likely represents coexistent rheumatoid arthritis. Antinuclear antibodies are no more prevalent in psoriatic patients than in the general population (5%). As in other inflammatory diseases, erythrocyte sedimentation rates, C-reactive protein, and anemia may vary with disease activity. Analysis of synovial fluid reveals inflammatory fluid with a neutrophilic predominance.

**16. What radiographic features help to differentiate psoriatic arthritis from other inflammatory diseases?**

Asymmetric involvement
Relative absence of juxta-articular osteopenia
Involvement of the DIPs
Erosion of the terminal tufts (acro-osteolysis)
Whittling of the phalanges
Cupping of the proximal portion of the phalanges (pencil-in-cup deformity)
Bony ankylosis distal to MCP joints
Osteolysis of bones (arthritis mutilans)
Polyarticular unidigit—MCP, PIP, and DIP of same finger involved
Sacroiliac and spondylitic changes (usually asymmetric)

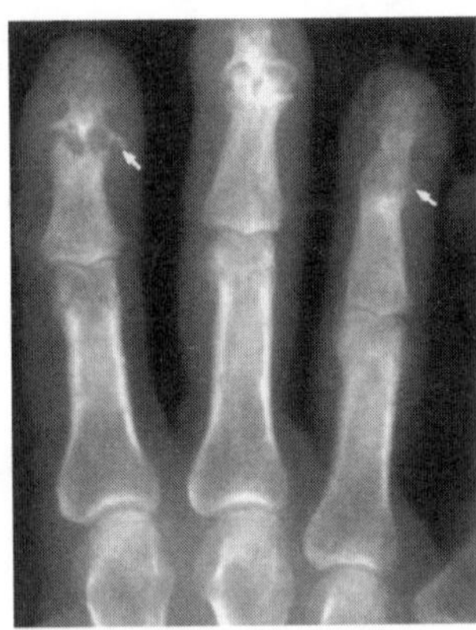

Psoriatic arthritis, showing erosions and ankylosis of DIP (arrows) and PIP joints. (From Perlman SG, Barth WF: Psoriatic arthritis: Diagnosis and management. Compr Ther 5:60–66, 1979; with permission.)

**17. How do you treat psoriatic arthritis?**

Most patients can be managed with NSAIDs alone. Intra-articular steroid injections are also helpful in joints that are resistant to NSAIDs and proven not to be infected. When NSAIDs fail to control the inflammation, disease-modifying agents should be considered. Parenteral gold, auranofin, D-penicillamine, sulfasalazine, methotrexate, cyclosporine, and other immunosuppressive agents have all been shown to be effective in some studies. Methotrexate is especially popular because of its efficacy in treating both the skin and arthritis. Due to large amounts of tumor necrosis alpha found in psoriatic arthritis synovium, anti-TNFα agents (infliximab, etanercept) have been shown to be effective therapy.

The role of antimalarials (hydroxychloroquine) is controversial. Exacerbation of the psoriasis and erythroderma can occur with antimalarials, and consequently some consider them to be contraindicated. Systemic glucocorticoids should also be used cautiously because of the risk of inducing a flare of skin disease if tapered too rapidly.

**18. How does the prognosis of psoriatic arthritis compare with that of rheumatoid arthritis?**

Psoriatic arthritis has a better prognosis than rheumatoid arthritis. Overall, 60% have erosive arthritis in five or more joints, whereas less than 5% experience arthritis mutilans. Up to 20% will develop ACR class III or IV functional impairment, and mortality appears increased. A younger age of onset, female gender, acute onset of arthritis, polyarticular disease, and elevated ESR predicted a poor prognosis.

**19. What other dermatologic conditions have been associated with arthritis?**

Palmoplantar pustulosis, acne conglobata, acne fulminans, psoriatic onycho-pachydermo-periostitis, and hidradenitis suppurativa. Note that acne vulgaris is not included.

**20. What musculoskeletal symptoms are associated with these cutaneous pustular lesions?**

- Anterior chest wall—pain and swelling in the sternoclavicular, manubrosternal, and sternocostal joints
- Axial skeleton—chronic cervical or lumbar pain. Symphysis pubitis common.
- Peripheral arthritis—least common type; usually involves < 3 joints (wrist, PIP, elbow, acromioclavicular, and MTPs are the most common)

**21. What is SAPHO syndrome?**

**S** Synovitis
**A** Acne—cystic acne
**P** Pustulosis—pustular psoriasis, palmoplantar pustulosis, or hidradenitis suppurativa
**H** Hyperostosis—especially of anterior chest well with sternocostoclavicular hyperostosis
**O** Osteitis—symphysis pubitis, sacroiliitis (50%), spondylodiscitis, anterior chest wall

The name was proposed in 1987 by Chamot et al. because they were impressed by the association of a sterile arthritis (frequently involving the anterior chest) and various skin conditions. Etiology is unclear, although *P. acnes* as a causative agent has been implicated. HLA B27 is positive in 33%. Therapy includes NSAIDs, sulfasalazine, doxycycline, IV pamidronate, and methotrexate.

**22. What is CRMO, and how does it relate to SAPHO?**

Chronic recurrent multifocal osteitis (CRMO) is a chronic sterile inflammatory and multifocal disease of bone that preferentially affects children, females (F > M 2:1), but with no racial predilection. Bone sites involved differ according to age of the patient. The metaphysis of the long bones is preferentially affected in children and adolescents whereas anterior thoracic, vertebral, and/or unilateral sacroiliac lesions predominate in adults. Bone biopsies are necessary to rule out bacterial osteomyelitis, tumor, and eosinophilic granuloma. Many patients with CRMO have psoriasis or skin lesions associated with SAPHO. Over time, most patients with CRMO evolve to satisfy criteria for a spondyloarthropathy, although they usually are HLA B27 negative.

## BIBLIOGRAPHY


1. Arnett FC, Reveille JD, Duvuc M: Psoriasis and psoriatic arthritis associated with human immunodeficiency virus infection. Rheum Dis Clin North Am 17:59–78, 1991.
2. Bennett RM: Psoriatic arthritis. In Koopman W (ed): Arthritis and Allied Conditions, 14th ed. Baltimore, Williams & Wilkins, 2001, pp 1345–1361.
3. Clegg DO, Reda DJ, Mejias E, et al: Comparison of sulfasalazine and placebo in the treatment of psoriatic arthritis. Arthritis Rheum 39:2013–2020, 1996.
4. Cuellar ML, Espinoza LR: Methotrexate use in psoriasis and psoriatic arthritis. Rheum Dis Clin North Am 23:797–809, 1997.

5. FitzGerald O, Kane D: Clinical, immunopathogenic, and therapeutic aspects of psoriatic arthritis. Curr Opin Rheumatol 9:295–301, 1997.
6. Gladman DD: Psoriatic arthritis. Rheum Dis Clin North Am 24:829–844, 1998.
7. Hayem G, Bouchaud-Chabot A, Benali K, et al: SAPHO syndrome: A long-term follow-up of 120 cases. Semin Arthritis Rheum 29:159–171, 1999.
8. McGonagle D, Conaghan PG, Emery P: Psoriatic arthritis: A unified concept twenty years on. Arthritis Rheum 42:1080–1086, 1999.
9. Mease PJ, Goffe BS, Metz J, et al: Etanercept in the treatment of psoriatic arthritis and psoriasis: A randomized trial. Lancet 356:385–390, 2000.
10. Vittecoq O, Ait Said L, Michot C, et al: Evolution of chronic recurrent multifocal osteitis toward spondyloarthropathy over the long term. Arthritis Rheum 43:109–119, 2000.
11. Winchester R: Psoriatic arthritis and the spectrum of syndromes related to SAPHO syndrome. Curr Opin Rheumatol 11:299–305, 1999.

# *VII. Arthritis Associated with Infectious Agents*

*As it takes two to make a quarrel, so it takes two to make a disease, the microbe and its host.*

Charles V. Chapin
(1856–1941)

## 42. BACTERIAL SEPTIC ARTHRITIS

*William* R. *Gilliland*, M.D.

**1. How do nongonococcal and gonococcal septic arthritis differ?**

| | GONOCOCCAL | NONGONOCOCCAL |
|---|---|---|
| Host | Young, healthy adults | Small children, elderly, immunocompromised |
| Pattern | Migratory polyarthralgias/arthritis | Monarthritis |
| Tenosynovitis | Common | Rare |
| Dermatitis | Common | Rare |
| Positive joint cultures | < 25% | > 95% |
| Positive blood cultures | Rare | 40–50% |
| Outcome | Good in > 95% | Poor in 30–50% |

**2. What clinical manifestations are typical of nongonococcal septic arthritis?**

An abrupt onset of swelling and pain involving one joint is the classic presentation. Many patients have serious underlying illnesses and may be febrile or have rigors. However, depending on the study of patients with septic arthritis, the presence of fevers over 38 degrees C ranges from 40–90% of cases and the percentage of cases with rigors ranges from 20–60%.

**3. How do organisms reach the synovium to cause septic arthritis?**

- Hematogenously from a remote infection (70%)
- Dissemination from adjacent osteomyelitis (especially in children)
- Lymphatic spread from infection near the joint
- Iatrogenic infections from arthrocentesis or arthroscopy (20%)
- Penetrating trauma from plant thorns or other contaminated objects

**4. What factors predispose an individual to develop septic arthritis?**

Impaired host defense (50%)
  Neoplastic disease
  Elderly (>65 years old) or children (<5 years old)
  Chronic, severe illness (i.e., diabetes, cirrhosis, chronic renal disease, HIV)
  Immunosuppressive agents (i.e., glucocorticoids, chemotherapy)
Direct penetration
  Intravenous drug abuse; puncture wounds; invasive procedures
Joint damage
  Prosthetic joints (over 50% occur in patients over 70 years old)
  Chronic arthritis (i.e., rheumatoid arthritis, hemarthrosis, osteoarthritis)
Host phagocytic defects
  Complement deficiencies; impaired chemotaxis

**5. Which joints are most commonly involved in nongonococcal septic arthritis?**

| | |
|---|---|
| Knee | 55% |
| Hip | 11% |
| Ankle | 8% |
| Shoulder | 8% |
| Wrist | 7% |
| Elbow | 6% |
| Others | 5% |
| Polyarticular | 12% |

**6. Which bacteria are usually responsible for nongonococcal septic arthritis?**

| | |
|---|---|
| *Staphylococcus aureus* | 61% (most penicillin resistant, up to 50% methicillin resistant) |
| Beta-hemolytic streptococci | 15% |
| Gram-negative bacilli | 17% |
| *Streptococcus pneumoniae* | 3% |
| Polymicrobial | 4% |

**7. Describe the trend in the bacteriology of septic arthritis over the past several decades.**

Over the past decade, gram-negative bacilli, non-group A streptococci, and anaerobes are being recovered more frequently. Pneumococci and *Haemophilus influenzae* are being recovered less frequently. Causative pathogens are documented by culture in approximately 70–90% of septic arthritis in most series.

**8. Why does *Staphylococcus aureus* cause most of the septic arthritis?**

*S. aureus* preferentially localizes to joints. A collagen adhesion factor, under the influence of a cna gene, has been found to be an important virulence factor contributing to joint localization.

**9. Which organisms are commonly involved in septic arthritis in children?**

Considerable institutional variation exists, but the most common organisms in various age groups are as follows:

| **Neonates** | **Age < 2 yrs** |
|---|---|
| *Staphylococcus aureus* (hospital-acquired) | *Haemophilus influenzae* (less common with immunizations) |
| | *Staphylococcus aureus* |
| Streptococci (community-acquired) | **Age 2–15 yrs** |
| | *Staphylococcus aureus* |
| Gram-negative bacilli | *Streptococcus pyogenes* |

**10. Name the organisms that are associated with underlying disorders in septic arthritis.**

| | |
|---|---|
| Rheumatoid arthritis | *Staphylococcus aureus* (frequently polyarticular) |
| Alcoholism/cirrhosis | Gram-negative bacilli |
| | *Streptococcus pneumoniae* |
| Malignancies | Gram-negative bacilli |
| Diabetes mellitus | Gram-negative bacilli |
| | Gram-positive cocci |
| Drug abuse | *Pseudomonas aeruginosa* |
| | *Serratia marcescens* |
| | *Staphylococcus aureus* |
| Dog/cat bites | *Pasteurella multocida* |
| Hemoglobinopathies | *Streptococcus pneumoniae* |
| | *Salmonella* spp |
| Raw milk/dairy products | *Brucella* spp |
| SLE | Encapsulated organisms (*Neisseria*, *Salmonella*, *Proteus*) |

**11. How helpful are synovial fluid analysis and culture in nongonococcal septic arthritis?**

Arthrocentesis with demonstration of the bacteria on Gram stain or culture establishes the diagnosis of septic arthritis. Of the tests that can be run on the synovial fluid, culture, Gram stain, and leukocyte (WBC) counts are the most helpful.

*Laboratory Tests in Nongonococcal Septic Arthritis*

| PROCEDURE | TECHNICAL ASPECTS | DIAGNOSTIC YIELD |
|---|---|---|
| Culture | Plate or inoculate culture bottles immediately | Nearly 100% positive in nongonococcal arthritis |
| Gram stain | May increase yield by centrifuging synovial fluid | 75% in gram-positive cocci, 50% in gram-negative bacilli |
| WBC count | Usually 50,000 cells/$mm^3$ but often 100,000 cells/$mm^3$ (> 85% PMNs) | Counts often overlap other inflammatory disease (gout, RA, Reiter's) |
| Glucose | < 50% of serum glucose | Helpful if present |
| Cell wall antigens | CIE or similar test | Only helpful in *H. influenzae* and *S. pneumoniae* |

CIE = counterimmunoelectrophoresis; RA = rheumatoid arthritis; PMN = polymorphonuclear leukocytes.

**Pearl**: Only 40–50% of all patients with septic arthritis have synovial fluid WBC counts100,000 cells/$mm^3$. So even if the synovial fluid WBC is not "classic" for septic arthritis, there can still be an infection even with WBC counts less than 30,000 cells/$mm^3$.

**12. Are any blood tests useful in septic arthritis?**

**Blood cultures** are probably the most useful, as approximately 50% (24–76%) of patients with nongonococcal septic arthritis have positive cultures. **Leukocytosis** and **elevated sedimentation rates** are seen in most individuals (60–90%) but are not usually helpful diagnostically. Quantification of elevations in C-reactive proteins (CRP) may also be helpful in distinguishing between an inflammatory and septic arthritis.

**13. Do plain radiographs play a role in diagnosing septic arthritis?**

Initial radiographs should be obtained to rule out adjacent osteomyelitis and to establish a baseline. However, definitive changes of septic arthritis may take several days to 2 weeks to develop.

**14. How can I remember the radiologic and/or pathologic changes in septic arthritis?**

Remember **A-B-C-D-E-S**.

| | RADIOGRAPHIC SIGN | PATHOLOGIC CORRELATE |
|---|---|---|
| **A** | Bony **ankylosis** | Fibrous or bony ankylosis (endstage) |
| **B** | Osteoporosis | Increased **blood** flow, inflammatory cytokines |
| **C** | Joint space loss | Pannus with **cartilage** destruction |
| **D** | Joint **deformity** | End stage of arthritic destruction |
| **E** | **Erosions** | Pannus with bony destruction |
| **S** | Joint effusion (the first sign), soft-tissue **swelling** | Edema of synovium with fluid production |

**15. Can other radiographic studies be helpful in septic arthritis?**

Other radiographic tests are especially helpful in visualizing joints that are deep or difficult to palpate (i.e., hip, sacroiliac, and sternoclavicular joints). They are also helpful early on in a septic process, when plain films do not yet demonstrate any abnormalities.

*Specialized Radiographic Studies in Septic Arthritis*

| PROCEDURE | UTILITY |
|---|---|
| Technetium bone scan | Often positive in 24–48 hrs, but not specific for septic synovitis |
| Gallium scan | More specific than bone scan but less sensitive. Especially helpful in children when there is difficulty in establishing abnormalities in growth plate areas. |
| Indium scan | Less sensitive than bone scan but more specific because it relies on direct labeling of WBCs that migrate to area of infection. Especially helpful in evaluation of prosthetic joints. |
| CT | Visualizes bony changes, such as erosions, prior to plain films. Especially helpful in sacroiliac and sternoclavicular joints. |
| MRI | Provides early detection of soft-tissue changes, such as edema and effusions. Also demonstrates osteomyelitis. |

**16. How do you treat nongonococcal septic arthritis?**

- Maintain a high index of suspicion in patients who are predisposed to septic arthritis.
- Choose effective antibiotic based on patient age, clinical situation, and Gram stain findings.
- Adequately drain the joint on a frequent basis (sometimes several times a day) by needle drainage unless open or arthroscopic drainage is required. Always send synovial fluid for cell count, Gram stain, and culture to make sure therapy is succeeding.
- Analgesics are useful as adjunctive therapy.
- Physical therapy is important.
  Immobilize the joint for first day or two.
  Passive range of motion after first 2 days.
  Active range of motion/weight-bearing as pain resolves.

**17. Which antibiotic should you choose? How long do you treat nongonococcal septic arthritis?**

Antibiotics should be started after cultures are obtained, with the choice of antibiotic determined by the organism and clinical situation. Parental therapy should be initiated for at least 2 weeks, followed by 2–4 weeks of oral therapy. The duration is variable and depends on the patient's clinical response.

*Antibiotic Treatment of Nongonococcal Septic Arthritis*

| ORGANISM | ANTIBIOTIC OF CHOICE | ALTERNATIVES |
|---|---|---|
| *Staphylococcus aureus* | Nafcillin | Cefazolin<br>Vancomycin<br>Clindamycin |
| Methicillin-resistant *S. aureus* | Vancomycin | — |
| *Streptococcus pyogenes* or *S. pneumoniae* | Penicillin | Cefazolin<br>Vancomycin<br>Clindamycin |
| *Enterococcus* | Ampicillin plus gentamicin | Vancomycin plus aminoglycoside |
| *Haemophilus influenzae* | Ampicillin | Third-generation cephalosporin<br>Cefuroxime<br>Chloramphenicol |
| Enterobacteriaceae | Third-generation cephalosporin<br>or<br>Levofloxacin | Imipenem<br>Aztreonam<br>Ampicillin<br>Aminoglycoside (not alone) |
| *Pseudomonas* | Aminoglycoside plus antipseudomonal penicillin | Aminoglycoside plus ceftazidime, imipenem, or aztreonam |

**18. When is surgical drainage absolutely indicated for a septic joint?**

- Infected hip joints and probably shoulder joints
- Vertebral osteomyelitis with cord compression
- Anatomically difficult-to-drain joints (i.e., sternoclavicular joint)
- Inability to remove purulent fluid by needle drainage because fluid is too thick or loculated
- Joints failing to respond to needle drainage (i.e., persistent positive cultures of synovial fluid or failure of synovial WBC to decrease)
- Prosthetic joints
- Associated osteomyelitis requiring surgical drainage
- Arthritis associated with foreign body
- Delayed onset of therapy (> 7 days)—irreversible cartilage damage starts within 1 week

**19. What is the prognosis in patients with nongonococcal septic arthritis?**

Despite better drainage and antibiotics, this remains a serious disease with a 5–15% mortality. Most of these patients (25–60%) have a chronic debilitating underlying disease that contributes to the mortality (i.e., rheumatoid arthritis, polyarticular sepsis, hemodialysis, and renal transplant). Of the surviving patients, between 30 and 50% have residual abnormalities (pain or limited motion of the joint).

**20. Do any factors suggest a poor outcome in nongonococcal septic arthritis?**

| | |
|---|---|
| Rheumatoid arthritis | Delayed diagnosis |
| Polyarticular sepsis | Immunosuppressive therapy |
| Positive blood cultures | Gram-negative organisms |
| Elderly age | Renal transplant/dialysis patients |

**21. How does septic arthritis differ in children?**

- Age of patient is very helpful in determining likely organism.
- Arthritis is often secondary to adjacent osteomyelitis.
- Children have a higher incidence of hip involvement.

**22. Discuss the important aspects in the association of rheumatoid arthritis (RA) and septic joints.**

Previously damaged joints and the use of **immunosuppressive agents** are probably responsible for the increased risk (≤ 3%) of septic arthritis in patients with RA. The patients are usually those with long-standing seropositive disease, marked disability, and a history of corticosteroid use. Unfortunately, the steroids may blunt the typical symptoms of septic arthritis, causing it to be mistaken for a "flare" of RA. **Gram-positive organisms**, especially *Staphylococcus aureus*, account for 75–90% of infections. Rare organisms and polymicrobial infections have also been reported. The most important feature is the poor **prognosis**. The mortality is 25%, with only half of those surviving attaining their preinfection level of functioning.

**23. Are there any peculiarities about septic arthritis in intravenous drug abusers?**

1. Higher incidence of gram-negative organisms, especially *Pseudomonas* and *Serratia*. However, *S. aureus* is the most common organism.
2. More insidious course with longer duration of symptoms.
3. Increased propensity to affect the axial skeleton (especially the lumbar vertebrae, sacroiliac joint, symphysis pubis, ischium, and sternocostal articulations).
4. In general, if given proper therapy have a very low risk of death and high likelihood of preserved joint function unless they have HIV.

**24. What is the incidence of prosthetic joint infections? What are the risk factors?**

The overall infection rate in total joint replacement is approximately 1%. Risk factors include impaired host defense, rheumatoid arthritis, revision arthroplasty (5–10× increased risk), increased operative time, and superficial joint replacements (i.e., elbow, shoulder, ankle).

**25. What are the most common organisms causing prosthetic joint infection?**

*S. epidermidis* is most commonly isolated from perioperative (< 6–12 months) infections and *S. aureus* from later postoperative infections. These organisms can get in the polysaccharide mucoid biofilm (glyco calyx) that forms on the prosthetic joint and provides a protective environment for bacterial growth.

**26. What symptoms and signs suggest prosthetic joint infections?**

Prosthetic infections occurring in first 6–12 months typically have pain, swelling, fever, and sometimes drainage. Late prosthetic infections present with a prolonged indolent course with increasing joint pain. Fever occurs in less than 50% and leukocytosis in 10%. Elevated ESR and CRP are common. The major differential is separating septic from aseptic joint loosening. Radiographs will show greater than 2 mm lucency between bone and cement, and bone scan/indium scan shows increased uptake around the prosthesis (bone scan should normally be negative 8 months after surgery). However, cultures of synovial fluid or tissue are needed to confirm the diagnosis.

**27. How are prosthetic joint infections treated?**

Prolonged antibiotics and surgical intervention. Less than 10% of large joint prosthesis infections can be treated without removal of prosthesis. Most surgeons favor prosthesis and cement removal, prolonged antibiotics, and delayed implantation with antibiotic impregnated cement. Rifampin use in conjunction with other antibiotics has been an effective additive therapy. Mortality rates are 5–20%.

**28. What is "pseudoseptic" arthritis?**

Pseudoseptic arthritis is seen in the setting of poorly controlled rheumatoid arthritis in which the patient presents with one or more inflamed joints with very high synovial fluid WBC counts (> 100,000 cells/mm$^3$). The cultures are negative, and patients respond to increased corticosteroids rather than antibiotics. However, infection always needs to be ruled out first! This presentation may also be seen in the crystal-induced arthritides and seronegative spondyloarthropathies.

**29. Who is at risk for disseminated gonococcal infection (DGI)?**

Unlike nongonococcal septic arthritis, the typical patient who develops gonococcal arthritis is a young, healthy person. Women are more commonly affected than men, and are more prone to develop DGI around menstruation, pregnancy, and postpartum. Other risk factors include urban residence, non-Caucasian race, low socioeconomic status, low educational status, prostitution, and previous gonococcal infection.

**30. How soon after infection do arthritic symptoms develop in DGI?**

Arthritis complicates 1–3% of patients with gonorrhea. Typically, symptoms develop 1 day to several weeks after the sexual encounter.

**31. What bacterial characteristics increase the potential for *Neisseria gonorrhoeae* to disseminate?**

1. Small, sharply bordered colonies with **surface pili** are more virulent than large colonies.
2. The presence of **outer surface membrane 1A protein** increases its virulence and also its ability to disseminate.
3. **Nutritional requirements**, in that organisms requiring arginine, hypoxanthine, and uracil (AHU) are more likely to disseminate.
4. Some strains have **resistance to bactericidal effects** of human serum.
5. **Antibiotic resistance** may be mediated by plasmids or chromosomal-mediated mutations.

**32. What host factors enhance susceptibility?**

1. High-risk sexual practices (i.e., multiple partners and prostitutes)
2. Local environment of the cervix (i.e., changes in pH that occur during menstruation)

3. Congenital or acquired complement deficiencies, especially of C6–C8, predispose to recurrent neisserial infections [**Pearl**: Always get a serum $CH_{50}$ level in a patient with recurrent neisserial infections. If it is 0, work up the patient for complement deficiency.]
4. Asplenia or reticuloendothelial dysfunction

**33. What patterns of arthritis are associated with gonorrhea?**

| | |
|---|---|
| Migratory polyarthralgia | 70% |
| Tenosynovitis | 67% |
| Purulent arthritis | 42% |
| Monoarthritis | 32% |
| Polyarthritis | 10% |

An important diagnostic clue is **tenosynovitis**. It most commonly affects the hands, ankles, wrists, and knees, but the pain is often out of proportion to what is seen on physical examination.

**34. Besides the articular complaints, what other symptoms are associated with DGI?**

Only 25% of patients with DGI have **genitourinary symptoms**. On the other hand, 67% or more present with **tenosynovitis**, **fevers**, and **dermatitis**. Classically, the dermatitis is maculopapular or vesicular. The lesions are often symptomatic and occur on the trunk and extremities. However pustules, hemorrhagic bullae, vasculitis, and erythema multiforme may be seen.

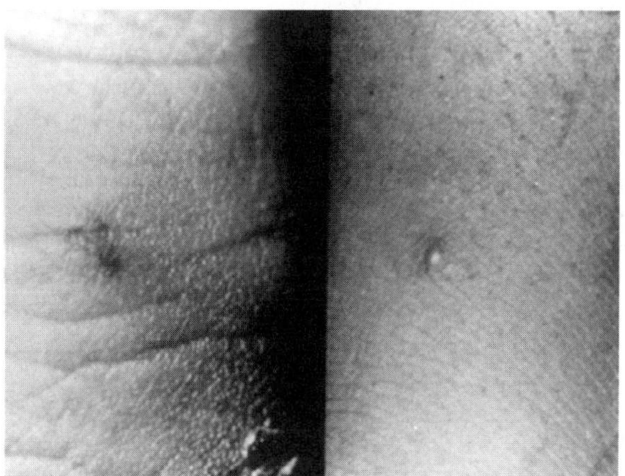

Vesicle and pustular rash of DGI. (From the Clinical Slide Collection on the Rheumatic Diseases. Atlanta, American College of Rheumatology, 1991; with permission.)

**35. How useful are cultures and Gram stains in diagnosing gonococcal septic arthritis?**

Unlike nongonoccal arthritis, in gonococcal arthritis the Gram stains of synovial fluid are positive in < 25%. Cultures improve the diagnostic yield. Because urethritis is often asymptomatic, appropriate smears and urethral cultures should always be obtained.

*Culture Positivity in DGI*

| SITE | ISOLATION RATE |
|---|---|
| Genitourinary | 80% |
| Synovial fluid | 25–70% |
| Rectum | 20% |
| Pharynx | 10% |
| Blood | 5–10% |
| Skin | Rare |

**Pearl**: Specimens obtained from contaminated sites (genitourinary tract, pharynx, and rectum) should be cultured on Thayer-Martin media. Specimens from noncontaminated areas (synovial fluid and blood) should be cultured on chocolate agar. Always use culture plates that have been warmed to body temperature and plate specimens immediately, often at bedside. This is because the neisserial organism causing DGI can be killed by vancomycin in Thayer-Martin media and cold temperatures.

**36. Are other laboratory tests helpful in DGI?**

Much like nongonococcal septic arthritis, in DGI leukocytosis and elevated sedimentation rates are common but nonspecific. Synovial fluid WBC counts range from 34,000–68,000 cells/mm$^3$ with a mean of 50,000/mm$^3$. Nested PCR can detect *N. gonorrhoeae* DNA in culture negative synovial fluid.

**37. How is DGI treated?**

In the past, a dramatic improvement on administration of penicillin was believed to be diagnostic of DGI. However, with the emergence of antibiotic-resistant strains, the initial drug of choice for gonorrhea has changed.

| | |
|---|---|
| Local (cervicitis) | **Ceftriaxone**, 250 mg IM, followed by **doxycycline**, 100 mg orally twice daily for 7 days |
| DGI | **Ceftriaxone**, 1–2 gm IM or IV per day until signs and symptoms resolve, followed by daily outpatient therapy to complete 7–10 days of treatment with **cefuroxime**, 500 mg orally twice daily, or **ciprofloxacin**, 500 mg orally two times daily |

Alternate antibiotics include spectinomycin (2 gm/12 hrs), ciprofloxacin (2 gm/day), or erythromycin (2 gm/day). If the strain is not resistant to penicillin, parental penicillin or amoxicillin (1 gm/8 hrs) may be used. Repeated joint aspirations are necessary until the synovial fluid WBC count decreases to low level.

Patients and their partners should also receive empiric treatment for coexistent and/or silent *Chlamydia* infections (doxycycline, 100 mg orally twice daily for 7 days, or erythromycin if the patient is pregnant). Patients should also be tested for syphilis (VDRL) and human immunodeficiency virus (HIV).

**38. Can *N. meningitides* cause a septic arthritis?**

Acute meningococcemia can cause arthralgias in up to 40% of cases. An acute purulent arthritis can later follow in a minority of cases. It usually involves the knee. Only 25% of patients have an associated meningitis. Many will have an associated maculopapular rash. Synovial fluid cultures are positive in 20% and should be kept for 7 days instead of the usual 3 days. Most patients respond well to antibiotics and joint drainage.

**39. Can syphilis cause an arthritis?**

Secondary syphilis can cause a polyarthritis that can be confused with multiple other connective tissue diseases such as SLE, RA, vasculitis, sarcoidosis, and spondyloarthropathies. One should suspect syphilis in patients with polyarthritis who have a maculopapular rash on the palms and soles (75–100%), generalized lymphadenopathy (75%), headache (50%), fever (50%), sore throat (33%), mucosal ulcers, and condyloma lata. The arthritis is symmetric and involves the knees and ankles more than small joints of the hands. Tenosynovitis may be present. Synovial fluid cell counts range from 4000–13,000/mm$^3$. Spirochetes cannot be seen in the fluid on dark field exam or cultured. Diagnosis is made by syphilis serologies (FTA-ABS) and clinical presentation. Therapy is penicillin.

**40. Can bursae become infected?**

The olecranon and prepatellar bursae are the most common sites of septic bursitis. Most septic bursitis occurs in patients who constantly traumatize the skin in these areas (carpenters, laborers). More than 50% also have a surrounding cellulitis. Over 80% of septic bursitis is due to *S. aureus*. Blood cultures are rarely positive because the organisms get to the bursa by transcutaneous spread through skin abrasions. Patients usually have abrupt onset of pain, swelling, and erythema. Diagnosis is made by aspiration, Gram stain, and culture of bursal fluid. Bursal fluid cell counts are elevated but not as much as septic joints. Antibiotics should be administered intravenously initially and the bursa aspirated repeatedly or incised and drained. This is especially important for febrile patients or those who are immunocompromised. After control of the infection, oral antibiotics are taken for an additional 2–3 weeks. Failure to respond is an indication for bursectomy.

**41. What is the difference between acute and chronic osteomyelitis?**

Acute osteomyelitis occurs predominantly in children. It is usually due to *S. aureus* (90%), which seeds the metaphysis of long bones by hematogenous spread. Patients typically present within a few days with fever, pain, and decreased range of motion of the involved bone/joint. Laboratory tests show leukocytosis and elevations of ESR/CRP. Blood cultures are positive in 50%. Radiographs are frequently normal or show mild periosteal reaction. Indium-111 labeled leukocyte scan (90%) or MRI (100%) are abnormal. Bone scans may be difficult to interpret as a result of growth plate activity. Therapy is with appropriate antibiotics for 4–6 weeks.

Chronic osteomyelitis usually occurs in adults secondary to an open wound or fracture. Localized bone pain, erythema, and draining sinus tract are typically seen. Radiographic changes are seen 2 weeks after onset of infection and reveal osteolysis, periosteal reaction, and sequestra. Bone scan, indium scan, CT scan, and MRI are abnormal. Specific bacterial diagnosis is made by bone biopsy. Culture of sinus tract is not reliable. *S. aureus* is the most common organism, but gram-negative bacteria are also isolated. Therapy includes antibiotics for 6 weeks and debridement of bone.

**42. What is the difference between a sequestra and Brodie's abscess?**

- Sequestra—segments of necrotic bone separated from living bone by granulation tissue. Must be removed by debridement, owing to inability of antibiotics to sterilize it.
- Brodie's abscess—bone abscess found during chronic stage of hematogenous osteomyelitis. It usually has a sclerotic margin on radiograph.

## BIBLIOGRAPHY

1. Baker DG, Schumaker HR Jr: Current concepts—acute monarthritis. N Engl J Med 329:1013–1020, 1993.
2. Cimmino MA: Recognition and management of bacterial arthritis. Drugs 54:50–60, 1997.
3. Donatto KC: Orthopedic management of septic arthritis. Rheum Dis Clin North Am 24:275–286, 1998.
4. Goldenberg DL: Bacterial arthritis. In Ruddy S, Harris ED, Sledge CB (eds): Kelley's Textbook of Rheumatology, 6th ed. Philadelphia, W.B. Saunders, 2001, pp 1469–1483.
5. Lew DP, Waldvogel FA: Osteomyelitis. N Engl J Med 336:999–1007, 1997.
6. Nair SP, Williams RJ, Henderson B: Advances in our understanding of the bone and joint pathology caused by *Staphylococcus aureus* infection. Rheumatology 39:821–834, 2000.
7. Perry CR: Septic arthritis. Am J Orthop 28:168–178, 1999.
8. Pioro MH, Mandell BF: Septic arthritis. Rheum Dis Clin North Am 23:239–258, 1997.
9. Zimmermann B, Mikolich DJ, Ho G: Septic bursitis. Seminars Arthritis Rheum 24:391–410, 1995.

# 43. LYME DISEASE

John Keith Jenkins, M.D.

**1. How was Lyme disease recognized as a distinct clinical entity?**

Lyme disease was first recognized as a distinct entity in Old Lyme, Connecticut, in 1975. A neighborhood outbreak of juvenile rheumatoid (chronic) arthritis (JRA) was reported to the state public health department by the mothers of the affected children because they believed the neighborhood clustering to be more than coincidence. The outbreak in this rural community was consistent with an infectious etiology transmitted by an arthropod vector. To put things in perspective, Lyme disease is the most common vector-borne disease in the United States and the second most common in the world (malaria being the most common).

**2. What is the etiology of Lyme disease?**

Lyme disease is caused by an infection with the tick-borne spirochete *Borrelia burgdorferi*, which was discovered in 1982. Only one of the three pathogenic species of *Borrelia* (i.e., *B. burgdorferi*) occurs in North America, while all three occur in Europe. There are many similarities to syphilis; it is a multisystem disease that occurs in stages that can mimic other diseases. *Borrelia* can only rarely be cultured from the blood or other infected tissues, and the incubation period is 3–32 days.

**3. What is the geographic distribution and seasonal occurrence of Lyme disease in the United States? In what other countries has it been reported?**

Lyme disease is tick-borne and is most prevalent from April or May to November in the endemic areas. The peak incidence is in the late spring and early summer months of June and July. Lyme disease has been reported in virtually all 48 contiguous states, but most cases occur in three regions:

- Northeast coast between Massachusetts and Maryland
- The Midwest in Wisconsin and Minnesota
- Western coast of northern California and Oregon.

The disease also occurs in Europe, Scandinavia, China, Asia, Japan, and Australia.

**4. Name the arthropod vector of *Borrelia burgdorferi*, its animal hosts, and describe how Lyme disease is transmitted.**

*Ixodes scapularis* (previously called *I. dammini*) was the tick first described to carry the causative organism and is the vector in the northeast and midwest United States. Up to 50% of adult ticks are infected in endemic areas. *Ixodes pacificus* is the vector on the West Coast, and its preferential host is the lizard, which is not a very good reservoir for *Borrelia*. Other *Ixodid* species are the vectors in other parts of the world: *I. ricinus* in Europe, where Lyme disease is common, and *I. persculatus* in the former Soviet Union and Asia. Small and large mammals are generally the preferred hosts.

The *I. scapularis* egg mass is laid in the leaf clutter at the bottom of the forest (consequently, this tick does not exist in dry climates). Larvae emerge in the summer and fall. They require a blood meal that they get from the white-footed mouse, which is an asymptomatic reservoir for *Borrelia*. The tick larvae acquire *Borrelia* with their blood meal, fall off the mouse, and molt. In late spring and summer of the following year, the larvae emerge as nymphs and again get a blood meal (and *Borrelia*) from the white-footed mouse. Infected nymphs can pass *Borrelia* on to other mice and humans when they take a blood meal. Later the nymphs become adults and the females feed on white-tailed deer (in the region of their shoulder, hence *I. scapularis*) to get blood nutrients to make eggs. The eggs are laid in leaf clutter. The eggs are not infected with *Borrelia* even if the female tick is. The deer does not remain infected with *Borrelia*. After the eggs are laid, the 2-year life cycle starts over again.

*Borrelia* infection occurs through the bite of the *Ixodid* tick, an event remembered by only half of patients with Lyme disease—a key point to remember when taking a history. The tick is also very small (size of a freckle) and often simply overlooked. The intestinal tract of the tick is the reservoir for *Borrelia*. The tick has a slow, extended feeding cycle, and hours after feeding it regurgitates transmitting *Borrelia* to the animal host. Other ticks have been shown to harbor *Borrelia*, including the Lone Star tick (*Amblyomma americanum*) and the American dog tick (*Dermacentor variabilis*). Whether or not these ticks can spread Lyme disease is unproven. In endemic areas, Lyme arthritis is one of the most common reasons for a lame dog.

**5. What organ systems are involved in Lyme disease?**

The disease is frequently thought of as a "rash-arthritis" complex, even though the arthritis may be a late manifestation. Not all patients have either rash or arthritis. In addition, the nervous system (both central and peripheral) and cardiac system may be involved. A patient infected with *Borrelia* who develops the typical skin rash, erythema chronicum migrans (ECM), and who is *not treated* with antibiotics has a 1–5% chance of developing cardiac manifestations, a 15% chance of developing neurologic manifestations, and a 60% chance of developing arthritis (50% migratory polyarthritis, 10% chronic monoarthritis).

**6. Describe the typical rash of Lyme disease.**

In 80–90% of patients with Lyme borreliosis, the disease begins with ECM, which usually occurs at the site of the tick bite. The ticks are attracted to warm, carbon dioxide–exhaling animals. The ticks prefer warm and moist areas to dine. Consequently, ECM is frequently found behind the knee or in the groin, beltline, or axilla. ECM begins as a red macule or papule that expands to form **a large annular lesion** up to 20 cm or more in diameter with **partial central clearing** and a bright red outer border (see figure). Atypical skin lesions can be seen and include diffuse erythema, urticaria, evanescent rashes, and a malar rash.

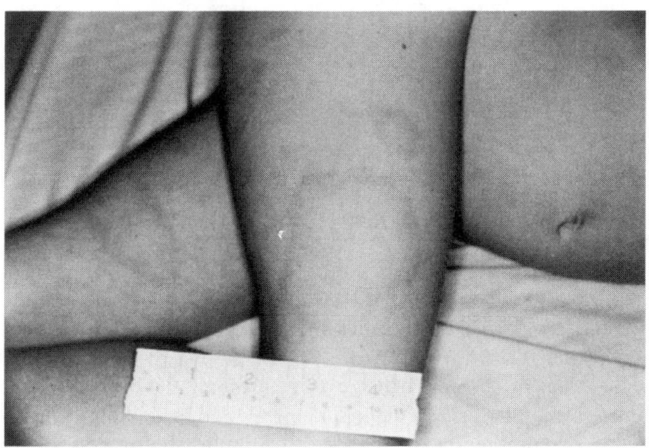

The lesions of erythema chronicum migrans. (From Steere AC, et al: Erythema chronicum migrans and Lyme arthritis: The enlarging spectrum. Ann Intern Med 86:685–698, 1977; with permission.)

**7. What are the stages of Lyme disease, their temporal relation, and which organ systems are involved in each stage?**

Lyme disease has three stages:

- Early localized ECM—skin (ECM)
- Disseminated infection—nervous and cardiac systems, skin and musculoskeletal (but potentially any organ) system

- Persistent infection (late disease)-musculoskeletal and nervous systems

After the incubation period (mean 7–10 days), the first stage of Lyme disease or ECM occurs. Regional lymphadenopathy (25%) may occur, leading to confusion with tularemia. "Flu-like" symptoms such as headache, fatigue, arthralgias, and fever (15%) may occur, but ECM usually fades in several days to a few weeks. The second stage, or disseminated infection, may begin within days to 10 months after ECM occurs and is due to hematogenous spread. The third stage occurs a mean of 6 months after disease onset but may occur as soon as 2 weeks or as late as 2 years after disease onset.

**8. What clinical manifestations occur in the second stage (disseminated infection) of Lyme disease?**

Characteristically, the central nervous system is involved. Symptoms include those of meningitis, headache, cranial neuritis (especially Bell's palsy), motor or sensory radiculoneuritis, encephalitis, and mononeuritis multiplex. Cardiac manifestations occur during the second stage and include varying degrees of atrioventricular block (usually temporary) and myo- or pancarditis. Secondary skin lesions are common. Arthralgias, bursitis, and tendon involvement are common and transient. Frank arthritis is usually not prevalent until the third stage.

**9. Describe the clinical manifestations of the third stage (late disease) of Lyme disease.**

The third stage of Lyme disease may represent persistent infection. It usually involves episodic attacks of an asymmetric oligoarticular arthritis in the large joints, especially the knee. With time, the arthritis becomes more persistent and chronic, leading to attacks that last months rather than weeks. Fatigue frequently accompanies the arthritis episodes, but in general fever and other systemic symptoms do not. Chronic nervous system involvement (5%) may occur in the third stage and is usually an encephalopathy (affecting memory, mood, and sleep) and/or a peripheral sensory neuropathy.

**10. What is the natural history of ECM?**

After the initial rash, secondary or satellite lesions (10% of cases) may occur that resemble the initial rash (i.e., erythematous and annular). ECM may be seen during both the first and second stages of the disease but is much less common during the third stage. More common in Europe, a chronic skin rash occurs during the third stage called acrodermatitis chronica atrophicans. It is a blue-red area of the skin with swelling that may lead to skin atrophy. Thickened patches of skin called morphea may also occur in this stage.

**11. How is ECM treated?**

When treating ECM, the physician needs to make sure that no other systemic manifestations suggesting disseminated infection are present (i.e., neurologic or cardiac). If none are present, oral antibiotics are adequate when given for 10 days but most physicians continue to use 3 to 4 week regimens for early Lyme disease. In general, *Borrelia* species are less sensitive to penicillin by in vitro testing than to amoxicillin, doxycycline, and second- and third-generation cephalosporins. The drugs of choice are doxycycline (100 mg PO bid) or amoxicillin (500 mg PO tid–qid). Azithromycin (500 mg) on the first day followed by 250 mg PO qd for 4 days is as effective as the other two oral regimens. In case of penicillin allergy, cefuroxime (500 mg PO bid), azithromycin, or erythromycin (250 mg PO tid–qid) may be used. Erythromycin may be less effective clinically. Overall, antibiotics cure more than 90% of patients with ECM.

**12. How is EMC treated in children and pregnant women?**

Doxycycline should be avoided in children less than age 8 and pregnant women, owing to effect on forming teeth. For children amoxicillin, 20 mg/kg/d in divided doses, and for pregnant women, amoxicillin 500 mg tid–qid for 20–30 days, are recommended. If penicillin allergic, erythromycin 30 mg/kg/d in divided doses for children and 250 mg tid–qid for pregnant women is used. Maternal-fetal transmission of *B. burgdorferi* is very rare.

**13. What diagnostic tests are available for Lyme disease?**

In addition to clinical diagnosis (tick bite followed by ECM and arthritis), serologic testing by ELISA is commonly used. This test measures antibodies to *Borrelia*. Serologic testing has problems because of interlaboratory variability and differences between the commercial tests that are available. Positives should be interpreted cautiously and are not definitive; and results are frequently misinterpreted. High positive rates occur in endemic areas. The height of the titer does not imply the activity of the disease. Western blot analysis can be used to detect antibodies in a patient's serum to the various specific *Borrelia* proteins and may discriminate between cross-reacting antibodies from other sources and those directed towards *Borrelia* proteins. Western blot analysis should not be used to screen for Lyme disease because of the cost and difficulty in interpreting the results. A PCR-based test may be useful in determining what type of treatment is needed in refractory or late disease. Somewhat better testing methods and an increase in tick populations in the US have probably accounted for the continued high rates of infection, which have even increased recently (late 1990s) in the US.

**14. Name the most common explanations for a false-negative Lyme test.**

Specific antibodies to *Borrelia* may not be present early (such as during the first stage of the illness), leading to a false-negative result. They may be detectable by a Western blot analysis but not by the ELISA. It is helpful to draw acute and convalescent sera in this case. Additionally, antibiotics, either complete and adequate therapy or partial therapy with residual infection, may halt the immune response and subsequent development of measurable levels of specific antibody if given early in the first stage of Lyme disease.

**15. Why might a false-positive serologic test for Lyme disease occur?**

In endemic areas, a large percentage of the population may have had a subclinical infection and be seropositive without acute or chronic illness. Adequately treated patients may remain seropositive long after an infection is eradicated. Antibodies directed towards other spirochetes may cross-react to the *Borrelia* antigen(s) used in the ELISA. For example, patients with antibodies to syphilis (*Treponema pallidum*) or Rocky Mountain spotted fever or those who recently had a dental procedure that exposed them to spirochetes in the oral cavity (*Treponema denticola*) may have IgM antibodies to these organisms that react positive in the Lyme ELISA. In addition, certain acute viral infections (EBV, CMV, parvovirus) and human granulocytic ehrlichiosis can give false-positive IgM seroreactivity to *B. burgdorferi*. Not recognizing a false-positive result will lead to a patient being treated for borreliosis while his or her underlying disease goes untreated. Interlaboratory variability and lack of standardization of the test may result in both false-positives and false-negatives. Serologic testing, though widely used, is of questionable value in diagnosing Lyme disease. The quality and nonspecificity of Lyme titers suggest that Lyme testing should only be used in a confirmatory manner in patients suspected of having clinical Lyme disease—not in screening patients with multiple vague complaints.

**16. Describe laboratory abnormalities that may be seen in Lyme disease.**

Antinuclear antibodies and rheumatoid factor are no more prevalent than in the general population. The neurologic manifestations of Lyme disease that occur during the second stage often involve symptoms of meningeal irritation. As one would expect, there may be a mild cellular pleocytosis and elevated protein in the CSF upon spinal tap. This may also occur in late stages of disease with chronic CNS symptoms that are not as suggestive of meningeal involvement. In these patients, a high IgG index and oligoclonal bands may be seen in the CSF. During episodes of arthritis, synovial fluid cell counts range from 1000 to 100,000/mm$^3$ and are predominantly polymorphonuclear leukocytes. Polymerase chain reaction (PCR) can detect *B. burgdorferi* DNA in skin, blood, spinal and synovial fluid, and synovial tissue. It is more sensitive than culture and more specific than ELISA but difficult to perform. *B. burgdorferi* can be cultured in early disease from ECM lesions but not from tissue in late disease (use PCR).

**17. How should the second (disseminated disease) and third (late disease) stages of Lyme disease be treated?**

There is not uniform agreement on how later stages of Lyme disease should be treated because the appropriate clinical trials have not been done. Before discovery of *Borrelia burgdorferi*, there were trials treating early disease with oral antibiotics and advanced disease with intravenous (IV) penicillin. In stage 2 and 3, intravenous antibiotics are generally indicated. For neurologic manifestations or a high degree of AV block, ceftriaxone (2 g IV qd for 2 to 4 weeks) or cefotaxime (2 g q 8hr for 2 to 4 weeks or 3 g q 12hr) is commonly used. Mild neurologic (Bell's palsy alone) or cardiac (first-degree AV block with a PR less than 0.3 seconds) disease may be treated with oral antibiotics as outlined in treatment for ECM above, but therapy should be for 3–4 weeks.

For stage 3 with chronic arthritis, there are no definitive prospective studies. Oral antibiotics may be used for 1 month if there is arthritis without neurologic manifestations: doxycycline (100 mg PO bid) or amoxicillin with probenecid (500 mg of each, PO tid–qid). Some physicians prefer the IV regimens for chronic Lyme arthritis. Other IV regimens include penicillin G (20 million U, 6 divided doses) and chloramphenicol (50 mg/kg/d, four divided doses) for 2–4 weeks. Late neurologic manifestations, which may occur after adequate treatment of arthritis with oral agents, definitely require IV antibiotics as outlined above for stage 2. Some consider ceftriaxone the drug of choice for any form of late Lyme disease, although doxycycline or amoxicillin plus probenecid for 1 month has been shown to work very well in arthritis.

**18. Why doesn't chronic Lyme arthritis respond well to antibiotic treatment?**

The response of the chronic arthritis to antimicrobials may be incomplete and may require up to 3 months. In some patients, the arthritis may be due to a chronic immune process resulting from the infection rather than persistent infection itself. Supportive evidence for this hypothesis is that there appears to be a genetic predisposition to the development of chronic arthritis in patients with particular class II MHC genes (HLA-DR4 and DR2). A rational approach is to treat chronic arthritis with 1 month of oral antibiotics. If there is no response in 3 months, try one more antibiotic course of ceftriaxone (2 g/d IV for 2–4 weeks). If this is ineffective, consider intraarticular steroids, hydroxychloroquine, or synovectomy.

**19. How can Lyme disease be prevented?**

Good tick bite prevention is, of course, necessary in endemic areas. Clothing that completely covers the body with shirts and pants legs tucked in should be worn. Light colored clothing allows detection and removal of ticks. Tick repellent should be used. There are no published recommendations on the use of antibiotics for tick bites once they occur, but a physician should use antimicrobial agents judiciously in this setting. Oral antibiotics are commonly used in endemic areas, but this may not be the correct approach. One study in an endemic area suggested that the chance of developing an adverse reaction to oral antibiotics for tick bites was as high as the likelihood of developing Lyme disease from the untreated bite. In non-endemic areas where most of the ticks probably do not harbor *Borrelia*, the prudent thing to do is remove ticks promptly (it takes several hours to engorge and then regurgitate *Borrelia*), have an appropriate index of suspicion, and recognize and treat disease in its early stages with appropriate antimicrobials.

**20. Is there a vaccine for Lyme disease?**

Two vaccines (LYMErix and ImuLyme) for prevention of Lyme arthritis have been studied in over 21,000 patients and been found to be effective for prevention of infection. They vaccinate the individual with one of the spirochete's outer surface proteins, OspA, and yield a positive ELISA result on serologic testing. LYMErix has been approved in the US. As commonly occurs in preventative medicine, the absolute risk reduction is low despite high vaccine efficacy because the infection rate, even in endemic areas, is relatively low. Large numbers of people would need to be vaccinated to prevent cases of clinical disease, perhaps as many as 4000 to prevent one serious case of multisystem Lyme disease. For this reason, it is recommended the vaccine "be considered" for people between the ages of 15 and 70 who reside, work, or pursue recreational areas of high or moderate risk of exposure and who engage in activities that result in frequent or prolonged exposure to tick-infested habitat. Also recall that 23% of Lyme disease occurs in children and the vaccine is not approved for this population, although this is likely to change soon. Persons with a history of Lyme disease may be immunized.

**21. How does the Lyme disease vaccine work?**

The Lyme disease vaccine is a recombinant outer-surface protein A (Osp A) with adjuvant. It is administered in a series of three shots. The person vaccinated forms protective antibodies. When the *Borrelia*-infected tick takes its blood meal from a vaccinated individual, the protective antibodies attack the *Borrelia* in the tick. Any *Borrelia* that escape this will be killed at the tick bite site.

## DIFFICULT CLINICAL SITUATIONS

**22. A patient reports she has had diffuse arthralgias/myalgias for many months and has a diagnosis of fibromyalgia. She reports she used to visit New York, although never went camping or hiking. Her physician ordered a Lyme test, and the IgM ELISA returned positive. Should she get antibiotics?**

No. The ELISA tests give many false-positives. The IgM Western immunoblots also give some false-positive results and are useful only in the first few weeks of an infection. Patients with symptoms for greater than 1 month who have a negative IgG ELISA and/or IgG Western blot do not have Lyme disease. In other words, seropositivity is virtually universal in late Lyme disease.

**23. A patient with a history of definite Lyme disease in the past has been treated with two courses of appropriate antibiotics for 1 month each time. She persists with myalgias and has been diagnosed with fibromyalgia. Should she receive another course of therapy with a different antibiotic?**

No. Post Lyme disease fibromyalgia occurs in 15–25% of patients (especially those with history of neurologic involvement) but does not respond to antibiotics. The patient should receive standard treatment for fibromyalgia. It should be noted that both IgM and IgG antibodies to *Borrelia* may persist in the serum for years after therapy and are not an indication for retreatment.

**24. A mother brings her child in and reports he was bitten by a tick the day before. The tick was not engorged. Should the child receive antibiotics prophylactically?**

Controversial. The risk of contracting Lyme disease is 1–3% if the tick has not been attached for 48 hours or not engorged. The bite site should be observed for the development of ECM and the child treated if ECM develops. A patient claiming a bite within 72 hours by an engorged tick in an endemic area should receive prophylactic antibiotics (doxycycline 200 mg one dose) since risk of infection is 25% and can be prevented with prophylactic antibiotics.

**25. How can you tell if a patient has been infected with other *Ixodes*-transmitted pathogens in addition to *B. burgdorferi*?**

*I. scapularis* can transmit other parasites at the time it transmits *B. burgdorferi*. The two most common are *Babesia microti* (babesiosis) and *Ehrlichia phagocytophila* (human granulocytic ehrlichiosis). Any patients with suspected Lyme disease who have leukopenia or thrombocytopenia should be investigated for coinfection with one of these pathogens.

Babesiosis causes hemolysis, thrombocytopenia, and elevated liver-associated enzymes. Intraerythrocytic organisms may be seen on peripheral blood smear. Treatment requires therapy with azithromycin or atovaquone (Mepron). Human granulocytic ehrlichiosis causes fever, headache, arthralgias, leukopenia, and thrombocytopenia. If it is misdiagnosed as Lyme disease, it still responds to doxycycline but not to amoxicillin therapy.

**26. A patient is going camping in Minnesota next week and wants to know if he should get the Lyme vaccine.**

No. The FDA endorses a dosing schedule of giving three doses of vaccine including an initial dose, a dose 1 month later, and the third dose 12 months after the first dose. This gives an efficacy of 80–90%. Although shorter schedules are being tested, the patient going camping cannot get the vaccine in the required amount of time. He should follow the tick precautions outlined in question 19.

## BIBLIOGRAPHY


1. American College of Physicians: Guidelines for laboratory evaluation in the diagnosis of Lyme disease. Ann Int Med 127:1106–1108, 1997.
2. Costello CM, Steere AC, Pinkerton RE, Feder HM Jr: Prospective study of tick bites in an endemic area for Lyme disease. J Infect Dis 159:136–139, 1989.
3. Klempner MS, Hu LT, Evans J, et al: Two controlled trials of antibiotic treatment in patients with persistent symptoms and a history of Lyme disease. N Engl J Med 345:85–92, 2001.
4. Lightfoot RW, Luft BJ, Rahn DW, et al: Empiric parental antibiotic treatment of patients with fibromyalgia and fatigue and a positive serologic result for Lyme disease: A cost effective analysis. Ann Intern Med 119:503–509, 1993.
5. Logigian EL, Kaplan RF, Steere AC: Chronic neurologic manifestations of Lyme disease. N Engl J Med 323:1438–1444, 1990.
6. Luft BJ, Gardner P, Lightfoot RW: The appropriateness of parenteral antibiotic treatment for patients with presumed Lyme disease—joint position paper of the American College of Rheumatology and the Council of the Infectious Diseases Society of America. Ann Intern Med 119:518, 1993.
7. Magid D, Schwartz B, Craft J, Schwartz J: Prevention of Lyme disease after tick bite: A cost-effective analysis. N Engl J Med 327:534, 1992.
8. Malawista SE: Lyme disease. In Koopman WJ (ed): Arthritis and Allied Conditions, 14th ed. Baltimore, Williams & Wilkins, 2001, pp 2629–2648.
9. Mitchell P, Reed KD, Hofkes JM: Immunoserologic evidence of coinfection with *Borrelia burgdorferi*, Babesia microtic, and human granulocytic *Ehrlichia* species in residents of Wisconsin and Minnesota. J Clin Microbiol 34:724, 1996.
10. Nadelman RB, Nowakowski J, Fish D, et al: Prophylaxis with single-dose doxycycline for the prevention of Lyme disease after an *Ixodes scapularis* tick bite. N Engl J Med 345:79–84, 2001.
11. Nocton JJ, Dressler F, Rutledge BJ, et al: Detection of *Borrelia burgdorferi* DNA by polymerase chain reaction in synovial fluid from patients with Lyme arthritis. N Engl J Med 330:229–234, 1994.
12. Sigal LH: Persisting complaints attributed to Lyme disease: Possible mechanisms and implications for management. Am J Med 96:365, 1994.
13. Sigal LH: The Lyme disease controversy: The social and financial costs of the mismanagement of Lyme disease. Arch Intern Med 156:1493, 1996.
14. Sigal LH: Special article: Pitfalls in the diagnosis and management of Lyme disease. Arthritis Rheum 41:195, 1998.
15. Sigal LH: Lyme disease. In Ruddy S, Harris ED, Sledge CB (eds): Kelley's Textbook of Rheumatology, 6th ed, Philadelphia, W.B. Saunders, 2001, pp 1485–1942.
16. Sood SK, Salzman MB, Johnson BJB, et al: Duration of tick attachment as a predictor of the risk of Lyme disease in an area in which Lyme disease is endemic. J Infect Dis 175:996–999, 1997.
17. Steere A: Lyme disease. N Engl J Med 345:115–125, 2001.
18. Steere AC, et al: Erythema chronicum migrans and Lyme arthritis: The enlarging spectrum. Ann Intern Med 86:685–698, 1977.
19. Steere AC, Dwyer E, Winchester R: Association of chronic Lyme arthritis with HLA-DR4 and HLA-DR2 alleles. N Engl J Med 323:219–223, 1990.
20. Thanassi WT, Schoen RT: The Lyme disease vaccine: Conception, development, and implementation. Ann Intern Med 132(8):661–668, 2000.
21. Tugwell P, Dennis DT, Weinstein A, et al: Laboratory evaluation in the diagnosis of Lyme disease. Ann Int Med 127:1109–1123, 1997.
22. Warshafsky S, Nowakowsky J, Nadelman RB, et al: Efficacy of antibiotic prophylaxis for prevention of Lyme disease. J Gen Intern Med 11:329, 1996.
23. Wormser GP, Nadelman RB, Dattwyler R, et al: Infectious Disease Society of America practice guidelines for the treatment of Lyme disease. Clin Infect Dis 31(suppl 1):S1–14, 2000.

# 44. MYCOBACTERIAL AND FUNGAL JOINT AND BONE DISEASES

*William R. Gilliland*, M.D.

**1. What percentage of patients with tuberculosis have bone or joint involvement?**

The number of cases of tuberculosis has risen because of its association with human immunodeficiency virus (HIV) infections. Extrapulmonary disease is now disproportionately represented (now seen in 16–18% as opposed to 7.8% in 1964). Approximately **1–3%** of current cases have osteoarticular involvement.

**2. How does tuberculosis disseminate to the bone and joint?**

Hematogenous spread
Lymphatic spread from distant focus
Contiguous spread from infected areas

Although joint involvement may be secondary to hematogenous spread, it usually is secondary to adjacent osteomyelitis. Therefore, tuberculous arthritis is usually a combination of bone and joint involvement.

**3. Who is at risk for osteoarticular tuberculosis?**

| | |
|---|---|
| Alcoholics | Drug abusers |
| HIV-positive patients | Elderly nursing home patients |
| Immigrants from endemic countries | Immunosuppressed patients |

**4. Which bones and joints are commonly affected with osteoarticular tuberculosis?**

**Spine involvement (Pott's disease)** accounts for 50% of cases. The thoracolumbar spine is more frequently involved than the cervical spine. It usually involves the anterior vertebral border and disc, ultimately progressing to disc narrowing, vertebral collapse, and kyphosis. Although tuberculosis may affect only the vertebral body, it usually will cross the disc and involve the adjacent vertebrae. Complications may include psoas abscess, sinus tract formation, and neurologic compromise. Sacroiliac joint involvement is unusual and usually unilateral when it occurs.

**Peripheral joint involvement** typically involves weight-bearing joints, usually the hip, knee, and ankle, and is monarticular. Subchondral bone involvement may precede cartilage destruction, so that joint space narrowing is often a late finding. Adjacent osteomyelitis is common. It accounts for approximately 30% of cases.

**Osteomyelitis** and dactylitis, tenosynovitis and bursitis, and Poncet's disease account for the remainder of cases. Osteomyelitis may only involve the appendicular skeleton; peripheral involvement is dependent on the age of the patient. In adults, metaphyseal regions of the long bones are commonly affected. In children, metacarpals and phalanges are more likely to be affected.

**5. What are the typical signs and symptoms of osteoarticular tuberculosis?**

| | |
|---|---|
| **Spinal tuberculosis** | Back pain (especially with movement), spasm, local tenderness, kyphosis, cord compression, mycotic aneurysm of aorta |
| **Peripheral joints** | Hip—pain in thigh, groin, or knee; limp (especially in children), muscle atrophy |
| | Knee—insidious pain, swelling, limp, stiffness |
| | Hand/wrist—carpal tunnel syndrome, swelling, pain |
| **Osteomyelitis** | Pain, lytic lesions on radiographs, dactylitis (especially in children) |

Constitutional symptoms often are not present.

**6. What is Poncet's disease?**

In patients with visceral or pulmonary tuberculosis, an acute polyarthritis (presumably reactive) may develop. Tuberculous organisms are not cultured from the involved joints. While any joint may be involved, knees, ankles, and elbows are most common.

**7. How do you diagnose osteoarticular tuberculosis (TB)?**

A definitive diagnosis is established by demonstrating *Mycobacterium tuberculosis* in tissue or synovial fluid. The yield for several common procedures is as follows:

| | |
|---|---|
| Synovial fluid smear for TB | 20% |
| Synovial fluid culture for TB | 80% |
| Synovial biopsy and culture | > 90% |

Synovial fluid analysis reveals elevated protein in virtually all patients with arthritis, while low glucose is seen in 60%. Cell counts are highly variable and range from 1000–100,000 cells/mm$^3$, but most fall in the 10,000–20,000 cells/mm$^3$ range. Polymorphonuclear cells predominate. Synovial membrane biopsies typically show caseating granulomas. Osteomyelitis is diagnosed by needle biopsy, which usually reveals granulomata that may or may not be associated with caseating necrosis.

**8. Does skin testing help in a patient with osteoarticular tuberculosis?**

Purified protein derivative (PPD) skin testing is positive in virtually all patients with osteoarticular disease. However, skin testing may be difficult to interpret if anergy is present (as it may be in many patients at risk for tuberculosis).

**9. What are the characteristic radiographic features of osteoarticular tuberculosis?**

No pathognomonic radiographic signs of tuberculosis exist. However, several signs may be helpful:

**Spine**

- Narrowing of joint space with vertebral collapse
- Anterior vertebral scalloping
- Extensive vertebral destruction with relative preservation of disc space

**Peripheral joint**

- Destructive lesions near joints with little periosteal reaction
- Soft-tissue swelling and osteopenia
- Subchondral erosions
- Joint destruction (late finding)

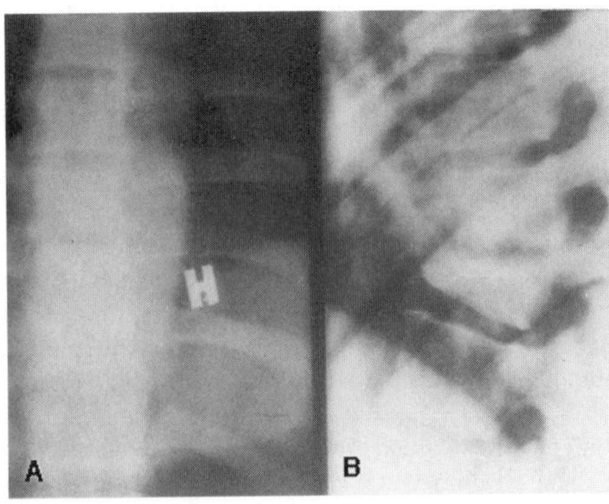


*A*, Abscess formation seen on anterior view of the thoracic spine. *B*, Vertebral collapse with angulation (Pott's disease) on lateral view. (From the Clinical Slide Collection on the Rheumatic Diseases. Atlanta, American College of Rheumatology, 1991; with permission.)

**10. How do you treat osteoarticular tuberculosis?**

Most information regarding treatment is derived from therapy for pulmonary disease. Although some authors still recommend long-term chemotherapy (1–2 years), many now recommend short-term (9 months) therapy as in pulmonary disease.

A typical long-term chemotherapy regimen includes **isoniazid** (5 mg/kg, up to 300 mg orally daily), **rifampin** (10 mg/kg, up to 600 mg orally daily), and **pyrazinamide** (15–30 mg/kg, up to 2 gm daily). Pyrazinamide is typically discontinued after 2 months. **Ethambutol** (15 mg/kg daily) should be added if there is a high likelihood of resistance or if the patient has previously been treated for tuberculosis.

For those with arthritis or minimal osteomyelitis, chemotherapy is often the only therapy needed. However, if bone involvement is extensive or there is neurologic compromise, surgery is often necessary to debride the abscess and hasten recovery.

**11. What musculoskeletal problems can be caused by "atypical" mycobacteria?**

Unlike *Mycobacterium tuberculosis*, the atypical mycobacteria have a propensity to involve the tendons and joints of the hands. In fact, 50% affect the hands, while only 20% affect the knees. Polyarticular disease is much less common.

*Mycobacterium avium–intracellulare* (MAI)

Most common systemic mycobacterial infection in patients with HIV (25% of AIDS patients)

Tenosynovitis, bursitis, and osteomyelitis are all well described

*Mycobacterium kansasii*

Found primarily in the southwestern United States

May cause all of syndromes listed in MAI plus reactivation after total hip replacement

*Mycobacterium marinum*

An aquatic organism that is an occupational hazard of oyster shuckers, aquarium enthusiasts, and others

Tenosynovitis of the hands or wrist is the classic presentation, although synovitis and osteomyelitis have been reported.

**12. What conditions predispose to infection with the atypical mycobacteria?**

- Prior surgery or trauma
- Intra-articular steroid injections
- Open wounds in the hands or fingers
- Immunosuppression

**13. Are any musculoskeletal conditions associated with leprosy?**

**Erythema nodosum leprosum**—It is seen in lepromatous leprosy and probably represents a "reactive" arthritis. Clinical manifestations include fever, subcutaneous nodules, arthralgias, and frank arthritis.

**Symmetric polyarthritis**—It is usually insidious and involves the wrist, small joints of the hands and feet, and knees. It is most often seen in tuberculoid or borderline leprosy. May be rheumatoid factor positive.

**Bony abnormalities** secondary to neuropathy—These include resorption of the distal metatarsals, aseptic necrosis, "claw" hands, and Charcot joints.

**Direct infection** of the bone—This typically affects the distal phalanges.

**Lucio's phenomenon**—Necrotizing vasculitis of skin due to lepromatous leprosy.

**14. How do fungal infections of the bones and joints present clinically?**

**Osteomyelitis** is the most common fungal musculoskeletal syndrome. **Septic arthritis** may arise from direct extension from bone or, less frequently, from inoculation or hematogenous spread. Generally, the monarthritis is indolent with delays in diagnosis of months to years. Acute arthritis is unusual except in *Candida* and *Blastomyces* infections.

**15. How helpful are synovial fluid analyses and cultures in a fungal septic arthritis?**

As in tuberculosis, **cell counts** are highly variable. Typically, WBC counts range from 10,000–60,000/mm$^3$ with either polymorphonuclear or mononuclear cells predominating.

**Culture** of synovial fluid is obviously important in establishing the diagnosis, but the colony counts are often low. Laboratory personnel must be alerted to the possibility of fungal disease so that they do not use inhibitory media.

Recently, polymerase chain reaction–based amplification techniques have been developed for many species of mycobacteria and fungi that may be useful diagnostic techniques in the future.

**16. What are the various fungi that can cause arthritis?**

| DEEP MYCOSES | OPPORTUNISTIC DEEP MYCOSES |
|---|---|
| *Histoplasma capsulatum* | *Sporothrix schenckii* |
| *Cryptococcus neoformans* | *Candida* species |
| *Coccidioides immitis* | *Aspergillus fumigatus* |
| *Blastomyces dermatitidis* | |
| Maduromycoses | |

**17. How and where are these fungi usually acquired?**

*Epidemiology of Fungi Causing Septic Arthritis*

| FUNGI | MODE OF INFECTION | GEOGRAPHIC AREA |
|---|---|---|
| *Histoplasma capsulatum* | Inhalation; aerosolized from soil rich in bird (esp. chicken) and bat feces | Worldwide, but highest in Ohio and Mississippi River valleys |
| *Cryptococcus neoformans* | Inhalation; aerosolized from pigeon droppings; also seen in immunosuppressed | Worldwide |
| *Coccidioides immitis* | Inhalation; especially in dry months; also seen in immunosuppressed and AIDS patients | Southwestern U.S., Central and South America (esp. in arid and semiarid regions) |
| *Blastomyces dermatitidis* | Usually inhalation, but rare case of dog-to-human, human-to-human, and inoculation reported; male to female ratio of 9:1 | Mississippi and Ohio River basins, Middle Atlantic states, Canada, Europe, Africa, and northern South America |
| *Sporothrix schenckii* | Cutaneous disease from scratch or thorn prick; systemic disease probably due to inhalation; also seen in immunosuppressed, alcohol abusers, and gardeners | Worldwide |
| *Candida* species | Endogenous; common in premature infants and other compromised hosts (malignancies, indwelling catheters, immunosuppression, wide-spectrum antibiotic use) | Worldwide |
| *Aspergillus fumigatus* | Inhalation of decaying matter or hospital air; also seen in surgical or trauma patients and immunocompromised | Worldwide |
| *Madurella* species | Implantation of aerobic bacteria or true fungi into uncovered feet | Worldwide, but typically in tropical climates where no shoes are worn (rare in U.S.) |

**18. How frequently is bone or articular involvement seen with these fungi? At what locations?**

*Histoplasma capsulatum*—In the acute setting, polyarthritis with or without erythema nodosum can be seen. In the chronic setting, it is very rare.

*Cryptococcus neoformans*—Osteomyelitis occurs in 5–10% of infections. Arthritis is very rare and almost always involves the knee.

*Coccidioides immitis*—Bone and joint involvement is seen in 10–50% with extrathoracic disease. Osseous involvement may involve multiple sites. Monarthritis of the knee is the most common arthritis.

*Blastomyces dermatitidis*—Bone and joint involvement is seen in 20–60% of patients with disseminated disease. Osseous involvement typically affects vertebrae, ribs, tibia, skull, and feet. Synovitis is usually monarticular.

*Sporothrix schenckii*—Seen in 80% of systemic cases. Arthritis is mon- or pauciarticular.

*Candida* species—Rare, but the number is increasing with greater use of broad-spectrum antibiotics and indwelling catheters.

*Aspergillus fumigatus*—Osteomyelitis and arthritis are both rare.

*Madurella* species—Bone and joint involvement is common with spread of the soft-tissue infection to the bone, fascia, and joint.

**19. How do you treat fungal septic arthritis?**

**Amphotericin B** has historically been the most effective therapy for most fungi but is limited by its renal toxicity. To limit this toxicity, liposomal amphotericin (AmBisome) and most recently caspofungin have been introduced. One of these drugs is indicated for all severe fungal infections or in fungi resistant or not responding to one of the oral antifungal agents. One of these agents is typically used first until antifungal sensitivities have returned, especially in seriously ill or immunocompromised patients.

Oral antifungal agents may be used for treatment of osteoarticular mycotic infections. These include fluconazole (cocci, crypto, *Candida albicans*) and itraconazole (blasto, sporo, *Aspergillus*, histo). Length of treatment is 6–12 months. In immunocompromised patients (i.e., HIV), oral antifungal agents may be used lifelong, owing to high frequency of recurrence.

## BIBLIOGRAPHY


1. Almekinders LC, Greene WB: Vertebral *Candida* infections: A case report and review of the literature. Clin Orthop 267:174–178, 1991.
2. Bocanegra TS: Mycobacterial, brucella, fungal and parasitic arthritis. In Klippel JH, Dieppe PA (eds): Rheumatology, 2nd ed. London, Mosby, 1999, pp 6.4.1–6.4.12.
3. Cuellar ML, Silveira LH, Citera G, et al: Other fungal arthritides. Rheum Dis Clin North Am 19:439–455, 1993.
4. Garrido G, Gomez-Reino JJ, Fernandez-Dapica P, et al: A review of peripheral tuberculous arthritis. Semin Arthritis Rheumatol 18:142–149, 1988.
5. Gibson T, Ahsan Q, Hussein K: Clinical review: Arthritis in leprosy. Br J Rheum 33:963–966, 1994.
6. Harrington JT: Mycobacterial and fungal infections. In Ruddy S, Harris ED, Sledge CB (eds): Kelley's Textbook of Rheumatology, 6th ed. Philadelphia, W.B. Saunders, 2001, pp 1493–1505.
7. Hirsch R, Miller SM, Kazi S, et al: Human immunodeficiency virus–associated atypical mycobacterial skeletal infections. Semin Arthritis Rheum 26:347–356, 1996.
8. Mahowald ML, Messner RP: Arthritis due to mycobacteria, fungi, and parasites. In Koopman WJ (ed): Arthritis and Allied Conditions, 14th ed. Baltimore, Williams & Wilkins, 2001, pp 2607–2628.
9. Marcus J, Grossman ME, Yunakov MJ, Rappaport F: Disseminated candidiasis, candida arthritis, and unilateral skin lesions. J Am Acad Dermatol 26:295–297, 1992.
10. Meier JL: Mycobacterial and fungal infections of bone and joints. Curr Opin Rheumatol 6:408–414, 1994.
11. Perez-Gomez A, Prieto A, Torresano M, et al: Role of the new azoles in the treatment of fungal osteoarticular infections. Semin Arthritis Rheum 27:226–244, 1998.

# 45. VIRAL ARTHRITIDES

Carolyn A. Coyle, M.D.

**1. List three general characteristics of viral arthritis.**

- Viral arthritis often occurs during the viral prodrome, at the time of the characteristic rash.
- The most common viral arthritides in the United States generally present with symmetrical small joint involvement, although different patterns of joint and soft tissue involvement occur with each virus.
- In all instances, the arthritis associated with viral infections is nondestructive and does not lead to any currently recognized form of chronic joint disease.

## HEPATITIS

**2. Is hepatitis A virus infection associated with any rheumatic manifestations?**

Hepatitis A virus infections are not commonly associated with extrahepatic manifestations. Arthralgias and rash have been reported in 10–14% of patients and usually occur early during the acute phase of the disease.

**3. Arthritis has been reported frequently with hepatitis B. Describe the general clinical course of hepatitis B virus (HBV) infection.**

The recognition of the "Australia antigen" as a marker for HBV infection in the 1960s has aided studies that characterized this infectious disease. HBV is a partially double-stranded DNA virus consisting of a nucleocapsid core with two antigenically distinct constituents, hepatitis B core antigen (HBcAg) and hepatitis Be antigen (HBeAg). The core is surrounded by a nucleocapsid coat, or surface antigen (HBsAg).

HBV is primarily transmitted parenterally and much less commonly through sexual contact. Most people exposed to it experience a clinically silent, self-limited infection resulting in an antibody response to HBsAg. Acute icteric infection occurs 40–180 days after exposure to the virus, though approximately 20% remain anicteric. Infection resolves in 90–95% with the remainder developing chronic infections. In approximately 5–10% of cases, HBV infection proceeds to a chronic phase characterized serologically by HBeAg, anti-HBcAg, and HBsAg. Of these patients, 30% proceed to chronic active hepatitis. Risk factors for chronicity include male sex, immunocompromised state, and infection at birth.

**4. What arthritic symptoms are associated with HBV infection?**

Arthralgias are estimated to occur in 20% of patients. Frank arthritis is less common, occurring in approximately 10%. Joint symptoms typically are present during the prodromal phase of acute HBV infection and may precede clinical jaundice by days to weeks. Articular symptoms usually have a rapid onset, occur in a symmetrical additive or migratory fashion, and primarily involve small joints of the hands and the knees. Early morning stiffness and pain are common, with symptoms persisting for 1–3 weeks. In patients with acute hepatitis, joint symptoms are self-limited and have not been associated with chronic joint disease or permanent damage. In patients with chronic active hepatitis, arthralgias and arthritis may be present or recur over long periods of time. Since the joint manifestations may occur in the setting of non-icteric hepatitis, only a high incidence of suspicion can lead to the diagnosis of HBV.

**5. How does HBV infection produce these arthritic symptoms?**

Arthritic manifestations are believed to be due to deposition of HBsAg–anti-HBsAg immune complexes in the synovial tissue, leading to a secondary nonspecific inflammatory response. This antibody response to HBsAg occurs earlier in the disease course in patients with arthritic symptoms compared with those without arthritic symptoms.

**6. Describe other rheumatologic manifestations of HBV.**
A variety of extra-hepatic manifestations are recognized to occur in addition to arthralgias/arthritis, including an arthritis-dermatitis syndrome, nephropathy, and systemic necrotizing vasculitis, in particular polyarteritis nodosa (PAN).

**7. Is there any association between the duration of articular symptoms and the development of systemic vasculitis?**
Prolonged articular symptoms may be a harbinger of systemic necrotizing vasculitis. It usually occurs within the first 6–12 months of HBV infection but occasionally can occur in late, chronic disease. It implies HBV antigenemia and persistent circulating immune complexes. Originally thought to be responsible for as many as 40% of PAN cases, HBsAg positivity is now found in only 5–10% of cases. In HBsAg-positive PAN patients, there appears to be a higher prevalence of malignant hypertension, bowel ischemia, and orchitis whereas glomerulonephritis is uncommon and the ANCA status is usually negative.

**8. What serum antibodies and other laboratory findings are commonly seen with HBV infection and arthritic symptoms?**
The diagnosis of HBV infection is made by confirming the presence of one or more HBV antigens or antibodies to these antigens in the sera of patients with HBV infection. Typically, during the period of joint involvement, free HBsAg is present in the serum. With the onset of jaundice and resolution of arthritic symptoms, the HBsAg titer falls and anti-HBsAg titer increases. Generally, liver function tests are abnormal; CH50, C3, and C4 may be normal or decreased; and synovial fluid appears inflammatory in nature with normal glucose levels, high protein, and high leukocyte counts. Patients may have a low-titer rheumatoid factor.

**9. How do you treat a patient with HBV-associated articular symptoms?**
Joint rest and anti-inflammatory therapy are the nonspecific therapies used to treat articular symptoms associated with acute HBV infection. One patient with chronic active hepatitis, persistent arthritis, and tenosynovitis was treated with interferon-alfa. After 14 weeks of therapy, the patient became HBsAg negative and anti-HBs positive, and resolution of his joint symptoms occurred several months later.

**10. Which rheumatic symptoms have been associated with hepatitis B vaccination?**
Although unusual, several rheumatic syndromes have occurred following recombinant hepatitis B vaccination: RA, erythema nodosum, uveitis, SLE, and others.

**11. Discuss the epidemiology of hepatitis C virus infection.**
Hepatitis C virus (HCV) was discovered in 1988 and is a linear, single-stranded RNA virus with extensive genomic variability. There are six different HCV subtypes. It is the most common blood-borne infection in the US, with a prevalence of 1–2% in the general population. Nationwide, HCV effects approximately 3.5 million people, with over 150,000 new lives affected each year. It is estimated that 8000–10,000 new deaths per year are related to HCV and is expected to exceed the deaths from HIV disease in 3–5 years.

**12. Describe the clinical manifestations of HCV.**
The incubation period for HCV is approximately 6 weeks, compared with 9–12 weeks for HBV. The initial infection is usually less clinically severe than HBV with only 25% of adult patients ever developing jaundice (compared with 80% in HBV). HCV causes more modest elevations in LFT's than HBV; however, more than 60% of acute infections lead to chronicity. 20–50% of HCV will ultimately lead to cirrhosis and with cirrhosis, an increased prevalence of hepatocellular

carcinoma. Like HBV, it is primarily transmitted parenterally by blood products or contact with contaminated needles, though the mode of transmission remains obscure in up to 50% of cases. Though HCV is found in saliva in up to 50% of infected patients, oral transmission has not been clearly demonstrated.

**13. Describe the diagnostic studies used in the diagnosis of HCV.**

Diagnostic testing for HCV infection usually begins with identifying anti-HCV antibodies in the sera of infected patients using enzyme immunoassay (EIA) and recombinant immunoblot assay (RIBA) methodology. The sensitivity of EIA studies is 80–90% but may be fairly non-specific. False-positives may occur in the setting of hypergammaglobulinemia, RF positivity, or recent influenza vaccine. The RIBA method is highly specific and sensitive, and in the presence of elevated transaminases is believed to be diagnostic of HCV infection. Among high-risk populations or EIA-positive patients, confirmation of HCV infection by RIBA approaches 95%. The gold standard of HCV detection remains the HCV RNA PCR test, which should be ordered in atypical cases of HCV and in situations that may influence therapeutic decisions.

**14. Discuss the autoantibodies that may be present in HCV infection.**

10–30% of chronically infected HCV patients have low-titer ANA, 60–70% have anti–smooth muscle antibodies, and 60–80% have a positive rheumatoid factor frequently associated with hypocomplementemia. These associations with HCV infection justify its consideration in the differential diagnosis of rheumatic disease patients. In fact, any patient suspected of having seropositive rheumatoid arthritis who has elevated liver-associated enzymes must be screened for HCV infection.

**15. Discuss the treatment of HCV hepatitis and its extrahepatic manifestations.**

The FDA-approved treatment for HCV infection includes IFN-alpha, 3 million units, three times per week, subcutaneously for 24 weeks, although longer therapy is recommended for the more resistant HCV genotype I. Combination therapy with ribavirin 1000–1200 mg/day is recommended and has been shown to give better response rates.

At this time, it appears that antiviral therapy alone may be adequate for patients with only mild extrahepatic disease. For patients with more active, severe vasculitic complications, a combined anti-viral and cytotoxic regimen is warranted. Glucocorticoids are indicated in organ-threatening disease despite the risk of increased viral loads, especially in doses greater than 20 mg/day (or approximately ½ mg/kg/day).

**16. Describe the rheumatologic manifestations of HCV.**

There is a clear association of HCV and "essential" mixed cryoglobulinemia. This syndrome has been applied to patients with type II or III cryoglobulins associated with a variety of distinctive features including palpable purpura, arthralgia, and multiple organ involvement such as glomerulonephritis and peripheral neuropathy. In recent years, it has been established that HCV infection is found in 80–90% of such patients with the disease and there is growing evidence to suggest that it is directly involved in pathogenesis.

There are scattered reports of a polyarthralgia/arthritis syndrome reported in patients with HCV, but numbers are small and a clinical syndrome has not been clearly defined. Sjögren's syndrome has been described in a number of HCV patients. These patients differ from patients with primary Sjögren's syndrome in that in HCV patients, there is a lower female predominance, absence of ANA and anti-SSA/SSB antibodies, and milder histology on salivary gland biopsy. Clinical symptoms are also less impressive with only 30% having xerostomia and virtually no xerophthalmia.

Several recent reports describe a possible association between fibromyalgia and HCV, and many believe the association is greater than would be expected by chance alone. In one study, 10% of HCV patients fulfilled the fibromyalgia diagnostic criteria compared with 2% of control patients. No relationship between the severity of HCV-associated liver disease and other immunological alterations was seen. HCV infection should be considered in selected patients with fibromyalgia, especially those with atypical features and particularly in the presence of elevated transaminases (even modest elevations) or risk factors for infections with blood-borne pathogens.

## RUBELLA

**17. Natural rubella infection or receipt of rubella vaccine is frequently associated with arthritic syndromes. When in the clinical course of natural rubella infection do the arthritic symptoms appear?**

Rubella virus infection is symptomatic in 50–75% of individuals and is characterized by an acute mild to severe viral exanthema, consisting of a maculopapular rash, and significant lymphadenopathy. The incubation period is approximately 18 days. The rash appears first on the face as a light pink maculopapular eruption and then spreads centrifugally to involve the trunk and extremities, sparing the palms and soles. The onset of joint symptoms occurs rapidly and within several days either before or after the skin rash.

**18. Who is usually affected by the arthritic manifestations?**

Rubella infection associated with joint symptoms is seen most commonly in women who are 20–40 years old. Approximately 30% of female patients and 6% of male patients with rubella have joint symptoms.

**19. What are the typical joint manifestations associated with natural rubella virus infection?**

Joint involvement is usually symmetrical and affects the small joints of the hands, followed by the knees, wrists, ankles, and elbows. Periarthritis leading to tenosynovitis and carpal tunnel syndrome is a well-recognized complication of rubella infection. Joint symptoms are usually self-limited; however, there are case reports of chronic arthritis, without joint destruction, lasting several years.

**20. Discuss the pathogenesis of the arthritic manifestations associated with rubella infection.**

Wild-type rubella and some vaccine strains have been shown to replicate in synovial organ cultures. A number of case reports of rubella-associated arthritis have also demonstrated persistent rubella virus infection of synovial tissue. These data and others support the belief that active viral replication in synovial tissues may be responsible for the joint symptoms. Immune complexes, however, have also been isolated from involved joints. More recently, rubella virus has been isolated from lymphocytes of patients who had experienced rubella-associated arthritis years earlier. Virus in these lymphocytes would serve as a source for later direct viral seeding of the joint or for antigen release and subsequent immune complex formation.

**21. Are any important laboratory abnormalities seen in rubella-associated arthritis?**

Diagnosis of rubella infection may be confirmed by direct viral isolation from nasopharyngeal cultures or serologic methods employing hemagglutination inhibition (HI) or complement fixation (CF) assays. There are no other distinctive laboratory abnormalities in patients with rubella-associated arthritis. Synovial fluid has occasionally yielded rubella virus, with mildly elevated protein levels and leukocyte counts (predominately mononuclear cells).

**22. How is it treated?**

As with all virus-associated arthritides, no specific therapy is available. Restriction of activity and anti-inflammatory therapy are effective in most patients.

**23. What are the arthritic symptoms associated with rubella vaccine?**

Arthritic symptoms occur approximately 2 weeks after rubella vaccination, a time coincident with seroconversion and the ability to isolate rubella vaccine from the pharynx of inoculated people. Joint symptoms are similar to natural infection, however, and involve the knees more frequently than the small joints of the hands. The rate of arthralgia or arthritis following vaccination is approximately 25% in seronegative adult women with far fewer women reporting more prolonged joint symptoms. In children, the frequency of joint manifestations is about 1–5%. Joint symptoms are usually self-limited, lasting 1–5 days, and most studies have failed to demonstrate the development of any form of chronic arthritis.

**24. What are the adverse side effects of the rubella vaccine?**

The Advisory Committee on Immunization Practices (ACIP) of the CDC currently recommends that all persons 12 months of age and older without evidence of rubella immunity, especially females of child-bearing age, be vaccinated against rubella to prevent rubella consequences and in particular the congenital rubella syndrome. Acute joint complaints following vaccination of females with RA 27/3 rubella vaccine (used in the US since 1979) occur in approximately 25% of seronegative adult female vaccines. Despite previous data suggesting a possible relationship between rubella vaccine and chronic arthritis in females, more recent data show no evidence of a causal relationship between immunization and persistent joint symptoms, neuropathies, or any other chronic conditions, which is in keeping with the general characteristics of viral-associated arthritides. In addition to joint symptoms, acute neurological adverse effects have been described following the rubella vaccine, including carpal tunnel syndrome and brachial and lumbar radiculopathies.

## OTHER VIRUS INFECTIONS

**25. What diseases are associated with human parvovirus (HPV) B19 infection?**

Parvovirus B19 was discovered in 1975 and is a small, single-stranded, species specific DNA virus that replicates in dividing cells and thus has a remarkable tropism for human erythroid progenitor cells. It is an emerging pathogen responsible for several diseases, including erythema infectiosum (fifth disease); transient aplastic crisis, especially in patients with underlying hematologic conditions such as sickle cell disease, thalassemia, and other bone marrow disorders; anemia in HIV disease; and fetal hydrops in infected mothers.

**26. What is the clinical course of HPV infection?**

In a clinical experiment in human volunteers, HPV caused viremia 6 days after inoculation in those volunteers without anti-HPV IgG antibodies. Viremic volunteers developed anti-HPV IgM antibodies by the second week after inoculation. The experimental infection was biphasic, with some individuals developing a flu-like illness during the viremic stage and some remaining asymptomatic. Onset of anti-HPV IgM antibodies was associated with clearance of HPV and a clinical illness characterized by rash, arthralgia, and arthritis. In addition, there was an areticulocytosis and, in some individuals, neutropenia, lymphopenia, and thrombocytopenia. In children, rash is common and appears as bright red "slapped cheeks." Joint symptoms are rare in children, occurring in only 5–10% of children. The opposite is true of adults, in whom rash is rare and joint symptoms occur in up to 60%.

**27. How is parvovirus B19 transmitted?**

Parvovirus B19 is presumed to be transmitted via respiratory secretions. The secondary attack rate among susceptible household contacts is about 50%. B19 can also be transmitted parenterally from contaminated blood products, especially clotting factor precipitates. Vertical transmission from mother to fetus has also been well documented, and the greatest morbidity to the fetus occurs when the infection is transmitted during the first or second trimester.

**28. Describe the arthritic symptoms in HPV infection.**

The arthropathy associated with HPV infection is similar to that seen after natural rubella or vaccine-associated infection. There is rapid onset of symmetrical polyarthritis in peripheral small joints, primarily of the hands and wrists. Joint symptoms are more common in adults than children and in women than men. In general, the symptoms are self-limited, but they may persist for months or even years in certain individuals. As with other viral arthropathies, no long-term joint damage or significant functional disability has been reported after HPV infection. The pathogenesis of joint symptoms appears to be secondary to immune-complex deposition and a nonspecific inflammatory response.

**29. How is the serologic diagnosis of HPV B19 infection made?**

The definitive diagnosis of B19 infection relies on detection of B19 IgM antibodies or viral B19 DNA. IgM antibodies occur early, increasing at about 1 month, but are often undetectable by 2–3 months. Detection of viral B19 DNA by PCR may persist even after IgM antibodies disappear. IgG persists for years and perhaps for life. Thus, the finding of IgG anti-B19 antibodies has little diagnostic significance and in fact are found in approximately 50% of the healthy adult population.

**30. Why is it important to make a diagnosis of HPV B19 infection?**

The clinical presentation of HPV B19 infection may resemble adult or juvenile rheumatoid arthritis, especially in patients who do not present with the typical HPV exanthema and who have a clinical course of greater than 2 months' duration. Many chronic B19 patients meet ACR criteria for the diagnosis of rheumatoid arthritis, some even having low to moderate serum titers of rheumatoid factor. In addition, B19 infection may mimic SLE. Both may present with rash, fever, myalgia, arthropathy, cytopenias, hypocomplemententemia, and a positive ANA. The symptoms and signs in B19 patients tend to be short-lived, though prolonged symptoms have been reported. The possibility of B19 should be considered in these patients, as diagnosis of HPV would avoid inappropriate treatment for other rheumatic conditions. Some patients with prolonged arthritis symptoms have responded to hydroxychloroquine or IV gammaglobulin.

**31. What five alphavirus infections have rheumatic complaints as a major feature?**

| ALPHAVIRUS | GEOGRAPHIC DISTRIBUTION |
|---|---|
| Chickungunya | East Africa, India, Southeast Asia, the Philippines |
| O'nyong-nyong | East Africa |
| Ross River | Australia, New Zealand, South Pacific islands |
| Mayaro | South America |
| Sindbis | Europe, Asia, Africa, Australia, the Philippines |

**32. Describe the clinical syndromes associated with alphavirus infection.**

The illnesses arising from infection by the five alphaviruses share a number of clinical features, of which fever, arthritis, and rash are the most constant and characteristic. Arthritis may be severe. The joints most frequently affected are the small joints of the hands, wrists, elbows, knees, and ankles. The arthritis is generally symmetric and polyarticular. In the majority of alphavirus infections, joint symptoms resolve over 3–7 days. Joint symptoms persisting for > 1 year have been reported, although there is no evidence of permanent joint damage.

**33. Describe the clinical features and course of mumps virus infection.**

Mumps virus is a member of the Paramyxoviridae family. It is a single-stranded RNA virus surrounded by a lipoprotein envelope. Subclinical infections with mumps virus are seen in 20–40% of patients. Some of the features of clinical infection include low-grade fever, anorexia, malaise, headache, myalgia, and parotitis. Epididymo-orchitis is the most common extrasalivary gland manifestation of mumps infections and is reported in 20–30% of postpubertal males. CNS involvement occurs in approximately 1 in 6,000 cases. Myocarditis is also not an uncommon finding.

**34. When do the rheumatologic manifestations occur in patients with mumps viral infection?**

Although rare, arthritis has been associated with mumps viral infection. Patients most commonly present 1–3 weeks after the clinical viral infection with a migratory polyarthritis that principally involves the large joints. The duration of symptoms is variable, usually resolving in approximately 2 weeks without residual joint damage.

**35. Are any rheumatic symptoms associated with enterovirus infection?**

Yes. Coxsackieviruses and echoviruses are among the enteroviruses causing a wide spectrum of clinical disease. Self-limited arthritis in both large and small joints has been reported in a limited number of patients with coxsackievirus or echovirus infections. Echovirus can cause myositis in patients with agammaglobulinemia.

**36. Is arthritis frequently associated with clinical infections by the herpetoviruses?**

Arthritis is rarely reported as a complication of these infections. The Herpetoviridae family includes herpes simplex virus, varicella-zoster virus, Epstein-Barr virus, and cytomegalovirus.

ACKNOWLEDGMENT

The author and editor wish to thank Cynthia Rubio, MD, for her previous contributions to this chapter.

## BIBLIOGRAPHY

1. Agnello V, Romain P: Mixed cryoglobulinemia secondary to hepatitis C virus infection. Rheum Clin North Amer 22:1–19, 1996.
2. Barkhuizen A, Bennett RM: Hepatitis C infection presenting with rheumatic manifestations. J Rheum Correspondence 24:1238, 1997.
3. Gran JT, Johnsen V, Myklebust G, Nordbo SA: The variable clinical picture of arthritis induced by human parvovirus B19. Scand J Rheumatol 24:174, 1995.
4. Gumber S, Chopra S: Hepatitis C: A multifaceted disease. Ann Int Med 123:615–620, 1995.
5. Inman R: Rheumatic aspects of hepatitis B infection. Sem Arth Rheum 4:406–420, 1982.
6. Maillefert JF, et al: Rheumatic disorders developed after hepatitis B vaccination. Brit Soc Rheum 38:978–983, 1999.
7. McHutchison JG, et al: Interferon alfa-2b alone or in combination with ribavirin as initial treatment for chronic hepatitis C. N Engl J Med 339:1485–1492, 1998.
8. McMurray RK: Hepatitus C infection and autoimmunity. Sem Arth Rheum 26:689–701, 1997.
9. McMurray RW: Hepatitis C–associated autoimmune disorders. Inf Arth 24:353–374, 1998.
10. Miki NPH, Chantler JK: Differential ability of wild-type and vaccine strains of rubella virus to replicate and persist in human joint tissue. Clin Exp Rheumatol 10:3, 1992.
11. Naides SJ: Rheumatologic manifestations of human parvovirus B19 infection in adults. Rheum Clin NA 24:375–401, 1998.
12. Naides SJ: Viral arthritis. In Ruddy S, Harris ED Jr., Sledge CB (eds): Kelley's Textbook of Rheumatology, 6th ed. Philadelphia, W.B. Saunders, 2001, pp 1519–1528.
13. Nesher G, et al: Parvovirus mimicking SLE. Sem Arth Rheum 24:297–303, 1995.
14. Nocton JJ, Miller LC, Tucker LB, Schaller JG: Human parvovirus B19–associated arthritis in children. J Pediatr 122:186, 1992.
15. Older SA, et al: Can immunization precipitate connective tissue disease? Report of five cases of systemic lupus erythematosus and review of literature. Semin Arthritis Rheum 29:131–139, 1999.
16. Ray P, Black S, et al: Risk of chronic arthropathy among women after rubella vaccination. JAMA 278:551–556, 1997.
17. Rivera J, et al: Fibromyalgia-associated hepatitis C virus infection. Brit J Rheum 36:981–985, 1997.
18. Scully LJ, Karayiannis P, Thomas HC: Interferon therapy is effective in treatment of hepatitis B–induced polyarthritis. Dig Dis Sci 37:1757, 1992.

# 46. HIV-ASSOCIATED RHEUMATIC SYNDROMES

*Daniel* F. *Battafarano,* D.O.

**1. What are the rheumatic manifestations associated with HIV?**

**Articular**
- Arthralgias (45%)
- Reiter's syndrome
- Psoriatic arthritis
- Undifferentiated spondyloarthropathy
- HIV-associated arthritis
- Painful articular syndrome (10%)

**Muscular**
- Myalgias
- Polymyositis
- Myopathy (i.e., HIV-wasting, zidovudine-induced, nemaline rod)

**Diffuse Infiltrative Lymphocytosis Syndrome (DILS) (5%)**

**Vasculitis**

**Infection**
- Septic arthritis
- Osteomyelitis
- Pyomyositis

**Other**
- Soft tissue rheumatism (i.e., tendinitis, bursitis)
- Fibromyalgia (30%)
- Avascular necrosis (due to protease-inhibitors)
- Gout

Adapted from Espinoza LR: Retrovirus-associated rheumatic syndromes. In McCarty DJ, Koopman WJ (eds): Arthritis and Allied Conditions, 13th ed. Philadelphia, Lea & Febiger, 2001, pp 2670–2683.

**2. Does HIV infection have a direct role in the pathogenesis of rheumatic syndromes?**

A wide spectrum of rheumatic syndromes/diseases has been described in HIV-positive individuals. Many of the rheumatic disorders are encountered in non-HIV populations, but some are unique to HIV infection such as DILS or HIV-associated arthritis. A direct role of the HIV infection in rheumatic syndromes has not been well established. Although the specific mechanism is unclear, many of the rheumatic syndromes (polymyositis, vasculitis, HIV-associated arthritis, and DILS) occur in the presence of profound immunodeficiency. Decreasing frequencies of rheumatic syndromes/diseases in HIV-infected individuals treated with combination anti-retroviral agents, nucleoside and nonnucleoside reverse transcriptase inhibitors, and protease inhibitors suggest at least an indirect role of HIV infection. In addition, the mechanism for rheumatic syndromes/diseases is CD4 T cell independent and CD8 T cells may play a more central role in the pathogenesis. Reiter's syndrome in AIDS was initially believed to be related to HIV infection but is now felt to be related to the sexually active nature of the population at risk for HIV. High levels of HIV messenger RNA (mRNA) directly correlate with opportunistic disease and death, and the high levels also correlate with declining CD4 T cell counts. The presence of high levels of mRNA in aspirates of parotid cysts suggests HIV-infected cells contribute at least to DILS.

**3. What role do autoantibodies have in AIDS-associated rheumatic syndromes?**

The most common laboratory abnormality is polyclonal gammopathy in up to 45% of HIV-infected individuals. Low-titer rheumatoid factor and antinuclear antibodies are found in up to 20%. The presence of IgG anticardiolipin antibodies may be observed in over 90% as HIV infection progresses to AIDS, but they are rarely of clinical significance since they are not associated with anti β2 glycoprotein I antibodies. Both cANCA and pANCA have been described in HIV-infected patients, although without characteristic vasculitis. Therefore, although autoantibodies are common, there is no clinical correlation with developing a particular rheumatic syndrome, although patients may be misdiagnosed as having a rheumatic disease and not AIDS.

**4. Name the rheumatic diseases that have a negative association with AIDS.**

Systemic lupus erythematosus (SLE) and rheumatoid arthritis (RA) are both mediated through a process involving the interaction of the MHC class II gene products and the CD4 T lymphocytes. Therefore, SLE and RA diseases may become quiescent with progressive HIV infection as a result of decreasing CD4 cell counts or will not even develop in HIV-infected individuals. Notably, however, some RA patients may not go into remission. When HIV-infected patients with previously diagnosed SLE or RA are being aggressively treated with combination medical therapy, it can be clinically challenging to distinguish symptoms from SLE or RA from complications of HIV infection.

**5. How does Reiter's syndrome typically present in an HIV patient?**

The incidence of Reiter's syndrome associated with HIV infection is 0.5–3%. The onset may precede the diagnosis of AIDS by up to 2 years, occur concomitantly, or most commonly present with severe immunodeficiency. Oligoarthritis of the lower extremities and urethritis are common, but conjunctivitis is rare. Enthesopathy, plantar fasciitis, dactylitis, stomatitis, and skin and nail changes are common, and balanitis may be seen. Axial skeletal involvement is unusual. Synovial fluid is inflammatory, and cultures are negative. The clinical course is typically one of mild arthritis with remissions and recurrences. Severe erosive arthritis does occur and can be very debilitating. The frequency of HLA-B27 in HIV-positive Reiter's patients is the same as that found in HIV-negative Reiter's patients of the same race.

**6. What is conventional treatment for Reiter's syndrome in AIDS patients?**

Nonsteroidal antiinflammatory agents (NSAIDs) are generally effective along with physical therapy modalities. Indomethacin has even been shown to inhibit HIV replication in vitro. Intra-articular and soft tissue cortisone injections are especially therapeutic for localized involvement. Low-dose corticosteroids (less than 10 mg per day) and sulfasalazine (1.5 g per day) may be effective agents for severe enthesopathy/arthritis. Hydroxychloroquine (up to 600 mg per day) and etretinate (0.5 to 1 mg/kg per day) have been useful additional second-line agents in refractory arthritis or cutaneous lesions. Methotrexate (less than 20 mg per week) and other immunosuppressive agents should be used with caution and be monitored closely because they may precipitate fulminant AIDS, Kaposi's sarcoma, or opportunistic infections.

**7. What is the association of psoriasis and HIV infection?**

Psoriasis and psoriatic arthritis tend to occur late in the course of HIV infection. The full spectrum of psoriaform skin manifestations can be observed in the same patient. Early descriptions of HIV infection with associated psoriasis and psoriatic arthritis were believed to be a harbinger for recurrent and life-threatening opportunistic infections. However, antiretroviral treatment is now very effective for either psoriasis alone or for psoriatic arthritis. In HIV-infected patients not taking antiretroviral therapy, this is still a significant clinical problem. Psoriatic arthritis may be specifically treated similar to the arthritis of Reiter's syndrome. Oral gold therapy has been successful in some patients for skin lesions and arthritis. Methotrexate, cyclosporine, and phototherapy are reserved only for refractory skin or joint involvement because they can precipitate worsening immunosuppression or the onset of Kaposi's sarcoma. Lastly, any patient with a severe unexplainable flare of psoriasis or the onset of psoriasis that is unresponsive to conventional therapy should be evaluated for HIV infection.

**8. Why are many HIV patients with arthritis categorized as having an undifferentiated spondyloarthropathy?**

Many patients develop oligoarthritis, enthesitis, dactylitis, onycholysis, balanitis, uveitis, or spondylitis without sufficient criteria to be classified as having Reiter's syndrome or psoriatic arthritis. These patients are ultimately given the diagnosis of an undifferentiated spondyloarthropathy. Local treatment, NSAIDs, intralesional cortisone injections, and sulfasalazine are the conventional approaches for treatment.

**9. What is HIV-associated arthritis? How does it differ from the painful articular syndrome?**

HIV-associated arthritis is characterized by extreme disability and pain in the knees and ankles. The synovial fluid is noninflammatory with negative cultures. The symptoms tend to last 1 to 6 weeks and respond to rest, physical therapy and NSAIDs, low-dose corticosteroids. Unlike Reiter's syndrome and undifferentiated spondyloarthropathies, there is no enthesopathy, mucocutaneous involvement, or HLA-B27 association and symptoms do not recur. Occasionally sulfasalazine may be necessary. Once the clinical disorder is resolved, the medications can be successfully discontinued.

The painful articular syndrome typically involves the knees, shoulders, and elbows and lasts only 2 to 24 hours. It is speculated that this may represent transient bone ischemia, since there is no evidence of synovitis.

**10. How is DILS associated with HIV infection different than idiopathic Sjögren's syndrome?**

Diffuse idiopathic lymphocytic syndrome (DILS) is diagnosed by (1) HIV-positive infection, (2) presence of bilateral salivary gland enlargement or xerostomia persisting for more than 6 months, and (3) histologic confirmation of salivary or lacrimal gland lymphocytic infiltration in the absence of granulomatous or neoplastic enlargement. The onset of symptoms usually presents with a mean period of 3 years before the diagnosis of HIV infection. It is characterized by xerophthalmia, xerostomia, parotid gland enlargement, persistent circulating CD8 T cell lymphocytosis, and diffuse visceral lymphocytic infiltration in an HIV-infected patient. Pulmonary involvement as a result of lymphocytic interstitial pneumonitis is the most serious complication of DILS and has decreased significantly since treatment with protease inhibitors. Neurologic manifestations consist of cranial nerve palsies, aseptic meningitis, and symmetric, peripheral motor neuropathy. Hepatomegaly, elevated liver-associated enzymes, and abdominal pain may be seen. Renal insufficiency, interstitial nephritis, hyperkalemia, and type IV renal tubular acidosis have been observed. Polymyositis and lymphoma have also been observed with DILS. Primary Sjögren's syndrome is contrasted with DILS below. Oral corticosteroids for glandular enlargement are beneficial. Topical treatment is usually satisfactory, but pilocarpine (5–10 mg three times per day) may be necessary for severe sicca symptoms.

| | SJÖGREN'S | DILS |
|---|---|---|
| Parotid swelling | Uncommon | Common |
| Sicca symptoms | Common | Common |
| Extraglandular manifestations | Uncommon | Common |
| Infiltrative lymphocytic phenotype | CD4 | CD8 T cell |
| Autoantibodies (RF, ANA, anti-SS-A/SS-B) | Common | Rare |
| HLA association | DRB1*0301 | DRB1*1102, 1301, 1302 |
| Corticosteroids for glandular symptoms | Rarely helpful | Beneficial |

**11. What are the HIV-associated muscle diseases?**

Muscle involvement in HIV-infected patients can range from myalgias to inflammatory myopathies. Skeletal muscle biopsies at autopsy commonly reveal muscle atrophy without inflammation. A noninflammatory necrotizing myopathy and HIV-related wasting syndrome has been described in over 40% of HIV patients diagnosed with myopathy. The pathogenesis is speculated to be immune mediated or may be related to metabolic or nutritional factors. Other myopathic diagnoses include asymptomatic sporadic creatine phosphokinase (CK) elevation, rhabdomyolysis, fibromyalgia, nemaline rod myopathy, pyomyositis, HIV-associated polymyositis, and zidovudine-associated myopathy.

HIV-associated polymyositis is clinically identical to idiopathic polymyositis with proximal muscle weakness, elevation of CK, a myopathic electromyography (EMG), and an inflammatory muscle biopsy. Most patients respond well to corticosteroid (30–60 mg/d) therapy for 8 to 12 weeks, and the dose adjusted based on the clinical course. Corticosteroids and zidovudine may also be useful in combination. Methotrexate may benefit selected patients as a second-line agent with persistent polymyositis but should be used with caution.

Zidovudine-induced myopathy occurs after a mean duration of therapy of 11 months. This syndrome is clinically indistinguishable from polymyositis. It is associated with an elevation of muscle enzymes, myopathic EMG, and inflammatory muscle biopsy. The muscle biopsy may reveal a zidovudine-induced toxic mitochondrial myopathy with the appearance of "ragged red fibers," which is indicative of abnormal mitochondrial and paracrystalline inclusions. In general, EMG and muscle biopsy are not necessary. The clinical recommendation for evaluating muscle weakness in a patient on zidovudine is to hold the drug for 4 weeks and reassess the patient with examination and CK level. Zidovudine-induced myopathy symptoms and lab tests will improve within 4 weeks, and the muscle strength will return 8 weeks after discontinuing the drug.

**12. List the forms of vasculitis that have been described with HIV infection?**

- Polyarteritis nodosa
- Giant cell arteritis
- Takayasu's arteritis
- Hypersensitivity angiitis
- Henoch-Schönlein purpura
- Wegener's granulomatosis
- Primary angiitis of the central nervous system
- Behçet's syndrome
- Kawasaki disease

**13. Is septic arthritis common in HIV-infected patients?**

No. Bone and joint infections from bacteria do not occur any more frequently in HIV-positive individuals compared with HIV-negative individuals. Intravenous drug abusers and hemophiliacs are clearly at increased risk for septic arthritis. The most common bacterial organism is *Staphylococcus aureus*. Atypical mycobacterium infections rarely occur except in advanced HIV infection. However, *Mycobacterium tuberculosis* arthritis can occur at any time in the course of HIV infection. Fungal musculoskeletal infections typically occur with severe immunosuppression. Osteomyelitis is rare and may occur independently or coexistent with septic arthritis.

**14. How does pyomyositis present clinically?**

Pyomyositis is rarely observed in developed countries but is still commonly diagnosed in Africa and India. It presents with fever, local muscle pain, erythema, and swelling. This uncommon infection typically involves the quadriceps muscle, and a single abscess is present in 75% of cases. *Staphylococcus aureus* is identified in the vast majority, although *Salmonella enteriditis*, *Microsporidia* species, and *Toxoplasmosis gondii* have been diagnosed. Patients respond to conventional surgical drainage and medical therapy.

**15. What other miscellaneous rheumatic syndromes are described with HIV?**

Fibromyalgia has been reported in up to 30% of HIV-infected patients. Tendinitis, bursitis, carpal tunnel syndrome, adhesive capsulitis, and Dupuytren's contracture may occur. Osteonecrosis has been reported in various joints. Recently, osteonecrosis has been reported in HIV patients treated with protease inhibitors.

**16. Do any other retroviruses cause rheumatic diseases?**

Human T lymphotropic virus type I (HTLV-I) is a complex type C retrovirus (RNA virus in subfamily Oncovirinae). It infects millions worldwide, particularly in the Caribbean, southern Japan, South Africa, and South America, especially Brazil. It is transmitted by breast milk, sexual intercourse, and blood products. The virus causes two types of disease: first, adult T cell leukemia/non-Hodgkin's lymphoma (5% lifetime risk) frequently with hypercalcemia and skin involvement; and second, a variety of chronic inflammatory syndromes (lifetime risk 2%). These inflammatory syndromes include a seronegative oligo or polyarthritis with tenosynovitis and nodules with fibrinoid necrosis. Other syndromes include polymyositis-like disease, dermatitis, uveitis, or transverse myelitis, also known as HTLV-1 associated myelopathy/tropical spastic paraparesis (HAM/TSP) . Diagnosis is made by detection of antibodies by ELISA with confirmation by Western blot and observing "flower cells" on peripheral smear. Treatment options are poor. Cases of this viral infection are being seen more frequently in the U.S. as a result of immigration and screening of donated blood.

## BIBLIOGRAPHY


1. Bangham CR: HTLV-I infections. J Clin Pathol 53:581–586, 2000.
2. Berman A, Cahn P, Perez H, et al: Human immunodeficiency virus infection/associated arthritis: Clinical characteristics. J Rheumatol 26:1158–1162, 1999.
3. Brannagan T: Retroviral-associated vasculitis of the nervous system. Neurol Clin 15:927–944, 1997.
4. Cornely OA, Huschild S, Weise C, et al: Seroprevalence and disease association of antineutrophil cytoplasmic antibodies and antigens in HIV infection. Infection 27:92–96, 1999.
5. Espinoza LR, Cuellar MC: Retrovirus-associated rheumatic syndromes. In McCarty DJ, Koopman WJ (eds): Arthritis and Allied Conditions, 13th ed. Philadelphia, Lea & Febiger, 2001, pp 2670–2683.
6. Font C, Miro O, Pedrol E, et al: Polyarteritis nodosa in human immunodeficiency virus infection: Report of four cases and review of the literature. Br J Rheumatol 35:796–799, 1996.
7. Hermann M, Neidhart M, Gay S, et al: Retrovirus-associated rheumatic syndromes. Curr Opin Rheumatol 10:347–354, 1998.
8. Kordossis T, Paikos S, Aroni K, et al: Prevalence of Sjögren's-like syndrome in a cohort of HIV-1 positive patients: Descriptive pathology and immunopathology. Br J Rheumatol 37:691–695, 1998.
9. Miro O, Pedrol E, Cebrian M, et al: Skeletal muscle studies in patients with HIV-related wasting syndrome. J Neurol Sci 150:153–159, 1997.
10. Reveille JD: The changing spectrum of rheumatic disease in human immunodeficiency virus infection. Semin Arthritis Rheum 30:147–166, 2000.
11. Reveille JD: Rheumatic manifestations of human immunodeficiency virus infection. In Ruddy S, Harris ED, Sledge CB (eds): Kelley's Textbook of Rheumatology, 6th ed. Philadelphia, WB Saunders, 2001, pp 1507–1518.
12. Stein CM, Davis P: Arthritis associated with HIV infection in Zimbabwe. J Rheumatol 23:506–511, 1996.


# 47. WHIPPLE'S DISEASE

*Carolyn A. Coyle, M.D.*

**1. What is Whipple's disease?**

Whipple's disease is an uncommon chronic systemic disorder caused by the gram-positive bacillus *Tropheryma whippelii*. It can present with polyarthritis, fever, malabsorption, and CNS manifestations. Because of its nonspecific presentation, the condition is usually diagnosed when it is in an advanced stage. The typical patient is in a middle-aged white man presenting with diarrhea, weight loss, and arthritis.

**2. When did Dr. Whipple first describe the disease and bacillus that now bears his name?**

In 1907, Dr. George Hoyt Whipple reported a "hitherto undescribed disease" in a 36-year-old medical missionary with migratory arthritis, cough, fever, diarrhea, malabsorption, weight loss, skin hyperpigmentation, and abdominal swelling with mesenteric lymphadenopathy. In Whipple's original case report, the patient's "first symptoms were attacks of arthritis coming on in several joints." At autopsy, Whipple noted "great numbers of rod-shaped organisms" in silver-stained sections of a mesenteric lymph node and speculated that this organism might be the causative agent of the disease.

**3. Describe the clinical presentation of patients with Whipple's disease.**

Whipple's disease is a systemic illness affecting primarily middle-aged, white men who usually present with a history of intermittent arthralgias/arthritis involving multiple joints over a period of years. Patients gradually develop diarrhea, steatorrhea, weight loss, and other organ involvement, including cardiac, central nervous system, and renal involvement. Hyperpigmentation of the skin is found in 50% of patients; low-grade fever and peripheral lymphadenopathy are common.

The multisystem manifestations of Whipple's disease can be remembered using the following mnemonic:

**W**asting/weight loss
**H**yperpigmentation (skin)
**I**ntestinal pain
**P**leurisy
**P**neumonitis
**L**ymphadenopathy
**E**ncephalopathy
**S**teatorrhea

**D**iarrhea
**I**nterstitial nephritis
**S**kin rashes
**E**ye inflammation
**A**rthritis
**S**ubcutaneous nodules
**E**ndocarditis

**4. Describe the arthritis associated with Whipple's disease.**

Seronegative migratory oligo- or polyarthritis primarily involving large joints and is characterized by brief episodic attacks lasting a few days and in a pattern akin to palindromic rheumatism. Arthritis is the presenting symptom in 60% of reported cases and is present in 90% of all patients. It does not correlate with intestinal symptoms and can precede other disease manifestations by a decade. Sacroiliitis is present in 7% and ankylosing spondylitis in 4% of cases. In addition, there is an increased association with HLA B27 (28% of Whipple's patients and 10% of healthy people); hence, Whipple's disease is often grouped among the spondyloarthropathies. Joint fluid examination may reveal PAS-positive material; however, joint fluid cultures are negative. Radiographs usually remain unremarkable.

**5. Describe the synovial fluid and microscopic results from arthrocentesis and synovial biopsies of patients with Whipple's disease.**

Arthrocentesis of patients with Whipple's disease and arthritis usually reveals an inflammatory fluid with white blood cell (WBC) counts between 2000 and 30,000/mm$^3$ with greater than 50% polymorphonuclear cells. Repeat arthrocentesis after antibiotic therapy shows resolution of inflammation with WBC counts between 100 and 300/mm$^3$ and less than 50% polymorphonuclear cells. Synovial biopsy also demonstrates an inflammatory picture with focal synovial lining cell hyperplasia and moderate perivascular hymphocytosis. Importantly, there are also PAS-positive granules in macrophages ("foamy" macrophages) within the synovial membrane most likely representing degenerated bacterial forms.

**6. What is the etiology of Whipple's disease?**

Multiple tissues show periodic acid–Shiff (PAS) staining deposits. These deposits contain rod-shaped free bacilli that can be seen using electron microscopy. Recently, investigators have used the polymerase chain reaction to amplify a unique 16S rRNA sequence from tissue specimens of patients with Whipple's disease. According to phylogenetic analysis, the bacterium is a gram-positive actinomycetes that is not closely related to any known genus. The name for the bacillus is *Tropheryma whippelii*. This microorganism has not been cultured in vitro, and the disease has not been reproduced in animals. Since Relman and colleagues identified the bacillus using molecular techniques in 1992, the use of polymerase chain reaction (PCR) technique now permits diagnosis of Whipple's disease in patients who never develop gastrointestinal involvement. In a recent study, synovial tissue and synovial fluid of two patients with histologically proven Whipple's were examined by PCR and DNA sequencing with positive results, leading the authors to propose that the range of arthritic presentations of Whipple's disease is due to the actual presence of the organism in the tissues rather than merely a reactive process.

**7. Describe the natural history of untreated Whipple's disease.**

In 1955, a report of four cases of Whipple's disease and review of the 59 cases previously reported in the literature described the disease as being a "fatal condition." Prior to that time, patients had been followed conservatively or treated with "radiation" with little impact on the disease course. With the advent of corticosteroids, patients were treated with ACTH gel or adrenocorticosteroid therapy, again with limited success. In 1964, antibiotics were used successfully in the treatment of the disease.

**8. How is the diagnosis of Whipple's disease most commonly made?**

Prior to the development of the PCR technique, the definitive diagnosis was established only when microscopic examination of a jejunal biopsy of small intestinal mucosa showed infiltration of the lamina propria by large macrophages that contained diastase-resistant inclusions that are positive by PAS staining. In 1961, electron microscopy demonstrated that the PAS-positive materials were rod-shaped bacilli. These bacilli can be found in multiple other tissues (lymph node, pericardium, myocardium, liver, spleen, kidney, synovium, and brain) and are located both intra- and extracellularly. With the advent of the PCR technique in the 1990s, diagnosis can now be made without biopsy, in cases who present with extraintestinal disease, or when biopsy results are inconclusive.

**9. Can a diagnosis of Whipple's disease be made by PCR of peripheral blood cells?**

PCR is a specific diagnostic test for Whipple's disease on biopsy material from small bowel, lymph node, cardiac, and synovial tissues. It also can be used to diagnose Whipple's in synovial, pleural, and cerebrospinal fluid. However, although genetic material has been found in peripheral blood cells in some patients, PCR has limitations as a diagnostic test if only used on peripheral blood.

**10. How commonly is the central nervous system involved in Whipple's disease?**

Up to 5% of Whipple's disease patients present with neurologic manifestations, and up to 40% will eventually develop CNS symptoms. Dementia is the most frequent symptom (70%), while oculomasticatory myorhythmia with supranuclear vertical gaze palsy is pathognomonic for CNS Whipple's but occurs only in 20% of cases. Brain biopsy and positive PCR of CSF are diagnostic in 90% of cases.

**11. What is the currently recommended therapy for Whipple's disease?**

There is no general consensus on the antibiotic regimen for treatment of Whipple's disease. An antibiotic that penetrates the CNS is generally favored and is the rationale for selection of trimethoprim/sulfamethoxazole, which is typically continued for at least 1 year. Empiric antibiotic therapy in several series of patients has included TMP/SMX, cephalosporins, penicillins, macrolides, and tetracyclines with varied durations and outcomes. In a case series of 29 patients with Whipple's disease, alleviation of symptoms and normalization of pathologic abnormalities were not related to the duration of antimicrobial therapy.

**12. How frequently do patients experience clinical relapses of disease following 1 year of treatment?**

Because Whipple's disease is uncommon, formal prospective studies of therapeutic regimens have not be done. A review of 88 patients with Whipple's disease who had long-term follow-up suggested that clinical relapse occurs in as many as 35% of cases; outcomes of treatment for relapse of CNS disease were particularly poor. The relapse rate may be 40% following long courses of tetracyclines alone, and many post-tetracycline relapses affect the brain. However, given the high relapse rate of Whipple's disease patients with almost any single drug combination, higher doses of a single drug or combination therapy, including oral rifampin, may be more effective. More long-term data are needed regarding choice and duration of antibiotic therapy. Polymerase chain reaction may also have a role in monitoring eradication or persistence of infection giving information to physicians regarding treatment decisions such as choice and alteration of antibiotic therapy and duration of therapy. In at least two studies, histological findings improved with therapy but did not predict recovery or relapse rate, whereas preliminary PCR studies show a correlation between persistent PCR positivity and relapse rate.

**13. How "rare" is Whipple's disease?**

Whipple's disease was first described in 1907. By 1988, there were more than 300 case reports in the literature, and another 2000 persons were estimated to have been afflicted during that same period. Though Whipple's disease is rare, a subset of patients who have seronegative arthritis with a relapsing or palindromic pattern may be found to have Whipple's disease instead. Probably the more relevant question is how many other rare diseases of unknown etiology will be found to have a definite infectious etiology susceptible to antibiotic therapy?

**14. A 57-year-old white man presents with a 6-year history of migratory polyarthritis, lymphadenopathy, abdominal pain, and an 18-kg weight loss over 3 years. A diagnosis of Whipple's disease is made, and the patient is treated with intravenous and then oral penicillin. During his initial treatment, the patient experiences a Jarisch-Herxheimer reaction. What does this mean?**

The Jarisch-Herxheimer reaction was initially described as a systemic reaction that occurs 1 to 2 hours after the initial treatment of syphilis with effective antibiotics, especially penicillin. It consists of the abrupt onset of fever, chills, myalgias, headache, tachycardia, hyperventilation, vasodilation with flushing, and mild hypotension. It has been well correlated with the release from the spirochetes of heat-stable pyrogens. It is self-limited; however, it can be prevented by the administration of oral prednisone. It has been reported after initial treatment of a number of infectious diseases besides syphilis, including leptospirosis, Lyme disease, relapsing fever, and rat-bite fever.


## Acknowledgment

The author and editor thank Cynthia Rubio, M.D. for her previous contributions to this chapter.


## BIBLIOGRAPHY


1. Chears WCJ, Ashworth CT: Electron microscopic study of the intestinal mucosa in Whipple's disease: Demonstration of encapsulated bacilliform bodies in the lesion. Gastroenterology 41:129, 1961.
2. Dobbin WO: Whipple's disease: An historical perspective. Q J Med 56:523, 1985.
4. Fleming JL, Wiesner RH, Shorter RG: Whipple's disease: Clinical, biochemical, and histopathologic features and assessment of treatment in 29 patients. Mayo Clin Proc 63:539, 1988.
5. Keinath RD, Merrell DE, Vlietstra R, Dobbins WO: Antibiotic treatment and relapse in Whipple's disease: Long-term follow up of 88 patients. Gastroenterology 88:1867, 1985.
7. O'Duffy JD, Griffing WL: Whipple's arthritis: Direct detection of *Tropheryma whippelii* in synovial fluid and tissue. Arth Rheum 42:812–817, 1999.
8. Ramzan NN, Loftus E Jr, et al: Diagnosis and monitoring of Whipple disease by polymerase chain reaction. Ann Int Med 126:520–527, 1997.
9. Relman DA, Schmidt TM, MacDermott RP, Falkow S: Identification of the uncultured bacillus of Whipple's disease. N Engl J Med 327:293–301, 1992.
11. Swartz Morton N: Whipple's disease—past, present, and future. N Engl J Med 342:648–650, 2000.
12. Whipple GH: A hitherto undescribed disease characterized anatomically by deposits of fat and fatty acids in the intestinal and mesenteric tissues. Bull John Hopkins Hosp 18:382, 1907.
13. Wollheim FA: Enteropathic arthritis. In Ruddy S, Harris ED, Sledge CB (eds): Kelley's Textbook of Rheumatology, 6th ed. Philadelphia, WB Saunders, 2001, pp 1081–1088.
3. Durand DV, Lecomte C, et al: Whipple's disease. Clinical review of 52 cases. Medicine 76:170, 1997.
10. Singer R: Diagnosis and treatment of Whipple's disease. Drugs 55:669, 1998.
6. Louis ED, Lynch T, Kaufmann P, et al: Diagnostic guidelines in central nervous system Whipple's disease. Ann Neurol 40:561–568, 1996.

# 48. ACUTE RHEUMATIC FEVER

*Carolyn A. Coyle,* M.D.

**1. What is acute rheumatic fever?**

Acute rheumatic fever (ARF) is a systemic inflammatory disease that occurs as a delayed complication of pharyngeal infection with group A streptococci (GAS). It involves multiple organ systems including heart, joints, central nervous system, skin, and subcutaneous tissues. Its most common clinical manifestations include migratory polyarthritis, fever, carditis, and, less often, chorea, subcutaneous nodules, and erythema marginatum. Although joint manifestations may be prominent enough to group it among the rheumatic diseases, its greatest significance relates to its adverse effects on the heart both acutely and chronically leading to rheumatic heart disease, a chronic condition caused by scarring and deformity of the heart valves.

**2. When were the first published studies on acute rheumatic fever (ARF) written? When was the association with group A streptococci made?**

The classic works in the field of ARF were published in 1836 by Jean-Bapite Bouillard and in 1889 by Walter B. Cheadle. They included extensive studies on "rheumatic arthritis" and carditis. The specific rheumatic lesion in the myocardium was described by Ludwig Aschoff in 1904. The introduction of Rebecca Lancefield's grouping system for beta-hemolytic streptococci in 1933 allowed clarification of the epidemiology of the disease by a number of investigators.

**3. How is the diagnosis of ARF established?**

The Jones criteria for guidance in the diagnosis of ARF were first published by T. Duckett Jones, M.D., in 1944 and have been revised over the years by the American Heart Association. The current guidelines are an update of these criteria and are designed to establish the initial attack of ARF.

| Major Manifestations | Supporting Evidence of Antecedent Group A Streptococcal Infection | Minor Manifestations |
|---|---|---|
| Carditis | Positive throat culture or rapid streptococcal antigen test | Clinical findings |
| Polyarthritis | Elevated or rising antibody titer | Arthralgia |
| Chorea | | Fever |
| Erythema marginatum | | Laboratory Findings |
| Subcutaneous nodules | | Elevated acute phase reactants |
| | | Erythrocyte sedimentation rate |
| | | C-reactive protein |
| | | Prolonged PR interval |

All patients should have evidence of a preceding group A streptococcal infection, with few exceptions, and the presence of two major manifestations or one major and two minor manifestations. Fulfillment of these criteria indicates a high probability of ARF. "These guidelines represent recommendations to assist practitioners in the exercise of their clinical diagnosis and are not a substitute for clinical judgment."[1] "In practice, the Jones criteria are most helpful in *ruling out* the diagnosis of rheumatic fever in patients suffering from one of the disorders that mimics it."[5]

**4. Is there an easier way to remember the major manifestations of the Jones criteria for ARF? (Submitted by Christopher T. Parker, D.O.)**

Yes. Simply use the word "Jones" and replace the "o" with heart-shaped symbol.

**J** = joints (75%)

♥ = carditis (40–50%)

**N** = nodules (< 10%)
**E** = erythema marginatum (< 10%)
**S** = Sydenham's chorea (15%)

Percentages listed in parentheses are the incidence of a particular symptom during a child's initial attack.

**5. In which situations can the diagnosis of ARF be made without strict adherence to the Jones criteria?**

There are three circumstances in which the diagnosis of rheumatic fever can be made without strictly adhering to the Jones criteria:

1. Chorea may occur as the only manifestation of ARF many months after the streptococcal pharyngitis and serologic evidence of an antecedent infection may be lacking. Anti-DNase B is the most likely antibody to be positive in a patient with chorea because it is the longest lasting.
2. Indolent carditis may also present as the only manifestation of ARF. Again, the prolonged latent period between clinical infection and the patient coming to medical attention may make documentation of antecedent streptococcal infection difficult.
3. In patients with a history of ARF or rheumatic heart disease, a new episode of ARF may be difficult to diagnosis. Although most of the patients fulfill the Jones criteria, a different heart lesion would need to be present to distinguish between old and new cardiac pathology.

**6. Describe the natural history of ARF and its relationship to the clinical and laboratory criteria necessary to establish a diagnosis.**

There is usually a latent period of approximately 18 days between the onset of streptococcal pharyngitis and ARF. It is rarely less than 1 week or longer than 5 weeks. A positive throat culture for *Streptococcus* is found in only about 25% of patients with ARF and may be negative owing to the latent period. Several rapid group A streptococcal antigen detection tests are commercially available. These tests are generally very specific but may not be very sensitive. Neither throat culture nor antigen test for group A streptococci distinguishes between a carrier state and infection. As many as one third of patients with ARF do not remember having any illness in the month preceding the onset of rheumatic fever.

Streptococcal antibodies may be more useful because (1) they reach a peak titer at about the time of onset of rheumatic fever, (2) they indicate true infection rather than transient carriage, and (3) by performing several tests for different antibodies, any significant recent streptococcal infection can be detected.

**7. What specific antibodies are used to help confirm a diagnosis of ARF?**

The specific antibody tests that have been used are directed against extracellular products found in the supernatant broth of streptococcal cultures. They include antistreptolysin-O (ASO), antideoxyribonuclease-B (antiDNase-B), antistreptokinase, antihyaluronidase, and antiDNase. The normal ranges for all of these antibody titers depends on several factors, including the patient's age, geographical location, epidemiologic circumstances, and the time of the year. The most commonly used tests are ASO, antiDNase-B, and antistreptokinase. Failure to demonstrate evidence of recent infection by a battery of these three serologic tests makes diagnosis of ARF doubtful.

As a general reference, an ASO titer is considered to be elevated at 240 Todd units in adults and 320 Todd units in children. AntiDNase-B titers of greater than 120 Todd units in adults and greater than 240 Todd units in children are also considered to be elevated. Samples should be drawn at 2- to 4-week intervals and all samples processed simultaneously.

The ASO test is the most widely used serological test for the detection of group A streptococcal (GAS) infections. Elevated ASO titers are found in approximately 80% of patients with clinical manifestations of ARF. The sensitivity can be increased even further to 90% using two serological tests and up to 95% using three serological tests. Elevated ASO titers should be interpreted with caution, however, because they are not very specific and other streptococcal groups (including groups C and G) and also other species of bacteria produce ASO-like products resulting in an elevated ASO titer but have no association with ARF. Therefore, when streptococcal infection is suspected, it is advisable to measure not only ASO but also a 2nd type of more specific streptococcal antibody such as the antiDNase-B titer.

**Pearl**: Clinicians should be aware that high ASO titers or other anti-streptococcal antibodies can also be found in patients (particularly children) with other known rheumatic diseases and no associated ARF. This is usually a result of nonspecific immune stimulation resulting in a polyclonal gammopathy demonstrating past streptococcal exposure.

**8. What about the Streptozyme test in diagnosis of ARF?**

The Streptozyme test is a slide hemagglutination test that detects antibodies to five or more streptococcal extracellular antigens. However, the nature of the antibodies assayed and the antigens they are directed against are not well characterized. There is also considerable lot-to-lot variability in the standardization of the reagent. Consequently, this is not a good test to confirm the diagnosis of ARF.

**9. What is the indirect evidence that the group A streptococcus causes ARF?**

Group A streptococcus is clearly implicated as the causative agent in ARF. Group A streptococcus has not, however, been cultivated from lesions of patients with ARF, nor is there a satisfactory experimental model of the disease. Epidemiologic data supporting group A streptococcus as the etiologic agent in ARF include careful military studies over a period of 20 years showing a clear sequential relationship of outbreaks of streptococcal pharyngitis and rheumatic fever. The attack rate of ARF following streptococcal pharyngitis averages 3%. Rheumatic fever does not occur without a streptococcal antibody response, and there is complete prevention of rheumatic recurrences by continuous chemoprophylaxis against streptococcal infection in rheumatic subjects and the prevention of initial attacks by prompt and effective penicillin therapy of streptococcal sore throat.

**10. What is known about the biology of group A streptococcus (GAS) and its relationship to ARF?**

*Streptococcus pyogenes* (group A streptococcus) is a ubiquitous human pathogen that causes a wide array of infections. Streptococcal infections at other sites, such as skin, wound infections, puerperal sepsis, or pneumonia, have not been associated with rheumatic fever. In addition, the so-called nephritogenic GAS very rarely if ever has been shown to cause ARF in well-defined epidemics of nephritis, i.e., the coexistence of ARF and acute glomerulonephritis in the same patient is quite unusual. The possibility that GAS differ in their propensity to elicit acute rheumatic fever was investigated as early as 1935. It has become clear that changes in the biologic properties and clinical virulence of prevalent streptococcal strains influence the rheumatogenic potential of GAS. The M protein is the chief virulence factor of GAS, and antigenic differences are used to divide the GAS into serotypes. Only streptococcal strains with certain M serotypes are known to be highly virulent and strongly associated with acute rheumatic fever. The degree of encapsulation varies greatly among strains of GAS, and GAS strains that are both rich in M protein and heavily encapsulated are readily transmitted from person to person and tend to produce severe infections.

**11. How does group A streptococcus cause ARF?**

Many hypotheses have been advanced to explain the occurrence of ARF and the exact genesis of rheumatic carditis and other clinical manifestations of disease. The most acceptable has been that the disease represents a damaging immune response on the part of the host to an antecedent group A streptococcal infection involving microbial antigens cross-reacting with target organs (molecular mimicry). The purification of the streptococcal M proteins and the identification of M protein peptides, which cross-react with cardiac myosin and are contained in some "rheumatogenic" M protein serotypes, may aid in confirming this hypothesis. Group A carbohydrate antibodies that cross-react with the glycoprotein of the human heart were found to decrease in ARF patients postvalvectomy, but not after valvotomy. These so-called heart-reactive antibodies (HRA) are found in higher titers in patients with rheumatic heart disease compared with those without. More recently, it has been demonstrated that M proteins of rheumatogenic streptococcal serotypes share certain epitopes with human cardiac myosin, cardiac sarcolemmal membrane, and articular cartilage and synovium. Immunoglobulin and complement have been found bound to the myocardium of children dying of rheumatic carditis, which suggests that circulating HRA may have pathogenetic significance. In addition, M protein and streptococcal pyrogenic exotoxin have been shown to function as "superantigens," capable of strongly activating a broad range of T lymphocytes. This suggests a potential mechanism mediating the unrestrained immunologic assault postulated to cause ARF.

**12. Which host factors contribute to the pathogenesis of ARF?**

ARF is most frequent among children in the 4- to 15-year-old group. Some observers have questioned whether repeated "primary" infections might be a prerequisite for the development of ARF. It is very rare in children less than 4 years old. There is no clear-cut sex predilection overall, though host factors including sex and age of GAS infection undoubtedly play some role. The incidence of chorea is equal among prepubescent boys and girls but is very rare in sexually mature men and is exaggerated during pregnancy. Other examples of sex predilection include the increased frequency of tight mitral stenosis in females and aortic stenosis in males. The attack rate of ARF after untreated streptococcal oxidative tonsillitis ranges from 1–3%, and the disease may cluster in families. A statistically significant association has been reported between certain HLA class II antigens (DR4 in whites and DR2 in blacks). Interestingly, a B lymphocyte alloantigen (designated D8/17) has been found in all of ARF patients and in only 15% of controls. This may explain why ARF is more likely to occur in family members, especially twins.

**13. Describe the arthritis associated with ARF.**

The arthritis of ARF usually involves the large joints, particularly the knees, ankles, elbows, and wrists, and occurs in 75% of patients. The hips, spine, and smaller joints of the hands and feet are less commonly involved. In the classic attack, several joints are involved in quick succession and each for a brief period of time, resulting in the typical picture of a migratory polyarthritis accompanied by signs and symptoms of an acute febrile illness. Acute polyarthritis occurs early in the course of ARF, and is almost always associated with a rising or peak titer of streptococcal antibodies. Patients are usually symptomatic for 1 to 2 weeks, and only rarely exceed a 4-week course. ARF never causes permanent joint deformities, with the rare exception of Jaccoud type deformity, which can occur in individuals who have had multiple attacks of ARF.

The pathologic changes of the joints in ARF include a serous effusion, with a thickened, erythematous synovial membrane covered by a fibrinous exudate. Microscopically, there is a diffuse cellular infiltrate of polymorphonuclear leukocytes (PMNs) and lymphocytes. Focal fibrinoid lesions and histiocytic granulomas may be late findings.

Subcutaneous nodules are similar to those found in rheumatoid arthritis and in systemic lupus erythematosus and are usually associated with severe carditis and not arthritis. The nodules are firm, painless, range from few millimeters to 2 cm, and can resolve within days.

**14. Is there a post-streptococcal reactive arthritis (PSRA) distinct from ARF?**

Several investigators have described the inverse relationship between the incidence and severity of carditis and the severity of joint involvement in ARF. Some investigators have described patients with a poststreptococcal "reactive" arthritis that occurs after a brief latent period, persists longer than the typical 4-week period that is typical of ARF, and that responds poorly to salicylates. It appears that this so-called post-streptococcal reactive arthritis (PSRA) is more common in females than males and that PSRA patients tend to be older than those who develop ARF. The arthritis has been described as predominantly non-migratory as opposed to the classic migratory arthritis described in ARF. Some have described PSRA as a *forme fruste* of ARF and hypothesize that it may be caused by different strains of GAS and have a more benign prognosis. However, because no clear data exist to distinguish PSRA from ARF, it is generally recommended that all episodes of poststreptococcal arthritis that fulfill the revised Jones criteria be assumed to represent ARF and be treated as such.

**15. What is St. Vitus' dance?**

St. Vitus' dance is Sydenham's chorea. It is a neurologic disorder characterized by emotional lability and rapid, uncoordinated, involuntary purposeless movements most notable in the face, hands, and feet. Sensation is not affected, but weakness can occur. The choreiform movements disappear during sleep. The latent interval between streptococcal pharyngitis and chorea onset may be prolonged, frequently greater than 6 to 8 weeks. Consequently, ASO titers may be normal although antiDNase-B may still be elevated. Brain MRI shows inflammation in the basal ganglia. Therapy is symptomatic. Symptoms can last 2 to 4 months and may be the only manifestation of ARF. Up to 33% of patients will develop rheumatic heart disease, particularly if a murmur is noted at time chorea presents.

**16. Describe the treatment of ARF.**

When the diagnosis of ARF is established, treatment with antibiotics adequate to eradicate the pharyngeal carriage of group A streptococci is indicated.

*Current Recommendations for Treatment of ARF*

| ANTIBIOTIC | DOSE |
|---|---|
| Benzathine penicillin G | 600,000 units for patients < 60 lb, IM, one dose<br>1,200,000 units for patients > 60 lb, IM, one dose **or** |
| Penicillin V | 250 mg 3 times daily by mouth for 10 days |
| For individuals allergic to penicillin: | |
| Erythromycin estolate | 20–40 mg/kg/day in divided doses (maximum 1 g/day) given by mouth for 10 days **or** |
| Erythromycin ethylsuccinate | 40 mg/kg/day in divided doses (maximum 1 gram/day) given by mouth for 10 days |

Note: Massive antibiotic therapy will not alter the course of ARF or the frequency or severity of cardiac involvement.

The other objectives of therapy of ARF are to quiet inflammation, decrease fever and toxicity, and control cardiac failure. Analgesics without anti-inflammatory properties are recommended for patients with mild disease. This allows complete expression of the clinical manifestations to aid in diagnosis and also avoids post-therapeutic rebounds. Most patients, however, require salicylates. Salicylate levels of 20–30 mg/dl are required to control the inflammatory response. Controlled trials with other NSAIDs are not available. Corticosteroids may be indicated to control the joint and systemic symptoms in more severe cases, with special consideration to dose tapering to prevent rebound symptoms. Most patients with severe carditis or heart failure are treated with corticosteroids; however, it is not clear that this therapy alters the course of their disease.

**17. What is the major sequela of ARF?**

Most of the manifestations of ARF are transient without long-term sequelae, with cardiac involvement being the exception. Damage to heart valves may occur that may be chronic and progressive. Severe cardiac failure, total disability, and death may ensue years after the acute attack. In fact, the earliest structural change of rheumatic inflammation—fibrinoid degeneration—is found in the collagen of the connective tissues of the heart. The characteristic Aschoff nodule is now believed to be derived from connective tissue elements. Rheumatic carditis is characteristically a pancarditis involving the pericardium, myocardium, and free borders of valve cusps.

**18. What is the recommended therapy for prevention of ARF?**

Prevention of ARF in patients without a prior history of ARF (primary prevention) involves antimicrobial therapy consisting of a single injection of 1.2 million units of benzathine penicillin G, or oral therapy with penicillin V, 250 mg 2–3 times a day for patients < 60 lb (27 kg) and 500 mg 2–3 times a day in adolescents and adults for 10 days. In penicillin-allergic patients, the dosage is erythromycin estolate, 20–40 mg/kg/day (maximum 1 g/day), or erythromycin ethylsuccinate, 40 mg/kg/day (maximum 1 g/day), administered in two to four equally divided daily doses for 10 days. Unfortunately, many patients fail to continue oral treatment for the full 10 days needed to eradicate the infecting organism because they are asymptomatic after the first few days of treatment. It is also important to keep in mind that no single regimen eradicates GAS from the pharynx in 100% of even fully treated patients.

Patients with a prior history of ARF (secondary prevention) are at progressively increased risk of developing recurrent ARF with each streptococcal infection and require continuous prophylaxis to prevent intercurrent streptococcal infections. The recurrence rate per infection may be as high as 50% in the 1st year and decreases sharply until 4–5 years after the attack when it levels off to 10% per year. The recommended regimens are as follows:

*ARF Prophylaxis*

| ANTIBIOTIC | DOSE |
|---|---|
| Benzathine penicillin G | 1,200,000 units, IM, every 4 w **or** * |
| Penicillin V | 250 mg twice daily **or** |
| Sulfadiazine | 0.5 g once daily for patients < 60 lb |
| | 1.0 g once daily for patients > 60 lb |
| For individuals allergic to penicillin and sulfadiazine: | |
| Erythromycin stearate | 250 mg twice daily |

* In high-risk situations, administration every 3 weeks is justified and recommended.

Note that sulfa medications can be used for prophylaxis but not for primary treatment of streptococcal infections. Patients with a history of ARF with cardiac involvement should receive lifelong antibiotic prophylaxis. Patients with a history of ARF without cardiac involvement should receive antibiotic prophylaxis for 5 years or until age 21, whichever is longer. If the ARF patient without cardiac involvement has frequent exposure to children (mother, day-care worker), he or she should receive prophylaxis for as long as this exposure continues.

It is hoped that as we learn more about the virulence factors of various GAS strains, we will be able to develop an effective vaccine resulting in eradication of ARF.

**19. What is a reasonable differential diagnosis when confronted with a patient with migratory polyarthritis?**

Gonococcal polyarthritis, subacute bacterial endocarditis, persistent viremias, rubella, hepatitis B, and sarcoid arthritis.

It is important to bear in mind that ARF does not cause urticaria, angioneurotic edema, or clinically overt glomerulonephritis. In addition, serum complement levels are increased and antinuclear and other autoantibodies do not appear in the course of ARF, no matter how persistent the disease.

**20. What is the worldwide impact of ARF?**

The frequency and severity of ARF have been declining rapidly in North America, Europe, and Japan (though a series of unexpected outbreaks in the US occurred in the mid-1980s). These declining trends were beginning even before the widespread use of antibiotics, and changes in social conditions and improved access to health care have undoubtedly contributed to the decline. ARF is, however, rampant in the Middle East, the Indian subcontinent, and selected areas of Africa and South America. It has been estimated that there are 20 million new cases of ARF each year, and rheumatic heart disease accounts for 25–40% of all cardiovascular disease in many developing countries.

### Acknowledgment

The author and editor thank Cynthia Rubio, M.D., for her contribution to this chapter in the previous edition.

## BIBLIOGRAPHY

1. Coburn AF, Pali RH: Studies on the immune response of the rheumatic subject and its relationship to activity of the rheumatic process. IV. Characteristics of strain of hemolytic streptococcus, effective and noneffective in initiating rheumatic activity. J Clin Invest 14:755, 1935.
2. Dale J, Beached EH: Epitomes of streptococcal M proteins shared with cardiac myosin. J Exp Med 162:583, 1985.
3. Diajani A, Taubert K: Treatment of acute streptococcal pharyngitis and prevention of rheumatic fever: A statement for health professionals. Pediatrics 96:758–764, 1995.
4. Diajani AS, Ayoub EM, Barman F, et al: Guidelines for the diagnosis of rheumatic fever: Jones criteria, updates 1992. Circulation 87:302, 1993.
5. Feinstein AR, Spagnuolo M; current commentary Bisno AL: The clinical patterns of acute rheumatic fever: A reappraisal. 1962 [classical article] with present day perspective, 1993. Medicine 72:262–283, 1993.
6. Gaasch WH, ed: Guidelines for the diagnosis of rheumatic fever. JAMA 268:2069–2073, 1992.
7. Jansen TL Th A, Jansen M, Van Riel PLCM: Acute rheumatic fever or post-streptococcal reactive arthritis: A clinical problem revisited. Brit J Rheum 37:335–340, 1998.
8. Stolerman GH: Rheumatogenic group A streptococci and the return of rheumatic fever. Adv Intern Med 35:1, 1990.
9. Tomai M, Kotb M, Majumdar G, et al: Superantigenicity of streptococcal M protein. J Exp Med 172:359, 1990.
10. Valtonen JMO, Koskimies S, et al: Various rheumatic syndromes in adult patients associated with high antistreptolysin O titres and their differential diagnosis with rheumatic fever. Ann Rheum Dis 52:527–530, 1993.
11. Williams RC: Rheumatic fever. In Ruddy S, Harris ED, Sledge CB (eds): Kelley's Textbook of Rheumatology, 6th ed. Philadelphia, W.B. Saunders, 2001, pp 1529–1540.
12. Zabriskie J, Lavenchy D, Williams RC, et al: Rheumatic fever–associated B cell alloantigens as identified by monoclonal antibodies. Arthritis Rheum 28:1947, 1985.

# VIII. Rheumatic Disorders Associated with Metabolic, Endocrine, and Hematologic Diseases

*Screw up the vise as tightly as possible—you have rheumatism; give it another turn, and that is gout.*

Anonymous

## 49. GOUT

Robert W. Janson, M.D.

**1. What is gout? How was the term derived?**

Gout is a disease in which tissue deposition of monosodium urate (MSU) crystals occurs as a result of hyperuricemia (MSU supersaturation of extracellular fluids), resulting in one or more of the following manifestations:

- Gouty arthritis
- Tophi (aggregated deposits of MSU occurring in articular, osseous, cartilaginous, and soft tissue)
- Gouty nephropathy
- Uric acid nephrolithiasis

The term *gout* is derived from the Latin *gutta*, which means a drop. In the 13th century, it was thought that gout resulted from a drop of evil humor affecting a vulnerable joint.

**2. Hyperuricemia is defined as a serum uric acid concentration above what levels in males and in females?**

Serum uric acid concentrations are both age- and sex-dependent. Concentrations rise in association with the onset of puberty in males and menopause in females. Gout is rare in males under age 30 and in premenopausal females. The peak age of onset of gout in males is 40–50 years and in females is after 60 years. Hyperuricemia is defined as a serum uric acid concentration > 7.0 mg/dl in males and > 6.0 mg/dl in females.

**3. How prevalent is gout? What is the ratio of males to females afflicted with gout?**

Overall, the prevalence increases with age and increasing serum urate concentrations. The prevalence of gout is 5–28/1000 for males and 1–6/1000 for females. Thus, gout is the most common cause of inflammatory arthritis in men over 40 years of age. The male to female ratio is 2–7:1. Although only 15% of all patients with hyperuricemia develop gout, the risk increases to 30% to 50% if their serum uric acid concentration is > 10 mg/dl.

**4. Uric acid is a product of the metabolism of which group of nucleotides?**

Uric acid is the end product of the degradation of **purines**. Humans lack the enzyme uricase, which oxidizes uric acid to the highly soluble compound allantoin. The lack of this enzyme subjects humans to the potential risk of tissue deposition of uric acid crystals. Although humans possess the uricase gene, it is inactive. It is postulated that humans have acquired the propensity to become hyperuricemic because uric acid may have powerful antioxidant and free radical scavenger properties.

**5. What pathogenic processes are responsible for the development of hyperuricemia?**

- Overproduction of urate (endogenous or exogenous [dietary] purine precursors)
- Underexcretion of urate (abnormal renal handling of urate)

• A combination of both processes.

Most patients with hyperuricemia and primary gout (90%) are underexcreters of uric acid.

**6. How do you determine if a patient with gout is an overproducer or underexcreter of uric acid?**

A 24-hour urine collection is obtained for the determination of uric acid and creatinine excretion (to ensure an adequate 24-hour collection). On a regular purine diet, a urate value > 800 mg/24 hrs suggests overproduction of uric acid. A 24-hour urate value < 800 mg suggests underexcretion.

**7. Name the two inherited enzyme abnormalities in the urate biosynthesis pathway that can cause urate overproduction.**

- Superactivity of phosphoribosylpyrophosphate (PRPP) synthetase
- Partial deficiency of hypoxanthine-guanine phosphoribosyltransferase (HGPRT) (Kelley-Seegmiller syndrome)

These enzyme abnormalities, which cause uric acid overproduction, are inherited as X-linked traits. Patients with these abnormalities often present with early adult-onset gout (< 30 years of age) and a high incidence of uric acid nephrolithiasis. Complete deficiency of HGPRT results in the **Lesch-Nyhan syndrome** (mental retardation, spasticity, choreoathetosis, and self-mutilation). In addition, patients with **glucose-6-phosphatase deficiency** (von Gierke's glycogen storage disease) also exhibit urate overproduction due to an accelerated breakdown of ATP during hypoglycemia-induced glycogen degradation. Inhibition of renal tubular urate secretion can also occur in this disease as a result of competitive anions from lactic acidosis. Finally, patients with hereditary fructose intolerance caused by **fructose-1-phosphate aldolase deficiency** can develop hyperuricemia in part because of accelerated ATP catabolism.

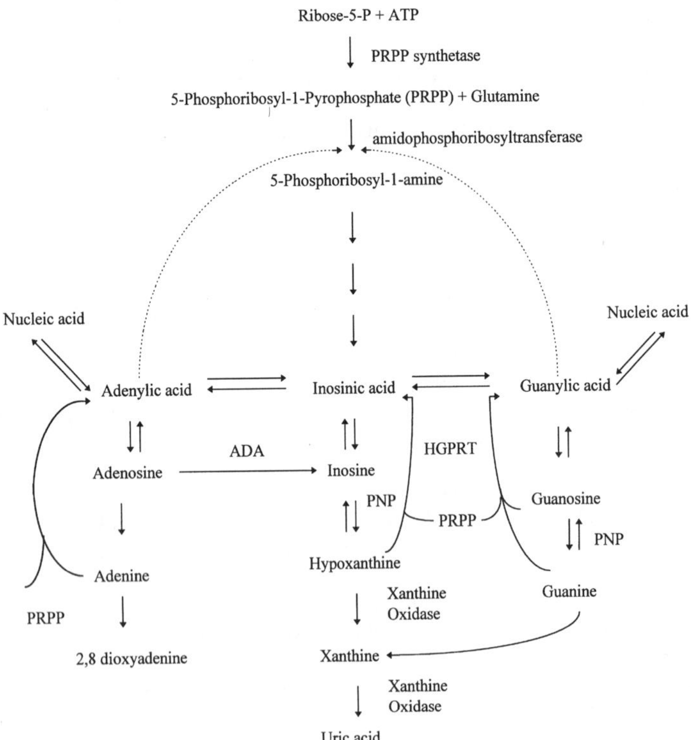


Urate biosynthesis. Broken arrows (- - - ->) represent feedback inhibition. HGPRT = hypoxanthine-guanine phosphoribosyltransferase; ADA = adenosine deaminase; PNP = purine nucleoside phosphorylase.

**8. What are the acquired causes of hyperuricemia?**

**Urate overproduction**: excess dietary purine consumption, accelerated ATP degradation in alcohol abuse, fructose ingestion in hereditary fructose intolerance, and increased nucleotide turnover in myeloproliferative and lymphoproliferative disorders.

**Urate underexcretion**: renal disease, polycystic kidney disease, lead nephropathy (saturnine gout), inhibition of tubular urate secretion (keto- and lactic acidosis), and miscellaneous causes such as hyperparathyroidism, hypothyroidism, and respiratory acidosis.

**9. Name the drugs that cause hyperuricemia due to decreased renal excretion of urate.**

The mnemonic **CAN'T LEAP** might be used to remember these drugs:

| | |
|---|---|
| **C**yclosporine | **L**asix (furosemide) (and other loop diuretics) |
| **A**lcohol | **E**thambutol |
| **N**icotinic acid | **A**spirin (low dose) |
| **T**hiazides | **P**yrazinamide |

Other drugs that can cause hyperuricemia by unknown mechanisms include levodopa, theophylline, and didanosine (ddI). In contrast, the new class of angiotensin receptor blockers (ARBs) have a hypouricemic effect.

**10. Why does excessive alcohol consumption often lead to hyperuricemia and gout?**

Alcohol consumption is associated with the production of lactic acid, which reduces the renal excretion of urate. In addition, it increases the synthesis of urate by accelerating the degradation of ATP. Finally, beer contains a substantial amount of the purine guanosine.

**11. What are the four stages of gouty arthritis?**

- **Asymptomatic hyperuricemia**. Elevated serum uric acid level without gouty arthritis, tophi, or uric acid nephrolithiasis.
- **Acute gouty arthritis**.
- **Intercritical gout**. The asymptomatic intervals between acute attacks of gout.
- **Chronic tophaceous gout**. Development of subcutaneous, synovial, or subchondral bone deposits of monosodium urate crystals.

**12. Describe the characteristics of an acute attack of gout.**

Early episodes of acute gouty arthritis are typically **monoarticular** (85%) and begin abruptly, often during the **night** or **early morning**. The affected joint becomes exquisitely painful, warm, red, and swollen. A low-grade fever may be present. The **periarticular erythema and swelling** may progress to resemble a noninfectious cellulitis termed gouty cellulitis. Acute gout may also occur in nonarticular sites, such as the olecranon bursa, prepatellar bursa, and Achilles tendon. Early attacks often spontaneously resolve over 3–10 days. Desquamation of the skin overlying the affected joint can occur with resolution of the inflammation. Subsequent attacks of gout can occur more frequently, become polyarticular, and persist longer.

**13. Which joints are most commonly involved in gout?**

The joints of the lower limbs are typically involved more often than those of the upper limbs. The **first metatarsophalangeal** (MTP) **joint of the great toe** is involved in > 50% of initial attacks and over time is affected in > 90% of patients. Acute gout of the first MTP is termed **podagra**. In order of frequency of involvement after the MTP joints are the insteps, ankles, heels, knees, wrists, fingers, and elbows. Attacks of gout at more axial sites (spine) are rare. Gout and tophi have a predilection for cooler, acral sites, where the solubility of monosodium urate crystals may be diminished as a result of the cooler temperature.

**14. What events may trigger an acute attack of gout?**

| | |
|---|---|
| Alcohol ingestion | Hemorrhage |
| Dietary excess of purines | Acute medical illness including infections |

| | |
|---|---|
| Exercise | Drugs |
| Trauma | Radiation therapy |
| Surgery (typically during postoperative days 3–5) | |

**15. Can symptomatic hyperuricemia (gout) be managed by diet alone?**

Unfortunately, it is often difficult to manage gout by diet alone because the purine content of the diet typically contributes only 1.0 mg/dl to the serum uric acid concentration. Patients should be advised to limit their consumption of the following purine-rich foods:

- Meats, particularly organ meats (liver, kidney, etc.)
- Seafood, particularly shellfish, sardines, anchovies
- Vegetables and legumes: asparagus, cauliflower, spinach, beans, peas, and mushrooms

**16. How is the diagnosis of gout established?**

Fresh synovial fluid must be evaluated for the presence of monosodium urate crystals. The intra- or extra-cellular crystals are typically needle-shaped and negatively birefringent (yellow when parallel to the axis of the red compensator) on polarized microscopy (see figure) (see Chapter 10). Extra-cellular crystals may be found in previously affected joints during the intercritical phases of gout.

The synovial fluid is inflammatory (typically 20,000–100,000 leukocytes/mm$^3$) with a predominance of neutrophils. Serum uric acid levels will be elevated at some time in almost all patients with gout, but the level can be normal at the time of an acute gouty attack in as many as 30% of patients. Since septic synovial fluids may contain urate crystals, synovial fluid cultures should be obtained if a clinical suspicion of a septic joint exists. Hematologic evaluation may show an elevated erythrocyte sedimentation rate, mild neutrophil leukocytosis, and possibly reactive thrombocytosis.

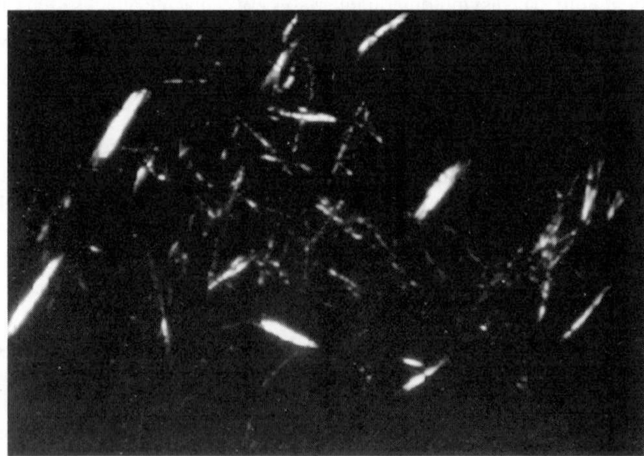

Polarized light microscopy showing needle-shaped uric acid crystals in synovial fluid.

**17. What are the typical radiographic features of gout?**

**Soft tissue swelling** around the affected joint can be seen in early acute attacks of gout. In chronic gout, **tophi** and **bony erosions** can be seen (see figure). Articular tophi produce irregular soft tissue densities that occasionally are calcified. Bony erosions in gout appear "punched-out" with sclerotic margins and overhanging edges, sometimes termed **rat bite erosions**. The joint space is typically preserved until late in the disease, and juxta-articular osteopenia is absent.

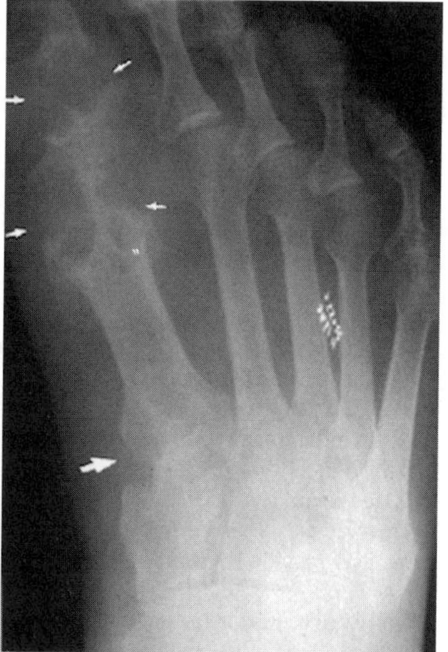

Radiograph of the foot showing erosive changes (arrows) of chronic tophaceous gout.

**18. How long is it from the initial attack of gout until the appearance of tophi? Where do tophi commonly occur?**

In untreated patients, tophi develop on average 10 years after the initial attack of gout. Tophi may occur at any site, with the common locations being the synovium, subchondral bone, digits of the hands and feet, olecranon bursa, extensor surface of the forearm, Achilles tendon, and, less commonly, the antihelix of the ear. Tophi can ulcerate through the skin and extrude a white, chalky material consisting of a dense concentration of monosodium urate crystals.

**19. What medical conditions associated with hyperuricemia and gout must be excluded as part of your evaluation of a gouty patient?**

The two most common medical conditions associated with hyperuricemia and gout:

- Obesity: weight loss can improve hyperuricemia
- Alcohol abuse

Other medical conditions and causes of hyperuricemia:

- Drugs (see Question 9)
- Renal insufficiency
- Hypothyroidism
- Myeloproliferative disease, lymphoproliferative diseases, hemolytic anemias, polycythemia vera
- Hyperparathyroidism, diabetic ketoacidosis, diabetes insipidus, Bartter's syndrome
- Polycystic kidney, lead nephropathy
- Sarcoidosis, psoriasis
- Others (e.g., dehydration)

Other common medical conditions frequently seen in gouty patients:

- Hypertension
- Hyperlipidemia
- Atherosclerosis

Consequently, in addition to a good history and physical examination, appropriate laboratory evaluation of a patient with gouty arthritis should include a complete blood count, SMA18 (chemistries, creatinine and blood urea nitrogen, calcium, liver enzymes, serum uric acid), thyroid-stimulating hormone, lipid profile, urinalysis, and a 24-hour urine for creatinine and uric acid.

**20. How do women with gout differ from male patients with regards to disease onset and clinical features?**

Female patients develop gout at an older age (typically after menopause). Polyarticular acute gouty attacks are more common. Female patients frequently have osteoarthritis, hypertension, and mild chronic renal insufficiency or are being treated with diuretics. Tophi are particularly common in previously damaged joints, including Heberden's nodes, and in the finger pads.

**21. Discuss the pathophysiology of acute gouty arthritis.**

Acute gouty arthritis is triggered by the precipitation of monosodium urate crystals in the joint. The inflammatory nature of the crystals is thought to be determined by certain proteins that coat the crystals; crystals coated with IgG react with Fc receptors on responding cells and promote an inflammatory response, whereas apolipoprotein-B coating of crystals inhibits phagocytosis and a cellular response. Urate crystals stimulate the production of chemotactic factors, cytokines (interleukins 1, 6, and 8 and tumor necrosis factor), prostaglandins, leukotrienes, and oxygen radicals by neutrophils, monocytes, and synovial cells in addition to activating complement and inducing lysosomal enzyme release.

**22. Why are early attacks of acute gouty arthritis often self-limited?**

The following mechanisms have been postulated:

- The cellular response may be modulated by different proteins coating the crystals.
- Phagocytosis and degradation of crystals by neutrophils decrease the crystal concentration.
- The heat associated with the inflammation results in increased urate crystal solubility.
- Enhanced ACTH secretion may suppress the inflammatory response.
- Proinflammatory cytokines (interleukin-1 and tumor necrosis factor) are balanced by the production of cytokine inhibitors and regulatory cytokines.

**23. Name the types of renal disease associated with hyperuricemia.**

- **Urate nephropathy**. Deposition of monosodium urate crystals in the renal interstitial tissue may cause mild and intermittent proteinuria and rarely causes renal dysfunction (associated hypertension is often the cause).
- **Uric acid nephropathy**. Precipitation of uric acid crystals in the collecting ducts and ureters results in acute renal failure, as in the acute tumor lysis syndrome.
- **Uric acid nephrolithiasis**. The frequency parallels the increase in serum and urinary concentrations of uric acid and in acidity of urine. Uric acid stones are radiolucent. The incidence of calcium stones is also increased in patients with gout, particularly those with hyperuricosuria. The uric acid serves as a nidus for calcium stone formation.
- **Other**. Polycystic kidney disease (one-third of patients have gout), lead intoxication, and familial urate nephropathy.

**24. When should treatment of asymptomatic hyperuricemia be considered?**

Asymptomatic hyperuricemia should only be treated in situations where there may be an acute overproduction of uric acid, as in the acute tumor lysis syndrome, or where severe hyperuricemia exists (serum uric acid > 12 mg/dl or 24-hr urinary uric acid > 1100 mg). The prevalence of uric acid nephrolithiasis is 50% in this latter population.

**25. Discuss the treatment options for acute gouty arthritis.**

**NSAIDs** and **colchicine** are effective in the treatment of acute gout. In patients with contraindications to these medications or with acute gout refractory to these therapies, **corticosteroids** may be used to suppress the inflammatory response. Drugs that alter serum uric acid levels (allopurinol, probenecid) should never be started until after complete resolution of the acute gouty attack, nor should they be stopped if an acute gouty attack occurs while the patient is on these medications.

*Medications Used in the Treatment of Acute Gouty Arthritis*

| TREATMENT OPTIONS | DOSAGE | COMMENTS |
|---|---|---|
| NSAIDs (indomethacin) | 50 mg po qid × 24–48 hr, then 50 mg po tid × 48 hr. Taper and discontinue after the attack subsides. | Indomethacin is the drug of choice. Other NSAIDs with short half-lives are probably as effective. |
| Colchicine* | 0.6 mg po qh until symptoms ease, GI toxicity occurs, or a maximum dose of 10 tablets (6 mg) is reached | Most effective within the first 24 hr of an attack. Nausea, vomiting, diarrhea develop in 80% of patients. Contraindicated in the elderly and those with renal or liver insufficiency. |
| Intra-articular steroids (triamcinolone or methylprednisolone) | 40 mg ia with lidocaine for large joints, 10–20 mg for small joints or bursae | Useful in the treatment of 1 or 2 involved joints or bursae. Effective within the first 12 hr of an attack in 90% of patients. |
| Systemic corticosteroids | Prednisone, 30–50 mg/day with taper over 7–10 days or triamcinolone acetonide (Kenalog) 60 mg im, can repeat once | Rebound arthropathy may occur. |
| Adrenocorticotropic hormone (ACTH) | 40–80 USP units im q12h as needed (1–3 doses typical) | More costly than alternative therapies |

* Colchicine (see Chapter 88) can also be given intravenously, although it is not recommended owing to its potential for severe toxicity. If the patient has normal kidney and liver function, the dose is 1.0–2.0 mg iv in 20 ml of normal saline infused slowly over 5–10 min. A dose of 1.0 mg iv can be repeated once in 6–12 hrs. Colchicine given iv is not associated with GI side effects, but can cause skin necrosis (if it extravasates from the vein), bone marrow depression, renal failure, DIC, arrhythmias, seizures, neuromuscular syndromes, multiorgan failure, and death. IV colchicine may soon no longer be manufactured, owing to its toxicities.

**26. What are the indications for chronic treatment of symptomatic hyperuricemia?**

Lifelong therapy with antihyperuricemic drugs is indicated in the following situations:

- > 2 or 3 acute attacks of gout within 1–2 years
- Renal stones (urate or calcium)
- Tophaceous gout
- Chronic gouty arthritis with bony erosions
- Asymptomatic hyperuricemia with serum uric acid > 12 mg/dl or 24 hr-urinary excretion > 1100 mg to decrease the risk of urate nephrolithiasis

The indications for allopurinol versus probenecid therapy, along with their dosing and side effects profiles, are discussed in Chapter 88.

**27. Acute gouty attacks can be precipitated with the initiation of antihyperuricemic therapy. How can this risk be minimized?**

The dose of the antihyperuricemic drug should be gradually increased, along with using either a low-dose NSAID twice daily or colchicine, 0.6 mg orally twice daily (normal renal and hepatic function) as prophylaxis for the first 6–12 months of therapy. If the patient is elderly or has a glomerular filtration rate (GFR) of 30 to 50 ml/min, colchicine should be dosed 0.6 mg/day or every other day. Acute or prophylactic colchicine should be avoided if the GFR is < 30 ml/min. In addition, these regimens are effective in reducing the overall frequency of acute attacks in patients with gout.

**28. What is the treatment for tophaceous gout?**

The goal of treatment is to lower the serum uric acid level substantially to permit urate resorption from the tophi. This result requires long-term treatment with allopurinol to keep the serum uric acid level ideally at least 1.0 mg/dl below the supersaturation threshold of 7.0 mg/dl. Sometimes probenecid is added to allopurinol in order to help the kidney excrete the uric acid load mobilized from the resolving tophi. Prophylaxis with oral colchicine or NSAIDs is often helpful in these patients to reduce the frequency of acute gouty attacks.

**29. Why is gout relatively common in organ transplant recipients?**

Therapy with cyclosporine, which reduces urinary urate excretion, is probably the most significant factor. Treatment of acute attacks and normalization of the hyperuricemia are often problematic. NSAIDs are relatively contraindicated in the setting of cyclosporine therapy or renal insufficiency, and allopurinol therapy with concomitant azathioprine may result in significant neutropenia. Intra-articular or systemic corticosteroids may be the safest treatment options for acute gouty attacks. Synovial fluid cultures should be performed routinely. Uricosurics are often ineffective in these patients as a result of a GFR < 50 ml/min. Allopurinol, at a dose adjusted for renal function, can be used if the patient is not on azathioprine (see Chapter 88). Even if the dose of azathioprine is reduced by 50–75% while the patient is on allopurinol, it is a dangerous combination that may result in severe leukopenia or bone marrow failure. Finally, colchicine should not be used in transplant patients taking cyclosporine because rare, severe cases of myoneuropathy have been reported.

**30. Who was Podagra?**

In mythology, Podagra was the foot-torturess born of the seduction of Venus by Bacchus. This terrible-tempered virgin goddess even inspired fear in Jove!

## BIBLIOGRAPHY


1. Agudelo CA, Wise CM: Gout: Diagnosis, pathogenesis, and clinical manifestations. Curr Opin Rheumatol 13:234–239, 2001.
2. Alloway JA, Moriarty MJ, Hoogland YT, Nashel DJ: Comparison of triamcinolone acetonide with indomethacin in the treatment of acute gouty arthritis. J Rheumatol 20:111–113, 1993.
3. Beutler A, Schumacher HR Jr: Gout and "pseudogout": When are arthritic symptoms caused by crystal deposition? Postgrad Med 95(2):103–116, 1994.
4. Clive DM: Renal transplant–associated hyperuricemia and gout. J Am Soc Nephrol 11:974–979, 2000.
5. Cohen MG, Emmerson BT: Crystal-related arthropathies: Gout. In Klippel JH, Dieppe PA (eds): Rheumatology, 2nd ed. London, Mosby, 1998, pp 8.14.1–8.14.14.
6. Edwards NL: Gout: Clinical and laboratory features. In Klippel JH (ed): Primer on the Rheumatic Diseases, 11th ed. Atlanta, Arthritis Foundation, 1997, pp 234–239.
7. Emmerson BT: Crystal-related arthropathies: The management of gout. In Klippel JH, Dieppe PA (eds): Rheumatology, 2nd ed. London, Mosby, 1998, pp 8.15.1–8.15.8.
8. Groff GD, Franck WA, Raddatz DA: Systemic steroid therapy for acute gout: A clinical trial and review of the literature. Semin Arthritis Rheum 19:329–336, 1990.
9. Janson RW: Diagnosis and management of acute gout and symptomatic hyperuricemia. Prim Care Case Rev 3:3–11, 2000.
10. Kerolus G, Clayburne G, Schumacher HR Jr: Is it mandatory to examine synovial fluids promptly after arthrocentesis? Arthritis Rheum 32:271–278, 1989.
11. Pratt PW, Ball GV: Gout: Treatment. In Klippel JH (ed): Primer on the Rheumatic Diseases, 11th ed. Atlanta, Arthritis Foundation, 1997, pp 240–243.
12. Puig JG, Michan AD, Jimenez ML, et al: Female gout: Clinical spectrum and uric acid metabolism. Arch Intern Med 151:726–732, 1991.
13. Schlesinger N, Schumacher HR: Gout: Can management be improved. Curr Opin Rheumatol 13:240–244, 2001.
14. Sells LL, German DC: An update on gout. Bull Rheum Dis 43:4–6, 1994.
15. Terkeltaub RA: Gout: Epidemiology, pathology, and pathogenesis. In Klippel JH (ed): Primer on the Rheumatic Diseases, 11th ed. Atlanta, Arthritis Foundation, 1997, pp 230–234.

16. Wallace SL, Singer JZ, Duncan GJ, et al: Renal function predicts colchicine toxicity: Guidelines for the prophylactic use of colchicine in gout. J Rheumatol 18:264–269, 1991.
17. Wortmann RL, Kelley WN: Crystal-associated synovitis: Gout. In Ruddy S, Harris ED Jr, Sledge CB (eds): Kelley's Textbook of Rheumatology, 6th ed. Philadelphia, WB Saunders, 2001, pp 1339–1376.

# 50. CALCIUM PYROPHOSPHATE DIHYDRATE DEPOSITION DISEASE

*Matthew* T. *Carpenter*, M.D.

**1. What is calcium pyrophosphate dihydrate (CPPD)?**

CPPD is a calcium salt ($Ca_2P_2O_2 \cdot 2H_2O$) that is deposited in cartilage, appearing as **chondrocalcinosis** on roentgenograms. CPPD can also be released as a crystal into a joint, causing an acute painful arthritis called **pseudogout**.

**2. How common is chondrocalcinosis?**

30% or more of the population has chondrocalcinosis on roentgenograms by the ninth decade of life. Asymptomatic chondrocalcinosis (or the "lanthanic" form of CPPD deposition disease) is the most common clinical presentation of CPPD deposition. In patients with CPPD, the most common sites for finding radiographic chondrocalcinosis are the knees and triangular fibrocartilage of the wrists (> 90%). Calcifications should be bilateral.

**3. Is all chondrocalcinosis caused by CPPD deposition?**

Calcium salts other than CPPD, such as calcium hydroxyapatite, can appear as chondrocalcinosis. For example, the calcification of the cartilage of intervertebral discs seen in ochronosis is largely calcium hydroxyapatite. Clinicians usually assume that certain radiographic patterns of chondrocalcinosis, such as the triangular fibrocartilage complex in the wrist or the hyaline cartilage and menisci in the knees, are due to CPPD deposition. Assuming isn't as precise a method as identifying the crystals in the laboratory.

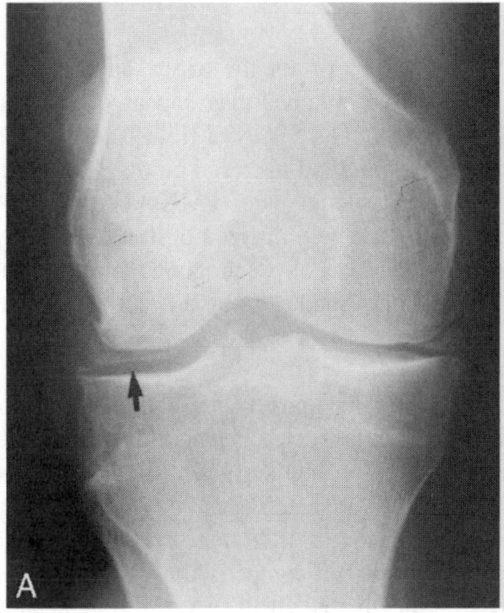


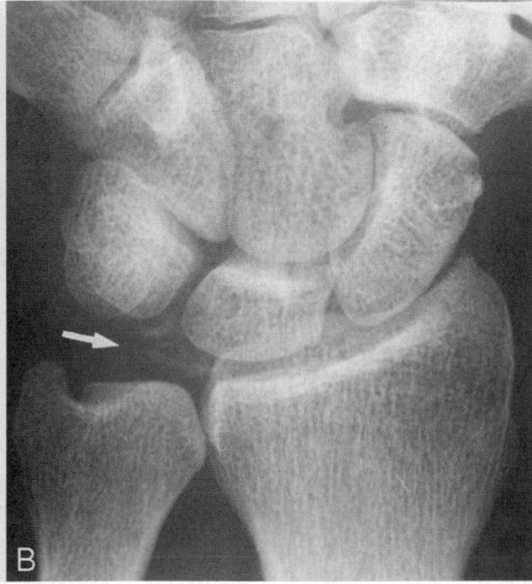


*A*, Chondrocalcinosis of the knee. *B*, Triangular fibrocartilage complex of the wrist.

**4. Do all patients with CPPD deposition have chondrocalcinosis?**

CPPD deposition can cause arthritis without showing up on roentgenograms as chondrocalcinosis. This is one reason that an acutely inflamed joint must be aspirated to identify the cause. An elderly patient who presents with an acutely inflamed knee could have gout or pseudogout as a cause of his or her arthritis, even if the roentgenogram is normal. The only way to tell is to aspirate the joint. The phrase "pyrophosphate arthropathy" has been used to describe structural damage to a joint associated with CPPD deposition, with or without chondrocalcinosis. Calcium pyrophosphate dihydrate deposition disease is the term for all problems associated with CPPD deposition, including chondrocalcinosis, pseudogout, and pyrophosphate arthropathy.

**5. How can CPPD disease present clinically?**

Pseudogout
Pseudo-rheumatoid arthritis
Pseudo-osteoarthritis without superimposed acute attacks of pseudogout
Pseudo-osteoarthritis with superimposed acute attacks of pseudogout
Asymptomatic (lanthanic) radiographic disease
Pseudo-Charcot or pseudo-neuropathic arthritis
These clinical presentations are frequently overlapping.

**6. What is pseudogout? How does it present?**

Pseudogout is an acute arthritis caused by release of CPPD crystals into the joint space. Polymorphonuclear leukocytes engulf the CPPD crystals and release cytokines and other mediators, which cause intense inflammation of the joint. Symptoms of acute pseudogout are the same as any acute arthritis, with rapid onset of pain and swelling. Physical examination reveals warmth, swelling with effusion, tenderness, and limited motion of the involved joint(s). Overlying erythema may simulate cellulitis. Occasionally systemic symptoms such as malaise and fever will also raise suspicion for infection.

The presentation of pseudogout can mimic gout, but the causative crystal is CPPD rather than monosodium urate. Attacks of pseudogout tend to be less painful and take longer to reach peak intensity than gout. Usually, only a single joint is affected, although oligoarticular and polyarticular pseudogout are described. Large joints are affected more commonly than small joints, with the knee being the most frequently involved joint. Untreated pseudogout is self-limited, resolving within a month. Patients are typically asymptomatic between attacks.

**7. How is pseudogout diagnosed?**

When a patient presents with an acute monarthritis or oligoarthritis, the critical and immediate diagnostic procedure is aspiration of the joint(s). The fluid obtained may appear yellow and cloudy or even opaque and chalky white from suspended crystals. Synovial fluid is sent to the laboratory for cell count and differential, as well as Gram stain and bacterial culture. Synovial fluid leukocytosis with a predominance of polymorphonuclear leukocytes (PMNs) is present. A specimen of synovial fluid is also promptly analyzed for crystals by **polarized light microscopy**. The presence of intracellular CPPD crystals confirms the diagnosis of pseudogout. Rarely, definitive diagnosis requires special methods of crystal identification such as x-ray diffraction.

**8. How is polarized light microscopy done?**

A drop of synovial fluid is placed on a clean microscope slide and covered with a cover slip. The slide is first examined under ordinary light microscopy. CPPD crystals tend to be rhomboid-shaped or rectangular. Compared with the monosodium urate crystals of gout, the ends of the CPPD crystals are blunt or square; monosodium urate crystals are needle-shaped or pointed.

Although a preliminary crystal identification may be made with light microscopy, definitive diagnosis requires polarized light microscopy with a first-order red compensator. CPPD crystals are referred to as **weakly positively birefringent**. This means that CPPD crystals appear blue when viewed under polarized light with the long axis of the crystal parallel to the *direction of* *slow vibration of light in the first-order red compensator.* (When rheumatologists talk about crystals, we just ask whether the crystal is aligned in the plane, rather than discussing the direction of slow vibration!) Usually, this axis is clearly indicated on the microscope to prevent confusion. Remember the mnemonic **ABC**—**A**ligned **B**lue **C**alcium—i.e., if the crystal is aligned with the red compensator and blue, then it is calcium pyrophosphate. CPPD crystals lying with their long axes at right angles to the direction of slow vibration will appear yellow rather than blue. If your microscope is equipped with a rotating stage, you can simply rotate the slide until the long axis of the crystal is properly aligned in order to see the expected color. (See Chapter 10.)

**9. What are the pitfalls to be wary of when diagnosing acute pseudogout?**

1. **Septic arthritis** can coexist with any acute crystalline arthritis, including CPPD. Enzymes that degrade cartilage can be released into the joint either from the infecting bacteria or the PMNs. These enzymes are able to "strip" crystals from the structures in and around the joint, causing an unwary clinician to miss a septic joint. This is why joint fluid is sent for Gram stain and culture on all arthrocenteses of acute arthritis.
2. It is possible for a patient to have simultaneous gout and pseudogout. Although rare, this condition is easily diagnosed with careful polarized light microscopy.
3. Acute pseudogout in the wrist of an elderly person may cause a carpal tunnel syndrome. Any patient with carpal tunnel syndrome requires a careful history and physical. Similarly, CPPD deposition has caused cubital tunnel syndrome.
4. Acute pseudogout is frequently precipitated by an urgent medical illness, such as myocardial infarction, or by a surgical procedure. Fluid shifts with fluctuations in serum calcium levels are thought to play a role in such attacks. An elderly hospitalized patient who complains of new joint pain should be investigated for pseudogout. Note that most patients with idiopathic pseudogout are older than 55–60 years old. Recently pseudogout has been reported after administration of intra-articular hyaluronate, which contains high concentrations of phosphate. Intravenous pamidronate has been implicated in attacks when hypercalcemia is rapidly normalized.
5. Up to 20% of patients with pseudogout may not have chondrocalcinosis on radiograph. You must examine synovial fluid for crystals.

**10. How is pseudogout treated?**

The principles of treating acute pseudogout are the same as those for treating acute gout, although the disease is not as well studied.

1. In some cases, **thorough aspiration** of the affected joint with removal of the offending CPPD crystals is said to halt the attack. Most rheumatologists would offer other therapy in addition to thorough aspiration.
2. **NSAIDs** in full doses are the next mode of therapy. **Indomethacin** can be administered in doses of 50 mg po three or four times a day for 1–2 days and then tapered as symptoms subside. Indomethacin is the classic treatment for acute crystalline arthritis, although other NSAIDs in full doses are just as effective. However, the population who suffers from pseudogout is often elderly with multiple chronic illnesses, such as renal insufficiency or peptic ulcer disease, which complicate the use of NSAIDs. It is always prudent to check a creatinine before starting an NSAID.
3. In the patient at risk for a side effect from NSAIDs, an option is **joint injection** with a long-acting corticosteroid preparation, such as **triamcinolone hexacetonide**. Triamcinolone hexacetonide is widely available in a 20-mg/ml solution. 20–40 mg is injected into large joints, such as the knee or shoulder. Smaller joints, such as the wrist, may be treated with 10–20 mg. Local injection is the best method to provide prompt, complete relief of the attack with little risk of systemic adverse effect. Because the patients are elderly and concomitant medical conditions often preclude other options, local injection is my favorite treatment.
4. If the patient is not already on chronic steroid therapy for another problem, such as asthma, an intramuscular or intravenous injection of 40 U of **ACTH** provides relief of symptoms

within 5 days. As in gout, ACTH is less likely to be helpful if the attack is well established (i.e., symptoms present for more than a few days).

5. One or two im injections of 60 mg **triamcinolone acetonide** have been shown to be as effective as indomethacin. This approach has been useful in hospitalized patients with contraindications to NSAIDs who decline local injection.

6. Oral **prednisone** is used for acute gout by some clinicians. This has not been studied in pseudogout but could be considered if intra-articular or intramuscular injection is not desirable, as in a patient with a bleeding diathesis. The patient is started on 40 mg of prednisone po daily, which is tapered to discontinue in 10–14 days. Of course, the side effects of any steroid preparation must be kept in mind, including the potential for temporarily worsening diabetic glucose control or exacerbating an infection.

7. Both oral and intravenous **colchicine** are known to interrupt acute pseudogout attacks, with intravenous colchicine being more effective. Colchicine is not favored by rheumatologists for pseudogout because it has significant potential toxicity in the elderly population affected, and the other therapies noted are well tolerated.

8. As in any acute arthritis, **resting the affected joint** is helpful, with gradual resumption of normal activities as the attack subsides.

9. Polyarticular attacks of pseudogout may be managed with NSAIDs, any of the systemic steroid regimens noted, or colchicine.

**11. Can any therapy prevent attacks of pseudogout from occurring?**

Fortunately, most patients only have a few attacks, which are widely separated in time, and thus require no prophylaxis against pseudogout. For patients with frequent attacks, colchicine, 0.6 mg twice a day, prevents recurrences. Some rheumatologists use daily low doses of an NSAID for the same purpose, although there are no reported studies of this approach.

**12. Does any treatment retard or reverse the deposition of CPPD that is causing the arthritis?**

Unfortunately, there is no therapy to prevent the deposition of CPPD or remove the CPPD deposits already present. Patients with chronic arthropathy from CPPD, in the pseudo-osteoarthritis or pseudo-rheumatoid pattern, are managed like those with osteoarthritis—with physical therapy, NSAIDs, or analgesics.

**13. What conditions are associated with CPPD deposition and need to be ruled out in a patient with CPPD deposition disease?**

*Disease Associations of CPPD Deposition*

| ASSOCIATION STRONG | ASSOCIATION LIKELY | ASSOCIATION POSSIBLE |
|---|---|---|
| Hyperparathyroidism (primary and secondary) | Osteoarthritis | X-linked hypophosphatemic rickets |
| Hemochromatosis | Amyloidosis | Ochronosis |
| Hypomagnesemia | Bartter's syndrome (secondary to resulting hypomagnesemia) | Paget's disease |
| Hypophosphatasia | Benign hypermobility | Wilson's disease |
| Aging | Hypocalciuric hypercalcemia | Acromegaly |
| Familial/hereditary forms | | Diabetes mellitus |
| Post-traumatic, including surgery | | Post-radiation therapy |
| | | True neuropathic joints |
| | | Gout |

* Adapted from Moskowtiz RW: Deposition of calcium pyrophosphate or hydroxyapatite. In Kelley WN, et al (eds): Textbook of Rheumatology, 4th ed. Philadelphia, W.B. Saunders, 1993.

**14. Describe the appropriate laboratory workup in a patient with newly diagnosed CPPD deposition disease.**

Most cases of CPPD deposition are sporadic or associated with normal aging. If the CPPD deposition is severe, affects many joints, or the patient is younger than 55 years, it is reasonable to search for a metabolic cause. Evaluations must be individualized for persons older than 55 years with hyperparathyroidism a primary consideration. Recommended laboratory studies include:

| | |
|---|---|
| Calcium | Ferritin |
| Magnesium | Iron |
| Phosphorus | Total iron binding capacity |
| Alkaline phosphatase | Thyroid stimulating hormone (controversial) |

**15. Can CPPD deposition disease be confused with rheumatoid arthritis?**

Differentiating CPPD disease and RA can be difficult. Up to 5% of patients with CPPD arthritis have involvement of multiple joints, particularly the knees, wrists, and elbows, with chronic low-grade inflammation persisting for weeks or months. This is called the **pseudo-rheumatoid pattern** of CPPD deposition disease. Joint involvement may be symmetric, and systemic symptoms such as fatigue or morning stiffness are present. Physical examination reveals synovial thickening, loss of joint motion, and flexion contractures. The ESR may be elevated.

Ten percent of patients with CPPD disease will test positive for rheumatoid factor (RF), as will healthy elderly patients. Usually RF is present in low titers in such individuals. Higher titers of RF, more widespread synovitis, involvement of the hands and feet, and characteristic erosions distinguish true RA from pseudo-RA.

Before making a diagnosis of seronegative RA, or RA with only a low positive RF, it is prudent to consider the possibility of CPPD deposition disease by reviewing roentgenograms and clinical features and by aspirating a joint to examine synovial fluid for crystals if necessary. This approach is particularly important in middle-aged men because about a third of patients with hemochromatosis present with arthralgias, which may be CPPD-associated. It is also important to remember that true seropositve RA with erosions and CPPD deposition have been reported to exist in the same patient.

Hydroxychloroquine 6.5 mg/kg po qd may be useful for patients with chronic CPPD associated arthritis.

**16. How do you distinguish a CPPD pseudo-neuropathic joint (or pseudo-Charcot joint) from a truly neuropathic joint?**

One feature suggestive of a true **neuropathic joint** is pain present in lesser degree than might be suggested by the severity of the clinical or roentgenographic findings. Patients with true neuropathic joints have abnormal neurologic examinations, with impaired sensation including vibration and proprioception. Patients with **pseudo-Charcot joints** from CPPD deposition have normal pain perception. The distinction is important because patients with true neuropathic joints are generally not offered total joint arthroplasties, while patients with pseudo-neuropathic joints are. Interestingly, patients with tabes dorsalis seem more likely to develop true neuropathic joints if they have underlying CPPD deposition.

**17. Do any features suggest that a patient has pseudo-osteoarthritis from CPPD deposition rather than typical osteoarthritis?**

Pseudo-osteoarthritis is seen in around half of patients diagnosed with CPPD deposition disease. The pattern of joint involvement is different from that seen in other types of osteoarthritis. CPPD pseudo-osteoarthritis results in severe degenerative changes in the metacarpophalangeal joints, wrists, elbows, and shoulders, as well as the knees. Of these joints, only the knees are typically involved in primary osteoarthritis.

In primary osteoarthritis the medial compartment of the knee is more commonly involved, resulting in varus changes or "bow legs." Pseudo-osteoarthritis is more likely to affect the lateral compartment, causing bilateral or unilateral valgus changes or "knock knees." Isolated patellofemoral osteoarthritis is also a common presentation. Flexion contractures in these joints are also said to be characteristic of CPPD pseudo-osteoarthritis. Pseudo-osteoarthritis is more likely to be symmetric than in primary osteoarthritis. Up to 50% of pseudo-osteoarthritis patients also suffer recurrent episodes of acute pseudogout. Radiographs typically show chondrocalcinosis and exuberant osteophyte formation.

BIBLIOGRAPHY


1. Concoff AL, Kalunian KC: What is the relationship between crystals and osteoarthritis? Curr Opin Rheumatol 11(5):436–440, 1999.
2. Fam AG: What is new about crystals other than monosodium urate. Curr Opin Rheumatol 12(3):228–234, 2000.
3. Jones AC, Chuck AJ, Arie EA, et al: Disease associated with calcium pyrophosphate deposition disease. Semin Arthritis Rheum 22(3):188–202, 1992.
4. Meed SD, Spillberg I: Successful use of colchicine in acute polyarticular pseudogout. J Rheumatol 8:689–691, 1981.
5 Reginato AJ, Reginato AM: Diseases associated with deposition of calcium pyrophosphate or hydroxyapatite. In Ruddy S, Harris ED, Sledge CB (eds): Kelley's Textbook of Rheumatology, 6th ed. Philadelphia, W.B. Saunders, 2001, pp 1377–1390.
6. Ritter J, Kerr LD, Valeriano-Marcet J, Spiera H: ACTH revisited: Effective treatment for acute crystal induced synovitis in patients with multiple medical problems. J Rheumatol 21:696–699, 1994.
7. Roane DW, Harris MD, Carpenter MT, et al: Prospective use of intramuscular triamcinolone acetonide in pseudogout. J Rheumatology 24(6):1168–1170, 1997.
8. Rosenthal AK, Ryan LM: Calcium pyrophosphate crystal deposition disease, pseudogout, and articular chondrocalcinosis. In Koopman WJ (ed): Arthritis and Allied Conditions, 14th ed. Philadelphia, Lea & Febiger, 2001, pp 2348–2371.
9. Rothschild B, Yakabov LE: Prospective 6-month double blind trial of hydroxychloroquine treatment of CPPD. Compr Ther 23:327, 1997.
10. Rull M: Calcium crystal-associated diseases and miscellaneous crystals. Curr Opin Rheumatol 9(3):274–279, 1997.


# 51. HYDROXYAPATITE AND OTHER CRYSTALLINE DISEASES

*Matthew* T. *Carpenter,* M.D.

**1. Are the crystals that cause gout and pseudogout the only crystals seen in synovial fluid?**

While monosodium urate crystals, which cause gout, and calcium pyrophosphate dihydrate (CPPD) crystals, which cause pseudogout, are the most commonly identified crystals in synovial fluid, many other crystals or particles may be encountered during polarized light microscopy. Some of these crystals cause disease, and some are just interesting incidental findings.

*Crystals and Particles Seen in Synovial Fluid*

| | | |
|---|---|---|
| Monosodium urate crystals | Starch from examination gloves | Hemoglobin |
| Calcium pyrophosphate dihydrate (CPPD) crystals | Cholesterol crystals | Aluminum |
| Calcium hydroxyapatite crystals (and other basic calcium phosphate crystals) | Lipid droplets | Cystine |
| Calcium oxalate crystals | Foreign organic matter (e.g., plant thorns) | Xanthine |
| Injectable corticosteroid crystals | Metallic fragments from prosthetic joints | Charcot-Leyden crystals |
| | Immunoglobulin crystals in cryolobulinemia | Amyloid |

**2. What is calcium hydroxyapatite?**

Calcium hydroxyapatite ($Ca_5(PO_4)_3{\cdot}2H_2O$) is a calcium-containing mineral found in bone. Hydroxyapatite and several other calcium-containing minerals may be found in soft tissue and tendon calcifications or in some forms of arthritis. Collectively, these calcium-containing minerals are referred to as **basic calcium phosphate** (BCP).

**3. Do BCP crystals cause arthritis?**

There are three groups of joint-related problems in which BCP may play a role:

Calcific tendinitis

Acute calcific periarthritis

BCP arthropathy (e.g., Milwaukee shoulder syndrome)

In acute calcific periarthritis, the BCP crystals are thought to cause the pain and swelling, much like monosodium urate crystals do in gout. In calcific tendinitis, it is not as clear whether the BCP crystals are the cause of the tendinitis or whether the BCP is deposited as a reaction to chronic strain in a poorly vascularized area (i.e., dystrophic calcification). BCP deposition in the soft tissues also occurs in the calcinosis syndromes seen in systemic sclerosis, dermatomyositis, tumoral calcinosis, chronic renal failure with elevated serum calcium and phosphorous product (> 70) (i.e., metastatic calcification), and hypercalcemia.

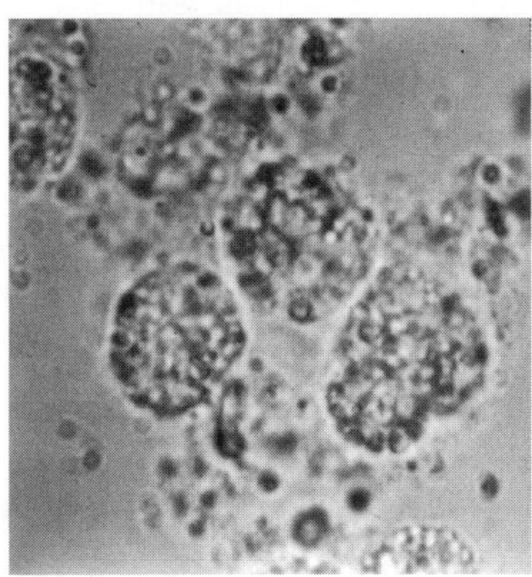

Aggregates of BCP crystals seen in neutrophils under light microscopy.

**4. How are BCP crystals identified if they are suspected of causing a joint problem?**

Identification of BCP crystals is difficult. If characteristic calcifications are observed on roentgenograms, BCP is often presumed to be the cause of symptoms. Aspiration of a calcific deposit may yield material that looks like toothpaste. Individual BCP crystals are so small that they cannot be seen. Ordinary light microscopy may reveal aggregated BCP crystals with an appearance described as "shiny coins."

BCP crystals are not birefringent and so are not seen on polarized light microscopy. Special stains, such as alizarin red, will confirm the presence of calcium in the aspirated material but are not widely available to clinicians and are not specific for BCP. Precise crystal identification requires techniques such as transmission electron microscopy, available only in large referral hospitals and not practical for the clinician.

**5. Where is calcific tendinitis most often seen?**

BCP deposition is common in the shoulder. Up to 5% of shoulder roentgenograms in adults will have periarticular calcium deposits, usually in the supraspinatus tendon. Tendons around other joints may also be affected, including hand, wrist, hip, knee, foot, and neck (longissimus colli muscle at insertion on anterior tubercle of the atlas).

**6. Are such calcifications symptomatic?**

Frequently, BCP deposits are noted as incidental findings. In the case of the supraspinatus tendon of the rotator cuff, the calcification is noted when a patient has a roentgenogram for symptoms of bursitis or impingement. The calcification may in fact be a *result* of chronic tendinitis rather than the cause.

**7. How do you treat calcific tendinitis?**

Of course, asymptomatic BCP deposits require no therapy. Patients with symptoms of bursitis or tendinitis are managed conservatively, with physical therapy and NSAIDs. Local injection with a short-acting corticosteroid such as betamethasone should be used sparingly, as steroids may promote calcification in the long-term. Occasionally, using a needle to disrupt the calcification causes more rapid dissolution of the deposit, by stimulating phagocytosis of the BCP. Surgical or arthroscopic debridement of very large or severely symptomatic calcific deposits may be necessary. Recently, pulsed ultrasound therapy has shown promise for dissolving BCP crystals.

**8. What is acute calcific periarthritis?**

When BCP crystals are shed from a calcific deposit, there is an intense local inflammatory reaction to the crystals, similar to other crystalline arthritides. If this occurs around a joint, the clinical picture is an acute arthritis with pain, warmth, loss of motion, and swelling. Roentgenograms reveal the BCP deposit and thus identify the crystal causing the problem.

In young women, acute calcific periarthritis can occur in the first metatarsal phalangeal (MTP) joint, causing podagra identical to that seen in gout. It may be distinguished from gout by the premenopausal status of the patient, the absence of monosodium urate crystals in synovial fluid, and the characteristic calcifications around the joint on roentgenogram. This particular type of acute periarthritis is called **hydroxyapatite pseudopodagra**. Attacks of calcific periarthritis can occur in the setting of calcific tendinitis in the shoulder or other joints, either spontaneously or after trauma. Symptoms subside over several weeks, either spontaneously or with treatment. Interestingly, the calcific deposit may dissolve during the acute attack, leading to disappearance of calcification on follow-up roentgenograms.

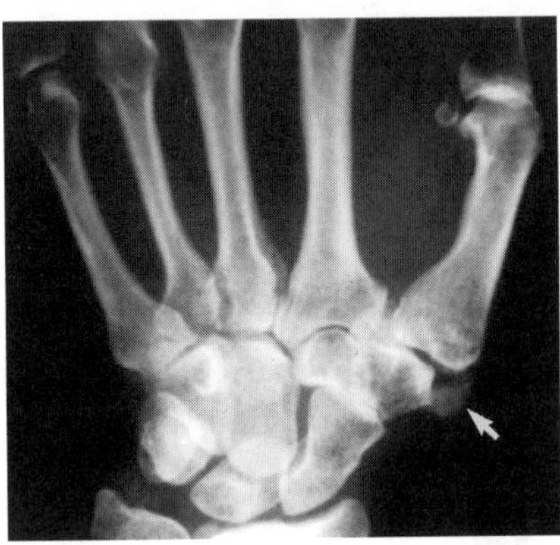

Amorphous homogeneous calcium deposits of BCP seen near the first CMC joint (arrow).

**9. Is any treatment for acute calcific periarthritis available?**

Attacks of calcific periarthritis may be managed similarly to other crystalline arthritides. NSAIDs given in full doses are the mainstay of therapy. For acute crystalline arthritis, indomethacin 50 mg po four times daily for 1–2 days, followed by tapering doses, is the classic approach. Other NSAIDs are probably just as effective. The age of the patient, underlying renal disease (which may be occult in the elderly), and history of peptic ulcer disease are factors that enter into the decision on whether to use NSAIDs. Colchicine, either oral or intravenous, is reported to be successful for acute calcific periarthritis. Aspiration of the joint with injection of a corticosteroid is often the most expedient way to provide relief. I favor triamcinolone hexacetonide for intra-articular injections and betamethasone for soft tissue injections.

**10. How does Milwaukee shoulder syndrome (BCP-associated arthropathy) present?**

Milwaukee shoulder syndrome is characterized by severe degenerative arthritis of the glenohumeral joint, with loss of the rotator cuff, associated with the presence of BCP crystals. Often, large joint effusions are present on physical examination. Patients with Milwaukee shoulder syndrome are usually women in their 70s. Bilateral shoulder involvement is common, with the dominant side more severely affected.

Symptoms vary from minimally symptomatic with shoulder motion to severe pain at rest. Physical examination reveals reduced active and passive range of motion with glenohumeral crepitus. Synovial fluid, which often has streaks of blood, is noninflammatory with few WBCs. Roentgenograms show severe osteoarthritis of the glenohumeral joint associated with upward migration of the head of the humerus, indicating a defect in the rotator cuff. Soft tissue calcifications may also be present.

BCP arthropathy can affect other joints as well, particularly the knees and hips. Lateral compartment joint-space loss in the knees distinguishes this from primary osteoarthritis, similar to CPPD-associated arthropathy. Rapidly destructive arthritis of the finger due to BCP has been called Philadelphia finger.

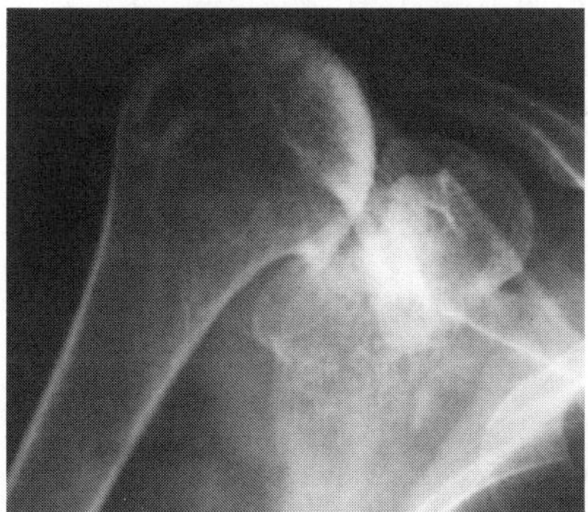

Milwaukee shoulder. Note upward migration of humeral head indicating rotator cuff tear.

**11. How do you treat Milwaukee shoulder syndrome?**

Treatment can be unsatisfactory. Some patients do well with a daily low dose of NSAIDs. Local heat is frequently beneficial. If large effusions are present, repeated arthrocenteses sometimes relieve symptoms. Joint usage needs to be reduced for severe symptoms. At the same time, physical therapy is vital to maintain range of motion and strengthen surrounding muscles. Surgical intervention may be considered for advanced degenerative changes.

**12. Describe the appearance and clinical presentation of other crystals in synovial fluid.**

- **Calcium oxalate crystals** are characteristically bipyramidal in appearance. They occur in effusions from patients with primary oxalosis or end-stage renal disease. Ascorbic acid is metabolized to oxalate, so dialysis patients taking ascorbate supplements are prone to this condition. So-called oxalate gout may cause both intra and extra-articular manifestations.
- **Cholesterol crystals** are found in synovial fluid from *chronic* joint effusions, usually rheumatoid arthritis. The crystals are square and plate-like with a single notched corner. Cholesterol crystals are beautifully birefringent, both positively and negatively. They do not cause inflammation. They are a sign of a chronic inflammatory effusion and form from the cholesterol in the neutrophils' cell membranes after they break down in the joint.
- **Steroid crystals** in synovial fluid may be confused with CPPD crystals because they are often small, irregularly shaped or rectangular, and weakly birefringent. Intracellular steroid crystals in synovial fluid are not uncommon. Careful polarized microscopy is necessary because steroid crystals may be positively or negatively birefringent (often both types are

seen in the same field), whereas CPPD crystals are always weakly positively birefringent. The patient will also have an antecedent history of joint injection with a corticosteroid, possibly weeks earlier. Patients sometimes do not volunteer this information, so a specific question about previous joint injection must be asked.

- **Talc (or starch) particles** from examination gloves are a common artifact during preparation of synovial fluid slides. They resemble little beach balls when viewed with polarized light microscopy.
- **Lipid droplets** have a "Maltese cross" appearance under polarized light microscopy. Lipid droplets in synovial fluid may represent a subchondral fracture or may be seen occasionally in medical conditions, including pancreatitis. Lipid droplets look like starch particles, although the size of starch particles is more variable.

There are many other types of particles or contaminants that can appear in synovial fluid, such as glass fragments from cover slips or specks of cartilage, so all synovial fluids must be examined carefully!

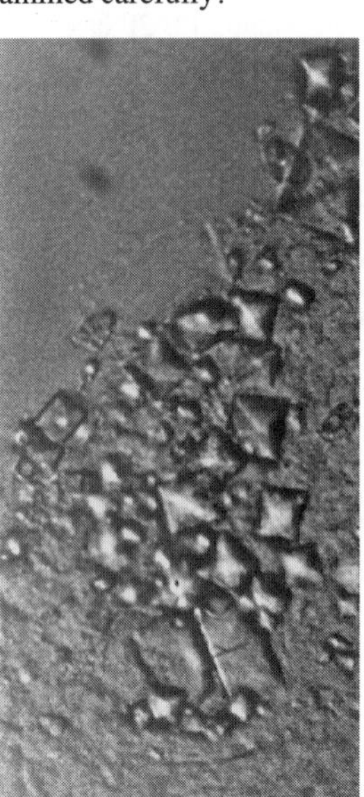
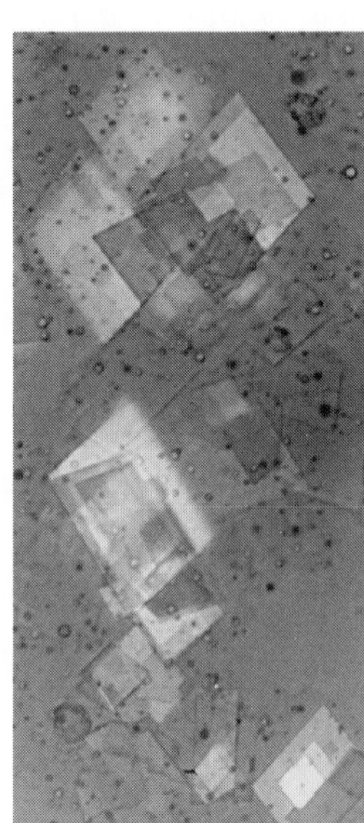
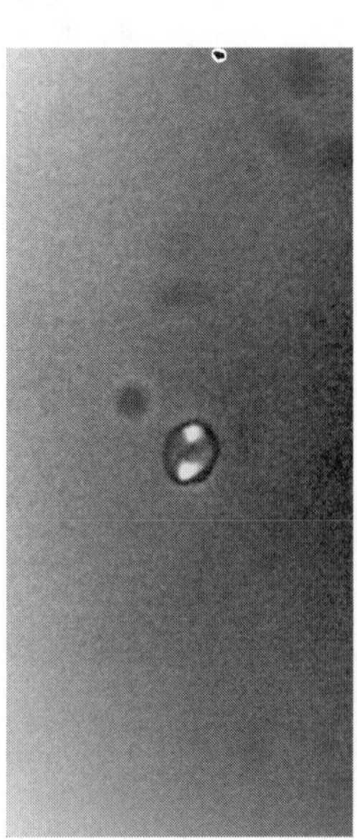

Other synovial fluid crystals. *Left*, Calcium oxalate crystals have a characteristic bipyramidal shape under ordinary light microscopy. (Courtesy of The Upjohn Company.) *Center*, Plane-shaped cholesterol crystals are strongly birefringent when viewed under polarized light microscopy. These crystals were obtained from aspiration of a knee effusion in a patient with rheumatoid arthritis. (Courtesy of Linda Sakai, M.D.) *Right*, Starch (talc) from examination gloves is a common artifact during slide preparation. (Courtesy of The Upjohn Company.)

## BIBLIOGRAPHY

1. Bonnefil PL, Demos TC, Lomasney L, Yetter EM: Radiologic case study. Hydroxyapatite crystal deposition. Orthopedics 24:517–520, 2001.
2. Fam AG, Stein J: Hydroxyapatite pseudopodagra in young women. J Rheumatol 19:662–664, 1992.
3. Halverson PB, Carrera GF, McCarty DJ: Milwaukee shoulder syndrome: Fifteen additional cases and a description of contributing factors. Arch Intern Med 150:677–682, 1990.
4. Halverson PB: Basic calcium phosphate (apatite, octacalcium phosphate, tricalcium phosphate) crystal deposition diseases and calcinosis. In Koopman WJ (ed): Arthritis and Allied Conditions, 14th ed. Philadelphia, Lea & Febiger, 2001, pp 2372–2392.
5. Reginato AJ: Calcium oxalate and other crystals or particles associated with arthritis. In Koopman WJ (ed): Arthritis and Allied Conditions, 14th ed. Philadelphia, Lea & Febiger, 2001, pp 2393–2414.

6. Reginato AJ, Reginato AM: Diseases associated with deposition of calcium pyrophosphate or hydroxyapatite. In Ruddy S, Harris ED, Sledge CB (eds): Kelley's Textbook of Rheumatology, 6th ed. Philadelphia, W.B. Saunders, 2001, pp 1377–1390.
7. Reginato AJ, Falasca GF, Usmani Q: Do we really need to pay attention to less common crystals? Curr Opin Rheumatol 11(3):446–452, 1999.
8. Rosenthal AK: Calcium crystal associated arthritis. Curr Opin Rheumatol 10(3):273–277, 1998.
9. Schumacher HR, Reginato AJ: Atlas of Synovial Fluid Analysis and Crystal Identification. Philadelphia, Lea & Febiger, 1991.

# 52. ENDOCRINE-ASSOCIATED ARTHROPATHIES

*Edmund* H. *Hornstein*, D.O.

**1. What signs or symptoms should prompt a search for an occult endocrinopathy?**

Entrapment neuropathy, particularly carpal tunnel syndrome
Calcium pyrophosphate dihydrate (CPPD) arthropathy
Diffuse myalgia with or without muscle weakness
Raynaud's phenomenon

**2. Which endocrine diseases have well-described rheumatologic manifestations associated with them?**

Diabetes mellitus
Hypothyroidism
Hyperthyroidism
Hypoparathyroidism
Hyperparathyroidism
Acromegaly
Cushing's syndrome

## DIABETES MELLITUS

**3. What rheumatologic syndromes are more common in patients with diabetes mellitus?**

- Intrinsic complications of diabetes mellitus
  - Diabetic hand syndrome of limited joint mobility (diabetic cheirarthropathy)
  - Neuropathic arthropathy (Charcot joint) and diabetic osteolysis
  - Diabetic amyotrophy
- Conditions with increased incidence in diabetes mellitus
  - Periarthritis of the shoulder (frozen shoulder)
  - Reflex sympathetic dystrophy (shoulder-hand syndrome)
  - Flexor tenosynovitis of the hands
  - Dupuytren's contractures
  - Carpal tunnel syndrome
  - Diffuse idiopathic skeletal hyperostosis (DISH)
  - Septic joint/osteomyelitis

**4. How does the diabetic hand syndrome of limited joint mobility (LJM) present?**

This syndrome, also known as diabetic cheirarthropathy, presents with the insidious development of flexion contractures involving the small joints of the hands, starting with the distal (DIPs) and proximal interphalangeal joints (PIPs) and moving proximally over time. This condition occurs in both insulin-dependent (IDDM) and non-insulin-dependent (NIDDM) diabetics and correlates with disease duration, glucose control, and renal/retinal microvascular disease. It may be seen in as many as 30–75% of long-term diabetics.

The "prayer sign" observed on physical examination reflects the inability to fully extend the joints of the fingers (see figure). These finger contractures are attributed to excessive dermal collagen and collagen crosslinks, as well as to increased dermal hydration resulting in indurated and thickened skin around the joints. This condition can be confused with scleroderma. Laboratory serologies and hand radiographs are unremarkable. Treatment is physical therapy and control of the underlying diabetes. Contractures usually progress slowly but rarely limit function significantly.

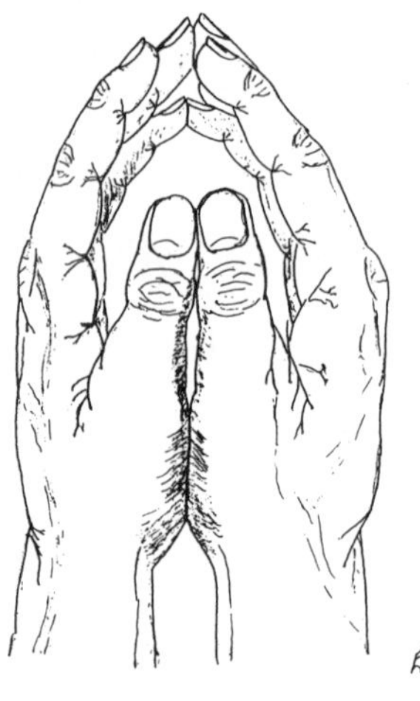

Prayer sign in a patient with LJM due to diabetes mellitus.

**5. Discuss the relationship between Charcot joint and diabetes mellitus.**

Charcot joint occurs in < 1% of all diabetics. It occurs in both males and females with equal frequency. Most patients (> 66%) are over age 40 and have had long-standing (> 10 yrs), poorly controlled diabetes complicated by a diabetic peripheral neuropathy. Patients present with painless swelling and deformity usually of the foot (most commonly tarsometatarsal joints) and ankle, although knee, hip, and spine can be involved. With progression of disease, the patient can develop "rocker bottom" feet due to midtarsal collapse. Skin over bony prominences can ulcerate and become infected without the patient's knowledge as a result of abnormal sensation resulting from the neuropathy.

Radiographs frequently show severe abnormalities characterized by the **5 Ds**: destruction, density (increased), debris, disorganization, and dislocation (see figure). The increased density and sharp margins of the bony debris help separate a Charcot joint from infection. Treatment includes protected weight-bearing, soft casts, good shoes, and aggressive treatment and prevention of skin ulcerations. Charcot joints, however, usually progress. There is no role for surgery (fusion, arthroplasty) other than amputation for severe cases. Diabetes mellitus has replaced neurosyphilis as the most common cause of a Charcot joint today.

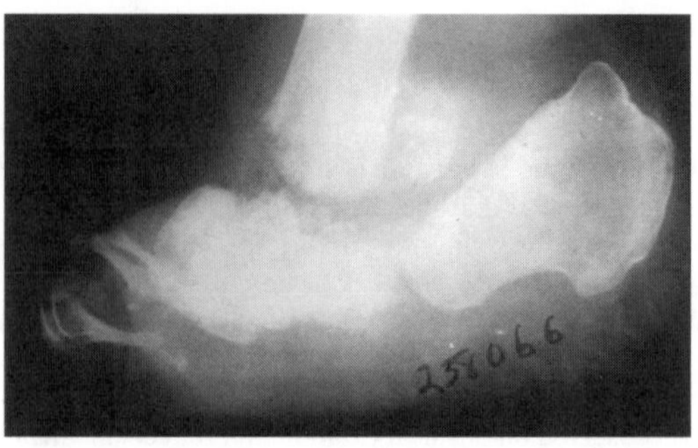


Charcot joints of foot and ankle.

**6. What is diabetic osteolysis?**

Diabetic osteolysis is a condition specifically occurring in diabetics. The osteolysis is characterized by osteoporosis and variable degrees of resorption of distal metatarsal bones and proximal phalanges in the feet. Pain is variable. Radiographs have a characteristic "licked candy" appearance. The pathogenesis is unclear, as this syndrome can occur at any time during the course of diabetes. The primary consideration in the differential diagnosis is osteomyelitis. Treatment is conservative and includes protected weight-bearing. The process may terminate at any stage and in some cases may completely resolve.

**7. How does diabetic amyotrophy present?**

Diabetic amyotrophy presents with severe pain and dysesthesia involving most commonly the proximal muscles of the pelvis and thigh. The condition may be bilateral in 50% of cases. Anorexia, weight loss, and unsteady gait due to muscle wasting and weakness may be seen. The typical patient is a 50–60-year-old man with well-controlled, mild NIDDM of several years' duration, although it can be the presenting sign of diabetes. Usually the patient has no evidence of diabetic retinopathy or nephropathy but may have a distal symmetric sensory neuropathy.

Laboratory evaluation is usually unremarkable except for an elevated cerebrospinal fluid protein. Electromyography/nerve conduction velocity (EMG/NCV) testing demonstrates changes compatible with a neuropathy, and muscle biopsy shows muscle fiber atrophy without an inflammatory infiltrate. The etiology is unclear but may be due to an acute femoral mononeuritis, and inflammatory vasculopathy may play a role. Treatment includes pain control and physical therapy. Increasingly, immunomodulating agents are being proposed. Over 50% recover within 3–18 months, though recovery is often incomplete. Some patients have recurrent episodes.

**8. What is diabetic periarthritis of the shoulder?**

Diabetic periarthritis of the shoulder is also known as **frozen shoulder** or **adhesive capsulitis**. It occurs in 10–33% of diabetics and is five times more common in diabetics than in nondiabetics. The typical patient is female with NIDDM of long duration who presents with diffuse soreness and global loss of motion of the shoulder. Up to 50% of patients have bilateral involvement, although the nondominant shoulder is frequently more severely involved. Laboratory studies and radiographs are unremarkable. Treatment includes NSAIDs, rarely intra-articular steroids, and vigorous physical therapy to improve range of motion. For unclear reasons, this syndrome may spontaneously remit after weeks to months.

**9. The shoulder-hand syndrome can be a complication of frozen shoulder. What is it?**

When a frozen shoulder is accompanied by vasomotor changes of reflex sympathetic dystrophy, it is known as shoulder-hand syndrome. (See Chapter 69.)

**10. How commonly does flexor tenosynovitis or Dupuytren's contractures occur in patients with diabetes mellitus?**

**Flexor tenosynovitis** occurs in 5–33% of diabetic patients. Females with long-standing diabetes are more commonly affected than males. Patients complain of aching and stiffness in the palmar aspect of the hand. Symptoms are worse in the morning. A "trigger" finger may occur as a result of an inflammatory nodule getting caught in the proximal pulley at the base of the finger. The thumb of the dominant hand is most commonly involved (75%), although multiple fingers on both hands can be affected. Laboratory findings and radiographs are unremarkable. Treatment includes NSAIDs, local steroid injections, and surgery.

**Dupuytren's contractures** occur in 33–60% of patients with IDDM. Patients present with nodular thickening of the palmar fascia, leading to flexion contractures usually of the fourth and fifth digits. Patients usually have long-standing diabetes, although there is no association with control of the diabetes. The pathogenesis is thought to be due to contractile myofibroblasts producing increased collagen secondary to microvascular ischemia. Treatment includes NSAIDs, physical therapy, vitamin E, local steroid injections, and rarely surgery.

**11. What is the relationship between diabetes mellitus and carpal tunnel syndrome?**

Carpal tunnel syndrome (CTS) commonly occurs in diabetic patients. Up to 15% of all patients with CTS will have diabetes. Patients present with numbness in the median nerve distribution. Nocturnal paresthesias, hand pain, and pain radiating to the elbow or shoulder (Valleix phenomenon) can also occur. Tinel's and Phalen's signs may be positive. Thenar atrophy is a late sign and indicates muscle denervation. The neuropathy may be from extrinsic compression or due to microvascular disease causing vasa nervorum ischemia. Treatment includes splints, NSAIDs, diuretics, local steroid injections into the carpal tunnel, and surgical decompression (see also Chapter 66).

**12. What is DISH? How commonly does it occur in diabetes mellitus?**

DISH is diffuse idiopathic skeletal hyperostosis, also known as Forestier's disease. It occurs in up to 20% of NIDDM patients who are typically obese and over age 50. Patients present with neck and back stiffness associated with loss of motion. Pain is not prominent. Radiographs are diagnostic and consist of at least four vertebrae fused together as a result of ossification of the anterior longitudinal ligament. Disc spaces, apophyseal joints, and sacroiliac joints are normal, helping to separate it from osteoarthritis and ankylosing spondylitis. Treatment is usually NSAIDs and physical therapy. (See Chapter 55.)

**13. What diabetes-associated rheumatologic syndromes have features in common with scleroderma?**

- The syndrome of limited joint mobility in which findings in the fingers are reminiscent of the sclerodactyly seen in the CREST syndrome.
- Scleroderma diabeticorum, also known as scleredema adultorum or Buschke scleredema, occurs as thickened, edematous areas of skin most commonly on the upper back and neck.

## THYROID DISEASE

**14. Describe the arthropathy associated with severe hypothyroidism.**

**Myxedematous arthropathy** usually affects large joints such as the knees. The patient presents with swelling and stiffness. Synovial thickening, ligamentous laxity, and effusions with a characteristic slow fluid wave (bulge sign) are common. The synovial fluid is noninflammatory with an increased viscosity giving a string sign of 1–2 ft instead of the normal 1–2 inches. Radiographs are typically normal.

**Osteonecrosis** can also occur (controversial). In adults, it typically involves the hip or tibial plateau. In children, abnormal epiphyseal ossification may occur, which can be confused with epiphyseal dysplasia or juvenile avascular necrosis (Legg-Calvé-Perthes disease) of the hip.

**15. What other common rheumatologic syndromes are associated with hypothyroidism?**

Think of **TRAP**:

**T**—**T**unnel (carpal) syndrome (7% of hypothyroid patients)

**R**—**R**aynaud's phenomenon

**A**—**A**ching muscles with findings indistinguishable from those of fibromyalgia

**P**—**P**roximal muscle weakness and stiffness with an elevated creatine kinase

Although chondrocalcinosis has also been ascribed to hypothyroidism, it probably does not occur more commonly than in age-matched controls.

**16. What is the relationship between Hashimoto's thyroiditis and other collagen vascular diseases?**

Hashimoto's thyroiditis occurs with increased frequency in several collagen vascular diseases. It has been described in SLE, Sjögren's, and rheumatoid arthritis, as well as mixed connective tissue disease, scleroderma, and polymyositis. The increased prevalence of HLA-B8, DR3 in patients with Hashimoto's thyroiditis accounts for its occurring with diseases that have similar

HLA associations. Any patient with a collagen vascular disease should be followed closely for development of hypothyroid symptoms.

**17. Which rheumatic problems occur in patients with hyperthyroidism?**

Thyroid acropachy

Painless proximal muscle weakness (70% of hyperthyroid patients)—more common in elderly patients with apathetic hyperthyroidism

Osteoporosis—most common musculoskeletal manifestation

Adhesive capsulitis of the shoulders (controversial)

**18. Describe thyroid acropachy.**

Thyroid acropachy is a rare (1%) complication of Grave's disease consisting of soft tissue swelling of the hands, digital clubbing, and periostitis particularly involving the metacarpal and phalangeal bones. Radiographs are characteristic (see figure). It is strongly associated with ophthalmopathy and pretibial myxedema. The symptoms usually occur after the patient becomes euthyroid. Pain is variable but usually mild. There is no effective therapy.

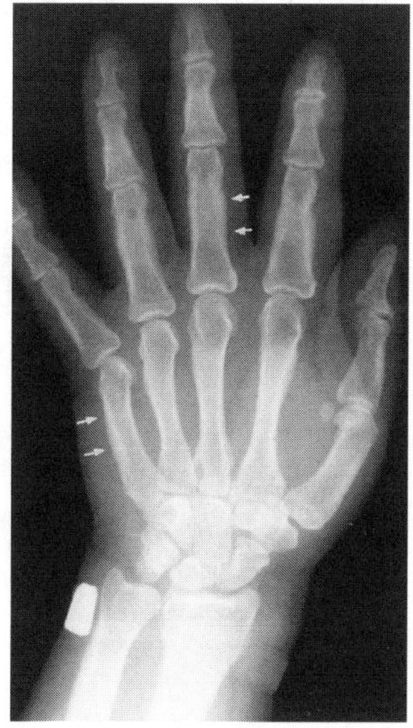

Thyroid acropachy. Note the periosteal reaction along shafts of the metacarpals and phalanges (arrows).

**19. How do you differentiate hyperthyroid myopathy from the myopathies of hypothyroidism and idiopathic inflammatory myopathy (polymyositis)?**

| | TSH | T4 | CK | PROXIMAL MUSCLE WEAKNESS | BIOPSY |
|---|---|---|---|---|---|
| Inflammatory myopathy | Normal | Normal | Increased | Mild-severe | Inflammation |
| Hypothyroidism | Increased | Decreased | Increased | Usually mild | Normal |
| Hyperthyroidism | Decreased | Increased | Normal | Usually mild | Normal |

TSH = thyroid-stimulating hormone; T4 = thyroxine; CK = creatine kinase.

**20. What medications used to treat hyperthyroidism can cause rheumatic syndromes?**

- Propylthiouracil—can cause a systemic vasculitis (pANCA positive)
- Methimidazole—lupus-like syndrome and a syndrome of diabetes mellitus due to anti-insulin antibodies

## PARATHYROID DISEASE

**21. List the rheumatic syndromes associated with primary hyperparathyroidism.**

- Painless proximal muscle weakness with normal muscle enzymes but a myopathic or neuropathic EMG
- Chondrocalcinosis with pseudogout attacks usually due to CPPD crystals
- Osteogenic synovitis due to subchondral bony collapse from thinning of bone (leading to osteoarthritis)
- Osteoporosis
- Ectopic soft-tissue calcifications

**22. What are the skeletal ramifications of primary hyperparathyroidism?**

Osteitis fibrosa cystica represents the classic sequela of prolonged hyperparathyroidism and is diagnosed by x-ray findings that are most prominent in the hands. Subperiosteal resorption with a blurring of the cortical margins is seen, accompanied by a decrease in bone diameter and resorption of the tufts of the distal phalanges (figure). **Diffuse osteopenia** is common, and erosions may be seen in the joints of the hands and at the ends of the clavicles. Discrete lytic lesions due to focal aggregates of osteoclastic giant cells and fibrous tissue with decomposing blood may occur and are known as **brown tumors**. Spinal compression fractures are common.

The full blown osteitis fibrosis cystica of primary hyperparathyroidism has become less common now that the diagnosis of this disorder is often made by the discovery of asymptomatic hypercalcemia on routine serum chemistry screen.

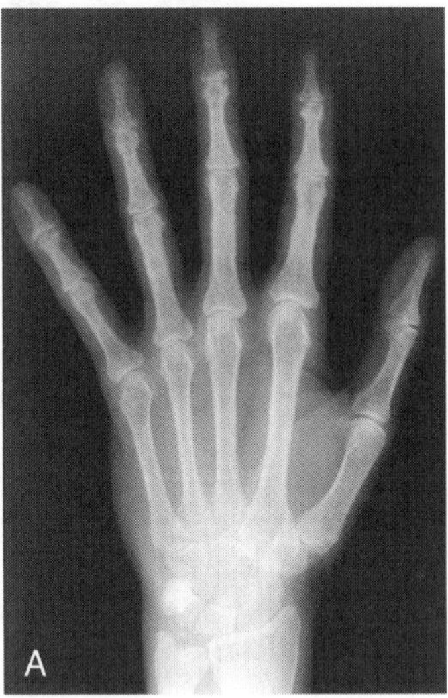


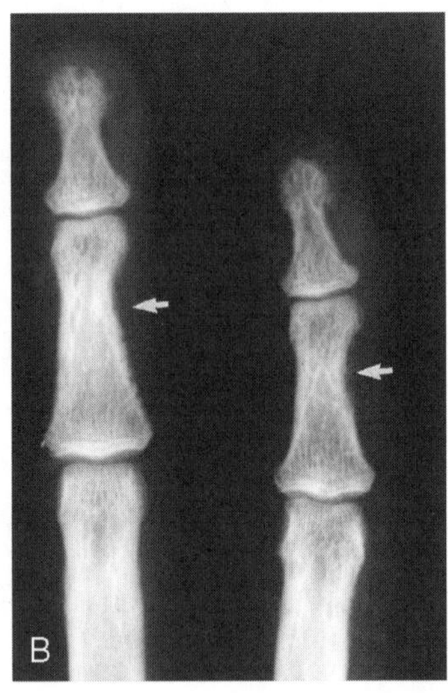


*A*, Radiograph of hand of a patient with hyperparathyroidism. *B*, Closeup of phalanges demonstrating subperiosteal resorption (arrows).

**23. What is the relationship between chondrocalcinosis and primary hyperparathyroidism?**

Up to 15% of patients with chondrocalcinosis will be found to have primary hyperparathyroidism. Conversely, over 50% of patients with long-standing primary hyperparathyroidism will have radiographic evidence of chondrocalcinosis.

**24. What is the knuckle, knuckle, dimple, knuckle sign?**

Patients with pseudo- and pseudo-pseudo-hypoparathyroidism may have a skeletal deformity with a short fourth metacarpal. When they clench their hand to form a fist, a dimple appears where the fourth knuckle should be, emphasizing the short fourth metacarpal bone. These patients also will have short stature and may have ectopic calcifications around weight-bearing joints.

## ACROMEGALY

**25. How often does arthropathy occur in acromegaly?**

It is common and may be seen in up to 74% of affected patients. Degenerative disease is the most common manifestation, and crepitus on exam the most common finding. The knees, shoulders, hips, lumbosacral spine, and cervical spine are the most frequently symptomatic areas, but the hands reveal the most characteristic radiographic changes.

**26. List the radiographic findings in the hands of patients with acromegaly.**

| | |
|---|---|
| Soft-tissue thickening | Deformation of epiphyses with squaring of phalanges |
| Enlarged terminal phalanx (spade-like) | Chondrocalcinosis (rare) |
| Increased joint space | Periosteal apposition of tubular bones |

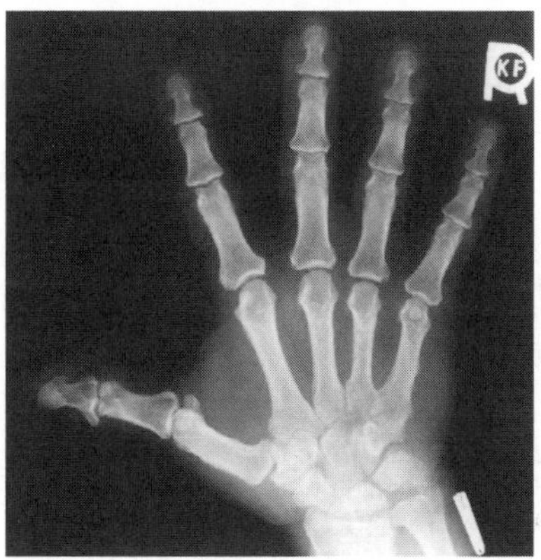

Acromegaly of the hand.

**27. What other rheumatologic syndromes may accompany acromegaly?**

Carpal tunnel syndrome (up to 50% of patients)
Proximal muscle weakness with normal EMG and normal muscle enzymes
Raynaud's phenomenon (up to 33% of patients)
Chondrocalcinosis (rare)

## CUSHING'S SYNDROME

**28. List the rheumatic syndromes associated with excessive glucocorticoids.**

| | |
|---|---|
| Proximal muscle weakness | Osteoporosis |
| Osteonecrosis | Steroid withdrawal syndrome |

**29. Describe the myopathy seen with excessive glucocorticoids.**

Proximal muscle weakness without muscle enzyme elevations can be seen in patients with Cushing's syndrome or in patients receiving > 10 mg of prednisone a day. EMG findings are usually normal or nonspecific. Muscle biopsy can show type 2b muscle fiber atrophy, which is nonspecific and can be seen with disuse atrophy. Patients should be treated with physical therapy, as muscle-strengthening exercises may delay the onset or improve this myopathy.

**30. What is the minimal dose of prednisone a person can take daily and not develop clinically significant osteoporosis?**

This is controversial. Clearly, > 10 mg of prednisone (or greater) a day will cause osteoporosis. Prednisone doses of 5 mg/day or less usually do not cause significant osteoporosis.

**31. Which is more likely to cause osteonecrosis: endogenous Cushing's or iatrogenic Cushing's syndrome?**

Iatrogenic Cushing's (i.e., prednisone therapy) is much more likely than Cushing's disease to cause osteonecrosis.

**32. What is the steroid withdrawal syndrome?**

This syndrome, sometimes called Slocumb's syndrome, is characterized by myalgias, arthralgias, and lethargy following too rapid a taper of corticosteroids. Sometimes patients can develop noninflammatory joint effusions, particularly in the knees. Low-grade fevers occasionally occur. This withdrawal syndrome can be confused with reactivation of the primary disease for which the corticosteroids were used. Increasing the corticosteroids, tapering the steroids more slowly, and using NSAIDs can all help the symptoms.

## BIBLIOGRAPHY

1. Bauer DC, Ettinger B, Nevitt MC, Stone KL: Risk of fracture in women with low serum levels of thyroid-stimulating hormone. Ann Int Med 134:561–568, 2001.
2. Dixon RB, Christy NP: On the various forms of corticosteroid withdrawal syndrome. Am J Med 68:224–230, 1980.
3. Forgacs SS: Acromegaly. In Klippel JH, Dieppe PA (eds): Rheumatology, 2nd ed. St. Louis, Mosby, 1998, Sect 8, Chapter 20, pp 20.1–20.6.
4. Forgacs SS: Diabetes mellitus. In Klippel JH, Dieppe PA (eds): Rheumatology, 2nd ed. St. Louis, Mosby, 1998, Sect 8, Chapter 23, pp 23.1–23.6.
5. Gray RG, Gottlieb NL: Rheumatic disorders associated with diabetes mellitus: Literature review. Semin Arthritis Rheum 6(1):19–34, 1976.
6. Igwe R, Kleerekoper M: Bone and joint abnormalities in thyroid disorders. In Klippel JH, Dieppe PA (eds): Rheumatology, 2nd ed. St. Louis, Mosby, 1998, Sect 8, Chapter 2, pp 21.1–21.4
7. Keerekoper M, Igwe R: Hyperparathyroidism. In Klippel JH, Dieppe PA (eds): Rheumatology, 2nd ed. St. Louis, Mosby, 1998, Sect 8, Chapter 22, pp 22.1–22.4.
8. Lieberman SA, Bjorkengren AG, Hoffman AR: Rheumatologic and skeletal changes in acromegaly. Endocrinol Metab Clin North Am 21:615–631, 1992.
9. McLean RM, Podell DN: Bone and joint manifestations of hypothyroidism. Semin Arthritis Rheum 24:282–290, 1996.
10. Sander HW, Chokroverty S: Diabetic amyotrophy: Current concepts. Semin Neurol 16(2):173–178, 1996.
11. Sergent JS: Arthritis accompanying endocrine and metabolic disorders. In Ruddy S, Harris ED, Sledge CB (eds): Kelley's Textbook of Rheumatology, 6th ed. Philadelphia, W.B. Saunders, 2001, pp 1581–1587.
12. Shagan BP, Friedman SA: Raynaud's phenomenon and thyroid deficiency. Arch Intern Med 140:832–833, 1980.
13. Turken SA, Cafferty M, Silverberg SJ, et al: Neuromuscular involvement in mild asymptomatic primary hyperparathyroidism. Am J Med 87:553–557, 1989.

# 53. ARTHROPATHIES ASSOCIATED WITH HEMATOLOGIC DISEASES

*Matthew* T. *Carpenter*, M.D.

**1. What is a hemarthrosis?**

Hemarthrosis is defined as extravasation of blood into a joint or its synovial cavity. The diagnosis may be readily apparent in the setting of hemophilia, but in other circumstances it is less clear. Streaks of blood, as opposed to the uniformly bloody fluid of a hemarthrosis, may be seen in the synovial fluid during routine arthrocentesis because of needle trauma to skin or other periarticular structures. Blood that appears in the synovial fluid at the end of an arthrocentesis is also because of trauma, particularly if the initial synovial fluid was not bloody. During an arthrocentesis, if frankly bloody fluid is seen initially on entering the joint, hemarthrosis must be suspected. The best option is to withdraw the needle and re-enter the joint at another site. If the original arthrocentesis was traumatic, synovial fluid obtained from the new site should become clear or be only blood-tinged. If diffusely bloody synovial fluid is seen again, hemarthrosis is likely. If you are still uncertain, check a hematocrit on the bloody synovial fluid. A hematocrit similar to peripheral blood is more likely from a traumatic arthrocentesis, whereas fluid from a hemarthrosis has a hematocrit less than peripheral blood. A synovial fluid hematocrit > 10% will make the fluid appear grossly bloody.

**2. What are causes of hemarthrosis?**

*Causes of Hemarthrosis*

| | |
|---|---|
| **Trauma** | **Miscellaneous** |
| Injury with or without fracture | Scurvy |
| Postsurgical | Sickle cell disease and other hemoglobinopathies |
| Post arthrocentesis | Myeloproliferative diseases with thrombocytosis |
| **Bleeding disorders** | Munchausen's syndrome |
| Hemophilia | Acute septic arthritis |
| von Willebrand's disease | Lyme disease |
| Thrombocytopenia | Arteriovenous fistula |
| Excessive anticoagulation | Ruptured aneurysm |
| Thrombolytic therapy for myocardial infarction | Charcot arthropathy |
| **Disorder of connective tissue** | Gaucher's disease |
| Ehlers-Danlos syndrome | Amyloid arthropathy |
| Pseudoxanthoma elasticum | Acute crystalline arthritis |
| **Tumors** | Post dialysis |
| Pigmented villonodular synovitis | |
| Tumors metastatic to joints | |
| Secondary tumors of synovium | |
| Hemangiomas | |

Adapted from Gatter RA, Schumacher HR: A Practical Handbook of Joint Fluid Analysis. Philadelphia, Lea & Febiger, 1991.

Any condition causing intense inflammation will cause synovial vessels to be congested and friable, predisposing patients to hemarthrosis after seemingly insignificant trauma.

**3. Is it safe to perform arthrocentesis when a patient has a prolonged prothrombin time from warfarin therapy?**

If a patient on warfarin develops an acute monarthritis, diagnostic aspiration is warranted, even if the prothrombin time is excessively prolonged. Some authorities report that reversal of anticoagulation is not necessary if proper technique is carefully observed and an appropriately small gauge needle is used. However, bleeding into the joint may occur following such arthrocenteses. Caution should be observed, particularly in large joints where it is difficult to apply direct pressure, like the shoulder or knee. There are no specific published guidelines for reversal of anticoagulation before arthrocentesis. Small doses of vitamin K, 1–2 mg, given intravenously have been noted to reverse rapidly the effects of warfarin to allow surgical interventions where significant bleeding is not expected; however, this has not been studied for arthrocentesis.

**4. What can be done for hemarthrosis in the setting of warfarin therapy?**

Spontaneous hemarthrosis in the setting of warfarin therapy is uncommon, and almost always occurs with an INR prolonged > 2.5 times control. The knee is the most commonly affected joint. Typically, there is an underlying arthritis in the joint, such as osteoarthritis, which may be occult. In fact, in the absence of knee arthritis, spontaneous hemarthrosis is rare unless the INR > 5. The affected joint is rested. Ice may be applied and analgesia provided with acetaminophen or narcotics. Symptoms usually subside spontaneously if the prothrombin time is reduced from supratherapeutic to simply therapeutic. If the patient's underlying condition permits, complete reversal of anticoagulation will hasten recovery. Occasionally, an intra-articular injection of triamcinolone hexacetonide will be needed to control symptoms. Chronic destructive arthritis resulting from warfarin therapy has been reported.

**5. Are there any rheumatologic manifestations of hemophilia?**

- Acute hemarthrosis
- Subacute or chronic arthropathy
- End-stage arthropathy
- Intramuscular or soft-tissue hemorrhage (may cause pseudotumor or compartment syndrome)
- Septic arthritis

**6. How does acute hemarthrosis present in a patient with hemophilia?**

Prodromal symptoms of stiffness or warmth occur in the affected joint. As the joint capsule distends, severe pain follows with swelling from effusion and decreased range of motion. The swelling will eventually tamponade the bleeding, and the hemarthrosis will gradually resolve over a matter of days to weeks. Almost all patients with severe hemophilia (< 5% of normal factor activity) will have recurrent hemarthroses spontaneously or following minor trauma. If factor levels are > 5% of normal, hemarthroses tend to be less frequent or occur following more significant trauma. Hemarthroses first begin to occur in weight-bearing joints when a child is just learning to walk.

**7. How do you treat an acute hemarthrosis in a patient with hemophilia?**

Treatment consists of placing the joint at rest in as much extension as can be tolerated, with applications of ice packs and other local measures. Analgesics are given for pain. Some authors have advocated glucocorticoids. Arthrocentesis, after appropriate factor replacement, may help relieve symptoms.

The mainstay of therapy for acute hemarthrosis in hemophilia is rapid replacement of deficient factor to achieve a level of ≥ 30%. A useful rule of thumb is that each IU of factor VIII or IX infused per kilogram of body weight causes a rise in factor levels by 2% or 2 IU/dl. More specific information on factor replacement has recently been published. Therapy can be promptly instituted by the family at the first symptoms of hemarthrosis to decrease the risks of sequelae. Patient education and involvement are critical for the success of any treatment program.

**8. When should a septic arthritis be suspected if a hemophiliac develops an acute monarthritis?**

If the pain of a suspected hemarthrosis fails to improve after factor replacement, concomitant septic arthritis must be suspected and aspiration of the joint becomes mandatory. It must be emphasized that HIV infection is the most significant risk factor for septic arthritis.

*Diagnostic Clues for Septic Arthritis Coexisting with Hemarthrosis*

| | |
|---|---|
| Failure of joint pain to resolve with factor replacement | Previous arthrocentesis in the same joint |
| Fever >38°C | Presence of arthroplasties |
| Peripheral leukocytosis | Underlying joint damage (chronic arthropathy) |
| HIV infection | Intravenous drug use |

Adapted from Ellison RT, Reller LB: Differentiating pyogenic arthritis from spontaneous hemarthrosis in patients with hemophilia. West J Med 144:42–45, 1986.

Any synovial fluid obtained on routine aspiration of a hemarthrosis should be submitted for Gram stain and culture.

**9. Do recurrent hemarthroses have any long-term consequences?**

As the patient approaches adulthood, acute hemarthroses become less frequent but chronic joint symptoms supervene. Recurrent hemarthroses lead to accumulation of hemosiderin in the joint lining tissues. Proliferative synovitis develops, and the joint cartilage is degraded. The end result is a chronically swollen joint, less painful than seen in acute hemarthroses, with decreased range of motion. Surrounding muscles become atrophic, and joint contracture is a frequent complication. Examination reveals bony enlargement, coarse crepitus, and deformity. Patients may be significantly disabled by chronic hemophilic arthropathy.

**10. Are there any characteristic radiographic findings?**

Radiographs in acute hemarthrosis will be remarkable only for soft-tissue swelling and effusion. Chronic arthropathy of hemophilia may have both inflammatory and degenerative features.

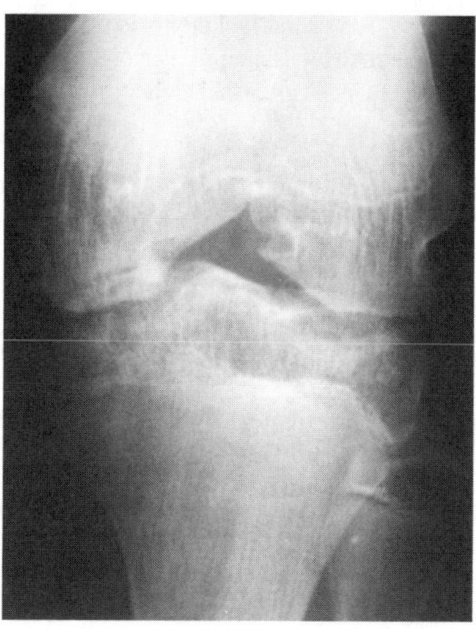

Knee of young patient with hemophilia. Note degenerative and erosive changes of both femoral condyles and the tibial plateau.

**11. What is the treatment of chronic hemophilic arthropathy?**

*Treatment Principles for Chronic Hemophilic Arthropathy*

| |
|---|
| Prophylactic infusions of factor VIII to prevent recurrences of hemarthrosis |
| Non-weight-bearing rest periods to allow synovitis to regress |
| Physical therapy to improve joint stability |
| Training in athletics to maintain muscle mass |
| Intra-articular glucocorticoids to reduce symptoms and recurrent hemarthroses |
| Nonacetylated salicylates for pain and swelling |
| Arthroscopic synovectomy for chronic synovitis unresponsive to conservative therapy |
| Total joint arthroplasty for end-stage joint disease |
| Consider rifampicin chemical synoviorthesis (particularly small joints) |
| Consider radioisotopic synovectomy (particularly if factor inhibitor present) |

Adapted from Upchurch and Brettler.[13]

Treatment programs must be individualized for each patient. Although in small studies ibuprofen and choline magnesium salicylate have both been shown to decrease joint pain in hemophiliacs without decreasing platelet function or increasing bleeding time, exercise caution when using these agents. The new Cox-2 inhibitors should theoretically be safe but have not been studied. Difficult patients are frequently referred to specialized treatment centers.

**12. Does sickle cell anemia have any rheumatologic manifestations?**

- Hand-foot syndrome
- Bone infarction
- Avascular necrosis of bone
- Noninflammatory joint effusions adjacent to areas of bony crisis
- Chronic inflammation of joints
- Hyperuricemia and gout
- Hemarthrosis
- Septic arthritis
- Osteomyelitis
- Focal muscle necrosis
- Rhabdomyolysis

**13. How does hand-foot syndrome present in a patient with sickle cell disease?**

Hand-foot syndrome, or sickle cell dactylitis, is a problem in infants with sickle cell disease. Children present with acute pain and swelling diffusely in the fingers or toes, usually as a first manifestation of sickle cell disease. Fever and leukocytosis may accompany the dactylitis. The etiology is thought to be local bone marrow ischemia. Periostitis may be seen on radiographs of the metacarpal or metatarsal bones 2 weeks after the acute episode. Symptoms generally subside spontaneously in a few weeks.

**14. Is avascular necrosis of bone a common problem in sickle cell disease?**

Bony tenderness and fever are common indications of sickle cell crisis causing a bone infarction. If there is sufficient microvascular occlusion by sickled cells, or an end artery is occluded, avascular necrosis of bone is the result. Avascular necrosis of the femoral head is seen in up to 10% of patients with sickle cell disease. Initially, radiographs may be normal. Radioisotope bone scanning and magnetic resonance imaging are more sensitive methods to detect early avascular necrosis of bone.

The following, in decreasing order of frequency, are sites of avascular necrosis in sickle cell disease:

- Femoral head
- Humeral head
- Tibial plateau
- Fibula
- Radius
- Ulna

**15. Can avascular necrosis be treated in the setting of sickle cell disease?**

Treatment is very unsatisfactory. The affected area should be put on non–weight-bearing status in an attempt to allow revascularization and prevent collapse of the affected bone. An orthopedic surgeon should be consulted promptly. Core decompression of the femoral head may be attempted, although this procedure has not been systematically studied in avascular necrosis due to sickle cell disease. Prosthetic joint replacement is often the treatment used when joint damage is advanced, although results are suboptimal. In one series, 19% of total hip replacements for avascular necrosis of the femoral head in sickle cell disease required revision within 5 years.

**16. Is gout seen frequently in sickle cell disease?**

In children with sickle cell disease, hyperuricosuria without hyperuricemia occurs, probably as a result of increased red cell turnover associated with crises. Up to 40% of adult sickle cell patients will have hyperuricemia, caused by renal tubular damage with decreased uric acid excretion. However, gout is surprisingly uncommon. Occasionally, gout may be seen, so crystals should be looked for in joint effusions seen during sickle cell crisis.

**17. What is the most common musculoskeletal infectious problem seen in sickle cell disease?**

Osteomyelitis is seen more than 100 times more frequently in sickle cell disease than in normal persons. Because of functional asplenia, *Salmonella* infections account for 50% of osteomyelitis in sickle cell disease. Gram-negative organisms are also common. Fortunately, septic arthritis is infrequent. (See table.)

*Factors Predisposing Sickle Cell Patients to Infection*

| | |
|---|---|
| Functional asplenia with decreased clearance of bacteria | Decreased opsonization |
| Tissue damaged by crisis | Decreased interferon-γ production |
| Decreased neutrophil function at lower oxygen tensions | Increased risk of nosocomial infection |

**18. What is the management of suspected osteomyelitis in sickle cell disease?**

*Management of Suspected Osteomyelitis in Sickle Cell Disease*

1. Admit patient to hospital for thorough evaluation.
2. Immobilize affected bones to avoid pathologic fracture.
3. Check baseline CBC and ESR.*
4. Consult hematology and infectious disease services.
5. Obtain blood cultures.
6. Order febrile agglutinins and stool cultures for *Salmonella.*
7. Obtain plain radiographs of all involved bones; repeat these in 10–14 days if the originals are normal.
8. Obtain a radionuclide bone or gallium scan.†
9. Aspirate for culture any bones that are suspected for infection.
10. After a diagnosis is established, preoperative measures are instituted to decrease the risk of surgical complications (transfusions to achieve hemoglobin A level 60% of total hemoglobin, maintenance of adequate oxygenation and hydration).
11. All abscesses in bones should be promptly decompressed to restore blood supply.
12. Avoid tourniquets for intraoperative hemostasis.
13. Do not start antibiotics until adequate specimens of blood, bone, and pus are obtained for culture and Gram stain.
14. Initiate antibiotics based on Gram stain results, considering the possibility of *Salmonella.*
15. Parenteral antibiotics are continued for 6–8 weeks.‡

Adapted from Epps CH Jr, Bryant DD, Coles MJM, Castro O: Osteomyelitis in patients who have sickle cell disease. Bone Joint Surg 73-A (9):1281–1294, 1991; with permission.

* Erythrocyte sedimentation rate is more useful to follow response to treatment than for differentiating sickle crisis from osteomyelitis. Note that sickle cell disease is associated with an abnormally low ESR because the sickled cells cannot form good rouleaux.

† Radionuclide scans are not as useful for differentiating bony infarction and osteomyelitis but will identify affected areas in the spine or pelvis, or unsuspected multifocal involvement.

‡ Prolonged therapy is necessary because both infection and sickle cell crisis impair blood flow to the affected bone.

**19. How does osteomyelitis present in sickle cell disease?**

Presentation of osteomyelitis may be subtle, mimicking sickle crisis or affecting multiple areas. Both sickle crisis and osteomyelitis may present with bone pain, fever, and leukocytosis, and radiographs may be identical. An absolute **band** neutrophil count > $500/mm^3$ is more suggestive of osteomyelitis than infarction; a band count > $1000/mm^3$ is even more specific for infection. The utility of radionuclide studies in distinguishing the two entities has not been firmly established. Combined technetium and gallium nuclear medicine scans performed over a period of 24 hours may identify all patients with osteomyelitis but are not specific. A recent study of 15 patients with osteomyelitis in sickle cell disease found that patients with osteomyelitis had a more striking clinical appearance than patients with simple bone infarction; they had more systemic signs and appeared more ill. In this study of osteomyelitis in sickle cell disease, findings included fever, malaise, and more severe localized bone tenderness, with pain and swelling of the affected area.

**20. Do the other hemoglobinopathies have any rheumatologic manifestations?**

Hemoglobin SC disease and sickle β-thalassemia may develop similar manifestations to sickle cell disease, including hand-foot syndrome and gout. Avascular necrosis of bone has been reported in both conditions. Generally, rheumatologic manifestations are less common in these other hemoglobinopathies. There are case reports of avascular necrosis occurring in patients with sickle cell trait, but the incidence is the same as in age-matched controls with normal hemoglobin. Patients with β-thalassemia may develop arthropathy from marrow expansion, and scoliosis is common in patients surviving two decades.

## BIBLIOGRAPHY


1. Anand AJ, Glatt AE: Salmonella osteomyelitis and arthritis in sickle cell disease. Semin Arthritis Rheum 24(3):211–221, 1994.
2. Andersen P, Godal HC: Predictable reduction in anticoagulant activity of warfarin by small amounts of vitamin K. Acta Med Scand 198(4):269–270, 1975.
3. Andes WA, Edmunds JO: Hemarthroses and warfarin: Joint destruction with anticoagulation. Thromb Haemost 49(3):187–189, 1983.
4. Avina-Zubieta JA, Galindo-Rodreiguez: Rheumatic manifestations of hematologic disorders. Curr Opin Rheumatol 10(1):86–90, 1998.
5. Birnbaum Y, Stahl B, Rechavia E: Spontaneous hemarthrosis following thrombolytic therapy for acute myocardial infarction. Int J Cardiol 40(3):289–290, 1993.
6. Dalton GP, Grummond S, Davidson RS, et al: Bone infarction versus infection in sickle cell disease in children. J Pediatr Orthop 16:540, 1996.
7. Ehrenfeld M, Gur H: Rheumatologic features of hematologic disorders. Curr Opin Rheumatol 11(1):62–67, 1999.
8. Ellison RT, Reller LB: Differentiating pyogenic arthritis from spontaneous hemarthrosis in patients with hemophilia. West J Med 144(1):42–45, 1986.
9. Epps CH Jr, Bryant DD, Coles MJM, Castro O: Osteomyelitis in patients who have sickle-cell disease. J Bone Joint Surg 73-A(9):1281–1294, 1991.
10. Porter DR, Sturrock RD: Rheumatological complications of sickle cell disease. Baillière's Clin Rheumatol 5(2):221–230, 1991.
11. Schumacher HR: Hemoglobinopathies and arthritis. In Ruddy S, Harris ED, Sledge CB (eds): Kelley's Textbook of Rheumatology, 6th ed. Philadelphia, W.B. Saunders, 2001, pp 1575–1580.
12. Shupak R, Teital J, Garvey MB, et al: Intra-articular methylprednisolone in hemophilic arthropathy. Am J Hematol 27(9):26–29, 1988.
13. Upchurch KS, Brettler DB: Hemophilic arthropathy. In Ruddy S, Harris ED, Sledge CB (eds): Kelley's Textbook of Rheumatology, 6th ed. Philadelphia, W.B. Saunders, 2001, pp 1567–1574.
14. Wild JH, Zvaifler NJ: Hemarthrosis associated with sodium warfarin therapy. Arthritis Rheum 19(1):98–102, 1976.
15. York JR: Musculoskeletal disorders in the haemophilias. Baillière's Clin Rheumatol 5(2):197–220, 1991.

# 54. MALIGNANCY-ASSOCIATED RHEUMATIC DISORDERS

*Daniel F. Battafarano*, D.O.

**1. Is there a causal relationship between malignancies and rheumatic disorders?**

It is uncommon for a rheumatic disease to mimic malignancy, but rheumatic syndromes have been associated with various malignancies, and patients with preexisting connective tissue disease (CTD) have developed malignancies. Approximately 15% of patients hospitalized with advanced malignancy will manifest a paraneoplastic syndrome. Endocrine syndromes secondary to ectopic hormone production account for one-third of all paraneoplastic syndromes followed by connective tissue, hematologic, and neuromuscular syndromes.

A causal relationship between some rheumatic syndromes and underlying malignancies has been established. For example, in patients with hypertrophic osteoarthropathy (HOA) secondary to malignancy, the musculoskeletal symptoms resolve after resection of the underlying tumor. However, the majority of rheumatic syndromes associated with malignancies do not demonstrate dramatic clinical relationships and therefore are indirectly related. It is generally accepted that an extensive search for occult malignancy is not cost-effective or recommended for common rheumatic syndromes.

**2. What are the clinical relationships of polyarthritis and malignancy?**

Polyarthritis can be the presenting manifestation of an occult malignancy. The association of polyarthritis and malignancy is suggested by:

1. A close temporal relationship (average, 10 months) between the onset of a seronegative arthritis and the diagnosis of malignancy
2. Improvement of the arthritis with treatment of the underlying cancer
3. Recurrence of the arthritis with tumor recurrence

Other clinical features suggesting an underlying malignancy are late age of onset of arthritis, asymmetric joint involvement, explosive onset, predominance of lower extremity involvement, and absence of rheumatoid factor or nodules.

**3. What musculoskeletal paraneoplastic syndromes are associated with malignancy?**

| PARANEOPLASTIC SYNDROME | MALIGNANCY | CLINICAL ASSOCIATION |
|---|---|---|
| **Myopathy** | | |
| Dermatomyositis-polymyositis | Adenocarcinoma | Cancer may precede, coincide, or follow diagnosis of myositis |
| **Arthropathy** | | |
| Hypertrophic osteoarthropathy | Various types | Lung cancer is most common |
| Amyloidosis | Multiple myeloma | 26% of primary (AL) amyloidosis is associated with multiple myeloma |
| Secondary gout | Myeloproliferative disorders | Tumor lysis syndrome |
| Carcinoma polyarthritis | Solid tumor or hematologic disorders | 80% of women will have breast cancer |
| Jaccoud's-type arthropathy | Carcinoma of lung | Painless, nonerosive, deforming arthropathy with rapid onset |

*(Table continued on next page.)*

| PARANEOPLASTIC SYNDROME | MALIGNANCY | CLINICAL ASSOCIATION |
|---|---|---|
| **Miscellaneous presentations** | | |
| Lupus-like syndrome (polyarthritis, serositis, pleural effusion, positive ANA) | Various types, primary or recurrent | May have history of previously treated malignancy |
| Necrotizing vasculitis | Lymphoproliferative disorders | Chronic unexplained necrotizing vasculitis |
| Cryoglobulinemia | Plasma cell dyscrasias, monoclonal gammopathies | Refractory Raynaud's syndrome |
| Immune complex disease | Hodgkin's disease | Nephrotic syndrome |
| Reflex sympathetic dystrophy syndrome (RSDS) | Ovarian is most common | |
| Shoulder-hand syndrome | | |
| Palmar fasciitis and polyarthritis | | |
| Scleroderma | Adenocarcinoma and carcinoid tumor | Women 3 times greater than men |
| Polyarteritis | Hairy-cell leukemia | Polyarteritis-like clinically and by arteriography |
| Polymyalgia rheumatica (PMR) | (Questionable relationship to various malignancies, as PMR shares similar clinical features and both have an elevated ESR | |
| Panniculitis | Pancreatic cancer | Subcutaneous modules and arthritis, eosinophilia |
| Polychondritis | Hodgkin's disease | Rarely associated with malignancy |
| Pyogenic arthritis | Colon cancer | Intestinal flora cultured |
| | Multiple myeloma | Rare cause of primary septic arthritis |
| Digital necrosis | Various types | Severe Raynaud's syndrome of short duration |
| Erythromelalgia | Myeloproliferative disorders | Severe burning pain, erythema, and warmth primarily in feet |
| **Oncogenic osteomalacia** | Solid tumors; tumors of mesenchymal origin | Bone pain, muscle weakness |

Modified from Caldwell DS: Musculoskeletal syndromes associated with malignancy. In Kelley WN, et al (eds): Textbook of Rheumatology. Philadelphia, WB Saunders, 1993, pp 1552–1566.

**4. What are the accepted direct associations between musculoskeletal syndromes and malignancy?**

Metastatic disease, leukemia, lymphoma, and primary synovial and bone tumors are directly associated with the pathologic mechanisms of the underlying tumor. **Bone metastases** typically involve the long bones, spine, or pelvis and generally arise from primary breast and lung neoplasms. The majority of skeletal metastases do not produce pain. Monoarthritis of the knee is the most common presentation of metastatic arthritis. Metastasis to the extremities can simulate gout, osteomyelitis, tenosynovitis, or acro-osteolysis.

**Leukemia** can present as a symmetric or migratory polyarthritis or as bone pain. Articular manifestations in acute leukemia occur in approximately 14% of children and 4% of adults. Joint pain has been attributed to leukemic synovial infiltration and usually involves the ankle or knee. The joint pain is disproportionally more severe than the clinical findings. Synovial effusions are uncommon and are only mildly inflammatory, and evidence of leukemic cells is rare. The WBC count is frequently normal, but lactic dehydrogenase (LDH) is always elevated, oftentimes to very high levels. Plain radiographs may be normal at the onset of the bone pain in at least 50%, but bone scintigraphy will detect osseous involvement early. At least 10% of patients with leukemia present with back pain. The joint or bone pain is optimally treated with systemic chemotherapy.

Nocturnal bone pain is the most common musculoskeletal complaint in patients with **lymphoma**. Arthritis occurs less commonly and usually exists as a consequence of adjacent bony invasion. Occasionally, patients with T-cell lymphoma may develop a chronic, nonerosive polyarthritis with erythroderma.

**5. Discuss the occurrence of cancer in patients with dermatomyositis (DM) and polymyositis (PM).**

There seems to be an association with DM (increased risk 3–6×) and malignancy, although this is much weaker for PM (increased risk 1.4–2×). This is especially true for DM the first 5 years after diagnosis. The onset of DM or PM may precede, coincide, or occur after the malignancy is diagnosed. Most patients have common malignancies such as breast, ovarian, colon, or lung cancer. Other associated cancers described include stomach, uterus, prostate, kidney, melanoma, lymphoma, leukemia, gallbladder, nasopharyngeal, and laryngeal. The association of DM and malignancy in childhood is rare. Creatine kinase and muscle biopsy data are not useful for distinguishing DM and PM in patients with or without malignancy. However, it has been noted that PM/DM with normal CPK but elevated aldolase are more likely to have a malignancy. It is recommended that all adult patients with new-onset PM or DM undergo an age-specific examination for occult malignancy. Some clinicians recommend an abdominal/pelvic CT scan owing to high incidence of lymphoma and ovarian cancer. All specific clinical symptoms should be thoroughly evaluated, and malignancy should be highly suspected in patients with treatment-resistant myositis. If initial cancer screen is negative, the physician should be alert for future development of cancer over next 3–5 years.

**6. What is the relationship of amyloidosis to multiple myeloma?**

Amyloidosis is a disease characterized by the deposition of an insoluble proteinaceous material in the extracellular matrix of one or several organs. Multiple myeloma–associated amyloidosis closely resembles primary generalized amyloidosis in its age distribution (mean age 55 years), sex predilection (M > F), and clinical presentation. The clinical features of both primary and multiple myeloma–associated amyloidosis are similar. Skin involvement is apparent in 50% of patients and manifests as waxy papules or plaques, nodules, or nonthrombocytopenic purpura. Renal failure and/or proteinuria is the next most common presentation, followed by restrictive cardiomyopathy. Neuropathic complications with sensorimotor symptoms occur in approximately 20% of patients and are frequently manifested by carpal tunnel syndrome. Hepatosplenomegaly, macroglossia, bronchioalveolar involvement, and an acquired factor X deficiency are also common. Most patients with myeloma-associated amyloidosis have both an intact paraprotein in the serum and Bence Jones proteins in urine. Twenty-six percent of all primary amyloidosis cases are associated with myeloma, and 6–15% of all multiple myeloma patients develop amyloidosis.

**7. What is hypertrophic osteoarthropathy?**

Hypertrophic osteoarthropathy (HOA) is a syndrome that includes (1) clubbing of fingers and toes, (2) periostitis of the long bones, and (3) arthritis. HOA is classified as primary or secondary. Primary HOA is hereditary and appears during childhood and is usually self-limited by early adult life. The secondary form can be subdivided into generalized or localized. The secondary generalized form is most often associated with neoplasms or infectious diseases but can be seen with congenital heart disease, inflammatory bowel disease, cirrhosis, or Graves' disease. The secondary localized form of HOA has been associated with hemiplegia, aneurysms, infective arteritis, and patent ductus arteriosus. The clinical course of secondary HOA is related to the nature and activity of the primary disease. The etiology of HOA is still unclear but appears to result from platelet-endothelial interaction with production of von Willebrand factor antigen, vascular thrombi, or antiphosphospholipid antibodies. Growth factors and immune mechanisms may contribute to the cause of HOA.

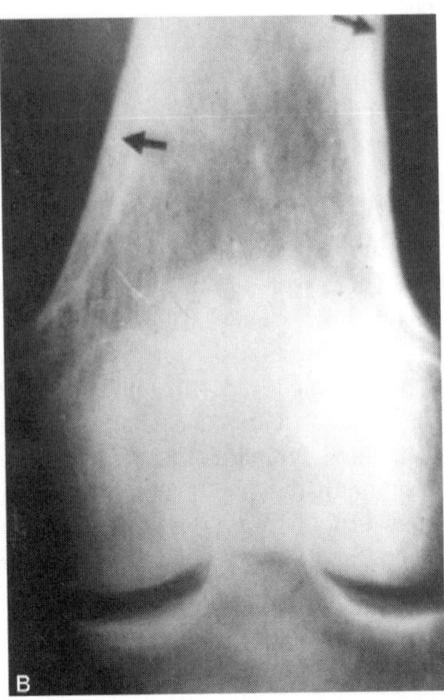


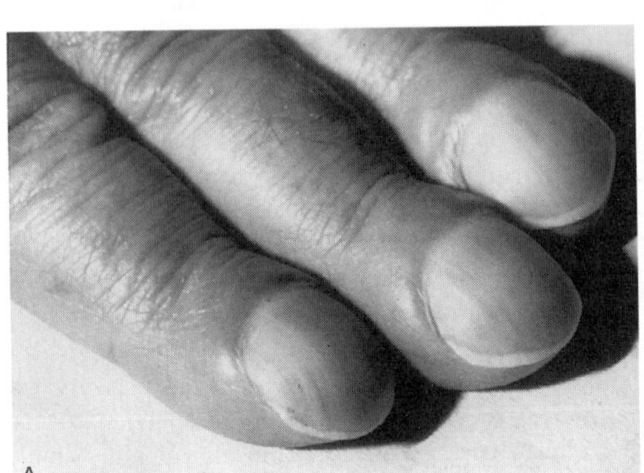


*A*, Clubbing of fingers. Soft tissue proliferation of the nailbed and distal tissues of the digits is seen. Usually the nail makes an angle of 20° or more with the projected line of the digit. When clubbing occurs, subungual proliferation causes diminution of the angle. *B*, Roentgenogram of the knee shows subperiosteal new bone formation of the lower femoral shafts (arrows). New bone is separated from the old cortex by a thin radiolucent line on the right; a later subperiosteal lesion is seen on the left. (From the Clinical Slide Collection on the Rheumatic Diseases. Atlanta, American College of Rheumatology, 1991; with permission.)

**8. Vasculitis occurs as a paraneoplastic syndrome with which malignancies?**

Vasculitis is most often associated with myelodysplastic disorders, leukemia, and lymphomas but may occur with other solid tumors. Leukocytoclastic vasculitis is the most common clinical paraneoplastic presentation. Henoch-Schönlein purpura, systemic vasculitis involving medium-sized vessels, and granulomatous vasculitis have also been described. A polyarteritis nodosa–like vasculitis is the most common rheumatologic manifestation of hairy-cell leukemia. Vasculitis may precede, coincide, or follow the malignancy diagnosis. Proposed mechanisms for vasculitis as a paraneoplastic syndrome include immune complex formation, direct vascular injury by antibodies to endothelial cells, and a direct effect of leukemic cells (i.e., hairy cells) on the endothelium. Malignancies associated with vasculitis include hairy cell leukemia, leukemia, multiple myeloma, non-Hodgkin's lymphoma, Hodgkin's disease, sarcoma, bronchogenic carcinoma, malignant histiocytosis, cervical carcinoma, breast carcinoma, prostatic carcinoma, renal cell carcinoma, melanoma, and colon cancer.

**9. What is Sweet's syndrome?**

Sweet's syndrome is also called acute febrile neutrophilic dermatosis and mimics vasculitis. It is associated with malignancy in at least 15% of patients. This is most commonly seen with acute myelogenous leukemia, but Sweet's has been described with many malignancies. It has been associated with acute, self-limited polyarthritis in 20% of cases. It is can be treated effectively with NSAIDs or corticosteroids. The cardinal features are:

- Abrupt onset of raised, often painful nodules or plaques on the extremities, face, neck, or trunk
- Fever

- Peripheral neutrophilic leukocytosis
- Dense dermal neutrophilic infiltrates without vasculitis on biopsy

**10. Which rheumatic syndromes have been described with ovarian carcinoma?**

Dermatomyositis-polymyositis
Palmar fasciitis and arthritis
Shoulder-hand syndrome
Lupus-like syndrome
Acute febrile neutrophilic dermatosis (Sweet's syndrome)
Carpal tunnel syndrome
Adhesive capsulitis
Fibromyalgia
Positive antinuclear antibody

**11. Describe the features of palmar fasciitis and arthritis and the shoulder-hand syndrome.**

Palmar fasciitis and arthritis and the shoulder-hand syndrome are considered to be clinical variants of reflex sympathetic dystrophy syndrome (RSDS).

Ovarian carcinoma is the classic malignant neoplasm associated with **palmar fasciitis and arthritis**, although this syndrome can be seen with other malignancies. The palmar fasciitis and arthritis syndrome has features of pain, swelling, limitation of motion, and vasomotor instability in the involved extremity similar to RSDS. The clinical characteristics of palmar fasciitis and arthritis that distinguish it from classic RSDS are (1) a severe symmetric inflammatory arthritis resembling rheumatoid arthritis, (2) bilateral extremity involvement (RSDS is bilateral in only 50%), and (3) its association with neoplasms. Plantar fasciitis can occur with lower extremity involvement. Histologic examination of the involved tissues reveals extensive fibrosis with increased fibroblast and mononuclear cell infiltration. There is no evidence of collagen deposition like that seen in scleroderma, and nailfold capillary examination is normal. Deposits of IgG in the palmar fascia and the presence of low-titer antinuclear antibodies in some patients suggest an immunopathologic mechanism. The response to NSAIDs, corticosteroids, ganglionic blockade, and/or physical therapy is variable. The presence of palmar fasciitis and arthritis portends a poor prognosis because it typically manifests after tumor metastasis. Successful removal of the underlying tumor may result in dramatic clinical improvement of the affected extremities.

The **shoulder-hand syndrome** is much milder than the palmar fasciitis and arthritis syndrome. This syndrome is most often described with ovarian carcinoma or with lung cancer localized to the superior sulcus (Pancoast tumor). Pain in the shoulder with loss of motion may result in adhesive capsulitis, and the hand of the involved side becomes puffy and stiff with vasomotor instability. Conventional treatment for RSDS provides variable relief.

**12. Which malignancies are associated with preexisting connective tissue disease?**

*Preexisting Connective Tissue disease Associated with Malignancy*

| CONNECTIVE TISSUE DISEASE | MALIGNANCY | CLINICAL ASSOCIATION |
|---|---|---|
| Systemic lupus erythematosus | Lymphoproliferative disorders | Adenopathy, splenomegaly |
| Discoid lupus erythematosus | Squamous cell epithelioma | Found in plaques >20 years |
| Sjögren's syndrome | Lymphoproliferative disorders (44 times normal risk) | May be primary or secondary Sjögren's |
| Rheumatoid arthritis (RA) | Lymphoproliferative disorders (2–5 times normal risk even in the absence of immunosuppressive therapy) | Longer disease duration, immunosuppression, Felty's syndrome, paraproteinemia |
| Scleroderma | Alveolar cell carcinoma | Pulmonary fibrosis, interstitial lung disease |
| | Nonmelanoma skin cancer | Areas of scleroderma/fibrosis |
| | ? Adenocarcinoma of esophagus | Barrett's metaplasia |
| | ? Breast cancer | Case reports of breast cancer near onset of scleroderma |

(*Table continued on next page.*)

*Preexisting Connective Tissue disease Associated with Malignancy (cont.)*

| CONNECTIVE TISSUE DISEASE | MALIGNANCY | CLINICAL ASSOCIATION |
|---|---|---|
| Dermatomyositis, polymyositis | Adenocarcinoma, melanoma, lymphoproliferative disorders | Older age, F > M |
| Osteomyelitis | Squamous cell carcinoma | Chronic osteomyelitis with cutaneous ulcer |
| Paget's disease | Osteogenic sarcoma | Occurs in 1% of preexisting Paget's lesions |
| Eosinophilic fasciitis | Lymphoproliferative disorders | Aplastic anemia, thrombocytopenia, Hodgkin's disease |
| Lymphomatoid granulomatosis | Lymphoproliferative disorders | At least 13% develop lymphoma |
| Remitting seronegative symmetric synovitis with pitting edema (FS3PE) | Lymphoproliferative disorders, myelodysplasia, endometrial carcinoma | — |

Modified from Caldwell DS: Musculoskeletal syndromes associated with malignancy. In Kelley WN, et al (eds): Textbook of Rheumatology. Philadelphia, WB Saunders, 1993, pp 1552–1566; with permission.

**13. How do malignancy and the drugs used to treat connective tissue disease (CTD) relate?**

Many of the immunosuppressive agents may decrease tumor surveillance and could subsequently lead to the development of a neoplasm. The common immunosuppressive drugs used to treat CTDs include alkylating agents (i.e., cyclophosphamide and chlorambucil), a purine analogue (i.e., azathioprine), a folic acid analogue (i.e., methotrexate), a pyrimidine synthesis inhibitor (i.e. leflunomide), and biologic response modifiers (i.e. etanercept). Prolonged daily treatment or a high cumulative dose of alkylating agents is clearly associated with an increased risk for hematologic malignancies years after the drug is discontinued. The prolonged use of oral **cyclophosphamide** also carries a significant increased risk for bladder carcinoma as a result of the acrolein metabolite excreted in the urine and this is clearly less with intravenous treatment. Patients treated with parenteral pulse cyclophosphamide for systemic lupus nephritis or cerebritis are being monitored to determine the risk for the development of hematologic malignancies; current data suggest that parenteral pulse (monthly) cyclophosphamide has minimal risk when compared with oral daily cyclophosphamide.

High-dose **azathioprine** (200 mg/day) increases the risk of lymphoproliferative malignancies in rheumatoid arthritis patients twofold over the risk due to rheumatoid arthritis alone. Low-dose oral weekly **methotrexate** has not been clearly associated with an increase in oncogenic potential, although a few case reports have suggested that there may be an increased risk of developing non-Hodgkin's lymphoma, which may regress when the methotrexate is discontinued. Leflunomide and entanercept have been commonly prescribed over the past few years, and there is no current evidence to suggest oncogenic potential. Total lymphoid **irradiation** and total body irradiation have been reserved for severe refractory rheumatoid arthritis. The risk of myeloproliferative disorders is increased in this subset of patients, but rheumatoid arthritis alone and prior immunosuppressive therapy (either before or after irradiation) may also contribute to this risk.

*Immunosuppressive Drugs/Agents Used in the Treatment of Connective Tissue Diseases and Their Potential Malignancies*

| TREATMENT | MALIGNANCIES |
|---|---|
| Cyclophosphamide | Bladder carcinoma, non-Hodgkin's' lymphoma, leukemia, skin cancer |
| Other alkylating agents | Acute myelogenous leukemia, non-Hodgkin's lymphoma |
| Azathioprine | Non-Hodgkin's lymphoma, skin cancer |
| Methotrexate | Immunosuppression-associated lymphoma |

(*Table continued on next page.*)

*Immunosuppressive Drugs/Agents Used in the Treatment of Connective Tissue Diseases and Their Potential Malignancies (cont.)*

| TREATMENT | MALIGNANCIES |
|---|---|
| Sulfasalazine | None |
| Penicillamine | None |
| Cyclosporine | Immunosuppression-associated lymphoma |
| Leflunomide | Not described |
| Biologic modifiers | Unknown (concern with infliximab at 10 mg/kg dose) |
| Radiation therapy | Basal cell carcinoma |
| Total lymphoid/total body irradiation | Myeloproliferative disorders, osseous sarcoma, solid tumors |

## BIBLIOGRAPHY


1. Asten P, Barrett J, Symmons D: Risk of developing certain malignancies is related to duration of immunosuppressive drug exposure in patients with rheumatic diseases. J Rheumatol 26:1705–1714, 1999.
2. Buchbinder R, Forbes A, Hall S, et al: Incidence of malignant disease in biopsy-proven inflammatory myopathy. Ann Int Med 134:1087–1095, 2001.
3. Carsons S: The association of malignancy with rheumatic and connective tissue diseases. Semin Oncol 24:360–372, 1997.
4. Fudman EJ, Schnitzer TJ: Dermatomyositis without creatine kinase elevation. Am J Med 80:329–332, 1986.
5. Genovese MC: Musculoskeletal syndromes in malignancy. In Ruddy S, Harris ED, Sledge CB (eds): Kelley's Textbook of Rheumatology, 6th ed. WB Saunders, 2001, pp 1595–1610.
6. Hutson TE, Hoffman GS: Temporal concurrence of vasculitis and cancer: A report of 12 cases. Arthritis Care Res 13:417–423, 2000.
7. M Abu-Shakra, Buskila D, Ehrenfeld M, et al: Cancer and autoimmunity: Autoimmune and rheumatic features in patients with malignancies. Ann Rheum Dis 60:433–441, 2001.
8. Naschitz JE, Rosner I, Rozenbaum M, et al: Rheumatic syndromes: Clues to occult neoplasia. Semin Arthritis Rheum 29:43–55, 1999.
9. Naschitz JE: Rheumatic syndromes: Clues to occult neoplasia. Curr Opin Rheumatol 13:62–66, 2001.
10. Sims RW: Less common arthropathies, hematologic and malignant disorders. In Klippel JH, Crofford LJ, Stone JH, Weyland CM (eds): Primer on the Rheumatic Diseases, 12th ed. Atlanta, Arthritis Foundation, 2001, pp 431–435.
11. Thomas E, Brewster DH, Black RJ, Macfarlane CG: Risk of malignancy among patients with rheumatic conditions. Int J Cancer 88:497–502, 2000.
12. Trapani S, Grisolia F, Simonini G, et al: Incidence of occult cancer in children presenting with musculoskeletal symptoms. Semin Arthritis Rheum 29:348–359, 2000.
13. Yazici Y, Kagen LL: The association of malignancy and myositis. Curr Opin Rheumatol 12:498–500, 2000.

# *IX. Bone and Cartilage Disorders*

*I cannot conceive why we who are composed of over 90 percent water should suffer from rheumatism with a slight rise in the humidity of the atmosphere.*

John W. Strutt (Baron Rayleigh)
(1842–1919)
British physicist, discoverer of argon

## 55. OSTEOARTHRITIS

*Scott Vogelgesang,* M.D.

**1. What is osteoarthritis?**

A slowly progressive musculoskeletal disorder that typically affects the joints of the hand (especially those involved with a pinch grip), spine, and weight-bearing joints (hips, knees) of the lower extremity. It is the most common articular disorder and accounts for more disability among the elderly than any other disease. It is characterized by joint pain, crepitus, stiffness after immobility, and limitation of motion. The clinical joint symptoms are associated with defects in the articular cartilage and underlying bone. There are no systemic symptoms, and joint inflammation, when present, is mild.

**2. Give five other names for osteoarthritis.**

Osteoarthrosis
Degenerative joint disease (DJD)
Hypertrophic arthritis
Degenerative disc disease (DDD, in the spine)
Generalized osteoarthritis (GOA) (Kellgren's syndrome)

**3. Under what circumstances can osteoarthritis develop?**

Osteoarthritis can develop when **excessive loads** (i.e., trauma) across the joint cause the articular cartilage or subchondral bone to fail. Alternatively, osteoarthritis may develop under **normal loads** if the cartilage, bone, synovium, or supporting ligaments and muscles are abnormal because of any one of a number of secondary causes.

**4. What are the pathologic features of osteoarthritis?**

**Early**

Swelling of articular cartilage
Loosening of collagen framework
Chondrocytes increase proteoglycan synthesis but also release more degradative enzymes
Increased cartilage water content

**Later**

Degradative enzymes break down proteoglycan faster than it can be produced by chondrocytes, resulting in diminished proteoglycan content in cartilage.
Articular cartilage thins and softens (joint-space narrowing on radiographs will be seen eventually).
Fissuring and cracking of cartilage. Repair is attempted but inadequate.
Underlying bone is exposed, allowing synovial fluid to be forced by the pressure of weight into the bone. This shows up as cysts or geodes on radiographs.

Remodeling and hypertrophy of the subchondral bone results in subchondral sclerosis and osteophyte ("spur") formation.

This pathology explains the joint-space narrowing, subchondral sclerosis, cysts/geodes, and osteophytes seen on radiographs in osteoarthritic patients.

**5. List the clinical features of osteoarthritis.**

1. Pain in involved joints
2. Pain worse with activity, better with rest
3. Morning stiffness (if present) < 30 minutes
4. Stiffness after periods of immobility (gelling)
5. Joint enlargement
6. Joint instability
7. Limitation of joint mobility
8. Periarticular muscle atrophy
9. Crepitus

**6. What is crepitus?**

A creaking, cracking, or grinding noise made by joints having irregular cartilage that moves against a similar surface. Crepitus may be painless but most often is uncomfortable.

**7. Name the joints typically involved in primary (idiopathic) osteoarthritis.**

- Distal interphalangeal (DIP) joints of the hands
- Proximal interphalangeal (PIP) joints of the hands
- First carpometacarpal (CMC) joints of the hands
- Acromioclavicular joint of shoulder
- Hips
- Knees
- First metatarsophalangeal (MTP) joints of the feet
- Facet (apophyseal) joints of the cervical and lumbosacral spine

**8. Name some joints *not* typically involved in primary (idiopathic) osteoarthritis.**

- Wrists
- Elbows
- Shoulders (glenohumeral joint)
- Ankles
- Metacarpophalangeal joints of the hands
- 2nd-5th MTP joints of the feet

Involvement of these atypical joints should prompt a search for secondary causes of osteoarthritis (see Question 22).

**9. What laboratory features are seen in osteoarthritis?**

Laboratory findings are nonspecific:

- Erythrocyte sedimentation rate (ESR) typically within normal limits
- Rheumatoid factor is negative
- Antinuclear antibodies (ANA) are not present
- Synovial fluid
  - High viscosity with good string sign
  - Color is clear and yellow
  - White blood cell counts typically < 1000–2000/$mm^3$
  - No crystals and negative cultures

**10. What are the radiographic "ABCDES" of osteoarthritis?**

**A**—No ankylosis

Alignment may be abnormal

**B**—Bone mineralization is normal
Bony subchondral sclerosis
Bony spurs (osteophytes)
**C**—No calcifications in cartilage
Cartilage space narrowing that is nonuniform (occurs in area of maximal stress in weight-bearing joints)
**D**—Deformities of Heberden's/Bouchard's nodes
Distribution: involvement of typical joints (see Questions 7 and 8)
**E**—No erosions
("Gull wing" sign in "erosive" osteoarthritis—see Question 18)
**S**—Slow progression over years
No specific nail or soft tissue abnormalities
Vacuum sign in degenerative disc disease (a collection of nitrogen in a degenerated disc space)

*Always obtain weight-bearing radiographs when evaluating for joint-space narrowing of lower extremity large joints (see figure).*

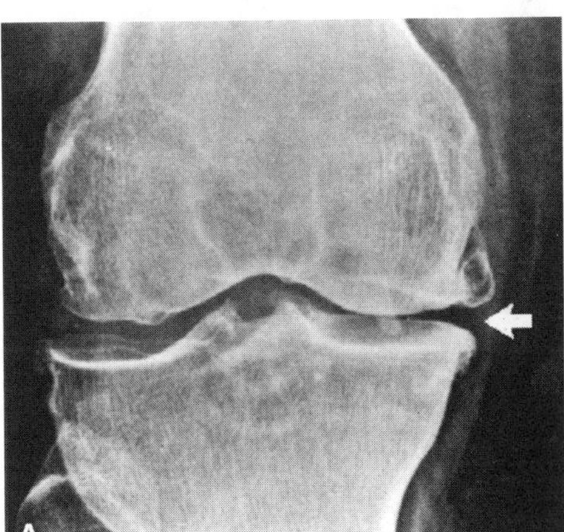


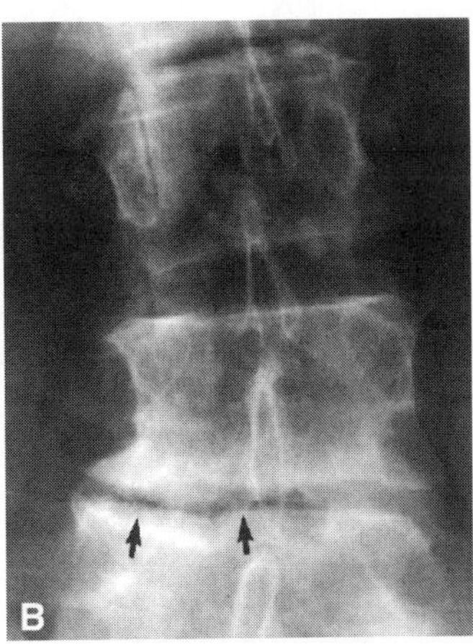


*A*, Radiograph of knee osteoarthritis, showing sclerosis, cysts, osteophytes, and medial joint space narrowing (arrow). *B*, Anterior radiograph of the lumbar spine with disc disease/osteoarthritis. Note disc space narrowing, osteophytes, and vacuum sign (arrows).

**11. How is osteoarthritis classified?**
- Primary, idiopathic osteoarthritis
  - Localized
    - Hands (DIP, PIP, and first CMC joints)
    - Hands (erosive, inflammatory)
    - Feet (first MTP joint)
    - Hip
    - Knee
    - Spine
  - Generalized (also called Kellgren's syndrome)
- Secondary osteoarthritis

**12. Name five epidemiologic features of primary (idiopathic) osteoarthritis.**
- More common in women than in men
- Association with increased age
- Symptomatic osteoarthritis in an estimated 2–3% of the adult population overall
- Symptomatic knee OA in 11% and hip OA in 5% of those > 65 years of age
- Radiographic evidence in > 50–80% of those > 65 years of age

**13. Where do Heberden's and Bouchard's nodes occur?**

Bony articular nodules (osteophytes or "spurs") located on the DIP joints are called **Heberden's** nodes. Such nodules on the PIP joints are **Bouchard's** nodes (see figure). Palmar and lateral deviation of the distal phalanx as a result of these nodules is not uncommon. Heberden's nodes are 10 times more frequent in women than in men. The tendency to develop Heberden's nodes may be familial, with one estimate suggesting that a woman whose mother has Heberden's nodes is twice as likely to develop similar joint changes as a woman without such a family history. The clinical importance of Heberden's and Bouchard's nodes is that they usually signify that the patient has primary osteoarthritis and does not have a secondary etiology for the osteoarthritis.

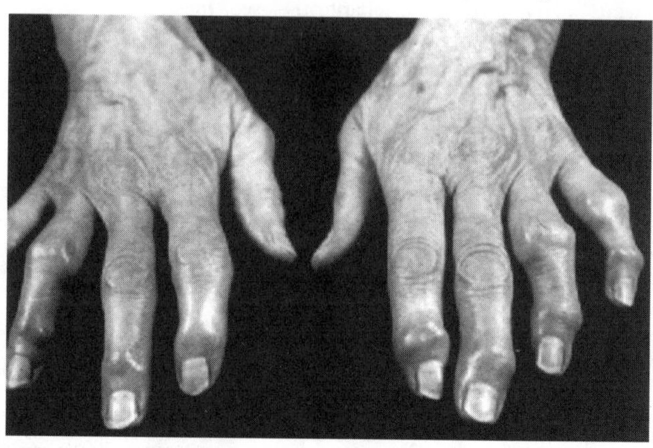

Heberden's (DIP joints) and Bouchard's (PIP joints) nodes in a woman with osteoarthritis. (From the Clinical Slide Collection on the Rheumatic Diseases. Atlanta, American College of Rheumatology, 1991; with permission.)

**14. Who was Heberden?**

William Heberden was an 18th-century physician who made substantial contributions to cardiology, preventive medicine, and rheumatology. He identified the interphalangeal nodular swellings seen in osteoarthritis that now bear his name. Heberden collected a set of clinical observations that became one of the first systems of differentiation of the arthritides.

**15. List seven risk factors for osteoarthritis.**

Obesity
Heredity (especially osteoarthritis of DIP joints)
Age
Previous joint trauma
Abnormal joint mechanics (i.e., excessive knee varus or valgus)
Smoking (may contribute to degenerative disc disease)
Certain occupations requiring bending and carrying heavy loads

**16. Does obesity predispose to osteoarthritis? (Controversy)**

Obesity is a clear risk factor for the development of osteoarthritis, especially of the knee but also, to a lesser degree, of the hand. Weight loss prior to the development of osteoarthritis is associated with a decreased risk of osteoarthritis. One theory to explain this association is that obesity increases the force across the joint and speeds degeneration of the joint. This explanation, although intuitive, is not universally accepted and would seem to be at odds with the fact that obesity is not strongly associated with osteoarthritis of the hip.

**17. Does running or jogging predispose to osteoarthritis?**

Previous joint injury and repetitive joint use predispose to the development of osteoarthritis, raising the question of whether runners are at increased risk for developing osteoarthritis in the knee and hip. Several studies attempting to address this question found no increase in the rate of knee and hip osteoarthritis or knee complaints in runners compared with controls. On the other hand, one uncontrolled study found that runners who developed osteoarthritis tended to have run more miles per week. Finally, one study found an increase of hip osteoarthritis in runners compared with controls. Although there is some disagreement in the literature, most of the present data suggest that in the absence of previous joint injury, runners do not develop osteoarthritis in the knee or hip at higher rates than others.

**18. What is erosive or inflammatory osteoarthritis?**

A subset of primary osteoarthritis, sometimes called Crain's disease, which occurs primarily in women > 50 years of age. The involved joints include DIPs, PIPs, first CMCs, and first MTPs. There is a component of joint inflammation that is superimposed on the degenerative osteoarthritic symptoms. Painful inflammatory "flares" of the involved joints can occur.

These patients are frequently misdiagnosed as having rheumatoid arthritis. However, unlike rheumatoid arthritis, this disease is not accompanied by systemic symptoms; does not involve the MCPs, wrists, or second to fifth MTPs; and serologically has normal sedimentation rates and negative rheumatoid factors and ANAs. Additionally, radiographs are characteristic, showing osteophytes and central "erosions" with a hallmark "gull wing" or "inverted-T" appearance (see figure). Note that these are not true synovial-based erosions, which occur in the periarticular "bare areas" in patients with inflammatory arthritides like rheumatoid arthritis (see Chapters 11 and 19). Patients with erosive osteoarthritis also need to have superimposed gout and crystal arthritis/pseudogout ruled out when they have "flares."

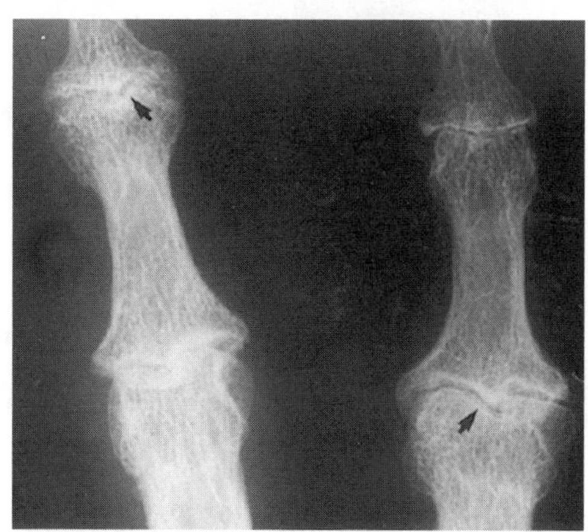

Radiograph of hands of a patient with "erosive" osteoarthritis of the DIP and PIP joints. Note "gull wing" sign (arrows), which is the hallmark of this disease.

**19. Define generalized osteoarthritis.**

A variant of osteoarthritis sometimes called Kellgren's syndrome in which individuals have several affected joints (≥ 4 joint groups) in the typical distribution for osteoarthritis. The disease frequently becomes manifest before age 40–50. Radiographic findings may be more severe than symptoms. Generalized osteoarthritis may simply be a more severe form of common osteoarthritis, although some researchers believe that a defect (such as an abnormal amino acid substitution) will be found in type II or IX collagens causing cartilage to degenerate more quickly.

**20. What is DISH?**

DISH stands for diffuse idiopathic skeletal hyperostosis, but this condition has also been called Forestier's disease and ankylosing hyperostosis. DISH can be confused with ankylosing spondylitis or osteoarthritis of the spine. It is, however, not an arthropathy in that there is no abnormality of articular cartilage, adjacent bone margins, or synovium. Instead, it is a bone-forming condition in which ossification occurs at skeletal sites subjected to stress. It occurs most frequently in the thoracic spine and can be associated clinically with pain or decreased motion. Involvement of the cervical spine can cause dysphagia. DISH occurs in approximately 12% of the elderly population and may coexist with other disorders, particularly type 2 diabetes mellitus.

**21. Describe the radiographic findings in DISH.**

Normal bone mineralization is seen in addition to "flowing" ossification of the anterior longitudinal ligament connecting at least four contiguous vertebral bodies. The calcification of the anterior longitudinal ligament is seen as a radiodense band separated from the anterior aspect of the vertebral bodies by a thin radiolucent line (see figure). Ossification of multiple tendinous or ligamentous sites in the appendicular skeleton may also be seen. Disc spaces, apophyseal joints, and sacroiliac joints are normal radiographically, helping to separate DISH from osteoarthritis and ankylosing spondylitis.

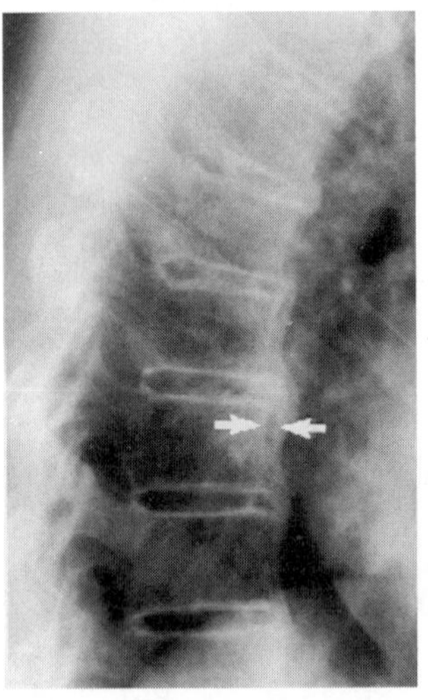

Lateral radiograph of thoracic spine showing calcification of the anterior longitudinal ligament connecting four vertebrae. Note the space between this calcified ligament and the anterior borders of vertebral bodies (arrows).

**22. How does secondary osteoarthritis differ from primary osteoarthritis?**

Secondary osteoarthritis has the same clinical features as idiopathic osteoarthritis except that it has an identifiable etiologic factor and may have a different joint distribution. Atypical joint involvement should prompt a search for an underlying disease process. A classic example is osteoarthritis seen in the MCP joints of the hands in association with hemochromatosis.

**23. List some causes of secondary osteoarthritis.**

- Congenital disorders
  - Hip
    - Legg-Calvé-Perthes
    - Congenital hip dislocation
    - Slipped capital femoral epiphysis
    - Congenital shallow acetabulum
  - Dysplasias
    - Epiphyseal dysplasia
    - Spondyloepiphyseal dysplasia
  - Mechanical features
    - Joint hypermobility syndromes
    - Leg-length discrepancy
    - Varus/valgus deformity
    - Scoliosis
    - Trauma

Metabolic diseases
- Hemochromatosis
- Ochronosis
- Gaucher's disease
- Hemoglobinopathy
- Crystal deposition disorders

Endocrine disorders
- Acromegaly
- Hypothyroidism
- Hyperparathyroidism

Neuropathic joints
- Diabetes mellitus
- Syphilis

Other
- End result of any infectious or inflammatory arthropathy
- Osteonecrosis
- Paget's disease
- Kashin-Beck disease

**24. Which medications are helpful in treating osteoarthritis?**

No medication has been shown to stop or reverse the disease process underlying osteoarthritis. Medications are used, therefore, to alleviate symptoms and increase function. **NSAIDs** are widely used. No single NSAID is more effective than another when evaluated in a large population, but efficacy in individuals may vary. Unfortunately, these medications may be associated with many side effects, some of which can be severe. Other therapeutic alternatives should be considered when possible. **Nonacetylated salicylates** can be useful and have much less gastrointestinal and renal toxicity. Analgesics such as acetaminophen may also be used effectively. A recent study has documented that **acetaminophen** was as efficacious as ibuprofen in the short-term treatment of osteoarthritis of the knee. NSAIDs with specificity for cyclo-oxygenase 2 are now available. It appears they are as effective as older, nonselective NSAIDs but likely have less gastrointestinal toxicity. There is no role for oral or parenteral corticosteroids.

**25. How would you initiate medical treatment in a typical patient with osteoarthritis?**

A reasonable approach to therapy in a patient with osteoarthritis is to start with acetaminophen, 650–1000 mg every 6 hours as needed. If this is unsuccessful, a trial of nonacetylated salicylates is warranted. Salsalate or choline magnesium trisalicylate can be used in typical doses of 1000 mg twice or three times a day. Salicylate levels can be followed to guide therapy. If unsuccessful, less-expensive, short-acting NSAIDs may be tried, such as ibuprofen or naproxen sodium. Using the smallest effective dose and/or intermittent dosing is prudent if possible. NSAIDs with specificity for cyclo-oxygenase 2 may be considered for those at higher risk of gastrointestinal ulceration.

**26. Are glucosamine and chondroitin effective in treating osteoarthritis?**

Glucosamine sulfate (or hydrochloride) and chondroitin sulfate (so-called nutraceuticals) are classified as dietary supplements and as such are not regulated by the federal government (i.e., FDA). Consequently, compound amount, purity, long-term safety, and product labeling are not guaranteed. Glucosamine is the principal component of glycosaminoglycans, which form the matrix of all connective tissue including cartilage. Glucosamine for nutraceuticals use is extracted from crab and lobster shells. Over 50% of an oral dose is absorbed through the small intestine, and 10–15% is retained in tissue with preference for cartilage. In vitro studies show glucosamine is incorporated into and increases synthesis of proteoglycans by chondrocytes. Glucosamine may also have some mild antiinflammatory effects. Chondroitin is derived from cartilage of bovine trachea. Only 10% of an oral dose is absorbed but preferentially distributes to joints. In vitro, chondroitin can stimulate proteoglycan synthesis and block certain proteases. Several published studies demonstrate benefit of glucosamine with or without chondroitin in osteoarthritis. These supplements are as effective as low-dose ibuprofen (400 mg TID) in relieving symptoms. A recent study suggests that glucosamine sulfate may slow cartilage space loss from the usual .1 mm/year to .02 mm/year. The usual dose is glucosamine 500 mg and chondroitin 400 mg three times a day. Symptomatic relief should be noted within 2 months if it is going to be effective. Monthly cost is $10–50, which is not usually covered by insurance. Side effects are minimal, although patients with shellfish allergies may react to glucosamine and crude preparations of chondroitin can have anticoagulant effects and potentially put a person at risk for mad cow disease.

**27. What is viscosupplementation?**

Viscosupplementation is a therapy for moderate (not end-stage) osteoarthritis for which standard medical management fails. The therapy consists of injecting hyaluronan into affected joints (approved only for the knee). Hyaluronan is a glycosaminoglycan found in synovial fluid that allows viscous lubrication at low loads and shock absorbency at high loads. In a normal joint's synovial fluid, there is 4–8 mg of hyaluronan with MW of 5 million daltons. In the osteoarthritic joint's synovial fluid, there is less hyaluronan with MW of 2–3 million daltons, making it less effective for lubrication/shock absorbency. There are two preparations available. Hyalgan has a MW of 500–730 thousand daltons and is derived from rooster combs. It comes prepackaged in 2-ml syringes and is administered weekly for 5 consecutive weeks. Synvisc has a MW of 6 million daltons, comes prepackaged and administered weekly for 3 consecutive weeks. Clinical trials suggest pain relief equivalent to NSAIDs without the gastrointestinal side effects. The therapy is more effective if effusions are aspirated dry before hyaluronan is injected. Intra-articular hyaluronan appears to be safe in the short-term, although reported side effects include local injection reactions (6%), systemic allergic reactions (especially in patients allergic to avian proteins, feathers, or eggs), and "pseudoseptic" reactions often times due to pseudogout. This injection therapy can be repeated every 3–6 months, although long-term safety is unclear. However, hyaluronan may have some chondroprotective (stimulates proteoglycan synthesis), anti-inflammatory (scavenger sink for inflammatory mediators), and anti-nociceptive effects, which explains its prolonged symptomatic benefit even though the hyaluronan can only be detected for a few days in the joint after the injection.

**28. Are there any surgical options for joints severely affected by osteoarthritis?**

Surgery is most often employed in hip and knee osteoarthritis but is also helpful for osteoarthritis involving the first CMC joint, first MTP joint, and, less commonly, the DIP and PIP joints. Approximately 50% of all hip and knee replacements are done for osteoarthritis. Pain relief and satisfactory function result in approximately 90% of patients who undergo total joint replacement. Failure rates after total joint replacement, requiring revision of the prosthesis, are variable and occur in 10–30% at 10 years.

**29. List the indications for total joint replacement for osteoarthritis of the hip or knee.**

- Severe pain unresponsive to medical therapy. For example:
  Consistently awakens from sleep due to pain
  Cannot stand in one place for > 20–30 minutes owing to pain
- Loss of joint function. For example:
  Cannot walk more than one block
  Had to move to single story house or apartment because of inability to climb stairs

**30. List other measures, beside medications or surgery, that may help someone afflicted with osteoarthritis.**

Weight loss
Rest of affected joints

Heel wedges, knee brace to unweight medial compartment of knee
Exercise for muscle strengthening and aerobic conditioning
Ambulatory aids (canes, crutches, walkers)
Splinting (CMC splints, knee sleeves)
Paraffin baths for hands (may be done at home)
Cervical collar
Cervical traction or distraction
Local corticosteroid injections (see Chapter 85)
Topical irritants
Topical capsaicin (different than topical irritants: it works by depleting nerve terminal of substance P, thereby decreasing pain)
Transcutaneous electrical nerve stimulator (TENS) (controversial but may help individual patients)
Superficial heat and cold
Patient education
Shock-absorbing insoles
Hydrotherapy

**31. What is the role of exercise in osteoarthritis therapy?**

A specific exercise program can play a significant role in improving joint range of motion and function and reducing pain. One recent study showed that a supervised program of fitness-walking resulted in improvement of pain and joint function. Other studies have shown participants also have improved psychological well-being. Caution is advised, however. Weight-bearing exercise may worsen the articular cartilage and subchondral bone.

The compromise should be an exercise that does not involve weight-bearing but does provide joint range of motion, muscle strengthening, and aerobic fitness. It is important that the individual select an exercise program that is enjoyable, easily done, and possible to accomplish. An ideal exercise for some is swimming. When done in a warm pool, the individual can move affected joints, strengthen periarticular muscles, and improve cardiovascular fitness, all without bearing weight on diseased joints. Other good options include bicycling, walking, and cross-country skiing.

**32. What is the natural history of osteoarthritis?**

Likely, the cartilage changes of osteoarthritis are asymptomatic for years. Despite this, osteoarthritis progresses with time in most individuals. The rate of progression (average .1 mm of cartilage/year), however, can be variable, and once symptomatic, the disease may seem to progress quickly. There may be rare individuals in whom the disease may remain stable or even improve somewhat. Nevertheless, osteoarthritis can lead to severe limitations in motion and eventual disability. Limitation in usual activities was noted by 60–80% of patients who reported having osteoarthritis according to the National Health Interview Survey.

**33. Are there any other therapies that may be available in the future?**

Metalloproteinase inhibitors, which are mainly tetracycline derivatives, at present are being studied to see if inhibition of proteases (collagenase, stromelysin, which can break down cartilage) can slow the progression of osteoarthritis. Cartilage growth factors and repair of cartilage by *in vitro* grown cartilage that is transferred back to the affected joint are also being investigated. Cartilage transplants from non–weight-bearing surfaces to fill defects in the weight-bearing cartilage surface also hold promise.

## BIBLIOGRAPHY

1. ACR Subcommittee: Recommendations for the medical management of osteoarthritis of the hip and knee: 2000 update. Arthritis Rheum 43:1905–1915, 2000.
2. Altman RD: Criteria for classification of clinical osteoarthritis. J Rheumatol 18(suppl 27):10, 1991.

3. Belhorn LR, Hess EV: Erosive osteoarthritis. Semin Arthritis Rheum 22:298, 1993.
4. Bradley JD, Brandt KD, Katz BP, et al: Comparison of an anti-inflammatory dose of ibuprofen, and analgesic dose of ibuprofen and acetaminophen in the treatment of patients with osteoarthritis of the knee. N Engl J Med 325:87, 1991.
5. Brandt KD, Smith Jr GN, Simon LS: Intraarticular injection of hyaluronan as treatment for knee osteoarthritis: What is the evidence? Arthritis Rheum 43:1192–1203, 2000.
6. Buckwalter JA, Lohmander S: Operative treatment of osteoarthritis: Current practice and future development. J Bone Joint Surg 76A:1405–1418, 1994.
7. Bunning RD, Materson RS: A rational program of exercise for patients with osteoarthritis. Semin Arthritis Rheum 21:33, 1991.
8. Crofford LJ, Lipsky PE, et al: Basic biology and clinical application of specific cyclooxygenase-2 inhibitors. Arthritis Rheum 43:4–13, 2000.
9. Deal CL, Moskowitz RW: Nutraceuticals as therapeutic agents in osteoarthritis. Rheum Dis Clin NA 25:379–394, 1999.
10. Felson DT, Zhang U, Anthony JM, et al: Weight loss reduces the risk for symptomatic knee osteoarthritis in women: The Framingham Study. Ann Intern Med 116:535, 1992.
11. Harris WH, Sledge CB: Total hip and total knee replacement. N Engl J Med 323:725, 1990.
12. Lane NE, Bloch DA, Jones JJ, et al: Long-distance running, bone density and osteoarthritis. JAMA 255:1147, 1986.
13. McKinney RH, Ling SM: Osteoarthritis: No cure, but many options for symptom relief. Cleveland Clin J Med 67:665–671, 2000.
14. Reginster JY, et al: Long-term effects of glucosamine sulfate on osteoarthritis progression: A randomized, placebo-controlled clinical trial. Lancet 357:251–256, 2001.
15. Resnick D, Shapiro RF, Wiesner KB, et al: Diffuse idiopathic skeletal hypertrophy (DISH). Semin Arthritis Rheum 7:153, 1978.

# 56. METABOLIC BONE DISEASE

*Michael* T. *McDermott*, M.D.

**1. What are the major components of bone?**

The main structural elements of bone are **osteoid**, which is a protein matrix, and **hydroxyapatite** (calcium phosphate) crystals, which are embedded in the osteoid. The major functional cells are **osteoclasts**, which resorb old bone, and **osteoblasts**, which form new bone.

**2. What is osteoporosis?**

Osteoporosis is a predisposition to skeletal fractures resulting primarily from a reduction in total or regional bone mass. Both hydroxyapatite and osteoid are reduced proportionately in osteoporotic bone.

**3. What fractures are most commonly associated with osteoporosis? What are their costs?**

Fragility fractures of the vertebrae, femoral neck, and distal radius (Colles' fractures) are characteristic, but any fracture may occur. A fragility fracture is defined as any fracture occurring due to a fall no greater than the person's standing height or with normal use. The lifetime risk of a fracture for a Caucasian woman is 20% for vertebral and 16% for hip. Lifetime risk for men is 6% for vertebral and 5% for hip. Thirty percent of vertebral fractures are asymptomatic. A loss of height of 1.5 inches is predictive of vertebral fractures. Over 75% of hip fractures are associated with falls in the home.

Only ⅓ of vertebral fractures come to medical attention due to acute pain. In these patients with clinically apparent fractures, survival decreases between 20–60% of age-adjusted norms. Much of this increased mortality is due to pulmonary infections. Each vertebral fracture decreases forced vital capacity by 9%. Kyphosis due to fractures leads to spinal malalignment and chronic pain with interference with activities of daily living in over 50% and depression in 40%.

All hip fractures are symptomatic. They are associated with a 15–20% increased mortality within 1 year, and 70% of survivors have compromised function.

**4. What are the major risk factors for osteoporosis?**

| **Non-modifiable** | **Modifiable** |
|---|---|
| Age | Low calcium intake |
| Race (Caucasian, Asian) | Low vitamin D intake |
| Female gender | Estrogen deficiency |
| Early menopause (< 45 yrs old) | Sedentary lifestyle |
| Slender build (< 127 lbs) | Cigarette smoking |
| Positive family history | Alcohol excess (> 2 drinks/day) |
| | Caffeine excess (> 2 servings/day) |
| | Medications (glucocorticoids, excess thyroxine) |

**5. What are the currently accepted indications for bone mass measurement?**

The National Osteoporosis Foundation has issued the following recommendations for screening:
- Women age 65 and older
- Postmenopausal women under age 65, with other risk factors
- Postmenopausal women with fractures
- Women considering therapy for osteoporosis
- Women on hormone replacement therapy for prolonged periods

Medicare considers the following to be indications for bone densitometry utilization:
- Estrogen deficiency plus one risk factor for osteoporosis
- Vertebral deformity, fracture, or osteopenia by x-ray
- Primary hyperparathyroidism
- Glucocorticoid therapy, ≥ 7.5 mg/day of prednisone for ≥ 3 months
- Monitoring the response to an FDA-approved osteoporosis medication

**6. How is bone density measured?**

Standard radiographs are inadequate for accurate bone mass assessment. The most accurate and widely used methods in current practice are **dual energy x-ray absorptiometry** (DEXA), computed tomography (CT), and ultrasound (US). In my opinion, DEXA offers the best accuracy and precision with the least radiation exposure in most patients. Radiation exposure is 2 uSv per site (a chest x-ray is 100 uSv).

Central densitometry measurements (spine and hip) are the best predictors of fracture risk and have the best precision for longitudinal monitoring. Peripheral densitometry measurements (heel, radius, hands), however, are more widely available and less expensive.

**7. Should bone densitometry screening be done at central or peripheral sites?**

Because of its availability and low cost, peripheral densitometry has gained great popularity as a screening tool. In many patients, screening with peripheral densitometry is adequate, but the technique is somewhat less sensitive in diagnosing osteoporosis than is central densitometry. Furthermore, densitometry values can vary greatly in the same individual at different skeletal sites. Therefore, even when peripheral bone densitometry values are normal, follow-up central densitometry must still be considered in the following circumstances.
- History of fragility fractures
- Two or more risk factors for bone loss
- Medical conditions associated with bone loss
- Medications that cause bone loss
- Postmenopausal women not on estrogens, who would consider treatment if bone density is low.

Since peripheral densitometry must be followed by central densitometry in many situations and because of the greater accuracy and precision during longitudinal follow-up, I prefer central measurements for all patients who meet the criteria listed in Question #5 above.

**8. How do you interpret a bone densitometry report?**

The most useful values on the bone densitometry report are the T-score, the Z-score, and the absolute bone mineral density (BMD).

**T-score**: a comparison of a patient's bone mass to that of young normal subjects (age 30). The T-score is the number of standard deviations (SDs) the patient's value is below or above the mean value for young normal subjects (peak bone mass). Thus, a T-score of –2.0 indicates that the patient is 2 SDs below normal peak bone mass. The T-score indicates whether or not the patient has osteoporosis.

**Z-score**: a comparison of a patient's bone mass to that of age-matched subjects. The Z-score is the number of SDs the patient's value is below or above the mean value for age-matched normal subjects. The Z-score indicates whether or not the patient's bone mass is appropriate for age or whether other factors are likely to account for excessively low bone mass.

**Absolute BMD**: the actual bone density value expressed in g/cm$^2$. This is the best parameter to use for calculation of percent changes in bone density during longitudinal follow-up.

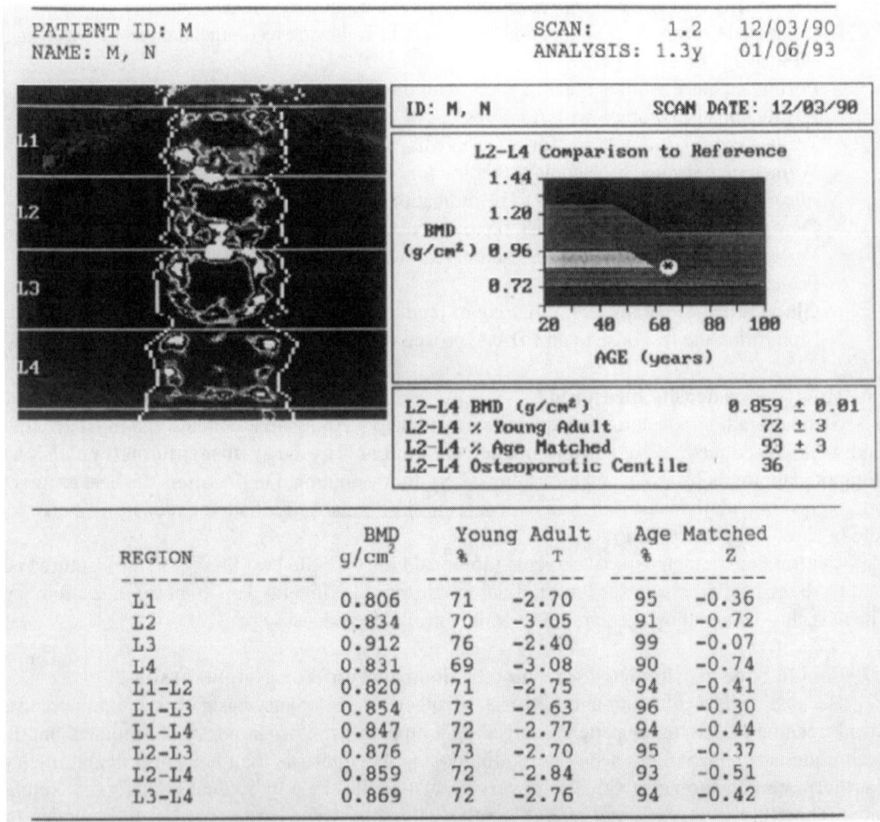

PATIENT ID: M
NAME: M, N

SCAN: 1.2 12/03/90
ANALYSIS: 1.3y 01/06/93



L2-L4 BMD (g/cm²) 0.859 ± 0.01
L2-L4 % Young Adult 72 ± 3
L2-L4 % Age Matched 93 ± 3
L2-L4 Osteoporotic Centile 36

| REGION | BMD g/cm$^2$ | Young Adult % | Young Adult T | Age Matched % | Age Matched Z |
|---|---|---|---|---|---|
| L1 | 0.806 | 71 | -2.70 | 95 | -0.36 |
| L2 | 0.834 | 70 | -3.05 | 91 | -0.72 |
| L3 | 0.912 | 76 | -2.40 | 99 | -0.07 |
| L4 | 0.831 | 69 | -3.08 | 90 | -0.74 |
| L1-L2 | 0.820 | 71 | -2.75 | 94 | -0.41 |
| L1-L3 | 0.854 | 73 | -2.63 | 96 | -0.30 |
| L1-L4 | 0.847 | 72 | -2.77 | 94 | -0.44 |
| L2-L3 | 0.876 | 73 | -2.70 | 95 | -0.37 |
| L2-L4 | 0.859 | 72 | -2.84 | 93 | -0.51 |
| L3-L4 | 0.869 | 72 | -2.76 | 94 | -0.42 |

Bone density report for a DEXA study of the spine. The L2–L4 region, the most frequently evaluated, shows a bone mineral density (BMD) of 0.859 gm/cm$^2$, a T-score of –2.84 , and a Z-score of –0.51. The very low T-score indicates osteoporosis with a significant fracture risk. The relatively normal Z-score indicates that age and menopause are likely the most important factors causing the low BMD.

**9. How is the diagnosis of osteoporosis made?**

The diagnosis of osteoporosis is made when a patient has a characteristic osteoporotic fracture or when the T-score on bone densitometry is sufficiently low. The World Health Organization (WHO) criteria for T-score interpretation are as follows.

| | |
|---|---|
| T-score > –1 | Normal |
| T-score between –1 and –2.5 | Osteopenia |
| T-score < –2.5 | Osteoporosis |

Thus, a T-score of less than –2.5 makes a diagnosis of osteoporosis even in the absence of a fracture. Before concluding that reduced bone mass or a fracture is due to osteoporosis, one must first rule out other causes of low bone mass.

**10. What estimates of bone loss and fracture risk can be made from a patient's bone mineral density measurement by DEXA?**

| T score | % Bone Loss* | Fracture Risk† |
|---|---|---|
| –1 | 12% | 2 times increased |
| –2 | 24% | 4 times |
| –3 | 36% | 8 times |
| –4 | 48% | 16 times |

* Note that one has to lose 30% of bone mineral density to see osteopenia on routine radiograph.

† If a person has had a previous fragility fracture, the risk of subsequent fracture doubles again, i.e., if T-score was –3, fracture risk is 2 × 8 = 16.

**11. What are the limitations of bone densitometry measurements?**

The WHO diagnostic criteria apply only to postmenopausal white women.
Disparities exist among bone density values at different sites and with different methods.
Low bone mass does not necessarily indicate on-going bone loss.
Low bone mass is not always osteoporosis.
Bone densitometry cannot distinguish among the causes of low bone mass.

**12. What other conditions must be considered as causes of low bone mass?**

| | | |
|---|---|---|
| Osteomalacia | Multiple myeloma | Chronic obstructive lung disease |
| Osteogenesis imperfecta | Rheumatoid arthritis | Inflammatory bowel disease |
| Hyperparathyroidism | Renal failure | Medications |
| Hyperthyroidism | Idiopathic hypercalciuria | Corticosteroids, cyclosporine, Dilantin, |
| Hypogonadism | Celiac disease | antiseizure meds, heparin, thyroxine, |
| Cushing's syndrome | Mastocytosis | others |
| Liver disease | Alcoholism | |

**13. Outline a cost-effective evaluation to rule out these possibilities.**

A complete history and physical examination should always be performed. Afterward, the following tests should be adequate in most patients:

Complete blood count with erythrocyte sedimentation rate
Serum calcium, phosphorus, alkaline phosphatase, creatinine, $CO_2$, chloride
Serum TSH
Serum testosterone (men)
24-hour urine calcium and creatinine (phosphorus if osteomalacia)

**14. What non-pharmacologic measures are useful for preventing and treating osteoporosis?**

1. Adequate calcium intake:
   1000 mg/day, premenopausal women and men
   1500 mg/day, postmenopausal women and men ≥ age 65 years of age
2. Adequate vitamin D intake: 400–800 units/day
3. Adequate exercise: aerobic and resistance
4. Smoking cessation
5. Limitation of alcohol consumption to 2 drinks/day or less
6. Limitation of caffeine consumption to 2 servings/day or less
7. Fall prevention

**15. How do you clinically assess a patient's dietary calcium intake?**

Although calcium is present in a variety of foods, the major bioavailable sources are dairy products and calcium-fortified drinks. Ask patients how much milk, cheese, yogurt, and calcium-fortified fruit juice they consume daily, and assign the following approximate calcium contents for their responses:

- Milk 300 mg/cup (8 oz)
- Cheese 300 mg/oz
- Yogurt 300 mg/cup (8 oz)
- Fruit juice with calcium 300 mg/cup (8 oz)

Total these amounts plus 300 mg for the general non-dairy diet and you have a reasonable estimate of that person's daily dietary calcium intake.

**16. How do you ensure an adequate intake of calcium and vitamin D? What is the best calcium supplement?**

A person absorbs only one-third of the calcium he or she ingests. Encourage the consumption of low-fat dairy products; this is the safest way to increase calcium intake without increasing the risk of kidney stones. Advise patients according to the estimated calcium content table in Question 15. Any shortfalls in dietary calcium intake should be supplemented with calcium tablets, elixirs, or multivitamins. Multivitamins contain 400 units of vitamin D per tablet; one or two tablets per day is sufficient for most patients.

Patients who require calcium supplements above their diet to reach adequate daily calcium intake should take either calcium carbonate (Ex: OS Cal, Caltrate, Tums) or calcium citrate (Ex: Citracal). Calcium carbonate is less expensive but needs acidification for best absorption. Because of the acid buffering capacity of calcium carbonate, it should be taken with meals and in split dose of no more than 500–1000 mg per dose (i.e., 500 mg TID). Calcium citrate may be a better alternative in patients with achlorhydria or on medication to limit acid in the stomach. It is important to make sure how much elemental calcium is in each pill (i.e., Citracal 1500 has only 315 mg of elemental calcium). To determine if a particular calcium supplement will be absorbed, put one pill in a glass of vinegar and see if it is dissolved in 30 minutes. If not, it isn't being absorbed. In patients who develop constipation due to calcium, a calcium/magnesium preparation can be recommended, since the magnesium may stimulate bowel motility. Finally, a chewable calcium that is chocolate-flavored (i.e., Viactiv) is well tolerated but contains vitamin K, which can affect Coumadin. A liquid form of calcium is available called Neo-Calglucon (330 mg/tablespoon).

**17. What are the most effective pharmacologic approaches currently available for the prevention and treatment of osteoporosis?**

Medications for the prevention and treatment of osteoporosis fall into two main categories: those that inhibit bone resorption, and those that stimulate bone formation.

| BONE-RESORPTION-INHIBITING AGENTS | BONE-FORMATION-STIMULATING AGENTS |
|---|---|
| Estrogen | Fluoride |
| Bisphosphonates | Androgens |
| Raloxifene | Growth hormone |
| Calcitonin | Parathyroid hormone |

The antiresorptive agents are in wide use because of their repeatedly demonstrated efficacy and safety. The formation-stimulating agents are still largely experimental. See Chapter 89 for a more comprehensive discussion of these agents.

**18. When should medical therapy be initiated for the prevention and treatment of osteoporosis?**

The non-pharmacologic measures discussed in Question #14 are appropriate for all individuals who want to reduce their risk of developing osteoporosis. The National Osteoporosis Foundation further recommends that pharmacologic therapy be initiated in any patient who has a

T-score of –2.0 or less and in patients with a T-score of –1.5 or less in the presence of other osteoporotic risk factors.

**19. When is a urinary *N*-telopeptide helpful?**

Measurement of the level of **N**-telopeptides (NTX) in the urine provides an estimate of activity of bone turnover. NTX is a breakdown product of type I collagen in bone. A 24-hour urine or second voided morning spot urine can be used. There is a 15% average difference between the value obtained between these two methods of urine collections. A normal urine NTX is 20–65 BCE/mmol Cr. However, a value greater than 50 predicts loss of bone mineral density over the next year while a value between 20 and 35 represents good control on present therapy. The cost of urine NTX is $65–70.

**20. What is considered a significant change in bone mineral density on DEXA scan?**

Owing to the precision error of a central DEXA, a change of ≥ 3% in the spine and ≥ 6% in the femur is considered significant. Note that osteophytes, vertebral fractures, and aortic calcifications can falsely increase values in the spine. Hip malposition and including the ischium in the field of measurement can affect femur measurements.

**21. How can falls be prevented?**

The major risk factors for falls include the use of sedatives, sensorium-altering drugs and antihypertensive medications, visual impairment, proprioceptive loss, and lower-extremity disability. Minimizing modifiable risk factors and removing obstacles to ambulation in the home are inexpensive and effective measures for reducing fractures due to falls. Simple measures such as carpeting slick surfaces and stairs, removing throw rugs and children's toys, and installing railings and night lights can have a significant preventive effect.

**22. How common is osteoporosis in men?**

Although it occurs more commonly in women, osteoporosis is not a rare disease in men. A 60-year-old man has a 25% lifetime risk of developing an osteoporotic fracture, and approximately 30% of all hip fractures worldwide occur in men.

**23. How is the diagnosis of osteoporosis made in men?**

Currently, there are no adequate data available to determine what level of bone loss significantly increases a man's risk of developing fragility fractures. Although the issue remains controversial, many investigators use the same criteria to diagnose osteoporosis in men as are used in women. According to these criteria, men with T-scores of –2.5 or less have osteoporosis, even in the absence of a preceding fragility fracture. Additional studies are clearly needed in this area.

**24. How do you treat osteoporosis in men?**

The same non-pharmacologic measures used to treat osteoporosis in women are also appropriate for the treatment of men with this condition. Therefore, men should have 1000–1500 mg/day of calcium, 400 units/day of vitamin D, and adequate exercise. They should be encouraged to discontinue smoking, to limit alcohol consumption, and to limit caffeine consumption. Men also respond well to bisphosphonates, and therefore these agents are appropriate for the treatment of osteoporotic men. Hypogonadal males with osteoporosis should be treated with androgen replacement therapy.

**25. How does glucocorticoid therapy cause osteoporosis?**

Glucocorticoids in supraphysiologic doses (prednisone dose > 7 mg/day) have several detrimental effects on bone. First, they directly inhibit osteoblastic bone formation. Second, they impair intestinal calcium absorption and promote renal calcium excretion, thereby lowering serum calcium levels sufficiently to increase the secretion of PTH, which then stimulates bone resorption. Finally, they impair secretion of gonadal steroids, which further increases bone resorption.

Because they both inhibit bone formation and stimulate bone resorption, glucocorticoids can cause significant bone loss and fractures within 6 months of therapy initiation. Patients on glucocorticoids fracture at T-scores that are not as low as patients with senile osteoporosis. Up to 30–50% of patients will experience fracture, with 15% in the first year if the T-score is less than –1.5.

**26. Can inhaled corticosteroids cause loss of bone density and fractures?**

Inhaled glucocorticoids at doses greater than 1200 μg of triamcinolone acetonide or equivalent can have mild increases in bone turnover markers but insignificant changes in spine and femoral neck bone mineral densities.

**27. When should osteoporosis prevention and treatment measures be instituted in patients taking glucocorticoid therapy?**

Non-pharmacologic measures, as discussed above, are indicated in all patients taking glucocorticoids. Pharmacological intervention should be considered for patients who will be on 7.5 mg/day of prednisone (or an equivalent dose of another glucocorticoid) for at least 3 months, particularly in postmenopausal women and in any individuals who have T-scores of –1.0 or less or who have had fragility fractures.

**28. What is the treatment for glucocorticoid-induced osteoporosis?**

Patients on glucocorticoid therapy should take calcium (1500 mg/day) and vitamin D (800 units/day). If urinary calcium excretion exceeds 300 mg/day, a thiazide diuretic may be added. Alendronate, risedronate, and etidronate all significantly increase bone mass in patients with glucocorticoid-induced osteoporosis and are the agents of choice for the prevention and treatment of this condition. Calcitonin may also be used in these patients, although its effects are less than those seen with bisphosphonates. Patients with hypogonadism should also receive gonadal steroid replacement.

**29. Describe vitamin D metabolism and action.**

Vitamin D has two sources: 90% of the body's vitamin D comes from the skin in response to sunlight exposure, while 10% comes from dietary intake. The cutaneous precursor of vitamin D (7 dehydrocholesterol) is converted by UV light/heat from sun into vitamin $D_3$ (cholecalciferol). It takes only 20–30 minutes of sun exposure to start this process. People with darkly pigmented skin, who use sunblocks, or who do not have exposure to sun (elderly, institutionalized) have less vitamin D production from the skin. Dietary sources of vitamin D are mainly from fortified cereals and dairy products. Other dietary sources are from animal and plant products. The main vitamin D from animal sources is vitamin $D_3$, while from plants it is vitamin $D_2$ (ergocalciferol). Vitamin $D_2$ and $D_3$ have equal potency and bioavailability. Because vitamin D is a fat-soluble vitamin, its absorption is dependent on emulsification by bile acids. Thus, malabsorption must be ruled out in patients with vitamin D deficiency.

After absorption, vitamin D is transported to the liver by vitamin D binding protein, where it is converted by 25 hydroxylase in the liver to 25 hydroxyvitamin D (25 OH vit D) (calcifediol). Severe liver disease and isoniazid can interfere with this process. Anticonvulsants and antituberculous drugs can accelerate the inactivation of 25 OH vit D after it is formed. The measurement of 25 OH vit D is the best test to determine total body vitamin D stores. When levels decrease to less than 15 ng/ml, secondary hyperparathyroidism develops. With levels ≤ 8 ng/ml, one is vitamin D deficient.

The 25 OH vit D is then hydroxylated by 1αhydroxylase in the kidney to 1,25 hydroxyvitamin D (1,25 OH vit D) (calcitriol). This is the active form of vitamin D, which binds to vitamin D receptors to promote, among other things, intestinal absorption of calcium and phosphorus. Renal insufficiency (CrCl < 30–40 ml/min) and ketoconazole decrease the 1αhydroxylation of 25 OH vit D, while increased parathyroid hormone levels and hypophosphatemia increase it. Consequently, measurement of 1,25 OH vitamin D levels is not a good indicator of total body vitamin D stores but can be measured in patients with severe renal insufficiency.

**30. What is osteomalacia?**

The word *osteomalacia* means "soft bones." The condition results from impaired mineralization (deposition of hydroxyapatite) in mature bone.

**31. What causes osteomalacia?**

Osteomalacia results from an inadequate concentration of extracellular fluid phosphate and/or calcium or from a circulating inhibitor of mineralization.

*Major Causes of Osteomalacia*

| | |
|---|---|
| Vitamin D deficiency | Hypophosphatemia |
| Low oral intake plus inadequate sunlight exposure | Low oral phosphate intake |
| Intestinal malabsorption | Phosphate-binding antacids |
| | Excess renal phosphate loss |
| Abnormal vitamin D metabolism | Inhibitors of mineralization |
| Liver disease | Aluminum |
| Renal disease | Bisphosphonates |
| Drugs (anticonvulsants, antituberculous drugs, ketoconazole) | Fluoride |
| | Hypophosphatasia |

**32. Describe the clinical manifestations of osteomalacia.**

Osteomalacia causes pain and deformity, particularly in the long bones and pelvis. Laboratory abnormalities may include low serum calcium and/or phosphorous, elevated serum alkaline phosphatase, reduced serum 25-hydroxyvitamin D levels, low urinary calcium excretion, and elevated parathyroid hormone levels. Any patient with a 24-hour urine calcium less than 50 mg/total volume should be investigated for vitamin D deficiency causing osteomalacia. Patients with osteomalacia due to phosphate wasting will have a low serum phosphorus and high urinary phosphorus excretion. Characteristic pseudofractures (milkman's fractures, Looser's zones) are seen radiographically at points where large arteries cross bones. Histologically, there is an increased amount of osteoid but significantly deficient hydroxyapatite deposition.

**33. What causes rickets?**

Rickets is a condition resulting from impaired mineralization of the skeleton during childhood. It may result from the same conditions that cause osteomalacia in adults as well as three congenital disorders:

1. Hypophosphatemic rickets is an inherited disorder, most commonly X-linked, in which excessive renal tubular phosphate losses result in serum phosphorus levels too low to allow normal bone mineralization. A person needs a calcium x phosphorus product of 24 to mineralize.
2. Congenital 1alpha-hydroxylase deficiency is caused by a genetic mutation in the 1alpha-hydroxylase gene. Deficiency of this renal enzyme results in inability to form 1,25 dihydroxyvitamin D, leading to inadequate intestinal calcium and phosphate absorption.
3. Congenital resistance to 1,25 dihydroxyvitamin D is caused by a genetic mutation in the vitamin D receptor gene. The defective or absent vitamin D receptor results in deficient 1,25 dihydroxyvitamin D mediated intestinal absorption of calcium and phosphorus.

**34. What are the clinical manifestations of rickets?**

The predominant clinical features are bone pain, deformities, fractures, muscle weakness, and growth retardation. Deformities differ depending on the time of onset:

| FIRST YEAR OF LIFE | AFTER FIRST YEAR OF LIFE |
|---|---|
| Widened cranial sutures | Flared ends of long bones |
| Frontal bossing | Bowing of long bones |
| Craniotabes | Sabre shins |
| Rachitic rosary | Coxa vara |
| Harrison's groove | Genu varum |
| Flared wrists | Genu valgum |

Laboratory abnormalities may be similar to those seen in osteomalacia. Radiologic findings include delayed opacification of the epiphyses, widened growth plates, widened and irregular metaphyses, and thin cortices with sparse, coarse trabeculae in the diaphyses. Histologically, there is increased osteoid but deficient mineralization.

**35. How are osteomalacia and rickets treated?**

*Treatment of Bone Deposition Disorders*

| ETIOLOGY | TREATMENT |
|---|---|
| Simple nutritional vitamin D deficiency | Vitamin D, 5000 U/day until healing, then maintain 400 U/day |
| Malabsorption | Vitamin D, 50,000–100,000 U/day |
| Renal disease | Vitamin D, 50,000–100,000 U/day, or calcitriol, 0.25–1.0 µg/day |
| Hypophosphatemic rickets | Calcitriol, 0.25–1.0 µg/day, and oral phosphate |
| 1alpha-hydroxylase deficiency | Calcitriol, 0.25–1.0 µg/day, and oral phosphate |
| Resistance to 1,25 dihydroxyvitamin D | Vitamin D, 100,000–200,000 U/day, or calcitriol, 5–60 µg/day, or IV calcium infusions |

**36. What other types of vitamin D are available, and when should they be used?**

Calderol (20 µg tablets) is 25 OH vit D and can be used in patients with severe liver disease or on medications that interfere with 25 hydroxylation of vitamin D. The usual dose is 20 µg three times a week, which can be advanced to daily. Serum calcium levels need to be followed.

Calciferol in oil (500,000 IU/ml) intramuscularly can be used in patients with malabsorption. If the patient has malabsorption and renal disease, 1,25 OH vit D (Calcijex) can be administered subcutaneously 1–2 µg three times a week. Again, calcium levels must be followed.

In the above therapies, it is important to not let 1,25 OH vit D levels get above the upper limit of normal, since this can actually contribute to bone loss by upregulating RANK ligand on osteoblasts, which in turn stimulates RANK on osteoclasts resulting in increased osteoclastogenesis.

**37. What is idiopathic hypercalciuria, and how is it treated?**

A 24-hour urine calcium should be obtained on all patients with osteopenia. A normal value is 100–300 mg/24 hours with the upper limit of normal being 3.5 mg/kg (women) to 4 mg/kg (men). Patients excreting excessive calcium in their urine need to be investigated for the etiology. If all known secondary causes are ruled out, the patient may have idiopathic hypercalciuria. This can be due to gut hyperabsorption or renal calcium wasting. On a low-calcium diet for 3 days, patients with gut hyperabsorption will markedly decrease their urinary calcium whereas they won't if they have renal calcium wasting. Patients with renal calcium wasting will have a high normal or elevated parathyroid hormone (PTH) to maintain a normal serum calcium. This can lead to osteoporosis and should be treated with thiazide diuretics (HCTZ 25 mg qd, not furosemide). This will increase distal renal tubular calcium absorption, which should lower PTH levels while keeping serum calcium levels normal. If the serum calcium increases on HCTZ, the patient most likely has mild primary hyperparathyroidism and not idiopathic hypercalciuria.

**38. What is hypophosphatasia?**

This rare congenital disorder is caused by mutations in the gene that codes for the alkaline phosphatase isoform found in cartilage and bone. Affected patients present with rickets or osteomalacia and low serum alkaline phosphatase levels. The mineralization defect appears to be due to inability to break down inorganic pyrophosphate, a known inhibitor of mineralization. The disorder is frequently severe and often fatal. Patients with milder forms may be relatively asymptomatic until adulthood. There is no known effective treatment.

**39. What is osteogenesis imperfecta?**

Osteogenesis imperfecta results from mutations in one of the two genes that code for type I procollagen. Osteoblasts produce abnormal osteoid, resulting in osteopenic, fragile bones. Although four subtypes of varying severity have been described, there is actually a continuum ranging from a fatal infantile form to a mild adult form. Associated abnormalities often include blue sclerae, dentinogenesis imperfecta, and deafness. The diagnosis is made on clinical grounds. Bisphosphonate therapy has recently been shown to significantly improve bone mass in these patients. Management also includes supportive, orthopedic, and rehabilitative measures.

**40. Define osteopetrosis.**

Osteopetrosis, or "marble bone disease," is caused by defective osteoclast function. One subset of patients have mutations in the gene for carbonic anhydrase II (CA II), resulting in CA II deficiency; osteoclasts in these patients are unable to generate the hydrogen ions (acidification) necessary for bone resorption. Another subset of patients may have *r*eceptor *a*ctivator of *n*uclear factor κ B (RANK-RANK ligand) deficiencies or excessive osteoprotegrin leading to ineffective differentiation of osteoclasts. Failure of osteoclasts to resorb bone normally produces dense, chalky, fragile bones and bone marrow replacement with pancytopenia. Generalized osteosclerosis is seen on skeletal x-rays. There is a severe, usually fatal, infantile form and a more benign form that allows survival into adulthood. The most effective treatment for the infantile type is bone marrow transplantation, which provides normal osteoclasts. High-dose calcitriol may also be effective in some patients.

## BIBLIOGRAPHY


1. Adachi JD: Management of corticosteroid-induced osteoporosis. Semin Arthritis Rheum 29:228–251, 2000.
2. Audan M: The physiology and pathophysiology of Vitamin D. Mayo Clin Proc 60:851, 1985.
3. Bauer DC, Ettinger B, Nevitt MC, Stone KL: Risk for fracture in women with low serum levels of thyroid-stimulating hormone. Ann Int Med 134:561–568, 2001.
4. Blake GM, Patel R, Fogelman I: Peripheral or axial bone density measurements? J Clin Densitometry 1:55–63, 1998.
5. Dawson-Hughes B, Harris SS, Krall EA, Dallal GE: Effect of calcium and vitamin D supplementation on bone density in men and women 65 years of age or older. N Engl J Med 337:670–676, 1997.
6. Eastell R: Treatment of postmenopausal osteoporosis. N Engl J Med 338:736–746, 1998.
7. Favus MJ (ed): Primer on the Metabolic Bone Diseases and Disorders of Mineral Metabolism, 4th ed. Philadelphia, Lippincott, Williams & Wilkins, 1999, pp 257–389.
8. Genant HK, Engelke K, Fuerst T, et al: Noninvasive assessment of bone mineral structure: State of the art. J Bone Min Res 11:707–730, 1996.
9. Gluer C-C: Quantitative ultrasound techniques for the assessment of osteoporosis: Expert agreement on current status. J Bone Miner Res 12:1280–1288, 1997.
10. Grisso JA, Kelsey JL, Strom BL, et al: Risk factors for falls as a cause of hip fracture in women. N Engl J Med 324:1326–1331, 1991.
11. Harper KD, Weber TJ: Secondary osteoporosis: Diagnostic considerations. Endocrinol Metab Clin North Am 27(2):325–348, 1998.
12. Israel E, Banerjee TR, Fitzmaurice GM, et al: Effects of inhaled glucocorticoids on bone density in premenopausal women. N Engl J Med 345:941–947, 2001.
13. Kelepouris N, Harper KD, Gannon F, et al: Severe osteoporosis in men. Ann Intern Med 123:452–460, 1995.
14. Klotzbuecher CM, Ross PD, Landsman PB, et al: Patients with prior fractures have an increased risk of future fractures: A summary of the literature and statistical synthesis. J Bone Miner Res 15:721–739, 2000.
15. Lane NE (ed): Osteoporosis. Rheum Dis Clinics North Am 27:1–268, 2001.
16. Manolagas SC, Jilka RL: Bone marrow, cytokines and bone remodeling. Emerging insights into the pathophysiology of osteoporosis. N Engl J Med 332:305–311, 1995.
17. Miller PD, Baran DT, Bilezikian JP, et al: Practical clinical application of biochemical markers of bone turnover. J Clin Densitometry 2:323–342, 1999.

18. Miller PD, Bonnick SL, Johnston CC Jr, et al: The challenges of peripheral bone density testing. Which patients need additional central density skeletal measurements? J Clin Densitometry 1:211–217, 1998.
19. Miller PD, Zapalowski C, Kulak CAM, Bilezikian JP: Bone densitometry: The best way to detect osteoporosis and to monitor therapy. J Clin Endocrinol Metab 84:1867–1871, 1999.

# 57. PAGET'S DISEASE OF BONE

*David* R. *Finger*, M.D.

**1. What is Paget's disease?**

Although evidence supports the existence of this disease in prehistoric times, it was not until the 19th century that Sir James Paget first described chronic inflammation of bone, using the term *osteitis deformans*. Paget's disease is a disorder of bone remodeling, with increased osteoclast-mediated bone resorption followed by increased bone formation. This process leads to a disorganized, mosaic pattern of woven and lamellar bone often associated with increased vascularity, marrow fibrosis, and mechanical weakness.

**2. Do we know what triggers the onset of Paget's disease?**

Many investigators suspect a viral infection, but this theory remains to be proven conclusively. Pagetic osteoclasts have been shown to contain intracellular particles resembling nucleocapsids of the Paramyxoviridae family of RNA viruses. Studies have linked canine distemper virus to Paget's disease, noting a three-fold higher incidence of Paget's disease in owners of unvaccinated dogs compared with owners whose dogs are vaccinated.

**3. Who gets Paget's disease?**

Paget's is more common in Caucasians of northern European ancestry. This disease is rare in the Far East, India, Africa, and the Middle East. It occurs more commonly in the northern United States, and men have a slightly higher risk (3:2) than women.

**4. How frequently does this disease occur?**

The incidence increases with age, occurring in 3–3.7% of patients over age 40 and approaching 90% after the 8th decade of life. It appears to be more common in England, with a prevalence of 5% compared to 1–3% in the United States.

**5. What is the evidence that Paget's disease is inherited?**

Paget's disease occurs seven times more often in relatives of patients than in controls. This risk is further increased if the affected relative has severe disease or was diagnosed at an early age. A positive family history is reported in 15–30% of patients, and HLA DQw1 and DR antigens have been found with increased frequency.

**6. Describe the clinical features of this disease.**

Only one-third of patients are symptomatic. **Pain** is the most common symptom (80%), followed by **joint pain** (50%), usually involving the knee, hip, or spine. Affected areas may feel **warm** to palpation as a result of increased blood flow. **Bone deformities**, such as tibial bowing and skull thickening, may occur in advanced cases. Spontaneous **fractures**, most commonly in the femur, tibia, humerus, and forearm, may also occur.

**7. Which part of the skeleton is most likely to be involved?**

Paget's disease can be polyostotic (80%) or monostotic (20%) and has been noted to occur in every bone in the skeleton. The most common locations for monostotic disease include the tibia and iliac bones. Overall, the most common sites (in descending order) include the pelvis, lumbar spine, femur, thoracic spine, sacrum, skull, tibia, and humerus.

**8. List some potential complications of Paget's disease.**

**Skeletal**

Bone pain
Bone and joint deformities (bowing, frontal bossing)
Fractures (7% of patients)

**Neurologic**

Deafness (auditory nerve entrapment) (13%)
Nerve entrapment (cranial nerves, spinal nerve roots)
Spinal stenosis
Basilar invagination
Headaches
Stroke (blood vessel compression)

**Vascular**

Hyperthermia
Vascular steal syndrome (external carotid blood flow to the skull at the expense of the brain)

**Cardiac**

High-output congestive heart failure (due to increased pagetic bone vascularity)
Hypertension
Cardiomegaly
Angina

**Malignancy**

Osteogenic sarcomas (0.2–1.0%)
Fibrosarcomas
Benign giant cell tumors

**Metabolic**

Hypercalcemia
Hypercalcuria
Nephrocalcinosis

**9. How is Paget's disease usually diagnosed?**

Asymptomatic patients are usually identified by an elevated alkaline phosphatase obtained on routine chemistry panels or by typical radiographic abnormalities noted on examination for some other complaint.

**10. Which laboratory tests are abnormal in Paget's disease?**

Paget's is characterized by accelerated bone turnover, with bone resorption and formation occurring simultaneously. Biochemical markers of each have been used in Paget's disease, but the most reproducible is **serum alkaline phosphatase**. These levels are often extremely elevated with skull involvement and high cardiac output, whereas other bony involvement (pelvis, sacrum, lumbar spine, femoral head) seems to be associated with lower levels. Alkaline phosphatase and **osteocalcin**, a less reliable index of disease activity, are markers of new bone formation. Levels correlate with the extent and activity of the disease process. Markers of bone resorption include urinary **hydroxyproline, pyridinoline cross-links**, and ***N*-telopeptide**, which are usually elevated in Paget's disease. **Hypercalcemia** can be seen, usually in the presence of fracture or immobilization.

**11. Identify the characteristic radiographic and scintigraphic findings seen in Paget's disease.**

Paget's can be evaluated both by plain radiography and technetium bone scanning ($^{99m}$Tc-bisphosphonate); however, there is some discordance. Roughly 12% of lesions seen on bone scan will not be seen on radiographs, and 6% of radiographic abnormalities are absent on bone scan.

**Plain radiographs** reveal osteolytic, osteoblastic, or mixed lesions. Cortical thickening is usually present, along with adjacent trabecular thickening. The edge of lytic fronts in long bones gives a "blade of grass" appearance. Significant trabecular thickening of the iliopubic and ilioischial lines may be seen along the inner aspect of the pelvis in a "brim sign" or "pelvic ring" (see figure), while "osteoporosis circumscripta" refers to extensive lytic involvement in the skull (see figure). Lytic lesions can progress, but usually at a rate of less than 1 cm/year.

Paget's disease classically produces regions of focal increased uptake on **bone scan** (see figure). Scintigraphy is useful for evaluating the extent of disease and for detecting relapses following treatment. This disease does not spread to adjacent bones or "metastasize" to distant regions.

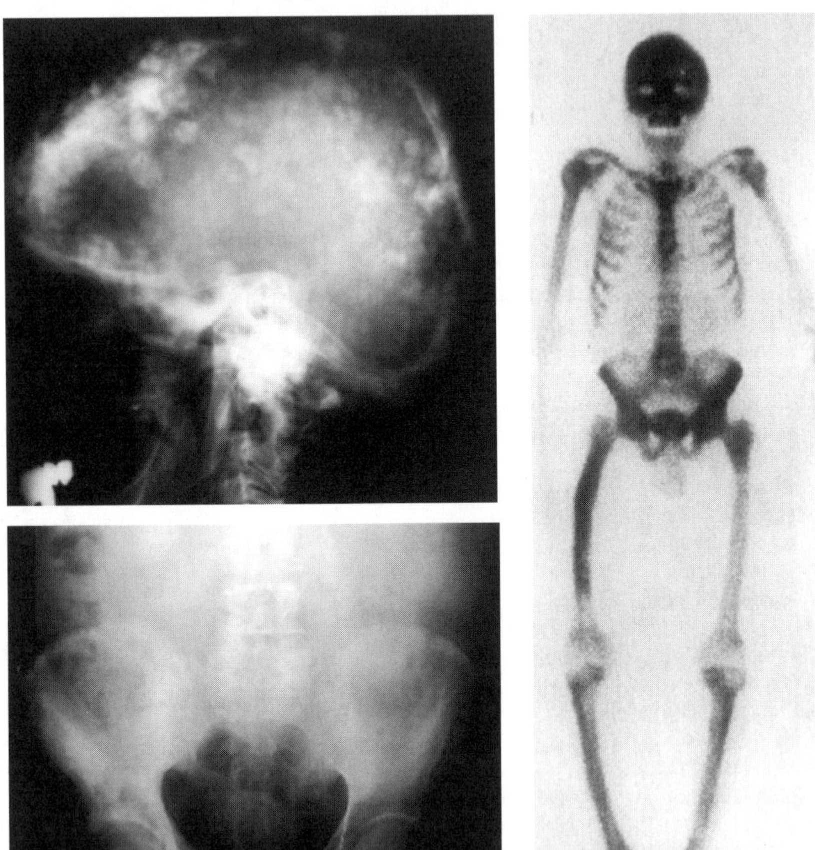

Skull radiograph showing a thickened cranium with regions of dense sclerosis and osteopenia resulting in a "cotton-wool" appearance. Pelvic radiograph showing right hemipelvic loss of normal trabeculation, sclerosis, and cortical thickening, along with sclerosis of the iliopectineal line. Full-body scintigraphy showing increased uptake in the skull, pelvis, lumbar spine, bilateral femurs with bowing of the right, tibias, scapula, and bilateral proximal humerus.

**12. What is the differential diagnosis of Paget's disease?**

Pagetic vertebrae may resemble lymphoma and metastatic cancers, especially adenocarcinoma of the prostate, but pagetic vertebrae are usually enlarged. In other affected bones, Paget's is often distinguished by the characteristic cortical thickening and adjacent thickened trabeculae.

The progression of Paget's through different stages (lytic to sclerotic) also helps to differentiate it from osteoblastic metastatic lesions. Focal increased uptake on scintigraphy can be seen in many conditions besides Paget's disease, including osteomyelitis, arthritis, metastases, and fractures.

**13. Describe the histopathologic findings seen in Pagetic bone.**

Initially there is increased bone resorption, mediated by giant multinucleated osteoclasts. This osteolytic phase is followed by a compensatory increase in bone formation, associated with accelerated lamellar and woven bone deposition in a disorganized fashion, producing the characteristic mosaic pattern. The areas of resorbed bone are replaced with fibrous tissue, and vascular hypertrophy occurs.

**14. What are the indications to treat Paget's disease?**

Bone or joint pain
Bone deformity
Bone, joint or neurologic complications
Preparation for orthopedic surgery
Immobilization hypercalcemia
Young patients
Active asymptomatic disease in sites at high risk for complication
  Skull (hearing loss, other neurologic)
  Spine (neurologic)
  Lower extremity long bones or areas adjacent to major joints (fracture, osteoarthritis)

**Note**: Because therapy is effective and safe, treatment should be withheld only in asymptomatic patients with disease located only in areas with no risk of complications.

**15. What treatments are available for Paget's disease?**

NSAIDs, calcitonin, bisphosphonates, plicamycin (previously mithramycin), gallium nitrate, and surgery have all been used successfully. **NSAIDs** are used to treat pain associated with osteoarthritis when Paget's occurs near joints. **Surgery** is sometimes needed to relieve nerve compression and increase joint mobility. Specific antipagetic therapy, however, consists primarily of **calcitonin** and **bisphosphonates**, as **plicamycin** has an unacceptable toxicity profile. Bisphosphonates are currently the treatment of choice because they are extremely effective, relatively inexpensive, well-tolerated, and (except for pamidronate) are given orally. **Calcitonin** is an alternative agent that is typically used when there is extensive lytic disease, severe pain, when a rapid response is desired (neurologic symptoms, high-output heart failure), or when bisphosphonates do not work or are poorly tolerated.

**16. How are bisphosphonates used in the treatment of Paget's disease?**

**Etidronate** was the first bisphosphonate to be approved for use in Paget's disease, but newer agents appear to be more effective and are not associated with osteomalacia. There are several bisphosphonates either in use currently or under development, to include alendronate, pamidronate, clodronate, tiludronate, risedronate, zoledronate, ibandronate, neridronate, and olpadronate. Bisphosphonates work by inhibiting osteoclastic activity, resulting in significant and prolonged inhibition of bone resorption. The vast majority of patients will experience a rapid reduction in symptoms as well as improvement in biochemical markers. Use of these agents can cause mineralization defect (etidronate), gastric symptoms (ulcerations, esophagitis, dyspepsia), and low-grade fever, transient leukopenia, and flu-like symptoms (pamidronate). Calcium (1000 mg) and vitamin D (800 IU) should be supplemented daily to prevent the development of secondary hyperparathyroidism.

**17. List bisphosphonates used for treating Paget's disease.**

*Bisphosphonates Used in the Treatment of Paget's Disease*

| DRUG | TRADE NAME | DOSE/TABLET | DOSAGE |
|---|---|---|---|
| Oral | | | |
| Etidronate | Didronel | 200 mg | 5 mg/kg/d for 6 months |

(*Table continued on next page.*)

*Bisphosphonates Used in the Treatment of Paget's Disease (cont.)*

| DRUG | TRADE NAME | DOSE/TABLET | DOSAGE |
|---|---|---|---|
| Oral (cont.) | | | |
| Tiludronate | Skelid | 200 mg | 400 mg/d for 3 months |
| Alendronate | Fosamax | 40 mg | 40 mg/d for 6 months |
| Risedronate | Actonel | 30 mg | 30 mg/d for 2 months |
| Intravenous | | | |
| Pamidronate* | Aredia | Vials of 30, 60, 90 mg | 30 mg weekly for 6 wk<br>60 mg every 2 wk for 3 doses<br>90 mg/wk for wk |

* Dilute in 500–1000 ml of normal saline and administer over 4–6 hours (15 mg/hour).

**18. How is calcitonin used in the treatment of Paget's disease?**

Calcitonin was the first successful therapy for Paget's disease. It is available in human and salmon parenteral preparations. A nasal spray is also available but has low bioavailability and is not approved for use in Paget's. Calcitonin is usually administered subcutaneously at 100 IU daily until clinical and biochemical improvement is seen, and then the dose is reduced to 50–100 IU every other day or three times a week. Injections may be associated with flushing, nausea, and transient hypocalcemia in as many as 20%. Starting at lower doses (25–50 IU) and gradually increasing every 1–2 weeks will minimize these side effects. Symptoms of Paget's disease usually diminish within a few weeks but return when therapy is discontinued. A plateau phenomenon may occur as a result of neutralizing antibodies to salmon calcitonin in 25% of patients, but human calcitonin will usually benefit these patients.

**19. How can you tell if a patient's pain is due to Paget's disease of bone or secondary osteoarthritis?**

In Paget's patients with joint involvement, bone pain from Paget's usually responds to bisphosphonate therapy (especially intravenous pamidronate) but secondary osteoarthritis will not respond.

**20. How do you follow a patient who has been treated for Paget's?**

Symptomatic patients should be monitored every 3–6 months for changes in symptoms. Disease activity can be effectively monitored by measurement of serum alkaline phosphatase and urinary *N*-telopeptide. Failure to normalize these markers results in development of new complications of Paget's in 60–70% of patients despite a favorable effect on pain. Therefore, therapy should be aimed at normalizing these markers, which usually occurs several months after the end of therapy. Recurrence of biochemical markers 20–30% above the upper limit of normal justifies retreatment.

## BIBLIOGRAPHY


1. Alvarez L, Guanabens N, Peris P, et al: Discriminative value of biochemical markers of bone turnover in assessing the activity of Paget's disease. J Bone Miner Res 10:458–465, 1995.
2. Burckhardt P: Biochemical and scintigraphic assessment of Paget's disease. Semin Arthritis Rheum 23:237–239, 1994.
3. Delaney MF, LeBoff MS: Metabolic bone disease. In Ruddy S, Harris ED, Sledge CB (eds): Kelley's Textbook of Rheumatology, 6th ed. Philadelphia, WB Saunders, 2001, pp 1635–1652.
4. Delmas PD, Meunier PJ: The management of Paget's disease of bone. N Engl J Med 336:558–566, 1997.
5. Hadjipavlou A, Lander P, Srolovits H, Enker IP: Malignant transformation in Paget disease of bone. Cancer 70:2802–2808, 1992.
6. Khan SA, Brennan P, Newman J, et al: Paget's disease of bone and unvaccinated dogs. Bone 19:47–50, 1996.
7. Raisz LG, Kream BE, Lorenzo JA: Metabolic bone disease. In Williams JD (ed): Williams Textbook of Endocrinology, 9th ed. Philadelphia, WB Saunders, 1998, pp 1231–1233.

8. Singer FR: Paget's disease of bone: Classical pathology and electron microscopy. Semin Arthritis Rheum 23:217–218, 1994.
9. Siris ES: Epidemiological aspects of Paget's disease: Family history and relationship to other medical conditions. Semin Arthritis Rheum 23:222–225, 1994.
10. Tiegs RO: Paget's disease of bone: Indications for treatment and goals of therapy. Clin Ther 19:1309, 1997.

# 58. OSTEONECROSIS

*Robert* T. *Spencer,* M.D.

**1. List some synonyms for osteonecrosis.**

Avascular necrosis (AVN), aseptic necrosis, and ischemic necrosis.

**2. How is osteonecrosis defined?**

Osteonecrosis refers to death of the cellular component of bone (osteocytes) and contiguous bone marrow resulting from ischemia. Although inciting factors for such ischemia are varied, their end results are clinically indistinguishable.

**3. What skeletal regions are predisposed to developing osteonecrosis?**

Bones are most vulnerable in those areas having both limited vascular supply and restricted collateral circulation, which are areas that are also typically covered by articular cartilage. The area most frequently affected is the **femoral head**. At risk areas include:

| | |
|---|---|
| Femoral head | Carpal bones (scaphoid, lunate) |
| Humeral head | Talus |
| Femoral condyles | Tarsal navicular |
| Proximal tibia | Metatarsals |

**4. Name some other common spontaneous osteonecrosis syndromes.**

- Navicular (Preiser's disease)
- Lunate (Kienböck's disease)
- Basal phalanges (Thiemann's disease)
- Capitulum of humerus (Panner's disease)
- Vertebral body (Calvé's disease)
- Femoral epiphysis (Legg-Calvé-Perthes)
- Navicular (Köhler's disease)
- Second metatarsal (Freiberg's disease)

**5. What is the etiology of this disorder?**

The etiology of osteonecrosis is most obvious and best understood in post-traumatic disruption of arterial blood supply. In those cases developing in the absence of trauma, various pathologic processes are capable of inducing hemostasis and, in turn, ischemia. Potential mechanisms include external vascular compression (due to marrow hypertrophy/infiltration, increased intraosseous pressure), thrombosis, embolization (fat/lipids, thrombi, sickle cells, nitrogen gas), osseous microfractures, and cytotoxic factors.

One etiologic factor theorized to be common to several associated conditions is that of fat/lipid embolization, which may occur in association with fatty liver (due to various causes), hyperlipidemia (particularly types II and IV), and disruption of fatty bone marrow (e.g., long-bone fracture). Conditions in which this is speculated to play a role include alcohol abuse, carbon tetrachloride poisoning, diabetes, hypercortisolism, hyperlipidemia, decompression illness, pregnancy, oral contraceptive use, hemoglobinopathies, and long-bone fractures.

**6. What clinical conditions are associated with osteonecrosis?**

*Conditions Associated with Osteonecrosis*

|  |
|---|
| **Nontraumatic** |
| Juvenile |
| Slipped capital femoral epiphysis |
| Legg-Calvé-Perthes |
| Adult |
| Corticosteroid administration |
| Cushing's disease |
| Alcohol abuse |
| Diabetes mellitus |
| Hyperlipidemia |
| Hypercoagulable states |
| Pancreatitis |
| Pregnancy |
| Oral contraceptive use |
| SLE and other connective tissue disorders |
| Renal transplantation |
| Sickle cell anemia |
| Hemoglobinopathies |
| Caisson disease/decompression illness |
| Gaucher's disease |
| Radiotherapy |
| Carbon tetrachloride poisoning |
| Tumor infiltration of marrow |
| Arteriosclerosis/vaso-occlusive disorders |
| **Traumatic** |
| Fracture of the femoral neck |
| Dislocation or fracture-dislocation of the hip |
| Hip trauma without fracture or dislocation |
| Hip surgery |

**7. Briefly describe the pathogenesis of osteonecrosis.**

Etiologic factors initiate hemostasis directly or trigger a cascade resulting in hemostasis. Histologic findings indicate that the final common pathway for the various inciting factors involves local intravascular coagulation and resultant tissue ischemia. The end result is that of cancellous bone and bone marrow death. With subchondral cancellous bone death, collapse of the articular surface may or may not occur, depending on the extent of involvement.

Pain, the earliest symptom of osteonecrosis, may occur in the early stages of involvement, before any radiographic changes are noted. This pain is likely due to elevated intraosseous pressure, since such pain can be relieved by decompression. In some individuals, no symptoms develop until late stages of the disease process when collapse of the articular surface occurs and secondary degenerative changes develop. Others, in whom the area of infarction is small enough that collapse does not occur, may never develop symptoms. Radiographs in these patients reveal sclerotic areas often referred to as "bone islands" or "bone infarcts."

**8. What is the suspected cause of idiopathic osteonecrosis?**

Osteonecrosis without an identifiable cause accounts for 30–40% of all cases. Extensive analysis supports that many of these patients may have a hypercoagulable state evidenced by elevated lipoprotein(a), low tissue plasminogen activator activity, and/or high plasminogen activator inhibitor levels. Others have been found to have high homocysteine levels, elevated antiphospholipid antibodies, low protein C or protein S levels, or the presence of Factor V Leiden.

**9. What clinical features would lead to suspicion of this disorder?**

The signs and symptoms stemming from osteonecrosis are nonspecific. **Pain** is what leads affected individuals to seek medical evaluation. For the hip, the joint most commonly involved, pain is unilateral at onset and localizes to the groin, buttock, medial thigh, and medial aspect of the knee. Occasionally, knee pain is the only complaint in an individual with late-stage osteonecrosis of the hip. Typically, morning stiffness is absent or of short duration (< 1 hour), allowing differentiation from inflammatory monoarticular arthritides. Range of motion is not affected, except as limited by discomfort, until late degenerative changes develop. Although these findings are common to other potential etiologies, their occurrence in the setting of a patient with a predisposing risk (e.g., recent trauma, high-dose steroid use) should suggest underlying osteonecrosis.

**10. What are the epidemiologic features of osteonecrosis?**

- An estimated 15,000 new cases develop each year in the United States.
- Of cases of nontraumatic osteonecrosis, steroid use and alcohol abuse may be responsible for 50% of cases; in up to 40%, there is no identifiable risk factor (idiopathic).
- Males are affected more frequently than females at a ratio of approximately 8:1, possibly reflecting a higher incidence of trauma in males.
- Most cases develop in the < 50-year-old age group. One exception to this observation is seen in osteonecrosis of the knee (femoral condyles, proximal tibia), to which women over age 50 are predisposed (F:M ratio of about 3:1).

**11. How much corticosteroids puts a patient at risk for osteonecrosis?**

A reasonable estimate is 20 mg of prednisone for over 30 days. The risk of osteonecrosis increases by 5% for every 20-mg increase in prednisone dose. Although controversial, high-dose pulse corticosteroids (i.e., 1 gm Medrol daily for 3 days) does not add to this risk. Patients who rapidly develop profound cushingnoid features are particularly likely to develop osteonecrosis.

**12. Are there any other medications that are associated with osteonecrosis?**

Recently, protease inhibitors, used to treat HIV infections, have been implicated in causing osteonecrosis. These medications have caused lipodystrophy, diabetes mellitus, hyperlipidemia, and hypercoagulability. The hyperlipidemia and hypercoagulable state may lead to osteonecrosis.

**13. What is SONK?**

*S*pontaneous *o*steo*n*ecrosis of the *k*nee (SONK) is an idiopathic form of osteonecrosis that affects primarily women (F > M 3:1) over the age of 50. Patients present with knee pain. MRI shows lesions that tend to be small on the medial more often than the lateral femoral condyle.

**14. What is the role of plain radiographs in the diagnosis of osteonecrosis?**

Initially, plain films are normal. Later, a region of generalized osteopenia may develop (a nonspecific finding). Eventually, after bone repair mechanisms have had time to work, a mottled appearance develops in the affected area as a result of the presence of "cysts" (regions of dead bone resorption) and contiguous sclerosis (regions of bone repair).

Early collapse of the cancellous bone beneath the subchondral plate is apparent as a pathognomonic radiolucent line frequently referred to as the **crescent sign**. (See figure, top of next page.) Once in this stage, further collapse is almost inevitable, and it thus represents the earliest irreversible lesion of osteonecrosis. Once the articular surface has collapsed and flattened, secondary degenerative changes develop, resulting in joint-space narrowing and secondary involvement of other bones within the articulation (e.g., acetabulum).

**15. How is radionuclide bone scanning used in the diagnosis?**

This technique is much more sensitive than plain radiography and is thus capable of detecting osteonecrosis at earlier and potentially treatable stages. However, the "hot spot" seen in osteonecrosis is nonspecific. On occasion, a "cold" area (representing necrotic tissue) is seen within

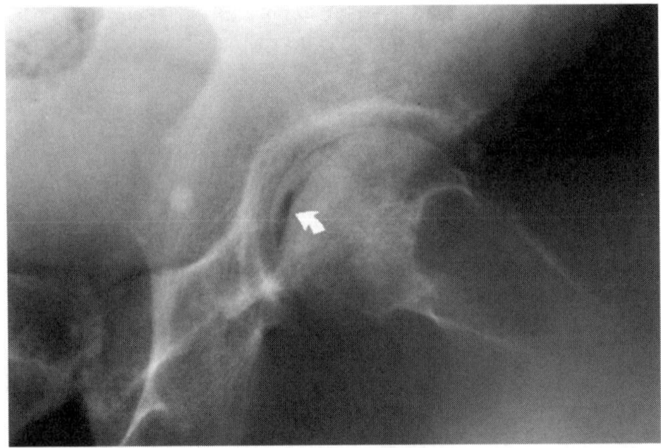

Plain radiograph of hip showing crescent sign (arrow) of osteonecrosis.

the area of enhanced uptake (a "cold-hot" lesion), and this finding is highly specific for osteonecrosis. Overall, the bone scan is being used less frequently in evaluation of this disorder owing to the enhanced specificity and sensitivity of MRI.

**16. How good is magnetic resonance imaging in the diagnosis of osteonecrosis?**

Compared with other diagnostic studies, MRI has been found to have the highest sensitivity and best diagnostic accuracy, thus obviating invasive diagnostic procedures such as biopsy and bone marrow pressure determinations. Sensitivity and diagnostic accuracy appear to be > 95%. The characteristic MRI finding is an area or **line of decreased signal** on both T1 and T2 images (see figure). This area appears to correspond with the demarcation between live regenerating bone and necrotic tissue.

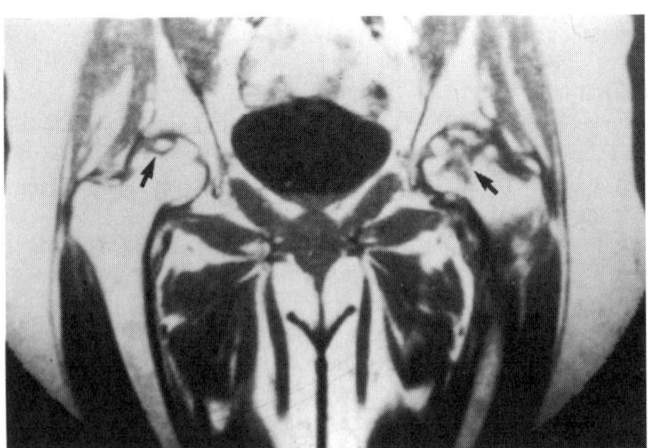

MRI of bilateral hips showing necrotic bone (arrows) in both femoral heads consistent with osteonecrosis.

**17. How often does osteonecrosis occur in a bilateral fashion?**

Approximately 50% of patients with symptomatic hip osteonecrosis have asymptomatic disease in the contralateral hip at the time of initial presentation. Two thirds of these asymptomatic hips will eventually progress to late-stage osteonecrosis. Consequently, bilateral hip MRI at time of presentation is recommended. Similar frequencies would be expected in osteonecrosis of humeral head and knee.

**18. Describe the staging scheme for osteonecrosis of the femoral head.**

*Steinberg Staging of Osteonecrosis of the Femoral Head*

| STAGE | PLAIN RADIOGRAPHIC FINDINGS | MRI/BONE SCAN |
|---|---|---|
| 0* | Normal | Normal |
| I | Normal | Abnormal |
| II | Osteopenia, bony sclerosis, cystic changes | Abnormal |
| III | Subchondral collapse (''crescent sign'') without articular surface flattening | Abnormal |
| IV | Flattening of the articular surface without joint-space narrowing | Abnormal |
| V | Flattening of the articular surface with joint-space narrowing and/or acetabular involvement | Abnormal |
| VI | Advanced degenerative changes | Abnormal |

* Stage 0 refers to an "at risk" asymptomatic, uninvolved hip in an individual with AVN on the contralateral side.

**19. Describe the medical management of osteonecrosis.**

The goal in treating osteonecrosis is to prevent bony collapse and subsequent deformity. Thus, effective treatment is contingent upon diagnosis while osteonecrosis is still in its early stages (stage II and less). Recommended medical management is limited to having the patient **discontinue weight-bearing** on the affected side for 4–8 weeks and administering **analgesics** for relief of associated pain. Unfortunately, hip survival rates with nonoperative management are only in the 13–35% range for stage I–IV disease. However, if the area of involvement of the femoral head is ≤ 15%, in which prognosis is more favorable, nonoperative management with close observation is definitely appropriate. There have been promising reports of results obtained utilizing pulsed electromagnetic field (PEMF) therapy, but this technique remains under investigation.

**20. Describe surgical management for this disorder.**

In **early, reversible stages** of osteonecrosis, several surgical procedures have been developed with the hope of preventing progression. Of these, **core decompression** of the femoral head has been most commonly performed and investigated. The rationale for this operation is that if increased intraosseous pressure can be relieved, vascular perfusion can then be enhanced and help prevent progression of the lesion. Several studies comparing core decompression to nonoperative management have shown favorable results, with success rates in the range of 47–84% for stage I–IV disease. **Vascularized fibula grafting** into the femoral head has been shown in several studies to be extremely promising, with 5-year hip survival rates of 81–89% for stage II–IV disease. Thus this procedure is a consideration in medical communities in which it is available.

In the **nonreversible stages** of osteonecrosis (particularly stages V–VI), the goal of surgical intervention is to restore joint function and relieve associated pain. The effectiveness and reliability of **total hip arthroplasty** (replacement) have made earlier procedures attempting to achieve these goals obsolete.

**21. Can osteonecrosis be prevented?**

Yes, to some degree. Modifiable risk factors can be manipulated—e.g., steroid dose, alcohol intake, speed of decompression (in divers and caisson workers), and control of diabetes and hyperlipidemia. As an example, the vast majority of cases of corticosteroid-related osteonecrosis occur in patients who have received the equivalent of ≥ 20 mg of prednisone/day, especially for prolonged periods. In rheumatoid arthritis, where prednisone doses rarely exceed 10–15 mg/day, osteonecrosis is uncommon. In contrast, in SLE in which higher doses of steroids are frequently used, 30–50% of patients may develop some degree of osteonecrosis.

**22. What is the bone marrow edema syndrome (BMES)?**

BMES, also known as transient osteoporosis of the hip, is a self-limited transitory clinical entity characterized by hip pain, osteopenia on radiographs, and bone marrow edema of femoral head and neck on MRI. This disorder typically affects women in the third trimester of pregnancy and middle-aged men. Usually one hip is involved, but 40% can have recurrence or involvement of other joints. Symptoms last an average of 6 months. Treatment is with analgesics and protective weight bearing. Core decompression is not indicated. BMES differs from osteonecrosis on MRI because it has both femoral head and neck abnormalities whereas osteonecrosis only involves femoral head.

## BIBLIOGRAPHY

1. Bonfonti P, Gabbut A, Carradori S, et al: Osteonecrosis in protease inhibitor-treated patients. Orthopedics 24:271–272, 2001.
2. Felson DT, Anderson JJ: A cross-study evaluation of association between steroid dose and bolus steroids and avascular necrosis of bone. Lancet 1:902–906, 1987.
3. Frankel ES, Urbaniak JR: Osteonecrosis. In Ruddy S, Harris ED, Sledge CB (eds): Kelley's Textbook of Rheumatology, 6th ed. Philadelphia, WB Saunders, 2001, pp 1653–1665.
4. Glueck CJ, Freiberg R, Tracy T, et al: Thrombophilia and hypofibinoysis: Pathophysiologies of osteonecrosis. Clin Orthop Rel Res 334:43–56, 1997.
5. Mont MA, Carbone JJ, Fairbank AC: Core decompression versus nonoperative management for osteonecrosis of the hip. Clin Orthop 324:169–178, 1996.
6. Urbaniak JR, Harvey EJ: Revascularization of the femoral head in osteonecrosis. J Am Acad Ortho Surg 6:44–54, 1998.
7. Urbaniak JR, Jones JP (eds): Osteonecrosis: Etiology, Diagnosis and Treatment. Rosemont, IL, American Academy of Orthopaedic Surgeons, 1997.

# X. *Hereditary, Congenital, and Inborn Errors of Metabolism Associated with Rheumatic Syndromes*

*The law of heredity is that all undesirable traits come from the other parent.*
Anonymous

# 59. HERITABLE COLLAGEN DISEASES

John Keith Jenkins, M.D.

**1. What are the most prevalent types of collagen in the body, and where are they located?**

Type I collagen accounts for 60–90% of the dry weight of skin, ligaments, and demineralized bone. Type II collagen accounts for 50% of the dry weight of articular cartilage. It is present in substantial amounts in the vitreous, nucleus pulposus, and nasal and auricular cartilages. Type III is found in blood vessels and in tissues that have type I collagen (except for bone). Type IV occurs in most basement membranes. Type VII collagen is also a basement membrane collagen found in the skin (see Chapter 3).

**2. Describe the important features of collagen synthesis relevant to inherited diseases of bone and connective tissue.**

Collagen synthesis is complex and requires normal expression of the different collagen genes in the right proportion. The molecules must also be functional. "Nucleated growth" of the newly formed procollagen fibrils requires the correct primary structure (amino acid sequence) as well as post-translational modifications of the procollagen molecules. For example, type I collagen is formed from two procollagen type I $\alpha_1$ chains and one procollagen type I $\alpha_2$ chain. The three chains combine at one end and twist together to form the triple helix (nucleated growth) after adequate post-translational modification of the proline residues. Fibrils are arranged in a quarter stagger array to form a large fiber. Disordering of any of these processes may result in poor collagen quality and clinical disease.

**3. How do abnormalities in collagen synthesis cause clinical disease?**

1. With mutations in collagen genes, the location of the collagen type that is abnormal determines which organs will be involved (see Question 1).
2. Mutations that simply diminish production of a particular collagen type may give a milder phenotype than does a high level of expression of a structurally abnormal protein.
3. The principle of nucleated growth explains why structurally abnormal molecules lead to devastating and potentially lethal clinical results.
4. Different amino acid substitutions in the same collagen gene may affect different functions of the molecule and lead to different clinical manifestations, but there may be significant overlap in the syndromes.

**4. Summarize the heritable disorders of collagen.**

- Type I collagen is important for strength of bone, ligaments, tendons, and skin. Diseases associated with type I collagen disorders include: osteogenesis imperfecta, Ehlers-Danlos syndrome, Marfan's syndrome, congenital contractural arachnodactyly, pseudoxanthoma elasticum, and cutis laxis.
- Type II collagen is important for compression of cartilage and growth. Diseases associated with type II collagen disorders include: achondroplasias (Stickler's syndrome and spinal chondrodysplasia), metaphyseal chondroplasia, and spondyloepiphyseal dysplasia.

- Type IV collagen and type VII collagen form barriers known as basement membranes. Abnormalities of type IV collagen include Alport's syndrome and of type VII collagen include epidermolysis bullosa.

## TYPE I COLLAGEN DISEASES

**5. What is osteogenesis imperfecta? Which organs are involved, and why?**

Osteogenesis imperfecta (OI), aka "brittle bone" disease, is actually a group of diseases defined by similar clinical manifestations (brittle bones and blue sclerae) occurring to various degrees with a similar etiology. The inheritance pattern and penetrance are variable. Most are autosomal dominant, but sporadic cases occur. A surprising result of recent research is that over 90% of all patients studied have a mutation in one of the genes encoding type I collagen, which is necessary for bone's structure and physical properties. The collagen abnormality results in osteopenia and brittleness, leading to frequent fractures. Diminished collagen in the sclerae leads to their translucency and apparent blueness. All the organs affected have a type I collagen problem. Clinical syndromes of brittle bone disease are variable. Affected individuals may experience *in utero* death to mildly brittle bones, blue sclerae, opalescent teeth, and hearing loss. The more severe forms allowing live birth have wormian bones, short stature, and multiple fractures.

Other "brittle" bone diseases may have molecular defects in type I collagen, namely osteoporosis. Familial osteoporosis in Europe and the United States is associated with collagen defects. Some investigators suspect that women at risk for osteoporosis may have an as-yet-undefined abnormality of collagen that predisposes them to "premature" osteoporosis. Bisphosphonates as used for osteoporosis may have some clinical utility in these diseases.

**6. How can a defect in type I collagen lead to brittle bone disease in one patient and familial osteoporosis in another?**

Collagen is a complex molecule containing multiple domains with different functions. The clinical manifestations of its abnormalities vary depending on the function or structure interrupted. In recent years, investigators have found overlap between milder OI and osteoporosis syndromes and between OI and Ehlers-Danlos syndromes. Defining the molecular defect in a specific collagen does not necessarily allow one to determine the precise clinical phenotype. These diseases demonstrate the Orwellian principle that some collagens are created more equal than others. The first corollary of this principle is that one still has to learn clinical syndromes for board examinations.

**7. What is the Sillence classification of OI?**

The Sillence classification groups OI into four clinical categories of severity. Multiple different collagen mutations may be responsible for each Sillence type.

**Type I OI** (mild) (50%): bone fragility, moderate number of fractures (wormian bones), blue sclerae, and short stature due to null allele causing underproduction of normal type I collagen.

**Type II OI** (usually lethal) (5%): multiple in utero fractures and blue or gray sclerae, *in utero*/neonatal death common

**Type III OI** (severe deforming) (20%): major skeletal deformities, variable bone fragility, scoliosis, joint laxity, gray or blue sclerae and osteopenia, not usually ambulatory

**Type IV OI** (moderate severity) (25%): variable fragility with a moderate number of fractures, wormian bones, normal (white) or gray sclerae, ambulatory.

Type III OI is autosomal recessive or sporadic, and types I, II, and IV are autosomal dominant. Dental abnormalities (dentinogenesis imperfecta) may accompany types I, III, and IV, and hearing loss may accompany forms I and IV. Types I and IV have A and B subtypes, opalescent or normal teeth, respectively. Bisphosphonate therapy may be beneficial, especially intravenous pamidronate.

**8. What is the significance of increased joint mobility? How do I diagnose benign joint hypermobility syndrome?**

Hyperflexible joints are common and do not necessarily indicate that someone has a heritable disorder of connective or elastic tissue. Some studies suggest that 10–25% of the population may have some hyperflexible joints. Increased joint mobility may be associated with a lack of stability leading to dislocation or injury. In the Ehlers-Danlos syndromes (EDS), this laxity results in congenital hip dislocation and habitual dislocation later in life or other injury. Arthritic disability may occur from recurrent dislocation with hemorrhage.

The benign hypermobility syndrome was formerly known as EDS type III. This syndrome is characterized by varying degrees of joint laxity without instability or disability and is an important cause of periarticular complaints. Arthralgias (hands, knees, and hips) occur with unusual physical activity, there is a familial tendency, and frequent ankle or wrist sprains may occur. Young girls are the most common patients with this disorder, and joint effusions do occur. A patient needs at least three of the six physical examination signs of hyperextensibility to diagnose this syndrome. There are six simple tests (Beighton criteria) for joint laxity, i.e., hyperextensibility, done during the physical examination:

1. Knee extension more than 10° past 180°
2. Extension of the elbow 10° or more past 180°
3. Extension of the thumb to touch the anterior surface of the forearm
4. Extension of fingers backward so that they are parallel with the posterior forearm
5. Trunk flexion so that the palms of the hands can be placed flat on the ground
6. Dorsiflexion of the foot more than 20° past a right angle

**9. Describe the clinical manifestations of the Ehlers-Danlos syndromes.**

The Ehlers-Danlos syndromes (EDS) comprise a group of uncommon disorders of elastic tissue primarily involving joint and skin laxity and arterial wall abnormalities. **Increased joint mobility** and **increased skin fragility and hyperextensibility** occur, though there is a wide variability in the joint, skin, and internal organ involvement. Hyperextensibility in EDS patients may be greater in the small joints than large joints and may diminish with age. Laxity/hyperextensibility in other organs include Gorlin's sign (ability to touch the nose with the tip of the tongue). Skin laxity and fragility may be manifest as easy bruisability, inability of stretched skin to return to normal resulting in papyraceous-appearing skin over the knees, gaping wounds from minor trauma, or the inability of skin to retain sutures. Arteries may develop aneurysms or rupture because of elastic tissue laxity. There are nine recognized types of EDS. Most involve some abnormality in collagen synthesis or enzymatic modification of collagen. The most common forms of EDS (type I and II) may be due to a defect of type V collagen leading to abnormal assembly of type I collagen.

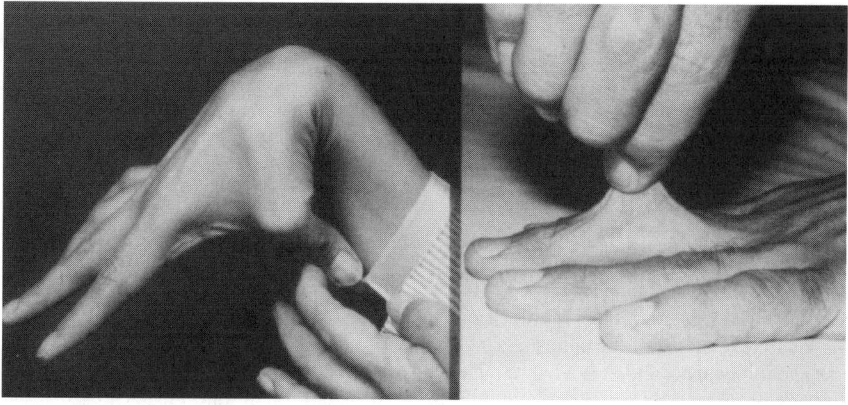

Patient with Ehlers-Danlos syndrome demonstrating hyperextensibility of joints and skin. (From the Clinical Slide Collection on the Rheumatic Diseases. Atlanta, American College of Rheumatology, 1991; with permission.)

**10. How is EDS inherited?**

In most cases, the defect is inherited in an autosomal dominant manner and results in diminished or defective collagen in some way. One exception is EDS type VI (oculo-scoliotic), which involves a recessive defect in lysyl hydroxylase, the vitamin C–requiring enzyme necessary for forming the hydroxylysine cross-links in collagen. In addition to joint and skin hyperextensibility, scoliosis and rupture of the ocular globe occur in this form. Pharmacologic doses of vitamin C may be beneficial for some forms of EDS and the benign hypermobility syndrome. The defect, though, still affects collagen.

**11. What is the arterial form of EDS?**

EDS type IV (arterial form) involves a defect in production of type III collagen, which is found in blood vessels. Skin and joint disease is less than with EDS types I and II, but arterial or bowel rupture may be dramatic and lethal. Defects in type III collagen have been shown to be a rather common cause of premature aneurysms in the cardiovascular (abdominal aortic) and cerebrovascular (proximal to the circle of Willis) systems. Rare diseases such as EDS and OI may simply represent the most severe phenotypes of mutations in structural proteins that otherwise manifest late in life as premature bone, joint, or vascular disease.

**12. What are the primary organ systems involved in the Marfan syndrome? Why?**

Marfan syndrome commonly involves primarily the ocular, skeletal, and vascular systems, but the skin and pulmonary systems are also involved. A defect has been found in the fibrillin-1 gene on chromosome 15 in all patients studied. Over 200 mutations of this gene have been reported. The inheritance pattern is autosomal dominant, although 25% are due to sporadic mutations.

Marfan syndrome was long suspected to be a defect in elastin, a specialized connective tissue providing elasticity and prominent in ligaments, but no abnormality in elastin has ever been found. Fibrillin, found in soft connective tissues, is a constituent of extracellular microfibrils that form the substructure for elastin. Organs involved in Marfan syndrome are those in which elastic fibers (and therefore fibrillin) are important, including the elastic wall of arteries (especially the aorta), zonula fibers of the eye, ligaments, skin, and lung parenchyma.

**13. Describe the phenotype and skeletal manifestations of Marfan syndrome.**

Patients with Marfan syndrome have a characteristic phenotype that is easily recognized: tall stature, long thin extremities, dolichostenomelia (abnormally low ratio of upper to lower body segments, $< 0.85$) (normal for whites $\geq .93$ and blacks $\geq .87$), and diminished subcutaneous fat. Skeletal manifestations include arachnodactyly (spider digits), pectus excavatum or carinatum, tallness, loss of thoracic kyphosis, and scoliosis. Other manifestations include a gothic (high, arched) palate and dolichocephaly (long, narrow face).

Several prominent athletes as well as Abraham Lincoln are said to have had Marfan syndrome. The Olympic sports in which persons with Marfan syndrome are said to excel are volleyball and basketball. In fact, a US Olympic volleyball star, Flo Hyman, is said to have died in 1986 of vascular complications of Marfan syndrome.

**14. How is arachnodactyly recognized?**

Look at the hands! However, there are three simple and more definitive methods to determine if it is present.

- The **thumb sign**, or Steinberg's sign, is a protrusion of the thumb past the hypothenar border when the hand is clenched in a fist.
- The **wrist sign**, or Walker-Murdoch sign, is overlap of the fifth finger and thumb when they encircle the wrist of the opposite hand.
- The **metacarpal index** is a radiographic measure of arachnodactyly. It is the average of the lengths divided by the midpoint widths of the second through fourth metacarpals (5.4–7.9 is normal, $> 8.4$ occurs in Marfan's).

All these signs indicate long, thin (spider-like) digits.

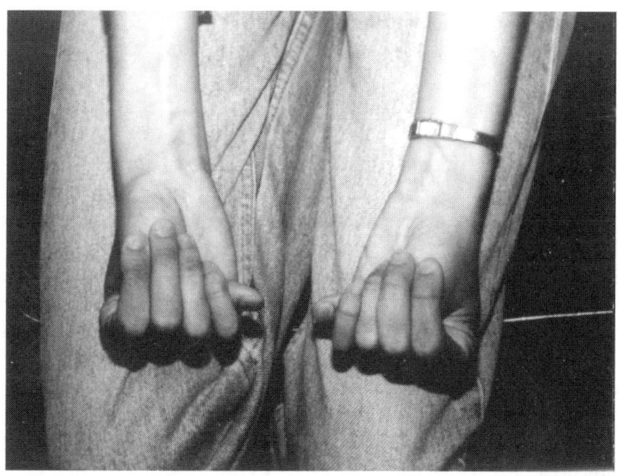

Patient with Marfan syndrome demonstrating Steinberg's thumb sign.

**15. Does the presence of arachnodactyly mean a patient has Marfan's? What is the differential diagnosis of arachnodactyly?**

Arachnodactyly is present in about 90% of cases of Marfan syndrome, is not diagnostic, and may be seen in other diseases. Nonasthenic Marfan syndrome may be a forme fruste of the disease; patients have a more normal-appearing phenotype with arachnodactyly but may have the same mutation as in other, more severely affected family members. Marfanoid hypermobility syndrome has skeletal features of Marfan phenotype, such as arachnodactyly, but also has hyperelastic skin and hyperextensible joints as in Ehlers-Danlos syndrome. Congenital contractural arachnodactyly is another autosomal dominant disease with tall stature, arachnodactyly, joint contractures, and unknown etiology. Homocystinurics may also demonstrate tallness, arachnodactyly, and spinal abnormalities.

**16. What are the nonmusculoskeletal manifestations of the Marfan syndrome? Which cause significant morbidity and mortality?**

Ectopia lentis (upward dislocation) occurs in over half of patients. Cardiovascular complications are multiple and common. Aneurysmal dilatation of the ascending aorta with dissection is the most common cause of death in patients. Mitral valve prolapse with regurgitation or aortic insufficiency is detectable in 60% of patients by auscultation and in > 80% by echocardiography. Pulmonary manifestations include cystic disease and spontaneous pneumothorax. The primary cause of morbidity is skeletal disease of the spine. Scoliosis is a major management problem and may be rapidly progressive during adolescence, requiring surgery.

**17. How is Marfan syndrome treated?**

Genetic counseling is indicated. Preventative measures are taken to monitor cardiovascular problems. Because the disease is autosomal dominant, 50% of offspring will be affected. Echocardiography is needed to determine the presence of mitral and aortic valvular disease. Infective endocarditis occurs in patients with mitral or tricuspid disease, and they should receive prophylaxis. Echocardiography is performed yearly to follow aortic dilatation; when the size exceeds 50% of normal (> 45 mm), echocardiography is recommended at 6-month intervals. Propranolol to keep exercise heart rate less than 100 beats/minute may retard progression of aortic dilatation. Vigorous exercise is contraindicated. Pregnancy is generally safe unless aortic dilatation is present. Surgery is indicated when aortic root exceeds 55 mm.

**18. What is congenital contractural arachnodactyly (CCA)?**

CCA is a disease due to mutations of the fibrillin-2 gene on chromosome 5. Patients have a marfanoid habitus but unlike Marfan's syndrome have stiff joints, "crumpled" ears, severe thoracic deformities, and no cardiac or eye abnormalities.

**19. What are the clinical features of pseudoxanthoma elasticum?**

Pseudoxanthoma elasticum is a rare disease that involves degeneration and calcification of elastic fibers in the eyes, skin, and arteries. The molecular defect is undefined but is somewhere in the structure of elastic fibers. There is moderate heterogeneity in the clinical findings. Both autosomal recessive and dominant forms occur. **Xanthomatoid papules** occur in flexural skinfolds and are the classic finding. **Angioid streaks** occur in the fundus owing to a break in Bruch's membrane. Visual loss may occur from a maculopathy and retinal lesions. **Calcific deposits** in the lungs and cardiac involvement mimicking cardiomyopathy may occur. **Arterial rupture** occurs in the gastrointestinal tract. Abnormal elastic fibers usually do not impair wound healing until late in life. Patients die of coronary artery fibrosis and calcification.

**20. What is cutis laxa?**

Cutis laxa refers to a group of disorders with a common finding of lax, redundant skin. The skin may appear wrinkled, aged, or sagging in loose folds. A similar skin appearance may occur after penicillamine use or subsequent to inflammatory skin diseases. The skin appears to have lost elasticity and does not recoil when stretched. In EDS, the skin does recoil. Cardiopulmonary manifestations may occur, including bronchiectasis and emphysema. There is no abnormality of skin fragility with bleeding, so surgery is safely performed (again, unlike Ehlers-Danlos syndrome).

## TYPE II COLLAGEN DISEASES

**21. What is the Stickler syndrome?**

The Stickler syndrome, or hereditary arthro-ophthalmopathy, is an hereditary disease of unknown etiology in which patients have skeletal and ocular abnormalities. It is thought to be relatively common (1 in 10,000), and the inheritance pattern is autosomal dominant. Half of families in one study were shown to have an abnormality in type II collagen (mutation in $\alpha_1$ (II) procollagen gene), the most common collagen in cartilage. The syndrome includes myopia, retinal detachment and other eye problems, cleft palate, mandibular hypoplasia, hyper- and hypomobile joints, epiphyseal dysplasia, and disability from joint problems. The diagnosis should be suspected in any young adult with degenerative hip arthritis or any infant with congenitally swollen joints (especially wrists).

Other clinical syndromes involving widespread cartilage disease that may be associated with abnormal type II collagen include primary generalized osteoarthritis, chondrodysplasia, and spondyloepiphyseal dysplasia.

## TYPES IV AND VII COLLAGEN DISEASES

**22. What is Alport's syndrome?**

Alport's syndrome includes hereditary glomerulonephritis and deafness. The defect is in a nonfibrillar basement membrane collagen, type IV collagen. Patients present with hematuria and sensorineural hearing loss. They eventually progress to renal failure.

**23. What is a disease due to mutation of type VII collagen?**

Epidermolysis bullosa is a skin disease leading to progressive blistering and bullae formation in the dermis. It is due to one of over 100 mutations found in type VII collagen, which forms the anchoring fibrils that tether dermis to basement membrane.

## BIBLIOGRAPHY

1. Kuivaniemi H, Tromp G, Prockop DJ: Mutations in collagens: Causes of rare and some common disorders in humans. FASEB J 5:2052–2060, 1991.
2. Mayne R: What is collagen? In Koopman WJ (ed): Arthritis and Allied Conditions, 14th ed. Baltimore, Williams & Wilkins, 2001, pp 187–208.
3. Milewicz DM: Molecular genetics of Marfan syndrome and Ehlers-Danlos type IV. Curr Op Card 13:198–204, 1998.
4. Pope FM, Narcisi P, Nicholls AC, et al: Clinical presentations of Ehlers-Danlos syndrome type IV. Arch Dis Child 63:1016–1025, 1989.
5. Prockop DJ: Osteogenesis imperfecta: Model for genetic causes of osteoporosis and perhaps several other common diseases of connective tissue. Arthritis Rheum 31:1–8, 1988.
6. Pyeritz RE: The Marfan syndrome. Ann Rev Med 51:481–510, 2000.
7. Pyeritz RE: Heritable and developmental disorders of connective tissue and bone. In Koopman WJ (ed): Arthritis and Allied Conditions, 14th ed. Baltimore, Williams & Wilkins, 2001, pp 1925–1961.
8. Shapiro JR: Heritable disorders of structural proteins. In Ruddy S, Harris ED, Sledge CB (eds): Kelley's Textbook of Rheumatology, 6th ed. Philadelphia, WB Saunders, 2001, pp 1433–1462.

# 60. INBORN ERRORS OF METABOLISM AFFECTING CONNECTIVE TISSUE

*John Keith Jenkins, M.D.*

**1. What are the homocystinurias?**

There are three clinically (and biochemically) distinct disorders of amino acid metabolism resulting in elevated serum and urine levels of homocystine. The most common form of homocystinuria is due to an autosomal recessive defect in methionine metabolism because of absence of activity of the enzyme cystathionine β-synthase. This enzyme is involved in the transsulfuration pathway from methionine to cysteine. Two other, less common forms are due to defective remethylation of homocystine to methionine.

**2. How common is homocystinuria, and how do I diagnose it?**

Cystathionine β-synthase deficiency probably occurs in about 1 in 200,000 (or less) live births in the United States, prompting some states to require newborn homocystine screening. In comparison, newborn screening for phenylketonuria, which most states require, detects 1 case in 10,000 livebirths. Heterozygotes for cystathionine β-synthase deficiency (1 in 70 in the general population) have been thought to be unaffected but may be at risk for premature peripheral and cerebral vascular disease.

Homocystine is increased in the blood and urine in all three known defects. The cyanide-nitroprusside test detects sulfhydryl-containing amino acids in the urine, so it is not specific for the particular enzymatic defect. The pathway is from homocystine to methionine to cysteine. Plasma methionine levels are high in cystathionine β-synthase deficiency but normal or low in the pre-methionine defects causing homocystinuria. The other known defects are in synthesis of the cofactors (methyl vitamin $B_{12}$ and methyltetrahydrofolate) needed for methionine synthesis. Consequently, patients with vitamin $B_{12}$ or folate deficiency can have high homocystine but low normal methionine levels. They get premature vascular disease but not the other manifestations of homocystinuria. A combination of homocystine and methionine levels in urine and blood must be measured. Precise tissue (e.g., cultured skin fibroblasts) enzyme assays can also be performed.

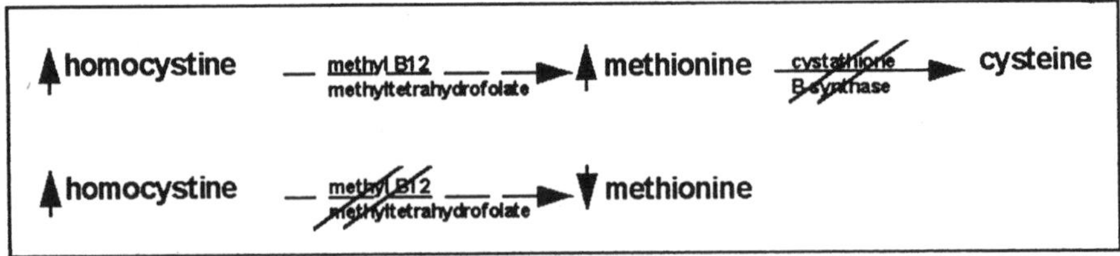


Biochemical pathways leading to homocystinuria. *Top*, Cystathionine β-synthase deficiency leads to increased homocystine and methionine levels. *Bottom*, Deficiency of other cofactors leads to decreased methionine and increased homocystine.

**3. List the major clinical manifestations of homocystinuria.**

Ectopia lentis (dislocated lens downward)—hallmark finding
Thromboembolism
Mental retardation
Connective tissue disorder similar to Marfan's syndrome

The musculoskeletal findings include tallness, arachnodactyly (dolichostenomelia), ectopia lentis, and chest wall and spinal deformity. Osteoporosis (generalized) and tight joints occur. Spinal osteoporosis occurs in up to 64% of affected individuals by age 15. Spinal disease is prominent and is usually a combination of osteoporotic fractures, degenerative disc/joint disease, and scoliosis.

**Pearl**: If you have a "mentally retarded Marfan's with stiff joints," think of homocystinuria.

**4. Why does homocystinuria affect connective tissue?**

Cysteine is deficient. However, cysteine is necessary for proper cross-linking (to cystine) of structural proteins such as collagen and fibrillin in connective tissue and bone, the suspensory ligament of the eye, and the extracellular milieu of endothelial cells. On this basis, altered collagen may be responsible for the lens dislocation and osteoporosis, while altered proteins in the elastomeric complex or its substructure (fibrillin) may be responsible for the phenotypic similarity to the Marfan syndrome. Altered endothelial ground substance is responsible for the thrombosis and subsequent mental retardation.

**5. How is homocystinuria treated? Which symptoms can be expected to respond?**

Effective treatment requires early diagnosis to prevent mental retardation, which is the basis of newborn screening for inborn errors of metabolism. $B_6$, $B_{12}$, and folate are cofactors for the different enzymes involved in methionine metabolism. One-half of patients are $B_6$-responders. Large doses of vitamin $B_6$ (15–500 mg of pyridoxine per day) lowers blood methionine, raises blood cysteine, and improves symptoms in patients with cystathionine β-synthase deficiency, presumably by augmenting a small amount of residual enzyme activity. Development of ectopia lentis, osteoporosis, and retardation may be mitigated with therapy, but they will not remit if already present.

**6. What causes alkaptonuria? What is the inheritance pattern?**

Alkaptonuria (also known as ochronosis) is a rare defect in tyrosine catabolism due to a deficiency in homogentisic acid oxidase. This enzyme catabolizes homogentisic acid to molecules that can be used in the TCA cycle. Deposition of homogentisic acid produces a gray to blue-black pigment in tissues; hence the name ochronosis. Alkaptonuria is a favorite board question because it was the first human disease shown to be autosomal recessive. Heterozygotes are unaffected even when challenged with high doses of the precursor amino acids.

**7. How is the diagnosis of alkaptonuria made?**

The clinical diagnosis is suggested by the typical triad of findings:

• Degenerative arthritis (premature)

- Abnormal pigmentation
- Urine that turns blue-black on standing (alkalinization or ferric chloride addition).

Homogentisic acid binds collagen and is therefore deposited in connective tissues. If you see blue-black (skin, ears, sclerae, cartilage), think ochronosis. A specific enzyme assay for homogentisic acid oxidase, as well as thin layer chromatography for homogentisic acid, can be performed.

**8. Describe the musculoskeletal manifestations of alkaptonuria.**

Degenerative joint disease occurs in the third decade with typical symptoms of pain, stiffness, and limited range of motion of large joints and spine. The most common site involved is the spine, followed by the knees, hips, and shoulders. Abnormal calcification and ossification occur. Tendinitis has been reported. Dense calcification of the intervertebral discs is said to be pathognomic. The vacuum sign is prominent in discs also. Synovial fluid does not darken on alkalinization as urine does, but it may have a characteristic ground-pepper appearance. Calcium pyrophosphate deposition disease has been noted to coexist with ochronotic arthritis.

**9. How is ochronotic arthritis treated?**

Symptomatic treatment of the arthritis as for osteoarthritis is the standard therapy: patient education, physical therapy and/or local therapy, analgesia, etc. Dietary restriction of phenylalanine and tyrosine are indicated. Surgical procedures (including arthroplasty) and arthroscopy have been of benefit for removal of osteochondral loose bodies in the knee. Large doses of vitamin C have been used, but there are no studies of its efficacy.

**10. What is Menkes' kinky hair syndrome? What is its inheritance pattern, and how does it affect the musculoskeletal system?**

Menkes' is an X-linked recessive disorder of copper metabolism in which the clinical abnormalities are primarily neurologic: seizures, abnormal reflexes, spasticity, mental retardation. Patients also have occipital horns and pili torti (beaded, brittle, and sparse hair). Abnormal copper metabolism due to a malfunction of ATPase dependent transport of copper affects copper-requiring metalloenzymes (lysyl hydroxylase) involved in collagen and elastin synthesis, thereby affecting connective tissues. The rheumatic manifestations may be either cutis laxa–like or Ehlers-Danlos–like with highly extensible skin and joints (used to be EDS IX).

**11. What are the musculoskeletal manifestations of the mucopolysaccharidoses (MPS)?**

The mucopolysaccharidoses are a group of diverse inborn errors of proteoglycan catabolism. Catabolites progressively deposit in various tissues and lead to skeletal dysplasia. Short stature is the rule. Thick calvaria, an enlarged J-shaped sella turcica, short and wide mandible, biconvex vertebral bodies, odontoid hypoplasia, short thick clavicles, coxa valga, short fingers, wide metacarpals with pointed proximal ends all occur. Many have mental retardation, corneal clouding, and organomegaly. The Hurler, Hunter Morquio and Maroteaux-Lamy syndromes (Types IH, II, IV and VI) have short trunk dwarfism. The diagnosis of MPS is made by fractionation of urinary mucopolysaccharides, enzymatic assays, and/or molecular genetics. Treatment is palliative and consists mainly of joint replacement and surgical stabilization of cervical instability. Bone marrow transplants have been successful in some forms of MPS.

## BIBLIOGRAPHY

1. Albers SE, Brozena SJ, Glass R, Fenske NA: Alkaptonuria and ochronosis: Case report and review. J Am Acad Dermatol 27:609–614, 1992.
2. Hunter T, Gordon D, Ogryzlo MA: The ground pepper sign of synovial fluid: A new diagnostic feature of ochronosis. J Rheumatol 1:45–53, 1974.
3. Mudd SH, Skovby F, Levy HL, et al: The natural history of homocystinuria due to cystathionine beta-synthase deficiency. Am J Hum Genet 37:1–31, 1985.
4. Pyeritz RE: Heritable and developmental disorders of connective tissue and bone. In Koopman WJ (ed): Arthritis and Allied Conditions, 14th ed. Baltimore, Williams & Wilkins, 2001, pp 1925–1961.

5. Sakkas L, Thomas B, Smyrnis P, Vlahos E: Low back pain and ochronosis. Int Orthop 11:19–21, 1987.
6. Shapiro JR: Heritable disorders of structural proteins. In Ruddy S, Harris ED, Sledge CB (eds): Kelley's Textbook of Rheumatology, 6th ed. Philadelphia, WB Saunders, 2001, pp 1433–1462.

# 61. STORAGE AND DEPOSITION DISEASES

Mark Jarek, M.D.

**1. What is the pattern of inheritance for hereditary hemochromatosis, Wilson's disease, and alkaptonuria (ochronosis)?**

All are inherited as autosomal recessive traits with heterozygotes being asymptomatic carriers. Wilson's disease occurs in about 1 in 30,000, and alkaptonuria in about 1 in 200,000 individuals. Alkaptonuria was the first human disease shown to be inherited as an autosomal recessive trait.

**2. What is the HFE gene, and what is its significance to hereditary hemochromatosis (HHC)?**

The HFE gene was identified in 1996 and is the gene responsible for most cases of HHC, accounting for approximately 80% of cases in the U.S. and 100% of cases in Australia. The gene is mainly expressed in crypt enterocytes where it codes for a protein that regulates brush border iron transport from the gut lumen. A single G-to-A mutation in the HFE gene resulting in a cysteine-to-tyrosine single amino acid substitution at position 282 (C282Y) is found in 85–90% of patients. A second less common mutation is an aspartate substituton for histidine at position 63 (H63D). The defective coded protein causes the crypt cell to misread the body's iron stores, and iron absorption is inappropriately increased.

The human body normally contain 3 to 4 grams of iron with two thirds contained in hemoglobin, myoglobin, and a variety of enzymes, and one third as storage iron in ferritin and hemosiderin within hepatocytes and macrophages of the liver, bone marrow, spleen, and muscle. Although the typical Western diet contains 10–20 mg of iron a day, only 1 to 2 mg is absorbed daily by the duodenal mucosa, which balances the iron loss from exfoliated GI epithelial cells and desquamation of the skin. In HHC, excess GI iron absorption ranges from 3 to 4 mg per day resulting in an accumulation of 15–35 grams of iron over a 35–60 year period.

**3. How common is HHC?**

Recent screening studies suggest that the HHC gene occurs in 5% of whites, giving a carrier (heterozygote) frequency of approximately 1:10 and a disease (homozygote) frequency of 1:400. There is a wide variation in gene frequency. The mutation frequency is highest in individuals of northwestern European descent and less common in southern and eastern Europe populations and is rarely found in indigenous populations of Africa, the Americas, Asia, and the Pacific Islands. Studies in Scandinavian families have identified the frequency of homozygosity to be as high as 1%. The global prevalence of the gene mutation is 1.9%, making this one of the most commonly inherited metabolic diseases. Given the frequency of HHC in the general population, many physicians recommend screening iron studies in all men by age 40. Odds ratio for developing HHC if homozygous for C282Y mutation of HFE gene is 2300, while homozygous for H63D is only 6.

**4. How does the typical patient with HHC present?**

Several factors, most notably physiologic blood loss in women and higher iron intake in men, modify expression of the disease. Accordingly, the symptomatic stage is approximately 10× more common in men than women and men tend to have onset of symptoms at an earlier age.

Clinical manifestations usually appear between ages 40–60 years, but the disease severity is quite variable. A few patients may develop full clinical expression as early as age 20, while 30% of HFE mutation homozygotes never develop clinical symptoms.

HHC typically presents with **asymptomatic abnormal liver function tests** with 95% having **hepatomegaly**. Liver disease usually progresses to hepatic cirrhosis in untreated cases. A characteristic **arthropathy** occurs in 20–50% of patients and may be the initial manifestation, although more often it occurs later in the disease and may even develop after treatment has been initiated. Other manifestations include a slate-gray skin due to iron in eccrine sweat glands and brown **skin pigmentation** due to melanin deposition (50%), **diabetes mellitus**, and **hypogonadism** manifested by decreased libido (20–40%), impotence, amenorrhea, or sparse body hair. **Constitutional symptoms** (80%) such as weakness or lethargy are also common. Cardiac involvement, manifested most commonly by **congestive heart failure**, is present in about 30% of patients and is a principal cause of death in untreated patients.

**5. What are some clinical features of the arthropathy of HHC?**

Most joints can be affected, but pain and stiffness affecting the second and third metacarpophalangeal joints (MCP) are the most characteristic complaints. Other joints affected are the proximal interphalangeal joints, wrists, knees, hips, ankles, shoulders, and occasionally metatarsophalangeal joints. Joint examination usually reveals firm swelling with mild tenderness, but warmth and effusions are absent, helping to distinguish it from rheumatoid arthritis. Arthritis may be the initial manifestation in 33% of patients with HHC.

**6. Describe the typical radiographic abnormalities seen in the arthropathy of HHC.**

Radiographs show osteoarthritis-like changes with sclerotic margins, joint-space narrowing, and osteophyte formation that is characteristically hook-like, particularly when found at the MCP joints. Chondrocalcinosis is present in 30–60% of patients and can occur without the degenerative arthropathy.

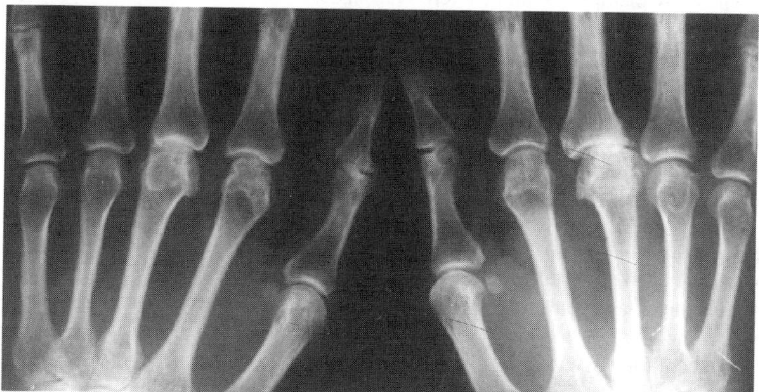

Hand radiographs of a patient with hemochromatosis. Note degenerative arthritis of the MCP joints with hook-like osteophytes.

**7. Generalized osteopenia is common in HHC. What are its possible causes?**

- Increased synovial iron (comparable with serum levels) directly inhibits bone formation.
- Pituitary iron infiltration decreases gonadotropin levels, leading to hypogonadism.
- Hepatic cirrhosis leads to testicular atrophy and hypogonadism. Also poor conversion of vitamin D to 25-OH vitamin D.

**8. How is the diagnosis of hemachromatosis made?**

In the fasting state, a transferrin saturation (iron/TIBC × 100) greater than 60% in men or 50% in women along with an elevated ferritin greater than 2 times normal is 95% sensitive and

85% specific for the diagnosis of hemachromatosis. Serum ferritin levels are an accurate measure of peripheral iron stores but may also be increased in the settings of acute liver injury, systemic inflammation, and neoplasia (i.e., lymphoma). The definitive diagnosis is made by direct measurement of iron in a liver biopsy. Additionally, synovial biopsies will show iron deposition in the type B synovial lining cells in patients with arthritis. However, biopsies may not be necessary in the setting of abnormal iron studies in a patient homozygous for the C282Y gene.

**9. Once a proband case of HFE-associated HHC is identified, who should be screened and by what method?**

All first-degree relatives of the patient should be screened for the disease using fasting transferrin saturation and testing for the C282Y and H63D mutations. Liver biopsy is not necessary for diagnosis unless severe fibrosis is suspected (serum ferritin > 1000 ng/L), or the diagnosis is in doubt, as in the case of persons heterozygous for the C282Y mutation with abnormal iron indices or liver function tests. Screening can be deferred until the second decade of life.

**10. Now that you have made the diagnosis of hemochromatosis, outline a treatment plan.**

Phlebotomy is performed twice weekly until the transferrin saturation is < 50% and ferritin level is < 50 ng/ml (up to 2–3 years) and then as required (usually every 3–4 months) to maintain low normal serum levels. Life expectancy of symptomatic patients is extended considerably by removal of excess iron stores (90% 5-year survival vs 33% survival without therapy). With therapy, hepatomegaly, liver function studies, and pigmentation all improve and cardiac function stabilizes or improves. Diabetes mellitus improves in about 50%. Phlebotomy has little effect on hypogonadism or arthropathy. Hepatic fibrosis may improve, but cirrhosis is irreversible. Hepatocellular carcinoma, a late sequela in one-third of those who develop hepatic cirrhosis (200× increased risk), is not diminished by phlebotomy and is the major cause (30–45%) of death in treated individuals. Because life expectancy of homozygotes diagnosed and treated before the development of cirrhosis is the same as that of the general population, the importance of family screening and early therapy cannot be overemphasized.

**11. Liver disease is the first clinical manifestation in approximately 50% of patients with Wilson's disease (hepatolenticular degeneration). What are the clinical presentations of liver involvement?**

Transient hepatitis, fulminant hepatitis, chronic active hepatitis, and cirrhosis. A clue to Wilson's disease as the etiology for fulminant hepatic failure is the disproportionately low aminotransferases (usually < 1500 u/L) and the marked increased bilirubin due to associated hemolysis.

**12. Are there other common clinical features in Wilson's disease?**

In addition to hepatic manifestations, Wilson's disease, which usually presents between ages 20 and 40, can also have neurologic manifestations, arthropathy (50%), and hemolytic anemia. The most common neurologic manifestations are either movement disorders arising from basal ganglion degeneration or rigid dystonia. Psychiatric disorders such as mood disturbances, neurosis, and hypophonia have also been described. Gynecologic manifestations can include amenorrhea and infertility. A kidney tubular disorder can also be seen.

**13. Describe Kayser-Fleischer rings. What is their significance?**

Kayser-Fleischer rings are green or brown deposits of copper in Descemet's membrane of the cornea that do not interfere with vision. They are present in 95% of cases with neurologic or psychiatric manifestations but are not specific for Wilson's disease. They have occasionally been seen in other causes of hepatic cirrhosis (primary biliary cirrhosis, sclerosing cholangitis, and autoimmune hepatitis) as well as occasionally in nonhepatic diseases.

**14. What is the biochemical defect in Wilson's disease? How is a diagnosis confirmed?**

Wilson's disease results from excessive copper accumulation in association with a ceruloplasmin deficiency. The capacity of hepatocytes to store copper is exceeded, and excessive copper is deposited in the liver and at extrahepatic sites such as the brain, kidneys, urine, and serum. Decreased serum ceruloplasmin (< 200 mg/L) and copper levels (< 70 μg/dL) with elevated urinary copper excretion (> 100 μg/day) are suggestive of Wilson's disease. An elevated hepatic copper concentration (> 250 μg Cu/g dry weight) is the most reliable test early in the course of the illness. Screening first degree relatives older than 6 years old should include a physical examination, liver functions, serum copper, ceruloplasmin, 24-hour urine copper, and slit lamp examination. The gene responsible for Wilson's disease (ATP7B) has been localized to human chromosome 13 and codes for an abnormal P-type adenosine triphosphatase. This is a membrane copper transport protein that normally transports hepatocellular copper into bile. The defect allows copper to build up in the hepatocytes. More than 60 mutations have been identified. Genetic testing using polymorphic DNA markers is helpful for testing presymptomatic siblings and recommended before treatment is initiated.

**15. A young person complaining of arthritis has been referred to you by an ophthalmologist who identified Kayser-Fleischer rings. What might you find on the musculoskeletal examination?**

Pain and swelling of the MCPs, wrists, elbows, shoulders, knees, and hips resembling hemochromatosis may occur, although asymptomatic radiographic changes are equally as common.

**16. Suspecting the diagnosis of Wilson's disease, you order radiographs of the involved joints. What are the radiographs likely to reveal?**

Subchondral and cortical fragmentation, as well as marginal, subchondral, and central bony sclerosis of the wrist, hand, elbow, shoulder, and knee, help to distinguish this arthropathy from primary osteoarthritis. Unlike hemochromatosis, involvement of the hip and MCP joints is uncommon. Less common radiographic findings include osteochondritis dissecans, chondrocalcinosis, chondramalacia patellae, and vertebral wedging. Generalized osteoporosis or osteomalacia may be present as a result of Fanconi's syndrome or renal tubular acidosis, both of which are common in Wilson's disease.

**17. How would you treat a patient with Wilson's disease?**

Life-long penicillamine chelation therapy is the preferred choice because it can prevent or improve virtually every manifestation of the disease. Side effects are common (30%). Other treatment options include trientine, zinc, and ammonium tetrathiomolybdate. Foods rich in copper such as organ meats, nuts, chocolate, and mushrooms need to be avoided. With early, effective chelation, most patients can live normal, healthy lives. Patients presenting with fulminant hepatic failure do not respond well to chelation and require urgent transplantation. This manifestation is more common than previously appreciated and accounts for a significant proportion of liver transplants each year.

**18. What is the biochemical defect underlying alkaptonuria (ochronosis)?**

Alkaptonuria is a disorder of tyrosine catabolism caused by a deficiency of homogentisic acid oxidase, leading to excretion of large amounts of homogentisic acid in urine and accumulation of oxidized homogentisic acid pigment in connective tissues (ochronosis). The tendency of the patient's urine to darken upon standing as a result of excessive homogentisic acid is characteristic.

**19. List five locations where ochronotic pigment may deposit.**

Foci of gray-brown ochronotic pigment can be found in the skin, sclera, arterial walls, prostate, and ear (concha, antihelix, and cerumen). These deposits can lead to aortic stenosis, conduction hearing loss, and prostatic calculi. Deposition in articular cartilage and intervertebral discs eventually leads to ochronotic arthropathy. Pigmented cartilage fragments are the nidus for chondral calcification and osteochondral loose bodies in the joints.

**20. Discuss the clinical features of ochronotic arthropathy.**

Ochronosis typically presents between ages 20 and 30 as a chronic progressive spondylosis with decreased range of motion of the lumbosacral spine. The posture of such a patient can be similar to that of a patient with ankylosis spondylitis (AS)—forward stoop, loss of lumbar lordosis, loss of height, flexed hips and knees, and wide-based stance—but patients lack the typical radiographic features of AS such as annular ossification or sacroiliac joint fusion. Ochronotic pigment deposition in the nucleus pulposus predisposes to herniation of the intervertebral disc, which can present as acute-onset low-back pain clinically indistinguishable from typical cases of herniated disc disease without alkaptonuria. A degenerative arthritis of the peripheral joints occurs less frequently than the spinal disease. Peripheral joints most commonly affected are the knees, shoulders, and hips. Pain, stiffness, and limited range of motion are the most common features, similar to hemochromatotic arthropathy. However, ochronosis spares the small joints of the hands, wrists, and feet.

**21. What are the characteristic findings on spinal radiographs in ochronosis?**

Lumbosacral radiographs show premature degenerative changes, dense calcifications of the intervertebral discs, and narrowing of the intervertebral spaces. Prominent intervertebral disc calcification can also be seen in hemochromatosis, hyperparathyroidism, calcium pyrophosphate deposition disease, paralytic poliomyelitis, and amyloidosis. The radiographic appearance of the large peripheral joints in ochronotic arthritis is virtually indistinguishable from that of primary osteoarthritis.

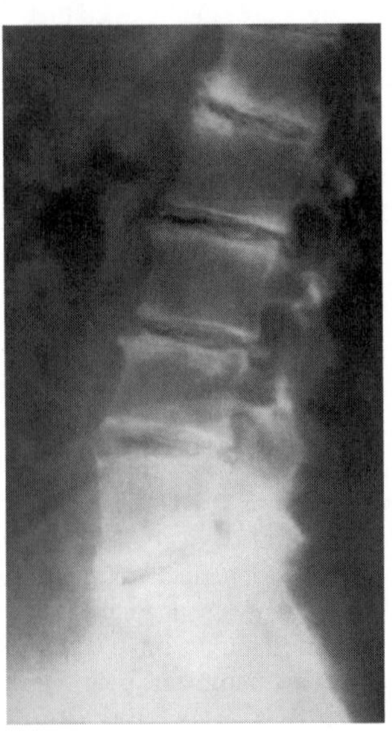

Lateral radiograph of the spine in a patient with ochronosis. Note the vertebral disc space calcification at multiple levels.

**22. Is there a beneficial treatment for patients with ochronosis?**

Numerous therapies, such as ascorbic acid, and diets low in protein, phenylalanine, and tyrosine have been studied, but to date no therapy has been proved to be beneficial. Symptomatic measures are most practical.

## BIBLIOGRAPHY

1. Bacon BR, Britton RS: Hereditary hemochromatosis. In Sleisenger & Fordtran's Gastrointestinal and Liver Disease, 6th ed. Philadelphia, WB Saunders, 1998, pp 1097–1103.
2. Gordon DA: Deposition and storage diseases. In Schumacher HR (ed): Primer on the Rheumatic Diseases, 11th ed. Atlanta, Arthritis Foundation, 1997, pp 328–333.
3. Hamdi N, Cooke TD, Hassan B: Ochronotic arthropathy. Internal Orthopaedics 23:122–125, 1999.
4. Lambert RE: Iron storage disease. In Ruddy S, Harris ED, Sledge CB (eds): Kelley's Textbook of Rheumatology, 6th ed. Philadelphia, WB Saunders, 2001, pp 1559–1566.
5. Niederau C, Fischer R, Sonnenberg A, Stremmel W, et al: Survival and causes of death in cirrhotic and noncirrhotic patients with primary hemochromatosis. N Engl J Med 313:1256–1262, 1985.

6. Powell LW, Isselbacher KJ: Hemochromatosis. In Wilson JD, et al (eds): Harrison's Principles of Internal Medicine, 14th ed. New York, McGraw-Hill, 1998, pp 2149–2152.
7. Powell LW, Yapp TR: Hemochromatosis. Clinics in Liver Disease 4:211–228, 2000.
8. Resnick D, Yu JS, Sartoris D: Wilson's disease. In Kelly WN, Harris ED, Ruddy S, Sledge CB (eds): Textbook of Rheumatology, 5th ed. Philadelphia, WB Saunders, 1997, pp 676–677.
9. Scheinberg IH: Wilson's disease. In Wilson JD, et al (eds): Harrison's Principles of Internal Medicine, 14th ed. New York, McGraw-Hill, 1998, pp 2166–2168.
10. Sternlieb I: Wilson's disease. Clinics in Liver Disease 4:229–239, 2000.

# 62. RHEUMATOLOGIC MANIFESTATIONS OF THE PRIMARY IMMUNODEFICIENCY SYNDROMES

*Mark Malyak*, M.D.

**1. Why are primary immunodeficiency syndromes of concern in rheumatology?**

Primary immunodeficiency syndromes may be associated with a variety of problems in addition to an increased risk of infection, including autoimmune manifestations, allergy, and increased risk of lymphoid and epithelial neoplasms. Autoimmunity may manifest as a recognized autoimmune disease, such as systemic lupus erythematosus in congenital deficiency of C4. Alternatively, various autoantibodies may be present in the absence of clinically expressed autoimmune disease, such as rheumatoid factor (anti-IgG antibodies) or anti-nuclear antibodies (ANA) in selective IgA deficiency.

**2. Which components of the immune system are involved in the primary immunodeficiency syndromes?**

- B cells (humoral immunodeficiency)
- T cells (cell-mediated immunodeficiency)
- Natural killer (NK) cells
- Phagocytes
- Complement proteins

The individual primary immunodeficiency syndromes may be due to dysfunction of a single component of the immune system, such as C4 deficiency, or dysfunction of multiple components, such as impairment of B-cell, T-cell, and phagocyte function in certain severe combined immunodeficiencies.

**3. The types of recurrent infection in a particular patient offer a clue to the underlying primary immunodeficiency syndrome. Which microorganisms are responsible for recurrent infection in B-cell immunodeficiency syndromes?**

B-cell immunodeficiency, such as X-linked (Bruton's) agammaglobulinemia, results in inadequate immunoglobulin production, leading to recurrent infection with extracellular, encapsulated, pyogenic bacteria, particularly *Streptococcus pneumoniae* and *Haemophilus influenzae*. These organisms typically cause acute and chronic infections of the upper and lower respiratory tracts, meningitis, and bacteremia.

**4. Which organisms are responsible for infections in primary T-cell immunodeficiency, such as thymic hypoplasia (DiGeorge syndrome)?**

- Viruses (e.g., herpesviruses)
- Intracellular bacteria (e.g., mycobacteria)

• Fungi (e.g., *Candida* species)
• Other (*Pneumocystis carinii*)

Primary T-cell immunodeficiency results in inadequate cell-mediated immunity, leading to infections similar to those encountered in patients with HIV infection, the prototypic acquired T-cell immunodeficiency state.

**5. What laboratory tests are performed to evaluate the integrity of the humoral immune system (B-cell function)?**

*Laboratory Evaluation of B-cell Function*

| CATEGORY | SPECIFIC TESTS | COMMENTS |
|---|---|---|
| In vivo functional tests (routine screening tests) | Isohemagglutinin titers (anti-blood group A and B) | Naturally occurring; predominantly IgM |
| | Diphtheria and tetanus booster immunization | Serum antibodies assayed prior to and 2 weeks later; assesses capacity to synthesize IgG antibodies against protein antigens |
| | Pneumococcal immunization | Serum antibodies assayed prior to and 3 weeks later; assesses capacity to synthesize antibodies against polysaccharide antigens |
| Immunoglobulin quantitation | IgM, IgG, IgA levels | Various immunoassays may be used; readily available |
| | IgG subclass, IgE levels | ELISA and RIA available (expensive) |
| In vitro tests (expensive) | Peripheral blood B-cell quantitation | Anti-Ig antibodies and specific monoclonal antibody may be used |
| | Bone marrow pre-B-cell quantitation | Measures surface Ig-negative, cytoplasmic μ-chain–positive cells |
| | In vitro immunoglobulin synthesis | Peripheral blood mononuclear cells stimulated in vitro with pokeweed mitogen |

ELISA = enzyme-linked immunosorbent assay; RIA = radioimmunoassay.

A reasonable screening evaluation of B-cell function is to determine the serum IgA level and perform the inexpensive in vivo functional tests. If all these tests are normal, clinically significant B-cell dysfunction may be excluded. If any of these tests is abnormal, quantitation of IgG and IgM levels, and possibly in vitro testing, will be necessary to determine the cause of the underlying primary immunodeficiency syndrome.

**6. What laboratory tests can be used to evaluate the integrity of the cellular immune system (T-cell function)?**

*Laboratory Evaluation of T-Cell Function*

| CATEGORY | SPECIFIC TESTS | COMMENTS |
|---|---|---|
| In vivo functional tests (skin testing for delayed-type hypersensitivity) (routine screening tests) | Candida skin test | Examine degree of induration 48–72 hr later |
| | PPD, *Trichophyton*, mumps, tetanus/diphtheria toxoid, keyhole-limpet hemocyanin | If *Candida* skin test is negative, testing with at least 4 of these antigens must be performed to determine if cell-mediated immunity is inadequate |
| Absolute lymphocyte count (routine screening test) | Determine from total WBC count and % lymphocytes | Severe cell-mediated immunity disorder unlikely in setting of normal lymphocyte count |

(*Table continued on next page.*)

*Laboratory Evaluation of T-Cell Function (cont.)*

| CATEGORY | SPECIFIC TESTS | COMMENTS |
|---|---|---|
| In vitro tests (expensive) | Quantitation of:<br>Total T cells<br>CD4+ cells<br>CD8+ cells<br>NK cells | Specific monoclonal antibody may be used |
| | Lymphocyte blastic transformation | Assessment of radiolabeled thymidine uptake following stimulation with lectins (such as PHA), specific antigen (such as *Candida*), or one-way mixed lymphocyte reaction |
| | Quantitate ability of T cells to synthesize IL-2 and IL-2 receptors | These and lymphocyte blastic transformation assay are indicators of successful T-cell activation. |

PPD = purified protein derivative (for tuberculosis); WBC = white blood cell; PHA = phytohemagglutinin; IL = interleukin.

A reasonable screening evaluation of T-cell function is to determine the absolute lymphocyte count and perform a *Candida* skin test. If these are both normal, clinically significant T-cell dysfunction may be excluded. If the *Candida* skin test is negative, negative delayed-type skin testing with at least four other antigens is necessary to demonstrate that T-cell function is inadequate. If these screening tests are abnormal, more sophisticated in vitro tests may be necessary to define the underlying primary immunodeficiency disorder. HIV testing should be performed as part of the screening evaluation to exclude this acquired T-cell disorder.

**7. Which organisms are responsible for septic arthritis in patients with hypogammaglobulinemia due to primary B-cell immunodeficiency?**

Selective IgA deficiency, X-linked (Bruton's) agammaglobulinemia, common variable immuno-deficiency, and immunoglobulin deficiency with increased IgM (hyper-IgM) account for > 99% of the primary hypogammaglobulinemic states (B-cell immunodeficiency). These patients are susceptible to septic arthritis owing to the usual organisms encountered in B-cell immunodeficiency states: *Streptococcus pneumoniae*, *Haemophilus influenzae*, and *Staphylococcus aureus*. In addition to these typical infectious agents, patients are also susceptible to joint infections with *Ureaplasma urealyticum* and other *Mycoplasma* organisms. The incidence of septic arthritis in these B-cell disorders is unknown but is less than that for the more frequently encountered infections of the upper and lower respiratory tract and gastrointestinal tract.

**8. Which primary immunodeficiency syndromes are most commonly associated with autoimmune phenomena?**

Selective IgA deficiency, common variable immunodeficiency, X-linked agammaglobulinemia, and hyper-IgM syndrome are the B-cell immunodeficiency syndromes commonly associated with autoimmune phenomena. Complete absence of certain complement components (C2, C4) is also associated with autoimmune phenomena, particularly systemic lupus erythematosus (SLE). Finally, chronic granulomatous disease, a primary disorder of neutrophils, is associated with the presence of ANA and, less commonly, SLE. For the most part, patients with predominantly T-cell immunodeficiency do not manifest autoimmune phenomena, owing at least in part to the fact that many of these patients do not survive infancy.

**9. What are the rheumatologic manifestations of X-linked agammaglobulinemia?**

*Rheumatologic Manifestations of X-linked Agammaglobulinemia*

| | |
|---|---|
| Septic arthritis<br>Extracellular, encapsulated bacteria (*S. pneumoniae*, *H. influenzae*, *S. aureus*)<br>*Mycoplasma*, particularly *Ureaplasma urealyticum*<br>Enteroviruses, particularly echovirus and coxsackievirus | Occurs in 20% of cases |
| Aseptic, possibly autoimmune, arthritis | Usually mono- or oligoarticular; involves large joints; rarely destructive; RF and ANA absent |
| Dermatomyositis-like syndrome associated with progressive enterovirus CNS infection | Presents with rash and muscle weakness |

X-linked (Bruton's) agammaglobulinemia is a rare disorder characterized by absent or near-absent levels of serum IgG, IgM, and IgA and by abnormal in vivo B-cell functional tests. Less severe forms of this disease have been identified. Cell-mediated immunity is intact. The molecular defect is mutation within the Bruton's tyrosine kinase gene, resulting in abnormal function of this signal transduction protein, which is normally present within B cells at all stages of development. This results in the characteristic cellular abnormalities: failure of maturation of the B-cell line and absence of B cells. Arthritis occurs in approximately 20% of patients, with half of these cases due to infection with the typical pyogenic bacteria. In addition, patients appear vulnerable to infections with enterovirus and *Mycoplasma*.

There are cases of arthritis in X-linked agammaglobulinemia in which an infectious agent cannot be detected despite rigorous evaluation. These cases may represent infection due to a fastidious organism that cannot be identified or may represent a true autoimmune disorder, such as juvenile rheumatoid arthritis. Overall, autoimmune phenomena occur much less frequently in X-linked agammaglobulinemia than in selective IgA deficiency or common variable immunodeficiency.

**10. What are the various rheumatologic manifestations of selective IgA deficiency?**

- Autoantibodies, particularly RF and ANA, in the absence of clinically expressed autoimmune disease
- Systemic autoimmune disorders (SLE, aseptic arthritis, etc.) occur in 7–36% of patients
- Organ-specific autoimmune disorders (diabetes mellitus type I, myasthenia gravis, etc.)

IgA deficiency is the most common primary immunodeficiency syndrome, with a prevalence of 1/700 in the general population. It is characterized by absent or near-absent levels of serum and secretory IgA, accompanied by normal levels of serum IgG and IgM. Cell-mediated immunity is intact. Patients may be asymptomatic, have recurrent respiratory and gastrointestinal tract infections, or manifest autoimmune phenomena. In most cases, IgA deficiency is likely a genetic disorder that is present at birth and remains persistent, but molecular defects have not yet been identified. Some cases may be acquired later in life, often associated with drug therapy (gold, D-penicillamine, sulfasalazine) or viral infection, and are often transient.

**11. List the autoantibodies seen in patients with selective IgA deficiency without clinically expressed autoimmune disease.**

The presence of autoantibodies in the absence of clinically expressed autoimmune disease commonly occurs in IgA deficiency. RF and ANA are most consistently observed. Other autoantibodies that may be present include antibodies against double-stranded and single-stranded DNA, cardiolipin, thyroglobulin, thyroid microsomes, smooth muscle, gastric parietal cell, striated muscle, acetylcholine receptor, and bile canaliculi. Autoantibodies against IgA occur in up to 44% of patients.

**12. What systemic and organ-specific autoimmune diseases are associated with selective IgA deficiency?**

| SYSTEMIC | ORGAN-SPECIFIC |
|---|---|
| Systemic lupus erythematosus* | Diabetes mellitus type I* |
| Juvenile rheumatoid arthritis* | Myasthenia gravis* |
| Rheumatoid arthritis* | Inflammatory bowel disease |
| Sjögren's syndrome | Autoimmune hepatitis |
| Scleroderma | Pernicious anemia |
| Dermatomyositis | Primary adrenal insufficiency |
| Vasculitic syndromes | |

* Most likely associations. Other conditions have been noted in case reports, but their true association with IgA deficiency remains to be proved.

**13. Describe the rheumatologic manifestations of common variable immunodeficiency (CVID).**

*Rheumatologic Manifestations of Common Variable Immunodeficiency*

Septic arthritis
- Extracellular, encapsulated bacteria (*S. pneumoniae*, *H. influenzae*, *S. aureus*)
- *Mycoplasma*, particularly *Ureaplasma urealyticum*

Aseptic, possibly autoimmune, arthritis

Organ-specific autoimmune disorders (pernicious anemia, autoimmune hemolytic anemia, idiopathic thrombocytopenic purpura)—occur in 20% of patients

CVID is an heterogeneous group of disorders characterized by IgG, IgM, and IgA hypogammaglobulinemia, often resulting in the very low levels seen in X-linked agammaglobulinemia. Features distinguishing CVID from X-linked agammaglobulinemia include equal sex distribution, onset of symptoms later in life, and presence of circulating B cells. Although the underlying immunologic defect is heterogeneous, most patients manifest a primary B-cell defect resulting in failure to maturate into Ig-secreting plasma cells. Like selective IgA deficiency, CVID is likely a genetic disorder in most cases, although some cases may be truly acquired and secondary to a viral infection or an adverse drug effect (i.e., cytotoxic therapy).

Septic arthritis due to *Staphylococcus aureus*, the usual extracellular encapsulated bacteria, and *Mycoplasma* species occurs with increased frequency in CVID. Because cell-mediated immunodeficiency sometimes occurs in CVID, fungi and mycobacteria must also be considered as potential pathogens.

The presence of autoantibodies in the absence of clinically expressed autoimmune disease appears less often than in selective IgA deficiency. Regardless, autoimmune disorders are not unusual in CVID. Polyarthritis in which an infectious agent cannot be detected despite rigorous evaluation has been described. Characteristics include involvement of the large and medium-sized joints with sparing of the small joints of the hands and feet. Rheumatoid nodules, erosions, and significant articular cartilage destruction are not features of this syndrome. This form of arthropathy often responds to treatment with intravenous gammaglobulin.

**14. What is the hyper-IgM syndrome?**

The hyper-IgM immunodeficiency syndrome is characterized by extremely low levels of IgG, IgA, and IgE and either a normal or markedly elevated concentration of polyclonal IgM. Patients develop both recurrent pyogenic infections and *P. carinii* pneumonia. There is also an increased frequency of autoimmune disorders and malignancy. The defect causing this x-linked syndrome is an abnormal gene resulting in a defective CD40 ligand (CD 154) on the surface of activated CD4+ T cells. This mutation results in failure of T cells to interact with CD40 on B cells. This lack of B cell signaling by T cells results in the B cell failing to undergo isotype switching and produce only IgM.

**15. What mechanisms may explain the presence of aseptic arthritis and other autoimmune phenomena in the primary immunodeficiency syndromes?**

The mechanisms responsible for autoimmune phenomena in the primary immunodeficiency syndromes remain unknown. The following possibilities exist:

1. Aseptic arthritis in the primary B-cell immunodeficiency states may be due to infection with a fastidious organism that cannot be identified by available methods.
2. Absence of secretory IgA in the primary B-cell immunodeficiency syndromes may lead to:
   - Excessive absorption of antigen from the gut, leading to the formation of immune complexes (in disorders other than X-linked agammaglobulinemia) and subsequent immune complex disease. Additionally, immune complexes may lead to the formation of rheumatoid factor.
   - Excessive absorption of superantigen from the gut, which may lead to activation of T cells containing particular $V_\beta$ families on their T-cell receptors. If one of these clones also reacts against self-antigen, an autoimmune state may result.
   - Excessive absorption of a particular antigen from the gut, leading to autoimmunity as a result of molecular mimicry.
3. Coexistence of primary immunodeficiency and autoimmunity may be coincidental rather than causal. Common HLA extended haplotypes often present in selective IgA deficiency and common variable immunodeficiency are also commonly present in autoimmune disorders such as SLE, diabetes mellitus type I, and myasthenia gravis. In fact, the prevalence of IgA deficiency in patients with SLE ranges from 1–5%, which is 10–20 times higher than the general population.

**16. Discuss the therapy for X-linked agammaglobulinemia, common variable immunodeficiency (CVID), and selective IgA deficiency.**

**X-linked agammaglobulinemia**: Intravenous immunoglobulin (IVIG) and aggressive treatment of bacterial infections with appropriate antibiotics are the recommended therapy. IVIG is usually administered in a dose of 200–600 mg/kg every month.

**CVID**: IVIG is also recommended for patients with CVID who have low IgG levels and recurrent infections. Occasionally, patients with CVID have complete absence of IgA, along with anti-IgA antibodies, placing them at risk for anaphylaxis with IVIG therapy.

**Selecive IgA deficiency**: The mainstay of therapy is rigorous treatment of active bacterial infections with antibiotics. IVIG should not be administered, since many patients have autoantibodies against IgA, including IgE anti-IgA, which may result in severe, occasionally fatal anaphylaxis. Patients should ideally receive blood products obtained from other patients with IgA deficiency.

**17. How do you screen for homozygous complement deficiency associated with a rheumatologic disorder?**

Homozygous deficiency of certain complement components is associated with a number of rheumatologic disorders. The **total hemolytic complement assay** ($CH_{50}$) assesses the integrity of the classic pathway of complement activation. Patient's sera is added to a standardized suspension of sheep red blood cells (RBC) coated with rabbit antibody. These "immune complexes" allow activation of the classic pathway, resulting in lysis of the sheep RBC. The $CH_{50}$ is the reciprocal of the serum dilution that lyses 50% of the sheep RBC. Because specific deficiencies that lead to rheumatologic manifestations are usually in the classical, rather that the alternative, pathway, $CH_{50}$ is the ideal, inexpensive screening test. Homozygous deficiency of a complement component in the classical pathway results in a $CH_{50}$ of 0; individual complement levels may then be determined by immunoassay. Complement component deficiencies of the classical pathway have an autosomal recessive pattern of inheritance.

**18. What are the rheumatologic manifestations of homozygous complement deficient states?**

Deficiencies of the early components of the classic pathway (C1, C4, C2) are associated with immune complex disease, particularly SLE. This may be due to inability to maintain circulating immune complexes in a soluble state and inability to remove circulating immune complexes. C2 deficiency is the most common deficiency.

Deficiencies of components of the membrane attack complex (C5–9) are associated with recurrent *Neisseria* infections, both *N. meningitidis* and *N. gonorrhoeae*. Patients with recurrent bouts of neisserial infection, particularly when systemic, should be evaluated for the presence of a complement deficiency.

## BIBLIOGRAPHY

1. Atkinson JP, Frank MM: Complement in disease: Inherited and acquired complement deficiencies. In Frank MM, Austen KF, Claman HN, Unanue ER (eds): Samter's Immunologic Diseases, 6th ed. Philadelphia, Lippincott Williams & Wilkins, 2001, pp 349–358.
2. Buckley RH: Primary immunodeficiencies of lymphocytes. In Frank MM, Austen KF, Claman HN, Unanue ER (eds): Samter's Immunologic Diseases, 6th ed. Philadelphia, Lippincott Williams & Wilkins, 2001, pp 317–328.
3. Itescu S: Adult immunodeficiency and rheumatic disease. Rheum Dis Clin North Amer 22:53–65, 1996.
4. Lee AH, Levinson AI, Schumacher HR Jr: Hypogammaglobulinemia and rheumatic disease. Semin Arthritis Rheum 22:252, 1993.
5. Liblau RS, Bach J-F: Selective IgA deficiency and autoimmunity. Int Arch Allergy Immunol 99:16, 1992.
6. Sneller MC: Common variable immunodeficiency. Am J Med Sci 321:42–48, 2001.

# 63. BONE AND JOINT DYSPLASIAS

*Edmund* H. *Hornstein*, D.O.

**1. What exactly is a bone or joint dysplasia?**

*Dysplasia* is a term literally meaning abnormal growth. Applied to the skeletal system, the term encompasses a group of conditions in which abnormalities of growth can affect the epiphysis, metaphysis, physis, or diaphysis of developing bone. These abnormalities may be devastatingly symptomatic or fatal, but they can also exist as mere radiologic curiosities. Broadly, these syndromes are grouped under the heading of **osteochondrodysplasias**. The vast majority of these syndromes are exceedingly rare and are not of practical importance in most clinical situations.

**2. Why should bone and joint dysplasias even be covered in a rheumatology text?**

- Dysplastic syndromes may present with musculoskeletal pain or dysfunction that mimics other rheumatologic disorders.
- Early recognition of some dysplasias may allow the initiation of therapy that can prevent or reduce later pain and disability.
- Many osteochondrodysplasias are inherited, and an accurate diagnosis may allow appropriate genetic counseling to be offered.

**3. How are the osteochondrodysplasias classified?**

By international consensus, these disorders are formally classified based on etiopathogenetic information concerning specific gene and/or protein deficits. It is useful and practical, however, to group these disorders by where the most prominent abnormalities in growth occur. The mnemonic **EMPD** (empty) can help to broadly group these syndromes.

**E** — **E**piphyseal dysplasias: The epiphysis is at the end of tubular bone and is formed as a secondary site of ossification. Normal development of the epiphysis is required if the joint surface is to be normal.

**M** — **M**etaphyseal dysplasias: The metaphysis is the wider part of a tubular bone between the diaphysis and physis.

**P** — **P**hyseal dysplasias: The physis, or epiphyseal cartilage plate, separates the metaphysis from the epiphysis during growth. It is the primary site responsible for elongation of tubular bones.

**D** — **D**iaphyseal dysplasia: The diaphysis is the shaft of a long or tubular bone. It is composed of the spongiosa and cortex and is covered with periosteum.

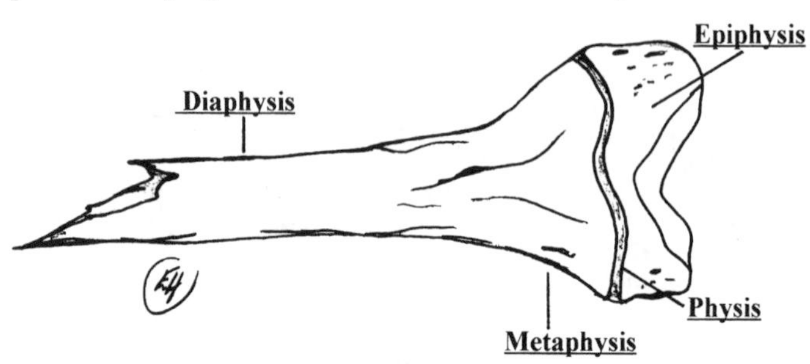


**4. What are the distinguishing features of the epiphyseal dysplasias?**

Epiphyseal dysplasia is characterized by abnormal ossification of the developing epiphysis. The resulting morphologic abnormalities of the ossification centers are used to differentiate the various subtypes within this category. The most important epiphyseal dysplasias from a rheumatologic standpoint are multiple epiphyseal dysplasia and spondyloepiphyseal dysplasia.

**5. How does a patient with multiple epiphyseal dysplasia present clinically?**

Usually, the patient complains of symmetric joint pain in the hips, knees, wrists, and ankles. These complaints are commonly accompanied by back pain. Limitation in range of motion of affected joints is frequent. Radiographs reveal irregular, flattened, small epiphyseal ossification centers during childhood and a deformed articular surface after physeal closure. The long bones of the legs and arms are most prominently affected. Vertebrae are often flattened (platyspondyly) with irregular appearing endplates. Adult stature is generally diminished and is proportionate to the severity of involvement. Disabling early degenerative arthritis is a common end result. Symptoms usually occur before adolescence but may not become apparent until early adulthood, depending on the severity of epiphyseal deformity.

**6. What other conditions can be confused with multiple epiphyseal dysplasia?**

**Inflammatory arthritis**: The pain and symmetry of involvement are sometimes mistaken for inflammatory arthritis. On closer evaluation, the absence of signs and symptoms of inflammation usually suffices to rule out this condition.

**Hypothyroidism**: Occult hypothyroidism can lead to developmental skeletal abnormalities that may closely resemble some of the hereditary epiphyseal dysplasias. Thyroid function should always be checked when a diagnosis of epiphyseal dysplasia is being considered.

**Juvenile osteochondrosis**: These disorders, including Legg-Calvé-Perthes disease, may have a radiographic appearance similar to epiphyseal dysplasia but are usually limited to a single joint.

**7. Describe the radiographic abnormalities typical for spondyloepiphyseal dysplasia.**

The spondyloepiphyseal dysplasias are a diverse group of disorders linked by the radiographic findings of marked **platyspondyly** (short flat vertebrae) in association with abnormalities of **epiphyseal ossification**. Spinal abnormalities are prominent, and impaired spinal growth often leads to the diagnosis.

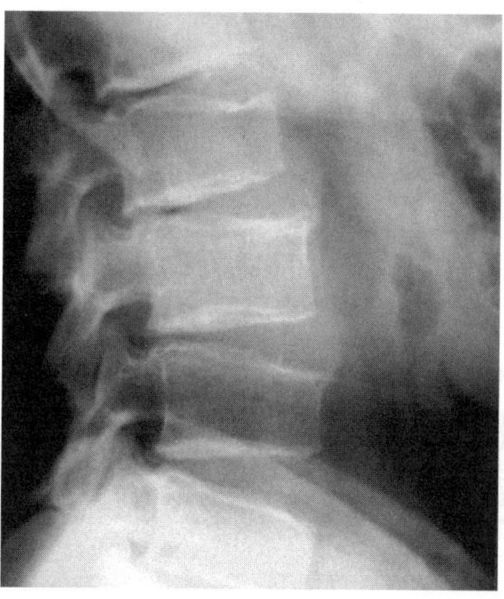

**8. Spondyloepiphyseal dysplasia tarda and spondyloepiphyseal dysplasia tarda with progressive arthropathy can sometimes be confused with juvenile rheumatoid arthritis. Why?**

Both of these X-linked recessive disorders are accompanied by enlargement of the ends of the tubular bones in the hands, which may be mistaken for JRA on visual inspection. Radiographic evaluation inevitably leads to the correct diagnosis.

**9. What abnormality characterizes the metaphyseal dysplasias?**

These dysplasias are characterized by a failure either to form or to absorb the spongiosa of developing bone. Important disorders from a rheumatologic standpoint within this category of dysplasias include the hypophosphatasias and craniometaphyseal dysplasias.

**10. What is the primary differential diagnosis in the hypophosphatasias?**

The hypophosphatasias may look like **rickets** in children and **osteomalacia** in adults. Subtle radiographic findings may allow the distinction to be made, but the diagnosis of hypophosphatasia is ultimately based on the findings of an exceptionally low serum alkaline phosphatase in conjunction with high urine and serum phosphorylethanolamine levels. Consideration of hypophosphatasia is warranted in any case of suspected rickets or osteomalacia.

**11. List the clinical findings that link the various forms of craniometaphyseal dysplasias.**

Joint pain, muscle weakness, scoliosis, pathologic fractures, genu valga, and Erlenmeyer-flask deformity of long bones. Cranial abnormalities include supraorbital bossing, a broad flat nose, hypertelorism, dental malocclusion, and a sclerotic thickened skull.

**12. One of the most common of the osteochondrodysplasias is considered a physeal dysplasia and leads to dwarfism. Name this syndrome.**

Achondroplasia. This physeal dysplasia is transmitted as an autosomal dominant trait, though spontaneous mutation is probably responsible for most cases. It is considered a disproportionate dwarfism with rhizomelic (shorter proximal compared with distal) short limbs, macrocephaly with prominent frontal bossing, and some midface hypoplasia. An exaggerated lumbar lordosis is usually seen as well as flexion contractures at the elbows and hips. Intelligence is normal. Mean adult height is approximately 52 inches in men and 49 inches in women. Rheumatologic complaints may stem from a narrowed spinal canal and symptoms of spinal stenosis or from ligamentous laxity of the knees, leading to complaints of pain and premature degenerative disease.

**13. Where is the abnormality of bone formation found in the diaphyseal dysplasias?**

Diaphyseal dysplasias result from abnormal formation of endosteal or periosteal bone. These dysplasias can be subclassified as hyperplasias or hypoplasias. Osteogenesis imperfecta is considered a hypoplastic diaphyseal dysplasia (see Chapter 59).

**14. A 21-year-old man complains of lower leg pain and swelling that has been gradually increasing. An x-ray is obtained and appears below. What is this disorder?**

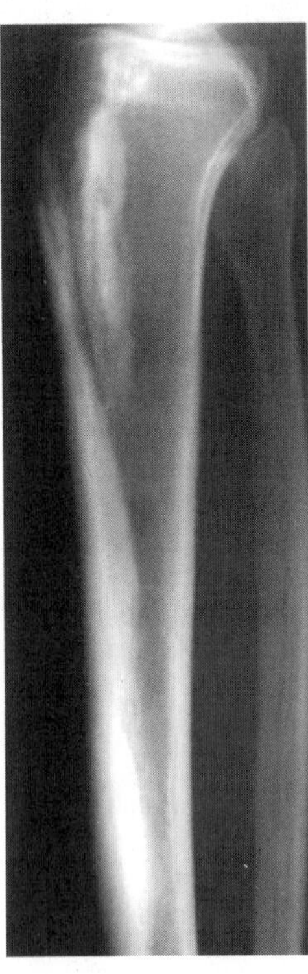

Melorheostosis, a nonhereditary idiopathic diaphyseal hyperplasia. Clinically, the patient complains of joint pain with onset usually in late childhood or early adulthood. Decreased range of motion, joint contracture or ankylosis, growth disturbances, foot deformities, and dystrophic skin, muscle, and soft tissue changes overlying affected bone are other features of this unusual disorder. The x-ray is characteristic and reveals dense, wavy, periosteal bony excrescences that have been described as resembling wax flowing down the side of a candle.

**15. Another diaphyseal hyperplasia has radiographic and clinical features in common with hypertrophic pulmonary osteoarthropathy, including clubbing of the digits, painful swollen joints, and periosteal bony apposition, but it is also associated with thickened, wrinkled elephant-like skin. Name this disorder.**

**Pachydermoperiostosis.** A literal translation of the term describes the major clinical manifestations of the disorder.

**16. A 15-year-old boy is seen complaining of thoracic back pain with no clear history of trauma. The pain is worse with activity, improves with rest, and is not associated with significant morning stiffness. Physical exam is remarkable only for a hint of increased thoracic kyphosis with some lower thoracic tenderness to palpation in the midline and mild paravertebral muscle spasm. Workup reveals a normal ESR, serum chemistries, and CBC. An x-ray report lists that the findings are most consistent with Scheuermann's disease. What the heck is that?**

Radiograph of the spine showing irregular vertebral endplates in a patient with Scheuermann's disease.

**Vertebral osteochondritis**, or Scheuermann's disease, is a developmental abnormality of ossification of the endplates of vertebrae seen most often in the thoracic spine but also seen in the thoracolumbar and lumbar regions. It occurs during adolescence and is symptomatic in up to 60% of those affected, though it may also be found by chance on plain spine or chest x-rays requested for other reasons. The x-ray shows anterior wedging of multiple vertebrae with Schmorl's nodes and irregular vertebral endplates. Though the pathogenesis is uncertain, a hereditary weakening of the vertebral endplates present in affected patients is believed to allow disc material to encroach into the vertebral bodies. This then leads to abnormal growth and the x-ray changes described. Therapy is usually symptomatic and aimed at minimizing the tendency toward kyphosis. Occasionally, surgical intervention is required.

**17. A newborn girl has a reproducible "click" as you flex and abduct her right hip (Ortolani's sign). You suspect that the child may have congenital dislocation of the hip. How can you verify this suspicion? What do you tell the parents?**

Congenital hip dislocation or dysplasia is screened for shortly after birth using physical exam maneuvers such as Ortolani's sign and by inducing dislocation and reduction of an unstable hip (Barlow's sign). Plain films may not be easily interpretable in the first weeks of life, and modalities such as ultrasound, CT, or MRI generally offer better sensitivity. Congenital hip dysplasia has an excellent prognosis if recognized soon after birth. Treatment usually involves splinting the legs in abduction, thus allowing the shallow acetabulum to fully contain the femoral head. If the diagnosis is missed, however, later therapy is often much more involved and may require extensive orthopedic surgery. Untreated, this condition leads to premature osteoarthritis and may require early total hip replacement.

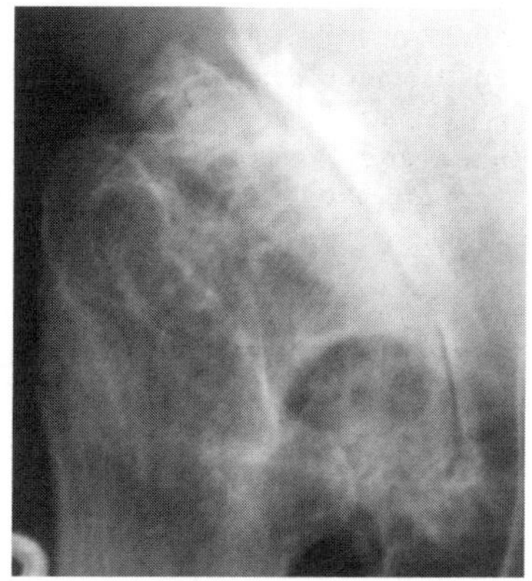

Hip radiograph from an adult with congenital hip dysplasia that was not treated during childhood. Note severe degenerative changes, shallow acetabulum, and malformed femoral head.

## BIBLIOGRAPHY

1. Altman RD, Tenenbaum J: Hypertrophic osteoarthropathy. In Harris ED, Ruddy S, Sledge CB (eds): Kelley's Textbook of Rheumatology, 6th ed. Philadelphia, WB Saunders, 2001, pp 1589–1594.
2. Borenstein DG, Wiesel SW: Vertebral osteochondritis. In Borenstein DG, Wiesel SW, Boden SD (eds): Low Back Pain: Medical Diagnosis and Comprehensive Management, 2nd ed. Philadelphia, WB Saunders, 1994, pp 281–284.
3. Clark RN: Congenital dysplasias and dwarfism. Pediatr Rev 12(5):149–159, 1990.
4. Greenspan A, Azouz EM: Bone dysplasia series. Melorheostosis: Review and update. Can Assoc Radiol J 50(5):324–330, 1999.
5. Kornblum M, Stanitsk DF: Spinal manifestations of skeletal dysplasias. Orthop Clin North Am 30(3):501–520, 1999.
6. Lachman RS: International nomenclature and classification of the osteochondrodysplasias (1997). Pediatric Radiology 28(10):737–744, 1998.
7. Lateur LM: Bone and joint dysplasias. In Klippel JH, Dieppe PA (eds): Rheumatology, 2nd ed. St. Louis, Mosby, 1998, Sect 8, Chapter 52, pp 52.1–52.8.
8. Lowe TG: Scheuermann disease. J Bone Joint Surg 72A:940–945, 1990.
9. Spranger J: The epiphyseal dysplasias. Clin Orthop 114:47–59, 1976.
10. Townsend DJ, Tolo VT: Congenital dislocation of the hip. Curr Opin Rheumatol 6:183–186, 1994.
11. Whyte MP, Gottesman GS, Eddy MC, McAllister WH: X-linked recessive spondyloepiphyseal dysplasia tarda. Medicine 78:9–25, 1999.

# XI. Nonarticular and Regional Musculoskeletal Disorders

*The lower back is at the crossroads where the psyche meets the soma.*
Voltaire
(1694–1778)

# 64. APPROACH TO THE PATIENT WITH NECK AND LOW BACK PAIN

Richard T. Meehan, M.D.

**1. Which rheumatic disorders commonly involve the neck?**

| DISORDER | FEATURE |
|---|---|
| Rheumatoid arthritis | C1–C2 (atlantoaxial) subluxation, cranial settling |
| Juvenile chronic arthritis | C2–C3 fusion, C1–C2 subluxation |
| Ankylosing spondylitis | Ankylosis, C5–C6 fracture |
| Diffuse idiopathic skeletal hyperostosis | Anterior longitudinal ligament ossification |
| Osteoarthritis | C5–C7 spondylosis |
| Polymyositis | Flexor muscle weakness |
| Polymyalgia rheumatica | Pain and stiffness |
| Fibromyalgia | C2, C5–C7 tender points |

**2. When assessing range of motion of the cervical spine, what does partial versus global loss signify?**

*Global* loss of range of motion is suggestive of *total* joint involvement, which is a feature of *inflammatory* rheumatic diseases (e.g., rheumatoid arthritis. spondyloarthropathies). In contrast, *mechanical* or *degenerative* disorders (e.g., osteoarthritis) will *partially* limit range to a few planes of movement. The same principle applies to the lumbar spine.

**3. When evaluating a patient with neck pain, how can you differentiate between a bony or muscular disorder?**

Comparison of *active* and *passive* range of motion is useful for differentiating articular from soft-tissue disorders. *Passive* neck range of motion is best performed by supporting (cradling) the head while the patient is supine. Full range of the cervical spine may then be tested: flexion, extension, rotation, and lateral bending. During rotation and lateral bending, *ipsilateral* discomfort elicited in the direction of movement is suggestive of *bony* pain. Pain and/or tightness produced on the *contralateral* side usually implicates a muscular disorder. Finally, palpable tenderness of the spinous processes may indicate *bony* pathology whereas local tenderness of paraspinous muscles usually indicates myofascial pain.

**Passive range of motion should *not* be performed if instability of the cervical spine is suspected!**

**4. What is Spurling's maneuver?**

Spurling's maneuver is a test for nerve root compression within the foramina of the cervical vertebrae. With the patient seated, downward pressure is uniformly applied to the patient's cranium while the head is gently rotated or flexed toward the side of the suspected lesion. The immediate development of pain and/or paresthesias with radiation to the upper limb (see below) is indicative of cervical radiculopathy.

**Spurling's maneuver should *not* be performed if cervical spine instability or fracture is suspected.**

**5. What physical findings enable you to identify the *approximate* level of common, cervical nerve root lesions?**

| NERVE | SENSORY LOSS | *MOTOR WEAKNESS | REFLEX |
|---|---|---|---|
| C5 (5%) | Lateral arm | Deltoid, biceps | Biceps |
| C6 (35%) | Lateral forearm, thumb, index finger | Wrist extensors, biceps | Radial# |
| C7 (35%) | Middle finger | Wrist flexors, finger extensors, Triceps | Triceps |
| C8 (25%) | Medial forearm, ring finger, Little finger | Finger flexors, thumb extensor | None |
| T1 (rare) | Medial arm | Finger abductors | None |

* Weakness of upper extremity muscles is often difficult to assess since innervations usually occur by two or more nerve roots.
# Radial reflex is also called the supinator jerk (tap on distal end of radius).

**6. What is Lhermitte's sign?**

Lhermitte's sign is the reported sensation of an electric-like shock propagating down the spine as a result of brisk neck flexion. This maneuver may also induce limb paresthesias and weakness. Lhermitte's sign is observed is some patients with spinal cord compression but also in patients with multiple sclerosis.

**7. Compare and contrast cervical myelopathy with cervical radiculopathy.**

| FEATURE | MYELOPATHY | RADICULOPATHY |
|---|---|---|
| Etiology | Spinal cord compression | Nerve root compression |
| Neck pain | Variable | Variable |
| Cranial nerve | Occasional | Never |
| Sensory loss | Stocking-glove paresthesias/numbness (all limbs) | Light touch/pinprick (upper limb dermatome) |
| Weakness (early) | All limbs (diffuse) | Upper limb myotome |
| Weakness (late) | Spastic paraparesis, quadriparesis | Upper limb myotome |
| Deep tendon reflexes | Upper limbs (decreased) lower limbs (increased) | Upper limb (decreased) |
| Pathologic reflexes | *Babinski's* sign, *Hoffmann's* sign | None |
| *Lhermitte's sign* | Occasional | Never |
| Bladder disturbance | Urine retention, urine incontinence | None |
| Spinal automaticity | Jumping legs | None |

**8. What are the major categories of low back pain?**

- Mechanical: degenerative disk disease, non-specific low back pain/strain (with or without psychogenic component), pregnancy, discogenic, spondylolisthesis, facet arthritis, fractures, etc.

- Radicular: foraminal nerve root compression, spinal stenosis
- Inflammatory: ankylosing spondylitis
- Infiltrative: cancer, infectious (osteomyelitis, abscess, and discitis)
- Referred: intra-abdominal pathology, i.e., abdominal aneurysm, nephrolithiasis

**9. How may back pain be categorized on the basis of historical symptoms?**

| FEATURE | MECHANICAL | INFLAMMATORY | SOFT TISSUE | INFILTRATIVE |
|---|---|---|---|---|
| Location | Diffuse | Diffuse | Diffuse | Focal |
| Symmetry | Unilateral | Bilateral | Generalized | Mid-line |
| Onset | Variable | Subacute | Acute or subacute | Insidious |
| Likely precipitant | Trauma<br>Degeneration | ±HLA-B27<br>Infection | Poor sleep<br>Stress | Infection, cancer |
| Morning stiffness | 30 min | > 1 h | Variable | None |
| Activity response | ↑ symptoms | ↓ symptoms | Variable | Persistent symptoms |
| Rest response | ↓ symptoms | ↑ symptoms | Variable | Persistent symptoms |
| Nocturnal pain | Mild | Moderate | Moderate | Severe |
| Systemic disease | No | Yes | No | Possible |
| Clinical conditions | Degenerative disc disease | Ankylosing spondylitis | Fibromyalgia | Cancer, infection |

**10. List the important questions that should be asked when obtaining a history from a patient with low back pain.**

One can use the helpful mnemonic **P-Q-R-S-T** (the components of an electrocardiogram tracing) when approaching any patient with pain:

**P** **Provocative and palliative factors**: sitting (worse with discogenic), walking (worse with spinal stenosis-relieved with forward flexion), supine (unrelieved with cancer or infection), Valsalva maneuver (worse with intrathecal or radicular process), lumbar extension (worse with spinal stenosis and facet arthritis) vs. flexion (worse with lumbar strain or fibromyalgia). What is position of maximal comfort, and does this reduce or eliminate pain or radicular symptoms?

**Q** **Quality of pain**: burning/tingling, numb, sharp, or dull?

**R** **Radiation of pain**: into leg (radicular), saddle area with bowel/bladder dysfunction (cauda equina syndrome), bilateral buttock or thigh (spinal stenosis, or referred from intra-abdominal pathology)?

**S** **Severity of pain or systemic symptoms**: pain scale 1–10, fever, weight loss, change in bowel habits, etc.

**T** **Timing of pain**: date of onset, associated trauma and prior similar episodes?

**11. What are the potential pain generators of mechanical low back pain?**

There are sensory nerve fibers in the discs, vertebral end plates, facet joints, ligaments, fascia blood vessels, spinal nerve roots, and muscles surrounding the lumbar spinal column. Therefore, non-specific mechanical low back pain could originate from any one or combinations of these sites.

**12. What are the RED FLAG signs and symptoms that indicate that a patient's low back pain may be from a serious cause?**

Most low back pain is mechanical in nature and should slowly improve over 2–6 weeks. The following are symptoms or signs that suggest a more serious etiology of low back pain:

- Unrelenting pain unaffected by change in position and not improved by supine position with hips flexed suggests infection, cancer, or infiltrative lesions.

- Fever, chills, weight loss suggests infection or cancer
- Patient writhing in pain on exam table and unable to lie still due to pain, consider retroperitoneal pathology: aortic dissection, nephrolithiasis, pancreatitis, or a ruptured viscus unless drug seeking behavior or psychogenic factors present.
- Pain and morning stiffness > 30 minutes that is improved with exercise in a patient less than 40 years of age suggest inflammatory spondyloarthropathy.
- Bilateral radiation of pain, which is progressive, suggests cancer, central disk herniation, or spondyloarthropathy
- Abnormal neurological exam: sensory/motor deficit (foot drop), loss of rectal tone, urinary incontinence, saddle anesthesia, Babinski sign, or ankle clonus suggests nerve root compression, cancer, or central disk herniation.
- Trauma or sudden onset of pain in a patient with risk factors for osteoporosis.

**13. What is sciatica?**

The simplest definition of *sciatica* is back pain that *radiates* down one leg below the knee. The character of the pain is usually sharp, or burning. Occasionally, dermatome numbness and paresthesias of the lower limb are also reported. *Valsalva* maneuvers or flexion and extension of the lumbosacral spine may exacerbate these symptoms. Sciatica pain is suggestive of nerve root irritation and usually occurs as a consequence of nerve root impingement by structures either within the central canal (disc protrusion, facet or ligament flavum hypertrophy, synovial cyst, etc.) or upon exiting the neural foramen (disc protrusion, congenital narrowing, spondylolisthesis).

**14. What physical findings enable you to identify the approximate level of common, lumbar nerve root lesions?**

| NERVE | SENSORY LOSS | MOTOR WEAKNESS | REFLEX |
|---|---|---|---|
| L4 | Anterior leg, medial foot | Tibialis anterior (ankle dorsiflexion) | Patellar |
| L5 | Lateral leg, web of great toe | Extensor hallucis longus (great toe extension) | None |
| S1 | Posterior leg, lateral foot | Peroneus muscles (foot eversion) | Achilles |

95% of nerve root impingement due to herniated disc disease occurs at the L5 or S1 level

**15. What maneuvers on physical exam suggest nerve root irritation?**

The *femoral stretch test* is performed to evaluate the upper lumbar roots (L2–L4). With the patient prone, the examiner maximally flexes the knee while gently extending the hip. Anterior thigh (L2, L3) or medial leg (L4) pain is suggestive of a lumbar root lesion. In contrast, *straight-leg raising* evaluates the sciatic nerve roots (L4–S1) and is performed with the patient supine. The examiner passively raises the extended leg, by the foot to 70° of elevation. Dermatome pain radiating below the knee upon raising the leg between 30° and 70° of elevation is a positive test for nerve root irritation. A positive test is more convincing if passive ankle dorsiflexion reproduces the pain after the leg has been lowered to an angle that abolished the radicular pain. A crossed-straight leg test is even more specific but less sensitive for nerve root irritation. This test causes contralateral radiating pain when the unaffected leg is elevated.

**16. What is Schober's test?**

Schober's test measures mobility of the thoracolumbar spine during maximum active lumbar flexion. Two midline marks are drawn originating from dimples of Venus (which are inferior to the posterior, superior iliac spines), and 10 cm proximal to that location in an upright patient. The distance between the marks is again measured with the patient's back at maximal flexion. A difference of less than 5 cm between neutral and flexion is suggestive of an inflammatory spondyloarthropathy. Limitation of lateral bending, reduced chest wall expansion during maximum inspiration, and restricted rotation of the thoracic spine with the pelvis held stable in a standing patient also support this diagnosis. See figure in Chapter 38.

**17. What exam suggests sacroiliitis?**

Pelvic compression, **Patrick's test**, and **Gaenslen's sign** may physically demonstrate sacroiliitis. Bilateral compression of the anterior iliac crests toward the midline, on a supine patient, may produce pathologic sacroiliac joint pain. Patrick's test is performed in a supine position by having the patient **F**lex, **AB**duct, and **E**xternally **R**otate (**FABER**) the hip such that the ipsilateral heel rests on the contralateral knee. Downward gentle pressure is then increasingly applied on the ipsilateral knee while stabilizing the contralateral anterior iliac crest. Pain arising from the contralateral pelvis is suggestive of sacroiliitis. Gaenslen's maneuver is performed with the patient supine and both hips and knees in flexion. The patient then moves one buttock off the examining table edge while extending the leg over the side. Sacroiliitis is suspected if the maneuver provokes sacroiliac discomfort. See figures in Chapter 38.

**18. What is lumbar spinal stenosis?**

Lumbar spinal stenosis is compression of nerve roots within the central lumbar canal that may clinically present as radiculopathy, pseudoclaudication, or cauda equina syndrome. Spinal stenosis results from narrowing of the normal oval spinal canal, which assumes a triangular appearance due to facet hyperostosis, ligamentum flavum hypertrophy, broad-based central disc protrusion and spondylosis or any combination. The typical patient has symptoms of lower limb claudication (neurogenic) in the absence of peripheral vascular disease. Symptoms are exacerbated by back extension and relieved with flexion, thus creating the classic simian posture. Patients will often report relief from walking-induced bilateral posterior buttock and thigh pain when they lean forward on their shopping carts. Symptoms can be produced by extending the patient's back (spinal Phalen's).

**19. What is cauda equina syndrome?**

Cauda equina syndrome is a serious clinical complex of low back pain, lower limb motor weakness, and saddle area anesthesia with bowel and/or bladder incontinence. The syndrome most commonly results from central intervertebral disc herniation into the sacral nerve roots. Rarely, advanced ankylosing spondylitis and malignancy may also cause cauda equina syndrome. The diagnosis of this rare syndrome requires an urgent MRI and a neurosurgical consultation.

**20. Define spondylosis, spondylitis, spondylolysis, and spondylolisthesis.**

**Spondylosis** refers to degenerative disease (e.g., osteoarthritis) of the intervertebral disc and/or the apophyseal (facet) joints. The natural, lordotic curves of the spinal column where maximum range of motion occurs at the C5–C7 and L3–L5 level predispose these segments to accelerated degenerative changes. Spondylosis of the cervical spine is the most common cause of neck pain.

**Spondylitis** literally means inflammation of the vertebral column, a classic feature of the spondyloarthropathies (e.g., ankylosing spondylitis). The inflammatory lesion of spondylitis occurs at the vertebral enthesis. Spondylolysis is characterized by a defective (separated) pars interarticularis, the bony bridge joining the superior and inferior articular processes of the vertebrae. The pars defect usually results from congenital dysplasia, degenerative disease, and/or trauma.

**Spondylolisthesis** occurs when the pars defect (spondylolysis) allows forward displacement (subluxation) of the proximal vertebra. Clinically significant spondylolisthesis (grade 2–4) is best identified on lateral radiographs and instability can be documented during maximum flexion and extension. **Spondylolysis**, with or without spondylolisthesis, is the most common structural cause of low back pain in older patients.

**21. What are the indications for obtaining a lumbosacral spine radiograph in a patient with low back pain?**

Image studies are always indicated If RED FLAGS are present because the yield is increased if you suspect cancer, fracture, or inflammatory spondyloarthropathy. Patients with back pain persisting > 4–6 weeks despite appropriate therapy for acute lumbar strain should also have spine films.

**22. Why not obtain x- rays on all patients with low back pain?**

Always ask yourself if you will treat the patient differently based upon this information. Age-related degenerative changes in the lumbar spine are often unrelated to the cause of the patient's myofascial pain. These images are often an unnecessary expense, and one lumbar series exposes the patient to the equivalent ionizing radiation dose of 40 chest x-rays!

**23. When should a MRI or CT myelogram be ordered for a patient with low back pain?**

Only if your approach will be altered. Patients with RED FLAGS for cancer, infection, or patients who are surgical candidates should have an MRI. Occasionally an MRI or CT of the sacroiliac joints is needed to diagnose early ankylosing spondylitis. The spine surgeon, if needed for operative planning, should order CT myelograms. MRI with gadolinium is indicated for patients who have undergone prior lumbar spine surgery to exclude infection or nerve root compression due to scar tissue. A history and physical examination consistent with lumbar radiculopathy in a patient who is improving with conservative therapy do not need an MRI. All imaging procedures must be interpreted in conjunction with the clinical history, physical examination, laboratory results, and electrophysiologic studies.

**24. When should an electromyogram (EMG) or nerve conduction velocities (NCV) be ordered for a patient with low back pain?**

An EMG is obtained in a patient with low back pain who has signs and symptoms of a radiculopathy if this information will change your approach. Usually MRI imaging has replaced the need for this EMG or NCVs. However, in complex cases, where the etiology of lower extremity pain or weakness is unclear despite careful neurological exam and imaging, NCV and EMG studies can be of value. The EMG is usually done at least 3 weeks after onset of symptoms. The results of an EMG are helpful only when combined with the clinical presentation, physical examination, and radiographic tests. Surgical removal of a disc has the greatest likelihood of improving symptoms if the physical examination, EMG, and radiographic studies all agree on the anatomic location of the disc compressing the nerve root.

**25. When should surgery be advised for a patient with radicular symptoms due to a herniated disc?**

The 1993 guidelines of the American Academy of Orthopedic Surgeons suggest before laminectomy, patients should have failed conservative therapy for 6 weeks (physical therapy and epidural steroids), or have incapacitating pain. They should also exhibit a positive straight leg-raising exam, which correlates with the same pathology identified on lumbar MRI, CT, or EMG/NCV studies.

**26. What are the sensitivity and specificity of the various diagnostic tests used to document a herniated lumbar disk? How often are they abnormal in individuals without low back pain?**

The diagnostic tests used to evaluate low back pain have the following sensitivity and specificity in patients with surgically documented herniated lumbar discs causing a compressive radiculopathy:

| | SENSITIVITY | SPECIFICITY |
|---|---|---|
| Electromyography | 92% | 38% |
| CT scans | 92% | 88% |
| Myelography | 90% | 87% |
| MRI scans | 93% | 92% |

It is important to note that a significant number of asymptomatic individuals without low back pain will have an abnormal CT scan or myelogram (30–40%). MRI studies have shown that 25-50% of individuals *without* low back pain will have a disc bulge or protrusion at one or more lumbar disc levels. Consequently, disc bulges/protrusions on MRI in patients with low back pain are *usually* coincidental, whereas disk extrusion, especially with compression of the lumbar nerve, is usually a significant cause of back pain.

**27. What exercises are good for patients with mechanical low back pain?**

Exercise is important in any rehabilitation program for mechanical low back pain. People who are more fit have fewer episodes of low back pain and recover from an episode of back pain more quickly. Exercise is important in maintaining the strength of the spinal segments.

Flexion exercises (Williams' exercises) are prescribed to decrease the load on the posterior facet joints and to open the intervertebral foramina. Extension exercises (MacKenzie's exercises) decrease compression load on the intervertebral disc and are consequently useful for patients with radiculopathies due to a herniated or degenerative disc. Spine stabilization exercises (correct abdominal strengthening and pelvic tilt) are important to decrease the load on pain sensitive structures and prevent recurrent episodes of mechanical low back pain/strain.

**28. What is the prognosis of patients with mechanical low back pain?**

It is estimated that up to 80% of all individuals will develop back pain during their life. Despite the potential number of people affected, the overall prognosis is good. Within 1 week of an acute episode, 50% of patients have symptomatic improvement; 75% will improve after 1 month; and 87% improve at 3 months. By 6 months, 93% are better. The remaining 7% have persistent symptoms and will develop chronic back pain.

**29. What are "Waddell's signs"?**

Although most back pain is organic, some patients present with complaints of low back pain that are due to a psychosomatic disorder. Other patients may complain of pain but are malingering to obtain secondary gain. To distinguish behavioral (nonorganic) from organic back pain, Waddell and colleagues found eight signs that identify nonorganic back pain. Patients should satisfy three or more of these signs if they have a behavioral cause for their low back pain.

- Superficial tenderness—discomfort to light touch to skin overlying back.
- Nonanatomic tenderness—tenderness that crosses multiple somatic boundaries or moves to various sites during the exam.
- Axial loading— report of low back pain when pressing down on the top of the head of a standing patient.
- Simulated rotation—when the shoulders and pelvis are rotated in unison less than 30 degrees (i.e., acetabular rotation test) in either direction, the structures in the back are not stressed. If patient reports pain with this maneuver, this test is considered positive.
- Distracted straight-leg raise—report of pain in low back or posterior thigh with less than 10 degrees of elevation of leg when supine, or pain with standard straight-leg raise test when patient recumbent but no pain when patient is sitting and knee is extended so that leg is at 90-degree angle with pelvis.
- Regional sensory change—"stocking" or global distribution of numbness, not in dermatomal distribution.
- Regional weakness—"breakaway" weakness in patient with normal strength on muscle testing.
- Overreaction—disproportionate grimacing, tremor, exaggerated verbalization, or collapse in a way not to hurt themselves during the exam.

**30. What other tests have been identified as suggesting a behavioral or nonorganic cause for back pain?**

- Sit-up—a patient with significant back pain can't do a sit-up. Patients with organic back pain will roll over to side and push up to sitting position. If patient can do sit-up, his pain is not severe.
- Shoes and socks sign—patients with significant organic back pain should have problems putting on shoes and socks. If no problem, back pain usually is not severe.
- Mankopf's test—pain should raise pulse rate 5% or more. Absence of this sign is a positive behavioral sign.
- O'Donoghue's maneuver—patients with true back pain should have greater passive range of motion than active range. If not, consider behavioral cause of pain.

ACKNOWLEDGMENT

The editor and author wish to thank Dr. Danny Williams for his contributions to this chapter in the previous edition.

## BIBLIOGRAPHY

1. Atlas SJ, Deyo RA, Keller RR, et al: The Maine Lumbar Spine Study, Part II: 1-year outcomes of surgical and nonsurgical management of sciatica. Spine 21:1777, 1996.
2. Bigos S, Bowyer O, Braen G: Acute low back problems in adults. Clinical practice guideline No 14, AHCPR Publication N.95-0642, Agency for Health Care Policy and Research, Public Health Services, US Department of Health and Human Services, Rockville, MD, 1994 (also available at http://text.nim.nih.gov)
3. Boden SD, Weisel SW, Laws ER, Rothman RH (eds): The Aging Spine. Essentials of Pathophysiology, Diagnosis and Treatment. Philadelphia, WB Saunders, 1991.
4. Borenstein DG: Chronic low back pain. Rheum Dis Clin North Am 22:439–456, 1996.
5. Casey PJ, Weinstein JN: Low back pain. In Ruddy S, Harris ED, Sledge CB (eds): Kelley's Textbook of Rheumatology, 6th ed. Philadelphia, WB Saunders, 2001, pp 509–524.
6. Cavanaugh JM: Neural mechanisms of lumbar pain. Spine 20:1804, 1995.
7. Deyo RA, Weinstein JN: Low back pain. N Engl J Med 344:363, 2001.
8. Hoppenfeld S: Physical Examination of the Spine and Extremities. New York, Appleton-Century-Crofts, 1976.
9. Jensen MC, Brandt-Zawadzki MN, Obuchowski N, et al: Magnetic resonance imaging of the lumbar spine in people without back pain. N Engl J Med 331:69–73, 1994.
10. Jonsson B, Annertz M, Sjoberg C, Stromquist B: A prospective and consecutive study of surgically treated lumbar spinal stenosis. Part I: Clinical features related to radiographic findings. Spine 22:2932, 1997.
11. Jonsson B, Annertz M, Sjoberg C, Stromquist B: A prospective and consecutive study of surgically treated lumbar spinal stenosis. Part II: Five-year follow-up by an independent observer. Spine 22:2938, 1997.
12. Kiester PD, Duke AD: Is it malingering, or is it real? Postgraduate Med 106(7):77–84, 1999.
13. Mannion AF, Muntener M, Taimela S, et al: A randomized clinical trial of three active therapies for chronic low back pain. Spine 24:2435, 1999.
14. Nakano KK: Neck pain. In Ruddy S, Harris ED, Sledge CB (eds): Kelley's Textbook of Rheumatology, 6th ed. Philadelphia, WB Saunders, 2001, pp 457–474.
15. Porter RW: Spinal stenosis and neutrogenic claudication. Spine 21:2046, 1996.
16. Saal JS: The role of inflammation in lumbar pain. Spine 20:1821, 1995.

# 65. FIBROMYALGIA

*Mark Malyak*, M.D.

**1. Define soft tissue rheumatism.**

Soft tissue rheumatism refers to a group of musculoskeletal pain syndromes that result from pathology of extra-articular and extraosseous periarticular structures. These "soft tissue" structures include bursae, tendons and their synovial sheaths, entheses, muscles, and fasciae. A major point conceptually is that pain from soft tissue rheumatism is not due to pathology of structures within the true joint (i.e., arthritis). Soft tissue rheumatism may manifest as well-defined pathology of a single periarticular site or a regional myofascial pain syndrome. Although fibromyalgia syndrome (FMS) is considered a form of soft tissue rheumatism in that patients experience soft tissue pain in the absence of articular disease, the underlying pathology is probably within the central nervous system.

Examples of involvement of **single periarticular sites** include bursitis, tendinitis, tenosynovitis, and enthesitis or enthesopathy (e.g., plantar fasciitis). Although diffuse connective tissue disorders, such as rheumatoid arthritis and seronegative spondyloarthropathy, may involve these soft tissue structures, involvement of a single or few periarticular sites in the absence of articular disease suggests the syndrome is due to chronic low-grade repetitive trauma or acute overexertion (e.g., the weekend warrior).

**Regional myofascial pain syndrome** is a localized soft tissue pain syndrome characterized by the presence of a trigger point within a muscle that upon palpation results in severe local tenderness and radiation of pain into characteristic regions. Though the discomfort of the myofascial pain syndrome remains regional, it is usually more widespread than bursitis or tendinitis. Regional myofascial pain syndrome most commonly involves the unilateral lower back, neck, shoulder, or hip region.

In the general population, 10% have chronic widespread pain, 20% have chronic regional pain, and 20% have chronic fatigue.

**2. Define FMS.**

*Criteria for Diagnosis of FMS*

| Always present | Often present |
|---|---|
| History | History |
| Chronic, diffuse pain | Morning stiffness |
| Physical examination | Fatigue |
| Characteristic tender points | Sleep disturbance |
| Otherwise unremarkable | Depression |
| Laboratory tests | Anxiety |
| All normal | Headache |
| | Paresthesias |
| | Raynaud's phenomenon |

FMS is a chronic (> 3 months) noninflammatory and non-autoimmune diffuse pain syndrome of unknown etiology associated with characteristic **tender points** detected on physical examination. In addition to diffuse chronic musculoskeletal pain, patients subjectively often have morning stiffness, severe fatigue, nonrestorative sleep, paresthesias, and Raynaud's phenomenon. Physical examination and pathologic investigation reveal no evidence of articular, osseous, or soft tissue inflammation or degeneration. FMS may occur alone (primary FMS) or may be associated with a number of other disorders. The absence of objective findings other than tender points refers to primary FMS. FMS associated with other disorders will exhibit physical exam and laboratory test abnormalities characteristic of the associated disorder.

**3. What are tender points? Where are they located in FMS?**

In normal individuals (and in patients with FMS), there exist specific regions on the surface anatomy that are more sensitive to applied pressure than other sites. FMS is a disorder of generalized pain amplification, and thus these regions are exceedingly tender, and are referred to as **tender points**. The classification criteria for FMS require chronic (> 3 months) presence of at least 11 of 18 tender points existing diffusely (above and below the waist). The amount of point pressure utilized to elicit tender points is 4 kg/cm$^2$ (enough pressure to blanch your thumbnail). Tender points in patients with FMS are more sensitive to pressure than in control patients and when compared with other, non-tender point sites (**control points**) in the same patient. (See figure, top of next page)

**4. What are control points?**

Control points are areas that are not normally painful when point pressure (4 kg/cm$^2$) is applied. They are located on the mid-forehead, thumbnail, volar surface of mid-forearm, and anterior mid-thigh. Control points are not tender in FMS patients but are frequently painful in patients with somatization disorders. It should be noted, though, that FMS is a generalized pain syndrome, and sites other than tender points (including control points) are more sensitive to point pressure than in normal individuals, though pressures greater than 4 kg/cm$^2$ are usually required.

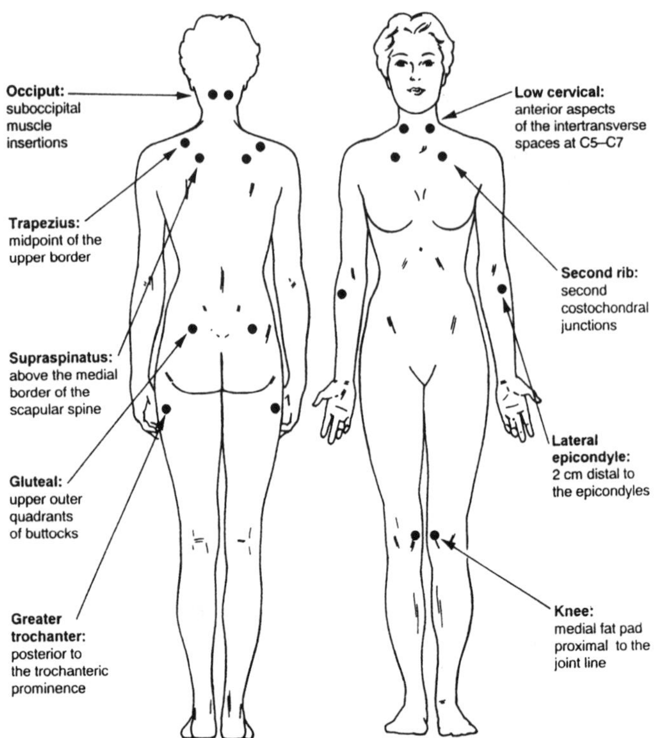


Location of the 18 (9 pairs) specific tender points in fibromyalgia patients. (From Freundlich B, Leventhal L: The fibromyalgia syndrome. In Schumacher HR Jr, Klippel JH, Koopman WJ (eds): Primer on the Rheumatic Diseases, 10th ed. Atlanta, Arthritis Foundation, 1993, pp 247–249; with permission.)

**5. Who generally develops FMS? At what age?**

Though there is lack of good population-based studies, the prevalence of fibromyalgia in the general adult population is probably 0.5–4% (3.4% of women, 0.5% of men). **Females** account for 70–90% of patients. The observation that **whites** represent 90% of patients with FMS may represent selection bias. The average **age of onset** is approximately 30–55 years, but ranges from childhood to the very old. FMS symptoms occurring for the first time in a patient older than 55–60 years, though, are usually due to a disease other than FMS (e.g., infection, neoplasia, arthritis).

**6. How can the pain of FMS be distinguished from the pain of widespread arthritis?**

Patients with FMS generally have diffuse pain that may be perceived to originate within joints, muscles, or both, and thus it may be confused with a diffuse arthritis syndrome, such as rheumatoid arthritis or ankylosing spondylitis. Pain involving the **axial skeleton** is universally present in FMS, with patients experiencing lower back, cervical spine, and/or thoracic spine pain. Patients with FMS also commonly experience **bilateral pain** in the upper and lower extremities. True arthritis may often be excluded by the physical examination, and therefore the joint exam in primary FMS reveals **absence of effusion**, synovial proliferation, deformity, and warmth. The multiple widespread **tender points** present in FMS are also helpful in distinguishing this disorder from a diffuse arthritis syndrome. Finally, laboratory and radiographic findings are normal in primary FMS.

Fibromyalgia may occur alone (primary FMS) or may coexist with numerous other medical syndromes, including arthritis. Therefore, the presence of an arthritis syndrome does not exclude the presence of coexistent FMS, and vice-versa. In these cases, the diagnosis of superimposed FMS may be considered if subjective pain and constitutional symptoms exceed that expected for the degree of objective arthritis as determined by physical examination, radiographs, and laboratory tests. The presence of diffuse tender points also suggests the diagnosis of coexistent FMS.

**7. Discuss the sleep disorder associated with FMS.**

Non-REM sleep progresses through four stages that can be identified by electroencephalography. Quiet wakefulness with closed eyes is characterized by alpha-waves (8–13 Hz), whereas alert wakefulness with eyes open and bright lights is characterized by beta-waves (14–25 Hz). Non-REM stage I sleep is a transition from wakefulness and is associated with predominantly theta-wave activity (4–7 Hz). As deeper sleep is reached, the frequency of brain waves slows further, so that by non-REM stage IV sleep, delta-waves (< 4 Hz) account for > 50% of brain wave activity. It is delta-wave, or non-REM stage IV, sleep that is responsible for restful and restorative sleep.

The sleep disturbance associated with FMS, termed **alpha-delta sleep**, is characterized by disruption of delta-wave sleep by frequent alpha-wave intrusion, such that non-REM stage IV sleep is significantly reduced. This sleep pattern is not specific for FMS and may be present during periods of emotional stress, in chronic painful conditions such as rheumatoid arthritis and osteoarthritis, in sleep apnea syndrome, and in some otherwise normal individuals. Alpha-delta sleep is clinically associated with nonrestorative sleep.

**8. Though FMS is a noninflammatory disorder, patients often have morning stiffness and other subjective findings suggestive of an inflammatory disorder, confounding the correct diagnosis. Discuss other subjective findings in FMS that are usually considered representative of inflammatory rather than noninflammatory disorders.**

Most patients with FMS have severe, often debilitating, fatigue. Fatigue is often most severe upon arising in the morning and is exacerbated by minor physical exertion. Confusion may arise because fatigue is a common constitutional symptom in systemic inflammatory disorders such as rheumatoid arthritis, and is usually absent in noninflammatory disorders such as osteoarthritis. Fatigue in chronic inflammatory disorders is likely due to circulating proinflammatory cytokines. Fatigue in FMS is probably a consequence of alpha-delta sleep disturbance.

Approximately 50% of patients perceive **subjective soft tissue swelling** of joints, suggesting a true arthritis. Physical examination, though, reveals no swelling or other evidence of arthritis in primary FMS.

**Paresthesias**, which may suggest impingement of neural structures or a neuropathy secondary to an inflammatory condition, are present in approximately 50% of patients with FMS. Paresthesias may be localized or diffuse and may or may not occur in dermatomal distributions. Subjective muscle weakness is also common. Neurologic examination is unremarkable in these patients, as is nerve conduction velocity/electromyographic examination.

**Raynaud's phenomenon** occurs in approximately 10% of patients. Though this symptom may occur in otherwise normal individuals, it is a characteristic finding in systemic sclerosis and may be present in other diffuse connective tissue diseases including rheumatoid arthritis and systemic lupus erythematosus.

**Dry eyes and mouth** occur in 15% of patients with FMS. Confusion arises because sicca symptoms are common manifestations of Sjögren's syndrome.

Other common subjective findings in FMS include manifestations of tension and migraine headache, irritable bowel syndrome, primary dysmenorrhea, and mood disorder.

**9. FMS often occurs independently, but there are well-described associations with other disorders. What are these associated medical disorders?**

FMS may occur in the setting of numerous **painful syndromes**, including rheumatoid arthritis, SLE (up to 25%), and osteoarthritis. Possibly, the chronic pain from the associated syndrome results in disruption of normal sleep patterns, which may be related to the pathophysiology of

FMS. In these cases, FMS may be truly secondary. In a similar fashion, FMS may be associated with **obstructive sleep apnea**.

FMS is also associated with **irritable bowel syndrome, tension headaches, migraine headaches, depression**, and primary **dysmenorrhea**. These conditions share a number of features, including female predominance, muscle pain, and lack of abnormal laboratory tests or pathologic features. These conditions may form a collection of disorders, labeled the affective spectrum disorders, that share common pathophysiologic mechanisms.

FMS also appears associated with the **chronic fatigue syndrome**, and in fact, these two syndromes may represent the same disorder. Other associations include **hypothyroidism** and chronic hepatitis C. Sleep disorders may be associated with FMS, probably through disruption of normal sleep patterns; these include obstructive sleep apnea, and possibly, nocturnal myoclonus and restless leg syndrome. Finally, **Lyme disease** may trigger FMS, which may persist despite eradication of the offending spirochete.

**10. What is the chronic fatigue syndrome (CFS)? How is it related to FMS?**

CFS is a disorder of unknown etiology and pathophysiology characterized by severe, chronic, and debilitating fatigue leading to an inability to perform usual activities. Numerous additional symptoms are commonly present, including joint and muscle pain, headache, and sleep disturbance. Like FMS, there is no evidence of chronic infection accounting for the symptoms. Numerous reports in the past have attempted to associate CFS with chronic active viral infection, most recently Epstein-Barr virus (EBV), but to date there is no evidence to suggest that viral infection is responsible in the vast majority of patients. Various studies have reported numerous but subtle immunologic abnormalities, including elevation of certain antibodies against EBV, abnormal T-cell subset ratios, reduced natural killer cell function and number, decreased immunoglobulin subset quantities, and reduced delayed-type hypersensitivity. Although not studied in detail, some of these abnormalities have also been detected in patients with FMS. Abnormalities of the hypothalamic-pituitary-adrenal axis have also been described.

Numerous hypotheses may explain the symptoms and observed immunologic findings in CFS. Chronic active viral infection remains a possible but unlikely explanation for most patients. Neuro-psycho-immuno-endocrine interrelations are now well-recognized, and dysfunction of any one aspect of this system may lead to abnormalities within the other three. Thus, a primary psychiatric disorder conceivably could lead to the symptoms and abnormal immunologic and endocrinologic findings in CFS. Finally, CFS and FMS may represent the same disorder or be manifestations of the affective spectrum disorders.

**11. Why is it important to recognize the coexistence of FMS and an underlying inflammatory disorder such as rheumatoid arthritis?**

The possibility of FMS should be ascertained to prevent overtreatment of rheumatoid arthritis. If articular pain and subjective joint swelling, morning stiffness, and fatigue are manifestations of active rheumatoid arthritis, antirheumatic treatment is inadequate, and more aggressive therapy should be considered to control these inflammatory symptoms and prevent articular destruction. If these same symptoms are due to coexistent FMS, treatment of this disorder should be instituted, thereby avoiding more aggressive and more toxic antirheumatic therapy.

**12. What laboratory tests should be obtained in patients with suspected FMS?**

In primary FMS, laboratory tests are normal. Thus, laboratory tests are performed to exclude disorders that may mimic FMS and to investigate for possible associated conditions.

- Complete blood count, erythrocyte sedimentation rate (ESR), creatinine, liver function tests, thyroid-stimulating hormone, creatine kinase, glucose, calcium, phosphorous, and urinalysis in all patients
- Rheumatoid factor and antinuclear antibody (ANA) (obtain only if there are supporting data for rheumatoid arthritis, SLE, or other diffuse connective tissue disease)
- Plain radiography (to check for underlying or coincidental arthritis or other pathology)

- Nerve conduction velocity (NCV), electromyography (EMG), MRI, CT, and muscle biopsy usually not necessary
- Formal sleep studies (to evaluate for obstructive sleep apnea in patients with compatible symptoms or signs)

**13. Discuss the differential diagnosis of FMS.**

*Differential Diagnosis of FMS*

| DISEASE | HISTORY | PHYSICAL EXAMINATION | LABORATORY TESTS |
|---|---|---|---|
| **Diffuse connective tissue disease** | | | |
| Rheumatoid arthritis | Morning stiffness<br>Peripheral joint pain, swelling<br>Fatigue | Synovitis<br>Joint deformities<br>Rheumatoid nodules | Rheumatoid factor<br>Inflammation indicators$^+$<br>Radiographs |
| Systemic lupus erythematosus | Fatigue<br>Peripheral joint pain, swelling<br>Raynaud's phenomenon<br>Rash, serositis, etc.* | Rash<br>Synovitis<br>Neuropathy | ANA<br>dsDNA, Sm, Ro antibodies<br>C3, C4<br>Urinalysis<br>Inflammation indicators |
| Systemic sclerosis | Raynaud's phenomenon<br>Fatigue<br>Peripheral joint pain, swelling<br>Esophageal, pulmonary symptoms* | Scleroderma<br>Edematous hands<br>Abnormal nailfold on microscopy | ANA<br>Centromere, Scl-70 antibodies<br>Esophageal motility studies<br>PFTs<br>Inflammation indicators |
| Sjögren's syndrome | Peripheral joint pain, swelling<br>Fatigue<br>Dry eyes, dry mouth<br>Raynaud's phenomenon | Enlarged salivary glands<br>KCS<br>Synovitis | ANA<br>Ro, La antibodies<br>Schirmer's and Rose bengal tests<br>Salivary gland biopsy<br>Inflammation indicators |
| Inflammatory and metabolic myopathies | Muscle weakness<br>Muscle pain<br>Fatigue | Muscle weakness | CK, aldolase<br>ANA<br>EMG/NCV<br>Muscle biopsy<br>Inflammation indicators |
| Polymyalgia rheumatica/giant cell arteritis (GCA) | Morning stiffness<br>Shoulder and hip girdle, and neck pain | Tender temporal artery with GCA | ESR<br>Inflammation indicators<br>Temporal artery biopsy |
| **Seronegative spondyloarthropathy** | | | |
| Ankylosing spondylitis | Morning stiffness<br>Lower back pain<br>Cervical spine pain<br>Peripheral joint pain/swelling | Limitation of motion of lumbar/cervical spine<br>Peripheral synovitis<br>Iritis | Sacroiliac joint radiograph<br>Spine, peripheral joint radiographs<br>Inflammation indicators |
| Colitic arthritis | Abdominal pain, diarrhea<br>Axial musculoskeletal pain<br>Peripheral joint pain/swelling | Peripheral synovitis<br>Limitation of motion of lumbar, cervical spine<br>Gross/occult blood in stool | Colonoscopy/radio-contrast studies<br>Spine, peripheral joint radiographs<br>Inflammation indicators |

(*Table continued on next page.*)

*Differential Diagnosis of FMS (cont.)*

| DISEASE | HISTORY | PHYSICAL EXAMINATION | LABORATORY TESTS |
|---|---|---|---|
| **Other** | | | |
| A miscellaneous group of other diseases including neurologic disorders (multiple sclerosis, myasthenia gravis), endocrine disorders (hypothyroidism, Addison's disease, Cushing's syndrome, hyperparathyroidism), infectious disorders (chronic hepatitis C, Lyme disease), and sleep disorders (obstructive sleep apnea, nocturnal myoclonus) may rarely be confused with FMS, and are usually easily distinguishable by routine laboratory tests, characteristic subjective findings, and abnormalities on physical exam. Psychological disorders that my mimic FMS are discussed below (see Question 14). | | | |

+ Inflammation indicators include anemia of chronic inflammation, elevated ESR, leukocytosis, thrombocytosis, hypoalbuminemia, and elevated serum globulins.

* Symptoms not present in FMS, whereas all other features under history are commonly present in FMS; not all listed subjective and objective findings are necessarily present in an individual patient with these disorders.

*Abbreviations*: KCS, keratoconjunctivitis sicca; PFTs, pulmonary function tests; CK, creatine kinase.

The fatigue and generalized pain of FMS are nonspecific symptoms common to many medical conditions. Though the symptoms of these other disorders may mimic FMS, objective data obtained from physical examination and laboratory evaluation will lead to the correct diagnosis. Except for the mandatory laboratory tests (see Question 12), other tests should be obtained only if the disorder being evaluated is clinically suspected through information obtained from the history, physical examination, and general laboratory tests.

**14. Which psychological disorders are sometimes confused with FMS? Why?**

**Functional psychiatric disorders**, such as the somatoform disorders, often result in symptoms identical to those of FMS. The term *functional* suggests the syndrome has no organic basis and is due to purely psychologic factors or conflicts. It is conceivable that in some patients FMS originates as a functional disorder, and subsequently the objective clinical, sleep, and neurotransmitter abnormalities become manifest as a result of neuro-psycho-immuno-endocrine interrelationships. Thus, although a "functional" psychiatric disorder may precipitate FMS, "organic" pathophysiologic mechanisms are likely responsible for the symptoms of FMS. The alternative possibility is that the chronic pain and fatigue of a somatoform disorder are purely functional in certain patients. It is unclear if these patients would have tender points on physical examination, alpha-delta sleep disturbance, or neurotransmitter abnormalities.

**Organic psychiatric disorders**, such as major depression, have also been associated with FMS, with up to 50–70% of patients with FMS having a history of major depression and up to 33% having major depression at time of FMS diagnosis. Alternatively, many patients diagnosed with major depression experience sleep disturbance, fatigue, and diffuse musculoskeletal pain. Three potential explanations may account for this association. (1) Depression and FMS may both be clinical manifestations of the affective spectrum disorders, and their presence in an individual patient is coincidental rather than causal. (2) Major depression may lead to alterations of the neuro-psycho-immuno-endocrine system such that it leads to the development of FMS. In a similar fashion, FMS may lead to the development of major depression. (3) FMS and major depression may represent a single syndrome, with the diagnosis in a particular patient dependent on the major clinical manifestations present.

Finally, the **anxiety** and **mild depression** often present in FMS may be a psychologic response to concerns regarding financial and personal independence in the setting of chronic pain and disability. This association may be present in any chronic pain or debilitating syndrome.

**15. Is the etiology of FMS known?**

No. Although patients often report no precipitating event prior to the onset of symptoms, FMS is occasionally preceded by an acute viral syndrome (parvovirus, hepatitis C), Lyme disease, physical (whiplash injury) or emotional trauma, a localized pain disorder such as myofascial pain syndrome, or withdrawal from certain medications (particularly glucocorticoids).

Although it is possible that these disorders may precipitate FMS, it is unlikely that they play a role in the maintenance or pathophysiology of the syndrome.

**16. What abnormalities in the central nervous system have been implicated in FMS?**

Most investigators believe that the pathophysiology of FMS primarily resides within the central nervous system, manifesting as amplified pain perception. Thus, physical stresses to the musculoskeletal system that in the normal individual are perceived as non-tender touch, position sense, non-tender temperature sensation, or are simply not noticed consciously, are perceived as pain in the patient with FMS. The underlying disorder within the CNS leading to amplified pain perception is not understood, but a number of specific abnormalities have been observed in some patients with FMS:

- Abnormalities within the descending analgesia system
- Alpha-delta sleep disturbance
- Abnormalities within the endorphin/enkephalin system
- Affective spectrum disorder
- Somatoform disorder

**17. Do FMS patients have any abnormalities on brain imaging to support a central mechanism for their amplified pain perception?**

Brain MRI is normal in FMS patients. However, functional imaging studies using SPECT scans have shown decreased regional cerebral blood flow to the thalamus and caudate nucleus. The caudate nucleus and thalamus signal noxious stimuli, and decreased blood flow to these areas has been demonstrated in other chronic pain disorders.

**18. Have any abnormalities of the autonomic or endocrine systems been found in FMS patients?**

Several studies have shown a global blunting of human stress response in FMS patients, owing to an attenuated response to stressors by the hypothalamic-pituitary-adrenal (HPA) and sympathetic nervous systems. This may explain some of the other symptoms FMS patients experience, including fatigue, vasomotor instability (livedo, Raynaud's), orthostatic hypotension, and sicca symptoms. Also up to 25% of FMS patients have low insulin-like growth factor–1 (somatomedin C) as a result of low production of growth hormone from the hypothalamus-pituitary area. This may affect muscle bulk and tone.

**19. Discuss the descending analgesia pathway and its potential role in the pathophysiology of FMS.**

The descending analgesia system is a physiologic mechanism by which the transmission of pain is inhibited at the dorsal horn and other locations within the CNS (see figure). Projections from the origin of this pathway within the hypothalamus, utilizing enkephalin as a neurotransmitter, reach the raphe magnus nucleus within the pons and medulla. The raphe nucleus sends projections into the dorsal horn, utilizing serotonin as a neurotransmitter, where they stimulate interneurons whose neurotransmitter is again enkephalin. These axons innervate the presynaptic region of incoming pain fibers, leading to the presynaptic inhibition of transmission of painful sensation to second-order pain fibers, most likely through the inhibition of calcium channels.

The implication of the descending analgesia system in the pathophysiology of FMS has been suggested by studies that have demonstrated decreased serotonin or serotonin availability within the CNS. It remains unclear if the observed serotonin abnormality is a primary dysfunction or secondary to another process within the neuro-psycho-immuno-endocrine system. It further remains unclear if the serotonin abnormality is in fact associated with dysfunction of the descending analgesia system.

Additionally, metabolites of norepinephrine are decreased in the CSF of FMS patients. This is important because there are norepinephrine-mediated pain-inhibitory pathways that descend to the spinal cord and thus may be abnormal in FMS patients.

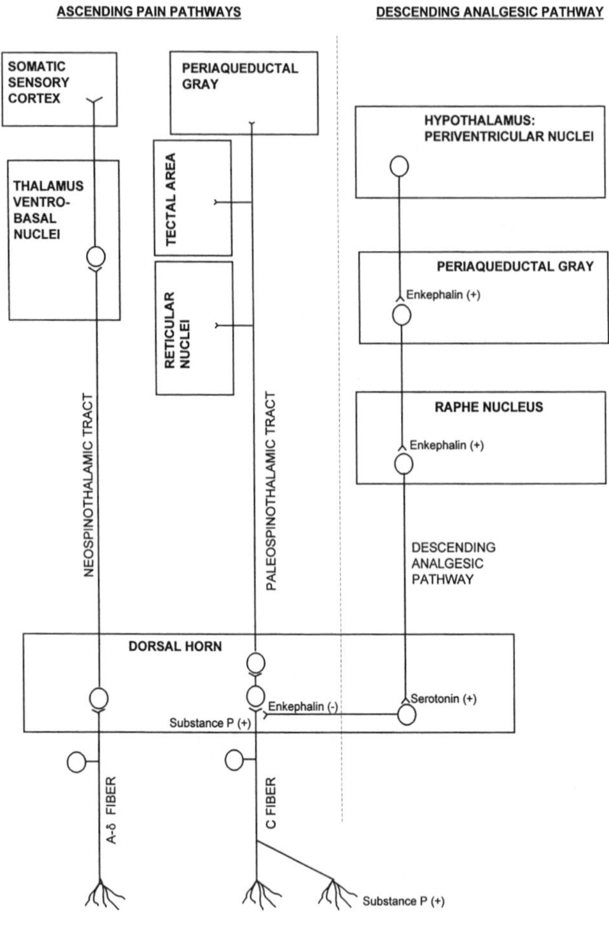


Pain pathways.

**20. What mechanisms originating in the peripheral musculoskeletal system may be important in the etiology and pathophysiology of FMS?**

- Muscle microtrauma
- Muscle deconditioning
- Substance P
- Alpha$_2$-adrenergic receptors

To date, there is no evidence that patients with FMS have an inflammatory or metabolic disorder of skeletal muscle. There is evidence that patients with FMS are deconditioned, which is likely due to disuse as a result of chronic pain resulting from a central pain amplification disorder. It is postulated that deconditioned muscle is more susceptible to microtrauma as a result of minor activity. This microtrauma may then result in greater pain that would further reduce activity, resulting in a vicious cycle of muscle inactivity, deconditioning, microtrauma, and pain.

Substance P is the neurotransmitter of type C pain fibers in the dorsal horn. In addition to transmitting "slow" pain, stimulation of type C fibers may also lead to the secretion of substance P from peripheral nerve fibers in an antidromic fashion, where it may lead to a localized inflammatory response. Excessive substance P, either as a primary or secondary disorder, conceivably could lead to a chronic pain syndrome. Interestingly, elevated substance P levels have been found in the cerebrospinal fluid of some FMS patients.

In patients with FMS, there appears to be a correlation between Raynaud's phenomenon and increased alpha$_2$-adrenergic receptors on platelets. This observation suggests that elevated concentrations of these adrenergic receptors within muscle, lacrimal glands, salivary glands, and peripheral digital vessels may lead to excessive adrenergic activity even in the presence of normal catecholamine levels, resulting in muscle pain due to relative ischemia, dry eyes, dry mouth, and Raynaud's phenomenon, respectively.

**21. List the six components of therapy for FMS.**

- Patient education
- Analgesia
- Correction of sleep disturbance
- Aerobic exercise
- Physical therapy
- Treatment of associated disorders

Although the etiology and pathophysiology of FMS remain unknown and many of the therapeutic interventions have been inadequately studied, a logical multidisciplinary approach to the treatment of this disorder is possible and necessary if meaningful results are expected.

**22. What three major points regarding the disease process should be emphasized in patient education programs?**

1. FMS is a "real" and objective disease. This fact provides relief to the many patients whose chronic symptoms were labeled as purely psychologic or imagined.

2. A serious underlying disorder such as malignancy or destructive arthritis is not responsible for the symptoms of FMS (unless FMS is secondary to one of these disorders).

3. Although FMS is a real disease, the patient has substantial control over many components that may modulate the resultant symptoms. Discussion of an hypothesis of FMS in lay terms is appropriate, emphasizing those components that may be modified by the patient, e.g., the roles of the sleep disturbance and muscle deconditioning in the positive feedback loop resulting in amplified pain (see figure). Provision of lay literature may also be helpful.

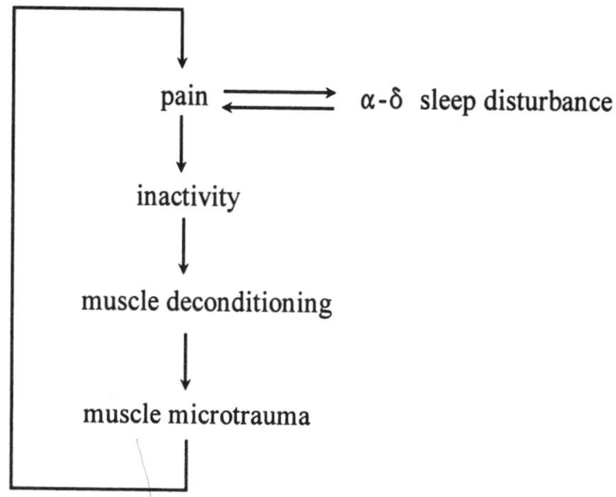


A simplified hypothesis of fibromyalgia may help patients better understand their disorder.

**23. What is the goal of exercise programs in FMS patients?**

Aerobic exercise improves muscle conditioning, which may lead to less muscle microtrauma and thus may interrupt the positive feedback loop. Aerobic exercise may furthermore improve restorative sleep and increase endogenous endorphins within the CNS. Because patients with FMS often experience severe postexercise pain, the intensity of exercise must be initially low and only gradually increased as tolerated. Exercise should be aerobic and nonimpact, such as swimming, water aerobics, walking with proper footwear, or bicycling. Some patients find group exercise programs to be beneficial. Physical therapy consultation may be helpful in designing the optimal exercise program for a particular patient.

**24. Which physical therapy modalities should be considered in treating a patient with FMS?**

It is reasonable to try safe, relatively inexpensive interventions such as massage and the application of local heat in patients with FMS. The more expensive interventions, such as transcutaneous electrical nerve stimulation, hypnotherapy, EMG biofeedback, and acupuncture, have been inadequately tested and cannot be recommended for routine use but may be considered in patients whose symptoms are resistant to more conventional therapy. In the unusual patient with FMS who is experiencing regional pain associated with a local very painful tender point (or trigger point) out of proportion to generalized pain, it is reasonable to treat as one would with a myofascial pain syndrome, including trigger point injection with a local anesthetic and possibly a glucocorticoid preparation followed by stretching of the muscle.

**25. Discuss the medicinal approach to therapy for FMS.**

1. **Tricyclic agents (TCA)**. Low-dose TCAs administered before bedtime have been objectively demonstrated to improve the sleep disturbance, pain, and tender points in a proportion of patients with fibromyalgia. An example of such a regimen is the administration of amitriptyline at a dosage of 10–25 mg 1–3 hours prior to bedtime. This dose may be increased by 10–25 mg increments at 2-week intervals; the usual effective dose is 25–100 mg daily. Adverse effects are common and are due to the TCA's anticholinergic and antihistamine activities. They include morning drowsiness, dry mouth, and constipation. If amitriptyline causes too many side effects, other TCA can be tried:

| | SEDATIVE | ANTICHOLINERGIC |
|---|---|---|
| Amitriptyline (Elavil, Endep) | ++++ | ++++ |
| Imipramine (Tofranil) | +++ | +++ |
| Doxepin (Sinequan) | +++ | +++ |
| Nortriptyline (Pamelor) | ++ | + |
| Desipramine | + | + |

Amitriptyline and imipramine are the most likely to cause orthostatic hypotension and cardiac toxicity (arrhythmias), although the others may also cause these problems. Cyclobenzaprine (Flexeril) is a weak TCA-like drug that can also be used at doses of 10–40 mg at night. Overall, 35% of FMS patients benefit from TCA. For patients who do not tolerate TCA, trazodone, clonazepam, and alprazolam have been used as alternatives.

Although the mechanism of action of the TCAs in the treatment of fibromyalgia remains unclear, the small dosages used and the rapid onset of action suggest it is not due to treatment of underlying depression. Since TCAs inhibit the reuptake of serotonin (and norepinephrine) at synaptic junctions, it is hypothesized that the greater availability of serotonin may be responsible for improved stage IV sleep in addition to providing a central analgesic effect through potentiation of the descending analgesic pathways. TCAs may also have an effect on CNS endorphins as well as on peripheral pain receptors.

2. **Analgesia**. It is reasonable to recommend **acetaminophen** to patients who do not respond to nonmedicinal interventions and TCAs. If acetaminophen provides no benefit and pain persists, low-dose **NSAID** therapy may be considered, keeping in mind that NSAIDs have common potentially life-threatening adverse effects and have not objectively been demonstrated to be of benefit in fibromyalgia. If low-dose NSAID therapy fails, there probably is no benefit but potential harm, in using anti-inflammatory doses of NSAIDs. Although the use of Cox-2

specific inhibitors in FMS have not been studied, it would be anticipated that efficacy would be similar to the conventional NSAIDs, while the risk of PUD and its complications of hemorrhage and perforation would be decreased. Tramadol and high-dose gabapentin have also been used for pain management. Narcotic analgesics should be avoided in the treatment of fibromyalgia.

3. **Selective serotonin reuptake inhibitors (SSRIs)**. SSRIs have not been studied to the extent of the TCAs and NSAIDs. One study demonstrated greater efficacy of combination therapy with fluoxetine 20 mg in the morning and amitriptyline 25 mg at bedtime than either of the agents alone. Theoretically, antidepressants with greater adrenergic and/or dopaminergic activity (nefazodone, venlafaxine) should work better than pure serotonincrgic drugs.

**26. What is the prognosis for fibromyalgia?**

Outcome studies suggest that the majority of patients continue to experience symptoms despite specific treatment. The poor outcome reported in these studies may reflect more severe disease, since they originate from tertiary care centers. The only community-based study reported that 25% of patients were asymptomatic and an additional 25% were substantially improved after conventional therapy. Despite these discouraging data, a sympathetic patient-physician interaction and an organized approach to therapeutic intervention will lead to substantial improvement in many patients with fibromyalgia.

**27. Should FMS patients be given disability? (controversial)**

It is estimated that as many as 25% of FMS patients in the United States receive some form of disability or injury compensation. However, disability awards do not result in clinical improvement and may actually contribute to a patient's inability to improve. Certainly, some patients need disability compensation but there should be an effort to not label FMS patients disabled.

## BIBLIOGRAPHY


1. Aaron, LA, Burke MM, Buckwald D: Overlapping conditions among patients with chronic fatigue syndrome, fibromyalgia, and temporomandibular disorder. Arch Intern Med 160:221, 2000.
2. Bennett RM: Fibromyalgia and the facts: Sense or nonsense. Rheum Dis Clin North Am 19:45–59, 1993.
3. Bennett RM: Fibromyalgia and the disability dilemma. Arthritis Rheum 39:1627–1634, 1996.
4. Carette S: Fibromyalgia 20 years later: What have we really accomplished? J Rheumatol 22:590–594, 1995.
5. Carette S, Bell MJ, Reynolds WJ, et al: Comparison of amitriptyline, cyclobenzaprine, and placebo in the treatment of fibromyalgia: A randomized, double-blind clinical trial. Arthritis Rheum 37:32–40, 1994.
6. Clauw DJ: Fibromyalgia. In Ruddy S, Harris ED, Sledge CB (eds): Kelley's Textbook of Rheumatology, 6th ed. Philadelphia, WB Saunders, 2001, pp 417–427.
7. Goldenberg DL: Fibromyalgia syndrome a decade later: What have we learned? Arch Intern Med 159:777, 1999.
8. Goldenberg DL, Mayskiy M, Mossey CJ, et al: A randomized, double-blind crossover trial of fluoxetine and amitriptyline in the treatment of fibromyalgia. Arthritis Rheum 39:1852, 1996.
9. Granges G, Zilko P, Littlejohn GO: Fibromyalgia syndrome: Assessment of the severity of the condition 2 years after diagnosis. J Rheumatol 21:523–529, 1994.
10. Hudson JI, Pope HG Jr: Fibromyalgia and psychopathology: Is fibromyalgia a form of "affective spectrum disorder"? J Rheumatol 16 (suppl 19):15–22, 1989.
11. Mountz JM, Bradley LA, Alarcon GS: Abnormal functional activity of the central nervous system in fibromyalgia syndrome. Amer J Med Sci 315:385–396, 1998.
12. Reichlin S: Neuroendocrine-immune interactions. N Engl J Med 329:1246–1253, 1993.
13. Roizenblatt S, Modlofsky H, Benedito-Silva AA, Tufik S: Alpha sleep characteristics in fibromyalgia. Arthritis Rheum 44:222, 2001.
14. Weigent DA, Bradley LA, Blalock JE, Alarcon GA: Current concepts in the pathophysiology of abnormal pain perception in fibromyalgia. Am J Med Sci 315:405, 1998.
15. Wilke WS: Treatment of "resistant" fibromyalgia. Rheum Dis Clin North Am 21:247–260, 1995.
16. Wolfe F, Anderson J, Harkness D, et al: A prospective, longitudinal multicenter study of service utilization and costs in fibromyalgia. Arthritis Rheum 40:1560–1570, 1997.

17. Wolfe F, Anderson J, Harkness D, et al: Health status and disease severity in fibromyalgia: Results of a six-center longitudinal study. Arthritis Rheum 40:1571–1579, 1997.
18. Wolfe F: The fibromyalgia syndrome: A consensus report on fibromyalgia and disability. J Rheumatol 23:534–539, 1996.

# 66. REGIONAL MUSCULOSKELETAL DISORDERS

*Scott Vogelgesang, M.D.*

**1. What is bursitis?**

- Bursitis is the condition when a bursa becomes inflamed or infected.
- A bursa is a sac with a potential space that makes it easier for one tissue to glide over another.
- Occasionally, a bursa may communicate with a nearby joint.
- Most bursae differentiate during development, but new ones may form in response to stress, inflammation, or trauma.

**2. What is tendinitis?**

Tendinitis occurs when at least one of the following occurs:

- Synovial tendon sheath (tissue that surrounds the tendon that resembles synovium or joint lining) becomes inflamed
- Trauma induces ischemia and subsequent inflammation
- Crystal deposition into the tendon [especially basic calcium phosphate (apatite) crystals] causes inflammation; called calcific tendinitis

Most of these conditions can be classified as "overuse" syndromes. Aging can decrease the integrity of the tendon, making it more prone to injury.

**3. Name three nonarticular causes of shoulder pain.**

- Impingement syndrome
- Subacromial bursitis
- Bicipital tendinitis

**4. Describe the shoulder impingement syndrome. How does it occur?**

The shoulder impingement syndrome is a chronic, painful condition of the shoulder that results from an encroachment of the tendons of the rotator cuff (most commonly the supraspinatus) occurring most commonly with shoulder abduction. Abduction elevates the greater tuberosity of the humerus and rotator cuff tendon insertions toward the coracoacromial arch. The coracoacromial arch is made up of the acromion, the coracoid process of the scapula, and the coracoacromial ligament. Etiologies include sporting or occupational overuse, degenerative changes of the tendons or surrounding skeletal structures, curved or hooked acromion, and a single traumatic episode with post-traumatic tendon inflammation. It can also be idiopathic.

In the normal functioning shoulder, the rotator cuff serves as a dynamic stabilizer of the joint. Its principal function lies in humeral head depression during shoulder abduction. The rotator cuff also assists with early abduction (to 0–30 degrees) as well as with internal and external rotation. When the rotator cuff is inflamed secondary to chronic, repetitive, microtrauma or acute post-traumatic tendon strain, it becomes relatively ineffective at shoulder depression, a characteristic called reflex inhibition. As a result, the humeral head moves closer to the coracoacromial arch (called superior translation) during contraction of the deltoid muscle (shoulder abduction). With continued motion and increased superior translation of the humeral head, there is impingement of the tendons on the coracoacromial arch, which leads to tendon inflammation and increased reflex inhibition. This is the *vicious cycle of impingement* and can lead to rotator cuff tears or voluntary decreased motion to avoid pain with resultant adhesive capsulitis (frozen shoulder).

**IMPINGEMENT CYCLE**

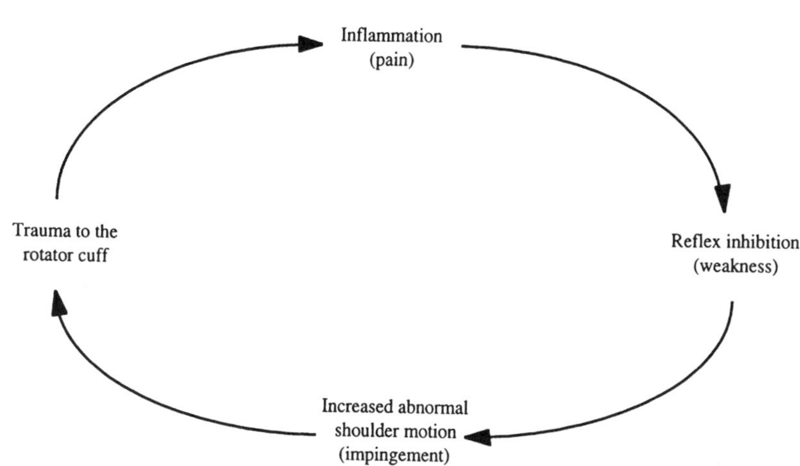


Vicious cycle in impingement syndrome.

**5. What are the three stages of shoulder impingement syndrome?**

- Stage I usually occurs under 25 years of age and is characterized by tendon hemorrhage and edema.
- Stage II usually occurs between 25 and 40 years and is characterized by tendinitis and fibrosis of the subacromial bursa.
- Stage III usually occurs over 40 years of age and is characterized by tears of the rotator cuff and biceps tendon.

Stages I and II are reversible with appropriate treatment.

**6. How is the impingement syndrome treated?**

The mainstays of management are physical therapy and anti-inflammatory medications. Regaining full shoulder motion and rotator cuff strength are the therapy goals. Inflammation in the tendons is treated with oral NSAIDs or a local injection of corticosteroid. Nonoperative management should be pursued for 9–12 months before consideration of surgical decompression, unless a full-thickness rotator cuff tear is present.

**7. Name the muscles of the rotator cuff.**

Remember the mnemonic **SITS**:

**S** — **S**upraspinatus
**I** — **I**nfraspinatus
**T** — **T**eres minor
**S** — **S**ubscapularis

**8. How does the impingement syndrome present clinically?**

- Pain with active shoulder movement (patient moves arm), especially flexion (between 60 and 120 degrees), abduction, and internal rotation
- Much less or no pain with passive movement (examiner moves arm)
- Absence of swelling, redness, or warmth at shoulder joint

- Radiographically, the space between the humeral head and inferior surface of the acromion may be < 8 mm

**9. What is the impingement sign?**

This maneuver produces pain in patients with the impingement syndrome. The examiner stands behind the patient. With one hand, the examiner prevents scapular movement and, with the other, moves the shoulder somewhere between flexion and abduction. If there is pain with this maneuver that is relieved with injection of local anesthetic, the diagnosis of impingement is supported.

**10. Describe the clinical aspects of subacromial bursitis.**

- Unusual to occur in the absence of the impingement syndrome
- Primary inflammation of the bursa may be due to crystal deposition or infection
- Clinical findings similar to those of the impingement syndrome
- Focal tenderness when area of bursa is palpated (see figure)

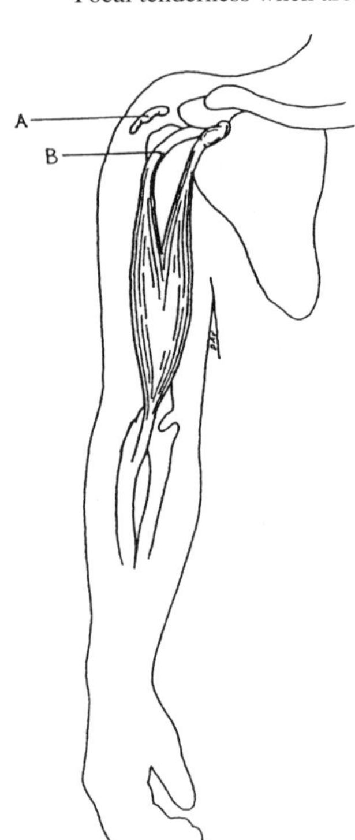


Shoulder anatomy. *A*, Subacromial bursa. *B*, Biceps tendon, long head.

**11. Describe the clinical aspects of bicipital tendinitis.**

- Anterior shoulder pain
- Pain worsened with active shoulder movement
- Positive Yergason's manuever and/or Speed's test
- Less pain with passive movement
- Absence of swelling, redness, or warmth at shoulder joint
- Focal tenderness when area overlying long head of biceps tendon is palpated (see figure)
- Frequently accompanies the impingement syndrome

**12. What are Yergason's maneuver and Speed's test?**

When one or both of these clinical signs are present, the diagnosis of bicipital tendinitis is supported:

**Yergason's maneuver**—Pain in the area of the long head of the biceps tendon is elicited by resisted supination of the forearm when the elbow is held at the side and flexed to 90 degrees.

**Speed's test**—Pain in the area of biceps tendon is elicited by resisted flexion of the upper arm with the elbow extended and the forearm supinated.

**13. What is a "frozen shoulder?"**

Also called adhesive capsulitis or pericapsulitis, frozen shoulder can occur after **any** cause of shoulder pain that leads an affected individual to limit the motion of the shoulder because of pain. With little movement, the shoulder joint capsule and surrounding structures contract, making range of motion physically restricted in addition to being painful. Arthrography shows decreased volume of the joint capsule. It is rarely seen before age 40 and, if not treated, can become permanent.

**14. Give three causes of nonarticular elbow pain.**

Lateral epicondylitis (tennis elbow)
Medial epicondylitis (golfer's elbow)
Olecranon bursitis

**15. List the clinical features of lateral epicondylitis.**

- Lateral elbow pain, especially with motions such as turning a screwdriver or shaking hands
- Pain is worsened with extension of the wrist, especially against resistance
- Pain is elicited by palpation at the origin of the wrist extensors (see figure)
- There may be swelling and warmth at the point of maximum tenderness
- Pain is caused by tendinitis of the wrist extensors

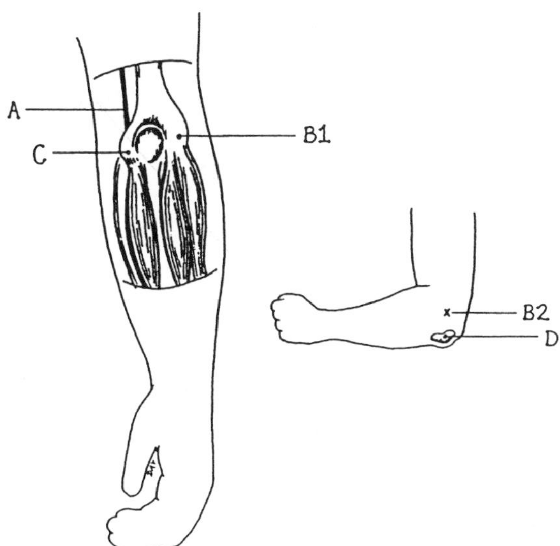


Anatomy of elbow. *A*, Ulnar nerve. *B1* and *B2*, Lateral epicondyle. *C*, Medial epicondyle. *D*, Olecranon bursa.

**16. List the clinical characteristics of medial epicondylitis.**

- Medial elbow pain
- Pain is worsened with flexion of the wrist, especially against resistance
- Pain is elicited by palpation at the origin of the wrist flexors (see figure)

- There may be swelling and warmth at the point of maximum tenderness
- Pain is caused by a tendinitis of the wrist flexors

**17. How is epicondylitis treated?**

- Avoid precipitating or exacerbating actions, if possible
- Forearm splint ("tennis elbow band")
- Nonsteroidal anti-inflammatory medications
- Ice (especially when symptomatic)
- Stretching and strengthening exercises directed at affected muscle groups
- Local corticosteroid injection
- Occasionally, splinting the wrist to prevent flexion and extension can help (*Caution*: the splint should be removed 2–3 times a day to allow wrist movement)

**18. Describe the clinical features of olecranon bursitis.**

- Pain, swelling, warmth at the location of the olecranon bursa on the extensor surface of the elbow (see figure)
- Bursa may be fluctuant and full
- Typically, elbow extension is normal but flexion may be limited
- Can be secondary to: trauma, rheumatoid arthritis, crystalline arthropathies (gout, CPPD), dialysis, or infection, especially if there is a break in the surrounding skin.

**19. What is deQuervain's tenosynovitis?**

- Tendinitis involving the abductor pollicis longus (APL) and extensor pollicis brevis (EPB) tendons
- Most frequently described as pain at the base of the thumb
- APL/EPB tendons form the palmar side of the anatomic snuffbox
- A positive Finkelstein maneuver supports the diagnosis

**20. What is the Finkelstein maneuver?**

The Finkelstein maneuver suggests the diagnosis of deQuervain's tenosynovitis when it reproduces the pain at the base of the thumb. To perform it, the patient touches the thumb to the base of the fifth finger, then wraps the other fingers around the thumb and abducts of the wrist (the fist moves toward the ulnar side).

**21. How is deQuervain's tenosynovitis treated?**

- Nonsteroidal anti-inflammatory medications
- Splint for the thumb and wrist called a *forearm-based thumb spica splint*
- Avoid precipitating or aggravating maneuvers
- Local corticosteroid injection
- Ice

**22. How does trochanteric bursitis present clinically?**

Patients complain of "hip pain." When asked to localize the pain, they point to the lateral aspect of the pelvis, with the area of greatest pain typically overlying the greater trochanter on the femur. Pain is exacerbated by lying on the affected side, walking, climbing stairs, and external rotation of the hip.

**23. What is "weaver's bottom"?**

- Also called ischial bursitis
- Bursa lies superficial to the ischial tuberosity
- Can be caused by prolonged sitting on hard surfaces, especially in thin individuals

**24. What is prepatellar bursitis?**

- Pain, swelling, and warmth in the prepatellar bursa
- Located superficial to the patella (see figure)

• Caused by repetitive trauma or overuse such as kneeling
• Can be infected, especially after breaks in the skin

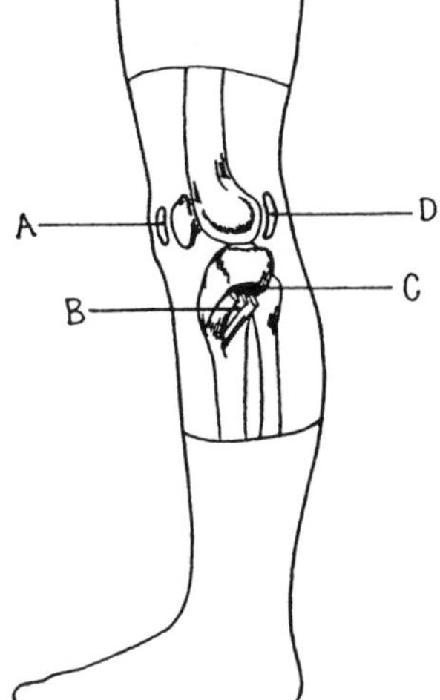


Anatomy of the knee. *A*, Prepatellar bursa. *B*, Conjoined tendons. *C*, Anserine bursa. *D*, Posterior fossa (where Baker's cyst will be felt).

**25. Give the common name for prepatellar bursitis.**
Housemaid's knee.

**26. What is anserine bursitis?**
Inflammation of the anserine bursa located at the medial aspect of the knee approximately 2 inches below the joint line. The bursa (see figure) lies between the tendons of the pes anserinus and the medial collateral ligament. It is frequently described as knee pain, but it is typically noticed when lying on one's side in bed when the knees are opposed. It is more common in obese individuals. Pain is elicited by palpating the bursa and may have associated warmth.

**27. Where do you find the pes anserinus?**
Literally meaning "goose's foot," it is the anatomic location of the conjoined tendons of the sartorius, gracilis, and semitendinosus muscles in the knee (see figure).

**28. What is Baker's cyst?**
Also called a popliteal cyst, this is swelling or fullness in the popliteal fossa with minimal tenderness (see figure). Its proposed etiology, in some individuals, involves a communication between the semimembranosus/gastrocnemius bursa and the knee joint. Some have postulated a one-way valve effect in which synovial fluid moves from the knee to the bursa. Baker's cysts can occur secondary to any process that produces synovial fluid (most commonly rheumatoid arthritis, osteoarthritis, or trauma). A ruptured cyst can occasionally dissect down the calf. It may be confused with deep venous thrombosis and is diagnosed with ultrasound or arthrography.

**29. Name five causes of heel pain.**
• Achilles enthesitis
• Achilles tendinitis
• Retrocalcaneal (Achilles) bursitis
• Plantar fasciitis
• Heel fat pad atrophy

**30. What is enthesitis?**

An **enthesis** is the place where a tendon or ligament inserts into bone. These areas can become inflamed in the spondyloarthropathies such as Reiter's syndrome or ankylosing spondylitis. Achilles enthesitis is a cause of heel pain and is characterized by swelling, warmth, and pain where the Achilles tendon inserts into the calcaneus (see figure).

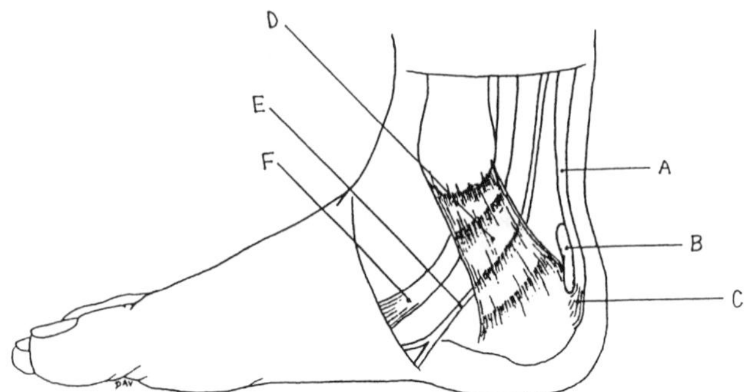


Anatomy of medial ankle and foot. *A*, Achilles tendon. *B*, Achilles bursa. *C*, Achilles enthesis. *D*, Flexor retinaculum. *E*, Posterior tibial nerve. *F*, Posterior tibial tendon.

**31. Describe the clinical features of Achilles tendinitis.**

- Heel pain, sometimes described as posterior leg pain
- Dorsiflexion increases the pain
- Area of most tenderness is 2–3 cm proximal to the insertion into the calcaneus (see figure)
- Tendon may be swollen with thickening, especially 2–3 cm proximal to the insertion
- May rupture spontaneously
  - Sudden onset of pain during dorsiflexion
  - Audible pop or snap
  - Positive "Thompson test"

**32. How is the Thompson test performed?**

The patient kneels on a chair with the feet extending back over the edge. As the examiner squeezes and pushes the calf toward the knee, normally plantarflexion of the foot should be seen but in rupture of the Achilles tendon, there will be no movement.

**33. How does retrocalcaneal (Achilles) bursitis present clinically?**

- Heel pain
- Fullness or swelling proximal and anterior to the insertion of the Achilles tendon into the calcaneus (see figure)
- Pain on palpation of the bursa

**34. Describe the clinical features of plantar fasciitis.**

Some may describe heel pain, but most affected individuals complain of pain along the plantar surface of the foot. The pain is worsened by pressure on the bottom of the foot (i.e walking, running, palpation). It is also worse with the first steps taken after getting out of bed in the morning. There is tenderness to palpation at the attachment site of the plantar fascia to the calcaneus.

**35. How is plantar fasciitis treated?**

- Initial therapy
  - Heel cup: consider custom orthotics if foot abnormalities are present
  - Nonsteroidal anti-inflammatory medications

Stretching exercises of the plantar fascia and Achilles tendon
Avoid weight-bearing exercise

- If no improvement after approximately 2–3 months, continue the plan above and add:
  Night splint: a removable splint to hold the foot in minimal dorsiflexion while sleeping
  Consider a local corticosteroid injection
- If no improvement after approximately 2–3 months, consider a referral for surgery

**36. What are the clinical features of heel fat pad atrophy?**

- Pain with prolonged standing or walking
- Pain with initial weight-bearing (i.e., in the morning)
- Tenderness to palpation in the central, plantar region of the heel
- Pain to palpation is improved with augmenting the fat pad (simultaneously squeezing the medial and lateral sides of the heel to force the subcutaneous tissue in a plantar direction)

**37. What is the significance of a heel spur?**

Heel pain is common. In many, it appears to be due to irritation of the subcutaneous tissue underneath the thick skin of the heel. It is worsened by pressure on the bottom of the foot (i.e., walking, running, palpation). Radiographically, an osteophyte (spur) can be seen to protrude from the calcaneus, and the pain is frequently attributed to the osteophyte irritating the surrounding tissue. Unfortunately, many people without heel spurs have similar pain, and some individuals with a heel spur seen radiographically are asymptomatic.

**38. What is posterior tibial tendinitis?**

Inflammation of the posterior tibial tendon and its synovial sheath. Pain is located more prominently on the medial side of the ankle. The pain and swelling are localized to the path of the posterior tibial tendon (see figure), with increased pain on resisted foot inversion.

**39. What are some clinical features of dysfunction or rupture of the posterior tibial tendon?**

- **Acquired pes planus**—Also called a flat foot, in which the normal contour of the longitudinal arch becomes flattened.
- **"Too many toes" sign**—Caused by hind-foot valgus and forefoot abduction. When the foot is viewed from behind the heel, you can see more toes over the lateral side of the affected foot than on the unaffected side.
- **"Heel-rise" sign**—The inability to rise to the ball of the affected foot while lifting the unaffected foot.

**40. How can the regional musculoskeletal syndromes be treated?**

- Avoid the precipitating movements or actions: bursitis and tendinitis can frequently be caused by repetitive motions or movements (e.g., biceps tendinitis caused by carrying a heavy briefcase daily).
- Rest the affected area: however, intermittent range of motion needs to be maintained, or the joint may contract or "freeze."
- Anti-inflammatory or analgesic medications: NSAIDs probably have a more important role than just analgesia.
- Splinting of the affected area (e.g., an elastic forearm band in epicondylitis).
- Local corticosteroid injections.
- Superficial heat and cold.
- Deep heat (ultrasound).
- Range of motion/flexibility exercises.
- Strengthening exercises.
- Ambulatory aids (cane, crutches, or walker).
- Surgery (bursectomy, tenosynovectomy, reattachment of ruptured tendons).

ACKNOWLEDGMENT

Illustrations by Debra Vogelgesang.

BIBLIOGRAPHY

1. Bland JH, Merritt JA, Boushey DR: The painful shoulder. Semin Arthritis Rheum 7:21–47, 1977.
2. Butcher JD, Salzman KL, Lillegard WA: Lower extremity bursitis. AFP 53:2317–2324, 1996.
3. Demaio M, Paine R, Mangine RE, Drez D Jr: Plantar fasciitis. Orthopedics 16:1153–1163, 1993.
4. Fulcher SM, Keifhaber TR, Stern PJ: Upper extremity tendinitis and overuse syndromes in the athlete. Clin Sports Med 17:433–448, 1998.
5. Neer CS II: Impingement lesions. Clin Orthop 173:70–77, 1983.
6. Salzman KL, Lillegard WA, Butcher JD: Upper extremity bursitis. AFP 56:1797–1806, 1997.
7. Smith DL, Campbell SM: Painful shoulder syndromes: Diagnosis and management. J Gen Intern Med 7:328–339, 1992.
8. Supple KM, Hanft JR, Murphy BJ, et al: Posterior tibial tendon dysfunction. Semin Arthritis Rheum 22:106–113, 1992.
9. Tisdel CL, Donley BG, Sferra JJ: Diagnosing and treating plantar fasciitis: A conservative approach to plantar heel pain. Cleveland Clinic J Med 66:231–235, 1999.

# 67. SPORTS MEDICINE AND OCCUPATIONAL INJURIES

*Donald G Eckhoff*, M.D., M.S.

**1. What is the difference between a sprain and a strain?**

A **sprain** is an acute traumatic injury to a **ligament**. There are three grades of sprains:

First-degree—mild pain due to tearing < 1/3 ligamentous fibers, < 5 mm laxity

Second-degree—moderate pain and swelling, 1/3–2/3 fibers of ligament torn, 5–10 mm laxity

Third-degree—severe pain from a complete rupture of the ligament causing joint instability

A **strain** is an acute traumatic injury to the **muscle-tendon junction**. It is commonly called a "pull." Strains are also classified according to three grades:

First-degree—mild

Second-degree—moderate injury associated with a weak and painful contraction of the involved muscle

Third-degree—complete tear of the muscle-tendon junction resulting in severe pain and an inability to contract the involved muscle

**2. How do overuse injuries and a sprain or strain differ?**

Strains and sprains are acute and traumatic in cause. Overuse injuries are nonacute injuries to the soft tissue structures due to chronic, repetitive microtrauma. Overuse injuries can involve the ligaments or the muscle-tendon junction. Microscopically, local tissue breakdown occurs with tissue lysis, lymphocytic infiltration, and blood extravasation.

Overuse injuries are reported to exist in 30–50% of the athletic population and are classified by four grades of injury:

Grade I—pain after activity only

Grade II—pain during and after activity but that does not interfere with performance

Grade III—pain during and after activity with interference with performance

Grade IV—constant pain that interferes with activities of daily living

**3. List some common overuse injuries of ligaments and tendons occurring in athletes.**

| Ligaments | Tendons |
|---|---|
| Little leaguer's elbow | Achilles tendinitis |
| Swimmer's knee | Suprapatellar tendinitis |
| Iliotibial band syndrome | Posterior tibialis tendinitis |
| Jumper's knee | De Quervain's tenosynovitis |
| Plantar fasciitis | Lateral epicondylitis (tennis elbow) |
| | Supraspinatus (rotator cuff) tendinitis |
| | Bicipital tendinitis |

**4. Is there any difference between tendinitis, tendinosis, and tenosynovitis?**

**Tendinitis** is usually due to tendon trauma with associated vascular disruption and acute, subacute, or chronic inflammation.

**Tendinosis** is noninflammatory, intratendinous atrophy and degeneration that is often associated with chronic tendinitis. Tendinosis can lead to partial or complete tendon rupture.

**Tenosynovitis** is inflammation of the paratendon, which is the outermost sheath that is lined in some tendons by a synovial membrane (e.g., extensor tendons of thumb in De Quervain's tenosynovitis).

**5. What is tennis elbow?**

**Tennis elbow**, better termed **lateral epicondylitis**, is an overuse syndrome that presents with lateral elbow pain. Etiologically, few patients who present with this disorder have acquired it through playing tennis. The differential diagnosis of lateral elbow pain includes local conditions, elbow arthritis, loose body in the elbow, nerve compression of the radial nerve or posterior interosseous nerve, and cervical spondylosis with radiculitis.

At present, lateral epicondylitis is believed to be an inflammatory process and/or microtearing involving the origin of the extensor carpi radialis brevis muscle. Provocative testing of forced middle-finger extension against resistance should reproduce pain, as the muscle in question inserts on the base of the middle-finger metacarpal. Treatment is conservative, with a tennis elbow band (Chopat strap) that anchors the muscle in the proximal forearm and unloads the true origin during activities; this is worn for 9–12 months. Oral NSAIDs are also used, as is local corticosteroid injection and physical therapy.

**6. Golfer's elbow and little leaguer's elbow sound similar mechanically to tennis elbow. Are they?**

**Golfer's elbow**, better termed a **medial epicondylitis**, results from an overuse injury to the tendinous origin of the flexor pronator muscle mass. This area is placed under valgus stress at the top of a backswing in golfing and proceeds through the downswing until impact with the golf ball. Pain is elicited over the elbow's medial epicondyle and is increased with resisted wrist flexion and forearm pronation. Management includes rest, ice, NSAIDs, and splints. Steroid injections and surgery are rarely required.

**Little leaguer's elbow** is a **medial apophysitis** seen mostly in young pitchers between ages 9 and 12 years. It occurs as a result of valgus stress, often from throwing curve balls. The person experiences microtearing of the flexor pronator muscle group and, in severe cases, fragmentation of the medial epicondylar apophysis. Treatment is 2–3 weeks of rest, no throwing for 6–12 weeks, and rarely surgery if the medial apophysis is displaced.

**7. What is impingement?**

Repetitive overhead activity, muscle imbalance, or deconditioning can lead to inflammation secondary to pinching the supraspinatus tendon, biceps tendon, and sub-acromial bursa between the acromion and humeral head. Chronic or recurring impingement leads to progressive degeneration and eventual failure (rupture) of the soft tissues (biceps and rotator cuff). The following table summarizes the natural history of shoulder impingement:

| STAGE | AGE | PATHOLOGY | DDx | CLINICAL COURSE |
|---|---|---|---|---|
| I | < 25 | Edema<br>Hemorrhage | Subluxation<br>Arthritic | Reversible |
| II | 25–40 | Fibrosis<br>Tendinitis | Frozen shoulder<br>Calcification | Recurrent |
| III | > 40 | Bone spurs<br>Tendon rupture | Radiculitis<br>Neoplasm | Progressive |

Charles Neer (1983)

**8. What clinical test is used to diagnose a rotator cuff tear (RCT)?**

The diagnosis is made by combining the epidemiology of RCT with the patient's history, physical examination, and imaging results. Cadaver and patient studies show that RCT is associated with the natural aging of the shoulder with 50% of patients > 59 years old having asymptomatic RCT. On the history, rotator cuff tear can present after a single traumatic event (shoulder dislocation) or as the end result of the impingement syndrome. If the tear is large, the rotator cuff will have lost its mechanical function and a positive **drop arm test** will result. A drop arm test is performed by allowing the patient to bring the arm down from a position of full abduction. When 90° of abduction is reached, the arm drops involuntarily toward the patient's side. Pain is not a part of this test.

If the cuff tear is small, as in early stage III impingement, the cuff will retain enough of its mechanical function so that the drop arm sign will not be positive; but patients may exhibit a similar response secondary to pain. Weakness can usually be demonstrated if the pain is removed. Therefore, to aid in diagnosis, a subacromial bursal injection of lidocaine is used to anesthetize the rotator cuff. Once done, strength of resisted abduction at 90° is tested. In addition, a small RCT will usually exhibit weakness in abduction and external rotation with the arm adducted to the side when compared with the opposite side.

**9. How is radiographic imaging used to diagnose rotator cuff tears?**

Imaging modalities are quite useful but not always required to make the diagnosis of RCT. **Plain films** may show superior migration of the humeral head toward the acromion, with an acromio-humeral distance of < 7 mm being suggestive of RCT. This is due to loss of the rotator cuff humeral head depression function. Signs of cuff-tear arthropathy may also appear on plain films. **Ultrasound** can be used to diagnose a RCT, but is operator-dependent. **MRI** can show full-thickness tears, tendinitis, and sometimes partial-thickness tears as well as other articular and peri-articular pathology. The once gold standard test for RCT, the **arthrogram**, is a test in which dye is injected into the joint. In a patient with a full-thickness RCT, dye will be visualized traversing the rotator cuff into the subacromial/subdeltoid bursae. Sizing tears and defining other pathology are limited with the arthrogram, limitations that combined with the morbidity of a contrast injection make this method less popular than MRI as the imaging modality of choice.

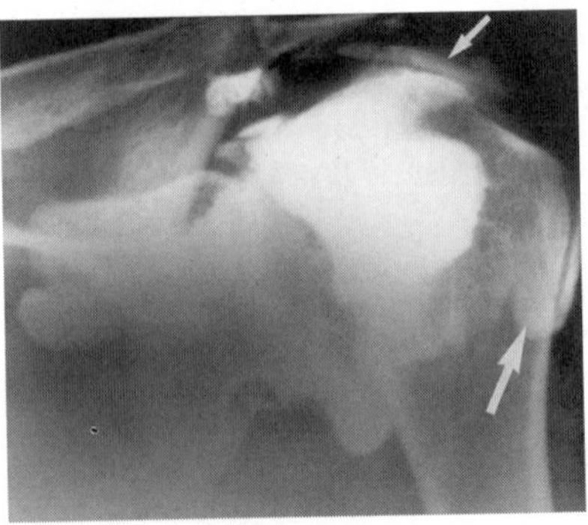

Rotator cuff tear with contrast extending into the subacromial (short arrow) and subdeltoid (long arrow) bursa.

**10. What is a stinger (burner) injury?**

The stinger is well known in football, resulting from forced lateral deviation of the neck and inferior force on the ipsilateral shoulder. This occurs with tackling, blocking, or ground contact. A traction injury to the brachial plexus results, predominately affecting the upper extremity. Players complain of significant shoulder and arm pain involving the lateral aspect of the entire upper extremity. Occasionally, shoulder pain is the only complaint. Motor weakness of the involved C5 and C6 root innervated muscles is commonly associated. A stinger should be managed by rest and avoidance of sports participation until normal strength has returned.

**11. What is a hip pointer?**

A hip pointer refers to a contusion of the iliac crest that usually results from a direct blow to the iliac crest during a contact sport (i.e., football). The athlete experiences severe localized pain, and an audible pop or snap commonly occurs at the time of injury. Frequently, the athlete cannot walk. Physical examination reveals tenderness, swelling, and often ecchymosis that can migrate down the leg. Treatment is ice, analgesics, and a supervised stretching program.

**12. Is a snapping hip the same as iliotibial band friction syndrome?**

A **snapping hip** occurs when the patient reports sounds or sensations of internal hip clicking with flexion and extension. This may reflect a torn acetabular labrum, or it may occur as the iliopsoas passes over the pelvic brim or as the iliotibial band moves over the greater trochanter. The patient usually does not have pain unless there is an associated bursitis. This usually occurs as a result of a tight iliotibial band or muscle imbalance.

The **iliotibial band (ITB) friction syndrome** causes lateral knee pain and is related to irritation and inflammation at the distal portion of the iliotibial band as it courses over the lateral femoral condyle. There is increased pain on palpation of this band distally and as the knee goes from flexion to extension. The patient usually has a positive **Ober test**. The Ober test is done by placing the patient on his or her side with the affected leg upward. The injured leg is flexed to 90° at the knee and fully abducted, following which the hip is extended. The leg is released and allowed to adduct. Pain or tightness (the knee will not cross the midline of the body) on adduction is considered a positive test.

The ITB syndrome is usually caused by running excessively or running uphill or on slanted surfaces. Treatment consists of stretching the iliotibial band, ice, modalities, NSAIDs, better training techniques, and rarely corticosteroid injections.

**13. How do swimmer's knee, jumper's knee, and runner's knee differ from each other?**

**Swimmer's knee** (breaststroker's knee) is knee pain due to the valgus stress placed on the knee by the whip kick used in swimming the breaststroke. This usually results in medial collateral ligament stress/strain causing pain.

**Jumper's knee** is an accepted term for **patellar tendinitis**. It is common in high jumpers and volleyball or basketball players. This injury is characterized by pain at the inferior pole of the patella at its attachment to the patellar tendon. It is due to repetitive stress whose frequency of occurrence exceeds the body's rate of natural repair or healing.

**Runner's knee** is more correctly called **patellofemoral syndrome**. This is the most common injury in runners and accounts for 30+% of running injuries. Pain is due to compression of nerve fibers in the retinaculum or in the subchondral bone of the patella or from a synovitis. It is not due to chondromalacia patellae (softening of the cartilage).

**14. How is a diagnosis of chondromalacia patellae made?**

By visually inspecting the cartilage surface of the patella at the time of surgery. The term *chondromalacia patellae* refers to a degenerative condition of the articular surface of the patella that progresses from softening, through fibrillar changes and full-thickness cracks, to exposed subchondral bone. It is graded from I to IV, according to the Outerbridge classification system, using the above descriptors, as well as the size of the lesion.

**15. List the differential diagnosis for anterior knee pain.**

For many years, chondromalacia patellae was used as a catch-all term for patients with anterior knee pain. Patellofemoral syndrome (PFS) was the next generalized title that evolved for this group of patients. The current accepted diagnosis is anterior knee pain. The differential diagnosis is extensive:

- Chondromalacia patellae
- Patellar malalignment
- Patellar tracking abnormality
- Tendinitis quadriceps/patellae
- Tight iliotibial band
- Meniscal pathology
- Painful bipartite patella
- Blunt trauma, occult fracture
- Osteochondritis dissecans (patella)
- Sinding-Larsen-Johansson syndrome
- Symptomatic plica of the knee
- Fat pad syndrome (Hoffa's disease)
- Bursitis, infrapatellar/prepatellar
- Pes anserine bursitis
- Retinacular neuroma
- Tight lateral retinaculum
- Post-surgical neuroma
- Referred pain from hip
- Radicular pain from lumbosacral spine

**16. What is the most common condition giving rise to anterior knee pain?**

Patellar maltracking due to a relative weakness of the vastus medialis portion of the quadriceps. This maltracking leads to increased pressure on the lateral facet of the patella and pain. With time, it can lead to chondromalacia. It is common in young adults and responds to directed rehabilitation of the quadriceps and stretching of the hamstrings. Adjunctive modalities of oral NSAIDs and patellar centralizing bracing or taping can also be effective.

Other common conditions that affect the patella and give rise to anterior knee pain are true patellar malalignment, limb malrotation, and tendinitis.

**17. What physical exam tests are most sensitive and specific for the diagnosis of an anterior cruciate ligament (ACL) injury?**

The best-known test for ACL deficiency is the anterior drawer sign, which measures anterior translation subjectively.

The most sensitive test is the **Lachman test**. The relaxed knee is placed in 20° of flexion, the distal femur is stabilized by one of the examiner's hands, and the proximal tibia is then translated anteriorly by the other hand. ACL-deficient knees exhibit increased translation and a soft or mushy endpoint, as compared with the opposite, uninjured knee.

The most specific test is the **pivot shift test**. It is performed by applying a valgus and internal rotation force on the tibia with the knee in full extension and hip abducted 10–20°. The knee is then gently flexed. A clunk of tibial rotation is appreciated as the knee passes 20–30° of flexion. This must be compared with the opposite side. The appreciable clunk occurs when the tibia, which is abnormally subluxated (anterior and internally rotated secondary to ACL absence), is pulled back into its normal position by the secondary restraints. This test is highly dependent on patient relaxation and is not recommended in the acutely injured, unanesthetized knee.

**18. How will a meniscal tear present, and what is the best test?**

The meniscus functions as a cushion between the femur and tibia on the medial and lateral sides of the knee. It is well suited to compression but tears when subjected to shear with a turning or twisting motion. The nutrition of the inner 2/3 meniscus is limited and predisposes the torn tissue to not heal once torn, a factor reflected by the typical chronic recurring history of symptoms. The torn tissue may create a mechanical block to the free motion of the knee, which will manifest symptomatically as clicking, popping, and locking, and be associated with pain and swelling at the joint line. These symptoms correlate, but often unreliably, to an audible/palpable pop with flexion/extension of the knee with the patient sitting (McMurray's test) and prone (Apley's test) on physical exam. The history and physical findings can be confused with patello-femoral pathology, particularly in the absence of a single precipitation event. Diagnosis is reliably confirmed by MRI or arthroscopy, and the problem is most efficiently remedied by arthroscopic repair or partial menisectomy.

**19. What is the "terrible triad" of knee injury?**

An ACL tear, complete medial collateral ligament tear, and a tear of the medial meniscus. This combination is almost always a result of sporting activities, particularly football. The knee in these injuries exhibits a markedly positive anterior drawer test, a positive Lachman's and pivot shift test, and marked valgus angulation with applied stress in full extension. The knee will be stable to varus stress testing because the lateral collateral ligament and posterior cruciate ligament remain intact. Effusion from hemarthrosis may be mild secondary to medial capsular tearing, which allows the traumatic bleeding to exit the knee joint. Suspicion of an injury of this magnitude should lead to the prompt referral to an orthopedic surgeon.

**20. Name two lower extremity tendon injuries commonly occurring in runners.**

Achilles tendinitis (see Chapter 66)
Posterior tibialis tendinitis (see Chapter 66)

**21. What is the best treatment for acute rupture of the Achilles tendon?**

Acute Achilles tendon rupture usually results from a forced contraction of the gastrocnemius muscle against resistance, which occurs either during sports participation or from a fall. It is not rare, and these are not subtle injuries. The patient usually presents with pain, most notable in walking, and with weakness in the push-off phase of gait. A positive Thompson test is common.

The best treatment remains controversial. Options include closed treatment with placement in a long or short leg cast with the foot in equinus (plantar-flexed by gravity). A percutaneous suture repair has been reported with good results but may risk some injury to the sural nerve. The third option is open direct primary surgical repair.

Many long-term studies have compared surgical versus nonsurgical treatment. The healing rate is excellent with all techniques. The closed technique requires longer cast immobilization and results in more ankle stiffness in the short-term. The biggest question revolves around the rate of rerupture. Rerupture rates are reported to be 1–5% with surgical treatment and 8–16% with closed-cast treatment. Therefore, selection of the best treatment option is individualized, with age, activity level, patient and surgeon interests, and experience as guiding parameters. The best treatment for rerupture is not controversial and universally accepted to be open surgical repair.

**22. What is the relationship of plantar fasciitis to the plantar heel spur seen on the lateral foot x-ray?**

This is an area of uncertainty. For years, the heel spur was believed to be a significant cause of heel pain, and surgical excision was common treatment. Now, with more information from anatomic dissection and clinical studies, the relationship, if any, becomes less clear.

Anatomically, the spur is located in the origin of the flexor digitorum brevis, located inferiorly on the anteromedial aspect of the calcaneal tuberosity just deep to the origin of the plantar fascia. Overuse of either of these two structures is thought to produce reactive inflammatory bone production or spur formation secondary to traction, but it is not clear which (if not both) mechanisms are responsible. In either case, the spur is secondary to an overuse phenomenon and treatment should be directed at the cause and not the result.

**23. What is a "turf toe"?**

Turf toe is a sprain of the plantar capsule ligament complex of the MTP joint of the great toe. It is more common on artificial turf and due to a hyperextension injury. Hyperflexion and valgus injuries to this toe can cause similar symptoms. Treatment includes rest, taping of the toe to restrict dorsiflexion, and stiffening of the sole of the shoe to prevent motion. Without proper therapy, hallux rigidus can result.

**24. How do a "shin splint" and a stress fracture differ?**

**Shin splint** is an overuse injury caused by chronic traction and inflammation of the tibial periostium. It may involve either tibialis muscles or the soleus muscle and is characterized by anteromedial or posteromedial leg pain of gradual onset. Pain occurs at the start of running, then decreases, and returns after the athlete stops running. Tenderness is found on palpation of the posterior medial border of the tibia, usually at the junction of the middle and distal thirds. Pain is increased with resisted dorsiflexion. Radiographs are normal, but a bone scan shows fusiform uptake of tracer. Shin splint is sometimes called **medial tibial stress syndrome**.

A **stress fracture** is an overuse injury that occurs when periosteal resorption exceeds bone formation. The tibia is the most common site for stress fractures (30%) in runners, but other areas can be affected depending on the activity or sport. A tibial stress fracture causes pain in runners the entire time they are running as well as afterward. There is often a focal area of tenderness along the anterior tibia. The pain is increased if a vibrating tuning fork is put over the site. Radiographs are usually negative at onset but become abnormal after 5 or more weeks. A bone scan shows uptake, and CT scan/MRI scans are abnormal. Avoidance of activity is necessary to permit repair and to prevent progression to complete fracture.

**25. What are some hand injuries that can occur in athletes?**

1. **Mallet finger**. Extensor tendon avulsion with or without fracture involving the distal interphalangeal (DIP) joint. The athlete cannot extend the DIP joint.
2. **Jersey finger**. Avulsion of the flexor digitorum profundus tendon causing inability to flex the DIP joint. Usually occurs from grabbing a jersey when tackling in football.
3. **Gamekeeper's thumb**. Rupture of the ulnar collateral ligament of the first metacarpophalangeal (MCP) joint. Frequent in skiing injuries.
4. **Boxer's knuckle**. Longitudinal tear of the extensor digitorum communis tendon or sagittal bands overlying the metacarpal head (usually the third MCP), resulting in extensor weakness of that finger.

**26. How common are occupational overuse injuries?**

Repetitive movements for prolonged periods can lead to overuse injuries in several professions. Approximately 10–20% of musicians, typists, keypunch/calculator/cash register operators, and assembly-line workers will experience a repetitive strain syndrome. The most common problems are bicipital tendinitis, carpal tunnel syndrome, and deQuervain's tendinitis. Patients presenting with tendinitis need to have a complete occupational history obtained to determine if their work is causing their problems.

**27. What occupations are associated with osteoarthritis?**

Several occupations can cause stress and trauma to joints, leading to early osteoarthritis. This occurs most likely in joints that have been previously injured, have an abnormal joint alignment, or are unstable as a result of ligamentous injury. Examples include ballet dancers (ankle, feet); farmers (hips); miners, riveters, or metal workers (elbows); pneumatic tool operators (hands or wrists); coal miners (knees); and cotton mill workers (hands). The relationship between osteoarthritis and sporting activities is less clear, owing to repeated joint injuries in addition to repetitive loading.

**28. Discuss the principles of treatment of tendinitis and overuse injuries.**

The general principles of management can be remembered with the mnemonic PRICES:

| Primary Therapies | Secondary Therapies |
|---|---|
| **P** — Protection | **P**hysical modalities |
| **R** — Rest | **R**ehabilitation |
| **I** — Ice | **I**njections |
| **C** — Compression | **C**ross-training |
| **E** — Elevation | **E**valuation and re-evaluation |
| **S** — Support | **S**alicylates |

Treatment of soft-tissue injuries with early control of pain and inflammation is critical. Sustained inflammation decreases soft-tissue healing and leads to gradual deconditioning and functional disability. With acute problems, relative rest is important. Ice is an effective anti-inflammatory in the first hours after an injury. Heat is often preferred after the acute injury. Orthotics, splinting, braces, or taping may be used to facilitate protected motion.

**29. When are medications useful?**

NSAIDs are often used, and all NSAIDs are equally effective. After acute injuries, there is little evidence to support using them for longer than 72 hours. More prolonged use is recommended for chronic overuse conditions.

Corticosteroid injections for chronic conditions are not definitive treatment but should be used to facilitate rehabilitation. Injections should be performed by clinicians experienced in performing these procedures and who are familiar with the side effects. Corticosteroids can increase the rate of collagen degradation, decrease new collagen formation, lower tendon tensile strength, and lead to tendon rupture if the procedure is performed incorrectly or too often. The patient should be advised to restrict activity of the affected area for 2–3 weeks after an injection.

ACKNOWLEDGMENT

The editor and author wish to thank John Reister, M.D., for his contributions to this chapter in the previous edition of this book.

## BIBLIOGRAPHY

1. Fulkerson JP: Patellofemoral pain disorders: Evaluation and management. JOAAOS 2:124–132, 1994.
2. Jobe FW, Ciccotti MG: Lateral and medial epicondylitis of the elbow. JOAAOS 12:1–8, 1994.
3. Lintner SA, Feagin JA, Boland AL: Sports medicine. In Ruddy S, Harris ED, Sledge CB (eds): Kelley's Textbook of Rheumatology, 6th ed. Philadelphia, WB Saunders, 2001, pp 439–456.
4. Neer CS: Impingement lesions. Clin Orthop 173:70–77, 1983.
5. O'Connor FG, Sobel JR, Nirschl RP: Five-step treatment for overuse injuries. Phys Sports Med 20(10):128–142, 1992.
6. Panush RS: Occupational and recreational musculoskeletal disorders. In Ruddy S, Harris ED, Sledge CB (eds): Kelley's Textbook of Rheumatology, 6th ed. Philadelphia, WB Saunders, 2001, pp 429—438.
7. Swain RA, Kaplan BK: Practice and pitfalls of corticosteroid injections. Phys Sports Med 23(3):27–40, 1995.
8. Torg JS, Glasgow SG: Criteria for return to contact activities following cervical spine injury. Clin J Sports Med 1:12–26, 1991

# 68. ENTRAPMENT NEUROPATHIES

*David* R. *Finger*, M.D.

**1. What are entrapment neuropathies, and how do they occur?**

Entrapment neuropathies occur when a peripheral nerve is compressed within an enclosed anatomic space. Entrapment can occur from increased pressure, stretch, angulation, ischemia, or friction; previously compromised nerves, such as from alcoholism or diabetes, are more vulnerable. The nerve damage is characterized by physiologic slowing, demyelination, and remyelination; intraoperative exposure of the involved nerve often reveals swelling proximal to the site of entrapment.

**2. Do entrapment neuropathies occur in rheumatoid arthritis?**

Inflammation and swelling of synovium, bursae, ligaments, or tendon sheaths all can cause pressure on adjacent nerves. Entrapment neuropathies have been reported to occur in nearly half of chronic RA patients at some point in their lifetime. Interestingly, there does not appear to be any correlation with duration of disease, positive rheumatoid factor, level of acute phase reactants (sedimentation rate), functional class, or extra-articular disease. Carpal tunnel syndrome (CTS) occurs with a reported frequency of 23–69% in RA.

**3. What are some other etiologies that should be considered when evaluating entrapment neuropathies?**

- Polyneuropathies
- Brachial plexopathy
- Radiculopathy
- Raynaud's phenomenon
- Reflex sympathetic dystrophy
- Vasculitis
- Tendinitis

**4. How are entrapment neuropathies usually diagnosed?**

The presence of characteristic symptoms along with provocative maneuvers (Tinel's sign) is usually adequate to support the diagnosis. Electrodiagnostic studies (nerve conduction velocities and electromyography) are often used to confirm and localize the site of entrapment, although this study can be normal in 10 to 25% of patients.

**5. When are electrodiagnostic studies indicated?**

- When the diagnosis is uncertain
- To exclude radiculopathy or polyneuropathy
- To follow the course of patients being treated conservatively
- Prior to surgery

**6. Describe characteristic clinical features of entrapment neuropathies.**

- Dysesthesias, usually localized to the sensory distribution of the involved nerve
- Symptoms described as burning, tingling, pain, or "pins and needles"
- Symptoms not use-related
- Tenderness of the involved area is usually not a feature
- Symptoms usually worse at night and while at rest
- Muscle weakness and atrophy are late findings
- Usually unilateral, with the exception of idiopathic CTS
- Swelling or vasomotor abnormalities absent

**7. Describe physical exam signs indicative of an entrapment neuropathy.**

A positive **Tinel's sign** occurs when tapping the nerve at the site of entrapment produces pain and dysesthesias radiating into the sensory distribution of the nerve distally. In CTS, this test has a reported sensitivity between 40 and 60% and specificity between 70 and 94%. **Phalen's test** can be performed to elicit CTS, with a positive test occurring when maximal passive wrist flexion for 1 minute produces or worsens paresthesias in the median nerve distribution. It has an approximate sensitivity of 75% and specificity of 50–80% for CTS. A recently described sign, the **volar hot dog** (swelling at the wrist on the ulnar side of the palmaris longus tendon), has been reported in over 90% of patients with CTS.

**8. What is the carpal tunnel syndrome (CTS)?**

Carpel tunnel syndrome (CTS) is easily the most common entrapment neuropathy, with a prevalence of 0.2–1%. CTS occurs when the median nerve is compressed by the flexor retinaculum at the wrist, producing characteristic nocturnal dysesthesias but occasionally progressing to sensory loss and weakness of thumb abduction (see figure, top of next page). This condition is bilateral in half of patients and occurs with increased frequency in occupations associated with high levels of repetition and force (meatpackers, shellfish packing, musicians).

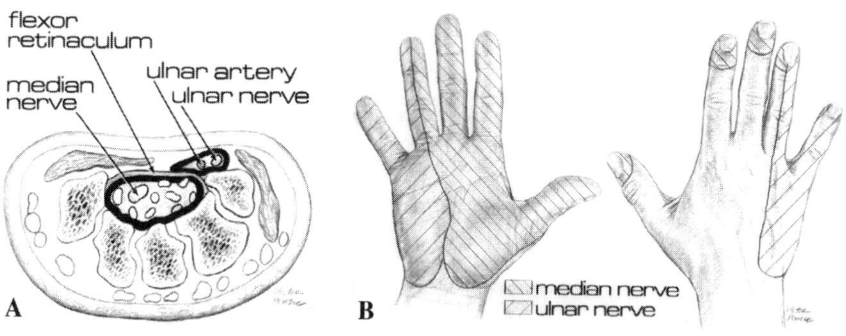


*A*, Wrist anatomy showing the median nerve through the carpal tunnel in close proximity to Guyon's canal, where the ulnar nerve passes. *B*, Median and ulnar nerve sensory distributions. (Illustration by Victor Powell.)

**9. List some diseases associated with CTS.**

Use the mnemonic **PRAGMATIC**.

**P**regnancy (20%)
**R**heumatoid arthritis (any inflammatory arthritis)
**A**cromegaly
**G**lucose (diabetes)
**M**echanical (overuse, occupational)
**A**myloid
**T**hyroid (myxedema)
**I**nfection (TB, fungal)
**C**rystals (gout, pseudogout)

**10. What are the treatment options for CTS?**

**Nonsurgical therapy** consists of avoidance of repetitive wrist motion, cock-up wrist splints at night (and for work), along with anti-inflammatory medications. Local corticosteroid injections result in excellent short-term relief in 80%. Indications for **surgical therapy** (sectioning of the transverse carpal ligament) include failure of conservative therapy, lifestyle limiting symptoms, and muscle weakness or atrophy. Surgical results are favorable in over 90% of patients. Complete recovery of nerve function occurs only if surgery is performed before evidence of denervation on EMG/NCV.

**11. Where else can median nerve entrapment occur?**

The **anterior interosseous nerve syndrome** occurs when this nerve, a purely motor branch of the median nerve, is compressed 6 cm distal to the lateral epicondyle. The resulting loss of distal thumb and index finger flexion produces a characteristic **flattened pinch sign** (inability to form an "O"). The **pronator teres syndrome** occurs when the median nerve is compressed by the pronator teres muscle at the forearm, resulting in proximal forearm pain that is worsened by grasping and pronation.

**12. Describe the various ulnar nerve entrapment syndromes.**

Ulnar nerve compression at the elbow, the second most common entrapment neuropathy of the upper extremity, can occur from external pressure at the medial epicondylar groove (synovitis, osteophytes, anesthetized patients with prolonged resting of the elbow on a flat surface), flexion dislocation, and compression at the aponeurosis of the flexor carpi ulnaris, the so-called cubital tunnel (see figure, next page). **Cubital tunnel syndrome** results in paresthesias in an ulnar nerve distribution, weakness in pinching and grasping, and hypothenar atrophy. Ulnar nerve entrapment is often exacerbated by elbow flexion. Therapy consists of avoidance of prolonged elbow flexion, local steroid injections (in RA), and surgical release in severe cases. **Ulnar tunnel**

**syndrome** occurs when the ulnar nerve is compressed in Guyon's canal at the wrist (see preceding figure), resulting in symptoms similar to those seen in the cubital tunnel syndrome. When ulnar nerve entrapment occurs insidiously, with few dysesthesias or sensory changes, this is referred to as **tardy ulnar palsy**.

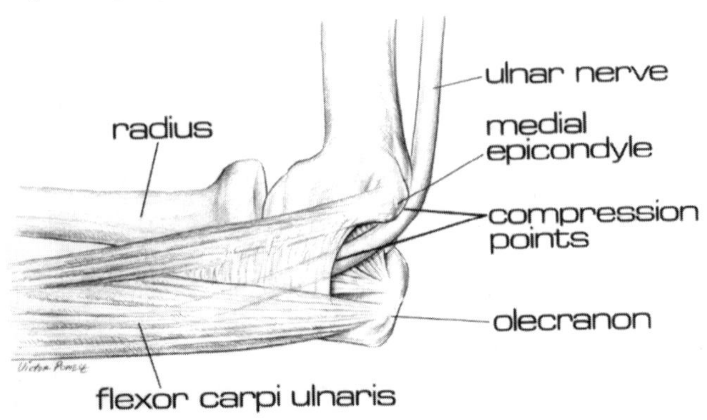


Anatomy of the ulnar nerve at the elbow, showing sites of common entrapment at the medial epicondyle and the cubital tunnel. (Illustration by Victor Powell.)

**13. What is the thoracic outlet syndrome (TOS)?**

This syndrome, which is often difficult to diagnose, can occur from either vascular or neurologic compression. Vasogenic TOS occurs when occlusion of the subclavian artery results in ischemic symptoms, or when venous occlusion results in edema, engorged superficial veins, and thrombosis. Neurogenic TOS occurs when there is brachial plexus impingement from a cervial rib (35%), fibrous tissue bands, scalene muscles, or an elongated transverse process of C7. This results in weakness of the intrinsic muscles of the hand along with sensory loss in the ulnar distribution over the hand and forearm. The **Adson maneuver** is performed by palpating the radial pulse while the patient inhales deeply and extends the neck, turning the head to the side being examined. A positive Adson maneuver occurs when there is diminution of the radial pulse and reproduction of symptoms. Another provocation test, the **hyperabduction maneuver**, is performed with the arm abducted to 180 degrees in external rotation. Electrodiagnostic studies are usually normal, and many normal people have false-positive physical exam provocation tests. Treatment consists of range of motion and strengthening exercises to improve posture, avoidance of hyperabduction, and surgery for those patients with severe, refractory symptoms (cervical rib or fibrous band resection).

**14. How does radial nerve entrapment occur?**

Improper positioning during anesthesia, sleeping on the arm, or improperly fitting crutches can result in prolonged compression of the nerve along the radial groove on the humerus. This results in wrist-drop, referred to as **Saturday night palsy** because it often occurs while the patient is intoxicated. The **posterior interosseous nerve**, a motor branch of the radial nerve, can be impinged at the elbow with resulting weakness in finger extension.

**15. What is meralgia paresthetica?**

Meralgia (Greek for "pain in the thigh") paresthetica results when the lateral cutaneous nerve of the thigh, a sensory nerve, is compressed at the inguinal ligament just medial to the anterior superior iliac spine. This syndrome results in burning pain and dysesthesia over the anteriolateral thigh (see figure). Common causes include obesity, pregnancy, trauma, surgical injury (appendectomy or inguinal herniorrhapy), tight-fitting clothing (belts), and diabetes mellitus. This syndrome usually is self-limiting, and treatment is conservative, involving weight loss, avoidance of tight clothing, and occasional local steroid injections at the site of compression.

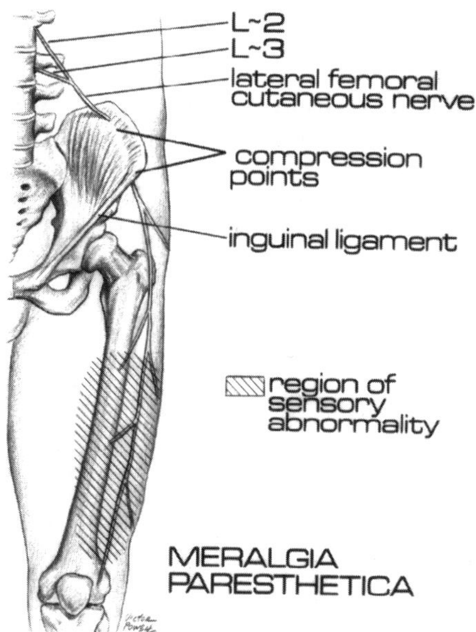


Anatomy of the lateral femoral cutaneous nerve. The inguinal ligament and the anterior superior iliac spine are most likely points of entrapment. (Illustration by Victor Powell.)

**16. Describe the piriformis syndrome.**

This controversial syndrome refers to sciatica that arises from entrapment of the sciatic nerve by the piriformis muscle. Symptoms include pain over the buttocks radiating down the back of the leg. It occurs more commonly in women and is usually precipitated by trauma. Physical examination reveals pain and sciatica on resisted hip external rotation (sometimes on internal rotation) along with tenderness of the piriformis muscle on rectal or vaginal examination. Local steroid injections can be beneficial.

**17. A 50-year-old woman presents with pain and burning between her third and fourth toe. Symptoms are worsened by walking on hard surfaces and wearing high heels. The region between her third and fourth metatarsal heads is tender to palpation. What is the most likely diagnosis?**

**Morton's neuroma**, caused by entrapment of the interdigital plantar nerve most commonly by the transverse metatarsal ligament, usually located between the third and fourth or second and third metatarsal heads. This occurs more commonly in women who wear tight-fitting shoes. Metatarsal compression may cause a palpable click as the neuroma is forced downward, where it may be felt on plantar surface. Treatment consists of wearing more supportive shoes, padding the metatarsal heads, and local steroid injections. Surgical removal is done if conservative therapy fails.

**18. Which nerve is most likely to be compressed in a patient presenting with a painless foot-drop?**

The common peroneal nerve. **Peroneal nerve palsy** usually occurs following compression over the head of the fibula from prolonged leg crossing, squatting, leg casts and braces. The distal lateral leg often has decreased sensation, and foot eversion (superficial peroneal nerve) and dorsiflexion (deep peroneal nerve) are affected because the lesion occurs proximally in the common peroneal nerve.

**19. A patient with rheumatoid arthritis presents with burning dysesthesias of toes and sole extending proximally to the medial malleolus; it is worse at night but somewhat relieved by walking. What syndrome does this patient most likely have?**

The tarsal tunnel syndrome. This syndrome occurs when the posterior tibial nerve is compressed at the flexor retinaculum, located posterior and inferior to the medial malleolus (see following figure). A positive **Tinel's sign** (obtained by percussing posterior to the medial malleolus) and a positive **tourniquet test** (applying pressure over the flexor retinaculum) will often reproduce the symptoms. This occurs more often in women, and is associated with trauma, fracture, valgus deformity, hypermobility, inflammatory arthritis (up to 25% of RA patients), diabetes, and occupational factors. Treatment consists of anti-inflammatory medications, local steroid injection, and orthotics. Surgical release is indicated when conservative measures fail.

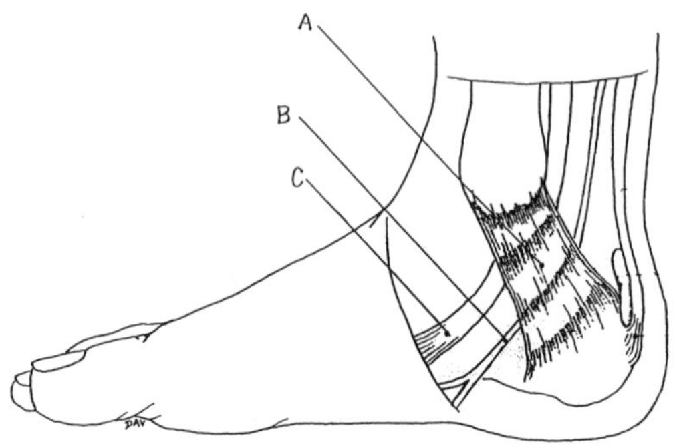


Diagram showing the posterior tibial nerve (*B*) and posterior tibialis tendon (*C*) as they descend inferior to the medial malleolus and underneath the flexor retinaculum (*A*). (Illustration by Debra Vogelgesang.)

## BIBLIOGRAPHY

1. Campbell WW: Diagnosis and management of common compression and entrapment neuropathies. Neurol Clin 15:549–567, 1997.
2. Chang DJ, Paget SA: Neurologic complications of rheumatoid arthritis. Rheum Dis Clin North Am 19:955–973, 1993.
3. Dawson DM: Entrapment neuropathies of the upper extremities. N Engl J Med 329:2013–2018, 1993.
4. Hadler NM: Nerve entrapment syndromes. In Koopman WJ (ed): Arthritis and Allied Conditions, 14th ed. Philadelphia, Williams & Wilkins, 2001, pp 2067–2074.
5. Katz JN, Larson MG, Sabra A, et al: The carpal tunnel syndrome: Diagnostic utility of the history and physical examination findings. Ann Intern Med 112:321–327, 1990.
6. Preston DC: Distal median neuropathies. Neurol Clin 17:407–424, 1999.
7. Rayan GM: Understanding and managing carpal tunnel syndrome. J Musculoskel Med 16:654–663, 1999.
8. Yassi A: Work-related musculoskeletal disorders. Curr Opin Rheumatol 12:124–130, 2000.

# 69. COMPLEX REGIONAL PAIN SYNDROME (REFLEX SYMPATHETIC DYSTROPHY SYNDROME)

*David H. Collier, M.D.*

**1. How is complex regional pain syndrome (CRPS) (reflex sympathetic dystrophy [RSD]) defined?**

There is no uniformly accepted definition for RSD. In November 1993, a consensus workshop of the International Association for the Study of Pain concluded that what was referred to as RSD may not involve abnormal sympathetic behavior and changed the name to CRPS. They divided this up into two types: CRPS type I and CRPS type II. These two types were defined as:

**CRPS type I (RSD)**

a. A syndrome that develops after an initiating noxious event.
b. Spontaneous pain or allodynia/hyperalgesia occurs, is not limited to the territory of a single peripheral nerve, and is disproportionate to the inciting event.
c. There is or has been evidence of edema, skin blood flow abnormality, or abnormal sudomotor activity in the region of the pain since the inciting event.
d. This diagnosis is excluded by the existence of conditions that would otherwise account for the degree of pain and dysfunction.

**CRPS type II (causalgia)**

a. Type II is a syndrome that develops after a nerve injury.
b. All of the above findings for CRPS Type I.

Previously, most definitions of RSD include four general criteria:

Diffuse pain, usually in a nonanatomic pattern and often unrelenting
Swelling in the involved extremity
Loss of function in the area due to pain and/or skin and bone changes
Autonomic dysfunction with vasomotor signs, including a cool or occasional warm skin temperature and moist/sweaty or dry/scaly skin

Some definitions include relief of pain by a sympathetic block. Others describe RSD in terms of signs and symptoms.

**2. What are the classic signs and symptoms of CRPS?**

- Pain and swelling in an extremity
- Trophic skin changes in the same extremity
  Skin atrophy or pigmentary changes
  Hypertrichosis
  Hyperhidrosis
  Nail changes
- Signs and symptoms of vasomotor instability
- Pain and/or limited motion of the ipsilateral shoulder
- A precipitating event, e.g., trauma, surgery, myocardial infarction, spinal disc disease

The pain is often described as burning and severe. It generally involves an entire area such as a hand or foot, although any site on the body can be involved. **Allodynia**, pain from a usually nonnoxious stimulation such as light touch or even a breeze, is commonly present. **Hyperpathia**, prolonged pain on stimulation, is also usually present. The vasomotor instability is manifested by a blue and cool area (but occasionally can be warm and erythematous) along with unusual sweating in the area (but occasionally can be dry and scaly). Dystrophic skin changes, such as atrophy of subcutaneous tissue with overlying tight, shiny, hairless skin, may develop later during evolution of CRPS. Contractures of the flexor surface of the hand may occur in the late stage of this disease, leaving a claw-like, nonfunctional hand.

**3. What are some synonyms for CRPS?**

Causalgia, major or minor
Acute atrophy of bone
Sudeck's atrophy
Sudeck's osteodystrophy
Peripheral acute toponeurosis
Traumatic angiospasm
Traumatic vasospasm
Post-traumatic osteoporosis
Postinfarctional sclerodactyly
Shoulder-hand syndrome
Reflex dystrophy
Reflex neurovascular dystrophy
Reflex sympathetic dystrophy
Sympathalgia
Algodystrophy
Algoneurodystrophy
Hyperpathic pain
Sympathetic maintained pain

**4. Who was Silas Weir Mitchell?**

Silas Weir Mitchell was a neurologist and an assistant surgeon in the U.S. Army during the Civil War. He was in charge of Turner's Lane Hospital, in Philadelphia, to which war-wounded with neurologic injuries were brought. In October 1864, during the beginning of Sherman's march from Atlanta to the sea and while Grant was besieging Petersburg, Dr. Mitchell and two colleagues, George Morehouse and William Keen, published one of the classics in medical literature, *Gunshot Wounds and Other Injuries of Nerves*. In this book are clear detailed descriptions of CRPS. He emphasized the association with trauma, yet the lack of direct injury to the nerve, and the articular nature of this syndrome. In 1867, Dr. Mitchell coined the word *causalgia* (from the Greek words for heat and pain) for this illness in an article in the *United States Sanitary Commission Memoirs*. He is the father of CRPS in the United States.

**5. Who gets CRPS?**

There is an equal incidence of CRPS in men and women. When individual inciting factors are examined that are more common in one sex than another (e.g., myocardial infarction in men), the statistics become skewed toward that sex. Adults get CRPS much more often than children. The highest incidence is in the 40–60-year age group with a mean age of 50 years. The incidence in children is thought to be under-reported because it often goes unrecognized, sometimes being diagnosed as a psychiatric condition. It is, in general, a more benign disease in children. About 75% of the time, there is a clear precipitating factor that causes the development of CRPS.

**6. What are some precipitating factors for the development of CRPS?**

**INCITING FACTORS**

Trauma (common cause)
Fractures
Lacerations
Crush injuries
Contusions
Sprains
Immobilization in a cast
Myocardial infarctions
Strokes and other CNS injury (common cause)
Pleuropulmonary diseases
Surgery (esp. for carpal tunnel and Morton's neuroma) (common cause)
Chemical burns
Electrical burns
Postherpetic neuralgia
Cervical spine pathology
Subcutaneous injections
Drugs (barbiturates)
Malignancies
Pregnancy
Peripheral nerve diseases
Emotional stress

**PREDISPOSING FACTORS**

Diabetes Mellitus
Hyperparathyroidism
Hyperthyroidism
Multiple sclerosis
Neurovegetative Dystonia
Hypertriglyceridemia
Alcohol abuse
Tobacco use

**7. How soon after a precipitating event, such as trauma, will a patient develop CRPS?**

CRPS usually begins days to weeks after the inciting event. In about 80% of cases, it occurs within 3 months of a traumatic episode, but in many cases, RSD begins over 6 months later.

**8. What is the shoulder-hand syndrome?**

This term was coined by Dr. Otto Steinbrocker in 1947 to describe the concomitant shoulder involvement seen with hand RSD. The ipsilateral shoulder will commonly become diffusely painful, develop limited range of motion in all directions, and may progress to adhesive capsulitis.

**9. What are the stages of CRPS ?**

Dr. Steinbrocker was the first to divide CRPS into three stages. Some recent authors may add a fourth stage:

**Stage 1** (acute stage): typically lasts 3-6 months after the development of RSD; characterized by:
Pain in the extremity or shoulder
Swelling in the extremity

Color change of the extremity (red or blue)
Movement painful and tendency for immobilization
Early osteoporosis on x-rays

**Stage 2** (dystrophic phase): persists an additional 3-12 months; characterized by:
Pain usually continues
Swelling changes to brawny hard edema
Beginning of atrophy of subcutaneous tissue and intrinsic muscles
Unilateral cold extremity
Progression of osteoporosis

**Stage 3** (atrophic stage): classically described beginning 9–18 months after the RSD starts; characterized by:
Pain remains constant or diminishes
Extremity becomes stiff
Swelling changes to periarticular thickening
Skin becomes smooth, glossy, and drawn
Brittle nails
May see spasm, dystonia, tremor
Progression of osteoporosis with pathologic fractures

**Stage 4** (psychological): occurs several months to years :
Loss of job
Unnecessary surgery
Orthostatic hypotension or hypertension
Neurodermatitis
Depression

Although these stages can be useful, it is often difficult to place an individual patient into one of them. Most often, stages 1 and 2 are merged or fluctuate back and forth. A patient may stay in one stage for months or years, and another patient may progress rapidly through the stages. The earlier stages are much easier to treat than the later stages.

**10. What motor and movement disorders have been emphasized in recent series looking at CRPS?**

Incoordination, tremor, involuntary movement, muscle spasms, paresis, pseudoparalysis.

**11. What factors may maintain the pain syndrome through the stages?**

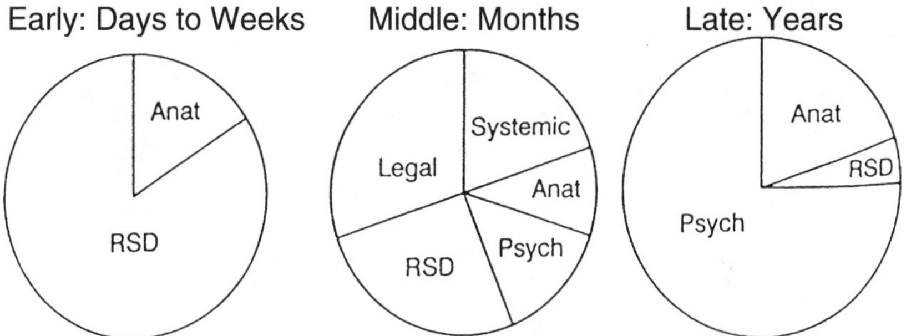


Anat = anatomic factors, such as the injury with which the RSD is associated; Psych = psychological factors; Systemic = systemic factors and associated diseases, such as diabetes mellitus, stroke, or myocardial infarction; Legal = litigation involving personal injury suits, worker's compensation, and other forms of secondary gain. (From Amadio PC, Mackinnon SE, Merritt WH, et al: Reflex sympathetic dystrophy syndrome: Consensus report of an ad hoc committee of the American Association for Hand Surgery on the definition of reflex sympathetic dystrophy syndrome. Plast Reconstr Surg 87:371–375, 1991; with permission.)

**12. Discuss the patterns of spread of CRPS.**

CRPS can spread from the initial site of presentation. Three patterns of spread have been defined: (1) Contiguous spread (CS) characterized by an enlargement of the initial area. (2) Independent spread (IS) characterized by spread of CRPS to a noncontiguous distant site. (3) Bilateral or mirror-image spread (MS) characterized by symptoms and signs on the opposite side that mirror the area and location of the initial presentation of CRPS. CS is the most common type of spread and is seen in most cases. Bilateral involvement in patients with CRPS has been described in 18–100% of patients, depending on the type of measurements and criteria used. Using an algometer on involved joints may demonstrate abnormalities bilaterally in almost all patients, whereas using bone scans may show bilateral involvement in 22% of cases of CRPS. The side secondarily involved tends to have less signs and symptoms than the originally involved side. Bilateral involvement is usually symmetric, with the same area of involvement on each side, but the side secondarily involved can occasionally have a patchy pattern of involvement.

**13. Are there notable plain radiographic findings in CRPS?**

The characteristic radiologic appearance is soft tissue swelling and regional patchy or mottled osteopenia. This appearance is especially evident when comparing the involved side with the contralateral side. This x-ray pattern was first described by Sudeck in 1900 and is often referred to as **Sudeck's atrophy**. This patchy osteopenia is helpful in making the diagnosis but is actually seen in less than half the patients in most series.

Fine-detailed radiography has actually revealed five patterns of bone resorption:

1. A thinning of the trabecular or cancellous bone of the metaphyseal regions, producing bandlike, patchy, or periarticular osteoporosis.
2. Subperiosteal cortical bone resorption resulting in a corrugated appearance of the outer margins of the diaphyses.
3. Endosteal bone resorption resulting in irregularity of the endosteal surface and variation in the thickness of the cortices.
4. Intracortical bone resorption resulting in excessive striation or tunneling within the cortex paralleling the longitudinal axis.
5. Subchondral and juxta-articular erosions visible as small periarticular erosions and intra-articular gaps in the subchondral bone.

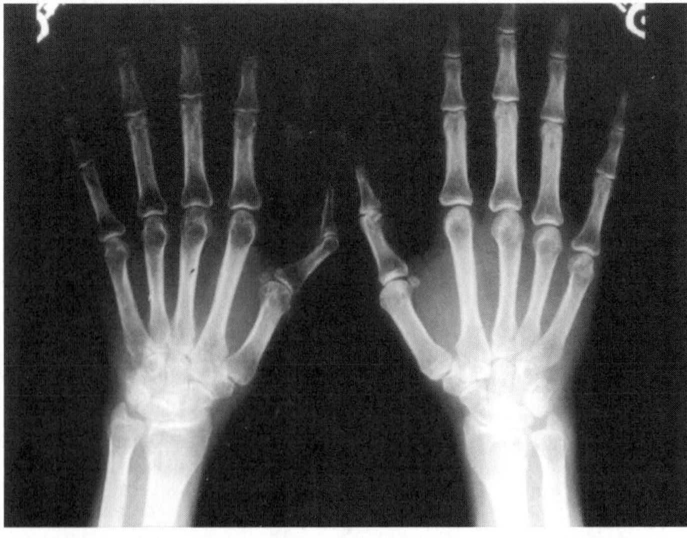

Radiograph of the hands showing RSD of left hand. Note marked periarticular osteoporosis compared with right hand.

**14. What are the scintigraphic findings in CRPS?**

The three-phase bone scan has emerged as an objective diagnostic test, used to determine if a patient has CRPS but without firm evidence to support such a conclusion. The results of a three-phase bone scan using technetium-99m pertechnetate can vary greatly depending on how early in the course of the disease the study is performed. In **stage 1**, there is an increase in blood velocity and blood pooling with early and delayed hyperfixation. The bone scan is abnormal about 80% of the time in this stage. In **stage 2**, there is normalization of blood velocity and blood pooling but a persistence of early and delayed hyperfixation. The bone scan is abnormal about half the time in this stage. In **stage 3**, there is reduced blood velocity and blood pooling, and a minority of patients have early and delayed hyperfixation. Thus, a bone scan performed early in the disease is usually abnormal, but as the disease progresses, scans can be normal. A normal bone scan does not exclude the diagnosis of CRPS. An abnormal (i.e., hot) bone scan may predict response to corticosteroids.

**15. Discuss the use of a thermogram and magnetic resonance images (MRI) in CRPS.**

Some authors believe that infrared thermography is the most sensitive test in the diagnosis of CRPS (90% accuracy). It documents the temperature differences and subtle temperature gradients in different parts of the skin. If the sympathetic nervous system is behaving abnormally due to CRPS, the thermogram picks up these cold or hot areas, usually in a regional pattern. Most patients will have a decrease of subcutaneous temperature associated with the CRPS, but some patients have an increase especially early in the syndrome.

Other authors emphasize the nonspecificity of the thermogram. Vascular problems unrelated to sympathetic abnormalities can give regional coolness. Secondly, sympathetic hyperfunction is not a prerequisite for the diagnosis of CRPS, and patients may have normal or even subnormal levels of sympathetic function.

MRI can demonstrate soft-tissue abnormalities in CRPS and may also help stage CRPS, but is not useful for the diagnosis of CRPS.

**16. Does synovial biopsy yield any typical findings in CRPS?**

CRPS is an arthritic problem. The involved joints tend to be more tender than the periarticular areas. The synovium has been shown to be clearly abnormal. Findings include synovial edema, proliferation and disarray of synovial lining cells, proliferation of capillaries, fibrosis in the deep synovial layers, and occasional infiltration with chronic inflammatory cells (chiefly lymphocytes).

**17. What is the pathophysiology of CRPS? (Controversial)**

Over the years, various theories have explained specific findings in CRPS (e.g., allodynia, bilateral involvement), and both central and peripheral nervous system mechanisms have been evoked to explain sympathetically mediated pain. However, there is no one accepted theory to explain RSD. A synthesis of various hypotheses to explain the traditional therapeutic approach to CRPS is as follows:

The afferent nerves consist of A fibers (α, β, δ) and C fiber (polymodal nociceptors). The A fibers are mainly involved in nonpainful sensation (except for some A-δ fibers). The C fibers relay pain. The A fibers are myelinated, and current flows much faster in them than in the unmyelinated pain fibers.

Wall and Melzach have proposed a **gate control theory** in which dorsal horn cells of the spinal cord can modulate the transmission of sensory information. The pattern of impulses allowed to go through this "gate" determines the rate of firing of the "action system" or spinal transmission neurons. In certain laminae (3 and 4) of the dorsal horn are wide dynamic range fibers that can transmit painful or nonpainful information to the brain depending on information coming from the peripheral and central nervous systems. The stimulated A fibers are thought to inhibit information from C type polymodal nociceptors until a specific number C fibers firing at a rapid frequency can break through the gate and impart painful information. This system is designed so that normal touch is not perceived as pain. When polymodal nociceptors are stimulated, the neuropeptide substance P is released around the receptor where the painful stimulus began. Substance P is pro-inflammatory and causes histamine release, neutrophil migration, vasodilation and vasopermeability, and the release of bradykinin that can stimulate prostaglandin production. Thus, the stimulation of pain fibers can promote inflammation.

When afferent nerves are damaged, two responses can happen. Myelinated A fibers will not send information to the dorsal horns, thus not acting as inhibitory neurons. Unmyelinated C fibers behave oppositely. They will spontaneously fire and become sensitive to certain chemicals, such as norepinephrine, from sympathetic fibers. Thus, painful messages are sent to the dorsal horn. The wide dynamic range fibers then send messages of pain to the brain. The sympathetics become stimulated, releasing chemicals that stimulate the polymodal nociceptors, and thus we have CRPS.

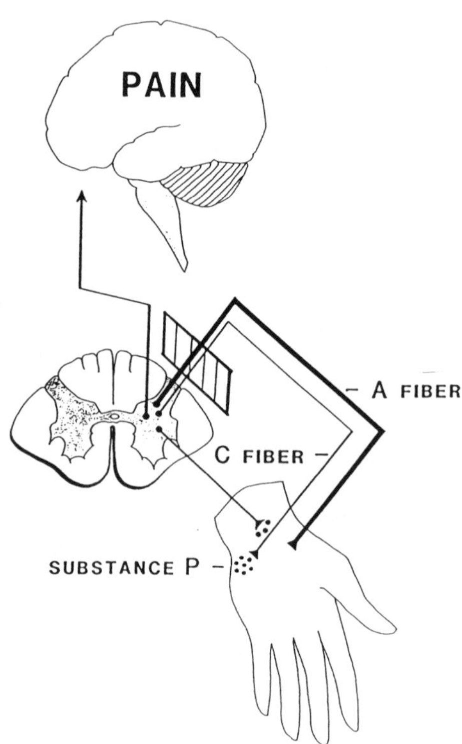


Recent and controversial studies have turned attention away from the hypothesis that the sympathetic nervous system behaves abnormally and more towards the abnormal behavior of α-adrenergic receptor activity on afferent neurons. This is due to the experimental findings of: (1) antisympathetic intervention is not always a successful treatment, and (2) pentolamine, an α-adrenergic receptor antagonist, can reduce the pain of CRPS in a similar fashion to a sympathetic block. Thus, the abnormality is in the C-type polymodal nociceptor and not in the sympathetic nervous system.

**18. Describe a rational approach to the treatment of CRPS.**

Stimulation of inhibitory neurons
- Physical therapy
- Massage, counterirritants
- Ultrasound

- Electroacupuncture
- Transcutaneous nerve stimulators
- Spinal cord stimulator

Anti-inflammatory agents
- NSAIDs
- Ketorolac in an IV regional block
- Corticosteroids (high dose then taper over 4-8 weeks)—use if abnormal bone scan

Sympathetic blocks
- Lidocaine, mepivacaine, bupivacaine, etc., into sympathetic ganglion
- Bier block with IV bretylium, guanethidine, phentolamine or reserpine
- Oral $\alpha$- and $\beta$-blockers
- Prazosin, terazosin
- Oral, patch, or epidural clonidine
- Sympathectomy
- Injection of opioid into sympathetic ganglion

Depletion of substance P in peripheral nerves
- Topical capsaicin

Anticonvulsants
- Phenytoin
- Carbamazepine
- Gabapentin
- Valproic acid

Antiosteoporotic therapy
- Calcitonin
- Intravenous pamidronate, alendronate, clodronate
- Oral alendronate

Treatment of dystonia
- Intrathecal baclofen

Other treatments
- Tricyclic antidepressants
- Calcium channel blockers
- Dimethyl sulfoxide (DMSO) topically

Psychological therapy
- Establish rapport with the patient
- Provide emotional support
- Assess for depression and treat with psychotherapy and medications if a problem
- Thermal biofeedback
- Relaxation training
- Stop alcohol and tobacco

**19. How might you prevent CRPS from occurring in a known susceptible individual who may undergo some trauma such as surgery?**

Perioperative sympathectomy or stellate ganglion block in patients with a history of CRPS has been shown to significantly reduce the recurrence rate of this disease process.

Vitamin C, 500 mg, was demonstrated in a prospective study to lower the risk of CRPS in patients who had wrist fractures.

## BIBLIOGRAPHY

1. Adami S, Fossaluzza U, Gatti D, et al: Bisphosphonate therapy of reflex sympathetic dystrophy syndrome. Ann Rheum Dis 56:201–204, 1997.
2. Amadio PC, Mackinnon SE, Merritt WH, et al: Reflex sympathetic dystrophy syndrome: Consensus report of an ad hoc committee of the American Association for Hand Surgery on the definition of reflex sympathetic dystrophy syndrome. Plast Reconstr Surg 87:371–375, 1991.

3. Awerbuch MS: Thermography—Its current diagnostic status in musculoskeletal medicine. Med J Aust 154:441–444, 1991.
4. Backonja MM: Reflex sympathetic dystrophy/sympathetically maintained pain/causalgia: The syndrome of neuropathic pain with dysautonomia. Semin Neurol 14:263–271, 1994.
5. Demangeat JL, Constantinesco A, Brunot B, et al: Three-phase bone scanning in reflex sympathetic dystrophy of the hand. J Nucl Med 29:26–32, 1988.
6. Genant HK, Kozin F, Bekerman C, et al: The reflex sympathetic dystrophy syndrome: A comprehensive analysis using fine-detail radiography, photon absorptiometry, and bone and joint scintigraphy. Radiology 117:21–32, 1975.
7. Harden RN: Complex regional pain syndrome. Br J Anaesth 87:99–106, 2001.
8. Jänig W, Stanton-Hicks M (eds): Reflex Sympathetic Dystrophy: A Reappraisal. Seattle, IASP Press, 1996.
9. Kozin F, Genant HK, Bekerman C, McCarty DJ: The reflex sympathetic dystrophy syndrome: II. Roentgenographic and scintigraphic evidence of bilaterality and of periarticular accentuation. Am J Med 60:332–338, 1976.
10. Kozin F, McCarty DJ, Sims J, Genant H: The reflex sympathetic dystrophy syndrome: I. Clinical and histologic studies: Evidence for bilaterality, response to corticosteroids and articular involvement. Am J Med 60:321–331, 1976.
11. Kozin F, Ryan LM, Carerra GF, et al: The reflex sympathetic dystrophy syndrome (RSDS): III. Scintigraphic studies, further evidence for the therapeutic efficacy of systemic corticosteroids, and proposed diagnostic criteria. Am J Med 70:23–30, 1981.
12. Phelps RG, Wilentz S. Review—Reflex sympathetic dystrophy. Int J Dermatol 39:481–486, 2000.
13. Reuben SS, Rosenthal EA, Steinberg RB: Surgery on the affected upper extremity of patients with a history of complex regional pain syndrome: A retrospective study of 100 patients. J Hand Surg (Am) 25:1147–1151, 2000.
14. Schott GD: Reflex sympathetic dystrophy. J Neurol Neurosurg Psychiatry 71:291–295, 2001.
15. Silber TJ, Majd M: Reflex sympathetic dystrophy syndrome in children and adolescents: Report of 18 cases and review of the literature. Am J Dis Child 142:1325–1330, 1988.
16. Steinbrocker O: The shoulder-hand syndrome. Am J Med 3:402–407, 1947.

# *XII. Neoplasms and Tumor-like Lesions*

*While there are several chronic diseases more destructive to life than cancer, none is more feared.*

Charles H. Mayo
(1865–1939), 1926

## 70. BENIGN AND MALIGNANT TUMORS OF JOINTS AND SYNOVIUM

*Edmund* H. *Hornstein*, D.O.

**1. Why should practicing physicians be concerned with tumors that affect the joints and synovium?**

Benign and malignant neoplasms affecting articular and periarticular structures may mimic inflammatory arthritis. Awareness of these conditions is crucial to prevent diagnostic delay and to avoid the initiation of ineffective and/or inappropriate therapy. Fortunately, primary neoplasms of the joint are rare.

**2. A young adult presents with a solitary, painless mass adjacent to a finger joint that has been slowly enlarging. What tumor is suggested by this scenario?**

This presentation would be typical for **pigmented villonodular synovitis** (PVNS). This benign condition, which occurs with a slightly increased predilection for females, is second only to the ganglion as a source of localized swelling in the hand and wrist. These nodular lesions usually occur in association with a tendon sheath (in which case it is called giant cell tumor of tendon sheath).

**3. PVNS exists in three forms: localized, diffuse, and as giant cell tumor of tendon sheath. How do these forms differ?**

In **diffuse PVNS**, the entire synovium of an affected joint or structure is involved. It affects individuals in their 30s and 40s with equal sex distribution. Grossly, the synovium is prolific with coarse villi, finer fronds, and diffuse nodularity. It is often darkly pigmented, ranging from dark yellow to chocolate brown. Diffuse PVNS is almost always monarticular. The most common locations include the knee (80%), hip (15%), and ankle. Swelling and effusion accompanied by moderate discomfort, decreased range of motion, and increased warmth to palpation are typical. Pain is frequently less than anticipated from the degree of swelling. **Localized PVNS** involves only a portion of a synovial surface in a joint, and the lesion is often pedunculated. It tends not to be as darkly pigmented and has less villous proliferation than is seen in the diffuse form. Giant cell tumor of tendon sheath has been discussed in Question 2 above. Histologically, all three forms of villonodular synovitis are remarkably similar. The etiology of PVNS is unknown.

**4. What does the synovial fluid analysis reveal in PVNS?**

Typically, the fluid is grossly **hemorrhagic**. This finding on joint aspiration should raise PVNS as a diagnostic consideration. However, up to 50% of cases will not have a hemorrhagic synovial fluid.

**5. What are the characteristic radiographic findings in a patient with PVNS?**

Plain radiographs are usually nonspecific except for mild increased density of the soft tissue of the joint due to blood and hemosiderin deposits. The tumor may invade into bone causing cysts or erosive changes mimicking gout. The MRI appearance of PVNS is diagnostic in most cases. Nodules with sufficient hemosiderin appear dark on T1-weighted images and even darker on T2-weighted images.

**6. Describe the histologic characteristics of PVNS.**

Grossly, the synovium looks like a tan to brown "shaggy carpet." Microscopically, PVNS is distinctive. It is characterized by a dense cellular infiltrate composed of histiocytes, lipid-laden cells, hemosiderin-containing cells, and scattered, frequent, multinucleated giant cells. Controversy exists as to the nature of this condition. DNA analysis is supportive of a neoplastic etiology for diffuse PVNS but not for the localized form of the lesion.

**7. How is PVNS treated?**

Surgical treatment with complete synovectomy is standard, either via open or arthroscopic approaches. Recurrences, particularly in diffuse PVNS, are not uncommon, occurring in 20–40%. Low-dose radiation is used in refractory cases.

**8. Synovial chondromatosis is another benign lesion of joints. Does it represent neoplasia?**

No. More appropriately considered a metaplastic lesion, this disorder is characterized by the development of multiple foci of cartilaginous metaplasia within the synovium. These foci form nodules that may calcify or ossify and that frequently are released as free bodies (**joint mice**) into the joint space.

**9. How is synovial chondromatosis diagnosed?**

Synovial chondromatosis is almost always monarticular. It usually occurs in the knee but can occur in the hip, ankle, elbow, or other joints. It can occur in any site of synovial tissue to include tendon sheath and bursa. Clinically, there is increasingly compromised range of motion with crepitus and often with unexpected locking. Effusion may occur. The x-ray examination may be diagnostic if the chondroid bodies are calcified resembling a calcified mulberry (see figure). If not, diagnosis may require arthroscopic biopsy.

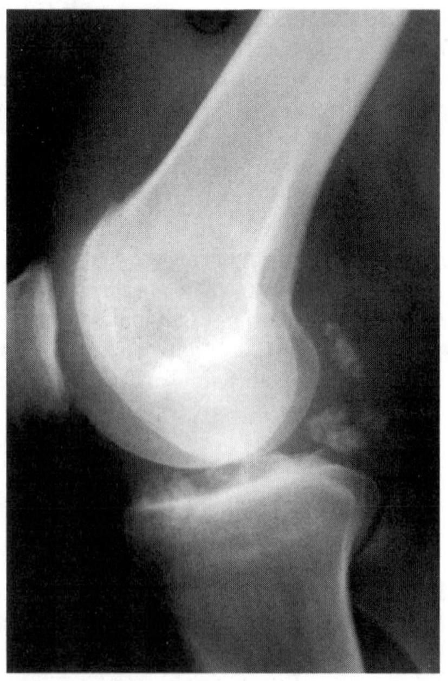

Synovial chondromatosis of the knee demonstrating multiple, calcified chondroid bodies.

**10. How is synovial chondromatosis managed?**

Treatment is via synovectomy. Though considered benign, this condition can result in extensive local joint destruction if left untreated. Occasionally, this lesion may be difficult to distinguish histologically from chondrosarcoma.

**11. What other benign tumor-like lesions can involve the joints?**

- **Lipomas** may occur within the joint capsule or synovium, but true intra-articular lesions are rare.
- Chondroma is an isolated mass of benign cartilage, usually in the knee.
- **Hemangiomas** are unusual intra-articular lesions that occur most frequently in the joints of children and young adults. The knee is the most common site. Recurrent hemarthrosis may occur. Diagnosis can be made by CT, MRI, or angiography.
- **Osteoid osteomas**, when occurring within the joint, have less of the "classic" pattern of nocturnal pain relieved by NSAIDs, and tend to involute spontaneously after 5–10 years.

**12. What is the most common primary malignant neoplasm involving the joints?**

**Synovial sarcoma**. This tumor constitutes up to 10% of all soft-tissue sarcomas. It is a highly malignant neoplasm and generally occurs in the lower extremities of young people. The tumor usually arises in the periarticular tissues of the knee or ankle. Only 10% of these malignancies arise directly within the joint itself.

**13. How does this tumor present clinically?**

A slowly growing, often minimally symptomatic mass adjacent to the joint is the typical presentation. Pain is reported by about 50% of patients with this tumor. Soft-tissue calcification on plain x-ray occurs in 30% of the cases, and this finding serves to provide a clue as to the underlying diagnosis (see figure).

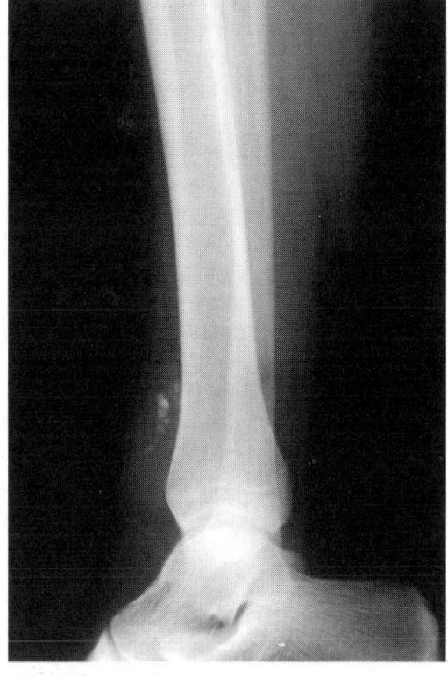

Synovial sarcoma adjacent to the ankle. Note the speckled calcifications.

**14. What is the cell of origin for synovial sarcoma?**

The histology of this tumor may be **biphasic**, in which epithelial cells arranged in clusters, tubules, and acini are interspersed in a spindle-cell stroma; or **monophasic**, in which either the epithelial or spindle cells predominate. Other morphologic types are recognized, however, including mixed and hemangiopericytic. Behavioral features include calcifying, ossifying, and poorly differentiated types. Though this tumor is called synovial sarcoma, ultrastructural and immunohistochemical studies have implicated an epithelial origin.

**15. How is synovial sarcoma treated? What is the prognosis?**

Treatment is an aggressive combination of radical surgery, radiation therapy, and chemotherapy. Prognosis depends in large part on tumor size at the time of discovery. The cause of death in progressive disease is usually due to extensive pulmonary metastasis. Other common sites of metastasis include regional lymph nodes, bones, skin, and brain.

*5-Year Survival in Synovial Sarcoma*

| | |
|---|---|
| All tumors | 40% |
| Tumor < 5 cm | 86% |
| Tumor > 10 cm | 22% |

**16. Clear-cell sarcoma is a rare highly malignant tumor of tendons, ligaments, and fascial aponeuroses. It usually presents as a slowly growing mass about the foot. What is its association with a malignancy more commonly thought of as a skin cancer?**

There are multiple lines of evidence suggesting, rather convincingly, that clear-cell sarcoma is a representation of **malignant melanoma**. This evidence includes an immunohistochemical staining pattern with S-100 and HMB-45, which are considered specific for melanoma, evidence of melanin by special staining, and the presence of characteristic pre-malanasomes by electron microscopy. Prognosis is generally poor.

**17. Which primary malignant tumor of joints may be difficult to differentiate from the benign cartilaginous metaplasia of synovial chondromatosis?**

Occasionally arising from **synovial chondromatosis**, synovial chondrosarcoma is an exceedingly rare malignancy that may be histologically difficult to differentiate from its benign cousin. Favoring a diagnosis of sarcoma is the loss of a differentiated clustering growth pattern, areas of necrosis, and spindling of cells in the periphery.

**18. In which malignant diseases can joint involvement occur as a secondary feature?**

Metastatic carcinoma
Lymphoma/myeloma
Leukemic infiltration
Contiguous spread of adjacent bone sarcomas

**19. What is the "classic" presentation of carcinoma metastatic to a joint?**

- Advanced lung or breast cancer is the most common etiology.
- Involvement is usually monarticular, with the knee the most common site.
- Effusion is often hemorrhagic.
- Synovial fluid cytology reveals the malignancy in approximately 50% of cases.

## BIBLIOGRAPHY

1. Abraham JH, Canoso JJ: Tumors of soft tissue and bone. Curr Opin Rheumatol 5:193–198, 1993.
2. Brodsky JT, Burt ME, Hajdu SI, et al: Tendosynovial sarcoma: Clinicopathologic features, treatment and prognosis. Cancer 70:484–489, 1992.
3. Burssens A, Dequeker J: Tumors of bone. In Klippel JH, Dieppe PA (eds): Rheumatology, 2nd ed. St. Louis, Mosby, 1998, Sect 8, Chapter 49, pp 49.1–49.14.
4. Choong PFM, Pritchard DJ: Neoplasms of the joints. In Klippel JH (ed): Primer on the Rheumatic Diseases, 11th ed. Atlanta, Arthritis Foundation, 1997, pp 344–350.

5. Convery FR, Lyon R, Lavernia C: Synovial tumors. In Klippel JH, Dieppe PA (eds): Rheumatology, 2nd ed. St. Louis, Mosby, 1998, Sect 5, Chapter 29, pp 29.1–29.8.
6. Fisher C: Synovial sarcoma. Ann Diagn Pathol 2(6):401–421, 1998.
7. Lin J, Jacobson JA, Jamadar DA, Ellis JH: Pigmented villonodular synovitis and related lesions: The spectrum of imaging findings. AJR Am J Roentgenol 172:191–197, 1999.
8. Paley D, Jackson RW: Synovial haemangioma of the knee joint: Diagnosis by arthroscopy. Arthroscopy 2:174–177, 1986.
9. Rosenberg AE: Tumors involving joints. In Harris ED, Ruddy S, Sledge CB (eds): Kelley's Textbook of Rheumatology, 6th ed.Philadelphia, WB Saunders, 2001, pp 1667–1690.
10. Ushijima M, Hashimoto H, Tsuneyoshi M, Enjoji M: Giant cell tumor of the tendon sheath (nodular tenosynovitis): A study of 207 cases to compare the large joint group with the common digit group. Cancer 57:875–884, 1986.

# 71. COMMON BONY LESIONS: RADIOGRAPHIC FEATURES

*Luis Gonzalez*, M.D.

**1. What are the radiographic characteristics of a nonaggressive, histologically benign bone tumor?**

1. **Geographic bone destruction**. A well-defined margin easily separated from normal surrounding bone is indicative of a slow-growing lesion. The zone of transition may be scalloped or sclerotic.

2. **Intact bony cortex**. The cortex usually provides an effective barrier to expansile growth, preventing penetration by nonaggressive, slow-growing lesions. While there may be cortical thinning or expansion, the cortex will remain intact and there will be no extension to the surrounding soft tissues.

3. **Lack of periosteal reaction**. If present, the periosteal response will be a singular, homogeneously expanding contour. Aggressive periosteal changes, such as the "onion-peel pattern" and the "radiating sunburst appearance" of Ewing's sarcoma and osteosarcoma, will not be seen.

4. **Slow growth over time**. Nonaggressive lesions are usually < 6 cm, with many being < 3 cm, and they show little change over a 6-month followup.

**2. What are the types of tumor matrix?**

1. Clear or cystic (Fig. 1)
2. Fibrous (Fig. 2)
3. Chondroid (Fig. 3)
4. Osteoid (Fig. 4)

The bony matrix refers to the internal architecture of the lesion. Tumors may be **clear or cystic**, or they can produce a matrix that calcifies or ossifies. Identifying the type of tumor matrix is extremely important to help differentiate lesions. **Fibrous** tumors demonstrate a uniform, homogeneous increase in radiodensity internally, known as a ground-glass appearance. **Chondroid** lesions frequently have a centrally located calcification described as ring-like, flocculent, or fleck-like. **Osteoid** tumors have a radiodense collection of variable size that may be hetero- or homogeneous.

*Types of Nonaggressive Primary Bone Tumors by Matrix Appearance*

| CLEAR | FIBROUS | CHONDROID | OSTEOID |
|---|---|---|---|
| Unicameral bone cyst | Fibroxanthoma | Enchondroma | Osteoma |
| Aneurysmal bone cyst | Fibrous dysplasia | Osteochondroma | Osteoid osteoma |
| Giant cell tumor | | Chondroblastoma | Osteoblastoma |
| Eosinophilic granuloma | | Chondromyxoid fibroma | |

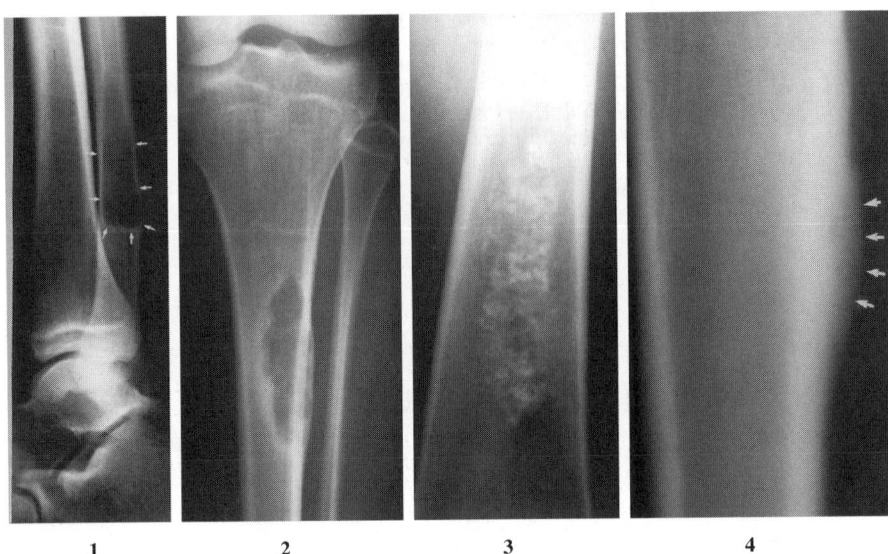


**3. A 30-year-old man presents with rectal bleeding and a well-circumscribed, geographic area of increased bone density seen on skull films in the left frontal sinus. What bone lesion is this?**

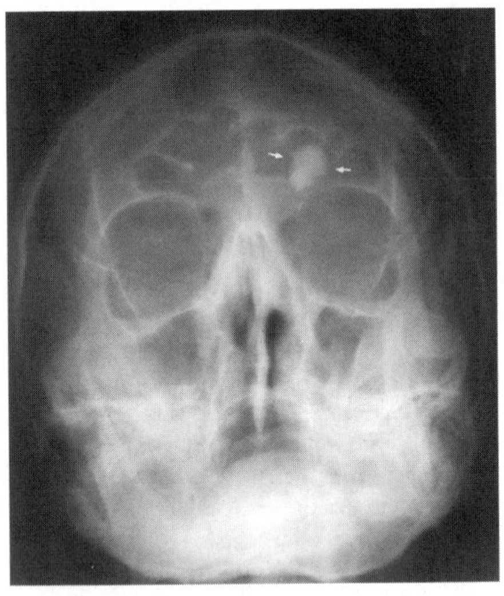

Osteoma. These tumors usually arise from areas of membranous bone formation such as the paranasal sinuses, skull, and mandible. The lesions are smooth, rounded, and often < 1 cm in size. Although they have no malignant potential, the tumors may become symptomatic according to their site of origin. Gardner's syndrome is a familial condition characterized by the triad of multiple osteomas, soft-tissue tumors, and colonic polyps.

**4. A 20-year-old man with leg pain at night has a round, sharply delineated radiolucent tumor, covered with a wide zone of uniform reactive sclerosis, on his upper tibia. What might this lesion be?**

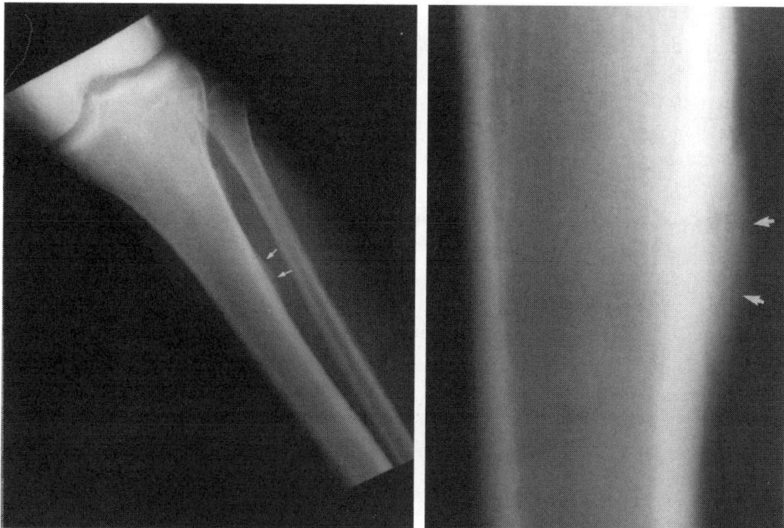

Osteoid osteoma. The round, sharply delineated radiolucent center or nidus measuring < 1 cm with a wide zone of uniform reactive sclerosis is characteristic of this lesion. Over 90% of patients with this lesion complain of nighttime pain relieved by aspirin. The area overlying the lesion is often tender to the touch. Tomography or CT scan may be helpful for demonstrating the nidus when it is obscured by the perilesional reactive zone. Because incomplete surgical excision of the nidus invites the recurrence of pain, radionuclide agents and the intraoperative use of a scintillation probe (Geiger counter) can help locate the intense focus of high radioactive counts associated with the nidus and guide the surgeon to complete removal of the lesion. Osteoid osteomas most frequently occur in the hip and occasionally the posterior spinous processes.

**5. Describe the characteristics of a chondroblastoma.**

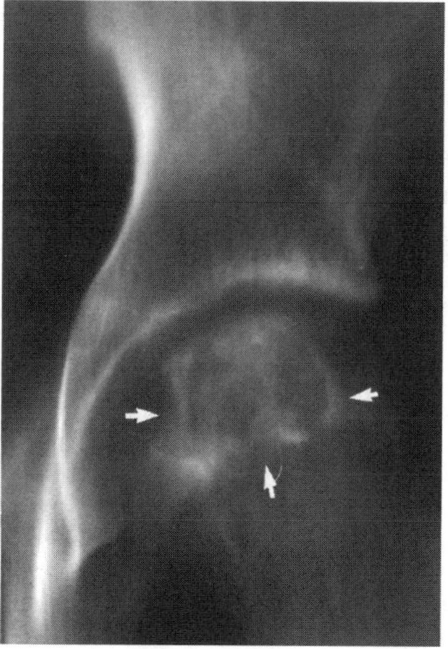

A chondroblastoma is an eccentric, lobulated lesion with a smooth geographic contour defined by a thin, discrete, marginal sclerosis. The internal matrix demonstrates flecks of stippled calcifications, making this a chondroid lesion. Chondroblastomas are the only nonaggressive chondroid lesions that originate in the epiphysis. Other nonaggressive lesions that originate in the epiphysis or that cross the physis to involve the epiphysis include aneurysmal bone cysts and giant cell tumors.

**6. A 31-year-old man with leg pain presented with an osseous tumor on the tibia, as seen in the following radiograph. What bone lesion does this represent?**

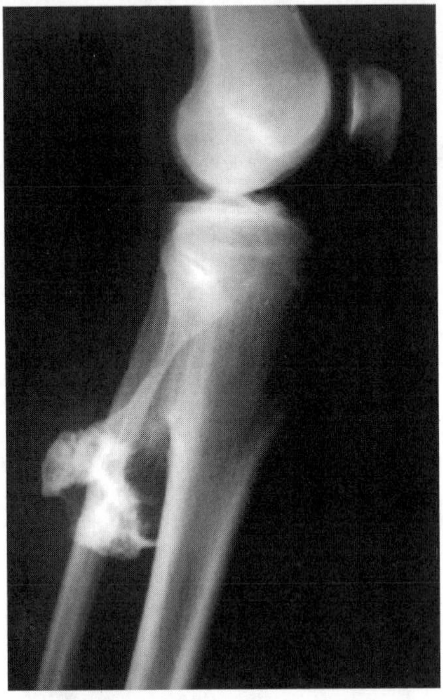

Osteochondroma. This osseous excrescence often arises from the metaphyseal region of a long tubular bone, such as the femur or tibia. The lesion is commonly pedunculated, directed away from the nearby joint along the path of ligamentous and tendinous insertion. The osteochondroma is continuous with the parent bone and contains both cortical and medullary elements.

Variable calcification is associated with the cartilaginous cap. This cap is usually less than 1 cm in diameter. If the tip is enlarged or has poorly defined, irregular calcifications, malignant transformation should be suspected. MRI is an excellent modality for assessing the cartilaginous cap. This transformation should also be suspected with unexplained pain (i.e., lesional pain in the absence of pathologic fracture or impingement of nerves or vessels), the presence of a soft-tissue mass, or the continued growth of the lesion after physeal fusion around the time of puberty. The incidence of malignant transformation to chondrosarcoma ranges from 1–25%, depending on whether the lesion is solitary or multiple. Multiple hereditary osteochondromatosis or diaphyseal aclasis is an autosomal dominant disorder.

**7. A 20-year-old woman has a painless soft-tissue swelling of the finger, as seen in the radiograph. What bone lesion is this?**

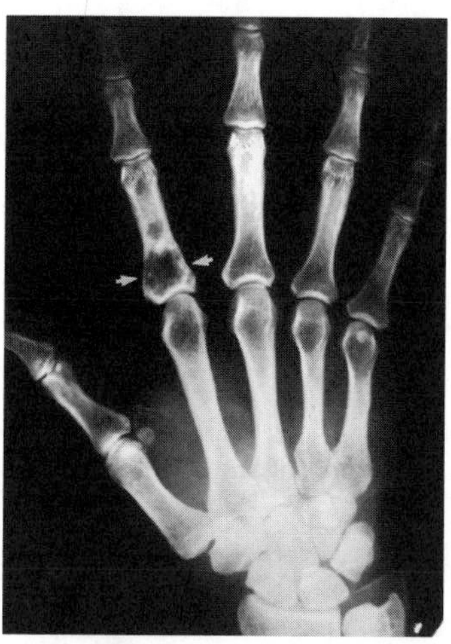

Enchondroma. This well-circumscribed, geographic lucency arises eccentrically within the diaphysis of the proximal phalanx. The lobulated contour is characteristic of cartilaginous lesions, as are the punctate, sharply defined calcifications. Endosteal erosion and bulging of the cortex are common.

Enchondromas are the most common, nonaggressive lesion of the hands. Greater than 50% of enchondromas occur in the diaphyses of the short, tubular bones of the hands and feet. The metaphysis is the site of origin when the long tubular bones are affected. Malignant transformation occurs in 1% of solitary enchondromas, usually arising in lesions of the long, tubular or flat bones.

Enchondromatosis (Ollier's disease) is a rare, nonhereditary disorder consisting of widespread involvement of predominantly one side of the body with multiple, asymmetrically distributed enchondromas. Often there is associated shortening and deformity of the long bones affected. Malignant transformation of an individual lesion in Ollier's disease is common, occurring in one-third to one-half of patients. Maffucci's syndrome is a rare, congenital disorder of mesodermal dysplasia characterized by enchondromatosis and soft-tissue hemangiomas.

**8. A 6-year-old boy with leg trauma presents with a 2-cm oval, geographic lesion on the lower tibia with erosion of the cortical surface and a sclerotic rim. What is it?**

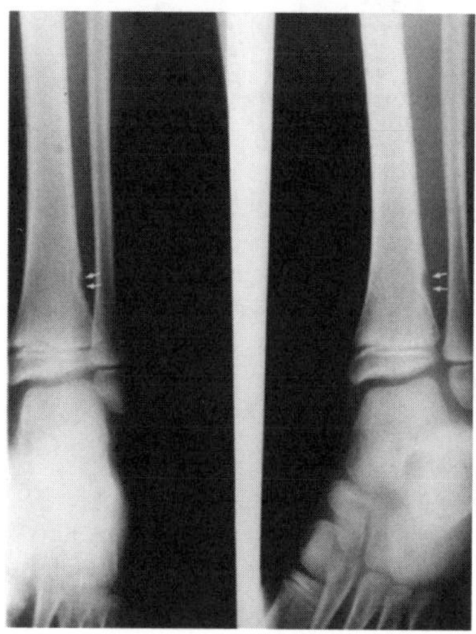

Fibrous cortical defect, or fibroxanthoma, is a common (30–40%) finding in children aged 2–8 years. These lesions occur predominantly in the lower extremities, especially within the metaphyseal region of the knee joint. The internal architecture, the matrix, is "ground glass," devoid of calcifications, and typical of a fibrous lesion. These lesions are usually asymptomatic, persist around 2 years, and then spontaneously regress.

Nonossifying fibromas are histologically identical, nonaggressive lesions. They tend also to occur about the knee but arise within the medullary cavity, unlike fibrous cortical defects that arise on the cortical surface. Nonossifying fibromas are far less common also. They occur in a slightly older population (6–10 year olds) and tend to be slightly larger (≥ 4 cm). Some radiopathologists combine these similar lesions, referring to them as fibroxanthomas.

**9. A 27-year-old woman with a previous history of precocious puberty presents with the bone lesions pictured in the radiograph. What does this bone lesion represent?**

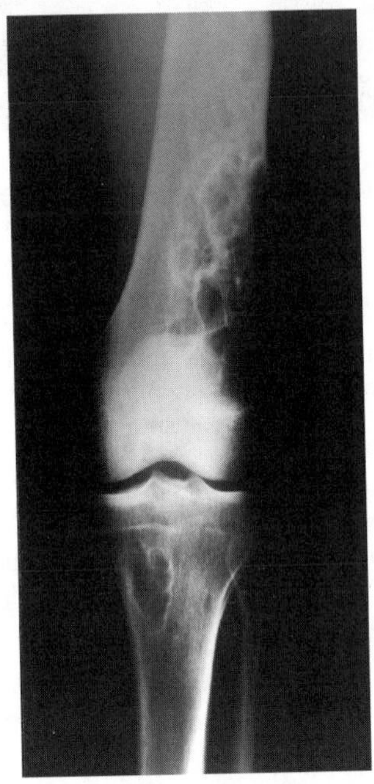

Fibrous dysplasia (FD). These large, geographic lesions with a homogeneous, ground-glass matrix and a thick rind of reactive bone are characteristic of this disease. As in this case, cortical expansion and deformities of bone, such as bowing or varus angulation (shepherd's crook deformity), are common. Histologically, FD represents a fibro-osseous lesion. Normal bone is replaced by abnormal fibrous tissue within an abnormally arranged trabecular pattern. This has led to speculation that FD may be a growth or developmental aberration rather than a true neoplasm. About 20–25% of patients with FD have multiple sites of involvement. The femur and tibia, skull and mandible, and ribs are commonly affected. McCune-Albright syndrome is identified by the triad of polyostotic, predominantly unilateral FD, café-au-lait macular lesions with irregular "coast of Maine" margins, and endocrine dysfunction, especially precocious puberty.

**10. A 9-year-old boy was injured during soccer practice and presented with a radiolucent lesion with mild cortical thinning and expansion, proximal to the shoulder. What bone lesion is this?**

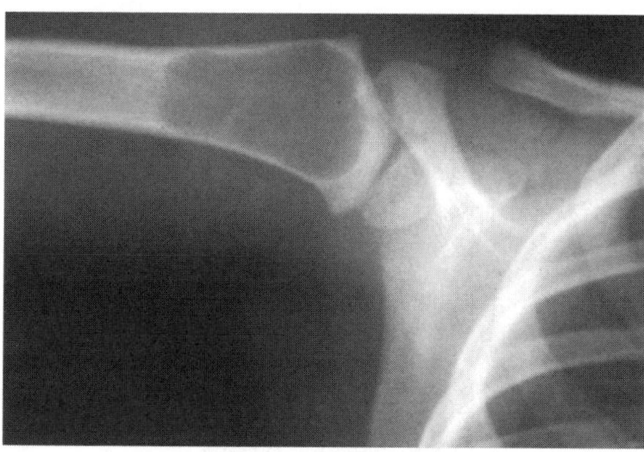

Unicameral (simple) bone cyst. On the radiograph, the short zone of transition of the lesion to normal bone is clearly defined by a thin, sclerotic margin. The internal matrix is clear or cystic. A vertical, bony density in the dependent portion of the lesion may represent a "fallen fragment" secondary to a pathologic fracture. Unicameral bone cysts generally occur in the long tubular bones, especially the proximal ends of the humerus and femur (up to 90%), and may represent a disturbance of growth at the physeal plate rather than a true neoplasm. Early intervention, either with surgical curettage and bone packing or steroid injection, is advocated to prevent a multiplicity of pathologic fractures and subsequent bone deformity and shortening. On radiographs, a favorable response is noted by a decrease in lesion size and an increase in radiodensity with adjacent cortical thickening.

**11. A 32-year-old man presents with a tender wrist. Radiographs show an expansile, lytic lesion that extends to the articular surface, involving both the epiphysis and metaphysis of the distal radius. The cortex is thinned. The internal matrix is clear with a delicate trabecular pattern. Any ideas?**

Giant cell tumor. These tumors may be differentiated from aneurysmal bone cysts because they tend to occur in the skeletally mature individual, after physeal closure, and involve the epiphysis extensively. Although soft-tissue involvement is suggested on plain films, CT or MRI is helpful to map the extent of bone and soft-tissue spread prior to resection. The prognosis with giant cell tumors is unpredictable: 50–60% recur; 10–15% undergo malignant transformation. Distal metastasis to remote sites such as the lungs has been reported.

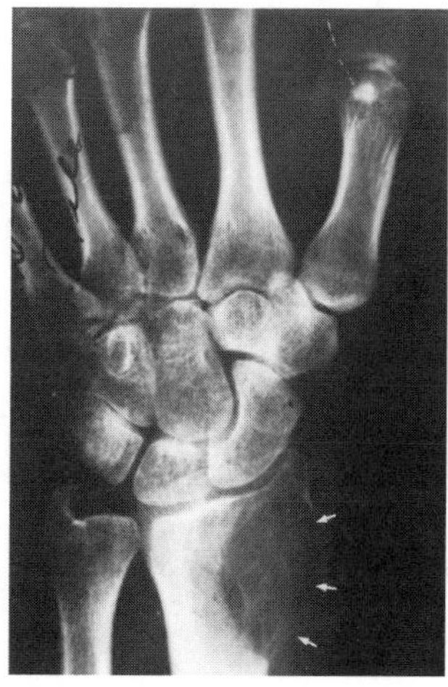

**12. A 6-year-old boy presents with leg pain. A radiograph shows ballooning of the cortical surface of the fibular metaphysis. What bone lesion does this represent?**

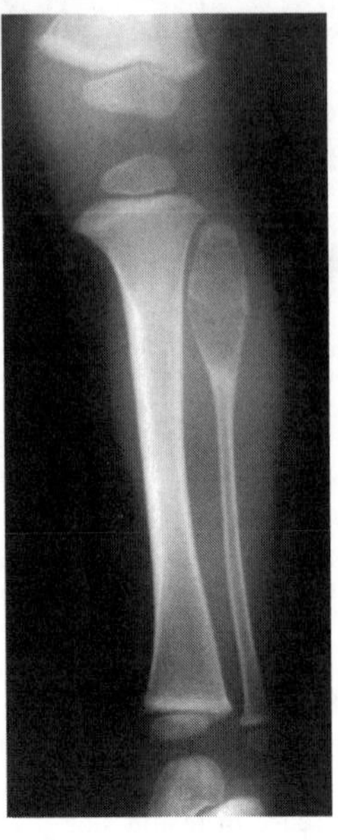

Aneurysmal bone cyst. This osteolytic lesion with occasional trabeculation arises from the fibular metaphysis. The cortical surface is markedly expanded or ballooned. The loss of cortical definition and suggestion of extension into the soft tissues are alarming features of a rapidly expansile lesion. Although histologically benign, aneurysmal bone cysts often simulate malignant tumors. They may be post-traumatic or reactive responses to preexisting bony lesions, possibly related to local alterations in hemodynamics (i.e., venous obstruction and arteriovenous fistulas). The blood-filled cavities of an aneurysmal bone cyst are exquisitely demonstrated by MRI, which delineates the fluid-fluid levels caused by the settling of red blood cells from the fluid blood. About 60–70% of aneurysmal bone cysts occur within the long tubular bones, usually originating from the metaphysis. These cysts also have a predilection for the posterior elements of the vertebral bodies, where they can be difficult to distinguish from other nonaggressive lesions that occur in this location (e.g., osteoblastomas and giant cell tumors).

**13. A 20-year-old man with head pain shows a single, lytic, "punched out" lesion on a skull film. What lesion is this?**

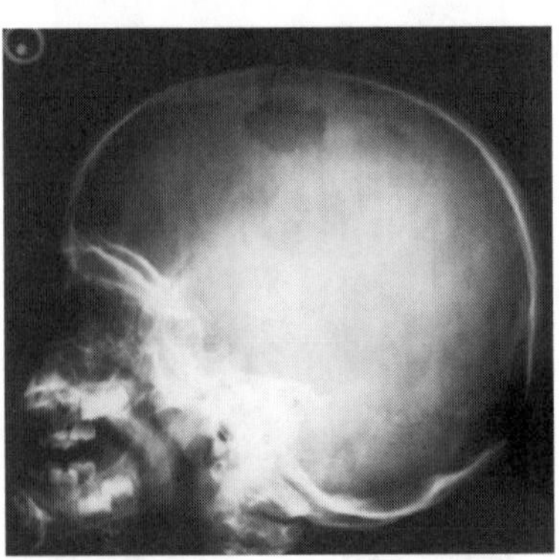

Eosinophilic granuloma (EG). The exquisitely well-circumscribed, "punched out" lesion in the skull with a clear matrix is characteristic of EG. Often, the margin appears beveled secondary to involvement of both the inner and outer tables of the calvarium. In the mandible, the loss of supporting bone results in the appearance of "floating teeth." When the metaphysis or diaphysis of the long bones is affected, the lesion is associated with both endosteal scalloping and extensive, thick, laminated periosteal reaction. EG is also one of the causes of complete collapse of a vertebral body, a condition known as *vertebra plana*.

Plain film remains the modality of choice for documentation of EG lesions, as 30–35% of lesions have no uptake of radionuclide and up to 10% result in "cold" areas of abnormally decreased uptake.

Letterer-Siwe and Hand-Christian-Schüller disease are EG syndromes reflecting a spectrum of bone and visceral involvement. Letterer-Siwe disease is an acute form of EG marked by rapid dissemination and poor prognosis. It tends to appear in children under 3 years old, causing bone lesions, hepatosplenomegaly, and occasionally "honeycomb" interstitial lung disease. Death usually occurs within 1–2 years from hemorrhage or sepsis. Hand-Christian-Schüller disease is an extremely varied form of EG associated with the chronic dissemination of osseous lesions. When it appears in a child 5–10 years old, visceral involvement may result in diabetes insipidus and exophthalmos. Ten to 30% of cases are fatal.

## BIBLIOGRAPHY


1. Hudson TM: Radiologic-Pathologic Correlation of Musculoskeletal Lesions. Baltimore, Williams & Wilkins, 1987.
2. Resnick D: Bone and Joint Imaging. Philadelphia, WB Saunders, 1989.
3. Resnick D, Niwayama G: Diagnosis of Bone and Joint Disorders. Philadelphia, WB Saunders, 1995.
4. Wilner D: Radiology of Bone Tumors and Allied Disorders. Philadelphia, WB Saunders, 1982.

# *XIII. Pediatric Rheumatic Diseases*

*Parents learn a lot from their children about coping with life.*
Muriel Spark (1918–), *The Comforter*

## 72. APPROACH TO THE CHILD WITH JOINT PAIN

Randy Q. Cron, M.D., Ph.D., and Terri H. Finkel, M.D., Ph.D.

**1. What is the differential diagnosis of joint pain in childhood?**

The rheumatic diseases of childhood are not rare and include at least 110 illnesses associated with arthritis or related musculoskeletal syndromes. The differential diagnosis can be remembered with the well-worn mnemonic "De patient is DE VICTIM." For completeness, we will use DE VICTIMNS:

**D** — Drug
- Serum sickness
- Drug-induced lupus

**E** — Endocrine
- Hypercortisolism
- Hypothyroidism

**V** — Vascular/hematologic
- Vasculitis
- Sickle cell anemia
- Hemophilia

**I** — Infectious/postinfectious
- Bacterial
  - Osteomyelitis
  - Discitis
  - Septic arthritis
- Viral
  - "Toxic" synovitis
  - "Transient" synovitis
  - Rubella vaccination
  - HIV

**C** — Collagen vascular
- Juvenile rheumatoid arthritis
- Juvenile ankylosing spondylitis
- SEA syndrome (seronegative enthesopathy and arthropathy)
- Juvenile psoriatic arthritis
- Reactive arthritis/Reiter syndrome
- Inflammatory bowel disease
- Rheumatic fever
- Systemic lupus erythematosus
- Dermatomyositis
- Mixed connective tissue disease
- Vasculitis
- Scleroderma
- Sarcoidosis

**C** — Collagen vascular (*continued*)
- Periodic fever syndromes
  - Familial Mediterranean fever
  - PFAPA
  - TRAPS
  - Hyper IgD syndrome
  - Cyclic neutropenia

**T** — Trauma/orthopedic/mechanical problems
- Chondromalacia patellae
- Osteochondritis dissecans
- Osteoid osteoma
- Osgood-Schlatter disease
- Slipped capital femoral epiphysis
- Legg-Calvé-Perthes disease
- Hypermobility syndromes

**I** — Idiopathic
- Reflex sympathetic dystrophy
- Fibromyalgia
- Growing pains
- Erythromelalgia

**M** — Metabolic
- Mucopolysaccharidoses
- Mucolipidoses
- Rickets (vitamin D deficiency)

**N** — Neoplastic
- Leukemia/lymphoma
- Neuroblastoma
- Bone tumors
- Synovial membrane tumors
- Metastases

**S** — PSychoSomatic
- Hysteria/conversion reactions
- School phobia

**2. What are the characteristics of an organic versus a nonorganic etiology for joint pain?**

| Organic | Nonorganic |
|---|---|
| Occurs day and night | Occurs only at night |
| Occurs during weekends and on vacation | Occurs primarily on school days |
| Severe enough to interrupt play and other pleasant activities | Child is able to carry out normal daily activities |
| Located in joint | Located between joints |
| Unilateral | Bilateral |
| Child limps or refuses to walk | Child is able to walk normally |
| Description fits with logical anatomic explanation | Description is illogical, often dramatically stated, and not consistent with known anatomic or physical process |

**3. What are the historical clues of an organic versus a nonorganic etiology for joint pain?**

**Organic**: Signs of systemic illness, including weight loss, fever, night sweats, rash, diarrhea
**Nonorganic**: Otherwise healthy child, may have history of minor emotional disturbances

**4. List the physical signs suggestive of an organic versus a nonorganic etiology for joint pain.**

| Organic | Nonorganic |
|---|---|
| Point tenderness<br>Redness<br>Swelling<br>Limitation of movement of affected extremity secondary to pain or anatomic restriction<br>Objective muscle weakness or atrophy<br>Signs of systemic illness: fever, rash, pallor, lymphadenopathy, and organomegaly | Normal exam or minor neurovascular changes, such as coolness or mottling of affected extremity |

**5. Which laboratory tests are helpful in differentiating causes of joint pain?**

| TEST | CONDITIONS IN WHICH TEST MAY BE HELPFUL |
|---|---|
| CBC, differential, platelets | Leukemia<br>Infections in bones, joints, muscles<br>Systemic collagen vascular diseases |
| Sedimentation rate | Infections<br>Collagen vascular diseases<br>Inflammatory bowel disease<br>Tumors |
| Radiographs | All bone tumors, malignant and benign<br>Osteomyelitis (chronic)<br>Discitis (late)<br>Fractures<br>Scoliosis<br>Rickets<br>Slipped capital femoral epiphysis<br>Legg-Calvé-Perthes disease<br>Leukemia |
| Bone scan | Osteomyelitis (acute and chronic)<br>Discitis<br>Osteoid osteoma<br>Malignant bone tumors and metastases<br>Infarction of bone<br>Reflex sympathetic dystrophy |

(*Table continued on next page.*)

| TEST | CONDITIONS IN WHICH TEST MAY BE HELPFUL |
|---|---|
| Muscle enzymes | Inflammatory muscle disease (idiopathic or viral)<br>Muscular dystrophy<br>Rhabdomyolysis |

**6. How does the number of affected joints help in sorting through the differential diagnosis of arthritis?**

Factors helpful in assessing the etiology of arthritis are the duration of disease at the time the child is evaluated, the sex and age of the child, and the onset type and pattern of joint involvement. The differential diagnosis of polyarthritis is considerably different from that of monarthritis or oligoarthritis. Juvenile rheumatoid arthritis (JRA) is the most common cause of chronic monoarthritis, especially in girls younger than 5 years of age.

| MONOARTHRITIS | POLYARTHRITIS |
|---|---|
| Acute onset of monoarthritis | Polyarticular JRA |
| Early rheumatic disease | Seronegative spondyloarthropathy |
| Oligoarticular JRA | Juvenile ankylosing spondylitis |
| Seronegative spondyloarthropathy | Juvenile psoriatic arthritis |
| Arthritis related to infection | Arthritides of inflammatory bowel disease |
| Septic arthritis | Systemic lupus erythematosus |
| Reactive arthritis | Polyarthritis related to infection |
| Lyme disease | Lyme disease |
| Malignancy | Reactive arthritis/Reiter syndrome |
| Leukemia | Rheumatic fever |
| Neuroblastoma | Other |
| Hemophilia | Sarcoidosis |
| Chronic monarthritis | Familial hypertrophic synovitis |
| Oligoarticular JRA | Mucopolysaccharidoses |
| Juvenile ankylosing spondylitis | |
| Juvenile psoriatic arthritis | |
| Villonodular synovitis | |
| Sarcoidosis | |

Adapted from Cassidy JT, Petty RE: Textbook of Pediatric Rheumatology, 3rd ed. Philadelphia, WB Saunders, 1995.

**7. How does the diurnal variation in joint pain aid in diagnosis?**

Stiffness and pain on range of motion (ROM) immediately upon arising in the morning (morning stiffness) and after periods of inactivity (gelling) are classic findings for the inflammatory arthritides. Morning stiffness will be relieved by heat and ROM exercises. The duration of morning stiffness is an excellent gauge of the severity of the arthritis and the efficacy of therapy. In contrast, mechanical joint pain will worsen over the course of the day and with activity. Finally, night time pain and/or awakening with pain are red flags for neoplasia or, on a less serious note, for "growing pains."

**8. In which rheumatic conditions are the affected joints erythematous?**

Septic arthritis, rheumatic fever, and neoplasia.

Red joints are very rare in JRA and in most other rheumatic conditions, and they should be a "red flag" for the above diagnoses. The arthritis of rheumatic fever is also characterized by its migratory nature and by pain often out of proportion to the apparent severity of findings on joint examination (e.g., degree of swelling, limitation of motion).

**9. In a child with a swollen joint, how is joint fluid helpful in determining the etiology of joint pain?**

| GROUP/CONDITION | WBC COUNT (/ML) | PMN (%) | MISCELLANEOUS FINDINGS |
|---|---|---|---|
| Noninflammatory | | | |
| Normal | < 200 | < 25 | — |
| Traumatic arthritis | < 2000 | < 25 | Debris |
| Osteoarthritis | 1000 | < 25 | — |
| Inflammatory | | | |
| SLE | 5000 | 10 | LE cells |
| Rheumatic fever | 5000 | 10–50 | — |
| JRA | 15,000–20,000 | 75 | — |
| Reiter syndrome | 20,000 | 80 | Reiter cells |
| Pyogenic | | | |
| Tuberculous arthritis | 25,000 | 50–60 | Acid-fast bacteria |
| Septic arthritis | 50,000–300,000 | >75 | Low glucose, bacteria |

Adapted from Cassidy JT, Petty RE: Textbook of Pediatric Rheumatology, 3rd ed. Philadelphia, WB Saunders, 1995.

**10. Describe the clinical characteristics of the three types of JRA.**

| | POLYARTHRITIS | OLIGOARTHRITIS (PAUCIARTICULAR DISEASE) | SYSTEMIC (STILL'S DISEASE) |
|---|---|---|---|
| Frequency of cases | 40% | 50% | 10% |
| Number of joints involved | ≥ 5 | ≤ 4 | Variable |
| Age of onset | Throughout childhood; peak at 1–3 yr | Early childhood; peak at 1–2 yr | Throughout childhood; no peak |
| Sex ration (F:M) | 3:1 | 5:1 | 1:1 |
| Systemic involvement | Moderate involvement | Not present | Prominent |
| Occurrence of chronic uveitis | 5% | 20% | Rare |
| Frequency of seropositivity | | | |
| Rheumatoid factors | 10% (increases with age) | Rare | Rare |
| Antinuclear antibodies | 40–50% | 75–85%* | 10% |
| Prognosis | Guarded to moderately good | Excellent except for eyesight | Moderate to poor |

* In girls with uveitis.
Adapted from Cassidy JT, Petty RE: Textbook of Pediatric Rheumatology, 3rd ed. Philadelphia, WB Saunders, 1995.

**11. How is leg length assessed in a child? Why is the affected leg often longer in a child with pauciarticular JRA?**

Leg length is measured from the anterior superior iliac spine to the medial malleolus. In a child with a joint contracture, the functional leg length may be shorter than the actual leg length, and therefore both must be measured.

The affected leg is often longer in a child with pauciarticular JRA (in particular, that affecting the knee) as a result of increased blood flow to the joint in response to localized inflammation and cytokine release. This increased blood flow may also lead to development of "macroepiphysis." A leg-length discrepancy may result in an abnormal gait, and correction with a lift on the bottom of the shoe of the shorter leg is recommended for a length discrepancy > 2 cm. The shorter, unaffected leg will usually "catch up" to the affected leg and may overgrow the affected leg, since the epiphysis of the inflamed joint will undergo accelerated fusion. Muscle bulk may also be affected in pauciarticular JRA. Interestingly, the muscles of the thigh or the calf may be affected in a particular patient with knee arthritis, and muscle bulk of the affected leg will rarely "catch up" to that of the unaffected leg, particularly if the arthritis has onset at < 6 years of age.

**12. What are "red flags" for neoplasia as the etiology of joint pain?**

- Joint redness
- Fever, weight loss, night sweats
- Night time pain
- Adenopathy
- Associated bone pain (i.e., pain between joints and on direct palpation) out of proportion to physical findings

Malignancy must be considered in any child in whom a diagnosis of systemic JRA is entertained, since the classic features of systemic JRA (i.e., fever, rash, and arthritis) are also seen in malignancy. Malignant infiltration of bone or synovium may mimic polyarthritis. In addition, joint effusions occur in children with malignancy, possibly owing to antigen-antibody complex deposition producing a serum sickness–like picture. This may also be responsible for the tremendous inflammatory response seen in some children with malignancy, again mimicking systemic JRA, with moderate to severe anemia, and elevation of the ESR.

Acute leukemia causing polyarthritis should be suspected in children with an elevated ESR but low platelet counts. Other frequent laboratory abnormalities are an elevated LDH, uric acid, and abnormal peripheral blood smear.

Radiographs of affected joints and/or whole body bone scans may be helpful in diagnosis. Bone marrow examination is recommended prior to initiation of high-dose corticosteroid therapy for systemic JRA, since inappropriate use of corticosteroids in malignancy can worsen prognosis.

**13. What neoplasms are most likely to have musculoskeletal complaints upon presentation in childhood?**

- Acute leukemia (especially ALL)—consider in any child with "painful" JRA.
- Neuroblastoma—70% in children with 85% less than 5 years old. Many have systemic symptoms.
- Ewing sarcoma—monoarticular pain.
- Lymphoma.

**14. Describe the characteristics of the childhood "pain amplification" syndromes: growing pains, primary fibromyalgia, and reflex sympathetic dystrophy (RSD).**

| | GROWING PAINS | PRIMARY FIBROMYALGIA | RSD |
|---|---|---|---|
| Age at onset | 4–12 yrs | Adolescence to adulthood | Late childhood and adolescence to adulthood |
| Sex ratio | Equal | F >> M | F >> M |
| Symptoms | Deep aching, cramping pain in thigh or calf<br>Usually in evening or during the night; never present in morning<br>Bilateral<br>Responds to massage and analgesia | Generalized fatigue, anxiety, depression<br>Disturbed sleep patterns | Exquisite superficial and deep pain in the distal part of an extremity<br>Exacerbated by passive or active movement |
| Signs | Physical exam normal | Tender points at characteristic sites (over 3 mos) | Diffuse swelling, tenderness, coolness and mottling<br>Bizarre posturing of affected part |
| Investigations | Laboratory exam normal | Laboratory exam normal | Osteoporosis, bone scan abnormalities<br>Laboratory exam normal |

Adapted from Cassidy JT, Petty RE: Textbook of Pediatric Rheumatology, 3rd ed. Philadelphia, WB Saunders, 1995.

**15. Describe the characteristics of the common non-rheumatic pain syndromes in childhood: patellofemoral pain syndrome (chondromalacia) and Osgood-Schlatter disease.**

| | CHONDROMALACIA | OSGOOD-SCHLATTER |
|---|---|---|
| Age at onset | Adolescence to young adulthood | Athletic adolescents |
| Sex ratio | F > M | M > F |
| Symptoms | Insidious onset of exertional knee pain<br>Difficulty descending stairs; need to sit with legs straight | Pain over tibial tubercle exacerbated by exercise |
| Signs | Patellar tenderness on compression<br>Quadriceps weakness<br>Inhibition sign<br>Joint effusion | Tenderness and swelling over attachment of patellar tendon |
| Investigations | — | Radiograph shows soft tissue swelling, enlarged and sometimes fragmented tubercle |

Adapted from Cassidy JT, Petty RE: Textbook of Pediatric Rheumatology, 3rd ed. Philadelphia, WB Saunders, 1995.

**16. What are the causes of hip pain in childhood?**

- Transient synovitis
- Bacterial infection
- Avascular necrosis (Legg-Calvé-Perthes disease)
- Slipped capital femoral epiphysis
- Protrusio acetabuli
- Arthritis
  - B27 arthropathy
  - JRA
  - Reactive arthritis/Reiter syndrome
  - Rheumatic fever
- Malignancy
  - Local
    - Benign (e.g., osteoid osteoma)
    - Malignant (e.g., Ewing sarcoma)
  - Generalized
    - Leukemia
    - Neuroblastoma

Arthritis of the hip joint is rare at the onset of pauciarticular JRA. Onset of apparent arthritis in the hip in a very young child should be considered first to be a septic process or congenital dislocation. Transient synovitis of the hip may cause very severe pain, but the process is self-limited, lasting one to a few weeks, and all laboratory and radiologic studies are normal. In the older child and adolescent, avascular necrosis (Legg-Calvé-Perthes disease) and slipped capital femoral epiphysis should be considered. In older boys, juvenile ankylosing spondylitis may present with unilateral or bilateral hip involvement, although distal joints are affected more commonly than proximal joints. Be aware that hip pain may be referred to the knee. In particular, hip pain in the infant may be misinterpreted by parents and physicians as knee pain.

**17. What causes back pain in childhood?**

Back and neck pain are relatively rare complaints in young children (unlike the situation in adolescents and adults) and should be taken very seriously. Although infection of an intervertebral disc space is rare secondary to osteomyelitis of an adjoining vertebral body, acute discitis should be considered. Discitis is an inflammatory process that occurs throughout childhood, with a peak at age 1–3 years. It may be caused by pathogens of low virulence (e.g., viruses, *Staphylococcus aureus*, Enterobacteriaceae, or *Moraxella*), although bacteria or viruses are seldom recovered by aspiration. Fever, refusal to walk, unusual posturing, stiffness, and point tenderness over the lumbar region are characteristic. The ESR is usually moderately elevated. Plain radiographs may show disc-space narrowing, although often not until late in the disease.

Earlier in the course, Tc-99m bone scan often shows increased uptake of isotope and is therefore valuable diagnostically at the time of presentation.

In addition, malignancy (e.g., metastases, primary bone tumors, or leukemia) should be considered, as well as juvenile ankylosing spondylitis (JAS). However, JAS generally presents as peripheral arthritis (75% of children at presentation), with back complaints (pain, stiffness, or limitation of motion of the lumbosacral spine or sacroiliac joints) only reported by 25% of affected children prior to the third decade. Back pain is uncommon in JRA. Spondylolysis, with or without spondylolisthesis, may cause chronic back pain. Scheuermann's disease or, rarely, herniation of an intervertebral disc results in pain in the lower thoracic or lumbar region.

**18. What medications are used to treat inflammatory arthritis in childhood?**

| MEDICATION | DAILY DOSE (MG/KG/D) |
|---|---|
| **NSAIDs** | |
| Salicylate | < 25 kg: 80–100<br>> 25 kg: 2.5 gm/m$^2$/d |
| Ibuprofen | 20–40 |
| Naproxen | 10–20 |
| Indomethacin | 0.5–3 |
| Tolmetin | 15–30 |
| Sulindac | 4–6 |
| Diclofenac | 2–3 |
| **DMARDs** | |
| Hydroxychloroquine | 5–7 |
| Sulfasalazine | 40–60 |
| Methotrexate* | 0.3–1.0 mg/kg/wk or 10–30 mg/m$^2$/wk (max: 15–30 mg/wk) |
| Etanercept* | 0.4 mg/kg/dose (given twice a week) |
| **Corticosteroids** | |
| Triamcinolone (into joints) | 1 |
| Prednisone | 1–2 |
| Pulse methylprednisolone | 30 |

* Methotrexate is given weekly (max: 1 gm/d), and etanercept is given bi-weekly, not daily. Methotrexate (25 mg/cc), ibuprofen (100 mg/5 cc), Naprosyn (125 mg/5cc), and indomethacin (25 mg/cc) come in suspensions as well as tablets. No dose should exceed the maximum dose recommended for adults. DMARD = disease-modifying antirheumatic drug.

**19. A child presents with a 1-week history of a single, hot, red, swollen, painful joint. The child is febrile and refuses to bear weight on the affected leg. Describe the work-up.**

Immediate joint aspiration is always indicated in such a patient to exclude septic arthritis or osteomyelitis. Gram stain should be performed; WBC and differential counts, glucose, and protein levels should be determined; and the synovial fluid should be cultured for *Haemophilus influenzae*, *Neisseria gonorrhoeae*, and gram-negative organisms. Special media and conditions are required if anaerobic organisms or mycobacteria are suspected. Cultures of blood and suspected sources of infection (e.g., cellulitis) are required in a child with suspected septic arthritis.

Although an organism can be identified in approximately two-thirds of children, no causative organism is identified in approximately one-third, with the diagnosis being made on the basis of a consistent history and the presence of pus on arthrocentesis. However, synovial fluid WBC counts may be low (< 25,000/mm$^3$) in up to one-third of patients with septic arthritis. Identification of an organism is particularly difficult in those patients who have received antibiotics. Supportive laboratory studies are an elevated WBC count with a predominance of PMNs and bands, and a markedly elevated ESR or C-reactive protein.

**20. Another child has an 8-week history of a single warm, swollen joint that is not very painful, tender, or red. The child has been afebrile and, with the exception of a mild upper respiratory infection, has been otherwise well. Describe the work-up.**

While any history of antecedent trauma should be elicited, trauma is very unlikely to cause a swollen joint persisting 8 weeks in the absence of significant pain. Interestingly, parents often date joint swelling to an acute event (such as a fall), although the event may serve only to bring their attention to an already swollen joint. The 8-week history of swelling meets the criteria of "> 6 weeks" required for a diagnosis of JRA. The first episode of JRA, and subsequent flares of arthritis are often precipitated by intercurrent illness, such as an upper respiratory infection.

The most useful finding on physical exam in this case would be the presence of a second (or more) affected joint(s), as this would argue strongly for a diagnosis of JRA. In particular, the small joints of the hands and feet should be examined carefully. If the knee is involved, a Baker's cyst would strongly indicate a diagnosis of JRA. Involvement of the wrists by JRA would be suggested if the child holds the hands still in the lap, supinated, with the wrists slightly flexed. Lack of neck movement, using only the eyes to follow the examiner, is a clue for neck involvement. Circumduction of the affected leg on gait examination may suggest a leg-length discrepancy, indicating a longer duration of arthritis than 8 weeks. Similarly, the presence of joint contractures would suggest a longer duration of arthritis.

In pauciarticular JRA, the CBC and ESR are often entirely normal. Radiographs, other than confirming the presence of effusion, also are normal, without evidence of loss of joint space or bony erosion. This form of JRA does not generally lead to joint destruction, and even in the more destructive forms (e.g., a subgroup of polyarticular JRA), bony erosion is rarely seen until after 2 years of disease. The anti-nuclear antibody (ANA) will be the most helpful laboratory test in suspected pauciarticular JRA. One-half of children with this diagnosis have a positive ANA, and one-half of children with a positive ANA have chronic anterior uveitis, a potentially blinding (yet almost invariably asymptomatic) inflammation of the eyes. Children with JRA only rarely have positive rheumatoid factors.

## BIBLIOGRAPHY

1. Ansell BM, Rudge S, Schaller JG: Color Atlas of Pediatric Rheumatology. St. Louis, Mosby–Year Book, 1992.
2. Cassidy JT, Petty RE: Textbook of Pediatric Rheumatology, 3rd ed. Philadelphia, WB Saunders, 1995.
3. Cron RQ, Sharma S, Sherry DD: Current treatment by United States and Canadian pediatric rheumatologists. J Rheumatol 26:2036, 1999.
4. Fernandez M, Carrol CL, Baker CJ: Discitis and vertebral osteomyelitis in children: An 18-year review. Pediatrics 105:1299, 2000.
5. Gedalia A, Brewer EJ: Joint hypermobility in pediatric practice—a review. J Rheumatol 20:371, 1993.
6. Johnson RP: Anterior knee pain in adolescents and young adults. Curr Opin Rheumatol 9:159, 1997.
7. Kocher MS, Zurakowski D, Kasser JR: Differentiating between septic arthritis and transient synovitis of the hip in children: An evidence-based clinical prediction algorithm. J Bone Joint Surg Am 81:1662, 1999.
8. Lovell DJ, Giannini EH, Reiff A, et al: Etanercept in children with polyarticular juvenile rheumatoid arthritis. N Engl J Med 342:763, 2000.
9. Peterson H: Growing pains. Pediatr Clin North Am 33:1365, 1986.
10. Prieur AM: Spondyloarthropathies in childhood. Bailliere Clin Rheumatol 12:287, 1998.
11. Sherry DD: Musculoskeletal pain in children. Curr Opin Rheumatol 9:465, 1997.
12. Sherry DD, Wallace CA, Kelley C, et al: Short- and long-term outcomes of children with complex regional pain syndrome type I treated with exercise therapy. Clin J Pain 15:218, 1999.
13. Southwood TR: Classifying childhood arthritis. Ann Rheum Dis 56:79, 1997.
14. Trapani S, Grisolia F, Simonini G, et al: Incidence of occult cancer in children presenting with musculoskeletal symptoms: A 10-year survey in a pediatric rheumatology unit. Semin Arthritis Rheum 29:348, 2000.
15. Wallace CA: The use of methotrexate in childhood rheumatic diseases. Arthritis Rheum 41:381, 1998.

# 73. JUVENILE CHRONIC ARTHRITIS

J. Roger Hollister, M.D.

**1. What are the main types of juvenile chronic arthritis [also called juvenile rheumatoid arthritis (JRA)]?**

1. **Polyarticular**, with involvement of many joints, large and small, in a symmetric fashion. Additionally, this type may be subgrouped on the basis of the presence or absence of rheumatoid factor in the blood. Rheumatoid factor positivity is a harbinger of a more-aggressive arthritis, with increased risk of joint damage, disability, and eventual need for surgery.

2. **Pauciarticular**, with one or a few (< 5) large joints, frequently asymmetric. There are two subgroups:

   a. Peak age of onset at 2–5 years, with a 3:1 female predominance and a high frequency of positive antinuclear antibodies (ANA). This subtype has a relatively benign prognosis with remissions likely, but it runs the greatest risk of the associated chronic iridocyclitis (iritis).

   b. Older age of onset (> 6 yrs), more often in males, and more often HLA B27 positive.

3. **Systemic onset**, which is characterized by high fevers, evanescent rash, polyarthralgia/arthritis, and extra-articular inflammation. Equal gender frequency and distribution throughout childhood characterize this type of juvenile chronic arthritis. This is also called Still's disease.

**2. What types of anterior uveitis are associated with juvenile chronic arthritis?**

*Anterior Uveitis in Juvenile Chronic Arthritis*

| | ACUTE UVEITIS | CHRONIC UVEITIS |
|---|---|---|
| Disease association | Spondyloarthropathy | Pauciarticular JRA |
| Lab markers | B27 antigen | Positive ANA |
| Symptoms | Hot, red, photophobic eye | None |
| Complications (if untreated) | Few | Synechiae, cataract, glaucoma, band keratopathy |
| Necessity of slit-lamp screening | No | Yes |

**3. Should ANA status affect the frequency of slit-lamp screening in pauciarticular JRA patients?**

Yes. ANA-positive patients with pauciarticular JRA have a 33% risk of developing chronic, asymptomatic uveitis, whereas ANA-negative children have a 10% risk. Therefore, ANA-positive patients should be screened every 3 months, and ANA-negative patients can be seen every 6 months.

**4. How long should slit-lamp screening be continued?**

One-half of children who will develop chronic uveitis will have it present at the first eye appointment. Uveitis incidence diminishes with each subsequent year after joint swelling develops. Five years after joint swelling develops, the risk of new-onset uveitis is so low that screening is no longer cost-effective. However, slit-lamp screening is necessary within the first 5 years even when the joint disease is in remission.

**5. In the differential diagnosis of arthritis in childhood, what is the significance of a migratory versus summating pattern of onset?**

**A migratory pattern**—i.e., one joint is subsiding as another becomes inflamed—is seen in rheumatic fever, post-streptococcal arthritis, and gonococcal arthritis. **A summating pattern**—

i.e., adding one inflamed joint to another—is characteristic of JRA, psoriatic arthritis, and spondyloarthropathy.

**6. Two fever patterns are represented below that may aid in the diagnosis of a fever of unknown origin (FUO). Which is characteristic of systemic JRA?**

The fever pattern of systemic JRA is characterized by fever spikes occurring at the same time each day, with spontaneous defervescence to normal or subnormal levels. In contrast, the fever spikes of bacterial sepsis are hectic and occur on an elevated temperature base. Normal temperatures are not found until adequate antibacterial treatment is initiated.

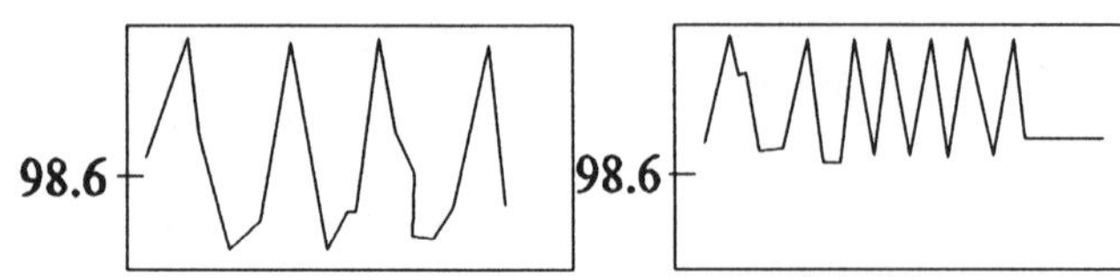


**7. In the diagnosis of FUO, what laboratory tests are specific for systemic JRA (Still's disease)?**

None. The laboratory tests demonstrate a chronic inflammatory process, and a normal sedimentation rate excludes the diagnosis of systemic JRA. The leukocyte count is often elevated to extraordinary, even leukemoid degrees, with a significant left shift. Platelet counts are often equally elevated, and thrombocytopenia is inconsistent with the diagnosis. A mild/moderate anemia of chronic disease is often present. Other acute-phase reactants, such as ferritin (> 1000 μg/L) and C-reactive proteins, are frequently increased. In perplexing cases, a normal lactate dehydrogenase level can add reassurance that a malignancy is not the cause of the FUO.

**8. Which rashes are specific to causes of juvenile arthritis?** (See figure, top of next page.)

The rash of **erythema marginatum** is pathognomonic of acute rheumatic fever, a condition that has diminished in frequency over the past several decades for unknown reasons. This circinate rash with central clearing appears at the time of the migratory arthritis, heart murmur, and subcutaneous nodules. It is one of the five major criteria for diagnosis of rheumatic fever.

The **ecchymotic, lower-extremity rash** characteristic of Henoch-Schönlein purpura may start as a maculopapular or even urticarial lesion. The rash usually precedes joint swelling but may follow it by a few days. It leaves no residue and rarely needs treatment.

The **"Still's" rash** of systemic JRA is present in 90% of cases. The pink macules are very evanescent, most common on the trunk and proximal extremities and rarely pruritic. They are frequently present during fever spikes. If the lesions are present for 24 hours in a single location, they are not the lesions of Still's rash.

**9. The child you are seeing with a single swollen knee has grandparents with what sounds to be rheumatoid arthritis. Is there a genetic relationship?**

Little, if any. The histocompatibility gene linked to seropositive rheumatoid arthritis, DR4, is actually found less often in the JRA population than in normal children. In pauciarticular JRA, DR5 and DR8 show an association in several studies but certainly not to the degree of B27 and the spondyloarthropathies.

**10. Which regions of the United States have the highest number of Lyme disease cases?**

Over 80% of reported cases of Lyme disease are found in only 5 states: New York, Massachusetts, Connecticut, Minnesota, and Wisconsin.

**11. In these regions, how does one clinically distinguish pauciarticular JRA from Lyme arthritis?**

**Lyme arthritis** is an episodic inflammation with attacks lasting, on average, 2–5 weeks. The inflammation of **pauciarticular JRA** is chronic and must be present for at least 6 weeks before the diagnosis is certain.

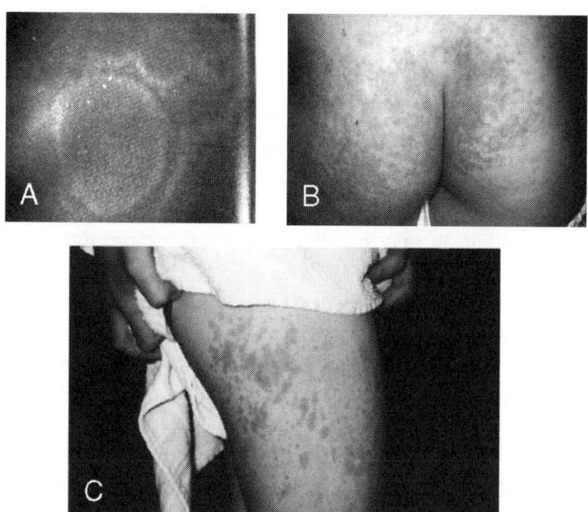

*A*, Erythema marginatum. *B*, Henoch-Schönlein purpura. *C*, Systemic JRA.

**12. A patient presents with poorly localized leg pain sufficient to interrupt sleep and cause a limp. Which malignancies must be considered in the differential diagnosis?**

**Leukemia** and stage IV **neuroblastoma** are the two neoplasms that can involve bone and simulate arthritis, even to the point of producing joint swelling, elevated sedimentation rate, and increased platelet counts. If an isolated lactate dehydrogenase level is elevated while other liver functions tests are normal, additional tests such as bone scans, ultrasound, or bone marrow biopsy may be warranted to rule out malignancy.

**13. A positive ANA is a prerequisite for the diagnosis of systemic lupus erythematosus (SLE) in childhood, and ANA is often seen in children with JRA. How specific is it to these diagnoses?**

Not very. Autoantibodies can be seen in a variety of situations in which the common denominator is prolonged antigen stimulation. Rheumatoid factors can be produced in experimental animals with immunization with irrelevant antigens. Similarly, they are found in patients with subacute bacterial endocarditis. A positive ANA that does not match a patient's clinical presentation is seen in children with a recent history of recurrent streptococcal infection and elevated levels of anti-streptococcal antibodies (unpublished observation).

**14. In a child with JRA, what is the risk that a sibling will develop the same illness?**

In several published series, there is a remarkable agreement that the risk is 1 in 100. The prevalence of the disease in the normal population is 1 in 1000. Therefore, there may be a genetic predisposition, although it clearly is not as strong as that for diseases such as hemophilia, cystic fibrosis, or diabetes. These facts suggest that an unidentified environmental agent may also be necessary for disease expression.

**15. The time-honored treatment for JRA was aspirin, but more recently, other nonsteroidal medications have supplanted aspirin. Why?**

As an NSAID, aspirin is as effective as other agents; however, with the increased public awareness about Reye's syndrome and the necessity of three or four doses a day, parents have become less accepting of this treatment. The relationship between Reye's syndrome and salicylate treatment during chicken pox or Asian flu is statistically valid. With the use of acetaminophen as an antipyretic, the incidence of Reye syndrome has dropped dramatically.

In addition, NSAIDs are now available in liquid form (naproxen and ibuprofen), which are much easier to administer to children < 5 years of age. For older children, naproxen, ibuprofen, and tolmetin are approved for use, although many rheumatologists use other NSAIDs with less frequent dosing to improve compliance.

**16. Prednisone may be necessary for the treatment of systemic JRA, pericarditis, or refractory iritis, but the side effects of high-dose prednisone are well-known. Is it possible to avoid untoward effects by using low-dose prednisone therapy?**

No. Osteoporosis and growth suppression can both be produced by as little as 5 mg of prednisone a day. The demineralization may be alleviated by a calcium intake of 1200 mg/day with 400 U of vitamin D.

Prednisone therapy has a profound effect on linear growth. However, alternate-day doses of prednisone up to 20 mg may still allow appropriate growth. Unfortunately, arthritis is more difficult to treat on an every-other-day basis in diseases such as SLE or dermatomyositis. Prednisone doses of less than .5 mg/kg may allow growth if underlying disease is controlled.

**17. Injectable gold salts was formerly the second-line treatment of JRA. In one subgroup of JRA, however, this treatment is relatively contraindicated. Why?**

In systemic JRA, a sufficient number of cases of disseminated intravascular coagulation due to macrophage activation syndrome have occurred with injectable gold salts (aurothioglucose or gold sodium thiomalate) to suggest a relative contraindication.

**18. School-aged children with JRA have legal rights to therapeutic resources in school. What are they?**

Under P.L. 94-142 (the Education for All Handicapped Act), children with arthritis are entitled to a free, public education that may require "special related services." These services may include physical and occupational therapy through the school system. This requirement depends on the financial status of the individual school district. However, if the school system provides such services for developmentally disabled children or those with cerebral palsy, they must provide them to children with arthritis.

**19. Advanced therapy for adult rheumatoid arthritis frequently includes low-dose weekly methotrexate therapy. Can this drug be used in children with JRA?**

Yes. In fact, methotrexate (MTX) has largely supplanted injectable gold as the second-line agent in the treatment of JRA. In numerous studies, methotrexate appears to be just as effective and safe in children as it is in adults. Furthermore, the injectable form of methotrexate (25 mg/ml), which is actually less expensive than the tablets, makes it easy to administer to children too young to swallow tablets. After 40 years of use, it is recognized that methotrexate carries very little oncologic risk and little to no risk to fertility. Liver function abnormalities and bone marrow side effects are similar to those in adults.

The starting dose should be 5 mg/wk in the smallest children and 7.5 mg/wk in older children. If no benefit is found after 3 weeks, the dose should be increased in 2.5-mg increments until a response is seen or the dose reaches 1 mg/kg/wk, at which point the patient should be considered as having a treatment failure. Doses greater than 0.6 mg/kg may need parenteral administration, owing to less gastrointestinal absorption above this dose. It is important to remind parents to continue to take their regular NSAID. MTX side effects include gastrointestinal and behavioral problems in some children.

**20. A 12-year-old boy develops knee pain during soccer season and is diagnosed with Osgood-Schlatter disease. Three months later, he is diagnosed with Achilles tendinitis. What form of juvenile chronic arthritis might he have?**

**Ankylosing spondylitis** or another **spondyloarthropathy**. More than 50% of young patients with this disease present with peripheral lower-extremity symptoms, including arthritis or enthesopathy, as was the case with this patient. Enthesopathy refers to inflammation at the site of tendon insertion into the bone. The B27 antigen is found in > 75% of patients. Long-term follow-up of these patients shows that about 30% will go on to develop sacroiliitis, the hallmark of the disease. Spondyloarthropathy is more episodic than JRA. Treatment with NSAIDs, especially indomethacin, permits most children to function quite normally.

**21. Can corticosteroid injections be used in children?**

Yes, particularly in older children who can understand the nature and reason for the injection. Published studies have shown good long-term results, especially with methylprednisolone acetate (Depo-Medrol) or triamcinolone diacetate (Aristocort). The dose to inject in a large joint like the knee is 1 mg/kg up to 40 mg. However, if synovitis recurs in several weeks, steroid injections should not be repeated because of untoward effects on growing cartilage. In very young children, the use of EMLA cream as a topical anesthetic may reduce the apprehension about the injection.

**22. Can the new biologic therapies be used in children with juvenile chronic arthritis?**

Yes. Enbrel (Etanercept) is the anti-TNFα inhibitor specifically FDA-approved for the treatment of children with juvenile chronic arthritis in whom methotrexate therapy fails. The starting dose is 0.4 mg/kg subcutaneous twice a week. It should not be used in children with a suspected progressive neurological condition. Side effects are remarkably few, mainly red marks at the site of injection. No laboratory supervision is necessary. Response is usually seen in 2–3 weeks. If there is no response, the dose can be increased up to the adult dose of 25 mg twice a week. It can be combined with methotrexate.

## BIBLIOGRAPHY


1. Dana MR, et al: Visual outcomes prognosticators in juvenile rheumatoid associated uveitis. Ophthalmology 104:236–244, 1997.
2. Giannini EH, et al: Methotrexate in resistant juvenile rheumatoid arthritis: Results of the U.S.A.-U.S.S.R. double-blind, placebo-controlled trial. N Engl J Med 326:1043–1049, 1992.
3. Hashkes P: The relationship of hepatotoxic risk factors and liver histology in methotrexate therapy for juvenile rheumatoid arthritis. J Pediatr 134:47–52, 1999.
4. Lovell DJ, et al: Etanercept in children with polyarticular juvenile rheumatoid arthritis. N Engl J Med 342:763–769, 2000.
5. Minden K, et al: Prognosis of patients with juvenile chronic arthritis and juvenile spondyloarthropathy. J Rheumatol 27:2256–2263, 2000.
6. Schaller JG: Juvenile rheumatoid arthritis. Pediatr Rev 18:337–349, 1997.
7. Wallendahl M, Stark L, Hollister JR: The discriminating value of serum LDH values in children with malignancy presenting as joint pain. Arch Pedriatr Adol Med 150:70–73, 1996.
8. Wargula JC, Lovell DJ: Use of etanercept in children. Bulletin on the Rheumatic Dis 49(12):1–4, 2000.
9. Woo P, Wedderburn LR: Juvenile chronic arthritis. Lancet 351:969–973, 1998.


# 74. JUVENILE SYSTEMIC CONNECTIVE TISSUE DISEASES

*Randy* Q. *Cron*, M.D., *Ph*.D., *and* *Terri* H. *Finkel*, M.D., *Ph*.D.

**1. What are the juvenile systemic connective tissue diseases (CTDs)?**

- Systemic juvenile rheumatoid arthritis (see Chapter 73)
- Systemic lupus erythematosus (SLE)
- Overlap syndromes, including mixed CTD
- Reactive arthritis, including Reiter's syndrome
- Sarcoidosis
- Inflammatory bowel disease
- Rheumatic fever
- Dermatomyositis
- Scleroderma
- Vasculitis

**2. Discuss the epidemiology of juvenile SLE.**

Data on the incidence and prevalence of SLE in children are few. The proportion of all patients presenting with SLE in childhood is ~15%. In childhood, the disease generally presents in adolescence and rarely before age 5 years. The ratio of girls to boys is about 2:1 before age 10 years and then, in adolescents, is similar to the ratio of women to men (5:1 to 10:1). SLE appears to be more common in children of black, Asian, and Hispanic origin. About 10% have one or more affected relatives, including siblings and twins.

**3. What are the criteria for the diagnosis of SLE in children?**

The same as in adults (Chapter 20). A child is considered to have SLE if any 4 or more of 11 criteria are present. Childhood-onset SLE is generally more severe than in adults, with a high incidence of nephritis, pericarditis, hepatosplenomegaly, and chorea.

**4. What are the clinical manifestations of SLE?**

SLE is characterized by multiple autoantibodies and multisystem involvement. An easy way to remember the complex array of systemic manifestations of SLE is to think from head to toe. Thus:

| | |
|---|---|
| General | Malaise, weight loss, fever |
| Skin | Butterfly rash, discoid lupus, vasculitic skin lesions, alopecia, photosensitivity |
| Brain | Headache, blurred vision, psychosis, chorea, seizures, neuropathies, cerebrovascular accident, transverse myelitis |
| Eye | Cotton-wool spots, retinitis, episcleritis, iritis (rarely) |
| Mouth | Oral ulcers |
| Chest | Pleuritis, basilar pneumonitis, pulmonary hemorrhage, shrinking lung syndrome |
| Heart | Pericarditis, myocarditis, Libman-Sacks endocarditis |
| Digestive system | Hepatosplenomegaly, mesenteric arteritis, colitis, hepatitis |
| Kidneys | Glomerulonephritis, nephrotic syndrome, hypertension |
| Extremities | Arthralgia or arthritis, myalgia or myositis, Raynaud's phenomenon, thrombophlebitis, aseptic necrosis |

**5. How does the ANA pattern and titer aid in the diagnosis and management of SLE?**

ANAs are present in the sera of almost all children with active SLE. In fact, the absence of ANAs, particularly at the time of symptomatic disease, essentially eliminates SLE as a diagnostic consideration. The average ANA titer in individuals with SLE is 1:320, although in active disease it may be considerably higher. Changes in the ANA titer are not a useful indicator of disease activity and are not followed subsequent to diagnosis.

The "rim" pattern on the ANA, in which fluorescence is seen rimming the nuclear membrane, is pathognomonic of SLE, though rarely seen. The "homogeneous" pattern, in which fluorescence is seen uniformly over the nucleus, is the pattern most commonly seen in SLE, while the "speckled" pattern is the least specific.

The ANA is a highly subjective test, and the pattern and titer vary greatly among laboratories. False-positives are not uncommon. False-negatives are rare, but if you are convinced of the diagnosis of SLE in a patient, repeat of the ANA is indicated in a different laboratory and/or at a future date.

**6. How does the ANA profile aid in the diagnosis and management of SLE and related juvenile systemic CTDs?**

As detailed in the table, while a negative ANA profile does not rule out any of the juvenile systemic CTDs, a positive ANA profile can be extremely useful in making a specific diagnosis. In particular, anti-DNA and anti-Sm antibodies are specific for SLE; high titers of anti-RNP antibody are suggestive of mixed connective tissue disease (MCTD); and anti-Ro and/or anti-La antibodies are found in Sjögren's syndrome, although this syndrome and antibodies are most commonly seen as a part of SLE. In addition, anti-histone antibodies may be seen in SLE and in drug-induced lupus. These two diagnoses may be distinguished by the presence of antibodies to specific histones. Finally, a positive ANA is essentially never found in systemic juvenile rheumatoid arthritis (RA, Still's disease).

| | ACTIVE SLE | MCTD | PSS | CREST | PRIMARY SJÖGREN'S | RA |
|---|---|---|---|---|---|---|
| ANA | 99% | 100% | 70–90% | 60–90% | > 70% | 40–50% |
| Anti-native DNA | 60% | Neg | Neg | Neg | Neg | Neg |
| Anti-SM | 30% | Neg | Neg | Neg | Neg | Neg |
| Anti-RNP | 30% | > 95% titer > 1:10,000 | Common (low titer) | Neg (low titer) | Rare | Rare |
| Anti-centromere | Rare | Rare | 10–15% | 60–90% | Neg | Neg |
| Anti-Ro (SS-A) | 30% | Rare | Rare | Neg | 70% | Rare |
| Anti-La (SS-B) | 15% | Rare | Rare | Neg | 60% | Rare |

PSS = progressive systemic sclerosis.

**7. Which other autoantibodies (other than ANA and ANA profile) can be helpful in the diagnosis of systemic juvenile CTD?**

Antibody reactive with Scl-70 is not typically measured in the standard ANA profile but is found in 15–20% of individuals with systemic sclerosis. Jo-1 and Mi-2 antibodies, while found in only a minority of children with juvenile dermatomyositis, may be useful in identifying those children at increased risk for complicating interstitial lung disease. Vasculitic syndromes associated with the presence of anti-neutrophil cytoplasmic antibodies (C-ANCA or P-ANCA) are polyarteritis nodosa, Wegener's granulomatosis, microscopic polyangiitis, Churg-Strauss syndrome, and crescentic glomerulonephritis.

**8. How are autoantibodies related to the pathophysiology of SLE?**

Autoantibodies to specific blood cells and vascular components are directly responsible for the hematologic manifestations of SLE, such as acute hemolytic anemia, thrombocytopenia, leukopenia, and coagulopathies. In addition, antigen-antibody complexes (in which the antigen is often an ANA) play a significant role in the pathogenesis of lupus vasculitis and nephritis. Lupus nephritis is caused by deposition of immune complexes composed of complement components, immunoglobulins, and DNA in the glomerular lesions. Elution techniques and fluorescence microscopy have demonstrated high titers of antibodies to native DNA in the renal glomeruli.

**9. Describe the management of children with SLE.**

- General
  - Counseling, education
  - Adequate rest
  - Use of sunscreens
  - Immunizations, especially pneumococcal
  - Management of infection
- NSAIDs for musculoskeletal signs and symptoms
- Hydroxychloroquine for cutaneous disease and as adjunct to glucocorticoids for systemic disease
- Glucocorticoids
  - Oral prednisone, 1–2 mg/kg/d
  - IV methylprednisolone initially for severe disease and then monthly for maintenance therapy

- Immunosuppressives
  Azathioprine, 1–2 mg/kg/d
  Cyclophosphamide
  Oral 1–2 mg/kg/d
  IV 500–1000 mg/m$^2$/mo

**10. Discuss the pathophysiology of neonatal lupus.**

Neonatal lupus is associated with the transplacental passage of IgG antibody to Ro (SS-A) and with maternal lupus or Sjögren's syndrome. The most frequent abnormalities are rash (lesions of discoid lupus or subacute cutaneous lupus) and thrombocytopenia, although congenital heart block is of most concern. The cutaneous and hematologic manifestations are transient, generally resolving within 2–6 months, while heart block is frequently permanent and may require a pacemaker.

**11. What is the differential diagnosis of Sjögren's syndrome in childhood?**

Sjögren's syndrome is characterized by dry eyes (keratoconjunctivitis sicca), dry mouth and carious teeth, and parotitis. Differentiating children with **benign recurrent parotid swelling** or **AIDS** from children with Sjögren's syndrome is important. As in adults, salivary gland biopsy of the lip is often helpful to confirm a suspected diagnosis of Sjögren's syndrome. Sjögren's is rare in childhood and is usually found in association with other CTDs, such as **SLE** or mixed **CTD**.

**12. What triad of signs and symptoms is associated with Henoch-Schönlein purpura (HSP) in children?**

Purpura
Colicky abdominal pain
Arthritis

HSP typically occurs in the spring, fall, or winter. The median age at presentation is 4 years, and the male to female ratio is about 1.5:1. About 50% of children have a history of preceding upper respiratory tract infection with a variety of organisms. 97% of children with HSP have a self-limited course, lasting 1–2 weeks. ~20% will recur during the first year. 3–5% of children will suffer persistent purpura with or without persistent renal disease. The purpura may be preceded by arthritis, edema, testicular swelling, and abdominal pain.

**13. List the clinical manifestations of HSP.**

HSP is a systemic vasculitis, and as a result, any organ may be affected.

| | % AT ONSET | % POST ONSET | NOTES |
|---|---|---|---|
| Purpura | 50 | 100 | Normal platelet count |
| Edema | 10–20 | 20–50 | Painful |
| Arthritis | 25 | 60–85 | Large joints |
| GI | 30 | 85 | Volvulus, ileal infarction |
| Renal | ? | 10–50 | — |
| GU | ? | 2–35 | Differential is torsion |
| Pulmonary | ? | 95 (by $DL_{CO}$) | Abnormal CO diffusion |
| Hemorrhage | ? | Rare | Fatal |
| CNS | ? | Very rare | Headache, encephalitis, seizures |

**14. What are poor prognostic factors in HSP at onset?**

| MANIFESTATION | COMMENT |
|---|---|
| Melena | 7.5-fold increase in renal disease |
| Persistent rash for 2–3 mos | Associated with glomerulonephritis |
| Hematuria with proteinuria > 1 gm/day | 15% progress to renal insufficiency |
| Nephrosis with renal insufficiency | 50% renal failure in 10 years |

**15. How should HSP be treated?**

- Arthritis responds to NSAIDs
- Edema responds to steroids
- Abdominal pain resolves within 72 hrs with or without steroids
- Evaluate for and treat infection (e.g., group A β-hemolytic streptococci)
- Aggressive treatment for children with poor prognostic signs

**16. Describe the physical exam of a child presenting with juvenile dermatomyositis (JDMS).**

JDMS is a myositis with characteristic skin rash and vasculitis. Muscle weakness, in particular of the proximal musculature (limbs, girdle, neck), is prominent. The Gower's maneuver is abnormal, and the child will be unable to do a sit-up as a result of weakness. The head may hang back as the child is lifted from a lying position, owing to weakness of the neck muscles. The eyelids and face are edematous, and a heliotrope or mauvish rash is noted around the eyes. Deep red patches, known as Gottron's papules, will be found over the extensor surfaces of the finger joints, as well as over the elbows, knees, and ankle joints. These patches may ulcerate as a result of vasculitis. Telangiectasias may be found around the eyelids and at the nailfolds. Arthralgia or arthritis may be found, sometimes with swelling and contractures of the fingers due to tenosynovitis. In severe chronic JDMS, nodules due to subcutaneous calcinosis may be found. Mobility may be impaired because of calcinotic lesions at the joints or due to involvement of musculature.

**17. How can the muscle weakness of JDMS be differentiated from that of other causes of weakness?**

The muscle weakness of JDMS predominantly involves the proximal musculature, and in general, the involvement is symmetric. The child gives a history of difficulty in climbing stairs or riding a bicycle. Some of the maneuvers detailed in the previous question (e.g., Gower's maneuver) can discriminate true muscle weakness from, for example, inanition. The palate and swallowing musculature may be weak in JDMS and may lead to choking, cough, or aspiration pneumonia. Serum muscle enzymes are elevated, but not to the degree seen in the muscular dystrophies. Assays for all four muscle-derived enzymes are required (aldolase, creatine kinase, SGOT/AST, lactate dehydrogenase) because only one may be elevated. Electromyography will show denervation and inflammatory myopathy. Muscle biopsy will show inflammation and/or fiber necrosis and small vessel vasculitis.

**18. How is JDMS distinguished from adult dermatomyositis or polymyositis?**

In children, dermatomyositis is distinguished by a generalized vasculitis. Chronic polymyositis, in which the rash is absent, is exceedingly rare in childhood. The documented association of adult dermatomyositis or polymyositis with malignancy has not been found in children.

**19. What forms of systemic vasculitis occur in childhood?**

Vasculitis is a component of many of the juvenile systemic CTDs, including HSP, systemic juvenile rheumatoid arthritis, JDMS, and SLE. Five percent of cases of polyarteritis nodosa occur in childhood and, as in adults, are characterized by rash, fever, weight loss, myositis, and cutaneous nodules. Life-threatening renal, GI, cardiac, and CNS involvements are often seen. Large vessel vasculitis, such as Takayasu's, is exceedingly rare in childhood. Wegener's granulomatosis occurs in childhood and may present initially mimicking HSP. The anti-neutrophil cytoplasmic antibodies (autoantibodies directed against enzymes in the neutrophil cytoplasmic granules) may be pathogenic and are of considerable use in the diagnosis and management of the childhood vasculitides.

**20. What is Raynaud's?**

In classic Raynaud's, a tricolor change of the fingers is seen, from white to blue to red. Only two colors, however, are required for diagnosis. Raynaud's involves the fingers only and not the whole hand. The thumb is frequently less involved.

**21. Raynaud's may be seen as primary Raynaud's disease or as Raynaud's phenomenon secondary to another condition. How can these be distinguished?**

Features of Raynaud's disease are:

Female sex

Symptoms for over 2 years

Normal physical exam including nailfold capillaries. No digital pits/ulcers.

Normal lab findings. In particular, absence of ANA or low-titer ANA, without centromere, nucleolar pattern, or specific antibody on ANA profile.

**22. Compare the occurrence and frequency of Raynaud's phenomenon and Raynaud's disease in children and adults.**

| CATEGORY | CHILDREN | ADULTS |
|---|---|---|
| Raynaud's disease | 5% | 70% |
| Raynaud's phenomenon with | | |
| Nonconnective tissue disease | 1 | 15 |
| Juvenile rheumatoid arthritis (or RA) | 1 | 7 |
| SLE | 60 | 4 |
| Scleroderma | 30 | 3 |
| Dermatomyositis | 3 | 1 |

Adapted from Cassidy JT, Petty RE: Textbook of Pediatric Rheumatology, 3rd ed. Philadelphia, WB Saunders, 1995.

Raynaud's phenomenon should be distinguished from normal vasomotor instability, particularly in young girls. It should also be distinguished from acrocyanosis, a rare vasospastic disorder of persistent coldness and bluish discoloration of the hands and feet, which may follow a viral infection.

**23. Describe the types of scleroderma that occur in childhood.**

- Scleroderma is characterized by abnormally increased collagen deposition in the skin and occasionally in the internal organs.
- **Localized scleroderma** occurs more commonly in children than adults. Localized scleroderma may take the form of morphea, with a single patch or multiple patches. Linear scleroderma may occur on the face, forehead and scalp (en coup de sabre), or on the limb (en bande).
- **Diffuse scleroderma** (systemic sclerosis) may be limited in its involvement, with a prolonged interval before the appearance of visceral stigmata, or as part of the CREST syndrome (calcinosis, Raynaud's phenomenon, esophageal dysmotility, sclerodactyly, and telangiectasias).

**24. What laboratory abnormalities are seen in the juvenile systemic CTDs?**

| | SYSTEMIC JRA | SLE | JDMS | SCLERODERMA | VASCULITIS | ARF |
|---|---|---|---|---|---|---|
| Anemia | ++ | +++ | + | + | ++ | + |
| Leukopenia | — | +++ | — | — | — | — |
| Thrombocytopenia | — | ++ | — | — | — | — |
| Leukocytosis | +++ | — | + | — | +++ | + |
| Thrombocytosis | ++ | — | + | — | + | + |
| ANAs | — | +++ | + | ++ | — | — |
| Anti-DNA antibodies | — | +++ | — | — | — | — |
| Rheumatoid factors | — | ++ | — | + | + | — |

(*Table continued on next page.*)

| | SYSTEMIC JRA | SLE | JDMS | SCLERODERMA | VASCULITIS | ARF |
|---|---|---|---|---|---|---|
| Antistreptococcal antibodies | + | — | — | — | — | +++ |
| Hypocomplementemia | — | +++ | — | — | ++ | — |
| Elevated hepatic enzymes | ++ | + | + | + | + | — |
| Elevated muscle enzymes | — | + | +++ | ++ | + | — |
| Abnormal urinalysis | + | +++ | + | + | ++ | — |

Adapted from Cassidy JT, Petty RE: Textbook of Pediatric Rheumatology, 3rd ed. Philadelphia, WB Saunders, 1995. JRA = juvenile rheumatoid arthritis; ARF = acute rheumatic fever.

**25. List some infections that can mimic childhood CTD.**

- Acute rheumatic fever—rare before age 4. Severely painful, migratory polyarthritis with fever (Chapter 48).
- Parvovirus infection—young children get erythema infectiosum ("slapped cheeks"). Older children and adults can get fever (50%), polyarthritis, and rash. Can mimic systemic or polyarticular JRA. IgM antiparvovirus antibodies can be negative for first 2–3 weeks, but polymerase chain reaction for parvovirus B19 DNA will be positive. Arthritis can last over 4 months (50%) (Chapter 45).
- Epstein-Barr virus infection—can mimic SLE. Monospot negative in children under 4 years old. Diagnose with IgM antibodies to VCA (viral capsid antigen) and negative antibodies to EBNA during initial acute infection.
- Immunodeficiency—humoral and combined immunodeficiency can present as infections including septic joints. Echovirus can cause a myositis and mycoplasma a chronic monoarticular arthritis. Consider immunodeficiency in any child with history of two previous bacterial pneumonias (Chapter 62).
- Lyme disease—can mimic pauciarticular JRA (Chapter 43). May start out as migratory arthritis.
- HIV infection—can present as muscle, skin, or joint problems in children. Generalized adenopathy, FUO with organomegaly, and thrombocytopenia are other presentations (Chapter 46).

**26. What bowel disease is most likely to present with arthritis and systemic symptoms?**

Up to 20% of children with Crohn's disease have arthritis, which is usually monoarticular or oligoarticular. Children won't volunteer information about their bowel habits, so they must be asked. Furthermore, some children with arthritis due to Crohn's disease will not have bowel symptoms or a positive stool guaiac. Consequently, Crohn's needs to be considered in any child with arthritis, weight loss, halt in linear growth, anemia, and elevated sedimentation rate.

**27. What are general principles of therapy of the juvenile CTDs?**

Although clearly therapy for the juvenile CTDs must be tailored to the specific diagnosis, certain therapeutic principles can be stressed. The principal drugs used are those that suppress the inflammatory and immune responses. The arachidonic acid metabolic pathways and the cells of the immune system are the primary targets of their therapeutic effects. An obvious difference in the use of these drugs in children, as compared with adults, is dosing on the basis of the weight of the child.

**28. Which anti-inflammatory agents are used to treat children with juvenile CTDs?**

**NSAIDs**. These agents have good analgesic and antipyretic properties, but are only weak anti-inflammatory agents. They are relatively safe when used long-term. Toxicities, particularly CNS and GI side effects, are less common than in adults and are seldom serious. There is considerable variation in patient response to the individual NSAIDs, and a trial of several may be necessary before finding one that is effective and well-tolerated.

**Disease-modifying antirheumatic drugs** (DMARDs), including the antimalarials, and sulfasalazine. Hydroxychloroquine is used in the management of SLE and dermatomyositis, as well as in JRA. D-Penicillamine is occasionally used to treat scleroderma. Sulfasalazine is used to treat the seronegative spondyloarthropathies and inflammatory bowel disease. Gold compounds were previously reserved for JRA, but their use has been largely supplanted by methotrexate.

**Glucocorticoids**. Glucocorticoid drugs are the most potent of the anti-inflammatory agents in the treatment of the juvenile connective system disorders. However, the doses required (often upwards of 2 mg/kg/d) frequently result in substantial toxicity. In addition to the potentially life-threatening complications of hypertension, susceptibility to infection, impaired carbohydrate tolerance, GI bleeding, cataracts, glaucoma, and osteoporosis, the marked growth suppression caused by prolonged use of high-dose glucocorticoids is particularly distressing in growing children. Even with cessation of therapy, catch-up growth often does not occur. In addition, the adverse cosmetic effects of glucocorticoids, including acne, hirsutism, obesity, and striae, negatively affect the already tenuous body image of the developing teenager. Thus, the goal of therapy is to use as little of these agents as possible and for as short a time as possible. Notably, steroid psychosis and osteonecrosis are rare in children treated with corticosteroids.

**Cytotoxic** or **immunosuppressive drugs**, including azathioprine, cyclophosphamide, methotrexate, and cyclosporine. Cytotoxic drugs prevent cell division or cause cell death of rapidly dividing cells, such as those of the immune system. Cytotoxic drugs have both anti-inflammatory effects, which act immediately, and immunosuppressive effects, which are delayed. Owing to the oncogenic potential and other serious toxicities of these agents, they are, in general, reserved for children with severe, potentially life-threatening disease and with inadequate response to less toxic therapy. However, the remarkable efficacy and relative safety of at least one of these agents (methotrexate) and the effectiveness of these agents in "steroid-sparing" have argued for their use at earlier stages of disease.

**29. Do biologic response modifiers have any role in the treatment of these children?**

Although a number of these are in experimental use, the predominant biologic response modifier in use clinically is intravenous gammaglobulin (IVIG). This agent has demonstrated efficacy in at least one inflammatory disease, Kawasaki's disease, and has been tried in a number of the juvenile systemic CTDs. The mechanism of action is not understood, but possibilities include clearance of an etiologic infectious agent and antibodies to inflammatory mediators. Although because IVIG is a blood product, transmission of an infectious agent must be considered, in practice the long-term side effects of IVIG are rare, and the short-term side effects (including fever, headache and chills during the infusion) can be readily managed. Recently, inhibitors of tumor necrosis factor and interleukin-1 have become available for use in treating rheumatic diseases in childhood.

## BIBLIOGRAPHY


1. Ansell BM, Rudge S, Schaller JG: Color Atlas of Pediatric Rheumatology. St. Louis, Mosby, 1992.
2. Arkachaisri T, Lehman TJ: Systemic lupus erythematosus and related disorders of childhood. Curr Opin Rheumatol 11:384, 1999.
3. Athreya BH: Vasculitis in children. Curr Opin Rheumatol 8:477, 1996.
4. Bauman C, Cron RQ, Sherry DD, et al: Reiter syndrome initially misdiagnosed as Kawasaki disease. J Pediatr 128:366, 1996.
5. Bont L, Brus F, Dijkman-Neerincx RH, et al: The clinical spectrum of post-streptococcal syndromes with arthritis in children. Clin Exp Rheumatol 16:750, 1998.
6. Cron RQ, Sharma S, Sherry D: Current treatment by United States and Canadian pediatric rheumatologists. J Rheumatol 26:2036, 1999.
7. da Silva NA, Pereira BA: Acute rheumatic fever. Still a challenge. Rheum Dis Clin North Am 23:545, 1997.
8. Guidelines for the diagnosis of rheumatic fever. Jones criteria, 1992 update. JAMA 268:2069, 1992.
9. Hirschl M, Kundi M: Initial prevalence and incidence of secondary Raynaud's phenomenon in patients with Raynaud's symptomatology. J Rheumatol 23:302, 1996.

10. Hochberg MC: Update the American College of Rheumatology revised criteria for the classification of systemic lupus erythematosus. Arthritis Rheum 40:1725, 1997.
11. Laxer RM, Feldman BM: General and local scleroderma in children and dermatomyositis and associated syndromes. Curr Opin Rheumatol 9:458, 1997.
12. Malleson PN, Sailer M, Mackinnon MJ: Usefulness of antinuclear antibody testing to screen for rheumatic diseases. Arch Dis Child 77:299, 1997.
13. Michels H: Course of mixed connective tissue disease in children. Ann Med 29:359, 1997.
14. Pisetsky DS: Anti-DNA and autoantibodies. Curr Opin Rheumatol 12:364, 2000.
15. Shetty AK, Gedalia A: Sarcoidosis in children. Curr Probl Pediatr 30:149, 2000.

# 75. KAWASAKI'S DISEASE

*J. Roger Hollister, M.D.*

**1. What are the diagnostic criteria for Kawasaki's disease?**

1. Fever (frequently > 40°C), usually high-grade for > 5 consecutive days, unresponsive to antibiotic treatment (100%)—mean 10 days (range 5–25)
2. Conjunctivitis, nonexudative, often dramatic (85%)
3. Cracking and fissuring of lips, with inflammation of mucosal membranes; "strawberry" tongue (90%)
4. Cervical lymphadenopathy (70%)—one or more enlarged nodes
5. Polymorphic rash involving trunk and extremities (80%)—frequently pruritic
6. Erythema (painful) of hands and feet, progressing to edema and finally desquamation (70%)

To meet the diagnosis, five of the above six criteria must be met, or four with echocardiographic demonstration of coronary artery dilatation.

**2. What complications may occur in the acute phase of the illness?**

**Cardiac**—Myocarditis, pericarditis, and arteritis predispose to aneurysms in approximately 20% of patients.

**Arthritis**—Short-lived, may involve small joints of hands and feet.

**Uveitis**—Acute, anterior.

**Hydrops of gallbladder**—Produces abdominal pain and jaundice.

**Gastrointestinal**—Vomiting and diarrhea.

**Others**—Meningitis, pneumonitis, sterile pyuria, transaminitis.

**3. Is there a diagnostic test for Kawasaki's disease?**

No. Laboratory tests show the findings of acute inflammation. However, a progressive increase in the platelet count, often to thrombocytotic levels (> 106/mm$^3$), is characteristic and is not seen in many other causes of fever of unknown origin.

**4. Name three epidemiologic factors that adversely affect the prognosis in Kawasaki's disease.**

Age < 1 year, male sex, Asian ancestry. This group is more likely to get coronary aneurysms (50%).

**5. Name a streptococcal illness in the differential diagnosis of Kawasaki's disease.**

**Scarlet fever** shares many of the features, including fever, conjunctivitis, mucous membrane involvement, and desquamating skin rash. Some authorities suggest that scarlet fever must be ruled out by appropriate cultures for streptococci before concluding that the diagnosis is Kawasaki's disease.

**6. What epidemiologic facts are known about Kawasaki's disease?**

- It is a disease of young children:
  Peak incidence at 9–12 months of age.
  50% cases in children < 2 years old.
  80% in children < 4 years old. Disease is rare after age 11.
- There is a 1–2% incidence in siblings.
- There is a 3% recurrence rate.
- Epidemics appear to be cyclic, occurring at approximately 2–3 year intervals, particularly in late winter and spring.
- More common among Japanese people and those of Japanese ancestry (17×).

**7. What symptoms and findings present in the acute phase of Kawasaki's disease suggest cardiac involvement?**

Obviously, in preverbal children, it may be difficult to communicate ischemic myocardial pain. Symptoms that may be helpful include restlessness, pallor, weak pulse, abdominal pain, and vomiting. A gallop rhythm with a third heart sound may be heard in 70% of cases. Friction rubs indicative of pericarditis are much less common. Coronary artery aneurysms are more common in patients with pericarditis. In one series, palpable axiliary artery aneurysms were highly predictive of coronary artery aneurysms.

**8. What tests are helpful in assessing cardiac involvement?**

Electrocardiograms may show ST-T wave changes indicative of pericarditis or myocarditis. Chest x-rays may show cardiomegaly. However, an echocardiogram is most useful to assess myocardial function, rarely valvular regurgitation, and most commonly coronary arterial dilatation and aneurysm formation (20% of all patients). Echocardiography should be done immediately on all children suspected of having Kawasaki's disease and should be repeated at 1, 6, and 12 weeks.

**9. Besides the fact that "giant" coronary aneurysms sound bad, what is the significance of finding coronary artery dilatations > 8 mm on echocardiography?**

"Giant" coronary artery aneurysms are the most prone to thrombosis and the least likely to regress with time. Their presence requires very close follow-up and perhaps longer term requirement for anticoagulation.

**10. What is the natural history of these lesions?**

From a peak incidence of 20% in the first 1–2 weeks of illness, most of the vascular dilatations will regress, so that only 2% can be found on echocardiography 1 year later. Antiplatelet therapy should begin with high-dose aspirin (80–100 mg/kg/day) split into three doses in the acute phase of the illness. This is followed by low-dose aspirin (5 mg/kg/d) once a day in the convalescent phase for an additional 2 months. In patients with aneurysms, low-dose aspirin should be continued indefinitely.

**11. What causes Kawasaki's disease?**

Unknown. It is believed that it is caused by an infectious agent. One theory suggests that staphylococcal enterotoxins, toxic shock syndrome toxin 1, or streptococcal pyrogenic exotoxins are elaborated and act as superantigens causing T cell expansion and activation of T cells, B cells, and monocyte/macrophages. Multiple cytokines such as 1L-1, IL-6, and TNFα are secreted from these activated cells, which in turn causes vascular endothelial cell activation. Endothelial cell activation results in adhesion molecule up-regulation accompanied by vessel wall infiltration by mononuclear cells. Circulating antibodies and cytokines that are cytotoxic against stimulated endothelial cells may cause endothelial cell damage predisposing to aneurysm formation and clot especially when patients develop thrombocytosis.

**12. Is there an effective treatment for Kawasaki's disease?**

Conclusive evidence from numerous multicenter, double-blinded, placebo-controlled series shows that intravenous immune globulin (IVIG) given within the first 10 days of illness is the treatment of choice in Kawasaki's disease. Two parameters have repeatedly been shown to be responsive to IVIG: resolution of the acute symptoms and prevention of coronary aneurysm formation. It is commonly observed that the fever lyses, the rash regresses, and the toxicity of the illness improves within 12 hours of IVIG administration.

**13. How effective is IVIG in preventing aneurysm formation?**

| | ANEURYSM AT 14 DAYS | ANEURYSM AT 30 MOS |
|---|---|---|
| ASA alone | 23% | 11% |
| ASA and IVIG | 8% | 2% |

**14. What dose of IVIG should be used?**

A single dose of 2 gm/kg of IVIG infused over 10–12 hours is as effective as various multiple-dose schemes that were previously employed. This therapy is most effective if started within the first 10 days of the illness.

**15. IVIG is a very expensive medication. Is it cost-effective to use this medication on all patients with Kawasaki's disease?**

Yes. In a comprehensive study, Klassen showed that the costs of acute care for Kawasaki's disease and the costs of the long-term sequelae of Kawasaki's disease (aneurysms, thromboses, etc.) were both significantly reduced by the administration of a single dose of 2 gm/kg of IVIG.

**16. Does IVIG have any side effects?**

The acute side effects include fever, chills, headache, and, rarely, aseptic meningitis. Most of these side effects respond to slowing the infusion. Fortunately, beyond the risk of all blood products, there are no long-term risks to IVIG.

**17. What is unique about IVIG that might explain its usefulness in Kawasaki's disease?**

IVIG is pooled material from 10,000 donors. When the antibody profile of IVIG was examined, it was found to have extraordinarily high titers of anti-staphylococcal, streptococcal, and toxic shock toxin antibodies. Many of the features of Kawasaki's disease (fever, rash, etc.) are reminiscent of toxin-mediated diseases.

**18. Can steroids be used to treat acute, refractory Kawasaki's disease?**

Recent studies have disproven a myth that existed for 20 years that steroids made the outcome worse for persistent aneurysms in Kawasaki's disease. The myth has been perpetuated based on a poorly controlled study in Japan. However, IVIG remains the initial standard of care. Steroid treatment should be reserved for patients in whom two or more courses of IVIG have failied.

## BIBLIOGRAPHY


1. Barone SR, Pontrelli LR, Krilov LR: The differentiation of classic Kawasaki disease, atypical Kawasaki disease and acute adenoviral infection: Use of clinical features and a rapid direct fluorescent test. Arch Pediatr Adolesc Med 154:453–456, 2000.
2. Burns JC, Kushner HI, Bastian JF, et al: Kawasaki disease: A brief history. Pediatrics 106:E27, 2000.
3. Dajani AS, Taubert KA, Takaheshi M, et al: Guidelines for long-term management of patients with Kawasaki disease. Circulation 89:916–922, 1994.
4. Leung DYM, Schlievert PM, Meissner HC: The immunopathogenesis and management of Kawasaki syndrome. Arthritis Rheum 41:1538–1547, 1998.
5. Newburger JW, Takahashi M, Burns JC, et al: The treatment of Kawasaki syndrome with intravenous gammaglobulin. N Engl J Med 315:341–347, 1986.
6. Noto N, Okada T, Yamasuge M, et al: Noninvasive assessment of the early progression of atherosclerosis in adolescents with Kawasaki disease and coronary artery lesions. Pediatrics 107:1095–1099, 2001.
7. Rauch A, Hurwitz E: Centers for Disease Control case definition for Kawasaki syndrome. Pediatr Infect Dis 4:702–703, 1985.

# XIV. *Miscellaneous Rheumatic Disorders*

*Sickness is a place, more instructive than a long trip to Europe, and it is a place where there's no company, where nobody can follow.*

Flannery O'Connor (1925–1963)

## 76. METABOLIC AND OTHER GENETIC MYOPATHIES

Ramon A. Arroyo, M.D.

**1. What are metabolic myopathies?**

Metabolic myopathies are conditions that have in common abnormalities in muscle energy metabolism that result in skeletal muscle dysfunction. Primary metabolic myopathies are associated with biochemical defects that affect the ability of the muscle fibers to maintain adequate levels of adenosine triphosphate (ATP). Secondary metabolic myopathies are attributed to various endocrine and electrolyte abnormalities. These conditions must be considered in patients who present with dynamic symptoms such as muscle pain, cramps, or myoglobinuria upon exercise, rather than static symptoms such as fixed weakness of a specific muscle group.

**2. Which conditions are considered primary metabolic myopathies?**

A. *Defects of glycogen metabolism*

Acid maltase deficiency (Pompe's disease)
Brancher enzyme deficiency (Andersen's disease)
Debrancher enzyme deficiency (Cori's-Forbes' disease)
Phosphorylase b kinase deficiency
Myophosphorylase deficiency (McArdle's disease)
Phosphofructokinase deficiency (Tarui's disease)
Phosphoglycerate kinase deficiency
Phosphoglyceromutase deficiency
Lactate dehydrogenase deficiency

B. *Defects in lipid metabolism that affect muscle*

Carnitine deficiency (CD) syndrome
  Primary muscle carnitine deficiency
  Systemic CD with hepatic encephalopathy
  Systemic CD associated with cardiomyopathy
Fatty acid transport defects
  Carnitine palmitoyltransferase defects I and II
  Carnitine-acylcarnitine translocate defects
Acyl-CoA dehydrogenase defects

C. *Mitochondrial myopathies*

Enzymes of b-oxidation deficiency
NADH-CoQ reductase deficiency
Cytochrome b deficiency
Cytochrome bc1 deficiency
Mitochondrial ATPase deficiency

D. *Disorders of purine metabolism*

Myoadenylate deaminase (MADA) deficiency

**3. What are secondary causes of metabolic myopathies?**

A. *Endocrine myopathies*

Acromegaly
Hyper- and hypothyroidism
Hyperparathyroidism
Cushing's and Addison's diseases
Hyperaldosteronism
Carcinoid syndrome

B. *Metabolic-nutritional myopathies*

| | |
|---|---|
| Uremia | Vitamin D and E deficiencies |
| Hepatic failure | Malabsorption and periodic paralysis |

C. *Electrolyte disorders*

| | |
|---|---|
| Elevated or decreased levels of sodium, potassium, or calcium | Hypophosphatemia |
| | Hypomagnesemia |

**4. What is the source of energy for muscle contraction?**

Hydrolysis of ATP. Intracellular concentrations of ATP are maintained by the action of enzymes such as creatine kinase, adenylate cyclase, and myoadenylate deaminase. The energy to replenish ATP after it is consumed during muscle contraction is provided by intermediary metabolism of carbohydrates and lipids by pathways of glycolysis, the Krebs' cycle, b-oxidation, and oxidative phosphorylation.

**5. How does ATP provide the energy for muscle contraction?**

The immediate source of energy for skeletal muscle during work is found in preformed organic compounds containing high-energy phosphates, such as ATP and creatine phosphate. Creatine kinase (CK or CPK) helps maintain intracellular ATP concentrations by catalyzing the reversible transphorylation of creatine and adenine nucleotides and by modulating changes in cytosolic ATP concentrations.

At rest, when there is excess ATP, the terminal phosphate of ATP is transferred to creatine, forming creatine phosphate (CrP) and adenosine diphosphate (ADP) in a reaction catalyzed by CK. The CrP serves as a reservoir of high-energy phosphate. With muscle activity and ATP utilization, CK catalyzes the transfer of those phosphates from CrP to rapidly restore ATP levels to normal. The stores of CrP are sufficient to allow the rephosphorylation of ADP to ATP for only a few minutes of exercise.

Thus, CK along with its products, creatine and creatine phosphate, serve as a shuttle mechanism for energy transport between mitochondria, where ATP is generated by oxidative metabolism (Krebs' cycle and respiratory/cytochrome chain), and the myofibrils, where ATP is consumed during muscle contraction and relaxation.

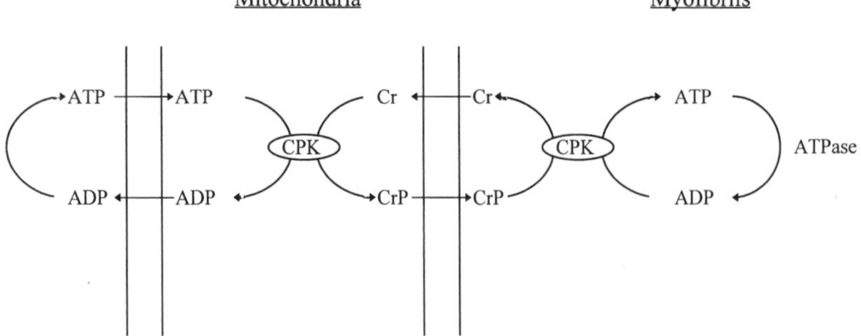


**6. What is the purine nucleotide cycle?**

When approximately 50% of creatine phosphate has been used during exercise, ATP levels in muscle begin to fall. When this occurs, the purine nucleotide cycle is activated.

During exercise, as ATP is hydrolyzed to ADP by ATPase and then to AMP by adenylate kinase, AMP accumulates. The first step of the purine nucleotide cycle is catalyzed by myoadenylate deaminase, which converts AMP to inosine monophosphate (IMP) with release of ammonia ($NH_3$) Both IMP and ammonia stimulate glycolytic activity in an attempt to generate more energy. As ATP levels fall, IMP levels rise until muscle activity decreases and recovery can occur. During recovery, oxidative pathways function and AMP is regenerated from IMP with the liberation of fumarate. Fumarate is converted to malate, which enters the mitochondria and participates in the tricarboxylic acid (Krebs') cycle. This helps to regenerate ATP by oxidative phosphorylation within the mitochondria.

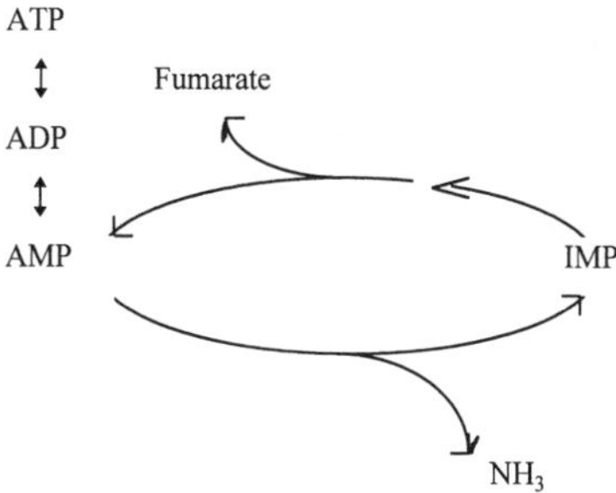


**7. What is the role of carbohydrate metabolism during muscle work?**

Glycogen, the major storage form of carbohydrate, is the major source of ATP generation when physical activity is of short duration and high intensity (lifting heavy weight) or when anaerobic conditions exist (sustained running).

Glycogen is mobilized to form glucose-6-phosphate (G-6-P) by glycogenolysis in a process started by the enzyme myophosphorylase. Glucose and glucose-6-phosphate are metabolized through a series of reactions in the glycolytic pathway to pyruvate. Under aerobic conditions, pyruvate enters the Krebs' (TCA) cycle and is metabolized to carbon dioxide and water. However, under anaerobic conditions, pyruvate is converted to lactate and does not enter the Krebs' cycle. Under these conditions, only two molecules of ATP are generated for each glucose molecule. Anaerobic glycogenolysis can supply energy to muscle for only several minutes until the muscle fatigues, whereas there are sufficient muscle glycogen stores to supply energy for up to 90 minutes under aerobic conditions.

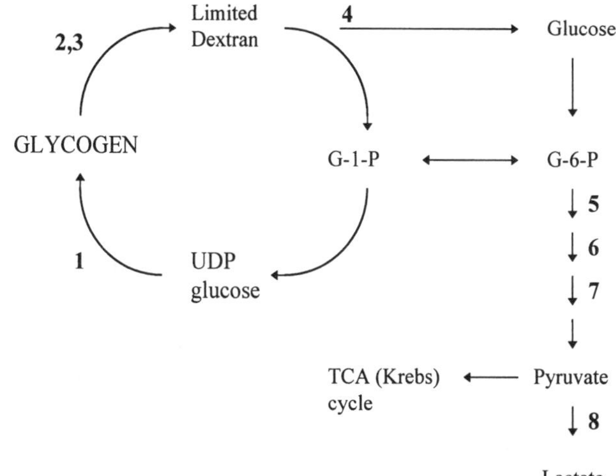


**Catalyst enzymes**: 1 = brancher enzyme, 2 = phosphorylase b kinase, 3 = myophosphorylase, 4 = debrancher enzyme, 5 = phosphofructokinase, 6 = phosphoglycerate kinase, 7 = phosphoglycerate mutase, 8 = lactate dehydrogenase, 9 [not shown] = acid maltase, which catalyzes release of glucose from glycogen and maltase in lysosomes.

**8. What is the role of lipid metabolism during muscle work?**

Lipids, in the form of fatty acids, constitute the major substrate for energy production (ATP) during fasting intervals, at rest, and with muscular activities of low intensity and long duration (more than 40–50 mins).

Long-chain fatty acids (L-cFA) from adipose tissues move through the bloodstream bound to albumin. These, plus medium and small chain fatty acids, move across endothelial cells and into the muscle cells (called fibers), where they are available for energy production, storage, or synthesis into membrane components. To be processed for energy, the free fatty acid must enter the mitochondria. Long-chain fatty acids must combine with carnitine to enter the inner mitochondrial matrix. The combination of long-chain fatty acids with carnitine and their release into the mitochondrial matrix are catalyzed by carnitine palmityl transferase (CPT) I and CPT II, respectively (1 and 2 in the diagram), which are located on the inner mitochondrial membrane (IM). Once in the mitochondria, the fatty acids are converted to their respective coenzyme A (CoA) esters and sequentially shortened by the process of β-oxidation, which release acetyl CoA that then enters the tricarboxylic acid (TCA, Krebs') cycle. At present, carnitine deficiency, CPT deficiency, and acylCoA synthetase deficiency have been described in patients with abnormal muscle function.

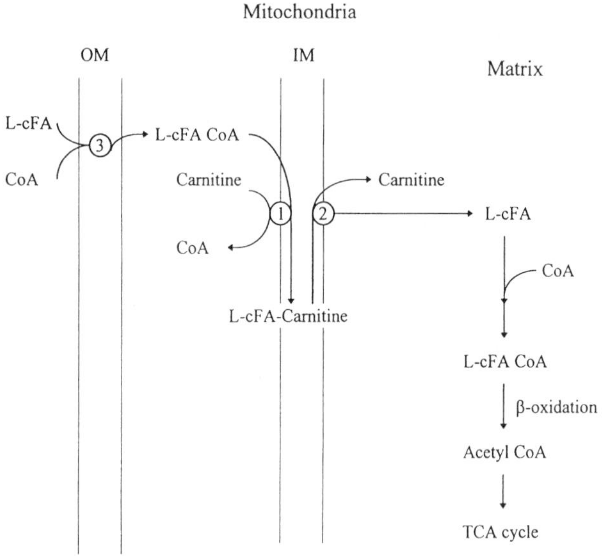

Mitochondria

OM
IM
Matrix
L-cFA
CoA
(3)
L-cFA CoA
Carnitine
Carnitine
(1)
(2)
L-cFA
CoA
CoA
L-cFA-Carnitine
L-cFA CoA
β-oxidation
Acetyl CoA
TCA cycle

**9. How do disorders of glycogen and glucose metabolism present clinically?**

Persons with a glycogen storage disease are well at rest and perform mild exercise without difficulty, because free fatty acids are the major source of energy under these conditions. The enzymatic block that interferes with the use of carbohydrates to generate ATP causes problems only when exercise reaches a level that produces anaerobic conditions. Typically, the patient starts exercising and within a few minutes the muscle fatigues (patients describe this as "hitting the wall"). In some cases, brief rest can result in improved exercise tolerance, referred as the "second wind" phenomenon. If they continue exercising, the muscle becomes painful and may develop a firm cramp. This could result in severe muscle damage and myoglobinuria. In children, defects in glycogenolysis may present with liver dysfunction, hepatosplenomegaly, or neurologic or cardiac involvement.

**10. Do all disorders of glycogen and glycolysis have the same clinical presentation?**

No, even though exercise intolerance is the most common presentation, there are some differences in clinical features according to the specific enzyme deficiency.

**11. Describe the clinical presentation seen in myophosphorylase deficiency (McArdle's disease).**

Myophosphorylase degrades glycogen to glucose-1-phosphate and hence is important in calling up stored energy for muscle use. The cardinal manifestation of this deficiency is exercise intolerance associated with pain, fatigue, or weakness. The degree of intolerance varies among affected individuals. Symptoms can follow activities of high intensity and short duration or those that requires less intense effort for longer intervals, but always resolve with rest. In fact, at rest, affected individuals function well and adjust their activities to a level below their threshold for symptoms. Some individuals experience the "second wind" phenomenon. For unknown reason, severe cramps and myoglobinuria are rare before adolescence. Elevated CK is a common finding in this myopathy. The forearm ischemic test is usually diagnostic, showing a flat venous lactate curve. Creatine monohydrate (5–10 mg/day) may improve exercise performance and tolerance in patients with this condition.

**12. How do deficiencies of brancher and debrancher enzymes (Andersen's and Cori's-Forbes' disease) present clinically?**

**Brancher enzyme** (UDP glucose to glycogen) deficiency causes fatal hepatic failure in childhood, which can be associated with hypotonia and contractures, or exercise intolerance and cardiomyopathy. In **debrancher enzyme** (limit dextran to glucose-1-phosphate) deficiency limit dextran accumulates in muscle, liver, and blood cells, causing hepatomegaly, fasting hypoglycemia, and failure to thrive in childhood. In adults, the main symptoms are progressive proximal or distal weakness and wasting, in some cases, with an associated peripheral neuropathy.

**13. How does phosphofructokinase deficiency (Tarui's disease) present?**

The clinical manifestations of phosphofructokinase (fructose-6-phosphate to fructose-1, 6-phosphate) deficiency can be identical to those of McArdle's disease. The second wind phenomenon is less common, and the exercise intolerance is likely be associated with nausea and vomiting. About one-third of affected persons develop myoglobinuria, and most have elevated CK at rest. The disease can also cause hemolytic anemia.

**14. And how does acid maltase deficiency present?**

Acid maltase catalyzes the release of glucose from maltose, oligosaccharide, and glycogen in lysosomes. Its deficiency is transmitted by autosomal recessive inheritance and produces three different clinical syndromes.

1. The infantile form causes symptoms of muscle weakness, hypotonia, and congestive heart failure that begins shortly after birth and progresses to death within the first 2 years of life.
2. The second form presents in early childhood with progressive proximal muscle weakness. Death is usually from respiratory failure and occurs before age 30.
3. The adult form presents in the third to fifth decades of life with insidious, painless limb-girdle weakness. The respiratory muscle can be affected. This form is frequently misdiagnosed as polymyositis, and a muscle biopsy is most helpful in differentiating them. Characteristically, there are muscle fibers with vacuoles filled with periodic acid-Schiff positive material with prominent acid phosphatase activity.

**15. How do disorders of lipid metabolism present clinically?**

In patients with disorders of lipid metabolism, symptoms such as muscle pain, tightness, or myoglobinuria are usually induced by events such as prolonged exercise, prolonged fasting, infection, general anesthesia, exposure to cold, and low CHO high fat diets. The heart, skeletal muscle, and liver depend on fatty acid oxidation for energy. Metabolic blocks in fatty acid oxidation result in accumulation of abnormal amounts of fatty acid in those tissues, leading to cardiomyopathy, weakness, and fatty liver. An increasing number of neurologic diseases have been associated with defects in fatty acid metabolism. Many of them cause abnormalities in the CNS. Few cases present as isolated instances of exercise intolerance. In contrast to patients with glycogen metabolic defects, patients with lipid metabolism defects do not experience muscle cramps or the second wind phenomenon.

**16. What is the syndrome of carnitine deficiency?**

The syndrome of carnitine deficiency is characterized by progressive muscle weakness that, with some exceptions, begins in childhood. The weakness is of the limb-girdle muscles, but facial and pharyngeal muscle involvement can be observed. Less common features are exertional myalgias, myoglobinuria, cardiomyopathy, and hepatic encephalopathy. Half or more of the patients have high CK levels, and most have myopathic changes on electromyography. The diagnosis is made by biochemical analysis of muscle tissue.

**17. How is it treated?**

Treatment includes L-carnitine supplementation in the diet, but the response is variable. Attempts at treatment should include a diet rich in carbohydrates and medium-chain fatty acids and avoidance of fasting. During acute attacks, therapy should be designed to avoid hypoglycemia and correct any electrolyte and acid-base imbalances that develop. The dose of L-carnitine for children is 100 mg/kg/day, and for adults it is 2–6 gm in divided doses. The D-isomer of carnitine should not be used because it is not effective and can cause muscle weakness. Some patients benefit from corticosteroids and propranolol.

**18. What is the syndrome of carnitine palmityl transferase (CPT) deficiency?**

CPT II deficiency is an autosomal recessive disorder characterized by attacks of exertional myalgias and myoglobinuria. Patients, most of whom are male, experience no difficulty with short bursts of strenuous activity. Indeed, the favorite recreational sport of the patient is often weight lifting. When prolonged exercise is demanded, particularly in the fasting state (when the body is dependent on fatty acid metabolism as a source of energy), muscle pain, fatigue, and myoglobinuria similar to that occurring in glycolytic disorders may ensue, but patients do not experience the "second wind phenomenon." The diagnosis is made by measuring CPT activity in biopsied muscle.

Treatment consists of education. Avoidance of prolonged strenuous exercise and fasting prevent most attacks. Myoglobinuria constitutes a medical emergency and should be treated as such.

**19. What are mitochondrial myopathies (MM)?**

These are a clinically and biochemically heterogeneous group of disorders that have morphologic abnormalities in the number, size, and structure of the mitochondria. The most typical morphologic change is the **ragged red fiber**, a distorted-appearing fiber that contains large peripheral and intermyofibrillar aggregates of abnormal mitochondria. These appear as red deposits on modified Gomori staining. MM are attributed to defects in mitochondrial DNA.

The syndromes associated with abnormalities of mitochondria have a variety of clinical manifestations. Many present multisystem problems with involvement of the CNS, heart, and skeletal muscle. The skeletal muscle involvement is manifested by progressive proximal muscle weakness, external ophthalmoplegia, inability to exercise, and severe fatigue. Dietary supplement with creatine monohydrate may be of benefit for some patients with MM.

**20. Are disorders in purine metabolism associated with any problems besides gout?**

Yes, myoadenylate deaminase (MADA) is an isoenzyme that catalyzes the irreversible deamination of AMP to IMP and plays an important role in the purine nucleotide cycle. Individuals with MADA deficiency complain of exercise intolerance, postexertional cramps, and myalgias. MADA deficiency is probably the most common metabolic abnormality of muscle, but the precise relationship between MADA deficiency and muscular symptoms is controversial. ATP is rapidly consumed during exercise in these patients, and the time to replenish ATP to normal concentration is prolonged. The expected rise in lactate during exercise occurs, but the corresponding change in ammonia concentration does not. CK and aldolase are usually normal in MADA deficiency, as are the electromyographic and muscle biopsy findings. Histochemical techniques are useful in establishing this deficiency.

**21. How do you clinically evaluate patients with suspected metabolic muscle disease?**

The evaluation begins with a careful history and thorough physical exam. The problem of diagnosing metabolic myopathies is confounded because at rest, patients are usually asymptomatic and have normal physical findings. The most significant complaints are related to exercise intolerance, such as severe prolonged cramps and **red-wine-colored urine**, indicating myoglobinuria. The physical findings may be entirely normal and at most may only show symmetrical proximal muscle weakness. The prime importance of the physical exam is to rule out other conditions that present with muscle weakness, especially those with a neurologic component.

**22. How are the metabolic myopathies diagnosed?**

Once a detailed history and physical examination are done, measurement of muscle enzymes and electrodiagnostic studies follow if complaints are suspicious for myopathy. Increased levels of CK, aldolase, liver transaminases, lactate dehydrogenase, carnitine, potassium, phosphorous, creatinine, ammonia, and myoglobin may be observed in the blood of patients with muscle diseases. Of these, CK is the most sensitive. Levels are usually increased in patients with glycogen storage disease but are usually normal in CPT or MADA deficiency.

The electromyogram (EMG) is useful in excluding a neuropathic process, demonstrating myopathic changes and indicating a preferential site for muscle biopsy. Elevated muscle enzymes and myopathic changes on EMG are variable and nondiagnostic. Measurement of venous lactate and ammonia before and after forearm ischemic exercise provides a useful tool for ruling out MADA deficiency and all myopathic forms of glycogen storage disease except acid maltase deficiency, phosphorylase kinase b deficiency, and brancher disease. A positive result should be confirmed by tissue analysis. A **muscle biopsy** provides the most important diagnostic information in the evaluation of a patient with a metabolic muscle disease. Magnetic resonance spectroscopy is another tool useful for the in vivo evaluation of muscle energetics. MRI has been used to identify sites of abnormal tissue and guide for muscle biopsy.

**23. What is the forearm ischemic test? How it is performed?**

The forearm ischemic test is a nonspecific tool used in individuals suspected of having myophosphorylase deficiency or a block anywhere along the glycogenolytic or glycolytic pathway. This test exploits the abnormal biochemistry that results in the absence of those enzymes. Normal muscle generates lactate from the degradation of glycogen when it exercises under ischemic or anaerobic conditions. When these pathways are blocked, no lactate is released into the circulation. In addition, ammonia, inosine, and hypoxanthine concentrations increase significantly. A protocol for forearm ischemic testing follows:

1. A blood sample for analysis of baseline lactate and ammonia concentrations is drawn through an indwelling needle in an antecubital vein, preferably without use of a tourniquet. Pyruvate can also be measured.
2. A sphygmomanometer cuff is placed on the upper arm and inflated. It is maintained at least 20 mm Hg above systolic pressure while the subject squeezes a tennis ball, or similar object, at a rate of one squeeze every 2 sec for 90 sec.
3. After 90 sec, the cuff is deflated and additional venous samples are obtained at 1, 3, 5, and 10 minutes thereafter.

In normal individuals, lactate and ammonia increase at least threefold from baseline values. The major reason for a false-positive result is insufficient work by the subject while exercising. This should be suspected if both lactate and ammonia fail to rise. If lactate (and pyruvate) does not rise but ammonia does, the patient may have a defect in glycolysis, such as McArdle's disease. If lactate rises but ammonia does not, the patient has MADA deficiency. If pyruvate rises but lactate does not, the patient has LDH-m subunit deficiency.

**24. Why is muscle biopsy the most important diagnostic tool in the evaluation of metabolic myopathies?**

Muscle biopsy for routine histologic, histochemical, and ultrastructural analysis (electron microscopy) is the most helpful tool in evaluating a suspected metabolic myopathy, primarily because it helps rule out other conditions that can cause muscle dysfunction and allows the specific enzyme defect to be determined. However, biopsy should be the final step in the clinical evaluation, done only after a preliminary diagnosis has been made. The most important histochemical studies are listed below:

| STAIN | CONDITION |
|---|---|
| Periodic acid-Schiff | Glycogen storage diseases |
| Sudan or Oil red O | Lipid storage diseases |
| Gomori | Mitochondrial myopathy |
| Acid phosphatase | Acid maltase deficiency |
| Histochemical for specific enzymes | Myophosphorylase, phosphofructokinase, lactate dehydrogenase, cytochromes, MADA |

**25. Describe the common muscular dystrophies that may be confused with childhood or adult polymyositis.**

**Duchenne dystrophy**. X-linked disease. Onset of shoulder and pelvic girdle muscle weakness by age 5. Elevated CK, myopathic EMG, and abnormal muscle biopsy showing fat and occasionally inflammation. Pseudohypertrophy of calf muscles. Inability to walk by age 11, and death from respiratory failure by age 20. Abnormal gene on X chromosome coding for the myocyte membrane protein dystrophin.

**Becker dystrophy**. X-linked disease. Similar to Duchenne dystrophy but milder, with patients able to walk beyond age 16 years.

**Fascioscapulohumeral dystrophy**. Autosomal dominant disease. Variable disease expression with disease onset between adolescence to middle-adult years. Presents with facial, shoulder, and proximal arm weakness. Lower extremities less involved. CK elevated up to 5 times normal, and inflammation can be seen on muscle biopsy.

**Limb-girdle dystrophy**. Autosomal recessive disease. Progressive upper and lower extremity proximal muscle weakness beginning in second to fourth decades. Facial muscles spared. This dystrophy is the one most readily confused with adult polymyositis.

**Myotonic dystrophies**. Autosomal dominant diseases. Facial weakness, ptosis, distal limb weakness, and systemic features (balding, cataracts, cardiorespiratory and gastrointestinal involvement). Characteristic physical finding is delayed relaxation and muscles stiffness (myotonia). Inability to relax handgrip when shaking hands and myotonic contraction of thumb when thenar eminence musculature is hit with a reflex hammer are commonly observed. EMG shows excessive insertional activity and a "dive bomber" sound with contraction of muscle. Ringed myofibers seen in 70% on muscle biopsy.

## BIBLIOGRAPHY

1. Darras BT: Energy metabolism in muscle. In 2000 Up To Date, Vol 8, No 2, Feb 1998.
2. Darras BT: Approach to metabolic myopathies. In 2000 Up To Date, Vol 8, No 2, Jul 1998.
3. Darras BT: Metabolic myopathies: Nonlysosomal and lysosomal glycogenoses. In 2000 Up To Date, Vol 8, No 1, May 1998.
4. Darras BT: Metabolic myopathies: Disorders of lipid metabolism. In 2000 Up To Date, Vol 1, No 8, Jan 2000.
5. Wortman RL: Inflammatory diseases of muscle and other myopathies. In Ruddy S, Harris ED, Sledge CB (eds): Kelley's Textbook of Rheumatology, 6th ed. Philadelphia, WB Saunders, 2001, pp 1273–1296.
6. Wortman RL: Metabolic and mitochondrial myopathies. Curr Opin Rheumatol 11:462–467, 1999.

# 77. AMYLOIDOSIS

James D. Singleton, M.D.

**1. What is amyloidosis?**

Amyloidosis is a condition in which an insoluble proteinaceous material is deposited in the extracellular matrix of tissue. The deposits may be localized to one organ or may be systemic. Amyloid deposition may be subclinical or may produce a diverse array of clinical manifestations.

**2. Why is it called amyloid? How does its deposition result in clinical disease?**

In 1854, Rudolph Virchow coined the term *amyloid* (starch-like) owing to the material's reaction with iodine and sulfuric acid. This designation has been retained despite the recognition of amyloid's proteinaceous nature. Amyloid deposits encroach on parenchymal tissues, compromising their function. Organ compromise is related to the location, quantity, and rate of deposition.

**3. Why is knowledge of amyloidosis important?**

Amyloidosis frequently mimics more common rheumatic diseases in its presentations. It also may occur as a potentially fatal sequela of long-standing inflammatory disease.

**4. Describe the structure of amyloid.**

All amyloid shares a unique ultrastructure as seen by electron microscopy. Thin, nonbranching protein fibrils constitute about 90% of amyloid deposits. Fibrils tend to aggregate laterally to form fibers. X-ray diffraction studies show that the polypeptide chains are oriented perpendicularly to the long axis of the fibril, forming a cross β-pleated sheet conformation. P-component, a protein composed of two pentagonal subunits forming a doughnut-like structure, makes up 5%. The remainder is composed of small amounts of carbohydrate and mucopolysaccharides.

**5. Describe the light microscopic appearance of amyloid.**

Without staining, amyloid appears as a homogeneous, amorphous, hyaline extracellular material. It is eosinophilic when stained with hematoxylin-eosin and metachromatic with crystal violet. Amyloid stains homogeneously with Congo red (congophilic) as a result of its β-pleated sheet configuration. Viewing of Congo red–stained tissue under polarized microscopy yields the pathognomonic apple-green birefringence.

**6. So isn't all amyloid the same?**

No. Although all amyloid shares a common structure and tinctorial properties, the major protein comprising the fibril varies from one disease to the next. Thus, there are many amyloidoses, each associated with a specific fibril protein. P-component is associated with all types of amyloid but is not essential for fibril formation.

**7. Where do the amyloid proteins come from?**

All fibrillar amyloid proteins are thought to derive from a larger serum precursor molecule. The amyloid protein is usually a fragment of the precursor molecule but may be an intact molecule (as it is with $\beta_2$-microglobulin). P-component is identical to a normal serum component, serum amyloid P (SAP). Although it is 50% homologous with C-reactive protein, an acute phase reactant, SAP is not an acute phase reactant.

**8. How are the amyloidoses classified?**

By the major protein component of the fibril. This also has become the basis for defining the clinical syndromes with certainty. However, routine stains do not identify the major fibril protein, and such testing is not used clinically.

| CLINICAL CATEGORIES | MAJOR PROTEIN TYPES | RELATIVE FREQUENCIES |
|---|---|---|
| Primary amyloidosis | AL | 56% |
| Myeloma-associated | AL | 26% |
| Secondary (reactive) amyloidosis | AA | 9% |
| Localized amyloidosis | Various | 8% |
| Hereditary amyloidosis | ATTR and others | 1% |
| Amyloidosis of dialysis | $A\beta_2M$ | — |

**9. What is primary amyloidosis?**

Formerly, systemic amyloidosis in the absence of multiple myeloma was called idiopathic or primary amyloidosis. It is now recognized that this amyloid, like that associated with myeloma, is composed of whole or fragments of immunoglobulin light chains. The designation AL was given to reflect the light chain source of this amyloid. AL amyloid appears to represent a spectrum of disease. At one end, the source of light chains is a malignant clone of plasma cells (myeloma-associated). At the other extreme, light chains are derived from a small, nonproliferative plasma cell population (immunocyte dyscrasia).

**10. How then is primary amyloidosis distinguished from amyloidosis associated with myeloma?**

The separation of AL amyloidosis into those with and without myeloma is not always clear-cut. Clinical judgment must play a role in distinguishing the two ends of the spectrum of one disease. Generally, multiple myeloma is considered to be absent when:

- There are no lytic bone lesions
- There is no hypercalcemia
- There is no anemia except that related to bleeding or renal insufficiency
- The serum or urine monoclonal component is small
- There are < 25% bone marrow plasma cells

These criteria have been applied in determining patient eligibility for participation in prospective treatment trials for amyloidosis. From a therapeutic standpoint, such distinction is not always necessary, as cytotoxic chemotherapy is used for both entities. However, treatment exclusively with noncytotoxic therapy should not be used for those with myeloma.

**11. Describe the demographic features of primary amyloidosis.**

AL occurs approximately twice as often in men as in women. The median age at diagnosis is 65 years, and 99% of patients are > 40 years of age. Caucasians are more frequently affected than other races. AL has been very rarely described in children.

**12. What are the most common initial symptoms in patients with primary amyloidosis?**

Fatigue (54%)
Weight loss (42%)
Pain (15%)
Purpura (16%)
Gross bleeding (8%)

Weight loss can be striking, exceeding 40 lbs in some patients and prompting a search for occult malignancy. Pain is more common in those with myeloma (40%) than those without (8%). In those without myeloma, pain is frequently due to peripheral neuropathy and/or carpal tunnel syndrome. Other symptoms are often present in patients with specific organ involvement (dyspnea; pedal edema with congestive heart failure; paresthesias with peripheral neuropathy; orthostasis; syncope with autonomic neuropathy or low-output congestive heart failure).

**13. What physical findings are common in patients with primary amyloidosis?**

Edema (most common)
Palpable liver (34%)

Macroglossia (22%)
Purpura (16%)

Edema may occur as a result of nephrotic syndrome, congestive heart failure, and rarely, protein-losing enteropathy. Hepatomegaly is usually of only modest degree. Macroglossia and purpura should particularly raise suspicion of amyloidosis; both may be a source of patient complaints and are easily overlooked. Increased firmness of the tongue and dental indentations are helpful in determining the presence of macroglossia. Cutaneous purpura is generally localized to the upper chest, neck, and face. Purpura of the eyelids is a clue that is seen only when the patient's eyes are closed.

**14. Since symptoms are nonspecific and physical findings insensitive, what clinical syndromes should suggest the presence of primary amyloidosis?**

| | |
|---|---|
| Nephrotic syndrome | Autonomic neuropathy |
| Congestive heart failure (CHF) | Carpal tunnel syndrome |
| Peripheral neuropathy | Hepatic disease |

The most common initial clinical manifestation is nephrotic syndrome. The major sign distinguishing it from other causes of nephrosis is the finding of a monoclonal protein in the serum or urine (electrophoresis *and* immunofixation should be done). Although overt CHF can occur in up to one-third of patients, amyloid cardiomyopathy, as revealed by echocardiography, is even more common. Peripheral neuropathy clinically resembles the neuropathy seen in diabetes, including the chronic course. Autonomic neuropathy may be superimposed on peripheral neuropathy or occur alone. A history of carpal tunnel syndrome is a very important clue to the presence of amyloidosis. It is typically bilateral, and surgical release may not provide complete relief.

**15. What clues should alert you to the presence of hepatic amyloidosis?**

- Proteinuria—high association with nephrotic syndrome
- Monoclonal protein in serum
- Howell-Jolly bodies in the peripheral blood smear due to splenic infiltration
- Hepatomegaly out of proportion to liver function tests (one-third with hepatomegaly will have normal test results)

**16. What are the echocardiographic findings in amyloid cardiomyopathy?**

Two-dimensional echocardiography has a high sensitivity for detecting amyloid. Symmetric thickening of the left ventricular wall or thickening of the interventricular septum may lead to an erroneous diagnosis of concentric left ventricular hypertrophy or asymmetric septal hypertrophy. Hypokinesis may suggest prior "silent" infarction. The combination of increased myocardial echogenicity and increased atrial thickness is 60% sensitive and 100% specific for the diagnosis of amyloidosis.

**17. So do most patients with primary amyloidosis display only one syndrome?**

No. Most patients have widespread disease and more than one syndrome. Carpal tunnel syndrome is seen more often in those with peripheral neuropathy and cardiomyopathy than in other syndromes.

**18. Name three presentations of amyloidosis that mimic other rheumatic diseases.**

Vascular involvement by amyloid can lead to claudication of the extremities and jaw as seen in temporal arteritis. Amyloid arthropathy can mimic rheumatoid arthritis. Clues are the lack of inflammation and frequent hip and shoulder involvement with periarticular amyloid infiltration, which leads to enlargement of the pelvic or shoulder girdle (shoulder pad sign). Synovial fluid analysis can be helpful in detecting amyloid deposits. Infiltration of amyloid into muscle may lead to weakness or pain, simulating polymyositis. Enlargement of involved muscles (pseudohypertrophy) can be striking and may not be associated with other symptoms.

**19. What is secondary (reactive) amyloidosis?**

Secondary amyloidosis is due to deposition of amyloid A (AA) and can complicate any chronic inflammatory disorder, whether infectious, neoplastic, or rheumatic.

**20. Name the infectious and neoplastic disorders most commonly associated with secondary amyloidosis.**

| Infections | Neoplasms |
|---|---|
| Tuberculosis | Hodgkin's disease |
| Leprosy | Non-Hodgkin's lymphoma |
| Chronic pyelonephritis | Renal cell carcinoma |
| Bronchiectasis | Melanoma |
| Osteomyelitis | Cancers of GI, GU tract, lung |
| Parenteral drug abuse | |

**21. What three rheumatic diseases are most commonly complicated by secondary amyloidosis?**

Rheumatoid arthritis, juvenile rheumatoid arthritis, and ankylosing spondylitis.

Older studies reported a 5–15% overall incidence of amyloid in rheumatoid arthritis, with an average disease duration of 16 years before the onset of amyloidosis. A frequency of 0.14% for amyloidosis in juvenile rheumatoid arthritis in the United States compares with an overall frequency of about 10% in Europe. The reasons for this difference are unknown. Ankylosing spondylitis has also been associated with secondary amyloidosis. Amyloidosis has been cited as a relatively common cause of death in patients with ankylosing spondylitis, and this disease has been relatively overrepresented in reports of secondary amyloidosis. With the new therapies available for RA, JRA, and ankylosing spondylitis, the frequency of secondary amyloidosis appears to be much less today (< 1%).

**22. Amyloid may occur in localized deposits, resembling tumors. The lung, skin, larynx, eye, and bladder are common sites. Most patients with localized amyloid do not have systemic disease. What histopathologic finding prompts investigation for systemic disease?**

Vascular involvement is common in primary and secondary amyloidosis, and if it is present in the biopsy of a localized form, further evaluation for widespread disease is required.

**23. Name two forms of amyloid localized to the brain and three localized to endocrine tissue.**

Aβ (β protein)—Alzheimer's disease, Down's syndrome

APrP (prion protein origin)—Creutzfeldt-Jakob disease, Gerstmann-Sträussler syndrome, kuru, scrapie

ACal (calcitonin)—medullary carcinoma of the thyroid

AANP (atrial natriuretic factor)—isolated atrial amyloid

AIAPP (islet amyloid polypeptide)—type II diabetes mellitus, insulinoma

**24. Study of many types of hereditary amyloidosis have shown them to be due to single amino acid variants of transthyretin (ATTR). What is their pattern of inheritance? How is it treated?**

Autosomal dominant. Treatment is liver transplantation, which removes the source of the variant TTR production and replaces it with normal TTR.

**25. Describe the features of amyloidosis of chronic dialysis.**

Serum $\beta_2$-microglobulin levels are elevated 50–100 times normal in patients on long-term dialysis. However, high levels alone do not predict the development of amyloid. Generally, patients with amyloidosis will have been on hemodialysis at least 5 years. Up to 80% of patients undergoing dialysis for more than 15 years will have evidence of amyloidosis. Carpal tunnel syndrome is the most common clinical presentation. Chronic arthralgias, especially of the shoulders, may also occur. Cystic bone changes and a destructive arthropathy can develop. Rarely, other areas (skin, gastrointestinal tract) are involved.

**26. How is the diagnosis of amyloidosis established?**

Polarized light microscopy showing the characteristic apple-green birefringence of Congo red–stained tissue.

**27. Which tissue should be biopsied?**

A screening biopsy should be performed first, as the sensitivity is good and complications are few. Abdominal fat pad aspiration may be the most useful, as it has a sensitivity near 90%. Screening sites and their yields are:

| | |
|---|---|
| Abdominal fat pad | 90% |
| Bone marrow | 30–50% |
| Rectal mucosa | 73–84% |
| Gingiva | 60% |
| Skin | 50% |

**28. What if the screening biopsies are negative?**

If screens are negative, biopsy of a clinically involved site may be undertaken, realizing that the risk of bleeding may be substantial. For this reason, do not biopsy a liver that is grossly enlarged. Yields for clinically involved sites are:

| | |
|---|---|
| Kidney | 90–98% |
| Carpal ligament | 90–95% |
| Liver | 92–96% |
| Sural nerve | 100% |
| Skin | 45–83% |

**29. What laboratory studies should be performed?**

All patients with systemic amyloidosis should be evaluated for evidence of an associated plasma cell dyscrasia using serum and urine protein electrophoresis *and* immunoelectrophoresis. Screening electrophoresis of serum and urine is insufficient to exclude the presence of a monoclonal band. Patients with amyloidosis associated with multiple myeloma will have a monoclonal protein in serum or urine. However, in up to 12% of patients with primary amyloidosis (not myeloma-associated), serum and urine studies will fail to show a monoclonal component.

**30. Describe the pathogenesis of amyloidosis.**

The pathogenesis is unknown, and there is no unified theory of pathogenesis. Little tissue reaction occurs around amyloid, and once deposited, amyloid resists proteolysis and phagocytosis. Features of the precursor proteins and/or host factors could result in abnormal processing by mononuclear phagocytic cells or ineffective degradation. Certain protein variants are "amyloidogenic," being more susceptible to the processing that leads to amyloidosis. The immunoglobulin light chain λ VI is highly associated with amyloidosis. Single amino acid variants of transthyretin are seen in many of the hereditary amyloidosis syndromes. Animal models suggest defective or inhibited enzymes may play a role in fibril deposition.

**31. How is primary amyloidosis treated?**

The control of light chain production by proliferating plasma cells has been the rationale for the use of cytotoxic agents. Melphalan-containing regimens have been shown to be superior to colchicine alone in the treatment of AL. High-dose chemotherapy with autologous peripheral blood stem cell transplantation can result in improvement of the patient's clinical condition, but treatment-related toxicity can be high. Noncytotoxic therapies (dimethyl sulfoxide [DMSO], vitamin E, and recombinant interferon α-2b) have no proven value.

**32. Describe the treatment of secondary amyloidosis.**

Mobilization and clearance of amyloid deposits are possible and are best recognized for patients with AA. A basic tenet is to control the underlying inflammatory disease. For example, treatment of osteomyelitis with amputation and aggressive surgical therapy for Crohn's disease have been reported to reverse or resolve nephrotic syndrome. Colchicine has also proved useful in treating renal amyloid complicating inflammatory bowel disease.

Many adults with AA suffer from rheumatoid arthritis or ankylosing spondylitis. The use of cytotoxic therapy in these patients remains controversial. Both DMSO and colchicine have been reported as useful. Chlorambucil is the most widely used therapy for amyloidosis complicating juvenile rheumatoid arthritis. Clinical remission of joint disease has been accompanied by lessened proteinuria and normal scan and plasma turnover studies of serum amyloid P, indicating regression of amyloid deposits. However, chlorambucil therapy carries a high incidence of azoospermia in males and risk of hematogenous malignancy in all patients.

**33. How is the amyloidosis of familial Mediterranean fever (FMF) treated?**

The excellent response of FMF to colchicine led to trials of colchicine in AL. Colchicine was first demonstrated to markedly decrease the attacks of polyserositis, completely suppressing attacks in some patients. Colchicine was then shown to be effective in the prevention of amyloidosis, decreasing the incidence of renal amyloidosis by two-thirds. In addition, colchicine can reverse the nephrotic syndrome in FMF patients and prevent recurrence of amyloid following renal transplantation in FMF patients who develop end-stage renal disease.

**34. Discuss supportive treatment for patients with amyloidosis.**

Supportive treatment including renal dialysis, cardiac pacemaker, and nutritional support can be lifesaving. Importantly, digitalis, calcium channel blockers, and β blockers are contraindicated owing to toxicity (arrhythmias) in amyloid patients.

**35. What factors are prognostic in AL amyloidosis?**

The presence of multiple myeloma reduces the median survival from 13 months to 5 months and the 5-year survival from 20% to 0. Grouping of patients by clinical manifestation (heart failure, nephrotic syndrome, peripheral neuropathy, and other) is a useful guide to long-term prognosis. The presence of heart failure is associated with the worst prognosis (median survival, 7.7 months). The best prognosis has long been associated with peripheral neuropathy when it occurs as the sole manifestation (median survival, 56 months). Although the 24-hour urinary total protein excretion does not affect survival, the presence of urinary free light chains and increased serum creatinine are powerful prognostic indicators. A trend has been noted for superior survival in female patients.

## BIBLIOGRAPHY


1. Comenzo RL, Vosburgh E, Falk RH, et al: Dose-intensive melphalan with blood stem-cell support for the treatment of AL amyloidosis: Survival and response in 25 patients. Blood 91:3662, 1998.
2. Falk RH, Comenzo RL, Skinner M: The systemic amyloidoses. N Engl J Med 337:898–909, 1997.
3. Gertz MA, Kyle RA: Amyloidosis: Prognosis and treatment. Semin Arthritis Rheum 24:124–138, 1994.
4. Husby G, Marhaug G, Dowton B, et al: Serum amyloid A (SAA): Biochemistry, genetics, and pathogenesis of AA amyloidosis. Amyloid 1:119, 1994.
5. Kyle RA, Gertz MA: Primary systemic amyloidosis: Clinical and laboratory features in 474 cases. Semin Hemat 32:45–59, 1995.
6. Sezer O, Eucker J, Schmid P, Possinger K: New therapeutic approaches in primary systemic AL amyloidosis. Ann Hematol 79:1–6, 2000.
7. Skinner M: Amyloidosis. In Ruddy S, Harris ED, Sledge CB (eds): Kelley's Textbook of Rheumatology, 6th ed. Philadelphia, WB Saunders, 2001, pp 1541–1549.
8. Westermark P: The pathogenesis of amyloidosis: Understanding general principles. Am J Pathol 152:1125, 1998.

# 78. RAYNAUD'S PHENOMENON

Marc D. Cohen, M.D.

**1. What is Raynaud's phenomenon (RP)?**

Raynaud's phenomenon is a vasospastic disorder characterized by episodic attacks of well-demarcated color changes with numbness and pain of the digits on exposure to cold. It may be primary (idiopathic) or secondary to an underlying condition. Primary RP is also called Raynaud's disease.

**2. How common is RP? Who gets it?**

The prevalence of RP is estimated to be 3 to 4% in most studies, although it may be higher (up to 30%) in colder climates and more common in women, younger age groups, and in patients with a family history of the phenomenon. The female:male ratio ranges from 4:1 to 9:1. RP appears to be equally distributed among ethnic groups.

**3. Which conditions are associated with secondary RP?**

Conditions associated with secondary RP may be grouped into six broad categories: (1) systemic, (2) traumatic (vibration) injury, (3) drugs or chemicals, (4) occlusive arterial disease, (5) hyperviscosity syndromes, and (6) miscellaneous causes (see table).

*Causes of Secondary Raynaud's Phenomenon*

| CATEGORY | CONDITION |
|---|---|
| Systemic rheumatic disorder | Systemic sclerosis, systemic lupus erythematosus, polymyositis-dermatomyositis, Sjögren's syndrome, rheumatoid arthritis, vasculitis, chronic active hepatitis, primary pulmonary hypertension |
| Traumatic | Rock drillers, lumberjacks, grinders, riveters, pneumatic hammer operators |
| Drugs or chemicals | Beta-blockers, ergots, methysergide, vinblastine, bleomycin, imipramine, bromocriptine, clonidine, cyclosporine, cisplatin, cocaine, interferon-alpha, vinyl chloride |
| Occlusive arterial disease | Postembolic/thrombotic arterial occlusion, carpal tunnel syndrome, thoracic outlet syndromes |
| Hyperviscosity diseases | Polycythemia, cryoglobulinemia, paraproteinemia, thrombocytosis, leukemia |
| Miscellaneous | Infections (bacterial endocarditis, Lyme borreliosis, infectious mononucleosis, viral hepatitis), reflex sympathetic dystrophy, fibromyalgia, peripheral arteriovenous fistula, carcinoma |

From Klippel JH: Raynaud's phenomenon: The French tricolor. Arch Intern Med 151:2389–2393, 1991; with permission.

**4. Discuss the relevant pathophysiology of RP.**

Digital artery blood flow is dependent on a pressure gradient that, in turn, is dependent on vessel length, blood viscosity, and vessel radius. The radius of a vessel is most subject to change and may be altered by variations in wall thickness, intrinsic smooth muscle tone, and sympathetic nervous system activity. A given reduction in radius results in a fourfold decrease in blood flow (law of Poiseuille).

Vasospasm of the digital arteries and cutaneous arterioles causes RP. Neural signals, circulating hormones, and mediators from immunomodulatory cells and endothelial cells all interact to control blood vessel reactivity. Neural signals from sympathetic, parasympathetic, and sensory motor fibers include epinephrine, vasopressin, bradykinin, histamine, leukotrienes, norepinephrine, acetylcholine, substance P, and calcitonin gene-related peptide. Mediators from circulating cells include serotonin and ATP/ADP. Mediators from endothelial cells include prostacyclin, endothelin, and other contractile factors.

Epinephrine acts directly on alpha-2 adrenoreceptors on the smooth muscle cells of small arteries causing vasoconstriction. Other substances may act indirectly by activating endothelial cells to produce vasodilators (e.g., nitric oxide) or vasoconstrictors (e.g., endothelin-1). Vascular smooth muscle may also react directly to circulating hormonal or environmental stimuli.

Vasospasm without any underlying arterial structural abnormalities is thought to result in primary RP. Vasospasm and structural arterial abnormalities are thought to cause secondary RP.

**5. Describe the triphasic color response of RP and briefly explain the pathophysiology of each phase.**

The sequential color changes of RP are white to blue to red. Initial digital artery vasospasm causes a **pallor** (blanching) of the digit (see following figure), which gives way to **cyanosis** as static venous blood deoxygenates. Reactive hyperemia causes the final stage, **rubor**. The classic triad in the classic order may not be seen in all patients. Pallor is the most definitive phase.

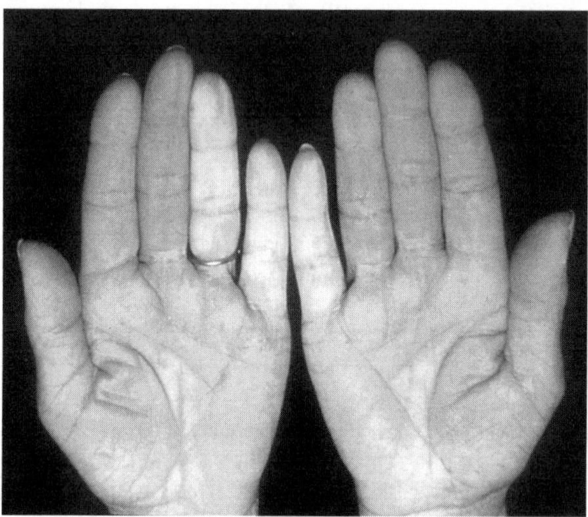

The pallor (blanching) stage of Raynaud's phenomenon. (From the Revised Clinical Slide Collection of the Rheumatic Diseases, copyright 1991. Used by permission of the American College of Rheumatology.)

**6. Contrast the clinical presentations of primary and secondary RP.**

The onset of primary RP usually occurs in women between the ages of 15 and 45 years. The fingers are most commonly affected, but 40% of patients have attacks in the toes as well. Ears, nose, tongue, and lips may also be involved. For reasons unexplained, the thumbs are frequently spared. The well-demarcated color changes involve part or all of one or more digits (never the "whole hand") on exposure to cold. The color changes may be accompanied by numbness during the ischemic phase and by a throbbing pain during the reactive hyperemic phase. The frequency, duration, and severity of attacks vary widely, with some patients having several attacks per day and other having two or three per winter. Rarely in primary RP do trophic complications such as digital ulceration, pitting, fissuring, and gangrene occur.

The onset of secondary RP is usually in the third and fourth decades and may be seen in either men or women depending on the underlying condition. The symptoms of digital vasospasm are the same as those of primary RP; however, secondary RP patients are more prone to trophic complications. Signs and symptoms related to an underlying condition may be seen on careful history and physical examination.

**7. Is cold the only precipitant of RP?**

Cold exposure is by far the most common precipitating cause of RP, especially when accompanied by pressure. Typical examples would be the gripping of a cold steering wheel, holding a cold soft drink can, or grasping items in the frozen food section of a grocery store. Other potential stimuli include emotional change, trauma, hormones, and certain chemicals such as those found in cigarette smoke. Additional "causes" like vibration injury are more correctly attributed to the associated conditions of secondary RP.

**8. Is the vasospasm of RP restricted to digital vessels?**

A large case control study has demonstrated an increased frequency of migraine headaches and chest pain in patients with primary RP. Other studies have implicated vasospasm of the myocardium, lungs, kidneys, esophagus, and placenta. Although definitive proof is lacking, RP probably is a systemic vasospastic disorder.

**9. In the evaluation of a patient with RP, what abnormalities may be noted on physical examination?**

Patients may occasionally present to the clinic with an ongoing attack of RP, thereby allowing a definitive diagnosis. Induction of an attack in the physician's office by submergence of hands in an ice water bath is frequently unsuccessful, seldom necessary, and sometimes dangerous.

The physical examination in primary RP is normal. The real goal in patients with RP is to discern the presence or absence of findings attributable to an underlying condition of secondary RP. A careful search for evidence of an underlying rheumatologic disease is required. Abnormal peripheral pulses or asymmetric involvement suggests peripheral vascular disease or perhaps thromboembolic disease. Puffy hands, tendon friction rubs, sclerodactyly, or telangiectasia suggest scleroderma or its variants. Examination for thoracic outlet syndrome (Adson's test) should be performed. Nailfold capillary microscopy may be useful.

**10. Describe the technique, clinical findings, and prognostic value of nailfold capillary microscopy (NCM).**

Along with the retina, the nailfold represents one of the only sites in the body where direct visualization of the vasculature is possible. NCM involves the placement of a drop of immersion oil on the cuticle of one or more digits (usually the ring or middle fingers), and visualization of the capillaries through an ophthalmoscope set at 40 diopters.

The normal nailbed demonstrates a confluent distribution of fine capillary loops (see following figure, top of next page). Dilated tortuous capillary loops and areas of avascularity ("dropout") are often demonstrated in patients with underlying rheumatologic diseases such as systemic sclerosis, dermatomyositis, and mixed connective tissue disease.

In patients with primary RP, normal NCM connotes an excellent prognosis and rheumatologic disease rarely develops in these patients. A small percentage of primary RP patients who demonstrate abnormal NCM may subsequently develop a rheumatologic disease, typically limited systemic sclerosis (i.e., CREST).

**11. Which laboratory studies are worthwhile in the evaluation of a patient with RP?**

To date, no laboratory test is pathognomonic of RP. In primary RP, laboratory tests should be normal or negative, although up to one-third of patients will exhibit low titer antinuclear antibodies in their serum. Less than 25% of these patients develop an autoimmune disorder. In patients with clinical evidence suggestive of an underlying collagen vascular disease, appropriate studies for the presence of a hypercoagulable state, cryoglobulins, hypothyroidism, and anticentromere and anti-toposomerase antibodies should be considered.

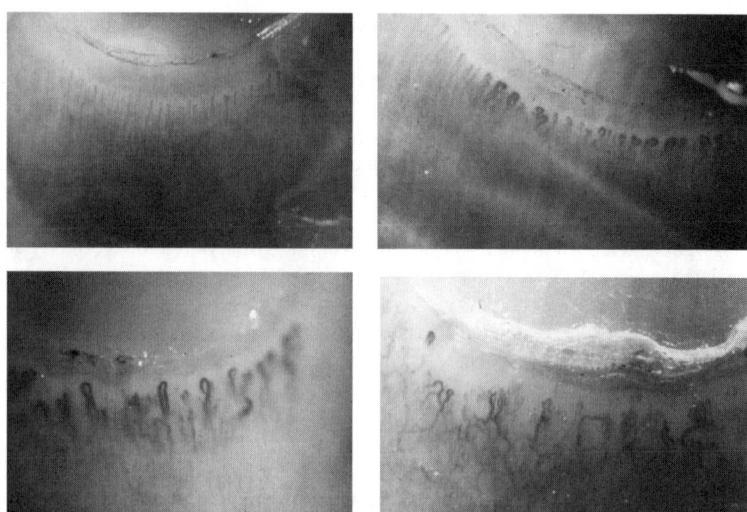

Nailfold capillary microscopy. *Upper left*, Normal pattern. *Upper right*, Dilated capillary loops in systemic sclerosis. *Lower left*, Dilated loops and avascularity in adult dermatomyositis. *Lower right*, Childhood dermatomyositis. (From the Revised Clinical Slide Collection of the Rheumatic Diseases, copyright 1991. Used by permission of the American College of Rheumatology.)

**12. Describe the usefulness of vascular or other studies in the diagnosis of RP.**

Doppler studies of vessels in the palmar arch may be helpful. Finger photoplethysmography and blood pressure studies at ambient temperature may also be useful, with abnormal waveforms or brachial-finger pressure gradients over 20 mmHg suggesting a proximal fixed obstruction.

Arteriography or magnetic resonance arteriography may reveal an embolic source but is usually not necessary. Similarly, nerve conduction studies may suggest a nerve compression syndrome and a chest radiography may demonstrate a cervical rib.

**13. List the "red flags" that would be worrisome for the potential presence or later development of a disease associated with secondary RP.**

- Onset of digital vasospasm after age 30
- RP in a man
- Trophic changes in the digits (ulcers, pits, gangrene)
- Abnormal nailfold microscopy
- Sclerodactyly, rashes, or other obvious evidence of an underlying condition
- Serologic presence of autoantibodies, especially anticentromere antibodies or antibodies against a specific nuclear antigen (SCL-70, RNP, Sm, SS-A, SS-B)

**14. Which general measures are important in the treatment of patients with RP?**

The majority of RP patients respond best to simple prevention measures. Careful planning of one's activities of daily living minimizes unnecessary exposure to cold. Because reductions in core temperature as well as peripheral temperature may induce digital vasospasm, it is important to promote "total body" heat conservation. Loose-fitting, layered clothing, warm socks, hats, and scarves should be worn in addition to gloves or mittens. Tobacco and beta blockers must be avoided. Temperature biofeedback training is also effective in some patients with primary RP.

**15. When is pharmacologic intervention indicated in the management of RP?**

Most patients with primary RP will not require pharmacologic therapy. Those with secondary RP more often require (but less often respond to) medication. Therapy of secondary RP should address the underlying disorder and the vasospasm. Pharmacologic intervention is indicated in patients who suffer frequent, prolonged, and/or severe episodes of RP in the setting of adequate preventative measure or with minimal provocation. Patients who manifest evidence of ischemic injury (digital pitting, etc.) should definitely be considered for medical management. Many patients who do require medication may only need it during the colder months of the year. Beta-blockers should be discontinued. Any evidence of digital infection should be treated with antibiotics. Analgesics may be necessary.

**16. Which medications have been useful in the management of the vasospastic component of RP?**

All available therapies work better in primary RP than secondary RP.

Calcium channel blockers, especially **nifedipine**, amlodipine, and diltiazem are best tolerated and most efficacious as vasodilators. Nifedipine also inhibits platelet activation, which may increase its effectiveness. Slow-release preparations are most commonly used. Potential side effects include edema, lightheadedness, and worsening gastroesophageal reflux. These drugs should not be used in pregnancy. Patients with compromised left ventricular function should use a calcium channel blocker of the dihydropyridine class (i.e., amlodipine).

Sympatholytic agents like prazosin or phenoxybenzamine have been beneficial particular with short-term use. They lose their effectiveness with long-term use. Postural hypotension may limit their usefulness. Presynaptic sympathetic inhibitors such as reserpine and guanethidine are rarely used because the other drugs are more effective and better tolerated.

Topical nitrates may be helpful. Patients use ¼ to ½ inch of topical 2% nitroglycerin ointment applied two times daily: once in the morning on arising and repeated 6 hours later. A rest from nitrates for 12 hours is necessary to prevent development of a refractory state. Dose can be increased. It is best to use topical therapy on only a few digits that are most severely involved. It is important to warn patients not to touch their eyes while it is on. Alternatively, a nitrate patch can be used. Headache is a common limiting side effect. Nitrates can be used in combination with calcium channel blockers.

Prostaglandins [($PGI_2$, (prostacyclin), $PGE_1$, $PGE_2$, iloprost] are vasodilators and platelet aggregation inhibitors. They are only available intravenously, and overall, their availability is limited, expensive, and not widely studied in RP. Iloprost (an analog of prostacyclin) is beneficial in patients with severe RP and may be tried to prevent severe vasospastic digital damage. Toxicity is common and includes chest pain, headache, and nausea. Oral iloprost and misoprostol (oral $PGE_1$) are no better than placebo.

Selective serotonin antagonists like ketanserin may also be helpful, but are not yet approved in the U.S. Anti-platelet drugs and pentoxifylline (Trental) have demonstrated minimal benefit, particularly in severe RP. Full anticoagulation is not recommended unless there is embolization or new thrombosis, although low-dose anticoagulation may be helpful in patients with systemic sclerosis. Thrombolytic therapy needs to be further studied.

Note that all vasodilators are nonselective and may vasodilate healthy vessels, stealing blood flow from diseased vessels and making Raynaud's worse in some digits. This must be monitored, especially in patients with secondary RP.

**17. Describe an approach to treatment of patients with RP.**

- Step 1—make sure to institute general measures.
- If general measures are not significantly effective, use medications. Try to use only during cold months.
- Step 2—Start nifedipine XL 30 mg/day, amlodipine 5 mg/day, or diltiazem (Cardiazem CD, Dilacor XR) 120 mg/day. If no response in 2 weeks, increase dose every 2–4 weeks until reach maximum (nifedipine XL 90 mg/day, amlodipine 10 mg/day, Cardiazem CD 360 mg/day, or Dilacor XR 480 mg/day) or get side effects.
- Step 3—Add topical nitrates or prazosin. Start prazosin with 1 mg test dose while lying down and increase it slowly to as high as 5 mg three time daily or side effects.

**18. What can be done medically in patients presenting with acute ischemic crisis that is digit threatening?**

- Step 1—put to rest in a warm environment in hospital.
- Step 2—Control pain. Chemical digital or limb sympathectomy preferable over narcotics, which can cause vasospasm. Sympathectomy helps open blood vessels so medication can get to the digits.
- Step 3—Start one of following vasodilator therapies:
  Calcium channel blocker—use amlodipine or short-acting nifedipine if not on them.
  Intravenous prostaglandins—epoprostenol (prostacyclin, $PGI_1$), alprostadil ($PGE_1$), or iloprost is available.
- Step 4—Antiplatelet therapy with aspirin 81 mg/day.
- Step 5—Anticoagulation with heparin during acute crisis can be considered especially if antiphospholipid antibodies.

**19. What surgical options can be done for patients who are refractory to standard therapy?**

Surgical sympathectomy may be considered in patients in whom more conservative measures have failed and who present with impending digital necrosis or evidence of recurrent ischemic complications. It can be performed at the cervical, lumbar, or digital levels. Permanent surgical ablation may be preceded by demonstrating efficacy using a bipuvicaine stellate ganglion block or epidural infusion. Sympathectomies may not provide long-term benefits, although digital sympathectomy may restore blood flow to fingers immediately. In patients with infarcted digits unresponsive to treatment, amputation for pain control is best option.

**20. What is the prognosis for patients with RP?**

The prognosis for patients with primary RP is excellent. In 10% of patients, attacks disappear completely. Digital vascular complications occur rarely. The vast majority of patients with primary RP never develop an underlying condition associated with secondary RP. This is especially true if nailfold capillary microscopy and autoantibody testing are negative.

The prognosis for patients with secondary RP is generally dependent on the underlying condition. Intrinsic vascular disease is often present. Complications arising from vasospasm such as digital ulcerations are common.

ACKNOWLEDGEMENT

The editor and author wish to thank Dr. Steven Older for his contributions to this chapter in the previous edition.

## BIBLIOGRAPHY

1. Belch JJ, Ho M: Pharmacotherapy of Raynaud's phenomenon. Drugs 52:682–695, 1996.
2. Cerinic MM, Generini S, Pignone A: New approaches to Raynaud's phenomenon. Curr Opin Rheumatol 9:544–556, 1997.
3. Ceru S, Pancera P, Sansone S, et al: Effects of five-day versus one-day infusion of iloprost on the peripheral microcirculation in patients with systemic sclerosis. Clin Exp Rheumatol 15:381–538, 1997.
4. Coffman JD: The diagnosis of Raynaud's phenomenon. Clin Dermatol 12:283–289, 1994.
5. Coffman JD: Raynaud's phenomenon. Curr Treat Options Cardiovasc Med 2:219–226, 2000.
6. Generini S, Matucci Cerinic M: Raynaud's phenomenon and vascular disease in systemic sclerosis. Adv Exp Med Biol 455:93–100, 1999.
7. Ho M, Belch JJ: Raynaud's phenomenon: State of the art 1998. Scand J Rheumatol 27:319–322, 1998.
8. Kahaleh B, Matucci-Cerinic M: Raynaud's phenomenon and scleroderma. Dysregulated neuroendothelial control of vascular tone. Arthritis Rheum 38:1–4, 1995.
9. Kahaleh MB: Raynaud's phenomenon and the vascular disease in scleroderma. Curr Opin Rheumatol 7:529–534, 1995.
10. Kirou KA, Crow MK: Raynaud's phenomenon. In Paget SA, Gibofsky A, Beary JFI, Pellici P (eds): Manual of Rheumatology and Outpatient Orthopedic Disorders: Diagnosis and Therapy, 4th edition. Philadelphia, Lippincott Williams & Wilkins, 2000.

11. Landry GJ, Edwards JM, McLafferty RB, et al: Long-term outcome of Raynaud's syndrome in a prospectively analyzed patient cohort. J Vasc Surg 23:76–85; discussion 85–86, 1996.
12. O'Keeffe ST, Tsapatsaris NP, Beetham WP Jr: Increased prevalence of migraine and chest pain in patients with primary Raynaud disease. Ann Intern Med 116:985–989, 1992.
13. Spencer-Green G: Outcomes in primary Raynaud phenomenon: A meta-analysis of the frequency, rates, and predictors of transition to secondary diseases. Arch Intern Med 158:595–600, 1998.
14. Sturgill MG, Seibold JR: Rational use of calcium-channel antagonists in Raynaud's phenomenon. Curr Opin Rheumatol 10:584–588, 1998.
15. Toumbis-Ioannou E, Cohen PR: Chemotherapy-induced Raynaud's phenomenon. Cleve Clin J Med 61:195–199, 1994.
16. Turton EP, Kent PJ, Kester RC: The aetiology of Raynaud's phenomenon. Cardiovasc Surg 6:431–440, 1998.
17. Wigley FM: Raynaud's phenomenon. In Weisman MH, Weinblatt ME, Louis JS (eds): Treatment of Rheumatic Diseases, 2nd ed. Philadelphia, WB Saunders, 2001, pp 382–389.
18. Yee AM, Hotchkiss RN, Paget SA: Adventitial stripping: A digit saving procedure in refractory Raynaud's phenomenon. J Rheumatol 25:269–276, 1998.

# 79. AUTOIMMUNE EYE AND EAR DISORDERS

*Raymond J. Enzenauer, M.D.*

## UVEITIS

**1. What is uveitis?**

The diagnostic term *uveitis* indicates the presence of inflammation in the uveal tract, which includes the iris, ciliary body, and choroid (see figure). Like arthritis, uveitis may be caused by many different diseases. Uveitis and iritis are used interchangeably.

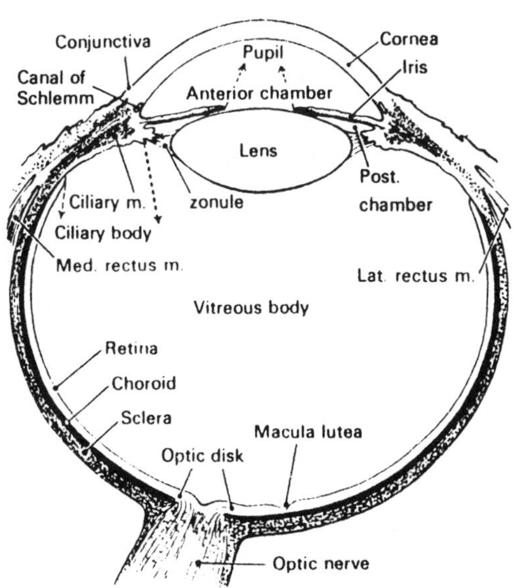


Diagram of a human eyeball. (From Stedman's Medical Dictionary, 23rd ed. Baltimore, Williams & Wilkins, 1976, p 500; with permission.)

**2. List the four primary parameters used to characterize subsets of uveitis.**

1. Anatomic location of inflammation (anterior, intermediate, posterior, panuveitis)
2. Laterality (unilateral, bilateral)
3. Onset (acute, insidious)
4. Duration (self-limited, chronic, recurrent)

The location, laterality, and onset of uveitis can assist in identifying a specific etiology of the uveitis. For example, HLA-B27–associated uveitis is almost always acute, anterior, and unilateral, while the uveitis associated with sarcoidosis may be a chronic, bilateral panuveitis.

**3. Which laboratory tests are of diagnostic value for a patient with unclassified uveitis?**

**Chest roentgenogram** and **fluorescent treponomal antibody absorption** (FTA-ABS). Because sarcoidosis and syphilis may have ocular inflammation without clinically apparent systemic disease, tests for these two entities are indicated in *all* patients with uveitis of unknown etiology. Specifically, one should obtain a serologic test for syphilis (FTA) and a chest roentgenogram to screen for sarcoidosis. Other laboratory tests should be ordered depending on the nature and setting of the uveitis.

**Antinuclear antibody** (ANA) testing is indicated only in the evaluation of pediatric patients with bilateral, chronic iritis, as this test is positive in up to 88% of patients with juvenile rheumatoid arthritis and iritis. It is not indicated for routine screening of adult patients with unclassified uveitis because a patient with uveitis and a positive ANA has a < 1% chance of having systemic lupus erythematosus.

Similarly, a patient with uveitis and a positive **purified protein derivative** (PPD) test has only a 1% likelihood of having tuberculosis. PPD testing in uveitis should be limited to patients having an appropriate exposure history or an abnormal chest roentgenogram suggestive of tuberculosis.

**HLA-B27 testing** is only appropriate for patients presenting with acute, anterior uveitis. It is not helpful in the evaluation of patients with chronic, intermediate or posterior uveitis.

**4. What percentage of acute anterior uveitis (AAU) is associated with HLA-B27? How does HLA-B27 affect presentation and outcome?**

In a white population, AAU is associated with HLA-B27 in 50% of cases. Of patients with HLA-B27–positive AAU, more than half suffer from an associated seronegative spondyloarthropathy (ankylosing spondylitis, Reiter's syndrome, psoriatic arthritis, or inflammatory bowel disease). Patients positive for HLA-B27 are often younger, are predominantly men, and have more frequent recurrences of AAU than patients negative for HLA-B27.

**5. List a differential diagnosis of anterior uveitis. Which is the most common cause?**

| | |
|---|---|
| Idiopathic | 52% |
| HLA-B27 (ocular only) | 36% |
| Ankylosing spondylitis | 8% |
| Reiter's syndrome | 3% |
| Juvenile rheumatoid arthritis | < 1% |
| Fuchs' iridocyclitis | < 1% |
| Psoriatic arthritis | < 1% |
| Inflammatory bowel disease | < 1% |
| Acute interstitial nephritis | < 1% |
| Kawasaki's disease | < 1% |
| Posner-Schlossman syndrome (glaucomatocyclic crisis) | < 1% |

Idiopathic anterior uveitis is probably the most common form of anterior segment inflammation, accounting for > 50% of cases.

**6. Define intermediate uveitis and pars planitis.**

**Intermediate uveitis** refers to an anatomic distribution of ocular inflammation primarily in the vitreous and peripheral retina just behind the lens. The condition is sometimes referred to as

**peripheral uveitis** because the inflammation involves, or is adjacent to, the peripheral retina in the area of the pars plana. When there is a large white opacity, or "snowbank," over the pars plana and ora serrata, this subset of intermediate uveitis is termed **pars planitis**.

**7. Define chronic uveitis. Describe the location of ocular inflammation and its etiology.**

**Chronic uveitis** is defined as intraocular inflammation persisting for 3 months or more. Most patients have chronic anterior uveitis (46%), with panuveitis in 25%, intermediate uveitis in 15%, and isolated posterior uveitis in 14%. An associated condition can be found in 60% of cases, with Behçet's disease being the most common etiology, particularly in panuveitis patients.

**8. What systemic diseases have been associated with intermediate uveitis?**

Although most cases are idiopathic, underlying systemic disease may occasionally be found to include **sarcoidosis** (2–10%), **multiple sclerosis** (10%), or **infection** (syphilis, Lyme disease, tuberculosis).

**9. List the rheumatic diseases most likely to be associated with uveitis. Compare their onset, laterality, and location.**

| RHEUMATIC DISEASE | ONSET | LATERALITY | LOCATION |
|---|---|---|---|
| Ankylosing spondylitis | Acute | Unilateral | Anterior |
| Juvenile rheumatoid arthritis | Insidious | Bilateral | Anterior |
| Psoriatic arthritis | Acute | Unilateral | Anterior |
| Reiter's syndrome | Acute | Unilateral | Anterior |
| Sjögren's syndrome | Insidious | Bilateral | Panuveitis |

Adult rheumatoid arthritis is *not* associated with uveitis. Early literature that described ankylosing spondylitis as "rheumatoid spondylitis" contributed to the mistaken impression that patients with rheumatoid arthritis are at increased risk for uveitis.

**10. How is the uveitis of juvenile rheumatoid arthritis (JRA) unique from all other causes of anterior uveitis?**

Unlike patients with almost all other causes of anterior uveitis, JRA patients with anterior uveitis usually are asymptomatic, and the involved eye is often white, without obvious evidence of inflammation. As a result, complications of uveitis may develop before the inflammation is detected. It is typically seen in ANA positive young girls with pauciarticular JRA.

**11. How do the typical presenting symptoms differ among anterior, intermediate, and posterior uveitis?**

**Anterior uveitis**. Patients usually present with complaints of **pain**, **redness**, and **photophobia**. Most cases are **unilateral**, but bilateral disease can be seen in patients with interstitial nephritis or Sjögren's syndrome.

**Intermediate uveitis**. Patients usually complain of the insidious onset of **floaters** or **mild haziness** of vision. Typically, the external eye is quiet, and there is no pain or photophobia. Although initial complaints are usually limited to **one eye**, evidence of mild inflammation in the contralateral eye is common.

**Posterior uveitis**. Patients usually complain of the insidious onset of **blurred vision**, **floaters**, and **scotomata**. As in intermediate uveitis, the external eye is quiet and there is no pain or photophobia.

**12. Define posterior uveitis. List the differential diagnosis of inflammation of the posterior uveal tract.**

Posterior uveitis describes inflammation that involves the retina and vitreous near the optic nerve and macula.

*Differential Diagnosis of Posterior Uveitis**

| | |
|---|---|
| Idiopathic retinal vasculitis (Eale's disease) | Acute posterior multifocal placoid pigment epitheliopathy |
| Sarcoidosis | Infectious posterior uveitis |
| Birdshot choroidoretinopathy | Herpes simplex—induced acute retinal necrosis |
| Behçet's disease | Cytomegalovirus retinitis |
| Vogt-Koyanagi-Harada syndrome | Toxoplasmosis retinochoroiditis† |
| Sympathetic ophthalmia | Syphilis |
| Serpiginous choroiditis | Histoplasmosis |
| | Tuberculosis |

* An etiology (other than infection) is more often found in patients with panuveitis than isolated posterior uveitis.

† Toxoplasmosis is now thought to account for 30–50% of all granulomatous inflammations of the posterior segment of the eye and is the leading cause of posterior uveitis.

**13. Which causes of uveitis have been associated with specific HLA types?**

| | |
|---|---|
| Reiter's syndrome | HLA-B27 |
| Behçet disease | HLA-B51 |
| Birdshot retinochoroidopathy | HLA-A29 |
| Pars planitis | HLA-DR2 |

**14. What are the indications for systemic corticosteroids in the management of uveitis?**

Bilateral moderate to severe ocular inflammation *or* vision-threatening anterior- or posterior-segment inflammation unresponsive to topically or periocularly administered corticosteroids. Systemic therapy is generally reserved for patients whose visual acuity has declined to 20/40 or worse because of an inflammatory condition and in whom recovery of vision is thought to be possible.

Usually, the initial dosage is 60 mg or 1–1.5 mg/kg/day, which is subsequently tapered slowly. A good approach is to taper the dosage to 15–20 mg over 3–4 weeks and to observe the patient carefully for any recurrence of symptoms. If the patient's condition remains stable, a slow taper off the medication may then be attempted.

**15. Discuss the indications and contraindications for cytotoxic therapy for uveitis.**

**Indications**: Sight-threatening uveitis unresponsive to corticosteroids or patients intolerant of corticosteroids because of side effects. Forms of uveitis commonly requiring cytotoxic therapy include sympathetic ophthalmia, posterior segment Behçet's disease, and ocular Wegener's granulomatosis.

**Contraindications**: Any uveitis of infectious origin.

**16. What is the drug of choice for uveitis associated with various etiologies?**

| | |
|---|---|
| Wegener's granulomatosis | Oral cyclophosphamide |
| Behçet disease | Oral chlorambucil |
| Reiter's syndrome | Topical corticosteroids |
| Vogt-Koyanagi-Harada syndrome | Oral corticosteroids |
| Sarcoidosis | Topical/oral corticosteroids |

**17. Which immunosuppressive drugs are reported to be effective in the treatment of uveitis?**

| | | |
|---|---|---|
| Cyclophosphamide | po | 1–2 mg/kg/day |
| | iv | 500–1000 mg/$M^2$/mo |
| Chlorambucil | po | 0.1 mg/kg/day |
| Methotrexate | po/im | 10–25 mg/wk |

| | | |
|---|---|---|
| Cyclosporine | po | 5–7 mg/kg/day |
| Bromocriptine | po | 2.5 mg 3–4 times daily |
| Dapsone | po | 25–50 mg 2–3 times daily |
| Colchicine | po | 0.65 mg 2–3 times daily |

Anti-TNFα therapy has shown some effectiveness in uveitis due to JRA or HLA-B27–related diseases.

**18. List the frequency of the common ocular presentations of sarcoidosis.**

| | |
|---|---|
| Anterior uveitis 54% | Posterior uveitis 15% |
| Panuveitis 27% | Intermediate uveitis 4% |

**19. What masquerade syndromes mimic uveitis? How can they be distinguished clinically?**

Masquerade syndromes include leukemia, lymphoma, retinitis pigmentosa, malignant melanoma, antiphospholipid antibody syndrome, and retinoblastoma. The diagnosis of a masquerade syndrome may be suggested by the appearance of the eye alone, age of the patient, or lack of response to standard uveitis therapy.

**20. What are some causes of an elevated serum angiotensin-converting enzyme (ACE) level in a patient with uveitis?**

Sarcoidosis, liver disease (primary biliary cirrhosis, granulomatous hepatitis, alcoholic liver disease), diabetes mellitus (especially with retinopathy), granulomatous infections (tuberculosis, coccidioidomycosis, leprosy, HIV), Wegener's granulomatosis, pneumoconioses (berylliosis, asbestosis, silicosis), Gaucher's disease, Hodgkin's disease, hyperthyroidism.

**21. What cause of uveitis classically presents with exudative retinal detachment?**

Vogt-Koyanagi-Harada syndrome.

## SCLERITIS/EPISCLERITIS

**22. What is the clinical classification of episcleritis and scleritis?**

- Episcleritis (33% of cases)
  - Simple 78.3%
  - Nodular 21.7%
- Scleritis (67% of cases)
  - Anterior 98%
    - Diffuse 40%
    - Nodular 44.5%
    - Necrotizing 14%
      - With inflammation 9.6%
      - Without inflammation 4.3% (scleromalacia perforans)
  - Posterior 2%

**23. How do symptoms and signs of scleritis and episcleritis differ?**

Episcleritis presents with injection along the exposed palpebral conjunctivae with or without pain. If present, pain is mild or dull.

Scleritis presents with severe, boring persistent pain. It frequently wakes the patient at night and resists analgesia. It is associated with injection, tenderness, photophobia, tearing, and decreased vision.

**24. How often is keratitis (corneal inflammation) and/or iritis (uveitis) associated with scleritis and episcleritis?**

Keratitis occurs in 50% of patients with scleritis and 15% of patients with episcleritis.

Iritis may present as a secondary phenomenon in 50% of patients with scleritis. With posterior scleritis, vitritis may be present.

**25. Describe the initial evaluation of patients with scleritis/episcleritis.**

The intensity of the initial evaluation is dictated by the severity of the condition or the presence of recurrent disease. General guidelines covering most evaluations include complete blood count (CBC), erythrocyte sedimentation rate (ESR), antinuclear antibodies (ANA), rheumatoid factor (RF), uric acid, antibodies to double stranded DNA (dsDNA), cryoglobulins, syphilis serology (FTA-ABS, MHA-TP), and antineutrophil cytoplasmic antibodies (C and P-ANCA).

Other studies in selected cases include B scan ultrasound (posterior scleritis), computed tomography (CT) of the chest and sinuses, PPD testing, and biopsy of other involved organs for evidence of systemic vasculitis.

Fluorescein angiography of the anterior segment (anterior scleritis) or fundus (posterior scleritis) may also be helpful.

**26. Describe the typical case of episcleritis.**

Episcleritis is typically sudden in onset, affecting women in two-thirds of cases. Attacks are transient, lasting < 10 days. Recurrent symptoms may be seen in 60% of patients in either eye. 75% of patients have no associated disease with 25% having a history of connective tissue disease, atopy, rosacea, or gout.

**27. Describe the typical case of scleritis**

Bilateral (though not necessarily simultaneous) disease is seen in 40–80% of cases with recurrence rates of up to 70%.

Diffuse scleritis is the most benign form with 50% of patients having an associated systemic disease, typically rheumatoid arthritis. 25% of patients will lose vision, and 33% may progress to other forms of scleritis.

Nodular scleritis is characterized by local inflammation with a tender immobile nodule. Nodules may have a dark red or violaceous hue. An associated systemic disease is typically seen with 20% of cases progressing to necrosis.

Necrotizing scleritis is the most destructive form with ocular and/or systemic complications in 60% of cases. Necrotizing scleritis may indicate increased activity of systemic vasculitis. 90% of patients with necrotic disease have an associated systemic disease. 45% of untreated patients will die from associated systemic vasculitis in 5 years.

Posterior scleritis is bilateral in 10–33% of cases and may be associated with anterior scleritis.

**28. What systemic diseases are associated with scleritis?**

Scleritis may be seen in a variety of rheumatic diseases to include rheumatoid arthritis, systemic lupus erythematosus, polymyositis, scleroderma, acute rheumatic fever, polyarteritis, systemic vasculitis, allergic granulomatous vasculitis, Wegener's granulomatosis, temporal arteritis, inflammatory bowel disease (ulcerative colitis and Crohn's disease), Behçet's syndrome, Cogan's disease, Eales disease, hypocomplementic vasculitis, cryoglobulinemia, hypereosinophilic syndromes, and hypersensitivity reactions.

Necrotizing scleritis with inflammation may be seen in a variety of rheumatic diseases to include Wegener's granulomatosis (WG), polyarteritis, rheumatoid arthritis, and relapsing polychondritis. Simultaneous corneal involvement typically is seen with WG or polyarteritis. Necrotizing scleritis without inflammation (scleromalacia perforans) classically appears in patients with rheumatoid arthritis. Posterior scleritis occurs with numerous rheumatic diseases such as rheumatoid arthritis, WG, and systemic lupus erythematosus as well as infections such as tuberculosis and syphilis.

**29. What rheumatic disease is most commonly seen in patients with scleritis?**

Almost half (48%) of patients with scleritis have an associated rheumatic disease. Rheumatoid arthritis (RA) is the most commonly associated with scleritis, usually occurring in the setting of severely disabling and well-established disease. Joint inflammation may be "burnt out," and patients often have other extra-articular complaints such as rheumatoid lung disease, cutaneous vasculitis, nodules, and neuropathy.

| | |
|---|---|
| Rheumatoid arthritis | 39% |
| Wegener's granulomatosis | 17% |
| Seronegative spondyloarthropathy (ankylosing spondylitis, Reiter's syndrome, psoriatic arthritis, and inflammatory bowel disease) | 16% |
| Relapsing polychondritis | 13% |
| Systemic lupus erythematosus | 8.5% |
| Polyarteritis | 2% |
| Behçet's disease | 1% |
| Temporal arteritis | 1% |
| Cogan's syndrome | 1% |

**30. How does ocular prognosis of scleritis vary with specific rheumatic diseases?**

Scleritis in spondyloarthropathies or in systemic lupus is generally a benign and self-limiting condition, whereas scleritis in Wegener's granulomatosis is a severe disease that can lead to permanent blindness. Scleritis in rheumatoid arthritis or relapsing polychondritis is a disease of intermediate severity.

**31. List some common extra-ocular manifestations of systemic vasculitis in patients with scleritis.**

Cutaneous (rash, erythema nodosum, purpura, ulceration), proximal muscle weakness, nephritis, sinusitis, tracheitis, asthma, arteritis (bruits, hemorrhage, purpura, biopsy, abnormal arteriography), and hematologic and serological abnormalities (leukopenia, thrombocytopenia, cryoglobulins, rheumatoid factor, and ANCA).

**32. What is the treatment of episcleritis?**

Initial symptomatic treatment includes cold compresses, cold irrigation, and pulsed topical vasoconstrictors. If required, systemic administration of nonsteroidal anti-inflammatory drugs (NSAIDs) is preferred to topical administration. Topical corticosteroids are the standard of care, typically frequent intensive topical administration on a short term pulsed basis.

**33. What is the treatment for scleritis?**

Systemic therapy is required for scleritis alone or in the setting of systemic disease. Pain is often the best indicator of whether or not inflammation is being controlled. Oral NSAIDs can be effective. If inflammation is not controlled, prednisone (60–120 mg/d) rapidly tapered over 2 weeks is indicated. A maintenance dose of 7.5 to 15 mg/day is frequently required. Cases unresponsive to oral corticosteroids or requiring maintenance doses of prednisone greater than 30 mg/day may require additional use of steroid-sparing immunosuppressive agents such as cyclosporine, azathioprine, methotrexate, or cytotoxic agents such as chlorambucil or cyclophosphamide (see Question 17).

## IMMUNE-MEDIATED INNER EAR DISEASE(IMIED)

**34. Define IMIED.**

Immune-mediated inner ear disease is a syndrome that includes the subacute onset of sensorineural hearing loss, often accompanied by vertigo and tinnitus.

**35. What are the sequelae of IMIED?**

Profound deafness and loss of vestibular function.

**36. What characteristics distinguish IMIED from other syndromes of inner ear dysfunction?**

- *Relatively rapid time course.* Progression to severe irreversible damage within 3 months of onset and often more rapidly.

- *Bilateral disease*. May be affected asymmetrically or asynchronously.
- *Fluctuating symptoms* over several months. Some cases of precipitous, unrecoverable hearing loss.

**37. What are the demographics of IMIED?**

Usually middle-aged, but cases have been reported in children and in the elderly. Two-thirds of patients are women.

**38. What are the etiologic categories of inner ear dysfunction?**

Aging, trauma, tumors, infections, ototoxic drugs, and immunologic.

**39. How is high-frequency hearing loss (HFHL) secondary to aging or chronic noise exposure distinguished from IMIED?**

Lack of vestibular symptoms.

**40. What is the principal criterion distinguishing Meniere's disease from IMIED?**

*Time course*. Hearing loss is several years in Meniere's disease rather than the weeks or months in IMIED.

**41. What systemic autoimmune diseases are associated with IMIED?**

Cogan's syndrome, Wegener's granulomatosis, relapsing polychondritis, polyarteritis nodosa, systemic lupus erythematosus, and Sjögren's syndrome. Note the similarity to diseases associated with scleritis (Question 28).

**42. What diagnostic tests are available in IMIED?**

Cochlear-specific antigens have low specificities for IMIED. Antibodies to a non-organ specific heat shock protein, a 68-kD antigen found in the inner ear, kidney, brain, and other organs, have a high specificity (58%) for IMIED.

**43. What is the treatment for IMIED?**

Until rapidly available and sensitive tests for IMIED exist, the decision to initiate immunosuppression for IMIED must be based on the patient's clinical characteristics and should proceed without delay.

Treatment is with corticosteroids, at least 1 mg/kg/day of prednisone. If significant improvement in auditory or vestibular function occurs within 2 weeks, prednisone is continued at this dosage for a total of 1 month, and then slowly tapered over 2 additional months. If hearing or balance deteriorate or do not significantly improve or if symptoms increase with tapering prednisone, cyclophosphamide may be added (2 mg/kg/d). If there is no evidence of relapse, cyclophosphamide may be discontinued after 3 months. Methotrexate may be a reasonable alternative to cyclophosphamide for patients in whom the precise duration of hearing loss is unclear. Patients with antibodies to the 68-kD antigen typically respond better to immunosuppressive therapy.

## COGAN'S SYNDROME

**44. What are the ocular and auricular symptoms of Cogan's syndrome?**

Nonsyphilitic interstitial keratitis and vestibuloauditory dysfunction. Ocular symptoms include redness, pain, photophobia and blurred vision. Vestibuloauditory symptoms include Meniere's-like vertigo, ataxia, tinnitus, nausea, vomiting, and hearing loss.

Hearing fluctuation coincides with disease exacerbation and remission.

**45. What are the demographics of Cogan's syndrome?**

Median age is 25 years, with most between 15–30 years, although cases in children and the elderly have been reported. Sexual distribution is equal between males and females. An upper respiratory infection precedes the onset in 40–60% of cases. Median duration of eye and ear involvement before diagnosis is 1 month.

**46. What are the long-term complications of Cogan's syndrome?**

Blindness in 8% and deafness in 40–60%.

**47. After eye and ear complaints, what additional symptoms are seen in patients with Cogan's syndrome?**

Musculoskeletal complaints are seen in up to 50% of patients with arthralgias and myalgias most common and arthritis in 16%. Additional symptoms include fever, weight loss, and fatigue in 50%; abdominal pain 30%; lymphadenopathy 18%; rash or nodules 15%; hepatosplenomegaly 15%; aortitis with aortic insufficiency 10%; and pleurisy 5%. Patients with systemic symptoms usually have an associated vasculitis.

**48. What is the differential diagnosis of Cogan's syndrome?**

Infection (syphilis, chlamydia, TB, herpes, rubella, rubeola, mumps), rheumatic diseases (rheumatoid arthritis, ankylosing spondylitis, sarcoidosis, Wegener's granulomatosis, relapsing polychondritis, temporal arteritis, vasculitis), toxins, Meniere's disease, Vogt-Koyanaga-Harada syndrome.

**49. Describe typical from atypical Cogan's syndrome.**

Typical Cogan's syndrome involves typical eye disease (interstitial keratitis or IK) and inner ear inflammation.

Atypical Cogan's syndrome involves ocular inflammation apart from IK (iritis, conjunctivitis) or if more than 2 years have elapsed between the development of ocular and vestibuloauditory difficulties.

**50. What is the treatment for Cogan's syndrome?**

The mainstay of therapy is corticosteroids, topical for ocular inflammation and systemically for vestibuloauditory manifestations.

Keratitis almost always responds to intensive corticosteroid therapy by the topical route (i.e., 1% prednisolone at a dosage of one drop every hour for 1–2 weeks). Occasionally, oral corticosteroids may be required for recalcitrant inflammation of the anterior or posterior segment.

Vestibuloauditory dysfunction may respond to oral prednisone 1 to 2 mg/kg/d. Initiating therapy as early as possible after onset of hearing loss improves the likelihood of a favorable outcome. The prednisone dose may be tapered within 2 to 4 weeks, relatively quickly for a rapid and complete response and more slowly for a delayed or incomplete response. Corticosteroid therapy should be discontinued within 3 months whenever possible.

Severe vestibuloauditory manifestations, vision-threatening eye disease, or large vessel vasculitis may warrant the addition of a steroid-sparing agent or treatment of corticosteroid-resistant disease. Anecdotal success has been reported using methotrexate, azathioprine, cyclophosphamide, and tacrolimus.

## RETINAL VASCULITIS

**51. Define retinal vasculitis.**

Retinal vasculitis is defined clinically as an abnormal appearance of the retinal vasculature due to inflammation.

**52. What are the symptoms of retinal vasculitis?**

Reduced visual acuity, cloudy vision, diminished color appreciation, a sensation of flashing lights (photopsia), or floaters.

By itself, it does not cause ocular pain or redness.

**53. What ocular findings are seen in patients with retinal vasculitis?**

One hallmark of retinal vasculitis is vascular "sheathing," which correlates with a perivascular infiltrate of inflammatory cells seen on pathologic specimens. Other non-specific findings include cotton-wool spots or cytoid bodies (indicative of retinal ischemia), Roth's spots (hemorrhages with a white center), macular edema, and optic disc edema.

**54. How is retinal vasculopathy classified?**

Retinal vasculopathy can be subdivided into noninflammatory and inflammatory causes.

Noninflammatory causes include atherosclerosis (the most common cause of abnormal retinal vessels), congenital abnormalities as in Coat's disease, and abnormal blood viscosity from hemoglobinopathies, leukemia, or paraproteinemias.

Inflammatory causes include (1) localized areas of chorioretinal inflammation associated with toxoplasmosis, cytomegalovirus, or acute retinal necrosis; (2) vaso-occlusive disease associated with antiphospholipid antibodies; (3) systemic diseases such as sarcoidosis, rheumatic diseases (Behçet's disease, polyarteritis, Churg-Strauss vasculitis, Wegener's granulomatosis, and systemic lupus erythematosus), multiple sclerosis, and Crohn's disease; and (4) primary retinal vasculitis with no apparent systemic disorder (Eales disease and frosted branch angiitis).

**55. What laboratory evaluation is indicated in the evaluation of retinal vasculitis?**

The laboratory evaluation of cases of retinal vasculitis is determined largely by the results of the patient's history and physical examination. Frequently obtained tests include a complete blood count, a chemistry screen that includes liver and renal function studies, quantitative immunoglobulins, serum glucose, a urinalysis (to exclude glomerular involvement), and an erythrocyte sedimentation rate (ESR). They are rarely useful in arriving at a specific diagnosis, however. Most patients with retinal vasculitis have no evidence of a disease process outside the eye (93%).

**56. Describe the treatment of retinal vasculitis.**

The treatment of retinal vasculitis depends on the detection of an associated condition, the severity of the disease, and whether the process is unilateral or bilateral. If its cause is infectious, the disorder should be managed with appropriate antibiotic therapy. In the absence of a specific infection, periocular corticosteroids may help control inflammation. If the disease is bilateral and interferes with activities of daily living, prednisone 40–60 mg/day is sometimes effective. Systemic immunosuppressive therapy beyond corticosteroids is reserved for patients with active inflammation, bilateral inflammation, and a best-corrected vision of no better than 20/50.

## BIBLIOGRAPHY


1. Allen NB, Cox CC, Cobo M, et al: Use of immunosuppressive agents in the treatment of severe ocular and vascular manifestations of Cogan's syndrome. Am J Med 88:296–301, 1990.
2. Banares A, Jovier JA, Fernandez-Gutierrez B, et al: Patterns of uveitis as a guide in making rheumatologic and immunologic diagnoses. Arthritis Rheum 40:358–370, 1997.
3. Bloom JN: Uveitis in childhood. Opthalmol Clin North Am 3:163–176, 1990.
4. Bodaghi B, Cassoux N, Wechsler B, et al: Chronic severe uveitis: Etiology and visual outcome in 927 patients from single center. Medicine 80:263–270, 2001.
5. de la Maza MS, Foster CS, Jabbur NS: Scleritis associated with systemic vasculitic diseases. Ophthalmology 102:687–692, 1995.
6. Dubord PJ, Chalmers A: Scleritis and episcleritis: Diagnosis and management. Focal Points 13(9):1–14, 1995.
7. Feltkamp TEW, Ringrose JH: Acute anterior uveitis and spondyloarthropathies. Curr Opin Rheumatol 10:314–318, 1998.
8. Forrester JV: Endogenous posterior uveitis. Br J Ophthalmol 74:620–623, 1990.
9. Hamideh F, Prete P: Ophthalmologic manifestations of rheumatic diseases. Semin Arthritis Rheum 30:217–241, 2001.
10. Jabs DA, Rosenbaum JT: Guidelines for the use of immunosuppressive drugs in patients with ocular inflammatory disorders: Recommendations of an expert panel. Am J Ophthalmol 131:679, 2001.
11. Malinowski SM, Folk JC, Pulido JS: Pars planitis. Curr Opin Ophthalmol 5:72–82, 1994.

12. Rosenbaum JT: An algorithm for the systemic evaluation of patients with uveitis: Guidelines for the consultant. Semin Arthritis Rheum 19:248–257, 1990.
13. Rosenbaum JT, Robertson JE, Watzke RC: Retinal vasculitis—a primer. West J Med 154:182–185, 1991.
14. Smith JR, Levinson RD, Holland GN, et al: Differential efficacy of tumor necrosis factor inhibition in the management of inflammatory eye disease and associated rheumatic disease. Arthritis Care Res 45:252–257, 2001.
15. St. Clair EW, McCallum RM: Cogan's syndrome. Curr Opin Rheumatol 11:47–52, 1999
16. Stone JH, Francis HW: Immune-mediated inner ear disease. Curr Opin Rheumatol 12:32–40, 2000

# 80. RHEUMATIC SYNDROMES ASSOCIATED WITH SARCOIDOSIS

*Daniel F. Battafarano,* D.O.

**1. What is sarcoidosis?**

Sarcoidosis is an inflammatory disorder with protean manifestations characterized by **noncaseating granulomas** in clinically affected organs and sometimes in asymptomatic organs.

**2. Who is affected by sarcoidosis?**

Sarcoidosis occurs worldwide but most frequently among African-Americans and northern Europeans. It typically appears in the third or fourth decade of life, and sex varies among ethnic groups.

**3. What are the immunologic features of sarcoidosis?**

Sarcoidosis is mediated primarily by CD4+ T-helper cells and cells derived from the mononuclear phagocytes. However, other inflammatory cells, epithelial cells, and endothelial cells contribute to increased tissue permeability and cell migration by the production of chemokines and the influence of adhesion molecules. In the early stages of alveolitis, there is an elevated lymphocyte count and increase in macrophage number with a marked increase in CD4/CD8 T lymphocyte ratio by bronchoalveolar lavage (BAL). Morphologic characteristics and immunohistologic patterns of the sarcoid granuloma suggest they are the result of an antigen-driven process. Although the antigens are unknown, type II alveolar cells, resident alveolar macrophages, and pulmonary dendritic cells in the lung appear to function as sarcoid antigen presenting cells. There is depression of delayed type hypersensitivity, imbalance of CD4/CD8 T-cell subsets, an influx of T-helper cells to sites of activity, hyperactivity of B cells, and circulation of immune complexes. Typical clinical observations include peripheral lymphopenia and a low CD4/CD8 T-cell ratio (0.8/1.0), cutaneous anergy (70%), polyclonal gammopathy, and autoantibody production (30%).

**4. What is the typical clinical presentation of sarcoidosis?**

More than 90% of patients will present with an abnormal chest roentgenogram revealing hilar adenopathy, pulmonary infiltrates, or both.

**5. Describe the stages of sarcoidosis and their prognosis.**

| STAGE | CHEST RADIOGRAPHIC FINDINGS | REMISSION RATE (%) |
|---|---|---|
| 0 | Normal | — |
| 1 | Bilateral hilar adenopathy | 60–80 |
| 2 | Bilateral hilar adenopathy with pulmonary infiltrates | 30–50 |
| 3 | Pulmonary infiltrates with lung insufficiency | < 20 |

**6. What are the extrathoracic clinical manifestations of sarcoidosis?**

The most common extrathoracic manifestations are **cutaneous** and **ocular involvement**. Cutaneous involvement occurs in 30% of patients and may be manifest as erythema nodosum in early sarcoidosis or as subcutaneous nodules, papules, plaques, and lupus pernio in chronic disease. Eye involvement can be seen in 20% and typically involves the conjunctiva, lacrimal gland, or uveal tract. Arthralgias and arthritis are present in up to 50%. Involvement of skeletal muscle occurs in 50–80%, although most patients are asymptomatic. Hepatomegaly (30%) and splenomegaly (10%) are common findings but rarely cause significant complications. Bilateral parotid enlargement is seen in 10% and is associated with xerostomia. Neurologic findings are observed in 5%, with unilateral facial nerve palsy being most common. Heart involvement (5%) presents with arrhythmias, left ventricular dysfunction, and pericarditis. The hypothalamic-pituitary axis may be involved and classically presents as diabetes insipidus. Kidney and gastrointestinal organs are rarely affected. Vasculitis of any size vessel has been described.

**7. Where are granulomas most commonly found on biopsy in sarcoidosis?**

Noncaseating granulomas are widely distributed and have been reported in many organs. They are most commonly found in the lung (86%), lymph nodes (86%), liver (86%), muscle (75%), spleen (63%), heart (20%), kidney (19%), bone marrow (17%), and pancreas (6%). Granulomas may produce elevated serum angiotensin-converting enzyme (ACE) levels and may significantly enhance production of 1,25-dihydrocholecalciferol responsible for clinical hypercalcemia.

**8. Is the serum ACE level useful for the diagnosis of sarcoidosis?**

No. The ACE level is elevated in 40–90% of all patients with sarcoidosis. Patients with Lofgren's syndrome frequently have a normal ACE level. It may also be elevated in miliary tuberculosis, histoplasmosis, Gaucher's disease, silicosis, asbestosis, leprosy, HIV infection, hepatitis, hyperthyroidism, and diabetes. The ACE levels can be useful in individual patients if elevated at the time of diagnosis. Serial levels in these patients tend to correlate with disease activity and will normalize in response to effective medical treatment.

**9. How do acute and chronic sarcoid arthritis differ clinically?**

| FEATURES | ACUTE | CHRONIC |
|---|---|---|
| Initial clinical manifestation | Common | Not seen |
| Joint involvement | Symmetrical; ankles, knees, wrists, PIP joints | Same as acute, dactylitis |
| Hilar adenopathy | Common, no pulmonary infiltrates | May be seen with pulmonary disease |
| HLA association | B8, DR3, in whites of Northern European ancestry | Not known |
| Synovial fluid | Mildly inflammatory; 3000 cells (80% mononuclear) | Inflammatory; 25,000 cells (90% neutrophil) |
| Synovial biopsy | Synovial hyperplasia, no inflammatory infiltrate | Sarcoid granuloma |
| Destructive bony lesions | Absent | Present |
| Clinical course | Benign, self-limited | Chronic |

Modified from Mathur A, Kremer JM: Immunology, rheumatic features, and therapy of sarcoidosis. Curr Opin Rheumatol 4:76–80, 1992.

**10. What is Lofgren's syndrome?**

This is a triad of acute arthritis, erythema nodosum, and bilateral hilar adenopathy in a patient with sarcoidosis. The arthritis typically involves the ankles and knees. These patients have an excellent response to corticosteroid therapy and have a greater than 90% remission rate.

**11. What are the rheumatic manifestations of sarcoidosis?**

| MANIFESTATION | FREQUENCY IN SARCOIDOSIS (% OF PATIENTS) | DIFFERENTIAL DIAGNOSIS |
|---|---|---|
| Arthritis | 15 | Rheumatoid arthritis, gonococcal arthritis, rheumatic fever, SLE, gout, spondyloarthropathies |
| Parotid gland enlargement | 5 | Sjögren's syndrome |
| Upper airway disease (sinusitis, laryngeal inflammation, saddle nose deformity) | 3 | Wegener's granulomatosis |
| Uveitis | 19 | |
| Anterior | 18 | Spondyloarthropathies |
| Posterior | 7 | Behçet's |
| Keratoconjunctivitis | 5 | Sjögren's syndrome |
| Proptosis | 1 | Wegener's granulomatosis |
| Myositis | 4 | Polymyositis |
| Mononeuritis multiplex | 1 | Systemic vasculitis |
| Facial nerve palsy | 2 | Lyme disease |

Modified from Hellman DB: Sarcoidosis. In Schumacher HR, et al (eds): Primer on the Rheumatic Diseases, 10th ed. Atlanta, Arthritis Foundation, 1993.

**12. How does muscular sarcoidosis present clinically?**

Sarcoid myopathy most commonly occurs in patients with multiorgan involvement. Although muscle involvement in sarcoidosis is usually asymptomatic, there are three clinical presentations: nodular, acute myositic, and chronic myopathic. The nodular presentation is the least common type, involving the musculotendinous junctions. Acute inflammatory myositis is rare and is indistinguishable from idiopathic myositis. Chronic myopathy is the most common form and is manifested by an insidious onset of proximal symmetrical muscle weakness. Muscle enzyme levels, electromyography, and muscle biopsies are necessary to differentiate the types of muscle involvement.

**13. What osseous changes occur in patients with sarcoidosis?**

The overall incidence of osseous sarcoid is reported in up to 14%. Bony lesions are associated with chronic skin and multiorgan involvement. The phalanges of the hands are most commonly involved. The metacarpophalangeal joints, metacarpals, and wrists are usually spared. Radiographic findings include soft tissue swelling, periarticular osteopenia, joint-space narrowing, cyst formation, eccentric/punched-out erosions, sclerosis and periosteal reactions, pathologic fractures, and phalangeal fragmentation.

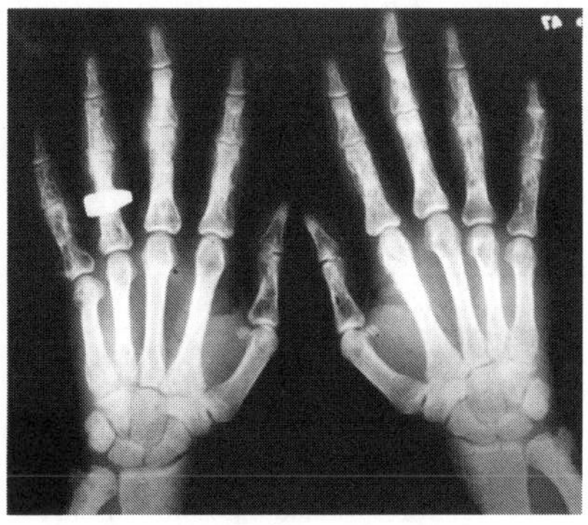

Osseous sarcoid involving the hands. The phalanges demonstrate a coarsened, reticulated, or lacelike trabecular pattern seen in chronic sarcoid bone involvement.

**14. Can sarcoidosis and other connective tissue diseases coexist?**

Yes. Several reports have described sarcoidosis in patients with other rheumatic diseases, including systemic lupus erythematosus, rheumatoid arthritis, Sjögren's syndrome, and spondyloarthropathies. This occurrence is believed to be a coincidence because there is not a known common etiopathogenesis.

**15. How is sarcoidosis usually treated?**

Corticosteroids (up to 1 mg/kg/day) are considered the most effective treatment for sarcoidosis. Significant impairment of vital organs (lung, heart, eye, kidney, or brain) or hypercalcemia is a clear indication for corticosteroid therapy. NSAIDs and/or lower corticosteroids dosages (less than 0.5 mg/kg/day) are used for joint and muscle involvement. Colchicine can be effective for acute arthritis. Chloroquine/hydroxychloroquine and low-dose methotrexate have been effective for long-term management of musculoskeletal involvement in selected patients. Cutaneous disease is typically treated with corticosteroids (topical or oral), but antimalarials, low-dose methotrexate, and azathioprine have been useful for chronic lesions. Cyclophosphamide (oral and intravenous) have been beneficial in treating cardiac or neurosarcoidosis that have failed combination corticosteroid and methotrexate treatment.

## BIBLIOGRAPHY


1. Abril A, Cohen MD: Rheumatological manifestations of sarcoidosis. Bul Rheum Dis 49:1–3, 2000.
2. Agostini MD, Adami F, Semenzato G: New pathogenetic insights into the sarcoid granuloma. Curr Opin Rheumatol 12:71–76, 2000.
3. Barnard J, Newman LS: Sarcoidosis: Immunology, rheumatic involvement, and therapeutics. Curr Opin Rheumatol 13:84–91, 2001.
4. Chatham WW: Sarcoidosis. In Ruddy S, Harris ED, Sledge CB (eds): Kelley's Textbook of Rheumatology, 6th ed. Philadelphia, WB Saunders, 2001, pp 1551–1566.
5. Conron M, DuBois RM: Immunological mechanisms in sarcoidosis. Clin Exp Allergy 31:543–554, 2001.
6. Fernandes SRM, Singsen BH, Hoffman GS: Sarcoidosis and systemic vasculitis. Semin Arthritis Rheum 30:33–46, 2000.
7. Hellman DB: Sarcoidosis. In Klippel JH, Weyand CM, Wortmann RL (eds): Primer on the Rheumatic Diseases, 11th ed. Atlanta, Arthritis Foundation, 1997, pp 325–327.
8. Hunnunghake G, Costabel U, Ando M, et al: Statement on sarcoidosis. Sarcoidosis Vasc Diffuse Lung Dis 16:149–173, 1999.
9. Jones CJ, Michele TM: The clinical management of sarcoidosis: A 50-year experience at the John Hopkins Hospital. Medicine (Baltimore) 78:65–111, 1999.
10. Newman L, Rose C, Maier L: Sarcoidosis. N Engl J Med 336:1224–1234, 1997.
11. Yee AMF, Pochapin MB: Treatment of complicated sarcoidosis with infliximab anti-tumor necrosis factor–α therapy. Ann Intern Med 135:27–31, 2001.


# 81. RHEUMATIC DISORDERS IN THE DIALYSIS PATIENT

*Mark Jarek*, M.D.

**1. What is renal osteodystrophy?**

The term *renal osteodystrophy*, which was introduced by Liu and Chu in 1943, refers to the full spectrum of musculoskeletal disorders associated with renal failure. Because the kidney plays a critical role in the overall regulation of mineral homeostasis, the development of renal failure has widespread consequences for the skeleton. Some of the musculoskeletal disorders that develop in chronic renal failure and dialysis can be recalled with the mnemonic **VITAMINS ABCDE**:

**V** — **V**ascular calcification
**I** — **I**nfections (osteomyelitis, septic arthritis)
**T** — **T**umoral calcifications
**A** — **A**myloid arthropathy ($\beta_2$-microglobulin)
**M** — **M**etabolic bone disease (osteomalacia, osteoporosis)
**I** — **I**nfarction (osteonecrosis)
**N** — **N**odules (tophi)
**S** — **S**econdary hyperparathyroidism

**A** — **A**luminum toxicity
**B** — **B**ursitis (olecranon)
**C** — **C**rystal arthropathy (gout, CPDD, hydroxyapatite)
**D** — **D**igital clubbing
**E** — **E**rosive spondyloarthropathy

**2. Why does secondary hyperparathyroidism develop in chronic renal failure? How does this lead to bone disease?**

Secondary hyperparathyroidism starts relatively early, when the glomerular filtration rate is in the range of 60–90 ml/min, as evidenced by increased levels of parathyroid hormone (PTH) and histological changes in bone. As renal function deteriorates, these changes become more dramatic. Several factors in patients with chronic renal failure contribute to the sustained increases in PTH secretion and, ultimately, to parathyroid gland hyperplasia.

- Hyperphosphatemia due to impaired renal excretion
- Impaired renal hydroxylation of 25-hydroxyvitamin D to 1,25-dihydroxyvitamin D
- Low calcium intake and absorption
- Insensitivity of the parathyroid gland to the suppressive effects of calcium on PTH secretion

The end result of each of these defects is a sustained increase in PTH release, which stimulates osteoclast activation and rapid bone resorption. Secondary hyperparathyroidism is usually asymptomatic but may cause bone pain and polyarthralgias.

**3. List the characteristic radiographic features of secondary hyperparathyroidism.**

**Early**

Subperiosteal resorption in the hands, wrists, feet, and medial tibia, particularly on the radial side of the middle phalanx of the index and middle fingers (see Chapter 52).

Osteoporosis

**Intermediate**

Subchondral resorption of sternoclavicular, acromioclavicular, discovertebral, and sacroiliac joints and symphysis pubis

Loss of the lamina dura around teeth

Acro-osteolysis of the phalangeal tufts

Chondrocalcinosis of knees, wrists, and symphysis pubis (see Chapter 50)

Periarticular and soft tissue calcification

**Late**

Bone cysts (single or multiple) (see figure)

Subligamentous bone resorption of trochanters, ischial tuberosities, humeral tuberosities, and calcanei

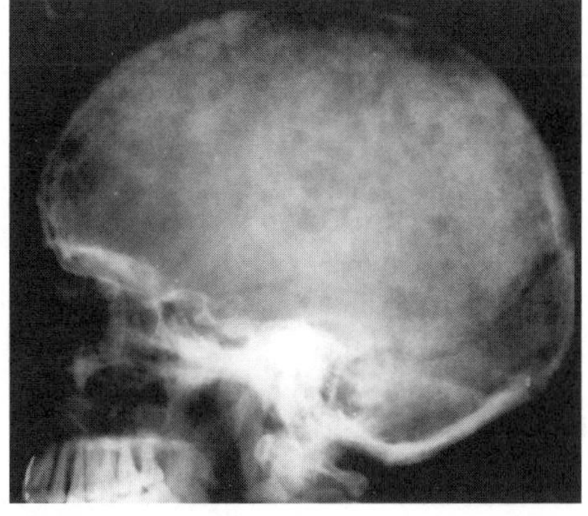

Skull radiograph of a patient with renal failure and secondary hyperparathyroidism. Note the bone cysts ("brown tumors") superimposed on a "salt and pepper" skull.

**4. What is a "salt and pepper" skull? "Rugger-jersey spine?"**

Both terms are descriptions of radiographic findings seen in hyperparathyroidism. Trabecular bone resorption creates a characteristic mottling of the cranial vault with alternating areas of lucency and sclerosis, producing the **salt and pepper** radiographic appearance. **Rugger-jersey spine** refers to band-like osteosclerosis of the superior and inferior margins of the vertebral bodies.

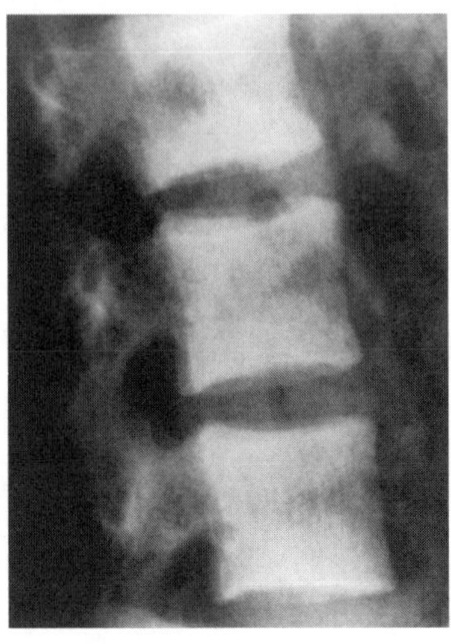

Rugger-jersey spine.

**5. How can you distinguish primary from secondary hyperparathyroidism on radiographs?**

**Osteitis fibrosa cystica** was the term applied to the characteristic subperiosteal erosions that were originally identified on radiographs in primary hyperparathyroidism. Today, routine serum chemistry screening provides for early detection of primary hyperparathyroidism in the asymptomatic stage, prior to the development of the characteristic bony findings. Therefore, osteitis fibrosa cystica has all but disappeared in primary hyperparathyroidism and is now seen only in renal osteodystrophy with secondary hyperparathyroidism.

*Primary Versus Secondary Hyperparathyroidism*

| FINDING | PRIMARY HYPERPARATHYROIDISM | SECONDARY HYPERPARATHYROIDISM* |
|---|---|---|
| Brown tumors | Common | Less common |
| Osteosclerosis | Rare | Common |
| Chondrocalcinosis | Not infrequent | Rare |
| Periostitis | Rare | Not infrequent |

Adapted from Resnick D, Niwayama G: Parathyroid disorders and renal osteodystrophy. In Resnick D, Niwayama G (eds): Diagnosis of Bone and Joint Disorders, 2nd ed. Philadelphia, WB Saunders, 1988, pp 2219–2285.

Additional findings of renal osteodystrophy are observed in secondary hyperparathyroidism, including osteomalacia and soft tissue and vascular calcification.

**6. What dietary modifications decrease PTH secretion and help to prevent the development of secondary hyperparathyroidism in chronic renal failure?**

Phosphate restriction

Calcium supplementation (calcium carbonate)

Adequate 1,25-dihydroxyvitamin D intake

Once hyperparathyroidism is advanced, it may be refractory to these dietary interventions, at which time high-dose intravenous 1,25-dihydroxyvitamin D may be beneficial. If these measures fail, subtotal parathyroidectomy is indicated to correct symptomatic hyperparathyroidism.

**7. What is amyloid arthropathy of renal failure?**

$\beta_2$-microglobulin is an endogenous structural protein (MW = 11 kD) that is poorly cleared by standard dialysis membranes and accumulates to extremely high levels in patients on long-term hemodialysis. It is deposited in and around joints, leading to chronic arthralgias and carpal tunnel syndrome. This chronic arthropathy most commonly involves the shoulder, hip, wrist and finger tendon sheaths, and rarely the spine. Rotator cuff and subacromial bursae deposition leads to impingement syndrome.

Synovial fluid is noninflammatory but may be hemorrhagic as a result of anticoagulation use during dialysis. Synovial fluid or biopsy will identify amyloid fibrils when stained with Congo red. Radiographs are notable for large subchondral bony cysts and erosions. The use of more permeable membranes may delay the onset of disease but does not prevent disease development.

**8. What role does aluminum play in renal osteodystrophy?**

In renal failure or hemodialysis, dietary aluminum is not adequately cleared and deposits in the osteoid lamellae of newly formed bone, inhibiting mineralization, which leads to osteomalacia. Clinically, osteomalacia presents as diffuse bone pain and predisposes to insufficiency fractures. Radiographic findings are osteopenia and Looser's zones. Deferoxamine chelation therapy is beneficial. Other common causes of osteomalacia, such as vitamin D deficiency, need to be considered, although this is now uncommon with the routine supplementation of vitamin D in dialysis patients. Secondary hyperparathyroidism, if present, needs to be treated aggressively to prevent concomitant osteoporosis.

**9. How çan you prevent aluminum-induced osteomalacia in renal failure?**

1. Avoid all aluminum-containing compounds (most phosphate binders, antacids).
2. Ensure adequate vitamin D intake.
3. Maintain normal plasma 25-dihydroxyvitamin D levels.
4. Maintain dialysate aluminum content < 20 mg/ml.
5. Monitor plasma aluminum levels frequently.

**10. A patient who is 3 months' post–renal transplant develops an acute knee arthritis. His current medications include cyclosporine, azathioprine, and prednisone. What is the most likely etiology for the knee pain?**

This is a common presentation of **acute gouty arthritis** associated with **cyclosporine** use. Cyclosporine blocks renal uric acid clearance, leading to marked hyperuricemia and gout. Polarized microscopy of the synovial fluid may identify numerous intracellular, negatively birefrigent, needle-shaped crystals, confirming the diagnosis of gout (see Chapter 49). Positive birefrigent rhomboid crystals of pseudogout also may be seen because of the association of secondary hyperparathyroidism and calcium pyrophosphate deposition (CPDD) disease. Septic arthritis needs to be considered in the differential diagnosis because of the potent immunosuppressive therapy used in this post-transplant patient. Therefore, joint fluid should be sent for Gram stain and cultures to include fungi and tuberculosis. Listeriosis also occurs in this setting.

**11. Which spondyloarthropathy is unique to dialysis patients?**

A **destructive spondyloarthropathy** (DSA) is found only in long-term dialysis patients and is defined by its radiologic picture. There is multilevel disc-space narrowing with erosions and cysts of adjacent vertebral end-plates without significant osteophytosis or sclerosis. Calcification of surrounding vertebral discs is common. The cervical and lumbar spine are most frequently involved. The erosions progress radiographically over a few weeks or more, followed by reactive endplate sclerosis. Diffuse spinal involvement is unusual, although multisegment involvement has been described.

This entity has been reported occasionally in uremic patients prior to dialysis but has not been reported following renal transplantation. Most patients are asymptomatic, which accounts for the rarity of its description. Neck pain or cervical radiculopathy is the most common complaint in symptomatic patients. Despite the severe radiologic picture, medullary compression has been reported only once. Biopsies reveal calcium crystals (CPDD or hydroxyapatite) or $\beta_2$-microglobulin. Hyperparathyroidism is usually also present and appears to play a role in the pathogenesis of DSA. Control of hyperparathyroidism, including subtotal parathyroidectomy, appears to prevent progression of DSA.

**12. What is tertiary hyperparathyroidism?**

Under normal homeostasis, a normal or elevated serum calcium level feeds back to inhibit PTH release, maintaining normal calcium levels. Tertiary hyperparathyroidism is the loss of this feedback inhibition on PTH release, which develops in long-standing secondary hyperparathyroidism. Renal transplantation often unmasks tertiary hyperparathyroidism, when PTH secretion remains elevated despite normalization of serum calcium with the improved renal function. This PTH release results in further bone resorption and hypercalcemia. In general, surgical treatment is indicated in symptomatic patients with nonsuppressible serum PTH levels. Symptoms may include those related to hypercalcemia, hyperparathyroidism, nephrocalcinosis, or nephrolithiasis. A subtotal parathyroidectomy is the treatment of choice.

**13. Where do soft tissue calcifications occur in renal osteodystrophy?**

Soft tissue calcification is common in renal osteodystrophy. Sites of soft tissue deposition are multiple, including the cornea and conjunctiva, viscera, vasculature, and subcutaneous and periarticular tissues. Calcification occurs in chronic renal failure when the concentration (mg/dl) product of plasma calcium and phosphorus exceeds 70. Periarticular and subcutaneous deposits may become quite large, particularly around the hips, knees, shoulders, and wrists, where they may cause pain, reduce range of motion, and predispose to infection. Vascular calcification may compromise blood flow leading to skin ulceration or tissue infarction. The chemical composition of the calcium depends on the site of deposition. In subcutaneous, vascular, and periarticular sites, hydroxyapatite is observed, while in viscera, magnesium Whitlokite-like material is found.

**14. What types of crystal deposition diseases occur in patients with renal disease?**

- Monosodium urate arthritis (**gouty arthritis**) occurs occasionally, although less frequently than one would expect considering how common hyperuricemia is in patients with chronic renal failure.
- **Calcium pyrophosphate deposition disease** (CPDD) is seen occasionally in secondary hyperparathyroidism (although less common than in primary hyperparathyroidism). CPDD is manifested by chondrocalcinosis (knee, wrist, symphysis pubis), acute pseudogout, and/or a degenerative arthritis.
- **Secondary oxalosis** rarely develops in long-standing renal failure. It is marked by oxalate deposition in visceral organs, blood vessels, bones, and articular cartilage, where it may contribute to chronic polyarthralgias. Oxalate is produced from ascorbic acid and is cleared very poorly in chronic renal failure and dialysis. Most cases of oxalosis can be prevented by limiting ascorbic acid intake. Treatment of established calcium oxalate arthropathy with NSAIDs, colchicine, intra-articular corticosteroids, or increased dialysis has produced only slight improvement.

**15. Describe what happens to the serum calcium, phosphate, 25-hydroxyvitamin D, and 1,25-dihydroxyvitamin D levels in osteomalacia and the hyperparathyroidism syndrome.**

| | Ca | $PO_4$ | 25-VIT D | 1,25-VIT D | iPTH | AlkPhos |
|---|---|---|---|---|---|---|
| Renal osteomalacia | ↓ | ↓ | ↔ | ↓ | ↔↓ | ↔↓ |
| Primary hyperparathyroidism | ↑ | ↓↔ | ↔ | ↑↓ | ↑ | ↓ |
| Secondary hyperparathyroidism | ↓↔ | ↓↔ | ↔ | ↓ | ↑ | ↓↔ |
| Tertiary hyperparathyroidism | ↑ | ↑ | ↔ | ↓ | ↑↑ | ↓ |

↓, decreased; ↑, increased; ↔, normal. Ca, calcium; $PO_4$, phosphate; 25-Vit D, 25-hydroxyvitamin D; 1,25-Vit D, 1,25-dihydroxyvitamin D; iPTH, immunoreactive parathyroid hormone; AlkPhos, alkaline phosphatase.

**16. What dose adjustments are needed for antirheumatic drugs in patients with renal insufficiency?**

Serum creatinine may be an inaccurate measurement of renal function because as renal function declines, less creatinine is excreted by glomerular filtration and more is excreted by tubular secretion. The use of cimetidine (400 mg QID for 2 days) blocks tubular secretion of creatinine and may improve accuracy of creatinine clearance measurements. Also, the Cockroft-Gault formula can be used to estimate creatinine clearance:

$$\text{CrCl (GFR)} = \frac{(140 - \text{age}) \times (\text{IBW in kg})}{72 \times \text{serum Cr} \times .85 \text{ (women)}}$$

Ideal body weight [IBW (men)] = 50 kg + 2.3 kg per inch over 5 feet tall
Ideal body weight [IBW (women)] = 45 kg + 2.3 kg per inch over 5 feet tall

After determining correct creatinine clearance, the following guidelines can be used:

- Antimalarials—avoid prolonged use in severe renal insufficiency glomerular filtration rate (GFR) < 30 ml/min. Not hemodialized. Watch for neuromyopathy.
- Allopurinol—GFR 30 ml/min, use 100 mg; GFR 60 ml/min, use 200 mg; GFR 90 ml/min, use 300 mg daily.
- Azathioprine—GFR 10–50 ml/min, reduce dose to 75%; GFR < 10 ml/min, cut dose 50%. Give after hemodialysis.
- Bisphosphonates—avoid in end-stage renal disease (ESRD). Use half dose in renal insufficiency.
- Colchicine—avoid prolonged use in patients with GFR less than 50 ml/min. Use only .6 mg daily in patients with renal insufficiency. Watch for neuromyopathy.
- Corticosteroids—no change in dose.
- Cyclophosphamide—GFR < 25 ml/min, reduce dose to 25% usual dose; GFR 25–50 ml/min, reduce dose to 50%. If patient in ESRD, give dose after hemodialysis.
- Cyclosporine—no dose adjustment for renal insufficiency. However, use of cyclosporine can worsen renal insufficiency. If creatinine rises, the cyclosporine dose needs to be lowered.
- Dapsone—GFR < 50 ml/min, give every other day.
- Etanercept, infliximab, anakinra = no dose adjustments.
- Gold—GFR 50–75 ml/min, use 50% usual dose. GFR < 50 ml/min, avoid gold.
- Leflunomide—insufficient data. 40–50% of drug is eliminated by kidneys.
- Methotrexate—reduce dose 50% with renal insufficiency. Should use with extreme caution owing to hematologic toxicity.
- Mycophenylate mofetil—hepatic metabolism. Reduce dose 25% for GFR < 25 ml/min. Do not exceed 2 grams per day.
- Narcotics—GFR 10–50 ml/min, use 75% usual dose; GFR < 10 ml/min, cut dose 50%. Avoid Darvon and meperidine.
- NSAIDs—most are metabolized by liver except for diflunisal. Note all NSAIDs except salsalate can make renal insufficiency worse. No need for dose adjustment for NSAIDs in ESRD except for diflunisal (decrease dose 50%). Avoid sulindac, owing to renal stone formation in patients with low urine output. Also avoid ketoprofen, since will be metabolized back to active drug if can't be renally excreted.
- Penicillamine—avoid if GFR < 50 ml/min.
- Probenecid—doesn't work if GFR < 50–60 ml/min. No dosage change for mild renal insufficiency.
- Sulfasalzine—no change in dose.
- Tacrolimus—same as cyclosporine.
- Tramadol—give dose every 12 hours instead of every 6 hours in renal insufficiency.

**17. What antirheumatic drugs are removed by hemodialysis?**

- Azathioprine
- Prednisolone

- Cyclophosphamide—removes 50%
- Penicillamine—removes 33%
- Tramadol—removes 70%

These drugs should be given after hemodialysis. Other antirheumatic drugs either are not removed by hemodialysis (NSAIDs, narcotics, cyclosporine, methotrexate, colchicine, gold, antimalarials) or it is unknown if they are.

## BIBLIOGRAPHY


1. Bardin T, Kuntz D: Dialysis arthropathy. In Klippel JH, Dieppe PA (eds): Rheumatology, 2nd ed. London, Mosby, 1998, section 8:29.1–4.
2. Bindi P, Chanard J: Destructive spondyloarthropathy in dialysis patients: An overview. Nephron 55:104–109, 1990.
3. Carpenter CB, Lazarus JM: Dialysis and transplantation in the treatment of renal failure. In Wilson JD, et al (eds): Harrison's Principles of Internal Medicine, 14th ed. New York, McGraw-Hill, 1998, pp 1520–1529.
4. Eastwood JB, Pazianas M: Renal bone disease. In Klippel JH, Dieppe PA (eds): Rheumatology, 2nd ed. London, Mosby, 1998, section 8:42.1–4.
5. Goodman WG, Coburn JW, Slatopolsky E, et al: Renal osteodystrophy in adults and children. In Favus MJ (ed): Primer on the Metabolic Bone Diseases and Disorders of Mineral Metabolism, 4th ed. Philadelphia, Lippincott–Raven, 1999, pp 347–366.
6. Indridason OS, SC, Quarles LD: Tertiary hyperparathyroidism and refractory secondary hyperparathyroidism. In Favus MJ (ed): Primer on the Metabolic Bone Diseases and Disorders of Mineral Metabolism, 4th ed. Philadelphia, Lippincott–Raven, 1999, pp 198–202.
7. Lazarus JM, Brenner BM: Chronic renal failure. In Wilson JD, et al (eds): Harrison's Principles of Internal Medicine, 14th ed. New York, McGraw-Hill, 1998, pp 1513–1520
8. Rafto SE, Dalinka MK, Schieber ML, et al: Spondyloarthropathy of the cervical spine in long-term hemodialysis. Radiology 166:201–204, 1988.
9. Resnick D, Niwayama G: Parathyroid disorders and renal osteodystrophy. In Resnick D (ed): Diagnosis of Bone and Joint Disorders, 3rd ed. Philadelphia, WB Saunders, 1995, pp 2012–2075.
10. Sergent JS: Arthritis accompanying endocrine and metabolic disorders. In Ruddy S, Harris ED, Sledge CB (eds): Kelley's Textbook of Rheumatology, 6th ed. Philadelphia, WB Saunders, 2001, pp 1581–1589.


# 82. RHEUMATIC DISEASE AND THE PREGNANT PATIENT

*Mark Jarek, M.D.*

**1. A young patient with recently diagnosed systemic lupus erythematosus is currently being treated with low-dose prednisone, hydroxychloroquine, and occasional nonsteroidal anti-inflammatory drugs (NSAIDs) with good disease control. She is considering pregnancy and asks about the optimal timing of a pregnancy and the potential maternal and fetal complications. What advice do you give her?**

Patients with systemic lupus erythematosus (SLE) should be advised to conceive while SLE is quiescent or at least under good control for 6–12 months. Patients who conceive with inactive SLE still are at increased risk for intrauterine growth retardation (IUGR), prematurity, and toxemia of pregnancy. There is a 20–30% likelihood of stable SLE relapsing during pregnancy, although the long-term disease outcome in these patients probably is not altered because most exacerbations are mild. Such patients need to be followed closely by a rheumatologist during pregnancy.

Patients with severe SLE, particularly active lupus nephritis, are at particularly high risk for maternal and fetal complications and should be cautioned strongly against conception. Fetal mortality in this group is increased at least 3-fold, and prematurity occurs in most of the successful pregnancies. In some studies, the fetal mortality rate did not improve even when the SLE nephritis was inactive. There is no increased rate of infertility for patients with SLE as long as the disease is under control.

**2. How can you distinguish lupus nephritis from toxemia of pregnancy?**

The **toxemia** syndrome (preeclampsia-eclampsia) usually occurs in the third trimester of primigravidas. It is manifested in mild cases by hypertension, proteinuria, and edema, with a consumptive coagulopathy, microangiopathic hemolytic anemia, and convulsions occurring in severe cases. The distinction between eclampsia and active **lupus nephritis** can be difficult, since both diseases can cause thrombocytopenia, hemolytic anemia, hypertension, seizures, and renal insufficiency with proteinuria. The absence of other clinical manifestations of SLE, such as arthritis, rash, and leukopenia, as well as the lack of red cell casts and stable anti-DNA antibodies, make the diagnosis of eclampsia more likely.

Complement values usually rise during a normal pregnancy but have been reported to decrease in SLE patients during pregnancy independent of a lupus relapse, and therefore complement values may not be helpful in distinguishing the two diseases. The ESR is usually elevated in both conditions and therefore is of no value. Proteinuria can occur during a normal pregnancy as a result of the physiologic increased renal blood flow but should be accompanied by a normal, pregnancy-associated rise in creatinine clearance and a corresponding fall in serum creatinine. Toxemia of pregnancy remits immediately following delivery and therefore usually requires no further therapy, whereas lupus nephritis requires high-dose corticosteroids frequently in combination with azathioprine during pregnancy or cyclophosphamide after completion of pregnancy.

*Clinical Findings Distinguishing Proteinuria Due to Pregnancy-Induced Hypertension (PIH) and Active Lupus Glomerulonephritis*

| ABNORMALITY | PIH | SLE |
|---|---|---|
| Blood pressure | High | Normal or high |
| Platelets | Low or normal | Low or normal |
| Complement | Elevated or normal | Normal or low |
| Uric acid | High | High or normal |
| Proteinuria | Present | Present |
| Hematuria | Macroscopic, no casts | Microscopic, with casts |
| Anti-DNA antibody | Normal or stable | Rising or high |
| Other SLE symptoms | Absent | Present |

**3. What is the significance of SLE developing during pregnancy?**

Fetal outcome is very poor when SLE develops during pregnancy, with a fetal death rate as high as 45%. In addition, the maternal course is frequently severe if lupus nephritis occurs for the first time during pregnancy.

**4. A patient whose SLE is well controlled on prednisone (5 mg/day), a NSAID, and hydroxychloroquine (400 mg/day) informs you that she is pregnant. What should you recommend regarding the current medications?**

The FDA classifies corticosteroids such as prednisone and methylprednisone, as category B in regards to risks of use during pregnancy. Placental enzymes metabolize 90% of these corticosteroids, and therefore low doses of prednisone (5–10 mg/day) are generally well tolerated during pregnancy and probably are protective against a flare of SLE during pregnancy or postpartum. Cleft lip (< 1–4%) and premature birth may occur with high-dose corticosteroids. NSAIDs have been used widely in pregnancy for preterm labor and have not demonstrated major adverse outcomes, although there are a few reports of premature ductus arteriosus closure, oligohydramnios, respiratory distress syndrome, pulmonary hypertension, and fetal death associated with indomethacin. Although congenital malformations, particularly cleft lip and palate, have been seen in animal studies, there is no evidence to suggest that aspirin, indomethacin, diclofenac, ibuprofen, or sulindac causes human fetal abnormalities. There are insufficient data on the newer NSAIDs to include COX-2 specific NSAIDs.

Low-dose aspirin (80 mg/day) is safe and may be effective prophylaxis for preeclampsia and IUGR. Full-dose aspirin use at the time of delivery is associated with prolonged labor, anemia, and increased maternal blood loss, along with a possible increased risk of neonatal hemorrhage in premature infants (pregnancy category D). Because of these concerns regarding aspirin and other NSAID use late in pregnancy, the First International Conference on Rheumatic Diseases in Pregnancy recommended switching to low doses of prednisone (< 20 mg/d) at least 2 months before delivery for management of most rheumatic complaints occurring during pregnancy.

Hydroxychloroquine and chloroquine are category C drugs. There were numerous reports of increased risk of miscarriages, retinal damage, and ototoxicity with these agents, but recent studies have suggested the risk is relatively low (4.5%) for these complications and the risk may be outweighed by potential benefits in some circumstances.

**5. Can aspirin, NSAIDs, corticosteroids, and antimalarial medications be used during breast-feeding?**

- **Aspirin** in doses greater than one 325-mg tablet results in high infant plasma salicylate levels and should be used cautiously during breast-feeding.
- Two **NSAIDs** (ibuprofen and naproxen) can be used during breast-feeding. Sulindac and indomethacin should be avoided, owing to enterohepatic circulation.
- **Corticosteroids** are excreted in the breast milk at a rate of 10–20% of the maternal dose. Some clinicians recommend that mothers wait at least 4 hours before nursing if the dose is > than 20 mg per day.
- **Antimalarials** (chloroquine/hydroxychloroquine) should be used with caution during breast-feeding, owing to potential accumulation in the infant causing retinal toxicity.

**6. Which disease-modifying antirheumatic drugs (DMARDs) can be considered relatively safe for use during pregnancy and lactation?**

Data on the use of immunosuppressive therapy are limited. Much of the information that is available is derived from anecdotal reports, not prospective studies.

**Sulfasalazine** (FDA category B) has been used safely throughout pregnancy and lactation in the treatment of inflammatory bowel disease. Therefore, although its safety in pregnant patients with rheumatic diseases has not been extensively studied, it is probably safe and can be used with caution during pregnancy and lactation. Folate supplementation is recommended. Sulfasalazine can cause reversible oligospermia, making conception difficult.

**Etanercept, infliximab, anakinra** (all FDA category B) can be used in pregnancy if clearly needed. There are little data available in humans, but etanercept appears safe in pregnant animals. Since they may be secreted in breast milk, women should not nurse while on these medications.

**Gold salts** (FDA category C) have frequently been associated with congenital malformations (10%). Although many healthy offspring have occurred, the data are too limited to recommend it routinely at this time. About 20% of a dose of gold is secreted into breast milk, but this has not been accompanied by any consistent complications in the newborn and therefore is considered to be relatively safe.

**Cyclosporine** (FDA category C) crosses the placenta and has been associated with IUGR and prematurity (40% rate). More serious effects such as teratogenesis have not been seen despite frequent use in pregnant transplant patients. Cyclosporine is secreted into breast milk. Owing to theoretical risks for immune suppression and growth retardation, use during lactation is not recommended.

**Azathioprine** has been used in patients with renal transplants, hematologic malignancies, inflammatory bowel disease, and lupus nephritis during pregnancy. Although placental metabolism may offer some protection to the fetus, various adverse effects to include fetal growth retardation, cytopenias, and opportunistic infections have been identified. Therefore, azathioprine (FDA category D) should be reserved for patients whose rheumatic disease is severe and life threatening (such as lupus nephritis). Close prenatal monitoring and long-term evaluation of the offspring are essential. Azathioprine has been detected in breast milk and therefore is not considered safe for use during breast-feeding. Azathioprine seems to be safe for men who are attempting to father children.

**7. Which drugs must be avoided during pregnancy?**

**Penicillamine** (FDA category D) has been studied most in patients with Wilson's disease and cysteinuria, during which severe adverse effects on the fetus, such as serious connective tissue disorders and neonatal sepsis, have been identified.

**Methotrexate** (FDA category X) is associated with increased spontaneous abortions and birth anomalies. Men and women on methotrexate should discontinue the drug at least 3 months before conception, owing to prolonged retention of methotrexate in tissues after discontinuation. Breast milk appears to be a minor route of excretion of methotrexate, but most physicians would recommend against breast-feeding if a patient is on methotrexate.

**Leflunomide** (FDA category X) is associated with increased fetal death and teratogenesis. Men and women on leflunomide desiring pregnancy should receive the standard protocol with cholestyramine (8 grams TID for 11 days) for drug elimination followed by two separate tests to verify negligible plasma levels. Without this elimination method, leflunomide remains at unsafe levels for up to 2 years.

**Cyclophosphamide** and **chlorambucil** (both FDA category D) are contraindicated during pregnancy because of the high risks of congenital malformation (22%, 33% respectively) if used during the first trimester. Neonatal bone marrow suppression, infection, and hemorrhage are concerns if used later in pregnancy. Cyclophospahmide is secreted into breast milk and has been associated with leukopenia in the offspring and therefore is not recommended for use during lactation. Chlorambucil has not been shown to pass into breast milk, but data are insufficient to recommend its use during lactation.

**8. Are combined oral contraceptives (COCs) safe in patients with SLE?**

The safety of COCs in women with SLE is controversial. Some studies have shown an increase in SLE flares with the use of COCs, while others have not. Most authorities would agree that women with lupus nephritis have an increased risk for SLE flare while taking COCs and women with antiphospholipid antibody syndrome have an increased risk for thromboembolic disease when COCs are prescribed. Other alternatives for contraception should be considered in these instances. In patients with active SLE, all of the potential risks as well as benefits of COCs need to be considered prior to initiating this treatment. **Progestin-only** contraceptive therapy (progestin-only pills, Depo-Provera injectable, and Norplant implant) lacks the risks and benefits of estrogen and therefore are considered safe in women with SLE with antiphospholipid antibodies. Drawbacks unique to these agents include reduction in HDL and lack of osteoporosis prevention. Both of these are frequently already present in women with long-standing SLE. The lower doses of estrogens used as **hormone replacement therapy** in postmenopausal women have not been proven to exacerbate SLE and therefore are recommended as long as there are no contraindication to their use.

**9. Describe the typical clinical presentation of infants with neonatal lupus erythematosus (NLE) and speculate on pathogenesis. What treatment options exist?**

The major clinical manifestations are dermatologic, cardiac, and hepatic. Hemolytic anemia and thrombocytopenia occur less commonly. The skin rash is similar to that of subacute cutaneous lupus erythematosus. Congenital heart block (CHB) is the most common cardiac manifestation and accounts for the major morbidity and mortality of NLE. CHB frequently is usually irreversible and permanent pacemaker therapy is required in about one-half of cases. Mortality in this subset is 20–30% as a result of myocarditis. The conduction defect is due to maternal IgG Anti-Ro (SS-A) or anti-La (SS-B) antibodies that cross the placenta and bind to fetal heart conducting cells, eliciting an inflammatory injury during the second trimester of pregnancy. Clinical manifestations of NLE occur in 5% of offspring of mothers with high circulating levels of these antibodies, with half of these (2.5%) having CHB.

Mothers with antibodies to SSA or SSB should have serial fetal echocardiography, focusing on 16 to 24 weeks' gestation. If complications such as recent onset complete heart block, incomplete heart block, or if signs of myocarditis, congestive heart failure or hydrops are present, treatment should be considered. Although no prospective clinical trials have been performed, treatment with either dexamethasone or plasmapheresis may offer some benefit. Dexamethasone (4 mg/day) is not metabolized substantially by the placenta and therefore crosses into the fetal circulation where it may be effective in treating the CHB. Postnatal treatment with high-dose corticosteroids or immune globulin may prevent progression to complete heart block. No therapy has been proven effective in reversing complete heart block once it is established. The risk of another fetus developing CHB in a mother with anti SS-A antibodies if a previous baby had CHB is 20–25%.

**10. How is the course of rheumatoid arthritis during pregnancy?**

Rheumatoid arthritis (RA) improves during pregnancy, possibly owing to immunomodulating effects of the gravid state. Seventy-five percent of women with RA experience remission during pregnancy, and thus treatment should be minimized to avoid unnecessary fetal exposure to medications. This improvement is unfortunately short-lived, as 90% develop a relapse by 6 months postpartum. This remission recurs with subsequent pregnancies. Rarely RA presents during pregnancy, although up to 10% have initial onset within 6 months postpartum. In patients with long-standing rheumatoid arthritis, joint involvement should be assessed prior to delivery. If the cervical spine is involved, care should be taken to not hyperextend the neck, and vaginal delivery may be precluded by significant hip involvement.

The relationship between RA and pregnancy, along with the female predominance of the disease during reproductive years (4:1), suggests a hormonal influence. Recent data suggest that COCs may protect against developing RA and decrease symptoms in women who have established RA.

**11. Does the presence of RA have an effect on fertility or pregnancy complications?**

Infertility is not increased in RA patients, and there is no significant increase in fetal or maternal complications except for risks associated with its therapy.

**12. How does systemic sclerosis affect fertility and pregnancy complications?**

Scleroderma was once considered to be associated with reduced fertility, but more recent data contradict this. A small percentage of women experience a worsening of their disease during pregnancy. The most feared complication, scleroderma renal crisis, does not appear to be increased during pregnancy. Pregnancy appears to have little overall effect on the course of scleroderma, though Raynaud's symptoms often improve and gastrointestinal reflux and arthralgias often worsen. Fetal complications, such as prematurity and IUGR in patients with scleroderma, are increased slightly, but miscarriage rates are not.

**13. What are some practical considerations for the pregnant scleroderma patient?**

Patients with systemic sclerosis need to be monitored closely for problems arising during pregnancy. Although successful pregnancies are common, the involvement of multiple organ systems by systemic sclerosis can greatly influence the postpartum course and subsequent child care.

*Difficulties of Pregnancy in Systemic Sclerosis*

| ORGAN INVOLVEMENT | DIFFICULTIES |
|---|---|
| Skin | Tight abdominal wall, venous/arterial access, oximetry, problems holding baby |
| Keratoconjuctivitis | Keratitis |
| Microstomia | Difficult oral intubation |
| Nasal telangiectasias | Bleeding |
| Skeletal muscle | Weakness, prolonged motor blockade with regional anesthetic |
| Heart | Cardiac failure |
| Lungs | Dyspnea, pulmonary hypertension |
| Kidneys | Renal failure, hypertension |
| Esophagus | Worsening dysphagia, aspiration risk |
| Small bowel | Malnutrition |
| Large bowel | Constipation, incontinence |

**14. What are the clinical features of the anti-phospholipid antibody (aPLA) syndrome?**

aPLA syndrome is clinically associated with thrombocytopenia, recurrent arterial and/or venous thrombosis, and recurrent fetal wastage. It can occur as a primary disorder (see Chapter 27) or occur in association with SLE or another rheumatic disorder. The syndrome is characterized by the production of autoantibodies against negatively charged phospholipids. These antibodies can be detected by different laboratory assays and may reflect different antibody activity and specificity:

- IgG or IgM anti-β2 glycoprotein I antibodies detected by ELISA
- IgG or IgM anti-cardiolipin antibodies (aCL) detected by ELISA
- Prolonged activated partial thromboplastin time that does not correct with a mixing study with normal plasma (lupus anticoagulant)
- Dilute Russell viper venom time (dRVVT) prolongation (lupus anticoagulant)
- False-positive rapid plasma reagin (RPR)

**15. How does the aPLA syndrome affect pregnancies?**

A recent prospective study found at least one aPLA present in 24% of low-risk patients at the first prenatal visit. However, only the presence of IgG aCL, which was present in 5% of mothers, was significantly associated with fetal loss (fetal loss 28%, RR 3.5). There was no increase in maternal complications, low birth weight, or low Apgar scores in mothers with IgG aCL. Therefore, routine screening in asymptomatic patients is currently not recommended. Primiparas and women with prior liveborns who are found to have aPLA need not be treated prophylactically, but the progress of their pregnancies (fetal growth and activity) should be monitored closely. Slowing of fetal growth or reduction in amniotic fluid volume may be warning signs. Though its prognostic value is less certain, a falling platelet count is taken by some authorities to indicate fetal involvement. In the presence of slow fetal growth or thrombocytopenia not explained by toxemia or SLE, prophylaxis treatment with aspirin (85 mg/day) or subcutaneous heparin (10,000–20,000 units twice daily) is recommended. High-dose (≥ 40 mg/day) prednisone is less beneficial for aPLA syndrome uncomplicated by active SLE and is associated with numerous potential side effects.

**16. A 35-year-old woman in her third trimester complains of unilateral hip pain that began 1 month ago. The pain is constant, dull, and unrelieved by rest or recumbency. Physical examination reveals an antalgic gait with normal range of motion, except for minimal pain with full flexion and internal rotation. The reflexes and sensory and motor examinations are unremarkable. Routine laboratory studies are normal, except for an ESR of 50 mm/hour. How do you proceed with your evaluation, and what is the most likely diagnosis?**

Although the ESR is elevated, this is a normal phenomenon of the third trimester of pregnancy and is not supportive of an infection in the hip. Septic hip arthritis is unlikely in this case because of the chronicity of the pain, presence of full range of motion, and a normal WBC count; arthrocentesis therefore is unnecessary. Plain radiographs with fetal shielding can be performed and would be diagnostic in this case. They probably would reveal marked unilateral osteopenia of the femoral head and acetabulum, indicating the diagnosis of **transient osteoporosis of pregnancy** (TOP).

TOP is a rare condition of unknown etiology that most commonly affects the hips (left more often than right) but can be seen in the knees or shoulders. It is more commonly seen in young women. Protected weight-bearing, rest, and acetaminophen offer some temporary benefit. The pain and osteopenia usually resolve after delivery. Magnetic resonance imaging may be helpful in excluding osteonecrosis of the femoral head, which may have a similar clinical presentation.

## BIBLIOGRAPHY


1. Abu-Shakra M, Shoenfeld Y: Azathioprine therapy for patients with systemic lupus erythematosus. Lupus 10:151–153, 2001.
2. Brucato A, Frassi M, Franceschini F, et al: Congenital heart block risk to newborns of mothers with anti-Ro/SSA antibodies detected by counter immunoelectrophoresis. A prospective study of 100 women. Arthritis Rheum 44:1832–1835, 2001.
3. Buyon J, Kalunian K, Ramsey-Goldman R, et al: Assessing disease activity in SLE patients during pregnancy. Lupus 8:677–684, 1999.
4. Carreira PE, Gutierrez-Larraya F, Gomez-Reino JJ: Successful intrauterine therapy with dexamethasone for fetal myocarditis and heart block in a woman with systemic lupus erythematosus. J Rheumatol 20:1204–1207, 1993.
5. Jansson NM, Genta MS: The effects of immunosuppressive and anti-inflammatory medications on fertility, pregnancy, and lactation. Arch Intern Med 160:610–619, 2000.
6. Lautenbach GL, Petri M: Women's health. Rheum Dis Clin North Am 25:539–565, 1999.
7. Levy RA, Vilela S, Cataldo MJ, et al: Hydroxychloroqine in lupus pregnancy: Double-blind and placebo-controlled study. Lupus 10:401–404, 2001.
8. Lynch A, Silver R, Emlen W: Antiphospholipid antibodies in healthy pregnant women. Rheum Dis Clin North Am 23:555–570, 1997.
9. Ostensen M: Treatment with immunosuppressive and disease modifying drugs during pregnancy and lactation. Am J Reprod Immunol 28:148–152, 1992.
10. Park-Wyllie L, Mazzotta P, Pastuszak A, et al: Birth defects after maternal exposure to corticosteroids. Teratology 62:385–392, 2000.
11. Petri M (ed): Pregnancy and rheumatic disease. Rheum Dis Clin North Am 23:1–28, 1997.
12. Ramsey-Goldman R, Schilling E: Immunosuppressive drug use during pregnancy. Rheum Dis Clin North Am 23:149–167, 1997.
13. Steen VD :Fertility and pregnancy outcome in women with systemic sclerosis Arthritis Rheum 42:763–768, 1999.
14. Tseng CE, Buyon JP: Neonatal lupus syndromes. Rheum Dis Clin North Am 23:31–54, 1997.
15. Waltuck J, Buyon JP: Autoantibody-associated congenital heart block: Outcome in mother and children. Ann Intern Med 120:544–551, 1994.
16. Welsch S, Branch DW: Antiphospholipid syndrome in pregnancy. Rheum Dis Clin North Am 23:71–84, 1997.


# 83. ODDS AND ENDS

*James D. Singleton, M.D.*

**1. Name the periodic syndromes. Why are they grouped together?**

Intermittent hydrarthrosis
Palindromic rheumatism
Familial Mediterranean fever (FMF)
Hyperimmunoglobulin D and periodic fever syndrome

Tietze's syndrome
RS3PE syndrome (see Chapter 19)

These syndromes are grouped together because they share four features: (1) intermittent arthritis followed by periods of remission; (2) complete resolution between attacks; (3) rare development of joint damage; and (4) unknown cause.

**2. Are all disorders with intermittent arthritis encompassed by the periodic syndromes?**

No. Many other disorders may include intermittent joint swelling and other characteristics of the periodic syndromes. Among these are mechanical and inflammatory disorders. Thus, a broad differential should be kept in mind in patients presenting with intermittent arthritis.

| | |
|---|---|
| Periodic syndromes | Spondyloarthropathies |
| Intermittent hydrarthrosis | Reactive arthritis |
| Palindromic rheumatism | Enteropathic arthritis |
| FMF | Infections |
| Crystalline arthropathies | Lyme disease |
| Gout | Whipple's disease |
| CPPD/pseudogout | Mechanical |
| Hydroxyapatite | Loose bodies |
| Sarcoidosis | Meniscal tears |

**3. Describe the typical clinical features of intermittent hydrarthrosis.**

Recurrent joint effusions occur at regular intervals, frequently paralleling menses in females. The knee or another large joint develops an effusion over 12–24 hours, with no or minimal discomfort or signs of inflammation. There are no systemic symptoms, no treatment is proven to prevent or abort attacks, and episodes may occur lifelong.

**4. What do laboratory studies and joint radiographs show in intermittent hydrarthrosis?**

Laboratory tests, including the erythrocyte sedimentation rate (ESR), are normal, even during an attack. Synovial fluid is normal or mildly inflammatory with a slight increase in polymorphonuclear leukocytes. An effusion may be seen on radiographs, but no other abnormalities are seen even after years of attacks.

**5. What is palindromic rheumatism? What does it mean?**

Palindromic rheumatism is a recurrent syndrome of acute arthritis and periarthritis. *Palindromic* means "recurring" and is derived from a Greek word which literally means "to run back." The term *palindromic* was introduced by Hench and Rosenberg in 1944 as descriptive of the syndrome. They preferred *rheumatism* to *arthritis* due to the frequent involvement of periarticular structures and occasional presence of subcutaneous nodules.

**6. How do the clinical features of palindromic rheumatism (PR) differ from those of intermittent hydrarthrosis?**

PR, like intermittent hydrarthrosis, affects both men and women, often begins in the third to fifth decade, and frequently affects the knees. Constitutional symptoms are uncommon in PR. However, attacks occur irregularly and may involve more than one joint (usually 2–5). The pattern of joint attacks tends to be characteristic in an individual patient. Symptoms may begin in one joint while waning in another. Attacks are sudden and pain may be intense, often reaching a peak within a few hours. Signs of joint inflammation (swelling, warmth, redness) can be noted soon after pain begins. Small joints of the hands and feet may be affected, and occasionally also the spine and temporomandibular joints. Also, unlike intermittent hydrarthrosis, periarticular attacks (occurring in one-third) and transient subcutaneous nodules may be seen.

**7. What do laboratory studies and joint radiographs show in PR?**

The ESR and other acute-phase reactants may be elevated during attacks but are normal between them. Rheumatoid factor (RF) and antinuclear antibodies (ANA) are typically negative;

positive results usually predict that the patient will progress to a connective tissue disease such as rheumatoid arthritis (RA). Serum complement levels are normal. There have been few studies of synovial fluid in PR. Leukocytes may vary from a few hundred to several thousand, with the magnitude poorly correlated with symptom severity. Radiographs show only soft-tissue swelling.

**8. How is PR treated?**

Nonsteroidal anti-inflammatory drugs (NSAIDs) may provide some relief from joint symptoms but do not reliably prevent attacks. A variety of other agents have been used; injectable gold salts are reported as the most consistently successful. Good clinical responses have also been reported with antimalarial agents, colchicine, sulfasalazine, and methotrexate.

**9. Describe the course of PR.**

Although the course is variable, fewer than 10% of patients experience a spontaneous remission. Some patients continue to have the disease for many years. However, 30–50% evolve into a chronic inflammatory arthritis, usually rheumatoid arthritis. Less commonly, a diagnosis of systemic lupus erythematosus (SLE) or other connective tissue disease is eventually made. Antimalarials have been reported to reduce the risk of subsequent development of RA or other connective tissue disease.

**10. What features are predictive of a patient with PR later developing RA?**

The presence of serum RF, persistent rheumatoid nodules, and HLA-DR4 positivity increase the likelihood of evolution to RA. Other factors that may be predictive are early involvement of the wrist and proximal interphalangeal (PIP) joints.

**11. What is familial Mediterranean fever (FMF)?**

FMF is an autosomal recessively inherited disorder (MEFV gene on chromosome 16 encoding the pyrin/marenostrin protein) characterized by irregular attacks, lasting 1–3 days, of fever and one or more inflammatory manifestations. FMF usually has its onset in childhood and is seen primarily in ethnic groups of east Mediterranean origin. Men seem to be affected more commonly than women. Amyloidosis is prevalent in certain ethnic groups with FMF and may be the sole phenotypic expression of the disease. Before the use of colchicine, amyloidosis was the cause of death in 99% of > 500 patients in one study; 90% of these deaths occurred before age 40.

**12. What are the clinical features of FMF?**

| | |
|---|---|
| Fever | 100% |
| Peritonitis | 85–97% |
| Arthritis | 50–77% |
| Pleuritis | 33–66% |
| Erysipelas-like rash | 46% |
| Lymphadenopathy | 1–6% |

Aseptic meningitis has been stressed as a clinical manifestation of FMF. Splenomegaly (33%) is believed to be due largely to amyloidosis. Rash is primarily on the lower extremities and histologically has a dermal neutrophilic infiltrate.

**13. Describe the arthritis of FMF.**

Intermittent monoarticular attacks of the knee or other large joint are most typical. Polyarthritis occurs in 20%. Arthritic episodes may be prolonged, lasting weeks or months in about 8% of patients, and subsequent attacks tend to follow the established pattern. Localized pain, exquisite tenderness, and joint dysfunction out of proportion to the degree of swelling should suggest the diagnosis of FMF. Joint erythema and warmth are notably absent.

**14. How is the arthritis of FMF treated?**

Recovery of joint function between attacks is the rule, and joint destruction is rare. However, in prolonged episodes involving the hip, functional recovery is less likely, and joint damage requiring surgical therapy may be needed. Temporary relief of joint pain may be achieved with analgesic therapy, but due to the recurrent nature of FMF, narcotics should be avoided. Glucocorticoids are ineffective, a feature that may assist in the differential diagnosis. Physical therapy is used to avoid muscle atrophy due to disuse.

**15. What hereditary periodic fevers have been defined other than FMF?**

Hereditary periodic fevers consist of a group of rare disorders characterized by intermittent self-limited inflammatory episodes with fever, synovitis/serosal inflammation, skin rashes, and conjunctivitis:

- Tumor necrosis factor (TNF) receptor-associated periodic syndromes (TRAPS, formerly called familial Hibernian fever), are autosomal dominant and due to abnormalities of the gene on chromosome 12 that encodes the TNF receptor 1 (p55). Both missense mutations in the extracellular domains of TNFRI and a defect in shedding this receptor from cell membrane have been described. This results in decreased soluble receptors to bind soluble TNFα and lymphotoxin. Therefore, more TNFα is available to bind to receptors on cell membranes, leading to inflammatory response. Clinically, patients can be identified by diffuse rash with mononuclear perivascular infiltrate, periorbital edema, and attacks lasting 7–21 days. Amyloidosis rarely occurs. Treatment is with anti-TNFα biologics; colchicine does not work.
- Hyperimmunoglobulin D syndrome (HIDS) is autosomal dominant and characterized by high serum IgD levels associated with attacks, lasting 3–7 days, of fever and abdominal pain starting in childhood. The rash can be polymorphic and is primarily on extremities. Cervical lymphadenopathy can be seen; amyloidosis is rare. Mutations have been found in the gene on chromosome 12 that encodes mevalonate kinase, an enzyme involved in metabolizing mevalonate (a cholesterol pathway intermediate). How this leads to inflammation is unknown.
- Other autosomal dominant recurrent fevers whose genetic defect remains undefined include Muckle-Wells syndrome, familial cold urticaria, and autosomal dominant cyclic hematopoiesis (cyclic neutropenia) as well as TRAPS-like syndrome without TNFRI defect.

**16. How does Tietze's syndrome differ from costochondritis?**

Tietze's syndrome is a syndrome of pain, tenderness, and swelling of joints of the chest wall, usually the costochondral joints. Costochondritis is a much more common syndrome characterized by costochondral joint pain and tenderness without objective signs of inflammation. Tietze's syndrome is more common in women, usually (80%) involves a single joint, and is rarely bilateral. Polyarticular disease affects neighboring articulations on the same side of the sternum.

**17. Define foreign-body synovitis.**

It is the inflammatory reaction of synovium (from joint, bursa, or tendon sheath) due to the introduction of a foreign material. Most commonly, it results from a traumatic event, but it may also follow surgical introduction of foreign material.

**18. Name the foreign bodies most commonly associated with foreign-body synovitis.**

Plant thorns, wood splinters, and sea urchin spines are the most common. Other recognized materials include fish bones, chitin fragments, stones, gravel, brick fragments, lead, glass, fiberglass, plastic, and rubber. Surgically implanted materials include metallic fragments, cement (methylmethacrylate), and silicone.

**19. Name five activities that are risk factors for foreign-body synovitis.**

Professional fishing, professional diving, marine recreational activities, farming, and gardening.

**20. Describe the clinical, laboratory, and radiographic features of foreign-body synovitis.**

The joints of the hands and knees are most commonly affected. There is sudden onset of pain at the site of injury, but it may be forgotten by the patient or overlooked by the physician. The patient may be seen with acute synovitis several days after the injury, ranging from months to years later, with chronic synovitis (particularly of the knee). The ESR is usually normal, and synovial fluid is inflammatory with a predominance of neutrophils. Radiographs may show soft-tissue swelling only and can be useful to detect radiodense particles (metal, fish bones, sea urchin spines) but not wood, plastic, or plant thorns. Chronic changes of periarticular osteoporosis, osteolysis, osteosclerosis, and periosteal new bone formation can mimic osteomyelitis or bone tumors.

**21. How is foreign-body synovitis diagnosed and treated?**

In the approximately two-third of patients with foreign-body synovitis due to exogenous particles who develop a chronic or relapsing course, diagnosis and treatment usually necessitate excisional biopsy with synovectomy. Ultrasound, CT, and MRI may be helpful in detecting particles that are small or radiolucent with conventional radiography. Bacteriologic studies (including mycobacterial studies) and histopathologic examination of tissue are essential. Polarized microscopy is useful in detecting birefringent fragments of plant origin, sea urchin spines, and polymethylmethacrylate.

**22. Multicentric reticulohistiocytosis (MRH) is a rare disease affecting the skin and joints. Describe its cutaneous features.**

Firm papulonodules, reddish-brown or yellow, occur most commonly on the face, hands, ears, arms, scalp, neck, and chest. These nodules may wax and wane and even disappear completely. A classic finding is "coral beads" around the nailbeds. In two-thirds of patients, the nodular skin eruption follows the onset of arthritis by months to years.

**23. How does the arthritis of MRH resemble that of RA? How does it differ?**

Like RA, the arthritis of MRH is inflammatory, usually chronic, symmetric, and polyarticular; it affects the joints of the hands and cervical spine; and it is destructive. Women are affected more frequently than men, and the onset is usually in middle age. However, unlike in RA, distal interphalangeal joint synovitis and destruction may be prominent, and severely deforming arthritis mutilans occurs in one-half of patients. Glucocorticoid therapy has little, if any, effect on the arthritis. Also in contrast to the case with RA, radiographs in MRH feature well-circumscribed erosions, widened joint spaces, and absent or disproportionately mild periarticular osteopenia for the degree of erosive change.

**24. Several disorders have been associated with MRH. Name them.**

- Tuberculin skin test positivity is seen in about 50%, but only two patients have been reported to have active tuberculosis.
- Xanthelasma occurs in one-third of patients.
- Malignant disease of various types has been reported in approximately 25%.

The cancer may precede, be concurrent with, or follow the development of MRH. Treatment of the malignancy has led to improvement of the MRH in some.

**25. What are the typical histologic findings of MRH on biopsy of skin or synovium?**

The characteristic finding is aggregates of multinucleated giant cells and histiocytes having a granular, ground-glass appearance. This ground-glass cytoplasm contains a periodic acid-Schiff-reactive material thought to be due to a mucoprotein or glycoprotein. This cellular tissue reaction has prompted the idea that MRH represents a histiocytic granulomatous reaction to an as yet unidentified stimulus. Fat stains, such as Sudan black, are also positive. MRH was once thought to represent a lipid storage disease, but no consistent abnormalities of lipids, serum or intracellular, have been discovered.

**26. How is MRH treated?**

No treatment has consistently shown benefit, and the rarity of the disease precludes a good prospective study. In patients with mild disease, symptomatic therapy with NSAIDs or nonnarcotic analgesics should be tried. Unfortunately, the arthritis in 40–50% of patients progresses to an arthritis mutilans. Cytotoxic therapy (cyclophosphamide, chlorambucil) has been reported to achieve partial and complete remissions. Topical nitrogen mustard therapy led to marked improvement in skin lesions in one patient.

**27. What is erythromelalgia?**

Erythromelalgia, primary erythermalgia, and secondary erythermalgia are three clinically similar syndromes with dissimilar etiologies and treatment. These syndromes are characterized by red, warm, swollen, and painful extremities. Erythromelalgia is associated with polycythemia vera and other chronic myeloproliferative disorders which may not manifest for months to years after the onset of cutaneous symptoms. Erythromelalgia is diagnosed on the basis of platelet counts exceeding 400,000, relief of symptoms lasting for days with low-dose aspirin, and histopathologic evidence of arterioles with fibromuscular proliferation. The symptoms may be asymmetric and can progress to gangrene. Primary erythermalgia is an autosomal dominant disease with onset by puberty. It is characterized by painful attacks of red, warm, swollen, bilateral hands and/or feet. Elevation and cold exposure give relief. There is no therapy. Secondary erythermalgia is similar to primary erythermalgia but typically has its onset during adulthood and is associated with various diseases or medications (calcium channel blockers). Treatment of the underlying disease or withdrawal of the offending medication is helpful. Neither primary nor secondary erythermalgia respond to aspirin.

**28. What is dystrophic calcification? What connective tissue diseases are associated with it?**

When calcification occurs in cutaneous tissues, it is called calcinosis cutis and can be divided into four categories: dystrophic, metastatic (high calcium x phosphorous product), idiopathic (tumoral calcinosis), and iatrogenic. Dystrophic calcification is the most common type and is secondary to nonmetabolic diseases like connective tissue diseases or to deposition of calcium salts in damaged tissue. The calcium is deposited either as numerous large masses (calcinosis universalis) or a few small, localized masses (calcinosis circumscripta). Dystrophic calcifications are most commonly associated with systemic sclerosis, dermatomyositis, SLE, pseudoxanthoma elasticum, panniculitis, and trauma.

**29. Described the histologic classification of the panniculitides and the most common connective tissue diseases associated with each.**

- Septal panniculitis: erythema nodosum
- Lobular panniculitis: Weber-Christian syndrome (relapsing febrile nodular nonsuppurative panniculitis), enzymatic panniculitis due to pancreatic enzymes or $alpha_1$-antitrypsin deficiency, and connective tissue panniculitis
- Mixed panniculitis: lupus profundus

**30. Discuss the musculoskeletal complications of cystic fibrosis.**

Cystic fibrosis (CF) is an autosomal recessive disease characterized by decreased mucous production leading to obstructive lung disease and malabsorption. Other organs, including sinuses, pancreas, liver, sweat glands, and reproductive tract, can be affected. It is due to a defect in the CF gene on chromosome 7, which encodes for a membrane glycoprotein (CFTR) that is a chloride ion channel. In cystic fibrosis, one of the chloride ion channels present on the apical membrane of the epithelial cell is either absent or defective. This leads to increased sodium absorption and decreased chloride secretion resulting in decreased extracellular water content. Patients get obstruction with infections in the lung and malabsorption from the gut. Due to this, patients are susceptible to osteoporosis due to poor calcium and vitamin D absorption. Additionally, 5–45% of patients get an episodic nondestructive oligoarthritis most commonly involving the fingers and lower extremity joints. The arthritis is felt to be due to immune complexes due to chronic lung infection. Attacks last for a few days and may be associated with fever and erythema nodosum. Rarely, a chronic erosive oligoarthritis, hypertrophic osteoarthropathy, and small vessel vasculitis can occur.

**31. What rheumatic and autoimmune syndromes are associated with the following medications?**

- Fluoroquinolones: Achilles tendinitis and rupture
- Minocycline: drug-induced lupus, autoimmune hepatitis, pANCA positivity
- Statins: myopathy
- Rifabutin: drug-induced lupus
- Zafirlukast: Churg-Strauss syndrome
- Interferon α: thyroiditis

**32. Describe the rheumatic disorders that may develop after hepatitis B vaccination.**

Various immunizations have been associated with causing demyelinating syndromes, reactive arthritis, and small vessel vasculitis. Recombinant hepatitis B vaccination has been associated with a higher than expected number of rheumatic disorders including vasculitis (especially central retinal vein occlusion), rheumatoid arthritis, SLE, reactive arthritis, as well as various demyelination syndromes. These rheumatic disorders occur within 1–2 months of the first, second, or third vaccination. Unlike other typical side effects of an immunization, these rheumatic disorders may not resolve.

**33. What are the genetic or immune defects in Canale-Smith and stiff-person syndromes?**

**Canale-Smith syndrome** (autoimmune lymphoproliferative syndrome [ALPS]): a rare autosomal dominant disorder presenting in the first two years of life and characterized by generalized lymphadenopathy (without fever), hepatosplenomegaly, and autoimmune hemolytic anemia and thrombocytopenia. Patients are diagnosed by increased numbers (≥ 5%) of circulating double-negative T cells (CD3+, CD4–, CD8–). Patients have mutations in the Fas gene (TNFRSF6), leading to abnormalities in the intracellular "death domain" of the Fas receptor (APO-1, CD95). This leads to the inability of the T cell to be signaled to undergo programmed cell death (apoptosis). Consequently, autoreactive T cells will down-regulate CD4 and CD8 molecules but cannot be disposed of by Fas-mediated apoptosis (similar to *lpr* mice), leading to autoimmune disease. Patients without Fas gene mutations have been found to have mutations in the Fas ligand gene (similar to *gld* mice) or enzymes involved in apoptosis (caspase 10). Corticosteroid therapy has variable effects and patients develop neoplasms in early adulthood.

**Stiff-person syndrome**—a disorder characterized by muscle rigidity and episodic muscle spasms, primarily involving the trunk. Episodes can be prolonged, painful, and precipitated by loud noises. There are three types. The most common (65%) type is associated with antibodies against glutamic acid decarboxylase (GAD65) and frequently with autoimmune diseases (e.g., type I diabetes mellitus, Graves' disease, hypothyroidism, pernicious anemia) due to its high association with HLA DQ-0201. It is postulated that the anti-GAD antibodies inhibit the enzymes in the CNS responsible for production of GABA, which is an inhibitory neurotransmitter. Consequently, neural transmission is unopposed and can lead to muscle rigidity. This type of stiff-person syndrome is treated with diazepam, immunosuppressives, and intravenous gammaglobulin. The other two types of stiff-person syndrome are not associated with anti-GAD antibodies or a certain HLA phenotype. One type (5%) is a paraneoplastic manifestation of cancers (lymphoma, breast, lung, colon), whereas the other type (35% of cases) is idiopathic. These two types do not respond to immune modulating therapies and are treated with high doses of muscle relaxants such as diazepam or baclofen.

**34. A patient presents with hemoptysis. He has a prior history of a deep venous thrombosis. Work-up of the hemoptysis reveals a pulmonary artery aneurysm. What does this patient have?**

Hughes-Stovin syndrome is a rare condition characterized by multiple pulmonary aneurysms and peripheral venous thrombosis. Patients typically have recurrent fever, chills, hemoptysis, and cough. Patients usually die of fulminant hemoptysis. The etiology is unknown but in some cases it is felt to be a forme fruste of Behçet's syndrome which is another syndrome associated with pulmonary aneurysm and venous clots. Pathologic tissue shows perivascular infiltrates of the vasa vasorum leading to loss of elastic tissue in the pulmonary vessels. The treatment is immunosuppression, arterial embolization, and/or surgical resection.

## BIBLIOGRAPHY

1. Hench PS, Rosenberg EF: Palindromic rheumatism. Arch Intern Med 73:293–321, 1944.
2. Gonzales-Lopez L, Gamez-Nava JI, Jhangri GS, et al: Prognostic factors for the development of rheumatoid arthritis and other connective tissue diseases in patients with palindromic rheumatism. J Rheumatol 26:540–545, 1999.
3. Maricic MJ: Foreign body synovitis. In Klippel JH (ed): Primer on the Rheumatic Diseases, 11th ed. Atlanta, Arthritis Foundation, 1997, pp 391–392.
4. Gorman JD, Danning C, Schumacher HR, et al: Multicentric reticulohistiocytosis: Case report with immunohistochemical analysis and literature review. Arthritis Rheum 43:930–938, 2000.
5. Ben-Chetrit E, Levy M: Familial Mediterranean fever. Lancet 351:659, 1998.
6. Drenth JPH, van der Meer JWM: Hereditary periodic fever. N Engl J Med 345:1748–1757, 2001.
7. Cohen J: Erythromelalgia: New theories and new therapies. J Am Acad Dermatol 43:841–847, 2000.
8. Johnson S, Knox AJ: Arthropathy in cystic fibrosis. Respir Med 88:567–570, 1994.
9. Van der Linden PD, et al: Tendon disorders attributed to fluoroquinolones: A study on 42 spontaneous reports in the period 1988–1998. Arthritis Care Res 45:235–239, 2001.
10. Drappa J, Vaishnaw AK, Sullivan KE, et al: Fas gene mutations in the Canale-Smith syndrome, an inherited lymphoproliferative disorder associated with autoimmunity. N Engl J Med 335:1643–1649, 1996.
11. Helfgott SM: Stiff-man syndrome: From bedside to the bench. Arthritis Rheum 42:1312–1320, 1999.
12. Herb S, Hetzel M, Hetzel J, et al: An unusual case of Hughes-Stovin syndrome. Eur Respir J 11:1191–1193, 1998.

# *XV. Management of the Rheumatic Diseases*

*As to diseases, make a habit of two things—to help, or at least to do no harm.*
Hippocrates (c460–377 BC)

# 84. NONSTEROIDAL ANTI-INFLAMMATORY DRUGS (NSAIDs)

David H. Collier, M.D.

*No drug is as good as the day it is first thought of.*
Sir William Osler

**1. Describe the general properties of the NSAIDs.**

The NSAIDs are weak organic acids that bind avidly to serum proteins (mainly albumin). The vast majority have ionization constants (*pKa*) ranging from 3–5, meaning that in the acidic environment of the stomach, NSAIDs are un-ionized, which can, with some NSAIDs, lead to local mucosal damage. Beneficially, acidic NSAIDs may become sequestered preferentially in inflamed joints, giving the NSAID a longer synovial half-life than plasma half-life. NSAIDs generally have anti-inflammatory properties, probably by inhibiting prostaglandin production but also by a number of other mechanisms.

**2. When were NSAIDs first used?**

Salicylates have probably been used for centuries. Hippocrates, Celsus, Galen, and many medieval herbalists recorded the use of willow bark and other plants known to contain salicylates to treat fever and pain. In more recent history:

1826—Salicylin, the active principle of salicylates, isolated from willow bark.
1838—Salicylic acid derived from salicylin.
1853—Acetylsalicylate (**aspirin**) first synthesized.
1899—Aspirin introduced in the United States (Bayer Company).
1949—Phenylbutazone, the first alternative to salicylates, introduced.
1965—Indomethacin introduced.
1970s and 1980s—Proliferation of NSAIDs.
1990s—Introduction of the specific cyclooxygenase-2 inhibitors.

Although it was first synthesized in 1853, aspirin was not used until late in the 19th century, when Felix Hoffman of the Bayer Company gave it to his arthritic father and it helped his arthritis. (This was essentially stage 1, 2, and 3 testing of this drug, which for new drugs today takes many millions of dollars and an average of 10 years.) Since the 1960s, a proliferation of NSAIDs has occurred. In some countries, there is a selection of up to 40 NSAIDs from which to choose.

**3. How often are NSAIDs used?**

It is estimated that > 100 million prescriptions for non-salicylate NSAIDs, costing > $1.7 billion in annual costs, were dispensed in the United States. One in seven Americans use NSAIDs. In the US, there are 17 million regular users, 50% over the age of 60.

**4. What are the beneficial effects of NSAIDs?**

**Analgesia**—These drugs are as analgesic as narcotics (in therapeutic doses) in acute pain.
**Antipyresis**—NSAIDs inhibit prostaglandins in the CNS, which reduces fever.

**Anti-inflammatory**—These effects are achieved by a number of mechanisms.

**Antiplatelet**—Most NSAIDs decrease platelet aggregation by preventing thromboxane $A_2$ production, which is important in activating platelets, and thus preventing the first step in coagulation.

**5. What is the structural classification of NSAIDs?**

Salicylates
- Acetylated—aspirin
- Nonacetylated—sodium salicylate, choline salicylate, magnesium salicylate, salsalate, salicylamide, diflunisal

Acetic acids
- Indole derivatives—indomethacin, tolmetin, sulindac
- Phenylacetic acid—diclofenac
- Pyranocarboxylic acid—etodolac

Propionic acids—ibuprofen, naproxen, fenoprofen, ketoprofen, flurbiprofen, oxaprozin

Fenamic acids—mefenamic acid, meclofenamic acid

Enolic acids
- Oxicams—piroxicam, meloxicam
- Pyrazolones—phenylbutazone

Pyrrolo-pyrrole—ketorolac

Nonacidic compounds
- Naphthylalkanone-nabumetone

Diaryl substituted pyrazole—celecoxib, rofecoxib, valdecoxib, paracoxib (injectable prodrug of valdecoxib)

**6. Why should you know the structural classification of the NSAIDs?**

The drugs in each class tend to have similar **side effects**. For example, the pyrazolones that were available in the United States at one time included oxyphenbutazone and phenylbutazone. Because of idiosyncratic aplastic anemia, oxyphenbutazone was taken off the market, and phenylbutazone was discontinued by its major manufacturer. The salicylates tend to have tinnitus as a consistent side effect. The propionic acid derivatives are generally a very safe group of drugs, and three of them are now available over-the-counter: ibuprofen, naproxen sodium, and ketoprofen. The diaryl substituted pyrazoles are all thought to be very safe for the stomach.

The second, and controversial, reason to know the structural classifications might be to select alternative treatments. If a drug in one classification is ineffective, you might try a different structural compound instead of repeatedly using drugs from one structural group.

**7. What is thought to be the major mechanism of action of the NSAIDs, and what advancement was made in the 1990s in our understanding of this mechanism?**

The major mechanism of action is thought to be the inhibition of cyclooxygenase, causing a decrease in prostaglandin production. We now realize there are two isoforms of cyclooxygenase—cylooxygenase-1 (COX-1) and cyclooxygenase-2 (COX-2). They both are 70-kd molecular weight, have similar but slightly different active sites, have 60% C-DNA homology, and are on different genes. COX-1 is on chromosome 9, lacks a TATA box and upstream transcriptional start sites, suggesting its role in producing a continuously transcribed stable message or "housekeeping gene." The COX-1 gene is constitutively made in the stomach, intestine, kidney, and platelet. COX-2 is on chromosome 1, contains a TATA box and bases upstream of the transcriptional start site that are a complex array of important transcriptional elements. These include binding sites for nuclear factor Kappa B, SP-1, GRE, PEA-3, AP2, nuclear factor IL-6, Ebox, and cAMP response elements. COX-2 is thought to be an inducible form involved in inflammation but is also found constitutively in the kidney and brain. It is this understanding of the different roles of COX-1 and COX-2 that led to the development of specific COX-2 inhibitors. The hope was that analgesic and anti-inflammatory NSAIDs could be made with little or no side effects.

**8. What are other mechanisms of action of the NSAIDs?**

Other mechanisms have been defined for various specific NSAIDs, including:
Inhibitory effects on lipoxygenase products (sulindac, meclofenamate, diclofenac)
Inhibition of superoxide formation (indomethacin, piroxicam)
Inhibition of neutrophil aggregation, adhesion, and enzyme release (salicylates, indomethacin)
Depression of lymphocyte transformation (salicylates)
Inhibition of rheumatoid factor production (piroxicam)
Inhibition of acidic and neutral degradative enzymes
Inhibition of cytokine production by inhibiting nuclear factor kappa B (salicylates)
Suppression of proteoglycan production in cartilage (salicylates, piroxicam, ibuprofen, fenoprofen, tolmetin)

**9. With our understanding of COX-1 and COX-2, how are NSAIDs mechanistically classified?**

They are classified by their ability to inhibit COX-1 and/or COX-2 in therapeutic doses. A classification system was described by a study group in the US and by another in Europe. This classification is:

| AMERICAN NOMENCLATURE | EUROPEAN NOMENCLATURE | NSAIDS IN THIS CLASSIFICATION |
|---|---|---|
| COX-1 specific | COX-1 selective | Low dose aspirin (binds to serine 530 on COX-1) |
| COX nonspecific | COX nonselective | Ibuprofen, naproxen, meclomen, indomethacin |
| COX-2 preferential | COX-2 selective | Etodolac, diclofenac, nabumetone, meloxicam |
| COX-2 specific | COX-2 highly selective | Celecoxib, rofecoxib, valdecoxib |

**10. What factors affect the choice of NSAIDs?**

| **Properties of the drug** | **Properties of the patient** |
|---|---|
| Efficacy | Individual variation |
| Tolerance | Disease being treated |
| Safety | Age |
| Convenience of dosage | Other diseases |
| Formulation | Other drugs |
| Cost | |

**11. What have efficacy studies of NSAIDs found?**

The effects of most NSAIDs are compared with aspirin and, more recently, naproxen, ibuprofen, diclofenac, and others. In general, there are no important differences among the various NSAIDs, although there are clear individual variations in response. The COX-2 inhibitors are similar in efficacy to the traditional NSAIDs. In certain arthritic diseases, one structural group of NSAIDs may be tried initially over another. For example, in gout and the seronegative spondyloarthropathies, indomethacin or tolmetin is usually the initial drug of choice. There is no clear relationship between the amount of cyclooxygenase inhibition and activity in arthritis. Although the pharmacodynamics of the drug are important in a given individual, there is no good correlation between the plasma level of the drug and efficacy except for salicylates.

**12. Who is at risk for a hypersensitivity reaction to NSAIDs?**

The patient most at risk is a severe asthmatic with nasal polyps; up to 78% may react to aspirin. Patients with nasal polyps, asthma, or chronic urticaria are also mildly at risk to react to NSAIDs usually with acute bronchospasm and shortness of breath. It is important to note that this is a sensitivity and not an allergy, because it is not IgE-mediated.

Two theories have been proposed to explain aspirin/NSAID-sensitive asthma. One suggests that asthma is caused by cyclooxygenase inhibition resulting in decreased production of prostaglandin $E_2$ which is important in maintaining bronchodilation in these patients. A second theory proposed that this type of asthma is a consequence of the 5-fold increased bronchial expression of leukotriene C4 synthetase. Thus, when aspirin or NSAIDs block cyclooxygenase, the arachidonic acid precursors are shunted down the leukotriene pathway resulting in excessive production of leukotrienes C, D, E (slow reacting substance of anaphylaxis). These theories are supported by: (1) salsalate does not inhibit cyclooxygenase and does not cause asthma attacks and so is the NSAID of choice for aspirin-sensitive asthma patients, (2) leukotriene inhibitors block bronchospasm provoked by NSAIDs in aspirin-sensitive patients, and (3) NSAID-induced asthma attacks are acute in onset, severe and prolonged, and can be resistant to glucocorticoids.

The selective COX-2 inhibitors have the same warning in their package inserts for this effect. However, two studies of aspirin-sensitive patients given rofecoxib did not demonstrate a hypersensitivity reaction, implying that the hypersensitivity reaction is a COX-1 effect, and rofecoxib can be used in these patients (**Controversial**).

**13. Discuss the hepatotoxicity of the NSAIDs.**

The clearance of NSAIDs is predominantly by hepatic metabolism, with the production of inactive metabolites that are excreted in urine. An elevation of liver enzymes, especially the aminotransferases (AST and ALT), can occur with all NSAIDs to some extent. This was first noticed with the use of aspirin in patients with systemic lupus erythematosus and juvenile rheumatoid arthritis. **Idiosyncratic severe hepatitis** has been reported with indomethacin, diclofenac, sulindac, and phenylbutazone. **Fatal hepatotoxicity** in children using indomethacin has been noted, prompting the recommendation that children under age 11 should not be given indomethacin for arthritis. **Cholestasis** has also been described. The NSAID-induced hepatotoxicity is usually evident during the first 6 months of use. Liver function studies should be obtained during the first month of use and every 3-6 months thereafter.

**14. Which NSAIDs are inactive drugs that must be metabolized by the liver to become the active metabolite?**

**Sulindac** and **nabumetone** are prodrugs. Sulindac is reversibly metabolized to sulindac sulfide, a potent cyclooxygenase inhibitor, and then converted back to the parent compound in the gut and kidney. Sulindac and its metabolites undergo extensive enterohepatic recirculation, which contributes to its long half-life of 16–18 hours. Nabumetone is non-acidic and is a poor inhibitor of prostaglandin production. It is metabolized to 6-methoxy-2-naphthylacetic acid, which is a potent inhibitor of prostaglandin synthesis. Nabumetone is hepatically, not renally, cleared and does not undergo enterohepatic circulation.

**15. What are the gastrointestinal (GI) side effects of NSAIDs?**

Dyspepsia, indigestion, and vomiting
Gastroesophageal reflux
Gastric erosions
Peptic ulcers
Gastrointestinal hemorrhage and perforation
Small and large bowel ulceration
Small bowel webs
Colonic diverticuli perforation
Diarrhea (especially with meclofenamate)

Although NSAIDs commonly cause GI symptoms, about one-half of all patients who develop significant peptic ulcers do not develop symptoms.

**16. How common are NSAID-induced gastritis and peptic ulcers?**

Gastritis and peptic ulcers are among the most common side effects of these drugs. NSAID injury to the GI tract is responsible for an estimated 103,000 hospitalizations and 16,500 deaths annually in the United States. Approximately 2% of patients treated with NSAIDs develop clinically significant, chronic peptic ulceration. Meta-analysis of pooled data suggests a threefold-increased risk of adverse GI events among NSAID users as compared with nonusers. The most common area for NSAID-induced ulcers to develop is the stomach, usually the antrum. Unfortunately, routine stool guaiac testing for blood is insensitive in detecting these lesions. The medical costs of GI complications from NSAIDs have been estimated to be $3.9 billion per year.

**17. Who is at risk for NSAID-induced gastroduodenal ulcer disease?**

Elderly people (> 60 yrs old)
History of peptic ulcer disease, with or without NSAIDs
Higher dosage of NSAIDs
Previous use of antacids, $H_2$-blockers, or proton pump inhibitors for GI symptoms
Chronic disease status such as RA, COPD, coronary artery disease
History of abdominal pain of unclear etiology, with or without NSAIDs
Anticoagulant therapy
Concomitant corticosteroid use (≥ prednisone 10 mg/d)
Tobacco use
Alcohol use
**Controversial**—Existing infection with *Helicobacter pylori*

**18. How do prostaglandins protect the gastric mucosa? What are the effects of NSAIDs on the stomach?**

**Prostaglandin $E_1$ and $E_2$ effect on gastric mucosa**

- Induce protective superficial mucous barrier
- Induce bicarbonate output
- Increase mucosal blood flow in the superficial gastric cell layer
- Inhibit gastric acid synthesis

**Effects of NSAIDs on the stomach**

- Decrease mucous secretion
- Decrease bicarbonate synthesis
- Decrease mucosal blood flow
- Increase gastric acid secretion
- Decrease glutathione synthesis, thus decreasing superoxide scavenging

**19. How can you decrease the incidence of NSAID-induced gastric and duodenal ulcers in high-risk individuals?**

1. When appropriate, use alternative analgesics.
2. Use the lowest dose of NSAID possible.
3. If NSAIDs are required, choose a COX-2 selective inhibitor. The COX-2 inhibitors, celecoxib and rofecoxib, have been shown in large multicenter studies to have less bleeds, perforations, or obstructions than traditional NSAIDs. The newest COX-2 inhibitor, valdecoxib, has also been shown to cause fewer ulcers than traditional NSAIDs.
4. If treating a high-risk patient, consider using misoprostol (a prostaglandin $E_1$ analog) that protects the gut from NSAID-induced ulcers and gastritis.
5. The preponderance of evidence is that the proton pump inhibitors, such as omeprazole, esomeprazole, rabeprazole, lansoprazole, and pantoprazole are protective of the ulcer inducing effect of NSAIDs.
6. It remains controversial whether the $H_2$ blockers (such as cimetidine, ranitidine, famotidine, and nizatidine), sucralfate, and antacids are protective of NSAID-induced ulcers. At this time, it is not recommended to use the $H_2$ blockers, sucralfate, or antacids to protect the gut, although they may help reduce NSAID-induced gastrointestinal discomfort.

**20. How nephrotoxic are the NSAIDs?**

Prostaglandins have relatively little effect on the normal kidney in the euvolemic person. However, in renal insufficiency or hypovolemic states, prostaglandins are important in maintaining adequate glomerular flow and pressure. Thus, prostaglandins can vasodilate renal arteries, increase sodium loss, and increase renin release. Nephrotoxic effects of NSAIDs include:

- Vasoconstriction decreasing glomerular filtration rate and increasing creatinine
- Increased sodium retention and blood volume (this can be important in patients with borderline congestive heart failure)
- Papillary necrosis
- Hyperkalemia
- Hyponatremia
- Acute allergic interstitial nephritis associated with fenoprofen
- Acute tubular necrosis with phenylbutazone
- Interstitial nephritis with aspirin, phenacetin, and caffeine (aspirin alone and other NSAIDs have been associated with interstitial nephritis in a few case reports)

**21. What NSAIDs would you use in a patient with mild renal compromise?**

The **nonacetylated salicylates** are poor prostaglandin inhibitors and may have less effect on glomerular filtration rate. **Sulindac** has been described as having less renal effects. The rationale for the use of sulindac is that this drug is a prodrug that gets activated to sulindac sulfide, the active compound; the kidney then can revert the active compound back to sulindac and thus not compromise the beneficial effects of prostaglandins. Studies have shown that, empirically, sulindac behaves similarly to other NSAIDs in the patient with renal insufficiency and offers no advantage. Thus sulindac should not be used preferentially in patients with renal compromise. The hope was that the selective COX-2 inhibitors would have less renal effects than the traditional NSAIDs. However, COX-2 is found in the glomeruli and renal vasculature in man. COX-2 appears to be the dominant contributor to salt and water homeostasis, and COX-1 has a more dominant role in the maintenance of glomerular filtration rate. Thus, in practice, the selective COX-2 inhibitors have similar effects on blood pressure and induction of edema as the traditional NSAIDs. Celecoxib appears to cause less edema and blood pressure problems than rofecoxib (**Controversial**).

**22. Do NSAIDs have adverse effects on the heart? (Controversial)**

Aspirin, by irreversibly inhibiting platelet activation, has been accepted therapy for the prevention of myocardial infarctions (MIs) in patients with known coronary artery disease. Other traditional NSAIDs that inhibit COX-1 can reversibly inhibit platelets, but their effect on preventing heart attacks is unknown. However, the selective COX-2 inhibitors have no effect on platelets. Controversy has surrounded the secondary analysis of a large multicenter study with rofecoxib (the VIGOR study group). A slight but significant increase in MIs was seen in patients on rofecoxib as compared with patients on naproxen. No aspirin was allowed in this study. A similar multicenter study with celecoxib (the CLASS study) compared with ibuprofen and diclofenac allowed aspirin to be used in patients at risk for an MI and did not see an increase in MIs. Thus, concern has been raised that patients with coronary artery disease maybe at a slightly greater risk for a MI than patients on traditional NSAIDs. Retrospective analysis of previous studies of rofecoxib and celecoxib have not demonstrated an increase risk for MIs. Also, a recent preliminary report has shown ibuprofen may block the beneficial effects of aspirin on the heart if given before the aspirin. Finally, as discussed above, all NSAIDs may increase blood pressure, cause edema, and induce congestive heart failure in susceptible individuals.

**23. Why would specific COX-2 inhibitors cause more thrombotic events than traditional NSAIDs?**

Since approval of the coxibs, over 200 thrombotic events have been reported to the FDA. The coxibs are specific COX-2 inhibitors and do not affect COX-1, which is critical for production of thromboxane $A_2$, a potent platelet activator. Abnormal blood vessels require COX-2 to produce prostaglandin $I_2$ (prostacyclin), which is antithrombotic. Consequently, a coxib by selectively inhibiting COX-2 may tip the natural balance toward prothrombotic thromboxane $A_2$ and away from antithrombotic $PGI_2$, resulting in thrombosis.

**24. What auditory complications can NSAIDs cause?**

Tinnitus is a relatively common complication of salicylates. Although tinnitus has been associated with a wide range of plasma levels of salicylates, it usually indicates that the plasma level is above the therapeutic range. Thus, tinnitus has been used as a "poor man's" way of monitoring salicylate levels. High levels of salicylates in children and the elderly may not induce tinnitus but instead may cause a reversible **hearing deficit**.

**25. Do NSAIDs cause any central nervous system problems?**

Headaches, dizziness, loss of concentration, depersonalization, tremor, and psychosis have been described in patients taking indomethacin and, to a lesser extent, tolmetin. Ibuprofen has been associated with aseptic meningitis, especially in patients with systemic lupus erythematosus.

**26. Your patient responds well to indomethacin but develops headaches. How can you decrease this side effect?**

**Probenecid** is a uricosuric and renal tubular blocking agent. Its co-administration increases the mean plasma elimination half-life of indomethacin, naproxen, ketoprofen, and meclofenamate. It may also interfere with indomethacin's passage through the blood-brain barrier. Thus, with the concomitant use of probenecid, you may be able to reduce the dose of indomethacin by as much as half and still get a good response without CNS side effects.

**27. List some rare adverse reactions to NSAIDs.**

1. Febrile reactions—ibuprofen
2. Drug-induced lupus—phenylbutazone
3. Vasculitis—indomethacin, naproxen
4. Mediastinal lymphadenopathy—sulindac
5. Pericarditis, myocarditis—phenylbutazone
6. Aplastic anemia—most NSAIDs, but most significantly phenylbutazone
7. Pure red cell aplasia—phenylbutazone, indomethacin, fenoprofen
8. Thrombocytopenia—most NSAIDs
9. Neutropenia—most NSAIDs
10. Hemolytic anemia—mefenamic acid, ibuprofen, naproxen
11. Stomatitis—most NSAIDs
12. Cutaneous effects (photosensitivity, erythema multiform, urticaria, toxic epidermal necrolysis)—most NSAIDs, especially piroxicam. Naproxen can cause porphyria cutanea tarda.
13. Aseptic meningitis (especially SLE patients)—ibuprofen, other NSAIDs less commonly
14. Small bowel webs—most NSAIDs but particularly piroxicam
15. Sulfa allergy—celecoxib

**28. Which of the NSAIDs have short plasma elimination half-lives, and which have long half-lives?**

| DRUG | HALF-LIFE (HRS) | DOSAGE |
|---|---|---|
| **Short half-life** (< 6 hrs) | | |
| Aspirin | 0.25 | |
| Diclofenac (Voltaren) | 1.1 | 25–50 mg bid–tid<br>75 mg bid |
| Etodolac (Lodine) | 3.0/6.5* | 200 mg tid–qid<br>400 mg tid |
| Fenoprofen (Nalfon) | 2.5 | 200–600 mg tid–qid |
| Flurbiprofen (Ansaid) | 3.8 | 50–100 mg bid–tid |
| Ibuprofen (Motrin) | 2.1 | 300–800 mg tid–qid |

(*Table continued on next page.*)

| DRUG | HALF-LIFE (HRS) | DOSAGE |
|---|---|---|
| **Short half-life** (< 6 hrs) (*cont.*) | | |
| Indomethacin (Indocin) | 4.7 | 25 mg tid–qid<br>50 mg tid<br>75 mg SR bid |
| Ketoprofen (Orudis) | 1.8 | 50 mg qid<br>75 mg tid<br>200 mg ER qd |
| Tolmetin (Tolectin) | 1.0/6.8* | 400–600 mg tid |
| **Long half-life** (> 10 hrs) | | |
| Diflunisal (Dolobid) | 13 | 250–500 mg bid |
| Nabumetone (Relafen) | 26 | 500–1000 mg bid<br>1000–2000 mg qd |
| Naproxen (Naprosyn) | 14 | 250–500 mg bid |
| Oxaprozin (Daypro) | 58 | 600–1200 mg qd |
| Phenylbutazone | 68 | 100–400 mg qd<br>100 mg tid–qid |
| Meloxicam (Mobic) | 17 | 7.5–15 mg qd |
| Piroxicam (Feldene) | 57 | 10–20 mg qd |
| Salicylate (Salsalate) | 2-15† | 750–1500 mg bid |
| Sulindac (Clinoril) | 14 | 150–200 mg bid |
| Celecoxib (Celebrex) | 11 | 200 mg qd to100–200 mg bid |
| Rofecoxib (Vioxx) | 17 | 12.5–25 mg qd, 50 mg qd (acute pain) |
| Valdecoxib (Bextra) | 8–11 | 10 mg qd, 20 mg bid (acute pain) |

* Elimination of this drug occurs in two phases, of which the first is generally more important.
† Elimination of this drug is dose-dependent. SR, sustained release; ER, extended release.

Patients are more compliant with single and twice-a-day regimens. The longer half-life drugs may have advantages in patients with morning pain and stiffness. Monthly costs range from generic ibuprofen (800 mg tid) at $3.60 to rofecoxib (25 mg qd) at $60.60 to celecoxib (200 mg bid) at $121.20. A generic NSAID plus misoprostol or a proton pump inhibitor costs over $110 a month.

**29. What are some different formulations of NSAIDs?**

1. **Enteric-coated tablets**. Enteric-coated aspirin are supposed to have less GI symptoms than regular aspirin, but there is no evidence that the enteric coating decreases gastritis or peptic ulcers.

2. **Liquid formulations**. Ibuprofen, naproxen, choline magnesium trisalicylate, indomethacin, and rofecoxib are available in liquid formulations that are designed for patients who have difficulty swallowing pills and for children.

3. **Slow release**. The slow-release formulation is designed to give a short-acting drug a longer half-life so that the drug can be taken only twice a day (indomethacin SR) or once a day (ketoprofen ER, naproxen CR, etodolac ER, diclofenac ER).

4. **Topical formulations**. Aspirin is the only readily available topical in the US, but other countries have topical forms of other NSAIDs.

**30. Are precautions needed when using NSAIDs in the elderly?**

Rheumatic diseases are common in the elderly, and this group of patients frequently use NSAIDs. The elderly have more complications from these drugs than any other group of patients, because of:

- Altered drug absorption. The gastric pH rises with age. Active absorption and transport of drugs may be altered.
- Reduced drug distribution.
- Decreased protein-binding. Plasma albumin decreases with aging, decreasing protein-binding sites.
- Hepatic metabolism and renal excretion may be altered.
- Polypharmacy. Some patient's medications may have drug interactions with NSAIDs.

Thus, to reduce the risk of NSAIDs in the elderly:

- Do not prescribe NSAIDs when they are not necessary. Do not continue treatment longer than necessary.
- Start at the lowest dose and follow up within a month for toxicity and therapeutic benefit.
- Increase the dose cautiously.
- Beware of high-risk drugs.
- Beware of high-risk patients.
- Maintain close supervision.

**31. List some drug-drug interactions involving NSAIDs.**

*NSAIDs Affecting Other Drugs*

| DRUG AFFECTED | NSAID IMPLICATED | EFFECT |
|---|---|---|
| Warfarin | Phenylbutazone | Inhibits metabolism of warfarin, increasing anticoagulant effect |
| | NSAIDs that inhibit COX-1 | Increases risk of bleeding owing to inhibition of platelet function and gastric mucosal damage |
| Sulfonylurea | Phenylbutazone | Inhibits sulfonylurea metabolism, increasing risk of hypoglycemia |
| | High-dose salicylate | Potentiates hypoglycemia by different mechanism |
| Beta-blocker | All PG-inhibiting NSAIDs | Blunts hypotensive but not negative chronotropic or inotropic effect |
| Hydralazine<br>Prazosin<br>ACE-inhibitor | All PG-inhibiting NSAIDs | Loss of hypotensive effects |
| Diuretics | All PG-inhibiting NSAIDs | Loss of natriuretic, diuretic, hypotensive effects of furosemide<br>Loss of natriuretic effect of spironolactone<br>Loss of hypotensive but not natriuretic or diuretic effects of thiazide |
| Phenytoin | Phenylbutazone | Inhibits metabolism, increasing plasma concentration and thereby risk of toxicity |
| | Other NSAIDs | Displaces phenytoin from plasma protein, reducing total concentration for the same active concentration |
| Lithium | Most NSAIDs | Increases plasma lithium level |
| Digoxin | Most NSAIDs | May increase digoxin levels |
| Aminoglycosides | Most NSAIDs | May increase aminoglycoside level |
| Methotrexate | Most NSAIDs | May increase methotrexate plasma concentration |
| Sodium valproate | Aspirin | Inhibits valproate metabolism, increasing plasma valproate concentration |

*Other Drugs Affecting NSAIDs*

| DRUG-IMPLICATED | NSAID AFFECTED | EFFECT |
|---|---|---|
| Antacids | Indomethacin<br>Salicylates<br>Other NSAIDs? | Aluminum-containing antacids reduce rate and extent of absorption<br>Sodium bicarbonate increases rate and extent of absorption |
| Cimetidine | Piroxicam | Increases plasma concentrations and half-life of piroxicam |
| Probenecid | Most NSAIDs | Reduces metabolism and renal clearance of NSAIDs |
| Cholestyramine | Naproxen<br>Probably others | Anion exchange resin binds NSAIDs in gut, reducing rate (and extent?) of absorption |
| Caffeine | Aspirin | Increases rate of absorption of aspirin |
| Metoclopramide | Aspirin and probably others | Increases rate and extent of absorption in patients with migraines |

**32. What might be future uses for NSAIDs?**

Treatment of familial adenomatous polyposis (celecoxib approved for use at 400 mg bid)
Prevention and treatment of colon cancer and other cancers
Prevention of Alzheimer's disease
Delay premature labor

## BIBLIOGRAPHY


1. Abramson SB, Weissmann G: The mechanisms of action of nonsteroidal antiinflammatory drugs. Arthritis Rheum 32:1–9, 1989.
2. Bombardier C, Laine L, Reicin A, et al: Comparison of upper gastrointestinal toxicity of rofecoxib and naproxen in patients with rheumatoid arthritis. VIGOR Study Group. N Engl J Med 343:1520–1528, 2000.
3. Brooks PM, Day RO: Nonsteroidal antiinflammatory drugs—Differences and similarities. N Engl J Med 324:1716–1725, 1991.
4. Catella-Lawson F, Reilly MP, Kapoor SC, et al: Cyclooxygenase inhibitors and the antiplatelet effects of aspirin. N Engl J Med 345:1809–1817, 2001.
5. Clive DM, Stoff JS: Renal syndromes associated with nonsteroidal antiinflammatory drugs. N Engl J Med 310:563–572, 1984.
6. Feenstra J, Heerdink ER, Grobbee DE, et al: Association of nonsteroidal anti-inflammatory drugs with first occurrence of heart failure and with relapsing heart failure: The Rotterdam Study. Arch Int Med 162:265–272, 2002.
7. Fitzgerald GA, Patrono C: The Coxibs, selective inhibitors of cyclooxygenase-2. N Engl J Med 345:433–442, 2001.
8. Golden BD, Abramson SB: Selective cyclooxygenase 2 inhibitor. Rheum Dis Clin North Am 25:359–378, 1999.
9. Hawkey CJ: COX-2 inhibitors. Lancet 353:307–314, 1999.
10. Hoppman RA, Peden JG, Ober SK: Central nervous system side effects of nonsteroidal antiinflammatory drugs. Arch Int Med 151:1309–1313, 1991.
11. Huang JQ, Sridhar S, Hunt RH: Role of *Helicobacter pylori* infection and nonsteroidal antiinflammatory drugs in peptic ulcer disease: A meta-analysis. Lancet 359:14–22, 2002.
12. Huskisson EC: How to choose a non-steroidal anti-inflammatory drug. Rheum Dis Clin North Am 10:313–323, 1984.
13. Mukherjee D, Nissen SE, Topol EJ: Risk of cardiovascular events associated with selective COX-2 inhibitors. JAMA 286:954–959, 2001.
14. O'Brien WM, Bagby GF: Rare adverse reactions to nonsteroidal antiinflammatory drugs [pts I and II]. J Rheumatol 12:13–20, 347–353, 1985.
15. Rich M, Scheiman JM: Nonsteroidal anti-inflammatory drug gastropathy: Mechanism and prevention. Semin Arthritis Rheum 30:167–179, 2000.
16. Rodriguez LAG, Williams R, Derby LE, et al: Acute liver injury associated with nonsteroidal anti-inflammatory drugs and the role of risk factors. Arch Intern Med 154:311–316, 1994.

17. Santana-Sahagun E, Weissman M: Nonsteroidal anti-inflammatory drugs (NSAIDs). In Ruddy S, Harris ED, Sledge CB (eds): Kelley's Textbook of Rheumatology, 6th ed. Philadelphia, WB Saunders, 2001, pp 799–822.
18. Silverstein FE, Faich G, Goldstein JL, et al: Gastrointestinal toxicity with celecoxib vs nonsteroidal anti-inflammatory drugs for osteoarthritis and rheumatoid arthritis. The CLASS study: A randomized controlled trial. JAMA 284:1247–1255, 2000.
19. Singh G, Triadafilopoulos G: Epidemiology of NSAID induced gastrointestinal complications. J Rheumatol 26(Suppl 56):18–24, 1999.
20. Steinbach G, Lynch PM, Phillips RKS, et al: The effect of celecoxib, a cyclooxygeanse-2 inhibitor, in familial polyrosis. N Engl J Med 342:1946–1952, 2000.
21. Stevenson D, Simon R: Lack of cross-reactivity between rofecoxib and aspirin in aspirin-sensitive patients with asthma. J Allergy Clin Immunol 108:47–51, 2001.
22. Tolman KG: Hepatotoxicity of antirheumatic drugs. J Rheumatol 17:6–11, 1990.
23. Veld BA, Ruitenberg A, Hofman A, et al: Nonsteroidal antiinflammatory drugs and the risk of Alzheimer's disease. N Engl J Med 345:1515–1521, 2001.
24. Whelton A: Renal aspects of treatment with conventional nonsteroidal anti-inflammatory drugs versus cyclooxygenase-2-specific inhibitors. Am J Med 110(3A):33S–42S, 2001.
25. Wolfe MM, Lichtenstein DR, Singh G: Gastrointestinal toxicity of nonsteroidal antiinflammatory drugs. N Engl J Med 340:1888–1899, 1999.

# 85. GLUCOCORTICOIDS—SYSTEMIC AND INJECTABLE

*Gregory J. Dennis, M.D.*

**1. List some general indications for implementation of glucocorticoid therapy.**

Glucocorticoids or corticosteroids are potent medications discovered in 1949 (Drs. Hench and Kendall won Nobel Prize in 1950) and since used for a variety of medical indications. In the management of rheumatic disorders, there are two primary indications for their use:

a. Suppression of the inflammatory cascade
b. Modification of the immune response

**2. How are the anti-inflammatory effects of glucocorticoids (GC) mediated?**

Steroids have beneficial anti-inflammatory effects through numerous mechanisms. Some of the most important are:

- Decrease in neutrophil margination, migration, and accumulation at inflammatory sites.
- Inhibition of neutrophil and macrophage phagocytosis, enzyme release, and pro-inflammatory cytokine production (especially interleukin-1 and tumor necrosis factor).
- Induction of lipocortin-1, which inhibits phospholipase A2 resulting in decreased arachidonic acid synthesis with a corresponding decrease in prostaglandin and leukotriene production. Steroids also inhibit cyclooxygeanse-2 (COX-2).
- Decrease in T-cell proliferation and interleukin-2 synthesis and secretion.

Many of GC antiinflammatory effects such as inhibition of up-regulation of adhesion molecules (ICAM-1i) and cytokine secretion (IL-1, TNFα, others) are due to transcriptional activation of the inhibitor of Kappa B (IκB) α gene, which results in inhibition of the nuclear transcription factor NFκB. GC also interfere with activity of Ap-1 and NF-AT transcription factors. This is done by GC binding to an intracellular GC receptor in the cytoplasm, which in turn promotes nuclear translocation and binding to GC response elements in the promoters of genes. GC inhibit Ap-1 activity through physical interference of GC receptor with AP-1 binding. GC can contribute to apoptosis of lymphocytes.

**3. Which methods of their administration may be effective in the treatment of rheumatic disease?**

While certain methods of administration clearly modify immune function and inflammatory reactions more rapidly, some conditions respond similarly to the various methods of administration. Common effective methods include:

a. Intrasynovial therapy (needle injection into joint, bursa, or tendon sheath) is generally used to control inflammatory reactions involving the synovial lining of articular surfaces.

b. Oral or alimentary therapy.

c. Parenteral: intramuscular and intravenous.

**4. How can a general clinical baseline be established for potential complications before instituting corticosteroid therapy?**

a. Some **chronic infections**, i.e., opportunistic, may not be immediately apparent on the initial physical examination and may progress rapidly when corticosteroid therapy is implemented. For a baseline, obtain a **chest x-ray** and a **tuberculin skin test**.

b. For **glucose intolerance**, a baseline **fasting glucose** is sufficient prior to the implementation of therapy, with periodic monitoring, especially with longer courses of therapy.

c. To assess one's risk for **osteoporosis**-related problems, a **bone mineral densitometry** should be performed. At a minimum, prophylactic therapy should be implemented in those on chronic therapy.

d. The activity of **gastrointestinal erosive disease** may be further aggravated by corticosteroid medications. A **stool guaiac** test and a **complete blood count** with mean cell volume should be performed prior to beginning therapy.

e. **Cardiovascular disease** and **hypertension** may be aggravated by corticosteroid medications. Attention should be given toward **blood pressure determination** as well as the presence of peripheral edema on physical examination, with periodic reevaluation.

f. Performing a **MiniMental status examination**, especially in those with a history of mental disturbance, to provide an objective baseline for future comparison.

**5. To minimize the risk of hypothalamic-pituitary-adrenal (HPA) axis suppression, when should patients take their daily dose of corticosteroid medication?**

Because natural cortisol secretion in humans has a circadian rhythm with the peak level in the morning, taking the corticosteroid at that time will have less of a suppressive effect on the release of cortisol-releasing factor. As such, taking the corticosteroid before approximately 10:00 AM will result in less suppression of the HPA axis. In patients on corticosteroids long term, this probably is less important.

**6. Is corticosteroid therapy the cornerstone of therapy for rheumatic disease?**

Yes, for several rheumatic diseases. In general, the rheumatic diseases for which steroids are used to rapidly gain control of the inflammatory process are listed in the accompanying table. Frequently, clinicians will use corticosteroid medications as an initial therapeutic agent and subsequently attempt to taper the medication more rapidly after the implementation of an additional agent as a steroid sparing drug. This approach is thought to minimize the potential consequences of more prolonged corticosteroid therapy.

*Examples of Steroid Responsive Rheumatic Diseases*

| | |
|---|---|
| A. | Selective complications of connective tissue diseases: |
| | Rheumatoid arthritis |
| | Systemic lupus erythematosus |
| | Polymyositis/dermatomyositis |
| | Sjögren's |
| B. | Vasculitis disorders (initial treatment) |
| C. | Polymyalgia rheumatica |

**7. List some important drug properties to consider when deciding which corticosteroid preparation to use.**

Biological half-life
Mineralocorticoid effects
Biological equivalency
Formulation of the preparation
Cost of the medication

**8. Does dosage scheduling influence the potency of corticosteroid therapy?**

Yes. The potency of corticosteroid therapy roughly correlates with the duration of hypothalamic-pituitary axis suppression. Listing the dosage schedules from the least to the most suppressive:

*Relative Potency of Corticosteroid Administration Schedules*

| | |
|---|---|
| Intermittent oral dosing | + |
| Alternate day | ++ |
| Single daily AM dose | +++ |
| Intermittent intravenous pulse therapy | ++++ |
| Multiple daily dosing | +++++ |

**9. How might corticosteroids be grouped in terms of biologic activity?**

Corticosteroids may be divided into three main groups according to their duration of biologic activity. They may be categorized as follows:

| SHORT-ACTING (HALF-LIFE 12 HRS) | INTERMEDIATE-ACTING (HALF-LIFE 12–36 HRS) | LONG-ACTING (HALF-LIFE 48 HRS) |
|---|---|---|
| Hydrocortisone | Prednisone | Paramethasone |
| Cortisone | Prednisolone | Betamethasone |
| | Methylprednisolone | Dexamethasone |
| | Triamcinolone | |

**10. What are some of the adverse consequences of corticosteroid therapy?**

Glucose intolerance
Growth suppression (less if dose ≤ .5 mg/kg)
Osteonecrosis (Chapter 58)
Cataract formation (even at prednisone 5 mg daily)
Skin disorders (bruising, striae, delayed wound repair)
Peptic ulcer disease (doses >10 mg/d with NSAIDs)
Obesity
Infection (doses ≥ .3 mg/kg)
Hirsutism
Abnormal menstruation
Depressed hormone levels (TSH, testosterone, FSH/LH)
Mental disturbance (doses ≥ 30 mg/d)
Muscle weakness (doses > 10–20 mg/d)
Osteoporosis (doses ≥ 5–7.5 mg/d)

**11. When establishing the patient's tuberculin reactivity status, why is it important to obtain skin testing before implementing corticosteroid therapy?**

Continuous administration of pharmacologic doses of corticosteroid is likely to result in suppression of the cellular response to skin testing within 2 weeks of therapy. Be aware, however, that the altered cellular response may selectively and only affect tuberculin reactivity. Thus, negative skin test results obtained after starting glucocorticoid medications are not totally reliable even when control skin testing is positive.

**12. Which group of corticosteroid medications results in the least amount of sodium retention?**

Sodium retention is dependent upon the mineralocorticoid effect of the preparation. It is insignificant in the usual doses of methylprednisolone, triamcinolone, paramethasone, betamethasone, and dexamethasone.

*Mineralocorticoid Properties of Glucocorticoid Preparations*

| GLUCOCORTICOID | MINERALOCORTICOID POTENCY* |
|---|---|
| **Short-acting** | |
| Hydrocortisone (cortisol) | 1 |
| Cortisone | 0.8 |
| **Intermediate-acting** | |
| Prednisone | 0.25 |
| Prednisolone | 0.25 |
| Methylprednisolone | ± |
| Triamcinolone | ± |
| **Long-acting** | |
| Paramethasone | ± |
| Betamethasone | ± |
| Dexamethasone | ± |

* Potency is expressed in milligram comparisons to cortisol reference value of 1.

**13. How do the glucocorticoid properties of the corticosteroids compare with cortisol?**

The glucocorticoid potency of medications correlates in part with the duration of biologic activity.

*Glucocorticoid Properties of Corticosteroid Preparations*

| GLUCOCORTICOID | GLUCOCORTICOID POTENCY* |
|---|---|
| **Short-acting** | |
| Hydrocortisone | 1 |
| Cortisone | 0.8 |
| **Intermediate-acting** | |
| Prednisone | 4 |
| Prednisolone | 4 |
| Methylprednisolone | 5 |
| Triamcinolone | 5 |
| **Long-acting** | |
| Paramethasone | 10 |
| Betamethasone | 25 |
| Dexamethasone | 30–40 |

* Potency is determined with cortisol as a reference value of 1.

**14. How common is adrenal atrophy in patients taking glucocorticoids?**

Exogenous administration of glucocorticoids is the most common cause of adrenal insufficiency, resulting from suppression of ACTH. In the complete absence of ACTH, the human adrenal cortex begins to atrophy in 1 week. Any patient who has received more than 20 mg of daily prednisone for more than a month in the preceding year or greater than 3–5 mg for more than a year should be considered to have a potentially suppressed hypothalamic-pituitary adrenal axis. The recognition that treatment with ACTH-suppressive doses may lead to functional adrenocortical atrophy is important, because when such patients are stressed by infection, trauma, or surgery, they are unable to respond with the usual cortisol output (up to 200–300 mg/day). Proper management during periods of physiologic stress aims to mimic the normal cortisol response.

Full recovery of the HPA axis may take 6–9 months after stopping glucocorticoid therapy. The adrenal responsiveness to ACTH is the last limb of the axis to recover. Some patients may develop steroid withdrawal syndrome with rapid tapering including arthralgias and myalgias. The responsiveness of the adrenal gland to stress can be tested with a short ACTH (Cortrosyn) stimulation test (.25 mg IM, measure baseline and 60-minute plasma cortisol). Normal response is doubling of baseline cortisol and 60 minutes level > 18 (g/dl).

**15. In the treatment of rheumatic disease, what is considered to be low-, medium-, and high-dose daily prednisone therapy?**

| | |
|---|---|
| Low dose | < 15 mg/d |
| Medium dose | 15–< 40 mg/d |
| High dose | > 40 mg/d |

**16. Are you able to list seven basic measures that should be done routinely for patients receiving glucocorticoids?**

1. Prescribe corticosteroids at the lowest possible dose and discontinue as soon as the disease activity permits.
2. Encourage physical activities and avoid immobilization (helps prevent myopathy).
3. Implement fall prevention program.
4. Prescribe calcium to achieve a minimum intake of 1500 mg/d.
5. Supply vitamin D at a minimum of 400 IU/d.
6. Consider bisphosphonate therapy implementation (if > 7.5 mg/day for > 3 months).
7. Patient education concerning the adverse effects of therapy.

**17. What are some drug interactions that need to be considered in patients on glucocorticoids?**

A large number of medications share with corticosteroids metabolism mediated by hepatic cytochrome P450 enzymes, particularly CYP3A4. Drugs that can up-regulate CYP3A4 levels resulting in reduced levels of glucocorticoids that could decrease glucocorticoids effectiveness in controlling disease are:

- Anticonvulsants—carbamazepine, phenobarbital, and phenytoin.
- Rifampin—if patient is on rifampin double the dose of corticosteroids to get same immune modulating effect.
- Phenylbutazone and sulfinpyrazone—no longer used or marketed.

Drugs that can inhibit metabolism of glucocorticoids and increase their effectiveness:

- Ketoconazole
- Macrolide antibiotics—erythromycin, triacetyloleandomycin

**18. Are corticosteroid medications ever used in rheumatic diseases for reasons other than their systemic effect?**

Yes, primarily in the form of local therapy. A variety of therapeutic modalities have been used for the local administration of corticosteroids; needle injection remains the most effective means of delivering medication to the musculoskeletal structures. Specific conditions for which corticosteroid injections are particularly effective include:

a. Intrabursal treatment of bursitis
b. Tendon sheath injection for tendinitis
c. Intra-articular injection for synovitis
d. Soft-tissue trigger point injection

**19. Name rheumatic disease syndromes likely to have an indication during their clinical course for corticosteroid injection therapy:**

| | | |
|---|---|---|
| Rheumatoid arthritis | Osteoarthritis | Tendinitis and epicondylitis |
| Systemic lupus erythematosus | Spondyloarthropathies | Bursitis |
| Crystal deposition disease | Tietze's syndrome | Entrapment neuropathies |

**Pearl**: The effectiveness of an injection ranges from 50–90% and lasts days to months.

**20. List some of the general indications for corticosteroid injection therapy in rheumatic conditions.**

- Monoarthritis or disproportionate joint inflammation (after joint infection is ruled out)
- Recurrent joint effusion
- Tendon sheath inflammation
- Bursitis or tendinitis refractory to NSAIDs

**21. What are the major benefits of intrasynovial corticosteroid injections?**

a. Alleviate inflammation in a joint, bursa, or tendon sheath
b. Avoid institution of systemic therapy

**22. Can you construct a summary table of corticosteroid preparations available for injection into a joint, bursa, or tendon sheath?**

*Corticosteroid Preparations Suitable for Joint or Other Injection*

| PREPARATION | STRENGTHS (MG/ML) | PREDNISONE EQUIVALENT (MG)* |
|---|---|---|
| **Short-acting, soluble** | | |
| Dexamethasone sodium phosphate (Decadron, Hexadrol) | 4 | 40 |
| Hydrocortisone acetate (Hydrocortone) | 25, 50 | 5, 10 |
| **Long-acting, less soluble** | | |
| Prednisolone tebutate (Hydeltra-TBA) | 20 | 20 |
| Methylprednisolone acetate (Depo-Medrol) | 20, 40, 80 | 25, 50, 100 |
| Dexamethasone acetate (Decadron-LA) | 8 | 80 |
| **Longest-acting, least soluble** | | |
| Triamcinolone acetonide (Kenalog, Aristocort) | 10, 40 | 12.5, 50 |
| Triamcinolone hexacetonide (Aristospan) | 20 | 25 |
| **Combination** | | |
| Betamethasone sodium phosphate/acetate+ (Celestone Soluspan) | 6 | 50 |

* Of 1 ml of injected steroid preparation. + Has longest-acting and short-acting steroid combined.

**23. Is there any other important characteristic(s) of corticosteroid preparations important to consider when determining which to use for injection therapy?**

Solubility of the corticosteroid preparation is an important factor when considering injection therapy. Reducing the solubility of a compound increases the duration of the local effect, since slower diffusion of the medication will occur. Thus, less soluble preparations have greater potency but are also more likely to result in adverse consequences.

**24. What volume of corticosteroid can be safely injected into a joint?**

The volume of corticosteroid that can be safely injected depends on the size of the joint. The physician must be aware of the volume to be injected into the joint. Attempts should be made to avoid overdistention of the surrounding joint capsule.

| SIZE OF JOINT | VOLUME (ML) |
|---|---|
| Large (knees, ankles, shoulders) | 1–2 |
| Medium (elbows, wrists) | 0.5–1 |
| Small (interphalangeal, metaphalangeal) | 0.1–0.5 |

**25. How do you determine the optimal dose of corticosteroid to be injected into synovial-lined spaces?**

The dose of corticosteroid to be injected into synovial-lined cavities depends on the:

a. Size of the joint
b. Degree of inflammation
c. Amount of fluid present (aspirate effusions dry before injections)
d. Concentration of corticosteroid used

**26. How often can a joint or tendon sheath be injected with corticosteroid medications?**

The main concern with frequent injections is accelerated deterioration of the joint due to cartilage breakdown or weakening of the tendon. The longer the interval between injections, the better. A minimum of 4–6 weeks between injections is recommended. Weight-bearing joints should not be injected more frequently than every 6–12 weeks. A good rule of thumb is not to inject the same joint or tendon sheath more than 3 times yearly.

**27. Can the corticosteroid for injection be combined with anesthetic to minimize the number of needlesticks to the patient?**

Yes, anesthetic preparations can be safely mixed with corticosteroid preparations. If the corticosteroid preparation contains a paraben compound as a preservative, flocculation of the suspension is likely to occur. Immediately prior to injecting, shake the syringe vigorously to minimize joint precipitation.

**28. Is there an optimal amount of corticosteroid that should be injected into a joint, bursa, or tendon sheath?**

It is generally recommended that short- or long-acting corticosteroids be injected into tendon sheaths, since they are more soluble and cause less soft tissue atrophy or chance of tendon rupture. The longest-acting, least-soluble corticosteroid preparations are typically injected into inflamed joints because they tend to be more effective.

*Guidelines for the Appropriate Dose of Corticosteroid to be Injected*

| SITE | PREDNISONE EQUIVALENT DOSE (MG) |
|---|---|
| Bursa | 10–20 |
| Tendon sheath | 10–20 |
| Small joints of hands and feet | 5–15 |
| Medium-sized joints (wrist, elbow) | 15–25 |
| Large joints (knee, shoulder, ankle) | 20–50 |

The dose for injection into a child's knee is 1 mg/kg.

**29. List some concerning problems and sequelae that may occur from corticosteroid injections.**

Infection (1 in 50,000 injections)
Skin hypopigmentation
Steroid crystal-induced synovitis (postinjection flare) (2%)
Subcutaneous tissue atrophy
Tendon rupture (never inject Achilles tendon)
Osteonecrosis (rare)
Erythroderma

**Pearl**: One corticosteroid injection transiently weakens a tendon (up to 40%) for up to 3–12 weeks. It can also suppress cortisol levels (HPA axis) by 30% for up to 7 days.

**30. How do you separate a postinjection flare from infection after a corticosteroid injection?**

Postinjection flares occur in 1–2% of patients who receive corticosteroid injections. It is most likely to occur with use of least soluble forms (i.e., long-acting) of corticosteroid preparations. Injections of the lateral epicondyle of the elbow are particularly prone to this complication. The flare occurs within 6–18 hours after an injection, which separates it from an infection, which usually won't manifest itself for 2–4 days after an injection. If need be, the joint can be aspirated and will show intracellular steroid crystals in a postinjection flare (look like CPPD crystals but polarize with first order red compensation like gout crystals), whereas bacteria will be seen with infection. Treatment is with ice, NSAIDs, and pain medication, and a postinjection flare should resolve within 24 hours.

**31. Are there any contraindications to intrasynovial corticosteroid injections?**

The physician must be aware of the contraindications to corticosteroid injection (whether relative or absolute) in order to decide if the injection is truly in the best interests of the patient. The following situations require serious consideration prior to injecting corticosteroid:

Periarticular and articular sepsis
Lack of response to previous injections
Inaccessible joints
Bacteremia
Intra-articular fracture
Excessive patient anxiety
Blood clotting disorders
Joint instability
Absence of suitable supplies

## BIBLIOGRAPHY


1. Axelrod L: Glucocorticoid therapy. Medicine 55:39–65, 1976.
2. Baxter JD: The effects of glucocorticoid therapy. Hosp Pract 27:111–134, 1992.
3. Bijlsma JWJ, Jacobs JWG: Hormonal preservation of bone in rheumatoid arthritis. Rheum Dis Clin North Am 26:897–910, 2000.
4. Chrousos GP: The hypothalamic pituitary-adrenal axis and immune-mediated inflammation. N Engl J Med 332:1351–1362, 1995.
5. Cupps TR: Therapeutic use. In Boumpas DT (moderator): Glucocorticoid therapy for immune-mediated diseases: Basic and clinical correlates. Ann Intern Med 119:1198–1208, 1993.
6. Feldweg AM, Leddy JP: Drug interactions affecting the efficacy of corticosteroid therapy. J Clin Rheumatol 5:143–150, 1999.
7. Hench PS, Kendall EC, Slocumb CH, Polley HF: The effect of a hormone of the adrenal cortex (17 hydroxy-11-dehydrocorticosterone: compound E) and of pituitary adrenocorticotropic hormone on rheumatoid arthritis: Preliminary report. Proc Staff Meet Mayo Clin 24:181–197, 1949.
8. Hoogwerf G, Danese RD: Drug selection and the management of corticosteroid-related diabetes mellitus. Rheum Dis Clin North Am 25:859–880, 2000.
9. Lazarevic MB, et al: Reduction of cortisol levels after single intra-articular and intramuscular steroid injection. Am J Med 99:370–373, 1995.
10. Moore JS: Flexor tendon entrapment of the digits (trigger finger and trigger thumb). J Occup Environ Med 42:526–545, 2000.
11. Sabir S, Werth V: Pulse glucocorticoids. Dermatol Clin 18:437–446, 2000.
12. Scheinman RI, et al: Role of transcriptional activation of NF-κB in mediation of the immunosuppression by glucocorticoids. Science 270:283–286, 1995.

# 86. SYSTEMIC ANTI-RHEUMATIC DRUGS

Kristin Bird, M.D., and James O'Dell, M.D.

*If many drugs are used for disease, all are insufficient.*
Sir William Osler

**1. What is meant by a disease-modifying drug in rheumatoid arthritis?**

Because there is no cure for rheumatoid arthritis (RA), the goal of treatment is to put the disease into remission. A category of drugs with some ability to do this is the disease-modifying antirheumatic drugs (DMARDs). To be designated a DMARD, a drug must change the course of RA for at least 1 year as evidenced by one of the following: sustained improvement in physical function, decreased inflammatory synovitis, slowing or prevention of structural joint damage.

**2. List the DMARDs and other medications currently available for treatment of RA.**

| DMARDs | Other Agents |
|---|---|
| Intramuscular (IM) gold (Solganal, Myochrysine) | Azathioprine (Imuran) |
| Hydroxychloroquine (Plaquenil) | Cyclosporine (Sandimmune, Neoral) |
| Sulfasalazine (Azulfidine) | Minocycline (Minocin, Dynacin) |
| D-Penicillamine (Cuprimine, Depen) | Etanercept (Enbrel) |
| Oral gold/auranofin (Ridaura) | Infliximab (Remicade) |
| Methotrexate (Rheumatrex) | Prednisone |
| Leflunomide (Arava) | |

**3. When should a patient with RA be started on a DMARD?**

Once the diagnosis of RA is established, all patients (with rare exception) should begin DMARD therapy. Bone erosions and joint space narrowing develop within the first 2 years of disease in most patients and are progressive from this point onward. Therefore, early, aggressive treatment with DMARDs is warranted. Additionally, patients with RA who have evidence of active disease (synovitis, morning stiffness, etc.), bony erosions or deformities, or extra-articular disease manifestations and are not already on DMARDs should begin treatment immediately.

**4. How quickly can DMARDs be expected to work?**

Most DMARDs used for the treatment of RA take several months (3–6) to achieve a significant response. It is important to educate patients about this time frame of response so they are not discouraged when results are not seen immediately.

**5. Describe the use of gold in RA.**

Intramuscular (IM) gold preparations are being used less frequently, but are effective and have been shown to result in short-term remissions. Long-term studies show clinical improvement, although erosions continue to develop. IM gold therapy is most commonly initiated with a test dose of 10 mg given IM. If no untoward reactions occur, this is followed by 25–50 mg 1 week later. Weekly injections are then given until the patient has a significant response or until a total of 1 gm has been given. If 1 gm has been given without improvement, therapy is usually abandoned because of lack of efficacy. If there has been an excellent response, gold injections can be given every 2 weeks for several months. If remission is maintained, they can be given every 3–4 weeks. IM gold is continued as long as it works. Unfortunately, less than 10% are still on it 5 years after initiation as a result of side effects or inefficacy.

Oral gold is rarely used because of its lower efficacy and frequent side effects, most notably **GI intolerance** and **diarrhea**. Its use is usually limited to early, mild RA or in combination with other medications.

**6. Describe the side effects of gold therapy and the parameters for monitoring its use.**

Side effects:
- Dermatitis, stomatitis, and/or pruritus
- Nitritoid reaction—flushing and hypotension, which occurs 15–30 minutes after receiving gold (especially Myochrysine)
- Proteinuria (due to membranous glomerulonephritis)
- Hematologic reactions [eosinophilia, leukopenia, thrombocytopenia (ITP), aplastic anemia]
- GI intolerance—IM gold can cause severe colitis, usually early in therapy. Oral gold can cause diarrhea but not colitis.

Monitoring: CBC with platelet count and urine dipstick looking for proteinuria are typically done prior to each injection.

**7. In which conditions might treatment with gold be indicated?**

Rheumatoid arthritis
Juvenile rheumatoid arthritis
Psoriatic arthritis
Palindromic rheumatism
Reactive arthritis (Reiter's syndrome)

**8. How are antimalarials used in the treatment of RA?**

The antimalarials are the **least toxic** of all DMARDs and can be safely combined with other DMARDs. They are particularly effective in early treatment of patients with mild to moderate or seronegative disease. Hydroxychloroquine is the main antimalarial used in the United States.

Dosage:
- Hydroxychloroquine (Plaquenil) 200–400 mg/day (≤ 6.5 mg/kg of ideal body weight)
- Chloroquine (Aralen) 250 mg/day (≤ 3.5 mg/kg of ideal body weight)
- Quinacrine (Atabrine), 100–200 mg/day

Side effects:
- Nausea and vomiting (less likely to occur if start at half dose and titrate up over 2–4 weeks)
- CNS effects—headache, dizziness
- Muscle—myopathy (in high doses or renal insufficiency)
- Aplastic anemia (quinacrine)—especially if develop lichen planus rash
- Hemolysis—in patients with G6PD deficiency
- Rash, hyperpigmentation of skin (gray-black with chloroquine, yellow with quinacrine), bleaching of hair
- Retinal toxicity (rare at currently recommended doses)

Monitoring: Ophthalmologic exam every 6–12 months

**9. What is the mechanism of action of the antimalarials?**

Unknown. Antimalarials are weak bases and accumulate in acidic vesicles such as lysosomes. By increasing lysosomal pH, it is thought there is a disruption in the normal assimilation of peptides with class II MHC molecules.

Other cellular effects of antimalarials are beneficial. For instance, they can increase lipoprotein (LDL) receptors, thus helping to lower lipid levels. They also decrease degradation of insulin, helping to prevent diabetes mellitus. Finally, they can inhibit platelet aggregation and adhesion, helping to prevent thrombosis.

**10. In which other rheumatic conditions is treatment with antimalarials indicated?**

Systemic lupus erythematosus (SLE)

Palindromic rheumatism

Psoriatic arthritis (controversial)—use with caution, since antimalarials may exacerbate psoriatic skin lesions

Sjögren's syndrome

Sarcoidosis

**11. Discuss the use of antimalarial therapy in SLE.**

Antimalarial therapy is very useful in treating patients with SLE. Skin manifestations, serositis, fatigue, and joint disease are especially responsive to treatment. Additionally, antimalarials are useful in **maintaining remissions** and **preventing flares** of disease. Lupus patients on antimalarial therapy are less likely to have flares of lupus nephritis or CNS manifestations. Antimalarials also have a mild antithrombotic effect and may decrease risk of thrombosis, especially in patients with antiphospholipid antibodies. Therefore, almost all patients who have demonstrated a significant tendency toward organ involvement from their lupus should be maintained on antimalarial therapy while they are believed to be at high risk for flares of their disease.

**12. How common is antimalarial retinopathy, and what steps can be used to decrease this toxicity?**

Chloroquine binds more avidly to corneal and retinal pigmented epithelium than hydroxychloroquine and thus causes more corneal deposits and retinopathy. Corneal deposits are not an indication to stop antimalarials, but retinopathy is an absolute indication to stop therapy. Retinopathy is very uncommon and occurs in less than 1–2% of individuals who have been on antimalarials for more than 2 years. It is extremely rare if dosed according to ideal (lean) body weight (see Question 8). Consequently, patients less than 66 inches in height should get 300 mg and less than 60 inches 200 mg of hydroxychloroquine and not the usual 400 mg. Likewise, patients less than 66–70 inches in height should get less than 250 mg of chloroquine a day. These doses must be decreased further if there is renal or liver dysfunction. Notably, owing to different chemical composition, quinacrine does not cause retinopathy. Consequently, quinacrine can be combined with chloroquine or hydroxychloroquine without added retinal toxicity.

An ophthalmologic examination should be done on all patients at 6 months after starting an antimalarial. Patients on chloroquine should continue every 6 month exams, while patients on hydroxychloroquine should be examined every 12 months. The first evidence of toxicity is loss of red light perception. If this is detected, the antimalarial can be stopped and there will be no loss of vision. However, if toxicity is allowed to progress to decrease in visual acuity and/or macular pigmentary changes, the patient may lose further vision even if the antimalarial is discontinued. An added inexpensive safety measure is to give a patient an Amsler grid and instruct in how to use it each day at home. If the lines become blurry, the patient should be examined immediately. Patients on higher than recommended doses, or who have coexistent eye disease, or have renal or liver dysfunction should be examined more frequently (i.e., every 3–6 months).

**13. What can interfere with antimalarial effectiveness?**

Smoking can induce hepatic cytochrome P-450 enzymes resulting in accelerated metabolism of antimalarials, causing them to be less effective. Cimetidine can decrease the clearance of antimalarials, while antimalarials can antagonize the effects of anticonvulsants and amiodarone.

**14. Discuss the use of D-penicillamine in the treatment of RA.**

D-penicillamine (cuprimine, Depen) is not routinely used in the treatment of RA because it takes 6 or more months for a significant response and has many adverse effects. It is useful in some patients with RA who have extra-articular manifestations such as vasculitis and Felty's syndrome.

| | |
|---|---|
| Dosage: | 125–250 mg/day increased stepwise (by 125–250 mg every 3 months) to 750–1000 mg/day |
| Side effects: | Hematologic disorders—leukopenia, thrombocytopenia (ITP) |
| | Nephropathy (membranous) |
| | Rash and/or pruritus |
| | Anorexia, nausea, dysgeusia |
| | Autoimmune syndromes such as myasthenia gravis, Goodpasture's syndrome, drug-induced lupus, and pemphigus |
| Monitoring: | Monthly CBC with platelets and urinalysis dipstick looking for protein |

**15. List the diseases treated with D-penicillamine.**

Rheumatoid arthritis
Systemic sclerosis
Wilson's disease
Cystinuria
Primary biliary cirrhosis

**16. Discuss the use of sulfasalazine in RA.**

Sulfasalazine (Azulfidine) is often used in early, mild disease because it acts quickly with measurable results in 4 weeks. For many years, this was the first and most commonly used DMARD in Europe. Its potential for toxicity is low, and it is often combined with other DMARDs. Sulfasalazine is a two-component drug, made up of sulfapyridine and 5-aminosalicylic acid (5-ASA).

Dosage: 1–3 grams/day in divided doses. Start at 500 mg and increase by 500 mg each week.

Side effects: Nausea and vomiting (less if dose is titrated up slowly, if taken with meals, and if enteric-coated tablets are used)
Rash (1–5%)
Headache and dizziness
Azoospermia (reversible on discontinuation of drug)
Neutropenia (1–5%)
Pulmonary infiltrates with eosinophilia
Hepatic enzyme elevation ± fever, adenopathy, rash

Monitoring: CBC with platelets and liver enzymes at baseline and monthly for the first 3 months of therapy and then every 3 months, creatinine at 1 month and then every third month

**17. In what rheumatic diseases is sulfasalazine used?**

Rheumatoid arthritis
Reactive arthritis (Reiter's syndrome)
Psoriatic arthritis
Ankylosing spondylitis (peripheral manifestations)
Enteropathic arthritis

**18. Discuss the role of methotrexate in RA.**

Methotrexate (MTX) is considered the most effective DMARD for RA. This is particularly true if one looks at the percentage of patients who remain on methotrexate after 3 to 5 years of therapy. Methotrexate acts relatively quickly after being started, often within several weeks. It has been found to suppress disease activity in a significant portion of patients with long-standing RA in whom other treatment has failed. In addition to providing efficacy clinically, methotrexate appears to retard appearance of new erosions in involved joints. Using other drugs in combination with methotrexate has resulted in improved efficacy over methotrexate alone without an additive increase in side effects.

**19. What dose of methotrexate is used to treat RA and what toxicities are associated with its use?**

Dosage: 7.5–25 mg PO, SQ, or IM weekly. Note that parenteral MTX gives serum levels 30% higher than oral MTX. After 20 mg is reached, no further MTX is absorbed orally and parenteral route should be used.
Folic acid 1 mg/day should always be given with methotrexate, and the dose can be increased to 2–5 mg/day if symptoms of toxicity (mouth sores) develop.
Folinic acid 5 mg given as one dose 24 hours after weekly dose of MTX can sometimes help mouth sores even if folic acid fails.

Side effects: Oral ulcers (folic acid helps prevent and/or decrease symptoms); photosensitivity. Nausea, vomiting, anorexia. Can worsen migraine headaches.
Hepatic toxicity (concern has lessened with further experience—see below).
Hematologic toxicity (leukopenia, thrombocytopenia, pancytopenia, megaloblastic anemia)—folic acid helps prevent this. Less likely to occur if normal renal function.
Pneumonitis (stop methotrexate and do not rechallenge, also need to rule out opportunistic infections such as *Pneumocystis carinii* pneumonia)
Lymphomas— some related to Epstein-Barr virus infection. May resolve if MTX is stopped.

**20. Discuss the precautions and monitoring required for patients taking methotrexate.**

Monitoring: Prior to starting methotrexate, CBC with platelets, hepatitis B and C serology, as well as AST, ALT, alkaline phosphatase, albumin, and creatinine should be obtained. A chest x-ray should be done if the patient has not had one in the last year. CBC with platelets, AST, ALT, albumin, and creatinine should then be followed every 4 to 8 weeks.

Precautions: Methotrexate should be avoided in patients with renal insufficiency. Patients should also avoid alcohol and trimethoprim-sulfamethoxazole (decreases excretion). Methotrexate is also contraindicated in pregnancy, and female patients of child-bearing age should use a reliable form of contraception. MTX should be stopped for 3 months in both males and females before attempting to get pregnant. MTX can accumulate in pleural effusions and be reabsorbed causing neutropenia. MTX should be used with caution if at all in patients with hepatitis B or C infections.

**21. When should a liver biopsy be done on patients receiving methotrexate?**

Routine liver biopsy in patients receiving methotrexate is not currently recommended. However, baseline liver biopsy is recommended in patients with risk factors for cirrhosis such as significant alcohol use, positive hepatitis serology, or elevated liver transaminase levels. Liver biopsy is also recommended if AST or ALT levels are persistently elevated (> 3 months) or if albumin levels decrease while on methotrexate.

**22. What is the mechanism of action for methotrexate's immunologic effects at the doses currently used?**

MTX has multiple effects on the immune system. At the low doses used to treat rheumatic diseases, it is unlikely that it significantly inhibits purine synthesis through inhibition of dihydrofolate reductase (resulting in a decrease in metabolically active reduced folates). However, MTX can inhibit AICAR transformylase. This leads to increases in the intracellular concentration of its substrate AICAR, which stimulates the release of adenosine. Adenosine is a potent inhibitor of neutrophil function and has potent antiinflammatory properties.

**23. In what other rheumatologic conditions is methotrexate used?**

Juvenile rheumatoid arthritis
Psoriatic arthritis
Reactive arthritis (Reiter's syndrome)
Ankylosing spondylitis (peripheral arthritis)
Polymyositis/dermatomyositis
Wegener's granulomatosus
Adult-onset Still's disease
SLE
Polymyalgia rheumatica/giant cell arteritis
Sarcoidosis
Uveitis

**24. Discuss the role of leflunomide in RA.**

Leflunomide (Arava) is a novel DMARD that inhibits pyrimidine synthesis and is approved for treatment of active RA. Studies conducted with leflunomide and sulfasalazine have demonstrated similar efficacy between the two agents in alleviating the signs and symptoms of RA. In another study, the efficacy of leflunomide was found to be comparable with low-dose methotrexate. Additionally, leflunomide has been shown to slow radiographic progression of RA. Leflunomide may be used in combination with methotrexate or in place of it, when methotrexate is contraindicated or not tolerated. It is often added to methotrexate in patients who have received benefit from methotrexate but still have active disease.

**25. Discuss the dosing and side effects of leflunomide.**

Dosage: 100 mg PO daily for 3 days, then 10–20 mg daily. To decrease side effects, the 100-mg loading dose can be given one day a week for 3 weeks. To save money, leflunomide 20 mg every other day works as well as 10 mg daily.

Side effects:
- Nausea, vomiting, and diarrhea (17%)—can lead to significant weight loss
- Skin rash (8%)/allergic reaction (usually occurs at higher doses)
- Neutropenia > thrombocytopenia
- Alopecia (reversible) (8%)
- Hepatic enzyme elevation
- Teratogenicity
- Does not cause pneumonitis like MTX

**26. What is the mechanism of action of leflunomide?**

The active metabolite of leflunomide, A77 1726, inhibits dihydroorotate dehydrogenase leading to a decrease in de novo synthesis of uridine resulting in a decrease in the synthesis of pyrimidines. Lymphocytes (B cells > T cells) have low pools of pyrimidine nucleotides, making them sensitive to this drug. When uridine is lowered below a critical level, the tumor suppressor p53 is activated, arresting lymphocyte cell division in the G1 stage of the cell cycle.

**27. Is leflunomide used in diseases other than RA?**

Yes. Although not FDA approved, leflunomide has been used in most of the diseases where MTX is used with similar results.

**28. What precautions and monitoring are required in patients taking leflunomide?**

Monitoring: Hepatitis B and C serology, AST, ALT, and creatinine should be obtained at baseline and monthly thereafter. If lab results are stable, monitoring can be done less frequently at the discretion of the clinician.

Precautions: Leflunomide should not be used in patients with hepatic impairment or positive hepatitis serology and is also contraindicated in pregnancy. Caution should be used in patients with renal impairment, as there are currently no clinical data available in this group of patients. Leflunomide has an extremely long half-life; in some cases, it may take up to 2 years to reach undetectable plasma concentrations. Because of this, an enhanced drug elimination procedure has been developed in cases of overdose, toxicity, or desire for pregnancy (both males and females). Cholestyramine 8 grams three times daily for 11 days (does not have to be consecutive days) will rapidly reduce plasma concentrations in these situations. In patients desiring to become pregnant, the active metabolite plasma level must be documented to be less than 0.02 μg/ml on two occasions 14 days apart. This is done through the company by calling 1-800-221-4023 to get the kit and instructions for blood draw.

Drug interactions: Rifampin increases serum level of active metabolite of leflunomide, which can increase toxicity.

**29. Discuss the management of hepatotoxicity due to leflunomide.**

There have been several reports of severe hepatotoxicity due to leflunomide. Some of these cases have resulted in liver failure and death. Most occurred in first several months of initiation of therapy. Most patients were taking additional medications (such as methotrexate) that are known to be hepatotoxic to the liver or had coexistent hepatitis B that was reactivated. Appropriate precautions can decrease the chance of this toxicity:

- Limit use of other drugs with potential for additive liver toxicity.
- Do not use leflunomide in patients with hepatitis B or C.
- Monitor ALT and AST monthly for first 6 months. If also on MTX or minor elevations of liver associated enzymes (LAE), continue monthly monitoring. Otherwise, monitor every 2 months.

The following are recommendations should LAE become elevated:

- Minor sporadic elevations [> 1 × and < 2 × upper limit of normal (ULN)]—follow with repeat testing.
- LAEs > 2 × ULN or persistent minor elevations—dose reduction.
- LAEs > 3 × ULN—stop leflunomide and consider drug elimination protocol that can be abbreviated (cholestyramine 4 grams tid for 5 days).

**30. When should DMARDs be stopped in patients with RA who are doing well?**

In most cases, DMARD therapy should be *continued indefinitely* in patients who are doing well. Spontaneous remissions in RA patients who have required DMARDs are very uncommon, and continued efficacy of all currently available DMARDs requires maintenance therapy. Flares that are severe may occur with discontinuation of most of these drugs.

**31. Can combinations of two or more DMARDs be used in the treatment of RA?**

The role of combination DMARD therapy in treatment of RA continues to evolve. With the addition of new medications, more therapeutic combinations are possible than ever before. Most clinical trials of combination therapy with DMARDs have included methotrexate. Several studies have shown combinations of DMARDs with methotrexate to be more beneficial than methotrexate alone. The following are combinations that have been studied:

- MTX and hydroxychloroquine
- MTX, hydroxychloroquine, and sulfasalazine
- MTX and leflunomide
- MTX and azathioprine
- MTX and cyclosporine
- MTX and etanercept
- MTX and infliximab

Although combinations of two or more DMARDs have been shown to be more efficacious than a single agent, one question that has not yet been answered is whether combination therapy should be the standard initial treatment in all patients with RA. Clinical trials comparing combination DMARD therapy with monotherapy using a rapid step-up or step-down approach are needed to help answer this question.

**32. Can patients on immunosuppressives be vaccinated?**

Patients on methotrexate, leflunomide, and/or medications listed in Chapter 87 should not receive live attenuated virus vaccines: yellow fever, measles/mumps/rubella, oral polio vaccine, and varicella. Furthermore, they should avoid contact with children recently vaccinated with oral polio vaccine, since the virus is shed in their stool. Patients on immunosuppressive medication can receive all other vaccinations without an increased chance of flaring their underlying disease. However, their protective antibody titers following vaccination may be blunted as a result of being on immunosuppressive medications.

**33. How is dapsone used in the treatment of the rheumatic diseases?**

Dapsone is a sulfone. It is poorly water-soluble, poorly absorbed through the gastrointestinal tract, and metabolized by the liver. It is used as an antimicrobial for treatment of leprosy.

However, it also has antiinflammatory effects and is particularly useful in dermatoses involving polymorphonuclear leukocytes. It is a free oxygen radical scavenger and impairs the myeloperoxidase system. In rheumatic diseases, it is particularly useful for skin vasculitis (leukocytoclastic, urticarial, or erythema elevatum diutinum, cutaneous PAN), skin lesions of Behçet's disease, SLE rashes (particularly bullous disease and panniculitis), relapsing polychondritis, and pyoderma gangrenosum. Doses range from 50 to 200 mg with average 100 mg a day. The major drug interaction is probenecid, which slows its renal excretion. Dapsone is also used as *Pneumocystis carinii* prophylaxis in patients allergic to sulfa antibiotics.

**34. What are the major toxicities of dapsone?**

All patients treated with dapsone will have some degree of hemolysis and methemoglobinemia and thus should be supplemented with 1 mg of folate daily. Patients with G6PD deficiency will have severe hemolysis, so all patients should be screened, particularly those of Mediterranean or African descent. The hemolysis is due to a metabolite of dapsone causing oxidation of glutathione, which is essential for erythrocyte membrane integrity. G6PD is necessary to produce NADPH, which is a cofactor for glutathione reductase, which reduces the oxidized glutathione back to an active form.

Other side effects can include leukopenia, hypersensitivity syndrome, liver toxicity, nausea, and peripheral neuropathy (on high doses). Monitoring should include CBC and reticulocyte count every month for 3 months, then every 3 months with renal and liver tests.

**35. How is thalidomide used in the treatment of rheumatic diseases?**

Thalidomide has antiinflammatory, immunomodulatory, and antiangiogenic properties. A major effect may be its ability to reduce tumor necrosis factor (TNFα) production by 40%. It is not immunosuppressive and has not been associated with opportunistic infections. At doses of 50 mg to 300 mg a day, it has been useful to treat inflammatory skin diseases associated with Behçet's and SLE that are resistant to standard therapy. It is particularly useful for severe oral and/or genital ulcerations. Major toxicities include sedation, constipation, rash, sensory polyneuropathy, and teratogenicity (phocomelia). Owing to these toxicities, the FDA requires registration for its use and following stringent regulations and guidelines for use (call 1-888-423-5436 to get application for use). Owing to the frequency of polyneuropathy (up to 50%), which is more common in women and not related to daily or cumulative dose, it is recommended that a baseline EMG/NCV be performed and repeated every 6 months. A decline in the sensory nerve action potential (SNAP) by 50% or development of subjective complaints at monthly follow-ups requires discontinuation of the drug, since the neuropathy is often progressive and nonreversible.

**36. What is the American College of Rheumatology (ACR) definition for improvement in rheumatoid arthritis treatment trials?**

An ACR study group determined that improvement for clinical trial patients with rheumatoid arthritis be defined as:

*Required:* ≥ 20% improvement in tender joint count
*and*
≥ 20% improvement in swollen joint count

*Plus*: ≥ 20% improvement in 3 of the following 5:
- Patient pain assessment
- Patient global assessment
- Physician global assessment
- Patient self-assessed disability (HAQ)
- Acute-phase reactant (ESR or CRP)

Patients who improve as defined above are said to have met criteria for ACR 20. If improved 50% or 70%, they have met criteria for ACR 50 or ACR 70.

**37. What are the monthly costs for these medications when used to treat RA?**

| MEDICATION | MONTHLY COST (DOLLARS) *Generic* | *Brand* |
|---|---|---|
| Minocycline (100 mg bid) | 51 | 215 |
| Hydroxychloroquine (200 mg bid) | 47 | 90 |
| Sulfasalazine (1000 mg bid) | 17 | 45 (Entabs) |
| Methotrexate (15 mg/week) | 6 liquid | 75 |
| Leflunomide (10 or 20 mg/d) | — | 280 |
| Dapsone (100 mg/d) | 6 | — |
| Thalidomide (100 mg/d) | — | 490 |

Note that liquid methotrexate is much less expensive than pills. Liquid MTX can be injected subcutaneously or mixed in juice and swallowed. Leflunomide 10 mg and 20 mg tablets cost the same. Owing to long half-life, a patient on 10 mg a day can be switched to 20 mg every other day, which is much less expensive.

## BIBLIOGRAPHY

1. Felson DT, Anderson JJ, Boers M, et al: American College of Rheumatology preliminary definition for improvement in rheumatoid arthritis. Arthritis Rheum 38:727–735, 1995.
2. Felson DT, Anderson JJ, Meenan RF: The comparative efficacy and toxicity of second-line drugs in rheumatoid arthritis. Arthritis Rheum 33:1449, 1990.
3. Felson DT, Alderson JJ, Meenan RF: Use of short-term efficacy/toxicity tradeoffs to select second-line drugs in rheumatoid arthritis: A metaanalysis of published clinical trials. Arthritis Rheum 35:1117, 1992.
4. Harris ED: Treatment of rheumatoid arthritis. In Ruddy S, Harris ED Jr, Sledge CD (eds): Kelley's Textbook of Rheumatology, 6th ed. Philadelphia, WB Saunders, 2001, pp 1001–1022.
5. Kremer JM: Rational use of new and existing disease-modifying agents in rheumatoid arthritis. Ann Int Med 134:695–706, 2001.
6. Landewe RBM, Boers M, Verhoeven AC, et al: COBRA combination therapy in patients with early rheumatoid arthritis: Long-term structural benefits of a brief intervention. Arthritis Rheum 46:347–356, 2002.
7. Lenardo TM, Calabrese LH: The role of thalidomide in the treatment of rheumatic diseases. J Clin Rheumatol 6:19–26, 2000.
8. O'Dell JR: Methotrexate use in rheumatoid arthritis. Rheum Dis Clin North Am 23(4):779–795, 1997.
9. O'Dell JR, Haire C, Erikson N, et al: Treatment of rheumatoid arthritis with methotrexate, sulfasalazine, and hydroxychloroquine, or a combination of these medications. N Engl J Med 334:1287–1291, 1996.
10. Paniker U, Levine N: Dapsone and sulfapyridine. Dermatol Clin 19:79–86, 2001.
11. Situnayake RD, Grindulis KA, McConkey B: Long term treatment of rheumatoid arthritis with sulphasalazine, gold, or penicillamine: A comparison using life-table methods. Ann Rheum Dis 46:177, 1987.
12. Smolen J, et al: Efficacy and safety of leflunomide compared with placebo and sulphasalazine in active rheumatoid arthritis: A double-blind, randomized, multicentre trial. Lancet 353:259–266, 1999.
13. Van Beek MJ, Piette WW: Antimalarials. Dermatol Clin 19:147–160, 2001.

# 87. CYTOTOXIC, IMMUNOREGULATORY, AND BIOLOGIC AGENTS

*Amy Cannella,* M.D., *and James O'Dell,* M.D.

*The physician without physiology and chemistry practices a sort of popgun pharmacy, hitting now the malady and again the patient, he himself not knowing which.*

Sir William Osler

1. **How is azathioprine (Imuran) supplied and used?**
    - Available formulations: 50 mg tablets, 100 mg/20 ml vial
    - Side effects: bone marrow depression, nausea, vomiting, skin rash, malignancy (lymphoma increased 2–5 times), hepatotoxicity, infections (herpes zoster), pancreatitis, hypersensitivity syndrome (within first 2 weeks of use)
    - Dosage: 50–200 mg/day (1–2.5 mg/kg/day). Start 50 mg/d and increase by 25 mg every 1-2 weeks to desired dose.
    - Cost: $150/month at 150 mg/day
    - Follow-up: complete blood count (CBC) and liver enzymes within 2 weeks with dose change, CBC monthly first 3 months, and then CBC every 1–3 months.
    - Precautions: avoid in pregnancy, avoid live vaccines, drastically reduce dose with allopurinol (reduce azathioprine dose by 75% or do not use at all). Sulfasalazine and bactrim/septra increase risk of leukopenia. Azathioprine may cause warfarin resistance.

2. **Describe the mechanism of action and metabolism of azathioprine.**

Azathioprine is a prodrug converted to 6-mercaptopurine (6-MP). 6-MP is then converted to thiopurine nucleotides which decrease de novo synthesis of purine nucleotides and are incorporated into nucleic acids of cells. This results in both cytotoxicity and decreased cellular proliferation. The patient is getting a maximum effect from azathioprine if the erythrocyte mean corpuscular volume increases by 5 cu μ.

The metabolism of 6-MP by two enzymes, xanthine oxidase and thiopurine methyl-transferase (TPMT), results in formation of inactive metabolites. Inhibition of xanthine oxidase (by allopurinol) or of TPMT (sulfasalazine) results in accumulation of 6-MP and in toxicity. In addition, TPMT activity is affected by genetic polymorphism with 90% having high activity, 10% intermediate activity, and 0.3% low activity. Blacks have less TPMT activity than whites. Patients with low TPMT activity are at risk for sudden onset of severe myelosuppression occurring between 4 and 10 weeks after starting azathioprine. Patients with intermediate activity have more frequent adverse side effects, particularly gastrointestinal. TPMT activity can be measured, but whether this is necessary prior to starting azathioprine is controversial.

3. **What rheumatic diseases are commonly treated with azathioprine?**
    - Rheumatoid arthritis
    - Systemic lupus erythematosus (particularly lupus nephritis)
    - Polymyositis/dermatomyositis
    - Behçet's syndrome
    - Many other rheumatic diseases (in an attempt to decrease corticosteroid dosage)

4. **How is mycophenylate mofetil (Cellcept) supplied and used?**
    - Available forumulations: 250, 500 mg capsules; oral suspension (200 mg/ml) and IV form (500mg/20 ml) available.

- Side effects: gastrointestinal (especially diarrhea 25%), leukopenia, anemia, hepatotoxicity, infections; less likely to cause lymphoproliferative malignancies than azathioprine (controversial)
- Dosage: 500–1500 mg 2 times/day
- Cost: 1000 mg 2 times/day is $1210/month
- Follow-up: CBC and liver enzymes weekly with dose change and then CBC every 1–3 months
- Precautions: avoid in pregnancy; avoid live vaccines. Cholestyramine and administration with food or antacids decrease bioavailability. Tacrolimus may potentiate effects of mycophenylate mofetil.

**Pearl**: good alternative to azathioprine in patients with gout who need allopurinol and in patients who need warfarin.

5. **What is the mechanism of action of mycophenylate mofetil (MMF)?**

MMF is an inactive prodrug that is hydrolyzed to the active mycophenolic acid (MPA). MPA is a reversible inhibitor of inosine-5'-monophosphate dehydrogenase (IMPDH), which is an enzyme necessary for the de novo synthesis of the purine, guanosine. Lymphocytes (T and B cells) depend on IMPDH to generate sufficient guanosine levels to initiate a proliferative response to antigen. Cytokine production is not affected. MPA also inhibits carbohydrate (fucose, mannose) transfer to glycoproteins, resulting in less production of adhesion molecules (VLA-4, ICAM-1). In summary, MPA inhibits lymphocyte proliferation and lymphocyte migration. The enterohepatic recycling of glucuronide-conjugated MPA contributes to gastrointestinal toxicity since gastrointestinal mucosal cells are 50% dependent upon de novo synthesis pathway of purines, which is inhibited by MPA.

6. **What rheumatic diseases have been treated successfully with mycophenylate mofetil?**

Use is similar to azathioprine. Some increased success has been seen in lupus nephritis (DPGN, membranous), cutaneous lupus (discoid and subacute cutaneous lupus), and vasculitis. Experience in rheumatoid arthritis is limited.

7. **Discuss the use of cyclophosphamide (Cytoxan) in the rheumatic diseases.**
   - Available formulations: 25 and 50 mg tablets; 100, 200, 500 and 1000 mg vials
   - Dosage: daily oral, 50–150 mg (0.7–3 mg/kg/day); monthly IV, 0.5–1 gm/m$^2$ body surface area (see Chapter 20, question 28).
   - Follow-up: daily dosing, CBC every 1–2 weeks until stable dose, then monthly; urinalysis monthly, urinalysis with cytology every 6–12 months after cessation of therapy. For monthly dosing, CBC with urinalysis before each dose, CBC 10–14 days after each dose.
   - Precautions: avoid in pregnancy, avoid live vaccines, use lower doses in elderly due to less bone marrow reserve (cellularity = 100%–age). Cimetidine and allopurinol increase frequency of leukopenia.

8. **Describe the mechanism of action and metabolism of cyclophosphamide.**

Cyclophosphamide is an inactive prodrug that is activated by hepatic cytochrome P-450 enzymes. The major active metabolite is phosphoramide mustard, which alkylates DNA and results in cross-linking of DNA, breaks in DNA, decreased DNA synthesis, and apoptosis. Cyclophosphamide synthesis has a marked effect on rapidly dividing cells and throughout the cell cycle, resulting in alterations in humoral and cellular immunity (B > T cells).

Liver disease does not increase toxicity of cyclophosphamide. Initial dose is decreased by 25% if creatinine clearance is less than 50 cc/min and by 50% if less than 25 cc/min. Cyclophosphamide is dialyzable and should be administered after dialysis.

Acrolein is a major metabolic product of cyclophosphamide metabolism. It is responsible for causing hemorrhagic cystitis and bladder cancer.

**9. In which rheumatic diseases is cyclophosphamide therapy indicated? How effective is it?**

- Wegener's granulomatosis
- Systemic lupus erythematosus (particularly lupus nephritis)
- Other systemic vasculitis syndromes
- Other rheumatic diseases refractory to conventional therapy

Cyclophosphamide is widely considered to be one of the most potent immunosuppressive drugs available. Its use has succeeded in almost all rheumatic diseases, particularly when other less potent and usually less toxic forms of therapy have failed. When preservation of renal function in patients with lupus nephritis is the desired result, cyclophosphamide has superior efficacy. However, because of its potentially severe toxicity, overall improvements in mortality have been more difficult to demonstrate. On the other hand, cyclophosphamide therapy is universally considered to be the cornerstone of therapy for patients with Wegener's granulomatosis who otherwise would have a fatal disease process.

**10. What are the major toxicities of cyclophosphamide? What can be done to prevent them?**

- Bone marrow suppression. The WBC nadir after a dose is 8–14 days later. Start at 50 mg/day and increase weekly while following CBC 1–2 times a week initially.
- Infection (all types, especially herpes viruses). Screen for hepatitis B and C, HIV, and tuberculosis prior to therapy. Keep WBC nadir above 3000/mm$^3$ and preferably at 4000/mm$^3$. Decrease prednisone dose to less than 20–25 mg/day as soon as possible. Prophylaxis for *Pneumocystis carinii* pneumonia with bactrim/septra, dapsone, or inhaled pentamidine. Pneumococcal vaccine should be administered.
- Hemorrhagic cystitis and bladder cancer. Nonglomerular hematuria occurs in up to 50% of patients with 5% developing bladder cancer (31-fold increased risk). Decrease risk by using monthly intravenous pulse therapy instead of daily oral therapy. Also can use mesna, a sulfhydryl compound that binds and inactivates acrolein in the urine. Stop smoking, which increases risk of bladder toxicity. With daily oral therapy, give cyclophosphamide in the morning and force fluids (> 2 L/day).
- Malignancy. Risk increased 2–4 fold. Increased risk if give daily oral vs. monthly intravenous; the higher the cumulative dose, the greater the risk.
- Infertility. The risk for ovarian failure ranges from 45–70% and varies depending on age of patient and cumulative dose. Risk may be slightly less with monthly intravenous than daily oral dosing. Women less that 20 years old have a 13% risk, age 20–30 a 50% risk, and over age 30 a 100% risk of premature ovarian failure. Ovarian failure is unlikely if women receive less than 6 monthly doses and common if they receive over 15 monthly pulses. Azoospermia is found in 50–90% of men. Various strategies have been tried to limit this toxicity. Banking ova and sperm can be done but is expensive. In women, using gonadotropin-releasing hormone analogue (Lupron depot, 3.75 mg IM monthly or 11.25 mg IM every 3 months plus estradiol 0.3 mg/day [or biweekly patch if patient hypercoagulable] to reduce hot flashes and protect the bone) may be protective. In men, testosterone, 100 mg IM every 15 days, may be protective.
- Pulmonary. Less than 1% get pneumonitis or pulmonary fibrosis.
- Others. Reversible alopecia, syndrome of inappropriate antidiuretic hormone secretion, nausea (use antiemetics), and teratogenicity.

**11. What other alkylating agents have been used to treat rheumatic diseases?**

Both nitrogen mustard and chlorambucil have been used to treat several rheumatic diseases. Chlorambucil is the more commonly used. The usual dose is 0.1 mg/kg/day (2–8 mg/day). It has been used primarily to treat the eye and neuropsychiatric complications of Behçet's disease. It has also been used in cryoglobulinemia, refractory polymyositis, lupus nephritis, and amyloidosis secondary to chronic inflammatory arthritis (rheumatic arthritis [RA], juvenile RA, ankylosing spondylitis). Major toxicities are myelosuppression and induction of leukemia and other malignancies.

**12. How is cyclosporine (Neoral) used in the treatment of rheumatic diseases.**

- Available formulations: 25 and 100 mg capsule; oral solution 100 mg/ml; IV solution 50 mg/ml
- Dosage: 2.5–5 mg/kg for most rheumatic diseases
- Cost: $200/month at 175 mg/day
- Follow-up: monthly creatinine, blood pressure, cyclosporine levels (controversial), magnesium, periodic CBC, liver function tests, potassium, and lipid levels.
- Precautions. Concurrent use of NSAIDs may contribute to renal insufficiency. Diltiazem increases cyclosporine levels causing toxicity. Cyclosporine is stopped if creatinine increases 30% over baseline. Concurrent use of colchicine can cause neuromyopathy.

Cyclosporine is a potent immunomodulating agent that works by inhibition of T cell activation. It does so by binding to a cytoplasmic protein (immunophilin), which is turn binds to calcineurin. This blocks the interaction of calcineurin with calmodulin which is necessary to dephosphorylate nuclear factor of activated T cells (NF-AT) which is a transcription factor needed to activate IL-2 and other T cell activation genes.

Cyclosporine was originally developed as an antifungal agent. Its primary use has been to suppress the immune system to prevent organ transplant rejection, but due to its potent immunosuppressive properties, it recently has been used to treat various rheumatic diseases that are refractory to other therapies.

**13. What affects cyclosporine absorption?**

Cyclosporine is poorly and variably absorbed from the gut with a bioavailability of 30% but with substantial variability among individuals. A high-fat meal can increase absorption. Grapefruit juice and marmalade from Seville oranges contain dihydroxy-bergamottin, which inhibits the cytochrome P450 enzyme in the small intestine, resulting in increased absorption and decreased metabolism of cyclosporine as well as statins and ACE inhibitors. St. John's wort decreases cyclosporine levels by inducing cytochrome P450 3A4, duodenal P-glycoprotein, and MDR-1 gene.

**14. What are tacrolimus (FK506, Prograf) and sirolimus (Rapamune)?**

Tacrolimus is a macrolide produced by a fungus. It has immunosuppressive effects similar to cyclosporine but at a dose 10-100 times lower. Both cyclosporine A and tacrolimus are potent inhibitors of T-cell activation and inhibit transcription of early T-cell activation genes, such as interleukin-2 (IL-2). It does so by interfering with the binding of nuclear regulatory factor, NF-AT, to its target region in the enhancer region of these inducible genes. Notably, tacrolimus causes less increase in uric acid than cyclosporine and it may be useful to switch from cyclosporine to tacrolimus in transplant patients with tophaceous gout.

Sirolimus inhibits T cell proliferation by binding to its cytoplasmic immunophilin which inhibits IL-2 receptor transduction events after the receptor has bound IL-2. This prohibits the T cell from responding to IL-2.

**15. What rheumatic syndromes have been treated with cyclosporine?**

- Rheumatoid arthritis (especially when combined with methotrexate)
- Polymyositis/dermatomyositis (especially with interstitial lung disease)
- Psoriatic arthritis
- Systemic lupus erythematosus (especially membranous glomerulonephritis)
- Uveitis

Studies have shown that cyclosporine is more effective in treating RA than placebo and has similar efficacy to that of some other disease-modifying drugs. It is more effective when combined with methotrexate. Patients with many other rheumatic disease syndromes have been treated with cyclosporine with improvement reported, but without good studies to confirm this improvement. Cyclosporine currently seems to hold promise in treating patients with refractory polymyositis/dermatomyositis and uveitis.

**16. What are the major toxicities of cyclosporine?**

- Decreased renal function (usually reversible)
- Infections
- Hypertension (treat with calcium channel blocker)
- Hyperpigmentation
- Anorexia
- Anemia (note that it does not decrease white blood cell count)
- Malignancies (lymphomas and skin cancers)
- Hyperuricemia and gout (switch to tacrolimus which causes less hyperuricemia)
- Headaches and tremors
- Bone pain (treat with calcium channel blockers and lower cyclosporine dose)
- Hepatotoxicity (rare)

The renal toxicity of cyclosporine has been particularly troublesome when treating patients with rheumatic diseases, many of whom already have renal problems. Of lupus patients, often we would most like to treat those with lupus nephritis with this drug but are limited by its renal toxicity. In the case of RA, the renal toxicity of cyclosporine has been heightened because many of these patients are on concomitant NSAIDs. Recently, in protocols in which cyclosporine has been used without NSAIDs in RA patients, the renal toxicity has been more manageable. A further significant consideration when prescribing cyclosporine is its cost, especially if the patient's medical insurance does not cover this cost.

**17. How significant is the risk of potential malignancies after use of azathioprine, cyclophosphamide, or cyclosporine?**

The possible induction of malignancies in these treatments should always be a major concern. Therefore, many clinicians have been reluctant to treat patients with so-called nonmalignant diseases with therapies that can induce malignancies. The risk/benefit ratio always needs to be kept in mind, but few can argue against use of cyclophosphamide therapy, which is life-saving for most patients with Wegener's granulomatosis, even if a small percentage of these patients develop non-Hodgkin's lymphomas after this therapy.

The risk of malignancy after treatment with immunosuppressive drugs is clearly greatest when using an alkylating agent, such as cyclophosphamide and chlorambucil, the two that are used most commonly in the treatment of rheumatic diseases. The use of azathioprine clearly increases (2–5 times) the risk for induction of malignancies, but this risk appears to be a much more significant problem in organ transplant patients than in RA patients. Studies have implicated cyclosporine in causing lymphomas in some patients. Some lymphomas (Epstein-Barr virus–associated) induced by these immunosuppressive therapies regress when the immunosuppressive therapy (i.e., cyclosporine, methotrexate) is stopped.

**18. What kinds of biologic agents are being studied for use in the treatment of inflammatory rheumatic diseases?**

With our increasing understanding of the pathogenesis of autoimmune rheumatic diseases, several biologic agents are being developed for treatment, especially for RA. These can be classified as follows:

Monoclonal antibodies
- Against T-cell surface molecules: CD4 (anti-CD4)
- Against B-cell surface molecules: CD20 (anti-CD20)
- Activation antigens: CD25 (anti-TAC)
- Against cytokines: TNF$\alpha$ (anti-TNF$\alpha$), IL-6 (anti-IL-6), IL-8 (anti IL-8)
- Against adhesion molecules: ICAM-1/LFA-1 interaction (anti-CD11$\alpha$ receptor)
- Against complement: C5 (anti-C5)
- Against costimulatory molecules: CD40L (anti-CD40L)

Biologics targeting T/B-cell collaboration molecules
- CD28/B7 interaction (CTLA-4 Ig)

Biologics targeting inflammatory cytokines
  Cytokine receptor antagonist proteins (IL-1 Ra)
  Soluble receptors (TNFα receptor)
Methods targeting antigen-MHC-TcR interaction
  Oral tolerance (Type II collagen in RA)
  TcR Vβ peptide vaccine
  MHC peptide vaccine
Other
  Antisense oligonucleotides (against ICAM-1)
  T-cell vaccination
  Gene therapy (IL-1Ra, Fas ligand)
  IL-10: an antiinflammatory cytokine

**19. Which biologic agents are currently available to treat rheumatic diseases?**

**Etanercept (Enbrel)**: a bioengineered molecule derived from Chinese hamster ovary cells which consists of a fusion protein created by linking the extracellular binding regions from two TNF-RII (p75) receptors to the Fc portion of human IgG1. This molecule is a dimeric soluble TNF receptor that binds soluble tumor necrosis factor α (TNFα) and lymphotoxin (TNFβ). Its half life is 72 hours.

**Infliximab (Remicade)**: chimeric mouse-human monoclonal antibody composed of the constant regions of human IgG1 heavy and partial kappa light chain domains coupled to the variable region of a mouse light chain with high-affinity for human TNFα. Infliximab binds both soluble and cell bound TNFα so has the ability to kill cells with TNFα bound to its surface. It does not bind lymphotoxin.

**Anakinra (Kineret)**: a recombinant, nonglycosylated form of the human interleukin-1 receptor antagonist (IL-1Ra). It blocks the biologic activity of IL-1 by competitively inhibiting IL-1 binding to the interleukin-1 type I receptor. The half-life is 4–6 hours.

**20. What is the rationale behind the use of these biologics?**

TNFα and IL-1 are key cytokines in the pathophysiology of inflammatory synovitis and destruction of bone and cartilage. TNFα is initially expressed as a transmembrane molecule on the surface of macrophages. The extracellular portion is cleaved by TNFα-converting enzyme (TACE) to form a soluble molecule that circulates as a homotrimer. TNFα (and TNFβ from T cells) binds to two receptors, TNF-RI (p55) and TNF-RII (p75), both of which are found on the surface of most cells. Binding of TNFα to its receptor triggers a variety of intracellular signaling events, inducing production of prostaglandins and proinflammatory cytokines, endothelial cell expression of adhesion molecules that help recruit neutrophils and monocytes into the synovial fluid, and synoviocyte/chondrocyte production of collagenase, which can destroy cartilage and bone.

Interleukin-1 (IL-1) is a proinflammatory cytokine which exists in two forms, IL-1α and IL-1β which are transcribed from closely related but distinct genes. IL-1α is in the cytosol and membrane bound. IL-1β is secreted into the extracellular space after cleavage of proIL-1β by interleukin-1β converting enzyme (ICE). Thus, IL-1β is the predominant form that binds to the IL-1 receptor triggering intracellular signaling leading to a proinflammatory response which is synergistic to that induced by TNFα, B cell activation and rheumatoid factor production, cartilage degradation by induction of synoviocyte/chondrocyte production of enzymes resulting in proteoglycan loss, and stimulation of osteoclasts causing bone resorption. Notably, cells producing IL-1 also produce IL-1Ra. However, in patients with inflammatory synovitis such as rheumatoid arthritis, the amount of IL-1Ra in the synovium is produced in insufficient amounts to neutralize the amount of locally produced IL-1.

**21. How is etanercept (Enbrel) used?**

• Available formulations: single use vial of 25 mg
• Dosage: 25 mg subcutaneous twice a week

- Follow-up: A complete blood count should be checked monthly for 3 months, then every 3 months. PPD prior to use.

**22. How is infliximab (Remicade) used?**

- Available formulations: single use vials of 100 mg
- Dosage: 3–10 mg/kg intravenous every 4–8 weeks
- Follow-up: CBC checked monthly for 3 months, then every 3 months. PPD prior to use.
- Precaution: Do not use in patients with congestive heart failure, (see Question 23).

**23. What are some of the side effects observed with the anti-TNFα biologic agents? How can these toxicities be limited?**

As of July 2001, over 270,000 patients have been exposed to etanercept or infliximab worldwide.

1. Hypersensitivity reactions
   - Etanercept: injection site reaction (50%) lasting 3–5 days usually resolves by 3 months of use. Treat with topical steroid or antihistamine. Rotate the injection sites.
   - Infliximab: infusion reactions such as hypotension, headache, dyspnea. Treat by stopping infusion and restarting at slower rate. If the patient has a reaction or ≥ 3 drug allergies, premedicate with Allegra, 180 mg, 45 minutes prior to infusion; may also premedicate with aspirin (better than acetaminophen) and, if necessary, Solu-Cortef.
2. Pancytopenia/aplastic anemia: total of 30 cases; usually with other medications, such as methotrexate. Check CBC every 3 months.
3. Demyelinating syndromes: 20 cases; reversible when biologic agent is stopped. Do not give to patients with history of multiple sclerosis or optic neuritis.
4. Opportunistic infections: tuberculosis (100 cases), fungal (35 cases), pneumocystis (17 cases), and listeria (12 cases). Infliximab is associated with tuberculosis and fungal infections more than etanercept, perhaps because of demographics of patients treated (many outside U.S., many Crohn's patients) or because infliximab is cytotoxic to cells with bound TNFα and etanercept is not. Patient must get PPD (no anergy screen) prior to starting these biologics. Get chest radiograph if risk factors or positive PPD is present. Prophylactic therapy with isoniazid (or equivalent) for 9 months in patients with latent tuberculosis. Do not start anti-TNFα until antituberculous therapy has been given at least 2 weeks.
5. Infections: serious infections occur in 2–3% of patients. Do not use biologics if predisposed to serious infections. Hold the anti-TNFα inhibitor during active infection.
6. Autoimmune phenomenon
   - Etanercept: Can develop non-neutralizing antibodies (16%), positive ANA (11%), and lupus-like syndrome (4 cases)
   - Infliximab: Human anti chimeric antibodies (HACA) develop in 17% unless infliximab used with methotrexate or other immunosuppressant. Positive ANA (20–30%), antiphospholipid antibodies, and lupus-like syndrome (4 cases) have been reported.
7. Malignancy: 28 cases of lymphoma; may be more common when high-dose (10 mg/kg) monthly infliximab is used. Use not recommended if less than 5 years from any cancer. The author does not use in patients with history of breast cancer and positive lymph nodes (controversial).
8. Others: seizures, colonic perforations, worsening congestive heart failure (infliximab).

**24. What diseases have been treated with the anti-TNFα inhibitors?**

- Etanercept has shown significant benefit in RA, polyarticular JRA, ankylosing spondylitis, and psoriatic arthritis.
- Infliximab has shown significant benefit in RA, Crohn's disease, ankylosing spondylitis, and psoriatic arthritis.
- Multiple other diseases are being investigated for treatment with these agents such as Reiter's syndrome, Wegener's granulomatosis, Still's disease, and temporal arteritis. These agents are probably contraindicated in lupus-like diseases.

**25. When is it appropriate to use biologic agents in RA?**

Treatment regimens need to be tailored to each individual patient. In clinical practice, if no contraindication exists, methotrexate is the first-line agent due to efficacy and well-established safety guidelines. If methotrexate alone does not control disease, combination therapy is employed, usually with hydroxychloroquine and sulfasalazine or leflunomide in addition to methotrexate.

Trials have shown superior efficacy both symptomatically and in decreasing radiographic damage when etanercept or infliximab is added to methotrexate vs. methotrexate alone in patients who responded suboptimally to methotrexate. However, they can be cost-prohibitive: etanercept costs \$1200–\$1600 per month and infliximab \$900–\$3000 a month. Additionally, the long-term consequences of TNFα suppression are unknown.

**26. How is anakinra (Kineret) used?**

- Available formulation: single use vial of 100 mg
- Dosage: 100 mg subcutaneously daily
- Follow-up: CBC monthly for 3 months, then every 3 months
- Adverse reactions: serious infections (2%), neutropenia (3%), injection site reaction (70%)
- Precautions: at present should not be used with anti-TNFα biologics. Do not use in patients with active infection.
- Indication: rheumatoid arthritis

**27. What is the relative cost for the biologics used to treat rheumatoid arthritis?**

| Biologic | Monthly Cost (dollars) |
|---|---|
| Etanercept | \$1200–1600 |
| Infliximab | \$620/100 mg vial; average 3 vials every 1–2 months = \$1860/month |
| Anakinra | \$925 |

**28. What other biologics are in the process of being tested which may help treat rheumatoid arthritis?**

- Adalimumab (D2E7): fully humanized anti-TNF monoclonal antibody. Given subcutaneously ever other week. Don't have to worry about neutralizing antibodies.
- CDP870: a long acting anti TNFα which can be given subcutaneously once very 4–8 weeks.
- TNFα-converting enzyme (TACE) inhibitors
- IL-1-converting enzyme (ICE) inhibitors
- Matrix metalloproteinase inhibitors
- MAP kinase inhibitors

**29. How is intravenous gammaglobulin used as an immunomodulator in the rheumatic diseases?**

- Available formulations: multiple suppliers; solution varies from 3–12% Ig; cost is \$25–\$60/gm
- Dosage: 1–2 gm/kg administered over 1–5 days
- Side effects: headache (2–20%), flushing, chest tightness, back pain/myalgias, fever, chills, nausea, diaphoresis, hypotension, aseptic meningitis, clot
- Follow-up: creatinine 24 hours after infusion
- Precautions: anaphylactic reaction in patients with hereditary IgA deficiency; transmission of infectious agents (rare)

Some side effects of gammaglobulin are avoided by premedicating patients with acetaminophen and diphenhydramine hydrochloride (Benadryl) or hydrocortisone sodium succinate (Solu-Cortef) and by slowing the rate of infusion. Infusion is started at 30 ml/hr and increased to a maximum of 250 ml/hr (sometimes higher).

**30. In which rheumatic diseases is IV gammaglobulin indicated? How does it work in these?**

- Autoimmune thrombocytopenia
- Kawasaki's disease
- Dermatomyositis and polymyositis
- Wegener's granulomatosis (controversial)
- Antiphospholipid antibody syndrome

The mechanisms by which IV immunoglobulin causes clinical improvement are debated. In autoimmune thrombocytopenia, IV immunoglobulin acts by Fc receptor blockade, reducing the efficacy of the reticuloendothelial system to remove antibody-coated platelets. Other effects include a reduction of autoantibody production and decreased autoantibody binding to platelets.

In Kawasaki's disease, IV immunoglobulin may work by reducing expression of adhesion molecules on endothelial cells, binding cytokines that can cause inflammation, reducing the number of activated T-cells, and binding staphylococcal toxin superantigens. In Wegener's, it may reduce the level of ANCA autoantibodies. Clearly, other mechanisms of action may play a role.

**31. When is plasmapheresis used in the treatment of rheumatic diseases?**

Theoretically, plasmapheresis should remove immune complexes and autoantibodies that contribute to the pathogenesis of some of the rheumatic diseases. There is good evidence for a beneficial effect of plasmapheresis combined with alpha-interferon (or other antiviral agent) in the treatment of hepatitis B associated polyarteritis nodosa and hepatitis B or C associated cryoglobulinemia. Anecdotally, plasmapheresis has been a useful therapy when used in conjunction with corticosteroids and cytotoxic medications in the treatment of severe lupus pneumonitis and neuropsychiatric lupus with coma. Plasmapheresis is usually used in combination with corticosteroids and/or cytotoxic therapy to decrease the risk of a rebound flare of the underlying immunologic disease once the pheresis is stopped. To date, little evidence supports its routine use in other rheumatic diseases.

Most plasma exchange protocols remove 2–4 liters (40 mg/kg) of plasma over a 2-hour period daily. Replacement fluid is generally albumin-saline or another protein-containing solution. To decrease the risk of infection and bleeding, 1–2 units of fresh frozen plasma are included as part of the replacement solution. If not, monitoring of coagulation studies and immunoglobulin levels are important. If the patient develops hypogammaglobulinemia, intravenous gammaglobulin needs to be given.

**32. Discuss the dosing of corticosteroids in the treatment of severe rheumatic diseases.**

The typical approach to treating severe presentations of rheumatic diseases is to give prednisone orally in doses of 1–2 mg/kg/day in divided doses. The reason for divided dosing is that the immunologic effects of prednisone typically last 8–12 hours before dissipating. Theoretically, prednisone given as a single daily dose would not be as immunomodulating as divided doses. Consequently, many clinicians start with divided dosing for the first 2–4 weeks, until the rheumatic disease is brought under control, and then consolidate the prednisone to a single daily dose before starting a taper schedule. There is no role for every-other-day corticosteroids in the initial treatment of severe rheumatic diseases.

**33. What about "pulse" corticosteroids?**

Many clinicians use intravenous pulse corticosteroids as the initial treatment of severe life-threatening or organ-threatening presentations of rheumatic diseases. This is typically methylprednisolone given in doses of 1 g/day for 3 consecutive days. This regimen of corticosteroid administration is felt to have more immunomodulating effects than high-dose daily oral corticosteroids (controversial). As the sole therapeutic intervention, pulse steroids probably have no role in long-term therapy. However, in combination therapy with a cytotoxic agent, pulse steroids may provide time for a second agent to achieve its therapeutic effect.

The effect of pulse steroids usually lasts 3–4 weeks. It has been used most often in the treatment of severe vasculitis, lupus nephritis, and neuropsychiatric lupus. Side effects include psychosis, arrhythmias (some from hypokalemia), and, rarely, sudden death. The risk of these adverse effects may be lessened by using a slow rate of infusion and ensuring that the serum potassium level is normal.

**34. What is the Prosorba column?**

The Prosorba column uses staphylococcal protein A covalently bound to an inert silica matrix. It can remove immunoglobulin G and IgG-containing circulating immune complexes. It is used to treat idiopathic thrombocytopenia purpura and rheumatoid arthritis that has failed multiple DMARDs. Its mechanism of action in the therapy of rheumatoid arthritis is unclear.

Procedure: apheresis of 1250 ml of blood through the column once a week for 12 weeks.

Cost: each column costs $1000 plus the cost of the pheresis.

Precautions: patients on angiotensin converting enzyme inhibitors can experience severe hypotension.

**35. Discuss the use of high dose immunoablative therapy with or without autologous hematopoietic stem cell transplantation for the treatment of severe autoimmune disease.**

Autologous (using patient's own stem cells) hematopoietic stem cell transplantation is a method of increasing the intensity of chemotherapy that can be given to a patient with a severe autoimmune disease who is failing standard therapy. By collecting stem cells (CD34+) prior to chemotherapy, higher doses of cyclophosphamide (200 mg/kg) can be given to ablate the immune system because the patient can be rescued from bone marrow failure by reinfusion of the patient's own stem cells. This strategy hopefully allows the patient to reconstitute their immune system without redeveloping their autoimmune disease. This strategy has been applied to patients with RA, SLE, systemic sclerosis, multiple sclerosis, and other autoimmune diseases with varying success rates and a 5–10% mortality at a cost of up to $100,000. Recently, high dose immunoablative therapy (50 mg/kg for 4 days) without stem cell transplantation has been done successfully since CD34+ stem cells express high levels of aldehyde dehydrogenase responsible for cellular resistance to cyclophosphamide enabling the bone marrow to repopulate itself without reinfusion of harvested stem cells. This strategy is less expensive and is potentially more effective since no autoimmune lymphocytes are infused which potentially occurs when harvested stem cells are reinfused during a stem cell transplant.

## BIBLIOGRAPHY


1. Leipold G, Schutz E, Haas JP, Oellerich M: Azathioprine-induced severe pancytopenia due to a homozygous two-point mutation of the thiopurine methyltransferase gene in a patient with juvenile HLA-B27-associated spondyloarthritis. Arthritis Rheum 40:1896–1898, 1997.
2. Fields CL, Robinson JW, Roy TM, et al: Hypersensitivity reaction to azathioprine. South Med J 91:471–474, 1998.
3. Havrda DE, Rathbun S, Scheid D: A case report of warfarin resistance due to azathioprine and review of the literature. Pharmacotherapy 21:355–357, 2001.
4. Sievers TM, Rossi SJ, Ghobrial RM, et al: Mycophenylate mofetil. Pharmacotherapy 17:1178–1197, 1997.
5. Adu D, Cross J, Jayne DR: Treatment of systemic lupus erythematosus with mycophenylate mofetil. Lupus 10:203–208, 2001.
6. Blumenfeld Z, Shapiro D, Shteinberg M, et al: Preservation of fertility and ovarian function and minimizing gonadotoxicity in young women with systemic lupus erythematosus treated by chemotherapy. Lupus 9:401–405, 2000.
7. Pilmore HL, Faire B, Dittmer I: Tacrolimus for treatment of gout in renal transplantation. Transplantation 72:1703–1705, 2001.
8. Weinblatt ME, Kremer JM, Bankhurst AD, et al: A trial of etanercept, a recombinant tumor necrosis factor receptor:Fc fusion protein, in patients with rheumatoid arthritis receiving methotrexate. N Engl J Med 340:253–259, 1999.
9. Bathon JM, Martin RW, Roy MF, et al: A comparison of etanercept and methotrexate in patients with early rheumatoid arthritis. N Eng J Med 343:1586–1593, 2000.

10. Lipsky PE, van der Heijde DMFM, St. Clair EW, et al: Infliximab and methotrexate in the treatment of rheumatoid arthritis. N Engl J Med 343:1594–1602, 2000.
11. Keystone EC: Tumor necrosis factor-α blockade in the treatment of rheumatoid arthritis. Rheum Dis Clin North Am 27:427–444, 2001.
12. Mease PJ, Goffe BS, Metz J, et al: Etanercept in the treatment of psoriatic arthritis and psoriasis: A randomized trial. Lancet 356:385–390, 2000.
13. Keane J, Gershon S, Wise RP, et al: Tuberculosis associated with infliximab, a tumor necrosis factorα-neutralizing agent. N Engl J Med 345:1098–1104, 2001.
14. Mohan N, Edwards ET, Cupps TR, et al: Demyelination occurring during anti-tumor necrosis factor alpha therapy for inflammatory arthritides. Arthritis Rheum 44:2862–2869, 2001.
15. Cohen S, Hurd E, Cush J, et al: Treatment of rheumatoid arthritis with anakinra, a recombinant human interleukin-1 receptor antagonist, in combination with methotrexate: Results of a twenty-four-week, multicenter, randomized, double-blind, placebo-controlled trial. Arthritis Rheum 46:614–624, 2002.
16. Moreland, LW: Potential biologic agents for treatment of rheumatoid arthritis. Rheum Dis Clin North Am 27:445–492, 2001.
17. Klassen LW, Calabrese LH, Laxer RM: Intravenous immunoglobulin in rheumatic disease. Rheum Dis Clin North Am 22:155–174, 1996.
18. Lewis EJ, Hunsicker LG, Lan SP, et al: A controlled trial of plasmapheresis therapy in severe lupus nephritis. N Engl J Med 326:1373–1379, 1992.
19. Felson DT, LaValley MP, Boldassare AR, et al: The Prosorba column for treatment of refractory rheumatoid arthritis: A randomized, double-blind, sham-controlled trial. Arthritis Rheum 42:2153–2159, 1999.
20. Brodsky RA, Petri M, Smith BD, et al: Immunoablative high-dose cyclophosphamide without stem-cell rescue for refractory, severe autoimmune disease. Ann Intern Med 129:1031–1035, 1998.
21. Snowden JA, Brooks PM: Hematopoietic stem cell transplantation in rheumatic diseases. Curr Opin Rheumatol 11:167–172, 1999.
22. Stein CM: Immunoregulatory drugs. In Ruddy S, Harris ED, Sledge CD (eds): Kelley's Textbook of Rheumatology, 6th ed. Philadelphia, WB Saunders, 2001, pp 879–898.
23. O'Neil EA, Sloan VS: A potential mechanism for cyclosporin-associated bone pain. Arthritis Rheum 41:565–566, 1998.

# 88. HYPOURICEMIC AGENTS AND COLCHICINE

*David* R. *Finger*, M.D.

**1. Identify the goals in the treatment of gout.**

The first goal is safe and rapid treatment of acute gouty attacks to alleviate pain and restore joint function. This is usually done with NSAIDs or colchicine, but corticosteroids can also be used. Once this is accomplished, the next goal is to prevent recurrent attacks and the future development of destructive arthropathy, tophi formation, and nephrolithiasis.

**2. What is colchicine?**

Colchicine, an alkaloid derivative from the plant *Colchicum autumnale*, has been used in the treatment of acute gout for nearly two centuries and for joint pain since the 6th century. It has long been believed that the clinical response of acute arthritis to colchicine was diagnostic for gout, though other inflammatory arthropathies such as pseudogout and acute sarcoid arthritis respond as well. Garrod stated over a century ago that "colchicine possesses as specific a control over the gouty inflammation as cinchona barks over intermittent fever. . . . We may sometimes diagnose gouty from any other sort of inflammation by noting the influence of colchicine on its progress."

**3. When is colchicine therapy indicated? What are the correct dosages?**

Colchicine can be used in the treatment of acute gouty attacks and as prophylaxis against future attacks, especially when hypouricemic therapy is initiated. Colchicine is available orally in 0.5- and 0.6-mg tablets and in a parenteral solution of 0.5 mg/ml.

The average dose for **prophylaxis** is 0.5 mg twice daily. This dosage either completely prevents attacks or significantly lowers their frequency in > 90% of patients followed long-term, with minimal toxicity. Prophylaxis doses usually do not cause gastrointestinal side effects and should be continued until the patient is without symptoms of gout for several months.

For **acute attacks**, colchicine is most effective if given in the first few hours. The dosage can be as high as 0.5 mg/hr orally until relief or side effects occur, not to exceed 12 tablets (except in the elderly and those with renal insufficiency, who should receive fewer tablets). Pain is usually gone within 24 hours in 90% of patients, but many will experience diarrhea with this regimen.

**4. How do you use colchicine intravenously?**

You shouldn't. Many countries, including most hospitals in the United States, have removed parenteral colchicine from their formularies owing to its narrow therapeutic window, which has led to several deaths. While associated with less gastrointestinal side effects than oral administration, it can cause irreversible bone marrow suppression. There is always an alternative treatment option available, such as corticosteroids (IV, IM, or intra-articular) or ACTH.

*Contraindications to the Use of Intravenous Colchicine*

| ABSOLUTE | RELATIVE |
|---|---|
| Preexisting bone marrow depression | Recent use of colchicine within 7 days |
| Creatinine clearance < 10 ml/min | Hepatic or renal insufficiency |
| Extrahepatic biliary obstruction | Advanced age |
| Sepsis | Localized infection |

**5. Discuss the mechanism of action and pharmacokinetics of colchicine.**

Colchicine has no effect on serum urate concentration or on urate metabolism. It functions as an anti-inflammatory agent by inhibiting neutrophil chemotaxis through irreversible binding to tubulin dimers, preventing their assembly into microtubules. Colchicine also interferes with membrane-dependent functions of neutrophils such as phagocytosis, and inhibits phospholipase $A_2$, which can lead to lower levels of inflammatory prostaglandins and leukotrienes. Colchicine is not bound to plasma proteins and is highly lipid-soluble, readily passing into all tissues. The half-life is 4 hours following oral administration and < 1 hour parenterally. It can be detected in neutrophils up to 10 days after a single dose. It is hepatically metabolized and excreted principally in the bile, with 20% excreted unchanged in urine.

**6. Describe the different manifestations of colchicine toxicity.**

Most adverse effects of colchicine are dose-related and more likely to be observed following intravenous rather than oral administration (except for gastrointestinal side effects). There are no antidotes to overdose, and hemodialysis is ineffective. Potential side effects include:

Gastrointestinal effects (diarrhea, nausea, vomiting, rarely malabsorption syndrome and hemorrhagic gastroenteritis)—usually seen following oral administration

Bone marrow suppression (thrombocytopenia, leukopenia)

Neuromyopathy (elevated creatine kinase, proximal weakness, peripheral neuropathy, lysosomal vacuoles on biopsy)—usually seen in renal insufficiency with chronic dosing

Alopecia

Shock, disseminated intravascular coagulation (parenteral)

CNS dysfunction

Cellulitis or thrombophlebitis (parenteral)

**7. What antihyperuricemic agents are available?**

Antihyperuricemic agents include uricosurics (probenecid and sulfinpyrazone), which reduce the serum urate concentration by enhancing renal excretion of uric acid, and **xanthine oxidase inhibitors** (allopurinol and oxipurinol), which inhibit uric acid synthesis by inhibiting xanthine oxidase, the final enzyme involved in the production of uric acid. These agents should be initiated only after an acute attack of gout has resolved entirely.

The risk of acute gouty attacks following the initiation of antihyperuricemic therapy can be minimized by gradual dose increases and by prophylaxis with colchicine or NSAIDs. The decision to use uric acid-lowering therapy is usually a lifelong commitment, so it is essential that these agents are initiated only when they are truly indicated. Uricosurics can be safely used concomitantly with allopurinol in some patients with severe tophaceous gout.

**8. Which patients with recurrent gouty arthritis are candidates for uricosuric therapy?**

- Hyperuricemia secondary to underexcretion of uric acid (< 700 mg of uric acid in a 24-hour urine collection, while on a regular diet)
- Age < 60 yrs
- Creatinine clearance > 50 ml/min
- No history of nephrolithiasis

**9. Identify some uricosuric agents and describe their mechanism of action.**

Many drugs have uricosuric properties, including high-dose aspirin or salicylates, but the two most common agents used clinically are **probenecid** and **sulfinpyrazone**. Uricosuric agents are weak organic acids, like uric acid, and they increase urinary excretion of uric acid by competitively inhibiting tubular reabsorption of urate. These agents are successful in lowering the serum uric acid to < 6.7 mg/dl in 75% of patients. Low doses of aspirin or salicylates should be avoided, since they inhibit urate secretion. Uricosurics work better when there is good urine alkalinization and flow (> 1500 ml/day) to minimize the risk of uric acid nephropathy and nephrolithiasis.

**10. How are probenecid and sulfinpyrazone dosed? How do these drugs differ?**

**Sulfinpyrazone** is an analogue of a phenylbutazone metabolite but possesses no anti-inflammatory properties. This drug is 98% bound to plasma proteins and has a half-life of 1–3 hours. Twenty to 45% is excreted unchanged in the urine, with most as a uricosuric metabolite. Unlike probenecid, sulfinpyrazone has antiplatelet activity through inhibition of thromboxane synthesis. It is available in 100-mg and 200-mg oral preparations, and is dosed initially at 50 mg twice daily but increased gradually to maintenance levels of 300–400 mg/day in three or four divided doses. Sulfinpyrazone is more effective than probenecid in patients with renal insufficiency and is 3–6 times more potent.

**Probenecid** has a longer half-life (6–12 hours) and is more extensively metabolized than sulfinpyrazone. Allopurinol prolongs the half-life of probenecid, while probenecid prolongs the half-life of penicillin, ampicillin, dapsone, indomethacin, and sulfinpyrazone by decreasing their renal excretion and prolongs the metabolism of heparin. Probenecid is available in 500-mg tablets. It is dosed initially at 250 mg twice daily but can be increased gradually up to 3 gm daily (average dose 1 gm/day) in 2–3 divided doses.

**11. What are the side effects of uricosuric therapy?**

Uricosuric therapy is generally well tolerated by > 90% of patients, and serious side effects only occur rarely.

**Preventable**
- Acute gouty attacks
- Urate nephropathy
- Urate nephrolithiasis

**Relatively common**
- Gastrointestinal symptoms (10%)
- Dermatitis (5%)
- Headache
- Drug fever

**Rare**
- Hemolytic anemia
- Aplastic anemia
- Nephrotic syndrome
- Hepatic necrosis
- Anaphylaxis

**12. Which inhibitors of uric acid synthesis are available?**

**Allopurinol**, a hypoxanthine analogue, is the most commonly used inhibitor of uric acid synthesis. **Oxipurinol** (Oxiprim) (100–600 mg/d), a xanthine analogue and the major metabolite of allopurinol, is used in Europe but is not yet widely available in the United States. Although it has poor gastrointestinal absorption, it can be used in patients who have allergic reactions to allopurinol, although up to 40% will have reactions to oxipurinol also.

**13. What are the indications for using allopurinol?**

Indications in patients with recurrent gout include:

1. Urate overproduction (uric acid > 700 mg in 24-hr urine collection on a regular diet)
2. Nephrolithiasis
3. Renal insufficiency (creatinine in clearance < 50 ml/min)
4. Tophi (may take several months to resolve)
5. Failure or intolerance of uricosuric agents

Other indications for allopurinol include:

1. Hyperuricemia with nephrolithiasis of any type
2. Prophylaxis against tumor lysis syndrome
3. Hypoxanthine phosphoribosyltransferase (HPRT) deficiency (Lesch-Nyhan syndrome)
4. Hyperuricemia due to myeloproliferative disorders
5. Serum urate > 12.0 mg/dl or 24-hr urine uric acid > 1100 mg

**14. Describe the mechanism of action and pharmacokinetic properties of allopurinol.**

Allopurinol lowers blood and urine urate concentrations by inhibiting the enzyme xanthine oxidase, thus leading to increases in the precursors xanthine and hypoxanthine. Allopurinol itself is metabolized by xanthine oxidase to the active metabolite, oxipurinol, which can be measured to assess compliance. Drugs that depend on this enzyme for their metabolism, such as 6-mercaptopurine and azathioprine, require a 50–75% dose reduction if they are given concomitantly with allopurinol. Allopurinol is well absorbed from the gastrointestinal tract and has a half-life of 40 minutes, while oxipurinol is poorly absorbed and has a much longer half-life (14–28 hours). The dosage of allopurinol must be lowered in the presence of renal insufficiency. The maximum antihyperuricemic effect is seen 7–14 days after starting allopurinol.

**15. How is allopurinol dosed?**

Allopurinol is available orally in 100- and 300-mg tablets, usually given in once-daily doses, to lower the serum urate < 6.0 mg/dl. The average dose needed to accomplish this is 300 mg/day but can be as high as 600 mg. One should investigate other correctable factors leading to hyperuricemia if it requires > 300 mg/day to achieve adequate uric acid levels, although non-compliance may be the most common cause. The dose should be reduced in the presence of renal insufficiency because oxipurinol is renally excreted. The dose should be lowered to 200 mg/day when the GFR approaches 60 ml/min and to 100 mg/day when it reaches 30 ml/min.

**16. List the major toxicities of allopurinol.**

The overall incidence of side effects is around 20%, but only 5% of all patients discontinue therapy as a result of drug toxicity.

**Common (rarely serious)**

Acute gouty arthritis
Maculopapular erythematous rash (risk three times higher if on ampicillin)
Nausea
Diarrhea
Abnormal liver-associated enzymes
Headache
Cataracts

**Uncommon (potentially serious)**

| | |
|---|---|
| Toxic epidermal necrolysis, exfoliative dermatitis | Oxipurinol xanthine nephrolithiasis |
| Allopurinol hypersensitivity syndrome | Cataracts |
| Bone marrow suppression | Sarcoid-like reaction |
| Hepatitis | Alopecia |
| Vasculitis | Lymphadenopathy |
| Peripheral neuropathy | Fever |
| Renal failure (interstitial nephritis) | Death |

**17. What can be done in a gouty patient who develops a maculopapular rash on allopurinol?**

An estimated 3% of patients on allopurinol, particularly those with renal insufficiency, will develop a pruritic maculopapular rash. After stopping the drug and the rash resolves, a gouty patient can undergo oral desensitization starting at 50 μg and slowly increasing to 100 mg by 1 month. Overall, this procedure is successful in 70–80% of patients. Desensitization is not done in patients who have had serious reactions such as Stevens-Johnson syndrome, toxic epidermal necrolysis, vasculitis, or allopurinol hypersensitivity syndrome.

**18. What is the allopurinol hypersensitivity syndrome?**

The allopurinol hypersensitivity syndrome can occurs in approximately 5–10% of patients who experience an allopurinol rash. Patients who develop this syndrome usually have associated renal insufficiency (75%) and are on diuretic therapy (50%). This typically occurs 2–4 weeks after initiating therapy, with significant morbidity and a mortality rate as high as 25%. Clinical manifestations of this syndrome include skin rash, fever, eosinophilia, hepatic necrosis, leukocytosis, and worsening renal function in most patients. Treatment includes high-dose steroids and hemodialysis (to remove oxipurinol).

**19. An organ transplant patient with recurrent gouty arthritis and tophi is referred to you for treatment. His medications include prednisone, cyclosporine, and azathioprine. Laboratories include creatinine 1.8 mg/dl and uric acid 12 mg/dl. What precautions must be taken when prescribing medications for his tophaceous gout?**

Acute gout attacks:

- NSAIDs can't be used, owing to renal insufficiency.
- ACTH can't be used, owing to lack of adrenal response since patient is on chronic prednisone.
- Best therapy is oral, IM, or IA steroids.

Chronic suppression

- Colchicine can be dangerous. Even one tablet a day can cause a severe neuromyopathy in a patient taking cyclosporine. The multidrug resistance ( MDR-1) transport system is important in hepatic and renal transport of colchicine. Cyclosporine is an inhibitor of MDR-mediated transport and as such will amplify the toxic effects of colchicine because it won't be excreted.

Hypouricemic therapy

- Uricosuric medications are ineffective in patients with low creatinine clearance.
- Allopurinol inhibits xanthine oxidase, which also breaks down azathioprine. Consequently, azathioprine toxicity is magnified unless its dose is decreased 75%. Another option is to switch from azathioprine to mycophenylate mofetil, which is not affected by allopurinol.
- Owing to renal insufficiency, allopurinol dose is adjusted to give 100 mg for each 30 cc/min of creatinine clearance. Can follow serum oxipurinol levels to titrate to therapeutic level.

**20. Identify the sites of action for drugs that are used to treat acute gout and to lower serum urate levels.**

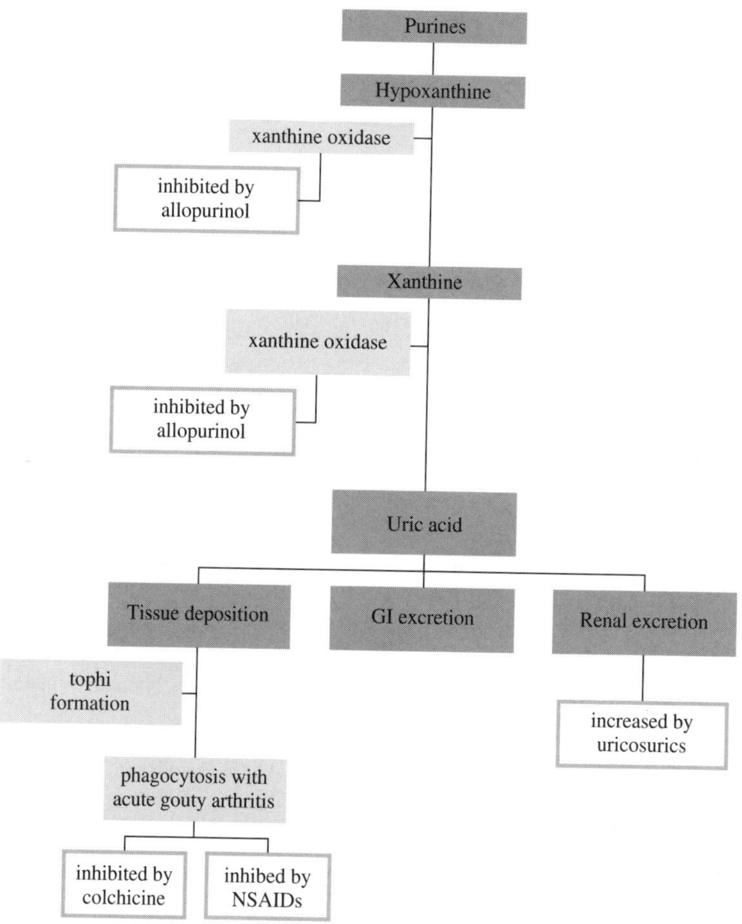


Drugs used in the treatment of gout and their sites of action. (Adapted from Klippel JH, Dieppe PA [eds]: Rheumatology. London, Mosby, 1994; with permission.)

**21. What therapies may be available in the future for gout?**

Benzbromarone is a uricosuric that is effective even in patients with creatinine clearance as low as 25 mg/min. Lisinopril, an angiotensin converting enzyme inhibitor, has a mild uricosuric effect. Oxipurinol is at present in trials and should be widely available in the future for allopurinol sensitive patients. Urate oxidase, or uricase, is an enzyme from *Aspergillus flavus* that catalyzes the conversion of uric acid to allantoin which is 10 times more soluble and easier for the kidney to eliminate. A parenteral recombinant uricase is at present in trials.

## BIBLIOGRAPHY

1. Agudelo CA, Wise CM: Crystal-associated arthritis in the elderly. Rheum Dis Clin North Am 26:527–546, 2000.
2. Ben-Chetrit E, Levy M: Colchicine: 1998 update. Semin Arthritis Rheum 28:48–59, 1998.
3. Emmerson BT: The management of gout. N Engl J Med 334:445–451, 1996.
4. Fam AG: Should patients with interval gout be treated with urate lowering drugs? J Rheumatol 22:1621–1623, 1995.
5. Fam AG, Dunne SM, Iazzetta J, Paton RW: Efficacy and safety of desensitization to allopurinol following cutaneous reactions. Arthritis Rheum 44:231–238, 2001.

6. Ferraz MB, O'Brien B: A cost effectiveness analysis of urate lowering drugs in nontophaceous recurrent gouty arthritis. J Rheumatol 22:908–914, 1995.
7. Perez Ruiz F, Calabozo M, Ferenendez Lopez J, et al: Treatment of chronic gout in patients with renal function impairment. J Clin Rheumatol 5:49–55, 1999.
8. Simkin PA, Gardner GC: Colchicine use in cyclosporine treated transplant recipients: How little is too much? J Rheumatol 27:1334–1337, 2000.
9. Singer JZ, Wallace SL: The allopurinol hypersensitivity syndrome: Unnecessary morbidity and mortality. Arthritis Rheum 29:82–87, 1986.
10. Terkeltaub RA: Pathogenesis and treatment of crystal-induced inflammation. In Koopman WJ (Ed): Arthritis and Allied Conditions, 14th ed. Philadelphia, Williams & Wilkins, 2001, pp 2329–2347.
11. Walter-Sack I, de Vries JX, Ernst B, et al: Uric acid lowering effect of oxipurinol sodium in hyperuricemic patients: Therapeutic equivalence to allopurinol. J Rheumatol 23:498–501, 1996.
12. Wortmann RL: Management of hyperuricemia. In Koopman WJ (ed): Arthritis and Allied Conditions, 14th ed. Philadelphia, Williams & Wilkins, 2001, pp 2314–2328.


# 89. BONE-STRENGTHENING AGENTS

*Michael* T. *McDermott*, M.D.

**1. Define bone remodeling.**

This is the process by which osteoclasts resorb old bone and osteoblasts secrete osteoid, which subsequently becomes mineralized with hydroxyapatite crystals to form new bone. Bone remodeling ensures that weak, older bone is removed and strong, new bone is formed in skeletal areas subject to the greatest mechanical stress.

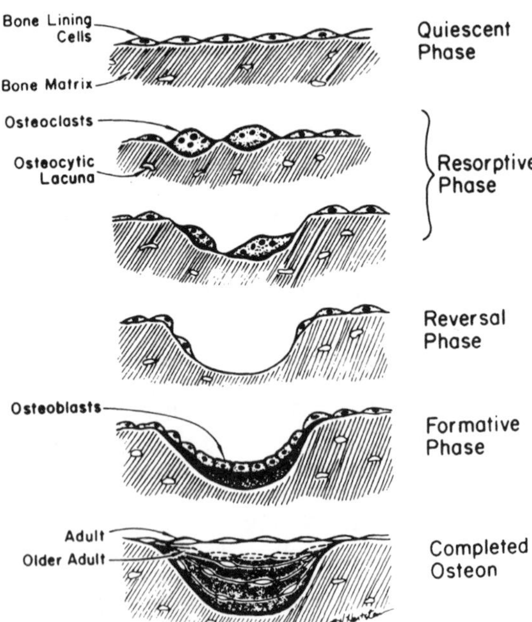


Bone remodeling. Osteoclasts resorb old bone, leaving an empty resorption pit. Osteoblasts then fill the pit by secreting osteoid, which is subsequently mineralized by calcium and phosphate from the extracellular fluid, forming new bone. (From Peck WA, ed: Bone and Mineral Research Annual 2. New York, Elsevier, 1984; with permission.)

**2. How does bone resorption occur?**

Bone resorption occurs when hematopoietic stem cells are recruited to form new osteoclasts. These multinucleated giant cells attach to bone surfaces by their ruffled borders and secrete acid and proteolytic enzymes that degrade bone. Osteoclastic bone resorption is stimulated primarily by circulating parathyroid hormone (PTH) and by locally produced cytokines, such as interleukin-6. It is inhibited by calcitonin, sex steroids, and other cytokines.

**3. How is bone formation regulated?**

Bone formation occurs when osteoblasts secrete osteoid that is subsequently mineralized by the deposition of hydroxyapatite (calcium-phosphate) crystals. Bone formation is stimulated by PTH, sex steroids, insulin-like growth factor 1, and locally produced cytokines.

**4. What markers are available to assess bone remodeling?**

| BONE FORMATION | BONE RESORPTION |
|---|---|
| Serum alkaline phosphatase | Urine N-telopeptides |
| Serum osteocalcin | Serum N-telopeptides |
| | Urine pyridinoline crosslinks |

**5. What therapeutic interventions effectively alter bone remodeling?**

| BONE-RESORPTION—INHIBITING AGENTS | BONE-FORMATION—STIMULATING AGENTS |
|---|---|
| Estrogen | Fluoride |
| Bisphosphonates | Androgens |
| Raloxifene | Growth hormone |
| Calcitonin | Parathyroid hormone |

**6. How do antiresorptive and formation-stimulating agents affect bone mass?**

Antiresorptive drugs characteristically increase bone mass during the first 12–24 months of treatment and then stabilize it at a constant level thereafter. Bone-formation—stimulating agents typically bring about a progressive linear increase in bone mass in most treated patients.

**7. Why do antiresorptive agents increase bone mass?**

These drugs significantly reduce bone resorption without affecting bone formation; as a result, bone formation temporarily exceeds resorption and bone mass increases. This phenomenon is referred to as the **bone remodeling transient**. After 12–24 months, bone formation gradually declines to the level of resorption and bone mass stabilizes.

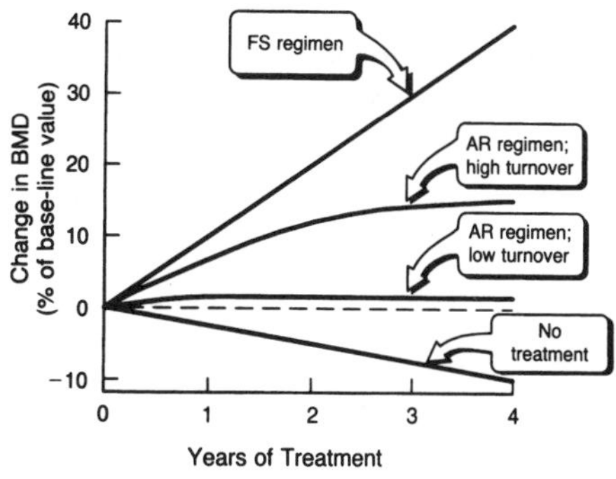


Bone mineral density (BMD) response to therapeutic interventions. Formation-stimulating (FS) agents produce a progressive linear increase in BMD. Antiresorptive (AR) agents transiently increase BMD 5–20% in high-turnover osteoporosis and 0–4% in low-turnover osteoporosis, after which they maintain BMD at a stable level. (From Riggs BL, Melton III LJ: The prevention and treatment of osteoporosis. N Engl J Med 327:620–627, 1992, with permission.)

**8. How effective are the antiresorptive agents in the treatment of osteoporosis?**

The efficacy of medications is best assessed by their effects on bone mass and on fracture reduction.

Reported bone mass increments observed over a 2–3 year period:

| MEDICATION | SPINE | HIP |
|---|---|---|
| Alendronate | 7–8% | 5–6% |
| Risedronate | 4–5% | 2–3% |
| Estrogens | 5–6% | 3–4% |
| Raloxifene | 2–3% | 2–3% |
| Calcitonin | 0–1% | 0% |

Observed reductions in fracture incidence:

| MEDICATION | SPINE | HIP |
|---|---|---|
| Alendronate | 47–50% | 51–56% |
| Risedronate | 33–46% | 8–58% |
| Estrogens | 42% | No data |
| Raloxifene | 31–49% | 0 |
| Calcitonin | 33% | 0 |

**9. Explain how bisphosphonates are used in the treatment of osteoporosis.**

The following bisphosphonates are clinically available, although only two (alendronate, risedronate) are currently FDA-approved for the treatment of osteoporosis because they are the only agents with proven anti-fracture efficacy at both the spine and the hip.

| MEDICATION | DOSE |
|---|---|
| Alendronate (Fosamax) | 10 mg p.o. q day or 70 mg p.o. q week |
| Risedronate (Actonel) | 5 mg p.o. q day |
| Etidronate (Didronel) | 200 p.o. BID 14 days every 3 months |
| Pamidronate (Aredia) | 30 mg IV every 3 months |

The oral bisphosphonates have very poor intestinal absorption that is further inhibited by the presence of food or medications in the gastrointestinal tract. Their major side effect is esophageal/gastrointestinal pain. In order to maximize intestinal absorption and to minimize gastrointestinal toxicity, they should be taken first thing each morning on an empty stomach with a full glass of water. The patient should then remain upright and take nothing by mouth for at least 30 minutes after medication ingestion. Alendronate is also available in a once-a-week preparation that may provide a more convenient dosing regimen with efficacy, toxicity, and cost that are similar to the daily dose regimen. Etidronate or pamidronate may be considered in patients who are unable to take one of the FDA approved agents.

**10. Discuss the use of hormone replacement therapy in the management of osteoporosis.**

The following hormone preparations are commonly used for hormone replacement therapy.

| MEDICATION | DOSE REGIMEN |
|---|---|
| Conjugated estrogens | |
| Premarin | .625–1.25 mg q day or days 1–25 |
| Estratabs | .625–1.25 mg q day or days 1–25 |
| Estradiol | |
| Estrace | .5–1.0 mg q day or days 1–25 |
| Estradiol patch | |
| Estraderm | .05–0.1 mg patch twice a week |
| Vivelle | .05–0.1 mg patch twice a week |
| Climara | .05–0.1 mg patch once a week |
| Combination pills | |
| Prempro | .625/2.5 mg or .625/5.0 mg (Premarin/Provera) q day |
| Premphase | .625 mg (Premarin) days 1–14, then .625/5.0 mg (Premarin/Provera) days 15–25 |

| MEDICATION | DOSE REGIMEN |
|---|---|
| Combination pills (*cont.*) | |
| OrthoPrefest | 1 mg (estradiol) q day for 3 days, then 1 mg/.09 mg (estradiol/norgestimate) q day for 3 days in repeat cycles |
| Combination patch | |
| Combipatch | .05/.14 mg or .05/.25 mg patch (estradiol/norethindrone) twice a week |
| Medroxyprogesterone | |
| Provera | 2.5–5 mg qd or 5–10 mg days 15–25 |

Unopposed estrogens significantly increase the risk of developing endometrial carcinoma. For this reason, women with an intact uterus must take estrogen in combination with progesterone, either cyclically (example: Premarin .625 mg days 1–25, Provera 5–10 mg days 15–25) or daily (example: Premarin .625 mg q day, Provera 2.5 mg q day). Hormone replacement therapy also appears to moderately increase the risk of developing breast cancer and thromboembolic disease. Counseling about and monitoring for these conditions are therefore indicated in patients on hormone replacement therapy.

**11. Discuss the use of selective estrogen receptor modulators (SERMS) in the management of osteoporosis.**

Selective estrogen receptor modulators (SERMS) are agents that function as estrogen agonists in some tissues and estrogen antagonists in other tissues. Raloxifene (Evista) is a SERM that has been shown to improve bone mass and to reduce spine fractures; it is FDA-approved for the treatment of postmenopausal osteoporosis. Raloxifene has also been shown to reduce the risk of developing breast cancer. The dose is 60 mg q day. Side effects include hot flashes, leg cramps, and an increased risk of thromboembolic disease similar to that seen with hormone replacement therapy.

**12. How is calcitonin used in the management of osteoporosis?**

Calcitonin is available as both intranasal (200 units q day) and injectable (100 units q day) preparations. This FDA-approved medication has been shown to modestly improve spinal bone mass and to reduce the incidence of spinal fractures. Potential side effects include nausea, nasal irritation (nasal spray) and skin irritation (injections). Calcitonin may also have some mild to moderate analgesic effects.

**13. Can the antiresorptive agents be used in combination with one another?**

Yes. Combinations of bisphosphonates and estrogens produce increments in bone mass that are greater than those observed when the drugs are used alone. Similar results have been reported when bisphosphonates are used with raloxifene. There have been no studies to date having sufficient power or duration to adequately demonstrate greater fracture reduction efficacy with combination therapy. Nonetheless, because bone histomorphometry is normal in patients treated with these regimens, it is predicted that they will likely reduce fractures to a greater degree than is seen with single drug therapy.

**14. How does PTH therapy stimulate bone formation and what effects does it have on bone mass?**

The most promising bone formation-stimulating agent on the horizon is parathyroid hormone (PTH). PTH is known to stimulate both bone formation and bone resorption in humans. Persistently elevated serum PTH levels, as seen in hyperparathyroidism, stimulate bone resorption more than formation and thereby cause bone loss. However, when PTH is given as single daily injections, the transient PTH bursts disproportionately enhance bone formation. Patients treated with PTH have been reported to have bone mass increments of nearly 15% in the lumbar spine and approximately 5% in the hip over 1–2 year study periods. Furthermore, vertebral fracture risk has been reported to decrease by as much as 65% in treated patients. There are no current studies that have been sufficiently powered to assess hip fractures, but based on bone densitometry changes and normal histomorphometry reports, it is likely that hip fracture risk will also be reduced. It is anticipated that PTH will soon be approved by the FDA and be available for the treatment of patients with osteoporosis.

**15. What are the skeletal effects of sodium fluoride?**

Sodium fluoride appears to directly stimulate osteoblasts and has been reported to increase bone mass by 16–20% over a 4-year treatment period. Although fracture reduction efficacy has been disappointing with daily sodium fluoride use, one study has reported both increased bone mass and a reduction of new vertebral fractures using an investigational intermittent slow-release sodium fluoride preparation. Because of lack of consistently demonstrated anti-fracture efficacy and long-term safety data, sodium fluoride is not currently approved by the FDA for osteoporosis treatment. Many experts agree, however, that we just have not yet discovered the best way to utilize this drug.

Symptomatic gastritis develops in 20–30% of patients on 50 mg/day dosages of sodium fluoride and in up to 50% of patients on 75 mg/day dosages. A painful lower-extremity syndrome, consisting of acute pain, tenderness, and swelling in the lower extremities, particularly the heels and ankles, also occurs in many patients. The disorder appears to be due to the development of stress fractures, probably related to rapid bone turnover. With rest and analgesia, resolution usually occurs in 6–8 weeks after the medication is discontinued. This syndrome tends not to recur if sodium fluoride is later re-instituted. A lower incidence of side effects has been reported with the investigational slow release sodium fluoride preparation.

**16. Are androgens useful as an osteoporosis therapy?**

Androgens are anabolic agents that also stimulate osteoblastic bone formation. Methyltestosterone (2.5 mg/day) given in combination with estrogens to postmenopausal women has been shown to increase bone mass significantly more than do estrogens alone. However, improved anti-fracture efficacy has not been demonstrated. Hirsutism, acne, and temporal balding are potential side effects with androgen treatment in women but are dose-related and therefore may be mild or absent with lower doses. Testosterone replacement therapy significantly increases skeletal mass in hypogonadal males but it has not been shown to have a beneficial effect in eugonadal males.

**17. How effective are growth hormone and insulin-like growth factor 1 therapy?**

Growth hormone (GH) is another anabolic agent that may promote bone formation. Although clearly beneficial in children and adults with GH deficiency, its effects in women with postmenopausal and senile osteoporosis have been moderate at best. GH therapy is also costly and may cause complications, such as arthralgias, acral enlargement, hyperglycemia, and hypertension. Studies with IGF-1 have only recently begun but its effects on bone remodeling appear to be beneficial.

**18. What is coherence therapy?**

Coherence therapy is a program in which an anti-resorptive medication is used in combination with or alternating with a bone formation-stimulating agent. Recently, combinations of alendronate with PTH and estrogens with PTH have been shown to increase bone mass significantly more than does any single agent alone. Although anti-fracture efficacy has not yet been demonstrated, these findings are very promising, particularly as a treatment approach for patients with very low bone mass.

**19. What is the role of exercise in osteoporosis management?**

Exercise stimulates bone formation and inhibits resorption. It may also reduce the incidence and severity of falls by improving muscular strength and coordination. Both aerobic and weight-training are beneficial.

**20. What percentage of patients sustaining an osteoporotic fragility fracture are evaluated for and/or placed on medical therapy for osteoporosis?**

Multiple studies have demonstrated that less than 25% are even put on calcium and vitamin D much less any other therapy. This represents a breakdown in medical care.

**21. What are vertebroplasty and kyphoplasty?**

New techniques to treat the pain and deformity of vertebral compression fractures. Vertebroplasty is the percutaneous injection under high pressure of polymethylmethacrylate (PMM) into a fractured vertebral body to relieve pain. Although successful for pain relief, it does not restore vertebral height and there is a high rate of cement leakage. Kyphoplasty involves percutaneous replacement of an inflatable balloon into the fractured vertebral body. Inflation results in the elevation of depressed vertebral body endplates, thereby restoring vertebral body height. The balloon is removed, and PMM is injected under low pressure (which results in less cement extravasation) into the void in the vertebrae. The ideal candidate is a patient with a recent vertebral fracture. Older vertebral fractures that show no evidence of bone marrow edema on MRI are less likely to respond.

## BIBLIOGRAPHY


1. Black DM, Cummings SR, Karpf DB, et al: Randomized trial of effect of alendronate on risk of fracture in women with existing vertebral fractures Lancet 348:1535–1541, 1996.
2. Chapuy MC, Arlot ME, Duboeuf F, et al: Vitamin $D_3$ and calcium to prevent hip fractures in elderly women. N Engl J Med 327:1637–1642, 1992.
3. Chesnut CH, Silverman S, Andriano K, et al: A randomized trial of nasal spray salmon calcitonin in postmenopausal women with established osteoporosis: The Prevent Recurrence of Osteoporotic Fractures Study. Am J Med 109:267–276, 2000.
4. Cummings SR, Black DM, Cummings SR, et al: Effect of alendronate on risk of fracture in women with low bone density but without vertebral fractures. JAMA 280:2077–2082, 1998.
5. Delmas P, Bjarnason NH, Mitlak BH, et al: Effects of raloxifene on bone mineral density, serum cholesterol concentrations, and uterine endometrium in postmenopausal women. N Engl J Med 337:1641–1647, 1997.
6. Eastell R: Treatment of postmenopausal osteoporosis. N Engl J Med 338:736–746, 1998.
7. Ettinger B, Black DM, Mitlak BH, et al: Reduction of vertebral fracture risk in postmenopausal women with osteoporosis treated with raloxifene. JAMA 282:637–645, 1999.
8. Harris ST, Watts NB, Genant HK, et al: Effects of risedronate treatment on vertebral and nonvertebral fractures in women with postmenopausal osteoporosis. A randomized controlled trial. JAMA 282:1344–1352, 1999.
9. Holloway L, Kohlmeier L, Kent K, Marcus R: Skeletal effects of cyclic recombinant human growth hormone and salmon calcitonin in osteopenic postmenopausal women. J Clin Endocrinol Metab 82:1111–1117, 1997.
10. Hosking D, Chilvers CED, Christiansen C, et al: Prevention of bone loss with alendronate in postmenopausal women. N Engl J Med 338:485–492, 1998.
11. Khovidhunkit W, Shoback DM: Clinical effects of raloxifene hydrochloride in women. Ann Intern Med 130:431–439, 1999.
12. Liberman UA, Weiss SR, Broll J, et al: Effect of oral alendronate on bone mineral density and the incidence of fractures in postmenopausal osteoporosis. N Engl J Med 333:1437–1443, 1995.
13. Lindsay R, Cosman F, Lobo RA, et al: Addition of alendronate to ongoing hormone replacement therapy in the treatment of osteoporosis: A randomized, controlled clinical trial. J Clin Endocrinol Metab 84:3076–3081, 1999.
14. Lufkin EG, Wahner HW, O'Fallon WM, et al: Treatment of postmenopausal osteoporosis with transdermal estrogen. Ann Intern Med 117:1–9, 1992.
15. Manolagas SC, Jilka RL: Bone marrow, cytokines and bone remodeling. Emerging insights into the pathophysiology of osteoporosis. N Engl J Med 332:305–311, 1995.
16. Overgaard K, Hansen MA, Jensen SB, Christiansen C: Effect of salcatonin given intranasally on bone mass and fracture rates in established osteoporosis: A dose-response study. BMJ 305:556–561, 1992.
17. Pak CYC, Sakhaee K, Adams-Huet B, et al: Treatment of postmenopausal osteoporosis with slow release sodium fluoride. Final report of a randomized controlled trial. Ann Intern Med 123:401–408, 1995.
18. Reginster J-Y, Minn HW, Sorensen OH, et al: Randomized trial of the effects of risedronate on vertebral fractures in women with established postmenopausal osteoporosis. Osteoporos Int 11:83–91, 2000.
19. Riggs BL, Hodgson SF, O'Fallon WM, et al: Effect of fluoride treatment on the fracture rate in postmenopausal women. N Engl J Med 322:802–809, 1990.
20. Riggs BL, Melton LJ III: The prevention and treatment of osteoporosis. N Engl J Med 327:620–627, 1992.
21. Rittmaster RS, Bolognese M, Ettinger MP, et al: Enhancement of bone mass in osteoporotic women with parathyroid hormone followed by alendronate. J Clin Endocrinol Metab 85:2129–2134, 2000.
22. The writing group for the PEPI trial: Effects of hormone therapy on bone mineral density. Results for the postmenopausal estrogen/progestin interventions (PEPI) trial. JAMA 276:1389–1396, 1996.

# 90. PAIN: THE FIFTH VITAL SIGN

Sterling G. West, M.D.

*The greatest evil is physical pain.*
St. Augustine (354–430 AD)

**1. What is the origin of the term *pain*?**

Pain is derived from the Latin *Poena*, meaning punishment. Our approach to pain has changed over the past decade and can be summarized by Kübler-Ross' statement, "There is not much sense in suffering, since drugs can be given for pain, itching, and other discomforts. The belief has long died that suffering here on earth will be rewarded in heaven."

**2. How is pain defined? Why does it vary among individuals?**

Pain is defined as "an unpleasant sensory and emotional experience associated with actual or potential tissue damage or described in terms of such damage." However, pain cannot be viewed simply as a stimulus followed by a similar response in all individuals. The neurons that transmit pain can be congenitally different between individuals and be significantly influenced by extrinsic input, including cognitive, emotional, and environmental factors. This helps to explain why there is a difference in pain sensation among individuals to the same noxious stimuli, i.e., we are not all "wired" the same. The clinical implications are clear. There will be differences in the amount of medications required to control pain, and behavioral modification and psychologic support can help modulate a patient's perception of pain.

**3. How do acute pain and chronic pain differ?**

**Acute**: sudden onset, clear-cut etiology, associated with autonomic nervous system hyperactivity, including tachycardia, increased blood pressure, and anxiety.

**Chronic**: pain that lasts for at least 3 months. Typically, there is an adaptation to sympathetic hyperactivity. Patients frequently have depression, social withdrawal, and personality and lifestyle changes.

**4. Discuss the different types of pain.**

1. Organic(identifiable cause)
   - Nociceptic: nociceptors are found in cutaneous or deep tissues like the musculoskeletal system (somatic pain) and organs (visceral pain). This pain results from direct stimulation of intact peripheral afferent nerve endings that are sensitive to noxious mechanical, thermal or chemical stimuli. Somatic pain is aching or throbbing and localized while visceral pain is dull, deep, and may be referred to a different region.
   - Neuropathic: caused by injury or disease affecting central (thalamic syndrome) or peripheral nervous system. Pain may be constant and steady or lancinating and described as burning, shooting, or tingling. Pain can be altered sensations (dysesthesias), electric shock sensation (paresthesias), hyperalgesia (extreme sensitivity to painful stimuli), or allodynia (pain with touch).
   - Complex regional pain syndrome: a syndrome of pain in an extremity mediated by sympathetic overactivity that does not involve a major nerve (see Chapter 69).
2. Idiopathic (psychogenic): somatoform pain disorder that lacks an identifiable organic cause.

**Pearl**: Each of these types of pain are treated differently.

**5. What is the epidemiology of chronic pain?**

- Affects 20% of adult population (15% regional, 5–8% widespread)
- Increased in women and elderly (> age 60).

- Third leading cause of lost work days.
- Low back pain, osteoarthritis, fibromyalgia, and peripheral neuropathy are most common causes of chronic musculoskeletal pain. Headache is also a common cause of chronic pain.
- Genetic polymorphisms and cultural influences explain differences between races and ethnic groups.

**6. Describe the neural pathways involved in pain perception.**

The pain signal from somatic and visceral tissues is transmitted from nociceptors on primary afferent nerves of the peripheral nervous system. These nociceptors can be activated by the chemical products of tissue damage and inflammation (e.g., prostaglandins, kinins, free radicals). These chemicals can directly activate these receptors or sensitize them to other mechanical, thermal, and chemical stimuli. The stimulated nociceptors generate signals that are transmitted along myelinated and unmyelinated nerve fibers. The small, myelinated A-delta fibers transmit pain signals rapidly (milliseconds to seconds) and are experienced as sharp pain such as when you first hit your thumb with a hammer. Unmyelinated C-fibers transmit signals and produce slow-building, dull (or burning) chronic pain, which is the prolonged aching after the initial hammer injury. Eighty percent of fibers in peripheral nerves are unmyelinated and more than 90% of those are nociceptive. Sodium and calcium channels in the nerve membrane are important in the activation of nociceptors and transmission of the pain signal.

Peripheral primary afferent nerves arise from cell bodies in the dorsal root ganglion. These cell bodies send central projections that terminate in the dorsal horn of the spinal cord gray matter, in an area called the substantia gelatinosa (levels I and II). Noxious stimuli activate the primary efferent peripheral nerves to release neurotransmitters of nociception within the dorsal horn, including the excitatory amino acids (EAAs, such as glutamate and aspartate) and a number of neuropeptides (e.g., substance P, calcitonin gene-related peptide, cholecystokinin, and neurokinin). EAAs act on N-methyl-D-aspartate (NMDA) as well as other receptors such as AMPA. Neuropeptides such as substance P act on neurokinin (NK) receptors. Stimulation of these post-synaptic receptors activates and sensitizes projection neurons that originate from level V in the dorsal horn by opening sodium and calcium channels and by increasing intracellular calcium stores. These spinal projection neurons traverse the spinothalamic and spinoreticular tracts to the pons/midbrain reticular formation and the sensory nuclei of the thalamus. The lateral part of the medial thalamic nuclei discriminates acute pain, whereas the medial part processes chronic pain. From the thalamus, neurons project pain impulses to the somatosensory regions within the post-central parietal cortex and other areas of the brain where pain is perceived. The anterior cingulate cortex is important in the affective and attentional components of pain perception.

Pain control pharmacology relies on an understanding of these pain pathways. NSAIDs counteract the chemical products released during inflammation and tissue damage. Abnormal ectopic activity of nociceptors can be inhibited by sodium channel blockers (i.e., lidocaine, mexiletine, anticonvulsants like carbamazepine). Finally, NMDA receptor antagonists (e.g., dextromethorphan, ketamine) can stabilize membrane excitability of the dorsal horn pain signaling neurons.

**7. What chemical mediators can contribute to the sensation of pain?**

Prostaglandins, histamine, bradykinin, serotonin, leukotrienes, and certain cytokines which are released at the site of tissue damage can stimulate or sensitize primary afferent nociceptive fibers making stimulation of the nociceptor easier. Bradykinin activates C fibers by activation of phospholipase C (PLC) which leads to production of protein kinase C which opens sodium channels resulting in influx of sodium, efflux of potassium, and change in charge along the cellular membrane (i.e., action potential). Activation of PLC also results in increased inositol triphosphate and diacylglycerol levels causing increased intracellular calcium resulting in release of neuropeptides (substance P, neurokinin A, etc.) which results in further inflammation (neurogenic inflammation). Indeed substance P which is located in the dorsal root ganglion neurons is transported to the periphery and released after activation of the primary afferent neurons. Substance P is the principal sensory mediator of pain. It activates C-fiber nociceptors and intensifies pain by mechanisms involving inflammation including prostaglandin release, cytokine stimulation, lysosomal enzyme release, and lymphocyte activation. For this reason NSAIDs, which decrease prostaglandin production, and capsaicin cream, which depletes peripheral afferent nerves of substance P, can be useful in pain management.

**8. Describe the nervous system pathways that downregulate pain perception.**

Pain signals transmitted by A-delta and C-fibers of peripheral afferent nerves terminate in the dorsal horn of the spinal gray matter. Notably, larger peripheral afferent nerve fibers (A-beta) which convey sensation of nonnoxious touch are myelinated fibers that terminate in the same area. Since A-beta fibers are larger, they transmit stimuli more quickly than A-delta or C-fibers. Consequently, signals from nonnoxious stimuli can prevent transmission of painful stimuli by inhibiting pain projection neurons of the dorsal horn. This is why rubbing your thumb after hitting it with a hammer makes it feel better. Also A-delta and C fibers synapse on excitatory interneurons in the spinal cord causing the spinal withdrawal reflex.

After a noxious stimulus causes activation of the spinothalamic tract, the input is transported up the spinal cord. The spinothalamic tract (and other tracts in the ascending anterolateral fasciculus) send projections to important areas in the medulla [nucleus raphe magnus (NRM), nucleus reticularis gigantocellularis (NGC), nucleus reticularis magnocellularis (NMC)], the medullary and pontine reticular formation, and the midbrain [periaqueductal gray (PAG), reticular formation, and nucleus raphe dorsalis (NRD)]. These areas in turn modulate the activity of the spinal afferent nociceptive neurons. Indeed, the PAG, reticular formation, and NRD contain enkephalin, dynorphin, serotonin, and neurotensin neurons. The reticular formation and NRD send axons to the NRM and NGC in the medulla. Here they synapse on primarily serotonergic neurons which descend in the dorsolateral funiculus of the spinal cord to terminate mainly in lamina I, II, and V of the dorsal horn, where they inhibit pain perception.

The PAG receives input from the cortex, limbic system, thalamus, locus cerulus, and hypothalamus. In turn, the PAG sends neurons to the pons (locus cerulus) and medulla (NMC). Here they synapse primarily on noradrenergic neurons which descend in the dorsolateral funiculus of the spinal cord to terminate in the dorsal horn laminae of the spinal gray matter where they inhibit pain perception. Stimulation of the PAG consistently relieves pain. The PAG also sends signals to the hypothalamus which mediates an autonomic and stress response to pain. In turn, the hypothalamus sends axons that release β endorphins to the PAG where they bind to opiate receptors which are numerous in this area. The PAG appears to be the key site for integration of behavioral, autonomic, and neuroendocrine response to painful stimuli.

The pharmacology of pain control relies on an understanding of the pathways that downregulate pain perception. Medications such as tricyclic antidepressants, which increase norepinephrine and serotonin in the nerve synaptic clefts, can modulate pain. Alpha-2-adrenergic agonists should have a similar effect. Opioid receptors and gamma-aminobutyric acid (GABA) receptors have been found throughout the central nervous system particularly the brainstem and spinal cord dorsal horn. Therefore, opioids (e.g., morphine) and procedures that increase endogenous opiates (endorphin release by acupuncture) as well as GABA agonists (topiramate, baclofen) will cause analgesia. Of these, the opioids are the most powerful and effective analgesic drugs.

**9. What is wind-up?**

Neural plasticity, or wind-up, implies that persistent nociception enlarges the receptive field of pain, producing allodynia and hyperalgesia in an ever-enlarging anatomic area. New painful synapses are created and become permanent. This concept suggests that untreated chronic pain eventually becomes a constant sensation because it "burns" its way into the central nervous system. Notably, EAA can induce central sensitization to pain by persistent stimulation of NMDA receptors along the entire pain perception pathway.

**10. What are the opiate receptors in the nervous system?**

Opiate receptors are concentrated in several regions, especially those regions involved in descending control of pain: PAG, medullary reticular formation, and spinal cord. There are also opiate receptors on the peripheral afferent nerves, brainstem, thalamus, hypothalamus, and limbic system. Five different opioid receptors have been proposed:

| ENDOGENOUS PEPTIDE | OPIOID RECEPTOR | EFFECT |
|---|---|---|
| Endomorphins | Mu ($\mu$) | Supraspinal and spinal analgesia |
| Enkephalin | Delta ($\delta$) | Spinal analgesia, short acting effect |
| Dynorphin | Kappa ($\kappa$) | Spinal analgesia, sedation, miosis, and dysphoria |
| B endorphin | Epsilon ($\varepsilon$) | Supraspinal analgesia, long-acting effect |
| — | Sigma ($\sigma$) | Dysphoria, hallucinations, respiratory and vasomotor stimulation |

The mu, delta, and kappa receptors have been confirmed. The epsilon and sigma receptors have been hypothesized but may not exist. There are two mu receptor subtypes, $mu_1$ and $mu_2$. $Mu_1$ stimulation results in analgesia while $mu_2$ receptor stimulation causes respiratory depression, physical dependence, slow gastric transit, nausea/vomiting, bradycardia, and euphoria. There are at least seven polymorphisms of the mu receptors accounting for individual differences in the sensitivity to analgesic and side effects of opioids. There may also be subtypes and polymorphisms of the delta (2 subtypes) and kappa (4 subtypes) opioid receptors.

**11. How do the opiate receptors modulate pain? What accounts for opioid tolerance and withdrawal symptoms?**

Spinal opiate receptors are 70% mu, 24% delta, and 6% kappa receptors. Presynaptic and postsynaptic mu and delta receptors have been identified and tend to co-localize. Stimulation of delta receptors may potentiate mu induced analgesia. Presynaptic receptors make up 70% of all mu and delta receptors. Kappa receptors are located on postsynaptic nerves. In accordance with localization in the dorsal horn, opioid receptors inhibit primary afferent nerve input into the spinal cord. Mu receptors are also localized on small primary afferent nerves, explaining why nociception is inhibited but touch is not.

Opioids bind to opioid receptors, which are coupled to G-proteins. Through G-proteins the opiate receptors can activate inwardly activating potassium channels and close calcium channels. This causes less neurotransmitter release presynaptically and makes it more difficult for postsynaptic neurons to reach their action potential thresholds. Additionally, opiate receptors through G-proteins (which bind GTP) inhibit adenylate cyclase and thus cAMP production which in turn results in inhibition of cAMP dependent protein kinase A. This causes suppression of terminal release of neurotransmitters such as substance P.

However, stimulated opioid receptors linked to G-proteins can also activate phospholipase C, resulting in increased inositol triphosphate and intracellular calcium, which in turn activates protein kinase C (PKC). PKC phosphorylates the opioid receptor and the NMDA receptor. Phosphorylation of the opioid receptor inhibits its function and may be the mechanism for tolerance to opioids and the need to increase doses. However, phosphorylation of the NMDA receptor can result in increased sodium and calcium influxes predisposing the nerve to depolarization. This may be the reason that with abrupt opioid withdrawal, symptoms of neuron hyperexcitability results (i.e. withdrawal symptoms) due to prolonged NMDA receptor hyperfunctioning. Tapering of opioid medication allows the NMDA receptor time to dephosphorylate and thus helps to abrogate withdrawal symptoms.

**12. What are the major classes of nonopioid analgesics used as primary or adjuvant therapies for patients with chronic pain?**

Nonopioid analgesics differ from opioids in that they do not bind opioid receptor sites in the central nervous system, tolerance and physical dependence do not develop, and they have a ceiling effect in that increasing the dose beyond a certain level does not produce additional analgesic effects. The major medications are:

- Acetaminophen: active metabolite of phenacetin. Mechanisms of action (MOA) may be inhibiting a new cyclooxygenase (? Cox-3) enzyme in the brain. Maximum single analgesic dose = 1000 mg. Maximum total daily dose = 1000 mg 4 times/day (4000 mg). Reduce total daily dose (≤ 2000 mg) or do not use if renal disease, hepatic disease, or chronic alcohol use is present.
- NSAIDs and Coxibs (see Chapter 84): Notably, cyclooxygenase-2 is constitutively expressed in the central nervous system and is upregulated by interleukin-1. Thus, NSAIDs can help inflammatory causes of pain although they are not very helpful for peripheral neuropathies. Ketorolac (Toradol) is a Cox-1/Cox-2 inhibitor used for short term (5 days) to control acute pain. Cox-2 inhibitors, especially rofecoxib and valdecoxib, are good alternatives for acute and chronic pain in individuals at high risk for gastrointestinal toxicity.
- Tramadol (Ultram): synthetic centrally acting (primarily at level of spinal cord) analgesic consisting of a mixture of two enantiomers. Tramadol and its M1 metabolite have both weak opioid and nonopioid properties. Tramadol binds to μ, δ, and κ opioid receptors with 6000 times less affinity than opiates. The M1 metabolite is 6 times more potent and binds with 200 times more affinity than the parent compound. The nonopioid properties refer to serotonin release (+ enantiomer) and inhibition of presynpatic reuptake of norepinephrine and serotonin (– enantiomer). Tramadol is not anti-inflammatory. Maximum single dose is 100 mg and maximum total daily dose is 400 mg in patients less than 75 years old without renal failure. Maximum daily dose in patients with cirrhosis is 100 mg/day and in patients with renal insufficiency 200 mg/day. Side effects include nausea, vomiting, somnolence and dizziness. Seizures occur in less than 1% with increased risk in patients with prior seizure disorder, history of head trauma, and concomitant use of drugs such as serum serotonin reuptake inhibitors (SSRI), tricyclic antidepressants (TCA), and opioids. Drug abuse risk is low although occurs in some patients with a prior history of substance abuse. Recently, a combination pill of tramadol (37.5 mg) and acetaminophen (325 mg) (Ultracet) has been introduced.
- Note that these medications can be used alone, in combination with each other, or in combination with opiates to increase analgesic effects.

**13. How can the side effects of tramadol be lessened?**

Slow introduction of tramadol reduces the incidence of side effects. Dose titration recommended is to start dosing at 25/day and increase by 25 mg every 3 days until desired dose is reached. This probably applies to all medications used for pain control. A person on tramadol who is taken off that medication should always be tapered off slowly since abrupt withdrawal can precipitate withdrawal symptoms.

**14. What are some other adjunctive medications used for chronic pain relief?**

**Antidepressants**. The tricyclic antidepressants (TCA) possess established efficacy for neuropathic pain. The MOA is hypothesized to be that TCA inhibit the reuptake of norepinephrine and serotonin at synapses resulting in enhanced central analgesia. All TCA except trazodone (desyrel) help relieve pain. Side effects include dry mouth, drowsiness, confusion, urinary retention, priapism (trazodone), cardiac conduction abnormalities, orthostasis, and weight gain. Desipramine (Norpramin) causes the least number of side effects. Dosing starts at 10–25 mg qhs and is increased every 5 days to average dose of 100 mg. SSRI antidepressants are effective for depression but of limited use as pain medications although venlafaxine (Effexor) does show some effect and paroxetine (Paxil) helps neuropathic pain and headaches.

**Anticonvulsants**: The newer antiepileptic drugs may become first-line agents for neuropathic pain. Carbamazepine, lamotrigine, phenytoin, and topiramate block the voltage-dependent sodium channels of neuronal membranes. Topiramate and tiagabine can potentiate GABA or inhibit its uptake enabling it to counteract the excitatory amino acid, glutamate, which is an important neurotransmitter. The MOA of gabapentin is unknown but it is highly effective for peripheral neuropathies and has no drug interactions. Side effects of these medications include dizziness, blurred vision, and ataxia which can be prevented by slow drug titration. Carbamazepine can cause neutropenia.

| Drug (Brand Name) | Tablet Doses (mg) | Daily Maintenance Dose |
|---|---|---|
| Carbamazepine (Tegretol) | 100, 200, 300, 400 | 800–1200 mg/d divided into 3 doses |
| Lamotrigine (Lamictal) | 25, 100, 150, 200 | 400 mg/d divided into 2–3 doses |
| Gabapentin (Neurontin) | 100, 300, 400 | 1800-3600 mg/d divided into 3–4 doses |
| Topiramate (Topamax) | 25, 100, 200 | 200 mg twice a day |
| Tiagabine (Gabitril) | 4, 12, 16, 20 | 32–56 mg/d divided into 2–4 doses |
| Phenytoin (Dilantin) | 100, 300 | 200–300 mg/d |
| Clonazepam (Klonopin) | 0.5, 1, 2 | 0.75–1.5 mg/d divided into 3 doses |

**Muscle relaxants**: Centrally acting muscle relaxants can help relieve musculoskeletal pain even if there is no overt muscle spasm. Cyclobenzaprine has a chemical structure similar to a TCA. Baclofen is an analogue of the inhibitory neurotransmitter GABA and exerts its action by activating the GABA beta receptors. It can inhibit synaptic reflexes at the spinal level and has an antispasmodic action.

| Drug (Trade Name) | Tablet Dose (mg) | Daily Dose |
|---|---|---|
| Baclofen (Liorexal) | 10, 20 | 20–60 mg/d divided into 3-4 doses |
| Carisoprodol (Soma) | 350 | 350 mg QID |
| Cyclobenzaprine (Flexeril) | 10 | 10 mg BID-QID |
| Methocarbamol (Robaxin) | 500, 750 | 1500 mg QID |
| Orphenadrine (Norflex, Norgesic) | 100 | 100 mg BID |
| Chlorzoxazone (Parafon Forte) | 250, 500 | 500 mg TID-QID |
| Metaxalone (Skelaxin) | 400 | 800 mg TID-QID |
| Dantrolene (Dantrium) | 25, 50, 100 | 25 mg BID-QID |
| Diazepam (Valium) | 2, 5, 10 | 2–10 mg TID |

Use these muscle relaxants with caution (if at all) in elderly and patients with urinary retention or narrow angle glaucoma.

**Tranquilizers**: Pain can cause significant anxiety which can heighten pain response. Use of benzodiazepines (alprazolam, lorazepam, diazepam) for patients with chronic pain should be limited due to side effects of depression, disruption of sleep physiology, and cognitive depression. To decrease anxiety, TCA and SSRI antidepressants are probably better choices.

**Hypnotics**: Pain can interfere with sleep which can lead to fatigue and decreased ability to tolerate pain. In addition to TCA, other agents used for sleep are listed below. Temazepam should be used sparingly in the elderly due to its long half life.

| Drug (Brand Name) | Tablet Dose (mg) | Typical Dosage |
|---|---|---|
| Temazepam (Restoril) | 7.5, 15, 30 | 7.5–30 mg qhs |
| Triazolam (Halcion) | 0.125, 0.25 | 0.125–0.5 mg qhs |
| Zaleplon (Sonata) | 5, 10 | 5–10 mg qhs |
| Zolpidem (Ambien) | 5, 10 | 5–10 mg qhs |

**Other drugs**

- Dextromethorphan: has an NMDA receptor antagonistic effect and helps to prevent central sensitization caused by excitatory amino acids in their transmission of pain from peripheral inflammation and tissue damage. Dextromethorphan given at same dose (1:1) as morphine can help prevent tolerance to opioid analgesia. SSRI antidepressants can raise blood levels of dextromethorphan causing CNS side effects.
- Mexiletine (Mexitil): useful for neuropathic pain by blocking neuronal membrane sodium channels. A response to IV lidocaine infusion (5 mg/kg over 1 hour) predicts a response to oral mexiletine. This drug is contraindicated in patients with second- or third-degree AV block. The dose should be slowly titrated to 150–600 mg/d or a maximum of 10 mg/kg/day divided into three doses. Nausea, dizziness, and tremors are common. Hallucinations and seizures can occur.
- Clonidine (Catapres) and tizanidine (Zanaflex): centrally acting alpha-2 adrenergic agonists that can have an antinociceptive effect on spinal transmission of pain. It is known that

norepinephrine binds to α2 receptors to decrease pain in spinal cord. Thus, alpha-2 adrenergic agonists should work through similar mechanisms. Side effects include CNS effects and hypotension. Clonidine dose is 0.1 mg 2 times/day; tizanidine dose is 8–16 mg daily divided into four doses.

- Bone agents: bisphosphonate can help cancer bone pain. Calcitonin may cause release of endogenous opiates.
- Dexamethasone: for acute neuropathic pain such as occurs with herniated disc. Dose = 4–8 mg 2 times/day

**15. What other therapies are available to treat musculoskeletal pain?**

**Physical therapy**: heat, cold, ultrasound, muscle strengthening, stretching.

**Injections**: intraarticular corticosteroids, epidural steroids (only for herniated disc or spinal stenosis with radiculopathy not for isolated neck or low back pain), trigger point injections, regional soft tissue corticosteroid injections (i.e., bursitis, tendinitis).

**Nerve manipulation**: diagnostic nerve block, transcutaneous electrical nerve stimulation (TENS; helps 30% of patients with chronic musculoskeletal or peripheral neuropathy pain), spinal cord stimulation (dorsal column) with implantable stimulator (helps 50% of chronic back pain patients), neurolysis (remove perineural adhesions), rhizotomy (destroy nerve by surgical division, radiofrequency waves, or chemical injection of phenol or glycerol).

**Topicals**: capsaicin (local joint pain or postherpetic neuralgia), methylsalicylate. Must apply capsaicin (hot chili peppers) 4 times/day for 2 weeks to deplete nerves of substance P.

**Psychologic support**: relaxation techniques, coping skills, treat anxiety and depression (present in 50–90% of patients with chronic pain).

**Acupuncture** (see Chapter 95): part of action due to stimulation of endogenous opioids.

**Ablative therapy**: central and spinal cord levels. Pain often recurs and possibly worse than prior to therapy.

**16. Which opioids should not be used for treatment of chronic pain especially in the elderly?**

**Propoxyphene (Darvon)**: weak analgesic. Long half-life may cause accumulation of its metabolite (norpropoxyphene), which can cause arrhythmias, seizures, and dizziness.

**Meperidine (Demerol)**: do not use more than 1–2 days. Accumulation of metabolites (normeperidine) can cause neurotoxicity. Contraindicated in renal disease or long term use.

**Pentazocine (Talwin)**: mixed agonist-antagonist. Stimulates κ receptors and blocks μ receptors; can cause hallucinations and disorientation due to κ receptor stimulation; has ceiling dose effect.

**Codeine preparations** (Fiorinal, Fioricet, Tylenol with codeine): 10% of population lacks enzyme to convert it to its active analgesic metabolite. Most constipating opiate. Oral codeine 100 mg is equivalent to oral morphine 30 mg.

**17. What opioids are available for treatment of acute and chronic pain?**

| OPIOID | DURATION OF ACTION (HRS) | STARTING DOSE | EQUIANALGESIC POTENCY (MG) |
|---|---|---|---|
| **Short-acting** | | | |
| Morphine sulfate | 3–6 | 15–30 mg q 4 hr (6 doses/day) | 30 oral, 10 parenteral |
| Hydrocodone (Lortab, Lorcet, Vicodin) | 2–4 | 5–10 mg q 3–4 hr | 30 |
| Oxycodone (Percodan, Percocet, Roxicodone, Roxicet, Roxilox, Tylox, OxyIR) | 2–4 | 5–10 mg q 3–4 hr | 20 |
| Hydromorphone (Dilaudid) | 2–4 | 7.5 mg q 3–4 hr (8 doses/day) | 7.5 oral, 1.5 parenteral |

(*Table continued on next page.*)

| OPIOID | DURATION OF ACTION (HRS) | STARTING DOSE | EQUIANALGESIC POTENCY (MG) |
|---|---|---|---|
| **Intermediate-acting** | | | |
| Levorphanol (Levo-Dromoran) | 3–6 | 1–4 mg q 6–8 hr | 4 acute oral<br>1 chronic oral<br>2 parenteral |
| Methadone (Dolophine) | 4–6 | 4–20 mg q 6–8 hr | 20 acute<br>2–4 chronic oral<br>10 parenteral |
| **Long-acting** | | | |
| Morphine–sustained-release (MS Contin, Oramorph SR, Kadian) | — | 15–30 mg q 8–12 hr | 30 |
| Oxycodone–sustained-release (OxyContin) | — | 10–20 mg q 12 hr | 20–30 |
| Transdermal fentanyl (Duragesic) | — | ≥ 25 μg/hr every 48–72 hr | N/A<br>0.1 mg parental (Innovar) |

**Note**: The only reliable indicator of pain relief is the patient's self-report. There is significant variability in opioid response. Patients that are opiate naive require less opioid than those patients who are on opiates (usually 50–66% less). "The dose that works is the dose that works."

**Pearl**: To give single IV dose use ¼ to ½ the listed parenteral dose.

**18. How can you convert from one opioid to another?**

Use the equianalgesic conversion equation:

$$\frac{\text{Current opioid (single conversion dose/route)}}{\text{New opioid (single conversion dose/route)}} = \frac{\text{Total 24-hr dose of current opioid}}{\text{Total 24-hr dose of new opioid}}$$

Example: If patient is taking morphine, 30 mg q 4 hours (180 mg/day), and wants to switch to Dilaudid:

$$\frac{\text{Morphine 30 mg oral dose}}{\text{Dilaudid 7.5 mg oral dose}} = \frac{\text{Total 24 hr morphine 180 mg}}{\text{X}}$$

X = Dilaudid, 45 mg orally per 24 hours. The patient should receive 6 mg q 3 hours.

For breakthrough pain, give 10–20% of the total 24-hour oral dose.

**19. Which opioids are combined with acetaminophen, aspirin, or ibuprofen?**

- Hydrocodone + acetaminophen = Lorcet, Vicodin, Zydone, Lortab, Anexsia
- Hydrocodone + ibuprofen = Vicoprofen
- Oxycodone + acetaminophen = Percocet, Roxicet (tablets), Roxilox (capsules), Tylox (capsules)
- Oxycodone + aspirin = Percodan

**Pearl**: It is important to not exceed recommended total daily acetaminophen dosage (4000 mg/d).

**20. When should you use a short-, intermediate-, or long-acting opiate?**

Short-acting opiates are best for acute pain. When the patient requires more than 4–5 doses/day and has chronic pain, it is best to use a long-acting opiate. Intermediate-acting opiates (methadone) are hard to use due to long half-life and accumulation of drug with side effects, especially in the elderly.

**21. List pearls related to the use of opiates.**

1. Available in many different forms: oral, IM, IV, rectal, transdermal, intranasal [butorphanol (Stadol)], sublingual. There is no ceiling effect for analgesia.

2. Morphine: all morphine products are not equivalent. Active metabolite is morphine-6-glucoronide. If liver disease with elevated prothrombine time, morphine may not be converted to

active form. Morphine causes neurotoxicity (the patient has hallucinations, tremor) in patients with impaired renal function.

3. Hydromorphone: no active metabolites; thus does not accumulate in patients with renal or liver failure. Major problem is need to redose every 3 hours if used orally.

4. Oxycodone: sustained release form gives smooth blood levels and may be best medication for chronic non-malignant pain.

5. Topical fentanyl: do not use in children or elderly patients less than 50 kg in weight. Onset of analgesia is 8–17 hours so only use for chronic pain. Peak analgesia in 24–72 hours. Thirty percent of patients require dosing every 48 instead of 72 hours.

6. Methadone: one of the best opiates for neuropathic pain at dose of 5–10 mg 2–4 times/day.

**22. Discuss the potential side effects of opioids.**

**Constipation** (100%): common side effect. Opiates slow gut motility and increase gut absorption of water. Prophylactic therapy should include a diet with fiber and a lot of water. Also use a wetting agent (docusate) and a motility agent: Senokot S BID and titrate to effect. Lactulose, 15–60 ml daily can also be used. Add 10 mg bisacodyl (Dulcolax) each night if no bowel movement during the day. Avoid bulk-forming laxatives (e.g.,metamucil) since they can cause impaction. Tolerance never develops to constipation, unlike other side effects.

**Nausea/vomiting** (10–40%): opioids cause this by sensitizing vestibular system or stimulating medullary chemoreceptor trigger zone. Tolerance can develop over 5–7 days. Treat with hydroxyzine for vestibular-related nausea and prochlorperazine or other antiemetic for other causes of nausea.

**Respiratory depression and sedation**: rare to develop significant respiratory depression without severe sedation. Be careful in patients with severe sleep apnea. Tolerance develops in 5–7 days. Treat acute, severe sedation with naloxone (Narcan), 0.4 mg IV.

**Pruritus** (parenteral > oral dosing): due to histamine release. Made worse if take opioids and alcohol. Histamine release can cause hypotension. Treat with chlorpheniramine.

**Urinary retention**: males more than females.

**Withdrawal**: if chronic opioid therapy is abruptly stopped the patient can develop a flu-like syndrome with chills, rhinorrhea, diarrhea, nausea, restlessness, fever, and diaphoresis. Most patients can be tapered off opioids by decreasing dose by 25% each week. Very sensitive patients may need clonidine, 0.2–0.4 mg/day for 2–3 weeks, to help with taper.

**23. Define the following terms.**

**Physical dependence**: physiologic state induced by chronic administration of a medication (e.g., opiates, glucocorticoids, antihypertensives) and characterized by a withdrawal syndrome if medication is abruptly stopped.

**Addiction**: abnormal, compulsive and deleterious use of a prescribed medication that grossly deviates from the physician's recommendations and from any approved medical and social standards. Between 5–10% of chronic pain patients may exhibit this behavior particularly if they have a history of other substance abuse. These patients need an opioid treatment contract and strict control of their prescriptions.

**Pseudoaddiction**: drug-seeking behavior in patients whose pain is poorly controlled. Behavior ceases when pain is controlled.

**Tolerance**: requirement for continued dose escalation to maintain same level of pain relief. Although common, this is not inevitable. Average is 10% escalation in opiate dose per 6–12 months of use.

**Pseudotolerance**: dose needs to be increased due to progression of disease, new reason for pain, lack of compliance, change in medication brand, addiction.

**Breakthrough pain**: transitory exacerbation of pain that occurs on a background of otherwise stable pain in a patient receiving chronic opioid therapy.

**24. What is the cost of opiate analgesia for chronic pain?**

Most long acting opiates cost between $20–25/week. Slow-release oxycodone costs $30/week, and the fentanyl patch costs $38/week.

**25. What is the analgesic ladder?**

The World Health Organization in 1990 recommended that pain be treated based on its severity with the following medications:

- Level 1 (pain score 1–3)
  - Acetaminophen
  - NSAIDs
- Level 2 (pain score 4–6)
  - Tramadol or Opioid for moderate pain (oxycodone, hydrocodone)
  - With or without nonopioid (NSAIDs)
  - With or without adjuvant (anticonvulsants, antidepressants, etc.)
- Level 3 (pain score 7–10)
  - Opioid for severe pain (morphine, hydromorphone, fentanyl)
  - With or without non-opioid
  - With or without adjuvant

**26. What is the minimal change in the 10 centimeter visual analogue pain scale that is considered significant?**

13 mm.

**27. Is it acceptable to use an opioid for nonmalignant pain if nonopioid analgesia is ineffective?**

Yes. In fact, there may be less serious side effects with opioids than NSAIDs, especially in the elderly.

**28. What are the major fears that prohibit doctors and patients from using opioids to control pain? What is the reality?**

**Physician**

1. Inadequate knowledge.
2. Fear of patient addiction—less than 10% of patients. Use opioid contract for high risk patients.
3. Concern about respiratory depression—rarely occurs and patient will develop tolerance.
4. Fear of regulatory control agencies—will not be a problem if document in chart reason for pain medication, how well it is working for the patient's pain, side effects, amounts prescribed, and frequency of visits.

**Patient**

1. Fear of addiction—physician needs to explain to the patient that he/she will be dependent on the medicine just like he/she is dependent on his/her anti-hypertensive (or other) medication and that this is not addiction.
2. Fear of side effects—physician needs to prophylax for constipation and tell patient about tolerance to other side effects. Doses should be started low especially in the elderly.
3. Fear of society branding them a "narcotic addict"—physician should refer to therapy as opioid analgesia and not as narcotic analgesia.

**29. Define the following terms.**

**Opium**: a bitter yellowish-brown drug prepared from the dry juice of unripe pods of the opium poppy (Papaver somniferum, originally from Asia Minor). Opium contains the natural alkaloids morphine, codeine, and papaverine. Other opiates used for analgesia are semisynthetic (dilaudid, hydrocodone, oxycodone) or synthetic (methadone, fentanyl).

**Laudanum**: tincture of opium usually added to brandy. Favorite of Edgar Allan Poe and others.

**Heroin**: diacetylmorphine originally developed by Merck as a nonaddicting form of morphine. This obviously was proved not to be true. Heroin, 4 mg is equivalent to morphine, 10 mg IM; lasts 3–5 hours.

**Narcotic**: derived from the Latin word *narcoticus* meaning "to make numb." Has been used in a negative connotation by the legal and judicial system that stigmatizes opiates.

## BIBLIOGRAPHY


1. Pisetsky DS, Bradley LA (eds): Pain management in the rheumatic diseases. Rheum Dis Clin North America 225:1–256, 1999.
2. Katz W: Pain Management in Rheumatologic Disorders. Drugsmartz Publications, 2000.
3. Garcia J, Altman RD: Chronic pain states: Pathophysiology and medical therapy. Semin Arthritis Rheum 27:1–16, 1997.
4. Fitzgerald GA, Patrono C: The coxibs, selective inhibitors of cyclooxygenase-2. N Engl J Med 345:433–442, 2001.
5. Lynch ME: Antidepressants as analgesics: A review of randomized controlled trials. J Psychiatry Neurosci 26:30–36, 2001.
6. Sindrup SH, Jensen TS: Pharmacologic treatment of pain in polyneuropathy. Neurology 55:915–920, 2000.
7. Waldman HJ: Centrally acting muscle relaxants and associated drugs. J Pain Symptom Manage 9:434–441, 1994.
8. Loeser JD (ed): Bonica's Management of Pain, 3rd ed. Philadelphia, Lippincott Williams & Wilkins, 2001.
9. Roth SH, Fleischmann RM, Burch FX, et al: Around-the-clock, controlled-release oxycodone therapy for osteoarthritis-related pain: Placebo-controlled trial and long-term evaluation. Arch Intern Med 160:853–860, 2000.


# 91. REHABILITATIVE TECHNIQUES

*Cliff A. Gronseth*, M.D.

**1. What is the goal of rehabilitation for patients with rheumatic disease?**

The goal of rehabilitation is to maintain or restore the individual's ability to function successfully in personal, family, and community life by developing that person to the fullest physical, psychological, social, vocational, avocational, and educational potential consistent with his or her physiologic or anatomic impairment and environmental limitations.

**2. Which functional areas may need to be assessed in a patient with a rheumatic disease?**

**Physical function assessment**

- History: pain and fatigue (can use visual analogue scales)
- Physical examination
  - Manual muscle strength testing
  - Range of motion (ROM, can use goniometers)
  - Transfers and ambulation
- Ability to perform activities of daily living (ADLs)
- Recreational (avocational) or leisure activities
- Occupational (vocational) activities including job, housework, and schoolwork
- Sexual activities
- Sleep history

**Psychological/cognitive function assessment**

- Affective function (depression, anxiety, mood)
- Coping skills
- Cognitive function
- Compliance with treatment plan

**Social function assessment** (family, friends, community)

- Social support systems
- Interpersonal relationships
- Social integration
- Ability to fulfill social roles
- Family functioning
- Socioeconomic/financial

**3. A quick screen of a rheumatic disease patient's functional abilities should include which areas?**

The most critical functional areas to be reviewed when time is limited can be remembered by using the mnemonic ADEPTTS-how well the patient "adapts" to his/her physical disability:

**A** — *A*mbulation
**D** — *D*ressing
**E** — *E*ating
**P** — *P*ersonal hygiene
**T** — *T*ransfers
**T** — *T*oileting
**S** — *S*leeping/*S*exual activities

**4. What health care personnel are available to help rehabilitate patients with rheumatic diseases? What rehab techniques do each use?**

**Physical therapist**—administers and instructs patients in the use of various therapeutic and pain-relieving techniques, including heat, cold, traction, diathermy, electrical stimulation, therapeutic exercise, stretching, transfer skills, ambulation methods, and joint ROM/function/strength.

**Occupational therapist** (OT)—responsible for optimizing function by instruction in joint protection and energy conservation. In addition, OTs provide or fabricate adaptive equipment and splinting, especially for upper-extremity functional activities. Some OTs, but usually **podiatrists**, provide orthotics for lower-extremity problems.

**Social workers** and **rehabilitation counselors**—assist in the management of social, economic, and psychological problems that create stress for the patient and family. This can include assistance in recreational activities as well as interpersonal and sexual relationships.

**Psychotherapists**—assist the patient with the psychological problems that arise from dealing with pain and loss of function.

**Vocational counselors**—can mobilize community resources to retrain and restore the patient to the workplace.

**Arthritis rehabilitation nurses** and **patient educators**—assist in instruction about the rheumatic disease and its therapy. Provide information, monitor compliance, and give emotional support to the patient and family.

## EXERCISE AND REST

**5. Name three forms of rest.**

Rest in an arthritic person may be done specifically to benefit an inflamed joint, to provide energy conservation, or, in specific disorders, to affect sedimentation rate and creatine kinase levels.

- **Local rest** is performed in a specific joint utilizing splinting techniques to reduce pain, inflammation, or to prevent contracture.
- **Systemic rest** is used for a period of up to 4 weeks if appropriate anti-inflammatory medication and outpatient rehabilitation management are ineffective in alleviating the manifestations of rheumatoid arthritis or polymyositis.
- **Short rest periods** are becoming increasingly popular, particularly in patients with rheumatoid arthritis. These are a preventive and proactive means of managing inflammation and fatigue. The patient interrupts daily activities of longer than 30 continuous minutes to take short breaks.

**6. How does exercise benefit a patient with arthritis?**

Fatigue, weakness, and decreased stamina or endurance are common symptoms in patients with rheumatic disease. Disuse or excessive rest and inactivity can be a major cause of lost muscle strength. Up to 30% of a muscle's bulk and 5–10% of its strength can be lost within a week if a joint is immobilized. In addition, joint immobility can lead to contractures with loss of ROM. Therapeutic exercise has the following goals and benefits in a patient with arthritis:

Maintaining or improving ROM
Preventing or reducing contractures
Increasing strength
Enhancing endurance
Preserving bone mineralization
Improving the ability for functional activities
Improving patient's overall feeling of well-being

**7. Which factors need to be considered in prescribing an exercise program for a patient with a rheumatic disease?**

Stage of disease
Extent of inflammation and deformity
Patient's general medical condition
Types of activities the patient enjoys (to improve compliance)

**8. Name three types of ROM exercise.**

1. **Passive ROM**—Motion is performed by the therapist or mechanical device without help of the patient.
2. **Active ROM**—The patient performs the movement.
3. **Active-assisted ROM**—The patient moves the limb with the assistance of the therapist.

**9. What is the minimum ROM of each joint that allows adequate function to perform activities of daily living?**

| JOINT | ROM |
|---|---|
| TMJ | 2.5 cm of jaw opening |
| Shoulder | Flexion 45, abduction 90, external rotation 20 |
| Elbow | Flexion 70 |
| Wrist | Dorsiflexion 5–10, supination 10–15 |
| MCP | Flexion > 30 |
| PIP | Flexion > 30 |
| DIP | Flexion > 30 |
| CMC | Internal rotation > 30 |
| Hip | Extension 0 to flexion 30 |
| Knee | Neutral to 60 flexion |
| Ankle | Plantar flexion 20 to 10 of dorsiflexion |

TMJ = temporomandibular joint. (Adapted from Hicks JE: Exercise in patients with inflammatory arthritis and connective tissue disease. Rheum Dis Clin North Am 16:845, 1990.)

**10. What types of active exercise are used to increase muscle strength and endurance in a patient with arthritis?**

1. **Isometric training**: A static muscle contraction in which the muscle length does not change and the limb does not move through ROM. Two to six contractions of each muscle are recommended, with each contraction held for 3–6 sec with 20–60 sec rest periods between contractions. This form of exercise is particularly good to maintain or increase muscle bulk and strength without increasing joint inflammation in a patient with active arthritis.
2. **Isotonic exercise**: A dynamic muscle contraction with movement through an arc of motion against a fixed resistance. It should be done when joint inflammation is under control. Isotonic training begins with 1–2-lb weights. Before increasing weight, patients should comfortably perform 12 repetitions.
3. **Isokinetic exercise**: The rate of movement is held constant, but the force produced by the individual may vary through the arc of motion. This form of exercise is rarely used in rehabilitation of arthritic patients.
4. **Aerobic and aquatic exercise programs**.

**11. How does strength training differ from endurance training?**

Strength is increased by isometric exercises and by isotonic exercises with increased resistance, resulting in fewer repetitions (7–10 repetitions). Endurance is increased by isotonic exercises with low resistance, enabling multiple repetitions (3 sets of 10 repetitions).

**12. In which aerobic activities can a rheumatic disease patient participate to increase cardiovascular fitness?**

Swimming, walking, stationary bicycling, and treadmill walking are recommended to increase cardiovascular fitness. The intensity should be sufficient to elevate the heart rate to 75% of maximum (220 – age) for 20–40 minutes.

**13. How often should a patient with arthritis exercise?**

All patients with arthritis should perform stretching for 10 minutes and ROM exercises daily. A patient with active joint inflammation or those with class III or IV functional capacity should also do isometric exercises and aquatic therapy for 30 minutes, 3–4 times a week. A patient whose disease is controlled and is functional class I or II should do isotonic exercises and aerobic exercises for 30 minutes, 3–4 times a week. Particular attention should be given to strengthening the shoulder and knee musculature.

**14. How can a patient with arthritis determine if he or she has done too much exercise?**

- Excessive pain during the exercise session
- Postexercise fatigue lasting > 1 hour
- Postexercise soreness lasting > 2 hours
- Increased joint pain or swelling the day following exercise

**15. What precautions should be taken before advising a patient to perform isometric exercise training?**

Isometric exercises, particularly of the upper extremities, increase systemic peripheral vascular resistance. These exercises are relatively contraindicated in patients with severe hypertension or a history of significant cardiovascular or cerebrovascular disease.

## PHYSICAL MODALITIES

**16. Which physical modalities are available for management of musculoskeletal pain?**

**Thermal agents**
- Superficial moist or dry heart
- Deep heat with ultrasound or diathermy
- Cryotherapy

**Electrotherapy**
- TENS
- Iontophoresis

**Traction**

**17. What is the main purpose of physical modalities in a patient with arthritis?**

To decrease pain so that the patient can participate in therapeutic exercises.

**18. How are superficial and deep heat used in the treatment of musculoskeletal problems?**

**Superficial heat** includes moist heat delivered by hot packs, whirlpool, paraffin baths, or aqua therapy and dry heat delivered by fluidotherapy. This heat only penetrates tissue to a depth of 1–1.5 cm, and its effects last for 30–45 minutes.

**Deep heat** is delivered by ultrasound or short-wave diathermy. Tissues at a depth of 3–6 cm can be heated to 41°C. The effect lasts for 30–45 minutes, during which time exercises should be done.

**19. What are some of the therapeutic effects of heat treatments?**

By warming tissue, several effects occur simultaneously: increased tendon and joint capsule extensibility, reduction in muscle spasm, production of analgesia, increased tissue blood flow, and increased tissue metabolism. Superficial joints are typically easier to heat by techniques such as hot packs, paraffin wax, fluidotherapy, hydrotherapy, and radiant heat. Heat treatments can be used palliatively to reduce pain and spasm, particularly in subacute and chronic conditions. To restore function, heat, both superficial and deep, is used in conjunction with formal therapy and therapeutic exercise; this improves joint ROM by way of reduction in tendon and joint capsule tightness and reduction of contracture.

**20. Are there contraindications to treating with heat?**

Tissue pain and damage commence with tissue temperatures of 113 (45°C). Increased collagenolysis has been found to occur with increased intra-articular temperatures. While there are potentially adverse implications for using heat in inflammatory conditions, such as rheumatoid arthritis, investigators have not found increased joint destruction to occur when heat is used.

Because pain is a critical warning sign of tissue injury, desensitized areas or patients with a reduction in mental status are contraindications to the use of heat. Other common contraindications include bleeding diathesis, malignancy, and tumor. Also, heat applications to the gonads or to a fetus should be avoided. Areas with inadequate vascular supply should not be heated because of their inability to dissipate heat appropriately or to meet the increased metabolic demands caused by the increased temperature. Deep heat should not be used if metal is in the area being treated.

**21. How is cryotherapy applied?**

Cold application can be very specific, as in the use of vapocoolant sprays, localized massage, or locally applied cold pack. Or it can be very generally applied, as in ice water immersion, refillable bladders, thermal blankets, or contrast baths. For subacute pain and spinal muscle spasm, it is typically applied as ice massage or cold pack. Cryotherapy is the treatment of choice following acute injury, particularly when combined with compression.

**22. Both superficial heat and cryotherapy reduce muscle spasm. How does the mechanism of cold differ from that of heat?**

**Cold** has its effect directly on the muscle, the intrafusal fibers of the muscle spindle mechanism, and sensory wrappings of the muscle spindles. **Heat** primarily affects muscle spasm indirectly by slowing the firing rate of secondary afferents, increasing the firing rate of Golgi tendon organs, and decreasing the firing rate of efferent fibers to the muscle spindle (gamma fibers).

**23. What is iontophoresis?**

It is the use of DC current to induce topically applied medications to migrate into soft tissues and nerves up to 3–5 mm deep. Common topical medications applied include lidocaine gel, dexamethasone gel, and analgesics. This therapy has been used in tendinitis (especially Achilles tendinitis), bursitis, and neuritis.

**24. When is traction useful for the management of cervical and lumbar spinal disorders?**

Traction involves applying force in a manner to distract the cervical or lumbar vertebral bodies. This increases the intervertebral foraminal area, allowing more space for the exiting nerve root. Cervical traction is set up in a specific position with weight from 10–15 lbs or more. Lumbar traction is applied with the patient supine and both hips and knees flexed to 90. The traction is 40–80 lbs. Both cervical and lumbar traction work best if applied two or three times a day until pain relief occurs. Failure to improve pain within 2–4 weeks and/or exacerbation of pain during traction are indications to stop this therapy.

## ORTHOSES, JOINT PROTECTION, AND ASSISTIVE DEVICES

**25. Why are splints and orthotics used in arthritis patients?**

Splints and orthotics are used in the treatment of inflammatory and degenerative arthritis to unweight joints, create stability in selected joints, decrease joint motion, increase joint motion, or support the joint in the position of maximal function. They can either be purchased over-the-counter or custom-formed to fit the individual patient.

**26. Name the major factor in patient noncompliance in the use of splints and orthotics.**

The **cosmetic appearance** of the splint is a major factor in nonuse. Fear of public attention to the device, including discrimination at work and in other environments, adds to a patient's unwillingness to use the device. Compliance with splints is increased when the splints significantly improve pain or function and when family or support groups reinforce the need to use the splint regularly. Cosmetic splints, particularly for the small digits of the hand, can be constructed of precious metals, and semiprecious stones.

**27. What are joint protection techniques?**

Techniques for joint protection and energy conservation include task modification, environmental design/modification, and adaptation. By reducing mechanical stress, joint integrity is preserved and inflammation is reduced. Minimizing static positions while emphasizing proper posture reduces stress on individual joints. Joint protection includes maintaining ROM, unloading painful joints, and adequate rest periods throughout the day.

**28. How can the use of adaptive devices and mobility aids benefit a patient with arthritis?**

Assistive devices that substitute for deficient function help a patient with arthritis conserve energy, decrease stress on joints, relieve pain, and be more functionally independent. Adaptive devices for kitchen, bathroom, and self-care are readily available and listed in many patient manuals. Mobility aids include canes, crutches, and wheelchairs.

**29. In which hand should a cane be placed to provide weight-bearing relief for a diseased hip?**

The cane is placed in the hand of the contralateral arm. This creates a moment arm that counteracts the patient's weight and significantly reduces the amount of force applied to the hip joint. Placing the cane on the same side as the involved hip actually increases loading on the hip joint and potentially exacerbates the discomfort, pain, or joint dysfunction. Note that with walking, the stress across the hip joint is equal to two to three times body weight.

**30. For an involved knee or ankle, which hand should hold the cane?**

Below the level of the hip, ground reactive force to an individual joint is relieved most effectively when the cane is held on the **ipsilateral side** as the involved joint. This position can be advantageous for climbing and descending stairs but can be disruptive to the normal rhythm of gait because of the reversal of the natural swing of the arm. The patient may find that the cane works well when held in the contralateral hand during normal ambulation, but then can change it to the ipsilateral side for specific actions or activities requiring direct force on the ankle and knee. With walking, the normal stress across the knee is 3–4 times body weight, whereas stress across the ankle can be as high as 4–5 times body weight.

**31. How can you tell if a cane or crutch has been properly fitted to the patient?**

A properly fitted cane or crutch should reach 8 inches lateral to the front of the foot when the patient is standing and holding the cane or crutch handle with the elbow flexed 15–30°. This position permits stability on standing and an easy reach to the ground ahead during walking.

**32. Describe shoe characteristics that should be recommended to patients with foot pain/arthritis.**

- High heels and pointy-toed shoes should be avoided. If must wear, should be for no longer than 3 hours a day three times a week.
- Floppy loafers or other shoes (i.e., can fold shoe toe to touch heel) will hurt feet.
- Tie lacing of several holes to secure foot and be able to loosen with foot swelling. If hand deformities prevent tying laces, consider Velcro closures.

- Need wide, deep toe box so toes aren't crowded. Leather should be soft with no rubbing from internal stitching.
- Heel height should be about 1 inch.
- Heel counter should be firm to prevent foot pronation or rolling.
- Soft cushioned sole (crepe sole) serves as a shock absorber.
- If significant bony foot deformity, may need custom made shoes.
- Recommend patient try on shoes and walk around store for 15–20 minutes before purchasing the shoes.

## SPECIFIC DISEASE REHABILITATION

**33. Name some general goals of therapeutic exercise for osteoarthritis.**

In addition to localized involvement of the joint and weakness of the directly associated muscles, patients with osteoarthritis who become inactive lose cardiovascular fitness and functional independence, and gain weight. The patients also progressively deteriorate in the performance of their activities of daily living and progressively lose independence. Exercise, as a part of treatment of osteoarthritis, attempts to counter this general decline. The general goals of an exercise program are to increase or maintain joint motion, normalize gait, build muscular strength and endurance, improve aerobic capacity, facilitate weight loss, improve functional capacity, and provide an opportunity for socialization.

**34. What kinds of exercise are available for a patient with osteoarthritis?**

Based on the general degree of dysfunction and specific involvement of individual joints, a physician may prescribe exercise that includes isometric, isotonic, aerobic, or aquatic exercise. The type of program should be individualized to the patient's interests, ability, and tolerance for exercise. The patient's compliance improves with his or her understanding of the exercise program and encouragement from physical therapists, group leaders, other patients, and family. Consistency in attendance to an exercise program is far more important than the intensity when the goals are more specifically directed to functional well-being than to increased performance.

**35. Describe a sample physical and occupational therapy prescription for a patient with rheumatoid arthritis who has recently recovered after an exacerbation requiring 2 weeks of bedrest.**

**Physical therapy**: Assess current function and commence progressive remobilization, including passive and active techniques, gait training, instruction in joint protective techniques, with goals of improved endurance, mobility, and reduction in pain. Three times per week for 4–6 weeks, 1–2 hours per session. Include aquatic therapy to enhance posture, gait, and strength 2 times per week. Transition this to a self-managed program.

**Occupational therapy**: Assess current functional activities and provide instruction for self-care activities, dressing, grooming, and hygiene. Progress to household activities as tolerated.

**Contraindications**: Avoid excessive stress to joints with residual inflammation, reduce activities if pain or fatigue occurs, provide adequate periods of rest, and avoid severe discomfort and pain.

**36. Can patients with rheumatoid arthritis benefit from a regular exercise program?**

Regular exercise can increase their functional levels, including endurance, activities of daily living, and mobility. Exercise programs must be adjusted specifically for the disease process. Patients benefit from low-repetition, low-resistance isotonic exercises, frequently undertaken through short arcs as compared with the entire arc of motion. The addition of swimming, bicycling, gardening, and other activities helps preserve and develop both type I and type II muscle fibers.

**37. What rehabilitative techniques can be used for some other rheumatic diseases?**

- Ankylosing spondylitis—spinal extension and hip and shoulder ROM exercises. Deep breathing exercises.

- Polymyositis/dermatomyositis—isometric exercises three times a week after inflammation is under control. ROM exercises to prevent contractures daily.
- Steroid-induced myopathy—active isometric and isotonic exercise program delay can decrease the severity of steroid myopathy.
- Systemic sclerosis—ROM exercises and splinting to decrease contractures. Finger flexion and extension exercises.
- Reflex sympathetic dystrophy—ROM exercises must be part of any program. Often, exercises must be performed after stellate ganglion blocks have been done to reduce the pain.

ACKNOWLEDGEMENT

The editor and author wish to thank Dr. Douglas Hemler for his contributions to this chapter in the previous edition

## BIBLIOGRAPHY

1. Biundo JJ, Rush PJ: Rehabilitation of patients with rheumatic diseases. In Ruddy S, Harris ED, Sledge CB (eds): Kelley's Textbook of Rheumatology, 6th ed. Philadelphia, WB Saunders, 2001, pp 763–776.
2. Braddom RL: Physical Medicine and Rehabilitation, 2nd ed. Philadelphia, WB Saunders, 2000.
3. Cameron MH: Physical Agents in Rehabilitation: From Research to Practice. Philadelphia, WB Saunders, 1999.
4. Cush JJ: Rheumatology: Diagnosis and Therapeutics. Baltimore, Williams & Wilkins, 1999.
5. Delisa JA, Gans BM: Rehabilitation Medicine: Principles and Practice, 3rd ed. Philadelphia, Lippincott–Raven, 1998.
6. Kesson M, Atkins E: Orthopaedic Medicine: A Practical Approach. Oxford, Boston, Butterworth-Heinemann, 1998.
7. Lennard TA: Pain Procedures in Clinical Practice, 2nd ed. Philadelphia, Hanley & Belfus, 2000.
8. Maddison PJ: Oxford Textbook of Rheumatology, 2nd ed. Oxford, New York, Oxford University Press, 1998.

# 92. PSYCHOSOCIAL ASPECTS OF RHEUMATIC DISEASES

*Elizabeth Kozora*, Ph.D., A.B.P.P.

**1. Name the most common psychosocial problems in rheumatic diseases.**

Depression and anxiety
Uncertainty and loss of control regarding the disease process
Altered body image and reduced physical ability
Decreased self-esteem and self-confidence
Fear of becoming physically dependent and disabled
Loss of independence and security in career and personal roles
Increased stress related to social changes and disability limitations

**2. Is there a relationship between psychological factors and the onset of illness?**

**Con**: In some studies, psychosocial stress has been associated with disease onset, but the mechanisms underlying this association are unclear. It is likely that there are multiple etiologies, and under heightened stress, disease activity may increase.

**Pro**: Studies to date suggest that stress can precede flare-ups of rheumatic disorders, such as systemic lupus erythematosus and rheumatoid arthritis. Psychosocial stressors, such as disrupted or conflictual relationships or lack of social support, have been associated with exacerbations.

There is also evidence suggesting that stress can lower a patient's pain threshold in certain medical disorders.

**3. Can features of the history identify psychosocial problems in rheumatic patients?**

- History of psychological problems prior to the illness
- Patient's self-report of significant emotional or social decline lasting > 2 weeks
- Prolonged negative and pessimistic attitude by the patient regarding his or her medical diagnosis
- Abrupt change in patient compliance toward medical treatment
- Perception by patient that disease and progression of symptoms are uncontrollable

**4. What factors are associated with depressive symptoms in rheumatic diseases?**

Increased disease severity and disability have been associated with increased depressive symptoms.

Increase in pain intensity.

The secondary consequences of severe medical disease may increase depression by perpetuating losses (i.e., career or social roles), increasing financial difficulties, and reducing access to social support.

Restricted activities/loss of valued activities.

Patients with lower socioeconomic status and education may be more susceptible to depression associated with medical disease.

Increased age is associated with increased depression in physically ill patients.

Although not consistently reported, female patients may experience greater depression.

**5. What are the most important symptoms associated with depression in rheumatic disease patients?**

Somatic symptoms that represent diagnostic criteria for major depression (e.g., fatigue, anorexia, weight loss, insomnia, sleep disturbance, loss of sexual interest) are common in both depressed and nondepressed medical patients. Thus, they may be less useful in identifying depression in rheumatic disease patients.

Some studies suggest that irritability, crying, sadness, dissatisfaction, discouragement about the future, and difficulty with decisions might be considered normal psychological reactions to illness. However, prolonged periods of these emotional states may signify depression.

Additional symptoms that help identify depression in rheumatic patients include:

| | |
|---|---|
| Guilt | Low self-esteem |
| Pessimism | Feelings of worthlessness |
| Sense of failure | Feelings of being punished |
| Poor body image | Suicidal ideation |

**6. Are there risk factors for developing depressive symptoms in rheumatic diseases?**

- Personal history or family history of depression prior to diagnosis of rheumatic illness
- Increased pain and physical discomfort
- Lack of satisfaction with current lifestyle
- Rapid decline in functional ability
- Loss of ability to participate in valued activities
- Learned helplessness—perceived inability to control a stressful or threatening situation

**7. How can you screen quickly for depression in a busy clinic setting?**

Studies have documented that between 33% and 50% of patients with chronic musculoskeletal problems (RA, fibromyalgia, etc.) have depression. A useful approach in identifying depression is through the following two-step process:

1. Screening question—During the past month, have you often been bothered by either of the following:

- Little interest or pleasure in doing things (anhedonia)
- Feeling down, depressed, or hopeless (depressed mood)

2. If one of the above is answered "yes," ask about the core symptoms of depression using the mnemonic "**SALSA**."

Have you experienced any of the following feelings nearly every day for the past two weeks or longer?

- **S**leep disturbance
- **A**nhedonia
- **L**ow **S**elf-esteem
- **A**ppetite decrease or change

3. The presence of two or more of the core symptoms correlated over 90% with diagnosis of major depression by DSM-IV diagnostic criteria.

**8. What can the physician do to decrease psychological problems in rheumatic disease patients?**

- Be honest about the nature of the illness, provide information to demystify the illness, and discuss treatment options openly.
- Any change in compliance should be directly addressed with the patient. For example, if the patient has not been taking prescribed medications, ask about the patient's perception of the medications and side effects.
- Know what is meaningful in a patient's life and how his or her self-esteem might be challenged. For example, if work is a primary source of identity for the patient, then loss of work may require increased sensitivity and additional intervention.
- Overmanaging these patients and making them more dependent may be detrimental to their overall development of adaptive coping styles.
- Provide direct recommendations for psychological or psychiatric treatment when significant emotional distress is apparent or reported by the patient.

**9. Do any individual psychological techniques appear most useful in treating psychological problems in patients with rheumatic diseases?**

Psychiatric consultation and possible medication should be considered in patients who demonstrate prolonged emotional distress that interferes with everyday functioning or full participation in treatment. **Individual**, **family**, or **group therapy** might be considered for mild psychological distress. The following techniques are commonly used in medical groups:

a. **Behavior therapy** focuses on modifying behavior-mediated aspects of illness. Therapy may be designed to alter personal or family behaviors that contribute to poor health habits.

b. **Cognitive therapy** focuses on changing faulty and distorted perceptions and thoughts that interfere with healthy adjustment.

c. **Relaxation therapies** (i.e., biofeedback, progressive muscle relaxation, and imagery) have been useful in decreasing pain and depression.

d. **Coping skills training** provides adaptive coping styles to improve problem-solving and reduce negative coping strategies such as catastrophizing and or wishful thinking.

e. **Stress management**: combined relaxation and coping styles training aimed to reduce learned helplessness and improve self-efficacy.

f. **Supportive therapy** can reduce feelings of isolation and helplessness and encourage expression of emotions related to illness.

g. **Educational** and **skills training** focuses on information and strategies for increasing patient involvement in treatment.

**10. What factors facilitate psychological adjustment to rheumatic diseases?**

1. Adequate social support, satisfaction in the quality of interaction with others, and the ability to overcome devaluating social attitudes.

2. Constructive cognitive appraisal of illness and the ability to restructure long-term goals toward realistic outcomes.

3. Using active coping strategies which include seeking information about disease, focusing on positive thoughts, and deriving personal meaning from illness experiences.
4. Positive affect can influence pain coping strategies and increase level of activities.
5. Perseverance, independence, intelligence, internal control, creativity, aggressiveness, and moral stamina.
6. Developing a broader scope of values with physical attributes subordinate to other values.
7. Obtaining alternate financial resources and maintaining a flexible work schedule.
8. Increase self efficacy, which is the belief that one can achieve specific health related goals.

**11. How do social factors influence the rehabilitation process associated with disability and pain in rheumatic diseases?**

Higher levels of education may benefit some patients in allowing them to have greater flexibility in their employment opportunities.

The loss of income associated with disability can dramatically affect family patterns as well as rehabilitation and therapeutic options. Social service agencies may be required for less economically advantaged.

Married patients may adjust better to disability by limiting the negative effects of social deprivation.

The age of disease onset may be associated with specific developmental phases that significantly impact the patient's life and choices.

Slowly progressing chronic illness is different than acute trauma. In general, the more responsibility a person had for the event, the better the adjustment. A degenerative prognosis requires continued reassessment and readjustment to conditions.

For many rheumatic disorders, the disability is invisible (i.e., pain and stiffness in rheumatoid arthritis), which may adversely affect rehabilitation and social awareness. The better individuals are able to integrate their disability into their lifestyle and self-concept, the greater their acceptance of limitations.

Patients with increased self efficacy (belief they can achieve their own goals) have better mental health. Therefore, social activities that allow the patient to develop and achieve personal goals can provide an avenue for improved self efficacy.

**12. What are the estimates of medical compliance in rheumatic disorders?**

**Long-term compliance** to therapeutic treatment in rheumatic disorders is about 50%, a rate consistent with other chronic illnesses. Estimates of noncompliance to **medications** in rheumatic disease range from 22–67%. Noncompliance to **physical therapy** ranges from 33–66%.

**13. What factors are related to compliance with medical treatment in the rheumatic disorders?**

Adherence declines when patients have significant **side effects** to medications or take medications that require **multiple dosages**. Compliance also declines when the patient doubts the effectiveness of the treatment.

Compliance increases when:

- The patient and physician agree on the problem, model of the disease, and goals of treatment. Shared information and decision-making, with the patient participating as a "co-manager" of his treatment, probably improves patient motivation and the patient-physician relationship.
- The patient is threatened by the disease symptoms and believes an effective treatment exists. The caregivers should inform patients about all aspects of the disease and its treatment. This facilitates the patients' ability to plan their lives efficiently, ease uncertainties, make wise use of available resources, and create better arrangements for a possible decrease in the ability to care for themselves.
- Simple self-monitoring techniques are used, and social reinforcement is appropriate. Encourage cooperation from patient and family members.
- The disease has a more recent onset, and the prescribed regimen is not disruptive to normal patterns of daily living.

**14. Do rheumatic diseases affect sexuality? How might that impact psychological function?**

In many rheumatic diseases, sexuality may be impaired as a result of the disease itself or the medications prescribed. Sexuality may be problematic when accompanied by pain, discomfort, fatigue, poor self-image, or side effects from medication. The partner of a rheumatic disease patient may also develop fears about sex (i.e., being too demanding of a sick person, causing pain), and changes in sexual functioning are likely to contribute to emotional distress. The physician should assess changes in sexuality by directly raising the issue and offering appropriate referrals (i.e., psychotherapy) if necessary.

**15. Can medications administered in rheumatic diseases affect psychological functioning?**

**Corticosteroids** are the most frequently reported medications associated with psychological abnormalities, which include psychosis, euphoria, and depression. They have also been correlated with cognitive difficulties. Group studies have not consistently reported dose-response associations, and individual differences have been strongly noted. In patients undergoing significant changes (increase or decrease) in prednisone, possible psychiatric and cognitive dysfunction should be monitored.

Psychological changes associated with other common antirheumatic medications are fairly infrequent, although there have been some documented changes. For example, **NSAIDs** have been associated with dizziness, vertigo, headaches, paranoia, depression, and hostility; **gold** and **chloroquine** have been previously associated with confusion, hallucinations, delirium, and nightmares; and **methotrexate** is known to cause behavioral abnormalities in high doses.

## BIBLIOGRAPHY


1. Ahles TA, Khan S, Yunus MB, et al: Psychiatric status of patients with primary fibromyalgia, patients with rheumatoid arthritis, and subjects without pain: A blind comparison of DSM-III diagnosis. Am J Psychiatry 148:1721–1726, 1991.
2. Badley EM, Rasooly I, Webser GK: Relative importance of musculoskeletal disorders as a cause of chronic health problems, disability and health care utilization: Findings from the 1990 Ontario Health Survey. J Rheumatol 21:505–514; 1994
3. Blalock SJ, DeVellis BM, Giorgino KB: The relationship between coping and psychological well-being among people with osteoarthritis: A problem-specific approach. Ann Behav Med 17:107–115, 1995
4. Brody DS, et al: Patients with depression in the primary care setting. Arch Int Med 158:2469–2475, 1998.
5. Burckhardt CS, Archenholtz B, Bjelle A: Quality of life of women with systemic lupus erythematosus: A comparison with woman with rheumatoid arthritis. J Rheumatol 20:977–981, 1993.
6. Hawley DJ, Wolfe F: Depression is not more common in rheumatoid arthritis: A 10-year longitudinal study of 6,153 patients with rheumatic disease. J Rheumatol 20:2025–2031, 1993.
7. Hudson JI, Goldenberg DL, Pope HG, et al: Comorbidity of fibromyalgia with medical and psychiatric disorders. Am J Med 92:363–367, 1992.
8. Katz D, Yelin EH: The development of depressive symptoms among women with rheumatoid arthritis. Arthritis Rheum 38:49–56, 1995.
9. Leibing E, Pfingston M, Bartmann, et al., Cognitive-behavioral treatment in unselected rheumatoid arthritis patients. Clin J Pain, 15:58–66, 1999
10. Magni G, Moreschi C, Rigatti-Luchini S, et al: Prospective study on the relationship between depressive symptoms and chronic musculoskeletal pain. Pain 56:289–297, 1994
11. Milgrom H, Bender BG: Psychological side effects of therapy with corticosteroids. Am Rev Respir Dis 147:471–472, 1993.
12. Nicassio PM, Radojevic V, Weisman MH, et al: The role of helplessness in the response to disease modifying drugs in rheumatoid arthritis. J Rheumatol 20:1114–1120, 1993
13. Rodin G, Graven J, Littlefield C: Depression in the Medically Ill. New York, Brunner/Mazel, 1991.
14. Sinclair VG, Wallson KA, Dwyer A: Effects of cognitive behavioral interventions for women with rheumatoid arthritis. Research in Nursing and Health 212:315–326, 1998.
15. Spitzer RL, et al: Utility of a new procedure for diagnosing mental disorders in primary care. The PRIME-MD 1000 study. JAMA 272:1749–1756, 1994.
16. Swan KL, Parker JC, Wright GE, et al: The importance of enhancing self-efficacy in rheumatoid arthritis. Arthritis Care Res 10:18–26, 1997

17. Wolfe F, Hawley DJ: The relationship between clinical activity and depression in rheumatoid arthritis. J Rheumatol 20:2032–2037, 1993.
18. Young LD, Bradley LA, Turner RA: Decreases in health care resource utilization in patients with rheumatoid arthritis following a cognitive-behavioral intervention. Biofeed Self-Regulat 20:259–268, 1995.

# 93. SURGICAL TREATMENT AND RHEUMATIC DISEASES

*Donald G. Eckhoff,* M.D., M.S.

**1. What are the major indications for joint replacement surgery in patients with arthritis?**

Pain that has failed to respond to non-operative management and is limiting activities of daily living. Pain relief is the most attainable result of surgery. Restoration of motion and function is less predictable.

**2. What medical factors require preoperative attention in patients undergoing total joint arthroplasty (TJA)?**

All surgical candidates for orthopedic reconstructive procedures require a comprehensive history and physical examination to assess the overall general operative risks. Patients should be examined for carious teeth, skin ulcerations (especially around the feet), and symptoms of urinary tract infection or prostatism, as these could increase the risk of postoperative infections. Women should have a urine culture to rule out asymptomatic bacteriuria. If patients are receiving NSAIDs, these medications should be switched to a COX-2 specific NSAID or stopped several days (at least five half-lives) before surgery to prevent bleeding due to their antiplatelet effects.

**3. What other factors must be addressed preoperatively in patients with rheumatoid arthritis (RA)?**

**Cervical spine**—An unstable cervical spine due to arthritic involvement places the patient at risk for catastrophic neurologic loss when the neck is manipulated during intubation. Preoperative lateral flexion and extension radiographs of the cervical spine are mandatory.

**Temporomandibular arthritis** (especially juvenile RA patients) and cricoarytenoid arthritis—May make intubations more difficult.

**Immune status**—Infection rates are significantly higher in RA patients, partly because of the disease process and partly because of the immunosuppressive drugs used to control it. Patients should be on the lowest corticosteroid dosage possible. It is recommended that methotrexate be withheld for the week of surgery and the week after surgery (**Controversial**).

**Nutritional status**—RA patients may be relatively malnourished, which predisposes them to infection. Patients with a total lymphocyte count >1500/mm$^3$ and albumin level > 3.5 gm/dl are less prone to infections.

**Hypothalamic-pituitary-adrenal axis**—Patients on chronic corticosteroid therapy are unable to respond normally to surgical stress. They must receive increased corticosteroids (stress dose) immediately preoperatively, intraoperatively, and postoperatively.

**4. Patients with RA frequently have multiple joints involved. What is the recommended sequence for reconstructive surgery?**

Lower-extremity surgery is done before upper-extremity surgery, since crutch use postoperatively would place excessive demands on any upper-extremity reconstructive surgery.

In the multiply involved lower-extremity, the hip is reconstructed before the knee to get the best possible alignment of the knee and relieve referred pain from the hip to the knee.

In the upper extremity, the preferred order is controversial. Usually proximal joints, nerve, and tendon problems are addressed before the hand and wrist. The wrist is done before the hand joints to help with alignment. For the shoulder and elbow, the most symptomatic joint is usually done first.

**5. What additional intraoperative and postoperative medical procedures are done to prevent postoperative complications following TJA of the hip or knee?**

Intraoperative **prophylactic antibiotics** are given to decrease the chance of infection. For lower-extremity TJA (hip, knee), compression stockings, early ambulation, and **anticoagulation** are done to prevent postoperative deep venous thrombosis. Deep venous thrombosis occurs in 50–60% of patients if postoperative anticoagulation (1–6 weeks) is not done. The prevalence of fatal pulmonary embolus is 0–3% in THA and TKA but studies have not been sufficiently powered to demonstrate an improvement with prophylaxis.

**6. What is Steel's rule of thirds?**

At the level of the first cervical vertebra (C1), the antero-posterior diameter is divided into thirds, allowing 1/3 for the dens, 1/3 for the spinal cord, and 1/3 for free space. Because there is significant free space at this level, small degrees of C1--2 subluxation (3–8 mm) usually do not compromise the cord. However, when the *anterior* atlanto-dens interval (measured from posterior part of anterior arch of C1 to the anterior aspect of odontoid) becomes > 10–12 mm, all the atlantoaxial ligamentous complex has usually been destroyed, and the space available for the spinal cord is usually compromised. Likewise, when the *posterior* atlanto-dens interval (measured from posterior aspect of the odontoid to the anterior aspect of the posterior arch of C1) is < 14 mm, the spinal cord is usually compressed. (See also Chapter 18.)

**7. When should the cervical spine (C1–2) be fused in patients with RA?**

This is an area of significant controversy. The presence of severe pain, myelopathic symptoms or signs, and/or basilar invagination > 5 mm seen on a lateral radiograph of the cervical spine are indications for surgical fusion. Recently, prophylactic arthrodesis regardless of symptoms and neurologic findings has been recommended for patients with anterior instability of C1–2 and a posterior atlanto-dens interval of 14 mm or less.

**8. Give the potential intraoperative and postoperative complication rates following cervical spine fusion in an RA patient.**

- Postoperative mortality: 0–10%. Has been as high as 33% for patients with severe neurologic compromise.
- Wound infections and dehiscence: up to 25% in older reports. Significantly less today.
- Nonunion rates: 0–50%. Average 20%.
- Late subaxial subluxation below previous fusion due to transfer of increased stresses.

**9. What surgical procedures are available for RA patients with shoulder involvement?**

Surgical procedures of the shoulder are performed predominantly for pain control. An increase in range of motion usually does not occur. Replacement arthroplasty can include the entire joint, termed total **shoulder arthroplasty**, or only the humeral head, termed **hemiarthroplasty**. The principal factor in choosing between the two is the status of the glenoid. For maximal functional use and stability of a total shoulder arthroplasty, soft-tissue tension from an intact rotator cuff plays an integral role. If the rotator cuff is not intact and cannot be repaired, then a constrained arthroplasty, bi-polar arthroplasty, or an oversized hemiarthroplasty is chosen.

**10. What are the surgical options for management of arthritis involving the elbow joint?**

In inflammatory arthritis not responsive to medical management, synovectomy will temporarily control the disease and reliably decrease pain, but it infrequently has any positive effect on joint motion. Open synovectomy may also include excision of the radial head if significantly involved.

In **osteoarthritis of the elbow**, the ulnohumeral articulation is predominantly affected, usually by osteophytes that develop on the coronoid process or olecranon. Surgically, these osteophytes are removed through an osteotomy in the distal humerus (Outerbridge-Kashiwagi). When the articular cartilage is lost, the joint surface can be resurfaced with autologous tissue, fascia lata most commonly.

In **post-traumatic arthritis** involving the radiohumeral or proximal radioulnar joint, a radial head excision can be performed with predictably good results, as long as the medical collateral ligament of the elbow is intact. Total elbow arthroplasty is becoming the surgical option of choice for most arthritic conditions of the elbow. This is due to the increasing reliability of the current prostheses and the magnitude of functional improvement for the patient.

Elbow arthrodesis should be a very last resort, as this procedure makes it impossible to position the hand for functional use. It is reserved for a septic elbow that has not responded to other treatments and when total elbow replacement is not feasible. Arthroscopy is used for diagnostic purposes, removal of loose bodies, and synovectomy for both biopsy and treatment purposes.

**11. How are the common problems of the wrist in RA managed surgically?**

RA has a predilection for the small joints of the hand and wrist. The wrist is almost universally involved and usually presents predictable patterns of involvement and resultant deformities. The goal of medical management lies in control of the inflammatory synovitis to prevent destruction of bony and soft-tissue structures. When this fails, surgery can be used to remove inflammatory synovium or correct deformity.

The dorsal wrist capsule and dorsal tendon sheath are commonly involved with synovitis and tenosynovitis that often lead to extensor tendon rupture. Prevention of tendon rupture is far better than tendon transfer, and therefore, if medical control is inadequate, early surgical synovectomy and tenosynovectomy are warranted. The term **Vaughn-Jackson syndrome** is applied when the extensor tendons of the ring and small finger have ruptured. Primary tendon repair is usually not possible, especially if the rupture occurred longer than a few days previously. Tendon transfer surgery is then required to restore function.

On the volar aspect of the wrist, tenosynovitis of the flexor tendons can cause compression of the median nerve in the carpal canal, leading to carpal tunnel syndrome. It can also lead to rupture of the flexor pollicis longus tendon, leading to inadequate thumb flexion and resting hyperextension at the interphalangeal joint. This is called the **Mannerfelt syndrome**. It usually requires tendon transfer or arthrodesis of the interphalangeal joint of the thumb.

The distal radioulnar joint is commonly involved by synovitis, which leads to laxity of this joint, osseous destruction of the ulnar head, and pain with forearm rotation. The ulnar head becomes dorsally prominent and adds to stress on the ulnar extensor tendons. This constellation of findings is called the **caput ulna syndrome**. Its surgical management entails aggressive synovectomy, ulnar head excision, capsulorrhaphy, and lateral tenodesis using a portion of the extensor carpal ulnaris tendon.

When the true wrist joint (radiocarpal joint) is involved, the deformity usually involves five components: radial translation, ulnar deviation, volar subluxation, intercarpal supination, and carpal collapse. Early on, reconstruction using an extensor carpi ulnaris tenodesis can be beneficial. With advanced changes, total wrist arthroplasty or wrist arthrodesis can be used to control pain and improve function.

**12. What are the surgical options for basilar thumb osteoarthritis?**

The carpometacarpal joint of the thumb, also known as the trapeziometacarpal or basilar thumb joint, is a saddle-shaped articulation with a high propensity for degenerative change. The older middle-aged to elderly woman is most at risk for degenerative arthritis in this region.

Surgical procedures include implant arthroplasty, tendon interposition arthroplasty, tendon suspension arthroplasty, and arthrodesis. Implants have a high rate of failure, and work continues on a better prosthetic design. Tendon interposition entails placing a wad of tendon into the cavity created by removal of some or all of the trapezium. Tendon suspension is similar, except after the trapezium is removed, a weave of tendon is created that supports the thumb metacarpal base like a sling. Arthrodesis is probably the best procedure for longevity of the reconstruction, but it does restrict metacarpal motion somewhat and it requires very precise positioning or function will not be optimal.

**13. How is a mucous cyst and osteoarthritis of the distal interphalangeal (DIP) joint managed?**

Mucous cysts are commonly associated with osteoarthritis of the DIP joints of the fingers. They present as a clear mucin-filled cystic mass, usually between the DIP joint and the proximal aspect of the nail. Historically, they may have had a number of spontaneous ruptures, resolution, and recurrences. This cycle may lead to thinning of the overlying skin, making surgical correction more risky.

Pathophysiologically, the mucous cyst results from chronic inflammation secondary to a dorsal osteophyte of the DIP joint. Therefore, appropriate evaluation includes an x-ray, and definitive management must be directed at removal of the osteophyte. If the DIP joint is significantly painful or unstable, fusion of the DIP joint in mild flexion becomes the treatment of choice.

**14. How are deformities of the proximal interphalangeal joints (PIP) surgically managed in RA patients?**

**Boutonniere deformities** result from synovitis within the PIP joints, causing extensor tendon elongation and rupture and leading to progressive flexion contractures. During early stages, synovectomy may be helpful.

**Swan-neck deformities** progress through four stages of deformity. During the first three stages, splinting, synovectomy, and surgical release of intrinsic muscle tightness and tendon adhesions are used. In the last stage, when the PIP joint is destroyed, surgical options include joint replacement or fusion.

**15. Describe the results of metacarpophalangeal (MCP) joint surgery in RA patients.**

Synovitis of the MCP joints ultimately leads to joint destruction, MCP subluxation, and ulnar deviation of the fingers. Early in the disease course, before significant radiographic joint destruction or deformity, synovectomy may be performed for pain relief if medical therapy has failed. There is little evidence that prophylactic synovectomy slows joint destruction, but it may postpone the need for joint replacement surgery.

MCP arthroplasty is indicated when synovitis has resulted in cartilage destruction, decreased motion, pain, ulnar drift, deformity, and loss of function. The most commonly used arthroplasty is made of silicone rubber (Swanson's implants). Common problems include breakage, stiffness, instability, and reactive synovitis to silicone debris. MCP arthroplasties, irrespective of design, result in 60° of motion which may decrease to 30° over time. Postoperative splinting and hand rehabilitation are extensive and last for several months. Consequently, a compliant and cooperative patient is necessary for optimal results.

Arthrodesis is not done except for the thumb MCP joint. This is because the thumb needs strength for pinch, whereas motion is less important.

**16. Name three symptoms that are indications for joint replacement surgery in a patient with arthritis of the hip or knee.**

1. Inability to walk more than one block due to pain.
2. Inability to stand in one place for longer than 20–30 minutes as a result of pain.
3. Inability to obtain restful sleep due to pain when rolling in bed at night.

**17. What does the term "low friction arthroplasty" mean?**

Sir John Charnley, a pioneer in total joint replacement, coined this term in 1979 when describing his prosthesis for total hip arthroplasty. It refers to the small size (22 mm) of the head of the femoral component. Because of the small surface area, friction between the prosthetic head and polyethylene socket was minimized. This reduced friction lead to less shear forces imparted to the acetabular cup, which decreased the rate of loosening and less *volumetric* wear on the polyethylene, which in turn decreased the amount of particulate debris created over time. However, the small femoral head concentrated the joint reactive force and over time produced an increase in creep deformation of the polyethylene with a corresponding increase in *linear* wear. Therefore, today's prosthetic head sizes range between 26–28 mm in an effort to reduce both forms of wear. Highly cross-linked polyethylene and alternative bearing surfaces including ceramic and metal-metal have also been introduced to decrease wear.

**18. How do cemented, cementless, and hybrid prostheses differ?**

The terms cemented and cementless refer to methods of fixation of total joint arthroplasty prostheses for the hip and knee. Most experience is with **cemented** prostheses where a self-curing acrylic cement, polymethylmethacrylate, is used to improve fixation between the prosthetic component and bone. Advances in cementing techniques over the years have lead to less problems with aseptic loosening.

**Cementless** prostheses include press fit and porous ingrowth prostheses. Press fit relies on a snug fit between prosthesis and bone without the use of cement. Porous ingrowth prostheses contain pores located on the proximal portion of the femoral component and acetabulum that allow ingrowth of bone. Hydroxyapatite or growth factors may be incorporated into the porous coating to stimulate bone ingrowth and better fixation. Overall, there is bone ingrowth into about 10% of the porous-coated surface.

Cementless acetabular components have demonstrated the best bony ingrowth into the porous-coated areas. Consequently, many centers use a cementless acetabular component with a cemented femoral component. This is termed a hybrid hip replacement.

**19. Who should get a cemented total hip arthroplasty (THA) and who should get a cementless prosthesis?**

This is an area of controversy. Conventional wisdom in the USA suggests that younger, active patients with good bone quality in whom intimate apposition of prosthesis to bone can be achieved intraoperatively are the best candidates for cementless THA. This is usually a patient < 50–60 years old with osteoarthritis of the hip. Cemented prostheses remain the "gold standard" and preferred in RA patients with poor bone stock and in the elderly with low activity levels.

**20. How commonly does aseptic loosening occur in THA? What causes this loosening?**

In cemented THA done using inferior techniques, the rate of aseptic loosening requiring revision was 10–15% at 10–15 years of follow-up (1% per year). Radiographic loosening of the femoral prosthetic component was as high as 30–40%. With contemporary surgical techniques embracing many of the techniques pioneered by Charnley, there is now < 3% loosening at 10 years, a rate that compares to the degree of loosening (3% at 10 years) occurring in the best porous-coated cementless prostheses. Patients who are young (< age 50), and heavy (> 200 lbs) have the highest incidence of loosening for both cemented and cementless methods.

Today, the cause of loosening is not primary cement failure. Most loosening is caused by particulate debris (polyethylene, methylmethacrylate, or metal) from the prosthetic joint. This debris stimulates macrophages in the membrane lining the bone-cement or bone-implant interface to produce prostaglandins and cytokines, such as interleukin-1 and tumor necrosis factor, which leads to endosteal bone resorption and a loose prosthesis for both cemented and cementless implants. Use of bisphosphonates such as alendronate may help to prevent this.

**21. What unique postoperative complication occurs in patients receiving cementless THA?**

Mild to moderate **thigh pain** occurs in approximately 20% of patients receiving the porous-coated THA. This pain is due to a bony stress reaction occurring at the tip of the femoral stem. It usually does not require medication and resolves in 12–18 months.

**22. How is arthroscopy used in the management of knee osteoarthritis?**

Arthroscopic debridement of the knee is indicated in early osteoarthritis if some of the patient's symptoms are due to an internal derangement, such as a meniscal tear. Arthroscopic debridement and/or lavage can provide several months of lessened pain in some patients with more advanced degenerative arthritic changes (**Controversial**).

**23. When should osteotomy about the knee be chosen over total knee replacement?**

In the young, active patient with unicompartmental arthritis. The high tibial osteotomy is the most commonly performed realignment procedure for the knee with degenerative changes limited to either the medial or lateral compartment. Involvement of the patellofemoral compartment, inflammatory arthritis, marked loss of motion, and older age are contraindications. This procedure is usually intended to relieve pain, preserve functional status, and delay the need for a total knee replacement. It is performed by realigning the mechanical axis (center of femoral head to center of the ankle mortise). The axis is moved from the involved to the uninvolved compartment by a wedge-shaped osteotomy of the tibia most commonly. If correction of the mechanical axis requires > 12° wedge, then the osteotomy should be performed in the distal femur to prevent the production of a laterally sloped joint line. The most common complications include under correction and peroneal nerve injury.

**24. What are the indications for unicompartmental arthroplasty of the knee?**

This is an area of some controversy, and many surgeons are opposed to unicompartmental arthroplasty. It is indicated in the older, thinner, sedentary patient with at least 90° of flexion arc and arthritic involvement of only one compartment of the knee. It is contraindicated in inflammatory arthritis, obesity, young age, < 90° arc of motion or 15° flexion contracture, and involvement of the patellofemoral compartment. It is accomplished by resurfacing the femoral and tibial joint surface in the involved compartment. Revision to total knee replacement is possible, but this is technically more difficult and has higher complication and failure rates than primary arthroplasty.

**25. Who should get a cemented total knee arthroplasty and who should get a cementless prosthesis?**

The cemented posterior-cruciate-retaining prosthesis, posterior-stabilized-condylar prosthesis and the total condylar prosthesis demonstrate 90–95% satisfactory results at 5–10 years for both RA and osteoarthritis patients. Cementless prostheses have not been as successful due to poor bone ingrowth and tibial component subsidence. At present, cementless components in total knee arthroplasty are generally reserved for the femur while tibia and patella components are cemented.

**26. Discuss the problems that can occur with a revision THA/TKA.**

Revision THA is technically more challenging than primary arthroplasty, and the outcome (longevity) of the revision is significantly shorter and attendant complications higher. One of the significant problems encountered during revision is loss of bone stock, irrespective of mode of fixation. Another problem is soft-tissue balance producing instability in the revised hip and altered mechanics in the revised knee.

**27. How frequently does infection complicate total hip and total knee arthroplasties?**

Early postoperative infection rates are typically < 0.5% with use of perioperative antibiotics. Late infections (> 1 year postoperatively) occur in 1% of RA patients and fewer patients with osteoarthritis.

**28. Should patients with total joint arthroplasties receive prophylactic antibiotics prior to having dental work done?**

Yes. Amoxicillin, cephalexin, or cephadrine, 2000 mg orally 1 hour before the procedure. If allergic to penicillin, patient should get clindamycin 600 mg orally 1 hour prior to the procedure.

**29. How is an infected joint prosthesis managed?**

**Early infections** (< 2 weeks postoperatively) can be managed with antibiotics and open syn ovectomy, thorough debridement, and retention of the prosthesis. Multiple surgical debridement are often necessary.

**Late infections** usually present with only pain but can present with obvious sepsis of the in volved joint. Once the diagnosis is made, treatment is removal of prosthetic components, thor ough debridement, and intravenous antibiotics for 6 weeks. If a low virulence organism i cultured, replantation with antibiotic-impregnated cement can be performed at 6 weeks. If gram negative organisms are cultured, a longer duration of resection arthroplasty is required, with oc casionally 12 months needed to reduce the reinfection rate.

**30. Name the two most common etiologies of ankle arthritis. How are they manage surgically?**

Post-traumatic arthritis and RA. The ankle joint very rarely becomes arthritic compared t the hip and knee, but when it does, it is most commonly related to post-traumatic changes Fractures that result in minimal amounts (1–2 mm) of lateral talar subluxation will produce de generative changes in a relatively short time because of decreased surface area contact and in creased joint reactive forces.

Regardless of the etiology, functional bracing should be pursued until the patient can n longer tolerate this form of management. Total ankle replacement arthroplasty has historicall had a high failure rate from infection and prosthetic loosening and cannot be recommended as procedure of choice. Ankle arthrodesis is currently the best salvage procedure for the end-stag arthritic ankle. The success rate of arthrodesis is better in post-traumatic arthritis than in RA where the rates of both infection and failure of fusion are significant. Technically, positioning c the talus properly under the tibia to facilitate walking is the key point of the surgical procedure t allow a relatively normal gait and prevent lateral metatarsal stress fractures.

**31. Which joints are fused in a triple arthrodesis?**

The subtalar, calcaneocuboid, and talonavicular joints. Both RA and juvenile RA affect th subtalar and transtarsal joints. These joint involvements can be isolated or combined, and ther has been a trend toward isolated arthrodesis of involved joints rather than triple arthrodesis whe possible. Particularly common is isolated talonavicular joint destruction. If this presents in a adult with RA, then isolated fusion is recommended. Conversely, if the involvement occurs at young age secondary to juvenile RA, then the entire transtarsal joint (talonavicular, calca neocuboid) should be arthrodesed because this will provide a longer term satisfactory result.

Isolated subtalar arthrodesis is commonly performed when the remaining articulations of th triple joint are uninvolved and supple. Triple arthrodesis requires similar precision in positionin as does ankle arthrodesis to maximize walking biomechanics. In general, insensate feet (usuall secondary to diabetes) are a contraindication to bony fusion due to the high likelihood of skin ul ceration and subsequent infection.

**32. What is hallux valgus and how is it evaluated for surgery?**

Hallux valgus is the most common affliction of the normal adult foot. It is a condition wher the large toe is deviated laterally with the first metatarsal head deviated medially causing bunio deformity. The hallux valgus angle is measured by a line drawn through the proximal phalanx o the large toe and through the first metatarsal. A normal angle is 0–15° with moderate (> 25°) an severe (> 35°) deformities commonly occurring.

The cause of hallux valgus can be due to heredity, especially in combination with a short bi toe relative to the second toe. Other congenital causes include pes planovalgus (flat feet) an metatarsus primus varus. The intermetatarsal angle between the first and second metatarsals i measured by a line drawn through the first and second metatarsals. The intermetatarsal angle i normally 0–10° while angles > 16° are moderate and > 21° severely deformed. The need for sur gical correction is considered if the painful deformity interferes with a patient's lifestyle or abilit to wear shoes and there is a failure of conservative management. There are over 100 different operations for correction of hallux valgus. The choice depends on the surgeon's skill and how the deformity needs correction (i.e., proximal metatarsal wedge osteotomy if intermetatarsal angle too great, etc.).

**33. What are the surgical indications for correction of the bunion deformity?**

On initial presentation, all patients with primary hallux valgus/bunion deformity should be managed conservatively. This includes wider toebox shoes or pressure-relieving alterations in existing shoe wear. If this fails to provide relief of pain or skin breakdown over the bunion after 2–3 months, surgery is planned. There are a number of surgical options, depending on the degree of deformity, congruence of the first MTP joint, and whether or not degenerative changes are present in the joint. In RA patients with hallux valgus/bunion deformity, arthrodesis (15° valgus, 25° dorsiflexion) is favored over soft-tissue reconstruction or osteotomy. Implant arthroplasty, once common, does not provide a reliable long-term result. Juvenile bunions, unfortunately not rare, have a > 50% recurrence rate after surgery.

**34. What is a Clayton-Hoffman procedure?**

A commonly performed salvage procedure for advanced rheumatoid forefoot deformity. The rheumatoid forefoot pattern of involvement usually includes degeneration and instability at the first MTP joint, leading to hallux valgus and bunion deformity. The lesser toes are also involved with synovitis, leading to subluxation and eventual dislocation at the remaining MTP joints. This results in prominent metatarsal heads on the plantar surface and the development of intractable plantar keratoses. This progressive deformation commonly involves all the MTP joints to some degree.

The Clayton-Hoffman procedure entails resection of all the metatarsal heads through either a plantar or dorsal approach. Rarely, only two metatarsal joints will be involved, and the procedure can be performed only on the involved joints. However, it is not recommended to remove only one or three involved metatarsal heads. Fusion of the first MTP joint is often done concurrently with the Clayton-Hoffman procedure.

**35. Differentiate between hammer toe, claw toe, and mallet toe.**

| FLEXIBLE TOE DEFORMITY | JOINT POSITION | | | |
|---|---|---|---|---|
| | MTP | PIP | DIP | SURGICAL MANAGEMENT |
| Hammer toe | Uninvolved, neutral | Flexion | Uninvolved, neutral | Flexible—flexor to extensor transfer<br>Fixed—hemiresection arthroplasty excision of distal portion of proximal phalanx |
| Claw toe | Fixed, extension | Fixed, flexion | Uninvolved, neutral or flexion | Resection of both sides of the PIP joint; joint dorsal capsulotomy and extensor tenotomy, flexor to extensor transfer |
| Mallet toe | Uninvolved, neutral | Uninvolved, neutral | Fixed, flexion | Excision of middle phalanx and/or flexor tenotomy if flexible |

**36. Discuss the indications for surgery in a patient with symptomatic disc herniation.**

Overall, about 1% of patients with herniated discs eventually require surgery. Absolute indications include disc herniation causing cauda equina syndrome, progressive spinal stenosis, or marked muscular weakness and progressive neurologic deficit despite conservative management.

Controversy arises over indications for surgery in patients with less severe symptoms and signs. Relative indications for laminectomy and disc removal include intolerable pain with sciatica symptoms unrelieved by nonsurgical treatment (including corticosteroid injections) and recurrent back pain and sciatica that fail to improve significantly so that the patient can participate in activities of daily living after 6–12 weeks of conservative nonsurgical therapy.

Overall, long-term relief of sciatica has been shown to be the same in operative versus nonoperative patients, although the operative patients achieve their degree of relief more rapidly. The best results from surgery are obtained in the emotionally stable patient who has unequivocal disc herniation documented by consistent symptoms, appropriate tension sign, and MRI of the spine or myelogram. The most common cause for surgical failure is poor initial patient selection. Patients should be warned that surgery will help the radicular symptoms but may not help the back pain.

**37. What is periprosthetic osteolysis?**

Osteolysis around prosthetic joints causing loosening of the components of the arthroplasty is the most important long term complication, particularly of total hip replacement surgery. It has been reported that between 30% and 70% of prosthetic components have evidence of periprosthetic osteolysis at 10 years post arthroplasty as evidenced by a radiolucent line > 3 mm in thickness around the prosthesis. The cause is believed to be polyethylene particles due to wear of the articulating surfaces of the prosthesis. The particulate debris tracks down along the side of the prosthesis where it is ingested by macrophages which release cytokines including IL-1 and TNFα as well as prostaglandins ($PGE_2$). This results in stimulation of osteoclasts possibly through RANK ligand upregulation. Treatment has included bisphosphonates (downregulates macrophages and osteoclasts), indomethacin (decreases prostaglandin production), anti-TNFα therapy, and aluminum.

ACKNOWLEDGMENT

The editor and author wish to thank John A. Reister, M.D., for his contributions to this chapter in the previous edition of this book.

BIBLIOGRAPHY

1. American Dental Association: Antibiotic prophylaxis for dental patients with total joint replacements. JADA 128:1004–1008, 1997.
2. Ayers DC, Short WH: Arthritis surgery. Clin Exp Rheumatol 11:75–84, 1993.
3. Boden SD: Rheumatoid arthritis of the cervical spine: Surgical decision making based on predictors of paralysis and recovery. Spine 19:2275–2280, 1994.
4. Brady OH, Masri BA, Garbuz DS, Duncan CP: Joint replacement of hip and knee—when to refer and what to expect. CMAJ 163:1285–1291, 2000.
5. Carette S, LeClaire R, Marçoux S, et al: Epidural corticosteroid injections for sciatica due to herniated nucleus pulposus. N Engl J Med 336:1634–1640, 1997.
6. Clayton ML, Winter WG (eds): The rheumatoid foot. Clin Ortho Related Res 340:July 1997.
7. Ferlic DC: Total elbow arthroplasty for treatment of elbow arthritis. J Shoulder Elbow Surg 8:367–378, 1999.
8. Friedman RJ (ed): Total should arthroplasty. Orthop Clin North Am 29:July 1998.
9. Gillespie WJ: Prevention and management of infection after total joint replacement. Clinical Infectious Diseases 25:1310–1317, 1997.
10. Gunther KP: Surgical approaches for osteoarthritis. Best Practice and Research Clin Rheumatol 15:627–643, 2001.
11. Hanley EN, David SM: Lumbar arthrodesis for the treatment of back pain. J Bone Joint Surgery 81A:716–730, 1999.
12. Hansraj KK (ed): Wrist and small joint arthroplasty of the hand. Clin Ortho Related Res 342:September 1997.
13. Harris WH: Wear and periprosthetic osteolysis: The problem . Clinical Ortho and Related Research 393:66–70, 2001.
14. Harris WH, Sledge CB: Total hip and total knee replacement (parts I and II). N Engl J Med 323:725–731 and 801–807, 1990.

15. Hull RD, Pineo GF, Stein PD, et al: Extended out-of-hospital low-molecular-weight heparin prophylaxis against deep venous thrombosis in patients after elective hip arthroplasty: A systemic review. Ann Int Med 135:858–869, 2001.
16. Jones RE, Blackburn WD: Joint replacement surgery: Preoperative management. Bulletin Rheum Diseases 47:5–8, 1998.
17. Linscheid RL: Implant arthroplasty of the hand: Retrospective and prospective considerations. J Hand Surgery 25:796–816, 2000.
18. Livesley PJ, Doherty M, Needoff M, et al: Arthroscopic lavage of osteoarthritic knees. J Bone Joint Surg 73B:922–926, 1991.
19. Loehr JF, Gschwend N (eds): Rheumatoid arthritis. Clin Ortho Related Res 366: September 1999.
20. Mehloff MA, Sledge CB: Comparison of cemented and cementless hip and knee replacements. Arthritis Rheum 33:293–297, 1990.
21. Merli GJ: Duration of deep vein thrombosis and pulmonary embolism prophylaxis after joint arthroplasty. Med Clin North Am 85:1101–1107, 2001.
22. Neufeld SK, Lee TH: Total ankle arthroplasty: Indications, results, and biomechanical rationale. Am J Orthopedics 29:593–602, 2000.
23. Peppelman WC, Krause DR, Donaldson WF, Agarwal A: Cervical spine surgery in rheumatoid arthritis: Improvement of neurologic deficit after cervical spine fusion. Spine 18:2375–2379, 1993.
24. Rathjen KW: Surgical treatment: Total knee arthroplasty. Am J Knee Surgery 11:58–63, 1998.
25. Weber H: Lumbar disc herniation: A controlled, prospective study with ten years of observation. Spine 8:131–138, 1983.
26. Wroblewski B: Cementless versus cemented total hip arthroplasty: A scientific controversy: Orthop Clin North Am 24:591–597, 1993.

# 94. DISABILITY

*Scott Vogelgesang,* M.D.

**1. What options are available for an individual who can no longer perform his or her job satisfactorily because of a musculoskeletal problem?**

- Adapt the workplace
  - Obtain or modify special equipment or devices
  - Modify work schedules
  - Job restructuring
- Consider switching jobs or reassignment to another position
- Vocational rehabilitation
- Apply for disability benefits.

**2. What is disability?**

Disability can be defined **generally** as *not being able to do something because of an illness or injury*. Most often, disability refers to an **individual** economic loss (by not being able to work at a previously acceptable level) because of a physical or mental condition. In insurance policies, laws, and regulations, the word disability has a more specific definition and needs to be distinguished from two similar, yet specific, terms: **impairment** and **handicap**.

**3. Give a specific definition of disability.**

*Disability is an alteration of an individual's capacity to meet personal, social, or occupational demands because of an impairment.* It is the gap between what an individual can do and what the individual needs or wants to do. The degree of disability is affected by not only the individual's impairment but also the economic and social aspects of that person's life (i.e., age, education, training). People with the same impairment do not necessarily have the same disability. Disability is assessed by nonmedical means.

**4. Define impairment.**

Impairment is a physical or mental **limitation to normal function** resulting from a disease process. Impairment is determined by a physician. An impairment does not necessarily mean that a person is disabled.

**5. What is a handicap?**

Handicap refers to the **social consequences** that relate to an impairment or disability. A handicap is present if an individual has:

1. An impairment or disability that substantially limits one or more of life's activities or prevents the fulfillment of a role that is normal for that individual;
2. Medical record of such an impairment;
3. Barriers to accomplishing life's tasks that can be overcome only by compensating in some way for the effects of the impairment. Such compensation involves things like crutches, wheelchairs, prostheses, or even the amount of time necessary to complete a task.

**6. List the important factors contributing to work disability in patients with a chronic musculoskeletal disease.**

*Disease*
- Type of musculoskeletal disease
- Disease severity
- Impairment severity

*Personal*
- Age
- Gender
- Education/training
- Personality

*Work*
- Occupation
- Job autonomy
- Work experience

*Social*
- Social support
- Peer and social pressures for or against disability

Most physicians concentrate on trying to alleviate the "disease" factors to decrease disability. The other factors may be just as important in determining whether a patient considers himself or herself disabled.

**7. What state and federal programs are set up to deal with disability?**

There are two major government programs that deal with a person's inability to work: **Social Security Disability** and **Worker's Compensation**. The Social Security Administration administers two programs that differ mainly in eligibility criteria: Social Security Disability Insurance (Title II) (SSDI, also called Disability Insurance Benefits) and Supplemental Security Income (Title XVI) (SSI).

**8. Describe Social Security Disability Insurance (SSDI).**

SSDI is a federally regulated program that was established in the 1950s. It is the largest disability insurance program in the world. In SSDI, employers and workers pay into a trust fund. Workers contribute through payroll taxes (FICA) and receive benefits (based on lifetime earnings) if they meet certain listed criteria.

The individual must be unable "to engage in any substantial gainful activity by reason of any medically determinable physical or mental impairment which can be expected to result in death or which has lasted or can be expected to last for a continuous period of not less than 12 months." It is expected that the individual cannot earn minimum wage because of the impairment. The Social Security Administration tries to take into account individual variations in impairment, vocational, and educational backgrounds. SSDI considers only global disability, so there are no partial awards. Persons may also qualify for Medicare to help cover medical expenses after receiving SSDI benefits for 24 months.

**9. What is Supplemental Security Income (SSI)?**

Individuals not qualifying for SSDI because of a lack of work experience may be covered by another program, SSI. SSI pays monthly sums to financially needy people who are either > 65 years of age or qualified persons of any age with documented disabilities. SSI requires an evaluation of assets, sometimes called a "means" test. Usually, those who receive SSI are eligible to have some medical expenses covered by Medicaid.

**10. Describe the workers' compensation program.**

Workers' compensation is primarily a state-based system, although there is also a program for federal employees under the auspices of the U.S. Department of Labor. Any worker who incurs an illness or sustains an injury during and because of employment is entitled to protection against financial loss. It is a "no-fault" insurance system that provides benefits to all workers who are covered and who meet criteria. It removes the necessity to sue the employer. Workers' compensation deals effectively with work-related traumatic accidents but has more difficulty with occupational illnesses. Workers' compensation can award partial disability.

**11. Who is eligible for Social Security disability?**

Any employee ≤ 65 years of age (with an appropriate work history—see Question 12 below)
Unmarried sons or daughters < 18 years old (can be 18 years of age if attending high school)
Unmarried son or daughter disabled before age 22
Spouse ≥ 62 years
Spouse who is:
  Caring for a child who is < 16 years
  Caring for a child who is disabled
Disabled widow or widower ≥ 50 years of age
Disabled, divorced widow or widower

**12. How much work is needed to be eligible for Social Security Disability?**

This is dependent on how long the individual has worked, how recently the individual was employed, and the age at which the individual became disabled. Currently, workers > age 31 must have contributed to the Social Security fund for at least 20 of the preceding 40 quarters. For younger workers, fewer years of contributions are required, older workers will need more contributions.

**13. What paperwork is necessary to apply for Social Security Disability?**

Social Security number
Birth certificate or other proof of age
Names and addresses of doctors, hospitals, clinics and institutions involved in medical care
W2 forms or tax return from previous year
Summary of work history for past 15 years
Date employee stopped working
Marital history (if spouse is applying)
Dates of military service

**14. For those who meet the eligibility criteria and assemble the required application items, the Social Security Administration then evaluates three major factors. Name them.**

- **Inability to perform substantial gainful activity** (work). Gainful activity is defined as earnings that average > $700/month (in 2000).
- **Severity and extent of impairment**. Objective evidence of a physical or mental impairment is required. Symptoms alone are never sufficient for a determination of disability. There must be corroborating physical, laboratory, and/or radiographic findings. The impairment must interfere with basic work-related activities.
- **Does the impairment meet or exceed listed criteria for disability for that impairment**? The patient's individual physician does not determine if the person is disabled. The Social Security Administration has a list of defined impairments under each body system. If the patient's disease meets the listed measurements of disease severity, then the patient is

assumed to have a disabling impairment. These listings make the system more objective and uniform. If the impairment is severe but does not meet the criteria for disability, the Social Security Administration will determine if the individual can perform the work they did previously. If not, the Social Security Administration will try to determine if other work could be done based on the medical condition(s), age, education, past work experience and transferrable skills.

**15. What is residual functional capacity?**

If an applicant's impairment fails to meet the listed criteria for automatic disability, a physician or vocational specialist employed by the Social Security Disability Determination Service must make a determination of the applicant's residual functional capacity (RFC). RFC is the degree to which the applicant has the capacity for sustained performance of the physical requirements of certain levels of work. The physical demands of work are divided into five categories: sedentary, light, medium, heavy, and very heavy.

**16. Outline the physical requirements for each of the five categories of work.**

These requirements are defined by the Department of Labor.

*Sedentary work*

Sitting most of the time
Occasional (up to one-third of an 8-hr day) lifting of ≤10 lbs
Occasional walking or standing

*Light work*

Lifting of ≤ 20 lbs
Frequent (up to two-thirds of an 8-hr day) lifting or carrying of ≤10 lbs
Frequent walking or standing
Sitting with push/pull arm or leg controls

*Medium work*

Occasional lifting of 20–50 lbs
Frequent lifting or carrying of 10–25 lbs
Physical demands in excess of those for light work

*Heavy work*

Occasional lifting of 50–100 lbs
Frequent lifting or carrying of 25–50 lbs
Physical demands in excess of those for medium work

*Very heavy work*

Occasional lifting of > 100 lbs
Frequent lifting or carrying of > 50 lbs
Physical demands in excess of those for heavy work

Other factors taken into account when determining a person's RFC are fatigue; ability to see, hear, and speak; adequate mental capacity; ability for social interaction with coworkers; and skills to adapt to changes in work routine.

**17. How does the Social Security Administration use the RFC in determining disability?**

The disability examiner determines the physical demands of the work previously done by the applicant and judges whether the individual has the RFC to do such work. If not, the examiner considers whether the applicant's RFC, coupled with the individual's age, education, and previous work experience, makes it possible for the applicant to do any work. If not, the applicant can be declared disabled, even though his or her impairment did not meet listed disability criteria.

**18. Are there ways to measure RFC apart from the Social Security System?**

Yes. Functional Capacity Evaluations can be performed by appropriately trained physicians or therapists. This is physical ability test that is specifically related to the indivdual's occupational requirements. Specific abilities and endurances are measured such as standing, sitting, crawling, lifting, bending, strength, flexibility, pushing, pulling and climbing stairs. These abilities and endurances are quantified according to Department of Labor standards according to weight and frequency of the activity (see Question 16).

**19. How is an application for disability benefits evaluated? Can a decision be appealed?**

An application to the Social Security Administration for disability benefits is first evaluated by a physician-panel without a personal appearance by the applicant. Approximately one-third of applications are approved at this point. However, an individual has the option of appeal at many stages, while the Social Security Administration does not. After initially being denied, an individual may have the application reviewed again by a separate physician-panel. However, few of these appeals are granted benefits. A denial at this stage may be appealed to a third level, an administrative law judge, where a personal appearance may first take place. Approximately 50% of the cases appealed to administrative law judges are subsequently approved, making this application step very important. Applications denied by the administrative law judge can be appealed to the Social Security Appeals Council and ultimately to a U.S. District Court. Few of these cases are ultimately approved. Overall, approximately 40–50% of all applications to the Social Security Administration are ultimately approved.

**20. If an individual who is receiving disability benefits returns to work, will their benefits be stopped?**

Disability recipients continue to receive full disability benefits for up to 9 months after returning to work. This 9-month period is called a trial work period. The 9 months need not be continuous, and only months count in which the individual earns > $200/month (in 2000). Disability benefits are reassessed after the trial work period. If it is decided that disability benefits are no longer needed, the individual receives three more monthly checks. Subsequently, benefits are paid for any month the individual is disabled and unable to perform substantial gainful activity (earn > $700/month in 2000) for up to 36 months after the trial work period ends. If disability payments end but the individual continues with impairment, the Medicare benefit can be continued for up to 39 months, even though the person is no longer receiving disability payments.

**21. What is vocational rehabilitation?**

Vocational rehabilitation (VR) is a service provided for by the Federal Rehabilitation Act of 1973. Funded by both state and federal governments, VR agencies assist people with disabilities to find and keep employment. Every state is required to have a VR program, although the range of services varies among states. Private vocational rehabilition agencies also provide a wide array of services to disabled and injured individuals.

Any person applying for disability is referred to and considered for vocational rehabilitation. The participating agencies provide counseling, interest/skills evaluation, basic living expenses, education expenses, transportation costs, purchase of special equipment, job training, and placement. These agencies may also acquire services from other public programs. Not all VR services are provided free of charge, but in some cases, VR does pay for all expenses when an individual has very limited resources. Disability benefits may be continued while an individual receives VR services, but refusal of VR services may stop disability benefits. If a person recovers while participating in VR services, disability benefits continue if they are likely to enable the person to work.

**22. What is the primary physician's role while the patient is applying for disability?**

The primary physician may be asked to fulfill several roles:

Information source for the patient

Details of the disability insurance system

Options to be pursued if the request is denied

Information source for the agency by documenting the impairment

Prior health status

Objective evidence of impairment (physical findings, radiographs, laboratory abnormalities)

Progression of symptoms
Impact the impairment has on the patient's activities of daily living
Response to therapy
Patient advocate, supporting the patient during the process of application
Monitor of on-going therapy
Independent validator of an impairment
Expert witness for litigation

Difficulties arise for both the physician and patient when these roles become contradictory. A physician who tries to be an effective patient advocate and an impartial adjudicator at the same time may be risking a strain of the physician-patient relationship.

**23. What are "activities of daily living"?**

Usual activities that need to be assessed and documented when evaluating or documenting impairments. Over 60% of patients with chronic musculoskeletal disorders report some limitation with one or more of these activities of daily living.

*Activities of Daily Living*

| CATEGORIES | SPECIFIC ACTIVITIES |
|---|---|
| Self-care and personal hygiene | Bathing, dressing, brushing teeth, combing hair, eating, toileting |
| Communication | Writing, speaking, hearing |
| Ambulation, travel, and posture | Walking, climbing stairs, driving, riding, flying, sitting, standing, lying down |
| Movement | Lifting, grasping, tactile discrimination |
| Sleep, social activities, and sexual function | — |

**24. Does the Americans with Disabilities Act of 1990 apply to musculoskeletal conditions?**

Yes. This Act makes it unlawful to discriminate in employment against a qualified individual with a disability. It also outlaws discrimination against individuals with disabilities in state and local government services, public accommodations, transportation, and telecommunications. To be protected, one must have a "substantial" impairment (one that significantly limits or restricts a major life activity) and must be qualified to perform the essential functions or duties of a job with or without reasonable accommodation. Reasonable accommodations include modifying work schedules, equipment or environment. An employer may deny providing reasonable accommodations for either financial hardship or business necessity.

## BIBLIOGRAPHY

1. American Medical Association: Guides to the evaluation of permanent impairment, 5th ed. Chicago, AMA, 2000.
2. Carey TS, Hadler NM: The role of the primary care physician in disability determination for Social Security Insurance and Worker's Compensation. Ann Intern Med 104:706, 1986.
3. Katz RT, Rondinelli RD: Impairment and disability rating in low back pain. Occup Med 13:213–230, 1998.
4. King PM, Tuckwell N, Barrett TE: A critical review of functional capacity evalutions. Phys Therapy 78:852–866, 1998.
5. Kennedy LD: SSI at its 25th year. Social Security Bulletin 62:52–58, 1999.
6. Minnigerode LK: Social Security and the physician. Missouri Med 97:156–158, 2000.
7. Stewart AL, Painter PL: Issues in measuring physical functioning and disability in arthritis patients. Arthritis Care Res 10:395–405, 1997.
8. Wolfe JS: De-mystifying social security disability adjudication: The physician's role. J Okla State Med Assoc 91:347–349, 1998.

Websites:
Department of Labor: http://www.dol.gov
Office of Administrative Law Judges: http://www.oalj.dol.gov
Social Security Administration Publication: http://www.ssa.gov/pubs

# *XVI. Final Secrets*

*Repetition is the key to good pedagogy. Read this book again.*
Thomas Brewer, M.D.
Senior resident who supervised the editor during his first month of internship (July 1976)

# 95. COMPLEMENTARY AND ALTERNATIVE MEDICINE

Alan R. Erickson, M.D.

*"I didn't say it was good for you," the king replied, "I said there was nothing like it."*
Lewis Carroll (1832-1898)
*Through the Looking Glass*

**1. What is the definition of complementary and alternative medicine?**

The term "complementary and alternative medicine (CAM)" describes therapies that have not been proven scientifically to be beneficial. This is not to be confused with quackery or fraud, which is a false claim made deliberately to promote a product or treatment.

**2. Just how widely used are CAM remedies?**

Over 130 unconventional modalities and more than 500 remedies to treat patients have been described. A 1999 survey conducted by *Arthritis Today* found that 28% of 790 patients were "highly interested" in alternative therapies and another 51% were "somewhat interested." Equally as revealing, only 40% of patients using these remedies told their physicians. In 1998, it was reported that 42% of adults had used at least one alternate therapy during the previous year. This is a 34% increase over 1990 data. In 1997, the percentage of patients with rheumatic disease who visited an alternative practitioner ranged from 25% to 54%, accounting for an estimated 629 million visits. It is estimated that patients with arthritis will spend over $3 billion annually on CAM remedies.

**3. Who uses CAM and why?**

There is no "typical patient profile" to predict who will be tempted by the promises of CAM remedies. Despite our scientific advances toward the understanding and treatment of rheumatic diseases, many of our therapies are empirical. Additionally, rheumatic illnesses are associated with significant pain. This, coupled with a lack of understanding by the lay public, psychosocial factors, and cultural practices, allows this huge market to succeed.

**4. Why should physicians care if patients use CAM remedies?**

Rheumatic diseases are confusing to both the medical community and lay public. CAM remedies often return to the patient a sense of understanding, responsibility, and hope. Unfortunately, not all CAM therapies are safe. Additionally, expenditures on CAM remedies can divert scarce health-care resources.

**5. List eight categories of CAM remedies.**

**Unconventional philosophies**

| | |
|---|---|
| Holistic medicine | Homeopathy |
| Naturopathy | New Age therapy |

| | |
|---|---|
| **Diet therapies** | |
| Dong diet | Elimination diet |
| Low-fat diet | Macrobiotic diet |
| Unpasteurized milk | Vegetarian |
| **Nutritional supplements** | |
| Amino acids | Antioxidants |
| Cod liver oil | Evening primrose oil |
| Fish oil | Green-lipped mussel |
| Propolis, royal jelly, bee pollen | Cartilage (shark, bovine, chicken) |
| Megavitamins and supplements | |
| **Herbal and natural remedies** | |
| Alfalfa | Chinese herbs (corydalis, genetian, paeonia, scutellaria, |
| Garlic | *Tripterygium wilfordii*, Hook F, and Ma-Huang) |
| S-adenosylmethionine (SAM-e) | Kelp |
| **Procedures** | |
| Acupuncture | Biofeedback |
| Chiropracty | Colon cleansing |
| Hypnotherapy | Massage and healing touch |
| Mineral baths | Hydrotherapy |
| **Diagnostic tests** | |
| Cytotoxic testing | Hair analysis |
| Iridology | Kinesiology |
| **Spiritual** | |
| Meditation | |
| Yoga | |
| Prayer | |
| **Miscellaneous** | |
| Copper bracelets | Dimethyl sulfoxide (DMSO) |
| Snake oil | Venoms |
| Antimicrobials | Exercise |
| Magnets | |

**6. Define holistic medicine, homeopathy, and naturopathy.**

**Holistic medicine** holds that people should try to maintain a balance between their physical and emotional processes while seeking harmony with the environment. Disease occurs when this balance is disrupted.

**Homeopathy** principles were set forth in the 1800s by German physician Samuel Hahnemann. They use dilute preparations of substances that cause the same symptoms the patient is experiencing to stimulate the body's natural defenses to fight disease.

**Naturopathy** claims that disease is an imbalance in the body that results from the accumulation of waste products. Natural therapies are said to remove the body's "poisons."

**7. Is there any evidence that diet affects arthritis?**

The subject of diet has attracted many claims of cures for patients with arthritis. This interest stems from various known facts. Autoimmune disease is a relatively current phenomenon and seems to correlate with our changing diet. In the late paleolithic period, the human diet was rich in protein, as opposed to our current diet, which is rich in fat. This increase in dietary fat can affect the composition of cellular membrane fatty acids. These membrane fatty acids are the source of arachidonic acid-derived prostaglandins and leukotrienes, which contribute to inflammation. It has been noted that some patients with inflammatory arthritis may be deficient in zinc, selenium, and vitamins A and C, which are involved in the scavenging or inactivation of oxygen free radicals. Though no convincing scientific evidence indicates that diet causes or cures arthritis, there are observations that diet may modulate the immune system.

**8. Can fatty acid ingestion alter our inflammatory response to rheumatic disease?**

Yes. Fatty acids (FA) are essential to the human diet, with omega-3 and omega-6 FAs being the two major groups. FAs are responsible for the composition of the phospholipids in cellular membranes, and thus these membranes can be altered by dietary intake of omega-3 or omega-6 FA. Additionally, FA are the precursors for leukotrienes (LT) and prostaglandins (PG), the agents (among many) responsible for our inflammatory response. Omega-3 FAs are the precursors of PGE3 and LTB5, a less inflammatory prostaglandin and leukotriene, compared with PGE2 and LTB4, which come from omega-6 FA.

**9. How do fish oils and evening primrose oil affect rheumatic diseases?**

It is known that ethnic cultures with diets rich in fish oils, which are primarily omega-3 FA, tend to have less autoimmune disease. Omega-3 FA diets can reduce arachidonic acid levels by 33% and increase eicosapentaenoic acid levels in cellular membranes by 20 times. This results in production of PGE3 and LTB5, which have less inflammatory potential than those agents made from omega-6 FA.

Evening primrose oil is gamma-linolenic acid (GLA), which is an omega-6 FA. In experimental animal models, excess dietary GLA results in more prostaglandin-1 compounds (PGE1) and less leukotriene production, leading to less inflammation. This conclusion has not been supported in human studies.

**10. What is the theory behind the use of antioxidants?**

Antioxidants interfere with the production of free radicals, compounds with an unpaired free electron that takes electrons from others, potentially affecting the immune system or cell membranes. One well-known free radical is superoxide, which is formed using NADPH. Superoxide is both a reducing and oxidizing agent and can spontaneously undergo a reaction to form hydrogen peroxide and oxygen. Hydrogen peroxide can also react with superoxide to produce a hydroxyl radical (the most reactive of the oxygen products) or chloride ions to form hypochlorous acid (the active ingredient in chlorine bleach).

A variety of antioxidants exist—including vitamins A, C, D, and E and the trace elements copper, zinc, iron, and selenium—which scavenge free radicals and protect cells against oxidation.

**11. The theory that arthritis is caused by an allergy to certain foods is the basis of several popular diets. What are the scientific studies to support this claim?**

Several anecdotal reports have described certain foods causing or worsening arthritis. Many of these are single case reports.

*Food Allergy*

| | |
|---|---|
| Rheumatoid arthritis | Dairy products<br>Wheat and corn<br>Beef<br>Nightshade foods<br>(tomatoes, potatoes, eggplant, peppers) |
| Behçet's disease | Black walnuts |
| Lupus in monkeys | Alfalfa (contains L-canavanine) |
| Palindromic rheumatism | Sodium nitrate |

There have been animal models of chronic synovitis induced with dietary changes. Apparently, food antigens can cross the gastrointestinal barrier and circulate not only as food antigens but also as immune complexes. Fasting appears to decrease disease activity in patients with rheumatoid arthritis. The postulated mechanisms are a reduction in immune activity, and a decrease in intestinal permeability potentially reducing arthrotropic bacterial exposure.

**12. Propolis, royal jelly, and bee venom have been claimed to cure arthritis. What is the science behind these claims?**

**Propolis** is a resin made by bees to seal the hives and is reportedly high in bioflavonoids. **Royal jelly** is a sticky substance secreted by the worker honeybees and fed to larvae; it is supposedly high in pantothenic acid. Both bioflavonoids and pantothenic acid are in the B-complex vitamin family, one of many vitamins said to cure and/or treat arthritis.

**Bee venom** has been said to cure arthritis in anecdotal reports. Patients receive the bee venom from bee stings or from a local injection in an affected joint. Adequate treatment of rheumatoid arthritis (RA) may require as many as 2000 or 3000 stings over the course of a year. Bee venom is rich in phospholipase and other anti-inflammatory agents. As expected, these remedies may lead to serious allergic reactions. None of these agents has been shown scientifically to be useful.

**13. A popular CAM remedy uses raisins and gin. What is the recipe and the origins?**

| *Recipe* |
| --- |
| 1. One box of golden raisins |
| 2. Cover the raisins with gin |
| 3. Let stand uncovered until the liquid disappears |
| 4. Eat 9 raisins per day |

Supposedly, as far back as biblical times the healing properties of juniper berries have been noted, and gin is made from juniper berries. Several of my patients with arthritis, both RA and osteoarthritis, have tried this remedy with mixed results.

**14. Many patients with rheumatoid arthritis wear copper bracelets. Why?**

Copper bracelets were used by the ancient Greeks for their healing powers. Copper salts have been used for the treatment of RA, achieving generally favorable responses, unfortunately along with significant side effects. Copper in bracelets is absorbed through the skin (turning the skin green) and is said to improve arthritis symptoms in some patients, perhaps by binding oxygen free radicals. Interestingly, d-penicillamine, a proven therapy for RA, binds copper, which would suggest that copper is not a useful therapy.

**15. Why is there so much interest in using antimicrobials for the treatment of rheumatic disease?**

For years it has been thought that arthritis, particularly RA, is caused by an infectious organism. Tetracycline was proposed for treating RA many years ago because it was thought that RA was caused by mycoplasmas. More recent research has shown that minocycline may be useful for RA, not because of its antimicrobial actions but because of its antiproliferative and anti-inflammatory properties. Yesterday's unconventional remedy may be tomorrow's new therapy. Remember, most stomach ulcers are now known to be due to *H. pylori* infections, which wasn't known 30 years ago. The following is a list of antimicrobials used for the treatment of rheumatic disease:

| | |
| --- | --- |
| Metronidazole | Minocycline |
| Clotrimazole | Ceftriaxone |
| Rifampin | Ampicillin |
| Tetracycline | Sulfasalazine |
| Dapsone | Hydroxychloroquine |

**16. Are herbal remedies used by patients with arthritis?**

Yes. Herbal products have been referred to as the most commonly used and abused form of alternative therapies. Herbs are claimed to treat arthritis and other diseases but, are there truths to the claim? Yes. Data does point toward a potential for phyto-anti-inflammation, likely through effects on eicosanoid metabolism. *Urtica dioica* (Nettle) is an example of a promising herb. In addition to inhibiting cyclooxygenase and lipoxygenase pathways, it suppresses cytokine release. Another common herb used especially in China is extract of thunder god vine (*Tripterygium wilfordii*), a Chinese plant. It's mechanism of action is anti-inflammatory and immunosuppressive through the inhibition of pro-inflammatory cytokines to include interleukin-2 and gamma-interferon and has been beneficial in rheumatoid arthritis.

**17. What are some other herbs and dietary supplements our patients are commonly using?**

- **Black cohosh**
  Uses: Treats hot flashes and moodiness at menopause.
- **Cayenne**
  Uses: Contains the chemical capsaicin that gives hot cayenne peppers their heat. When applied as a skin cream, it can deplete substance P from nerve endings, thus decreasing pain. Used for postherpetic neuralgia and rubbed on single joint with arthritis.
- **Coenzyme Q-10**
  Uses: Relieves chronic fatigue, immune stimulant, heart failure. Contains ubiquinone, which is a cofactor for metabolic pathways that generate ATP. Also a free radical scavenger and can act as an antioxidant.
  Drug interactions: Can decrease warfarin's effect.
- **Echinacea**
  Uses: Stimulate immune system, upper respiratory infections.
  Disease precautions: Liver disease.
  Drug interactions: Chemotherapy drugs for cancer treatment, HIV drugs, anticoagulants, immunosuppressive drugs, drugs that may be toxic to liver.
- **Feverfew**
  Uses: Migraine prophylaxis.
  Disease precautions: Pregnancy—uterine contraction causing abortion, ragweed allergy.
  Drug interactions: Anticoagulants, antiplatelet medications.
- **Garlic**
  Uses: Lower LDL cholesterol, platelet inhibition.
  Disease precautions: Surgery.
  Drug interactions: Anticoagulants, antiplatelet medications.
- **Ginger** (*Zingiber officinale*)
  Uses: Arthritis. Ginger inhibits prostaglandin and leukotriene production.
  Disease precautions: Gallstones, surgery.
  Drug interactions: Anticoagulants and antiplatelet medications.
- **Gingko biloba**
  Uses: Treatment of dementia, vertigo, ringing in ears. Can inhibit platelets and increase blood flow.
  Disease precautions: Intracranial bleeding, gastrointestinal bleeding, seizures, surgery, peripheral vascular disease. Gingko has anticoagulant effects and decreases platelet aggregation. Can cause GI upset.
  Drug interactions: Anticoagulants, antiplatelet medications, thiazide diuretics, tricyclic antidepressants, MAO inhibitors.
- **Ginseng**
  Uses: To fight fatigue, improve performance, reduce stress. Can inhibit platelets.
  Disease precautions: Heart disease, diabetes, pregnancy/nursing, surgery.
  Drug interactions: Caffeine (using both may cause high blood pressure), antiplatelet medications, insulin (ginseng may lower blood sugar), anticoagulants, MAO inhibitors, loop diuretics.
- **Goldenseal**
  Uses: It is not absorbed through GI tract. Used topically on canker sores.

- **Grape seed extract**
  Uses: Antioxidant similar to pycnogenol.
- **Green tea**
  Uses: Antioxidant, improve cardiovascular health.
  Disease precautions: Asthma, hypertension.
  Drug interactions: Decreases absorption of atropine, codeine, ephedrine, and asthma medications. Can cause hypertension.
- **Indian frankincense** (*Boswellia serrata*)
  Uses: Antiinflammatory by inhibiting leukotrienes.
  Disease precautions: None.
  Drug interactions: None.
- **Kava Kava**
  Uses: Reduce anxiety and insomnia.
  Disease precautions: Persistent depression—increased risk of suicide, withdrawal ??, pregnancy/nursing, surgery (potentiates anesthesia).
  Drug interactions: Alcohol, alprazolam, barbiturates, St. John's wort.
- **Ma-Huang (Ephedra)**
  Uses: For cough/bronchitis, as a stimulant and for weight loss.
  Disease precautions: Anxiety and restlessness, high blood pressure, heart disease, glaucoma, prostate adenoma, cardiac arrhythmias, surgery (causes high blood pressure).
  Drug interactions: Caffeine, decongestants, digoxin, MAO inhibitors.
  *This is a dangerous herb.*
- **Milk thistle**
  Uses: As a liver protectant.
  Disease precautions: None.
  Drug interactions: Phenothiazines.
- **Pycnogenol** (*Pinus pinaster*)
  Uses: Antioxidant because it is a bioflavonoid. Protects from heart disease and cancer.
- **Saw palmetto** (herbal catheter)
  Uses: Prostate and irritable bladder, stimulates libido.
  Disease precautions: Hormone-dependent cancer, pregnancy/nursing. Can cause diarrhea.
  Drug interactions: Hormone replacements, oral contraceptives (Propecia, Proscar).
- **St. John's wort** (*Hypericum perforatum*) (Nature's Prozac)
  Uses: Treatment of mild depression.
  Disease precautions: Can cause photosensitivity.
  Drug precautions: MAO inhibitors (Nardil, Parnate), SSRIs (Prozac, Zoloft, Paxil), digoxin, Ultram, oral contraceptives (decreased efficiency), photosensitizers (tetracycline, quinolones, Feldene), Dyazide, Bactrim, Septra, theophylline (decreased levels of theophylline), HIV protease inhibitors (decreased levels of Indinavir), cyclosporine
- **Turmeric** (*Curcuma longa*)
  Uses: Relieves inflammation by inhibiting prostaglandin production and stimulates cortisol production. Acts like capsaicin to deplete nerve endings of substance P.
- **Valerian root** (Nature's Ambien)
  Uses: Insomnia.
  Disease precautions: Can cause hepatitis.
  Drug interactions: Increased sedation with alcohol and other sedating medications.
- **Wild yam**
  Uses: Natural source of DHEA. Can't be utilized by body.
- **Yucca** (Adam's needle) and Devil's claw
  Uses: Contains saponin, which decreases abnormal fat content in blood and improves intestinal circulation. Claimed to have analgesic and antiinflammatory properties.

Disease precautions: Current or previous gastrointestinal ulcers. These stimulate gastric acid.

- **Zinaxin**—Ginger root extract called hydroxy-methoy-phenyl-33 (HMP 33). *See* Ginger.

**Pearl**: There is no standardization of herbal medicine in the United States. Consequently, a patient has little idea of how much active herb they are getting in what they buy over the counter. Daily cost of most herbs ranges between $.30 and 1.50 a day.

**18. What is DMSO, MSM, and SAM-e?**

- **Dimethyl sulfoxide (DMSO)**—It is a byproduct of wood pulp processing. There is medical grade that is safe and an industrial grade that is used in paint thinner and antifreeze. DMSO can be used as a solvent to transport molecules across cell membranes like the skin. DMSO taken internally or topically causes the person's breath to smell like garlic or oysters. DMSO is a prescription drug given by catheter to treat interstitial cystitis. Therefore, it can't be sold over the counter. Patients getting it from vendors are taking industrial-grade DMSO, which is unsafe. There are reports supporting DMSO's ability to relieve pain and reduce inflammation.
- **Methylsulfonylmethane (MSM)**—15% of DMSO is broken down to MSM. MSM doesn't cause oyster-garlic smell. Animal studies suggest it may be anti-inflammatory, but no scientific data to support its use. MSM has become popular since the actor James Coburn said that it works for his rheumatoid arthritis. Usual dose is 1000 mg BID.
- **S-adenosyl-L-methionine (SAM-e)**—This is already formed in the body from methionine and ATP. Plays a role in cartilage formation. SAM-e is equivalent to NSAIDs in therapy of osteoarthritis in controlled trials. Dose is 400 mg TID and costs $50 a month. Also used to treat depression.

**19. Are there any herbs believed to be unsafe?**

- **Carcinogens**—borage, calamus, coltsfoot, comfrey, life root, sassafras.
- **Hepatotoxicity**—chaparral, germander, life root, skullcap, Jin Bu Huan, comfrey.
- **Other**—licorice (electrolyte imbalance), Ma Huang (hypertension, strokes, seizures).

**Pearl**: Stop all herbs for at least 24 hours prior to surgery, since many have an anticoagulant effect.

**20. What other CAMs have people tried?**

- **Movement therapy**—Tai Chi has been shown to decrease falls in the elderly.
- **Magnets**—Static magnets cause a localized magnetic field. Theorized to interact with the body's nerve conduction and reduce pain perception. Magnet strength ranges between 300 and 4000 gauss (refrigerator magnet is 60 gauss). Little data to support use of this expensive therapy. May help localized joint pain.
- **Acupuncture**—Theory is that good health is maintained by circulation of vital energy (known as Qi) in the body. Illness is due to disruption of this flow. In order to correct this disruption, insertion of needles at defined points along meridians causes discomfort that is necessary to elicit Qi. Actually, it has been shown that acupuncture causes endorphin release, which can help pain.
- **Shark cartilage**—reported to have antiinflammatory properties and to inhibit angiogenesis. No data to support its use. Because it may inhibit angiogenesis, it should not be used in pregnancy, children, or patients undergoing surgery or with coronary artery disease.

**21. Are manipulation techniques useful for the treatment of rheumatic diseases?**

Yes. I recommend them everyday. Many patients with soft-tissue rheumatism respond positively to physical therapy and manipulation from chiropractors and osteopaths. Manipulation has been shown to decrease joint pain, although the mechanism of action is not well understood. I believe that if these modalities are used appropriately, it often leads to a decrease in the need for systemic anti-inflammatories. They also give patients a sense of participation in their treatment program.

**22. How does one report a potentially unsafe CAM remedy?**

The Office of Consumer Affairs publishes the *Consumer's Resource Handbook* that explains how to file a complaint. The publication is free by writing to Consumer's Resource Handbook, Pueblo, CO 81009.

**23. In summary, how should CAM remedies be approached?**

CAM remedies are widely used by patients with rheumatic diseases. Some are safe and harmless, and others can be deadly. Some remedies have therapeutic potential and may unlock the door to the next treatment for rheumatic disease; these deserve the attention of the medical community. I would encourage all health-care providers to discuss their use with patients. There are several internet resources to get additional information. One of these is the National Center for Complementary and Alternative Medicine at www.nccam.nih.gov.

## BIBLIOGRAPHY


1. Altman RD, Marcussen KC: Effects of a ginger extract on knee pain in patients with osteoarthritis. Arthritis Rheum 44:2531–2538, 2001.
2. Eisenberg DM, Kessler RC, Foster C, et al: Unconventional medicine in the United States: Prevalence, cost and patterns of use. N Engl J Med 328:246–252, 1993.
3. Gertner E, Marshall PS, Filandrinos D, Smith TM: Complications resulting from the use of Chinese herbal medications containing undeclared prescription drugs. Arthritis Rheum 38:614–617, 1995.
4. Kremer JM: Nutrition and rheumatic disease. In Kelley WK, Harris ED, Ruddy S, Sledge CB (eds): Textbook of Rheumatology, 4th ed. Philadelphia, W.B. Saunders, 1993, pp 484–498.
5. Lipsky PE, Tao XL: A potential new treatment for rheumatoid arthritis: Thunder god vine. Semin Arthritis Rheum 26:713–723, 1997.
6. Miller GE: Herbal medicinals. Arch Intern Med 158:2200–2211, 1998.
7. NIH Consensus Development Panel: Acupuncture. JAMA 280:1518–1524, 1998.
8. O'Hara M, Kiefer D, Farrell K, Kemper K: A review of 12 commonly used medicinal herbs. Arch Fam Med 7:523–536, 1998.
9. Panush RS: Complementary and alternative therapies for rheumatic diseases I. Rheum Dis Clin North Am 25:4, 1999.
10. Panush RS: Complementary and alternative therapies for rheumatic diseases II. Rheum Dis Clin North AM 26:1, 2000.
11. Tilley BC, Alarcón GS, Heyse SP, et al: Minocycline in rheumatoid arthritis: A 48-week, double-blind, placebo-controlled trial. Am Intern Med 122:81–89, 1995.
12. Yocum DE: Alternative therapies for arthritis. Rheum Grand Rounds 3:1–8, 2000.


# 96. HISTORY, THE ARTS, AND RHEUMATIC DISEASES

*James* S. *Louie*, M.D.

**1. What is the derivation of the word *rheuma*?**

*Rheuma* is derived from the Greek term indicating "a substance which flows," a humor that originates in the brain and causes various ailments. Guillaume Baillou claimed that "what arthritis is in a joint is what rheumatism is in the whole body," raising the idea that arthritis is but one manifestation of systemic processes. In 1940, Bernard Comroe coined the term *rheumatologist*, and in 1949, Hollander used the term *rheumatology* in his textbook *Arthritis and Allied Conditions*.

**2. Who described and named rheumatoid arthritis?**

Augustin-Jacob Landre-Beauvais (lahn-dray boh-vay) is credited with the first clinical description in 1800. He called it a variant of gout—"goutte asthenique primitif." Benjamin Brodie described the slow progression from a synovitis and bursal and tendon sheath involvement. A.B. Garrod (gair-roh) coined the term *rheumatoid arthritis* (RA) in 1858 and differentiated RA from gout in 1892.

**3. Which famous French painters were afflicted with RA?**

Pierre Auguste Renoir (1841–1919), the popular French impressionist, developed a severe form of RA beginning about 1890. Despite his increasing disabilities, he continued to paint, supported his family, and devised his own exercises and adaptive equipment. By 1912, he was bedridden and unable to transfer (class 4B). Just before his death, he developed vasculitis in his fingertips. Because he had rheumatoid nodules and vasculitis, one would guess his genotype was HLA-DRB 1*0401, homozygous.

Raoul Dufy (1877–1943), the talented Fauvist who explored "the miracle of imagination in color" in paintings, watercolors, ceramics, tapestries, and stage and mural designs, exhibited his first attack of RA at age 60. Within 13 years, when he became dependent on his crutches and wheelchair, he was invited to Boston to participate in one of the first drug studies that utilized different steroid preparations for the treatment of RA. He underwent a remarkable recovery, returned to his painting with vigor, but also suffered the consequences of the steroids, including a buttock abscess and a gastrointestinal bleed prior to his death.

**4. What other famous people had RA?**

Performers who developed rheumatoid arthritis include Edith Piaf, the French chanteuse, and motion picture actresses Rosalind Russell and Katherine Hepburn. The cardiac surgeon Sir Christian Barnard had RA, as did U.S. Presidents Thomas Jefferson, James Madison, and Theodore Roosevelt.

**5. Who is credited with the early descriptions of systemic lupus erythematosus (SLE)?**

1845 Ferdinand von Hebra described the butterfly rash on the nose and cheeks.

1895 Sir William Osler described the systemic features under the name *exudative erythema.*

1948 William Hargraves described the LE cell in bone marrow aspirates.

1956 Peter Miescher described the absorption of the LE cell factor by cell nuclei.

1958 George Friou described the method identifying anti-nuclear antibodies by labeling with fluorescent anti-human globulin.

**6. Name some famous people who had SLE.**

Famous persons who died of the complications of systemic lupus erythematosus include the Southern authoress Flannery O'Connor and the former Philippine President Ferdinand Marcos.

**7. Who is credited with the early descriptions of scleroderma?**

c. 400 BC Hippocrates described "persons in whom the skin is stretched, parched and hard, the disease terminates without sweats."

1842 English physician W.D. Chowne described a child with the clinical features.

1846 English physician James Startin described an adult with clinical features.

1860 French clinician Elie Gintrac coined the term *sclerodermie.*

1862 Maurice Raynaud described the vasospastic phenomenon of painful, cold-induced acrocyanosis.

1964 Richard Winterbauer, while a medical student, described the CRST syndrome of calcinosis, Raynaud's, sclerodactyly, and telangiectasia. The E for esophageal dysmotility was added subsequently (CREST).

**8. What famous Swiss painter and printmaker had scleroderma?**

**Paul Klee** (1879–1940), the complex and incredibly talented Swiss artist who completed more than 9000 works in diverse media, was stricken with scleroderma at age 56. His last paintings include "Ein Gestalter" (the Creator) as he recovered his desire and energy to paint; "Stern Visage," which described the skin changes; "Death and Fire," as he painted his requiem; and "Durchhalten" (Endure), a line drawing that described the dysphagia prompting his final admission to the sanitorium.

**9. Who is credited with the early descriptions of the spondyloarthropathies?**

In the late 1890s, the Russian physician Vladimir von Bechterew the German-Russian physician Adolf Strumpell, and the French physician Pierre Marie described ankylosing spondylitis. In the early 1900s, the German physician Hans Reiter and the French physicians Fiessinger and Leroy described the clinical characteristics of reactive arthritis or Reiter's syndrome. The association with the class I gene, HLA-B27, is credited to the Americans Lee Schlosstein, Rodney Bluestone, and Paul Terasaki, and the Englishmen Derrick Brewerton, Caffrey, and Nicholls.

**10. Which famous personages had ankylosing spondylitis?**

Olympic gold medalist swimmer Bruce Furniss

Television emcee Ed Sullivan

Renowned cellist Gregor Piatigorsky

Motion picture actor Boris Karloff (All of the stiff walking in his Frankenstein role may not have been acting!)

**11. What persons are credited with the early descriptions of gout?**

5th century BC: Although gout was reported in medieval medicine as *gutta*, Latin for "a drop" of a poisonous noxa, Hippocrates first described the clinical features of gouty arthritis following dietary excesses in sexually active men and postmenopausal women.

Late 1600s: Thomas Sydenham described the clinical features, and Anton van Leeuwenhoek described the microscopic appearance of uric acid recovered from a tophus.

1814: John Want reported the effectiveness of colchicine in the treatment of 40 patients with gout.

1857: A.B. Garrod developed an assay that detected uric acid in hyperuricemic states, demonstrated uric acid in cartilage of those with gout, and formulated the current hypotheses that lead to gouty arthritis.

1961: Joseph Hollander and Daniel McCarty demonstrated monosodium urate in the synovial fluid cells of those with gout.

1964: Michael Lesch, as a medical student, wrote the clinical description of a patient with neurobehavioral changes for his mentor, William Nyhan, who described the complete deficiency of hypoxanthine-guanine phosphoribosyl transferase (HGPRT), the enzyme that catalyzes the salvage reactions of purines (Lesch-Nyhan syndrome).

**12. Which famous Flemish painter had gout?**

**Peter Paul Rubens** (1577–1640), the portrayer of Baroque, developed attacks of fevers and arthritis that put him to bed at age 49. Within 10 years, his attacks were continuous, and he had difficulty painting and ambulating. He died of "ague and the goutte" at age 63. Some interpret the stylistic paintings of the hands as deformities that resembled rheumatoid arthritis.

**13. Which American Presidents suffered from gout?**

James Buchanan (1791–1868) and Martin van Buren (1782–1862).

**14. What was Beethoven's disease?**

Ludwig von Beethoven (1770–1827) noted hearing loss at age 26, was "stone deaf" at age 49, and died at age 57. His deafness is popularly attributed to otosclerosis, or 8th nerve compression from Paget's disease. More in-depth studies included records of attacks of rheumatism. A postmortem by Wagner and Rokitansky described "dense half-inch-thick cranial vault, shrunken auditory nerves, wasted limbs, with cutaneous petechiae, cirrhosis with ascites, a large spleen, and chalky deposits in the kidneys." These findings led to the differential diagnosis of meningovascular syphilis, sarcoidosis, and Whipple's disease.

**15. What were the rheumatic diseases in the Civil War era?**

Medical records of the American Civil War recorded 160,000 cases of "acute rheumatism," mainly acute rheumatic fever, perhaps infectious arthritis or gout. More than 260,000 cases of "chronic rheumatism" were recorded, probably chronic rheumatic fever and reactive arthritis, of which 12,000 were discharged. The validity of these clinical diagnoses on the war front may temper some of these data, and more recent data of war-related rheumatic syndromes gives a better perspective.

In 1863, General Robert E. Lee described paroxysms of chest pains radiating to the left shoulder and back, which was diagnosed as rheumatic pericarditis. He was given quinine. By 1870, because the pains occurred at rest, these attacks were probably advancing coronary atherosclerosis.

**16. Did Abraham Lincoln have a genetic disease?**

The debate on whether the American President Abraham Lincoln had **Marfan's syndrome**, the autosomal dominant disorder of connective tissue, reached national proportions when an advisory committee ruled on proposed molecular genetic testing of his tissue, which is preserved at the National Museum of Health and Medicine at the Armed Forces Institute of Pathology. Actually, the FBN1 gene on chromosome 15, which codes for fibrillin, the main component of extracellular fibrils, is the locus for mutations that result in a spectrum of true connective tissue diseases, including classical Marfan's syndrome. Because more than 20 different FBN1 mutations or abnormal fibrillin metabolism have been described in Marfan's and even in healthy relatives and normal controls, genetic testing will not be definitive for the diagnosis.

**17. What was Henri de Toulouse Lautrec's disease?**

Henri de Toulouse Lautrec (1864–1901) developed growing pains at age 8, was hospitalized for rehabilitation at age 10, and fractured his femurs following minimal trauma at ages 14 and 15. The clinical geneticists Maroteaux and Lamy noted the parental consanguinity and short stature and proposed the diagnosis of pyknodysostosis, an autosomal recessive disease characterized by mutations of the cathepsin K gene on chromosome 1. This retrospective diagnosis has been disputed.

**18. What musicians may have been "helped" by their proposed connective tissue disease?**

Nicolo Paganini (1782–1840) of Genoa, Italy was a violin virtuoso who had a flair for the dramatic and ostentatious. Although he had extraordinary musical talent, he also had extraordinary manual dexterity and hypermobility believed to be due to Ehlers-Danlos syndrome. This enabled him to play notes that most ordinary mortals could not.

Sergei Rachmaninov (1873–1943) was known to have hands so large that they "covered the keyboard like octopus tentacles." He was believed to have Marfan's syndrome.

## BIBLIOGRAPHY

1. Appelboom T, de Boelpaepe C, Ehrlich G, Famaey JP: Rubens and the question of antiquity of rheumatoid arthritis. JAMA 245:483–486, 1981.
2. Ball GV: The world and Flannery O'Connor. In Appelboom T (ed): Art, History and Antiquity of Rheumatic Diseases. Brussels, Elsevier Librico, 1987, pp 82–83.
3. Benedek T: History of the rheumatic diseases. In Schumacher HR (ed): Primer on the Rheumatic Diseases, 10th ed. Atlanta, Arthritis Foundation, 1993, pp 1–4.

4. Bollet AJ: Rheumatic diseases among Civil War troops. Arthritis Rheum 34:1197–203, 1991.
5. Brewerton D, Caffrey M, Nicholls A: Ankylosing spondylitis and HLA-27. Lancet i:904–907, 1973.
6. Francke U, Furthmayr H: Marfan's syndrome and other disorders of fibrillin. N Engl J Med 330:1384–1385, 1995.
7. Frey J: What dwarfed Toulouse-Lautrec? Nature Genet 10:128–130, 1995.
8. Gelb BD, Shi GP, Chapman HA, Dresnick RJ: Pycnodysostosis, a lysosmal disease caused by cathepsin K deficiency. Science 273:1236–1238, 1996.
9. Homburger F, Bonner CD: The treatment of Raoul Dufy's arthritis. N Engl J Med 301:669–673, 1979.
10. Louie JS: Renoir—his art and his arthritis. In Appelboom T (ed): Art, History and Antiquity of Rheumatic Diseases. Brussels, Elsevier Librico, 1987, pp 43–45.
11. Mainwaring RD: The cardiac illness of General Robert E. Lee. Surg Gynecol Obstet 174:237–244, 1992.
12. Maroteaux P, Lamy: The malady of Toulouse-Lautrec. JAMA 191:715–717, 1965.
13. Marx R: The Health of the Presidents. New York, G.P. Putnam's Sons, 1960.
14. Palferman TG: Beethoven: Medicine, music, and myths. Int J Dermatol 33:664–671, 1994.
15. Parish LC: An historical approach to the nomenclature of rheumatoid arthritis. Arthritis Rheum 6:138–158, 1963.
16. Schlosstein L, Terasaki P, Bluestone R: High association of an HLA antigen, w27, with ankylosing spondylitis. N Engl J Med 288:704–706, 1973.
17. Sharma OP: Beethoven's illness: Whipple's disease rather than sarcoidosis? Int J Dermatol 87:283–286, 1994.
18. Shearer PD: The deafness of Beethoven: An audiologic and medical overview. Am J Otol 11:370–374, 1990.
19. Smith RD, Worthington JW: Paganini. The riddle and connective tissue. JAMA 199:820–824, 1967.
20. Young DAB: Rachmaninov and Marfan's syndrome. Br Med J 293:1624–1626, 1986.

# 97. SIR WILLIAM OSLER, I PRESUME

*Sterling* G. *West*, M.D.

*When a patient with arthritis walks in the front door, I feel like leaving out the back door.*
Sir William Osler

**1. A patient with osteoarthritis of his hand joints wants to know if "popping" his knuckles when he was younger caused him to develop arthritis. What is your answer?**

The joint cavity is a potential space with a negative pressure compared with ambient atmospheric pressure. Joint synovial fluid acts as an adhesive seal that permits sliding motion between cartilage surfaces while effectively resisting distracting forces. During knuckle cracking or popping, there is a fracture of this adhesive bond. A gas bubble is created within the joint, which cavitates with a cracking sound, liberating energy in the form of heat and sound. This radiologically obvious bubble of gas can require up to 30 minutes to dissolve before the synovial fluid adhesive bond can be reestablished and the joint can be "cracked" again. Although knuckle cracking looks and sounds obnoxious, there are no data to support that it leads to osteoarthritis of the finger joints.

**2. A 39-year-old man presents to the emergency room with a 3-day history of right shoulder pain. The pain came on after he painted his house. Physical examination shows he is afebrile. He has full but painful range of motion of his right shoulder. There is no heat, erythema, or swelling. Palpation of the tendon anterior to the humerus elicits pain. Speed's test and Yergason's maneuver are positive. What is the diagnosis? What further tests, if any, are necessary to establish the diagnosis?**

This patient has bicipital tendinitis following overuse. The full range of motion of the joint, lack of inflammatory physical examination findings, and increase in symptoms with stressing maneuvers confirm the diagnosis. No additional laboratory or radiographic tests are necessary to establish the diagnosis prior to treatment. (See Chapter 66.)

**3. A 62-year-old woman presents with a 5-year history of increasing left leg pain. Read the description and decide the diagnosis.**

She describes the pain as a dull ache in her groin that radiates to her medial thigh. She also notes pain in her hands, feet, knees, neck, and low back, although to a lesser degree than in her leg. These pains have been present for about 10 years and have not been associated with swelling, redness, or warmth of the joints. Examination of her joints reveal bony swelling of DIP and PIP joints, limiting her ability to close her fist completely. She has a bony prominence at the base of her thumbs on both sides. Examination of the hips reveals normal right hip motion but pain when she flexes her left hip beyond 75°. Both hips externally rotate to 50° without pain. Internal rotation of the right hip to 15° is asymptomatic, but the left hip has only about 5–10° of internal rotation that produces pain. Both knees have crepitus without effusion or warmth. Patellar grinding is present. Her feet reveal bilateral great toes that are angulated and overlap the other toes. The first MTP is prominent and slightly tender but not red or warm. Her gait is remarkable for a noticeable limp. CBC, electrolytes, liver transaminases, and urinalysis are normal. Hand and hip radiographs are shown below. **What is the diagnosis?**

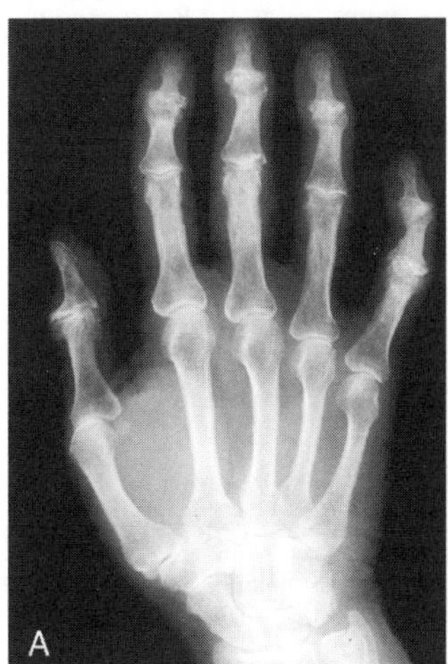


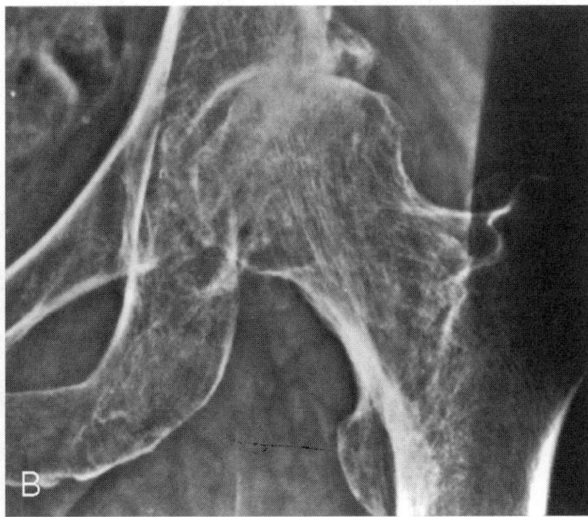


This patient has primary generalized osteoarthritis. Her major symptom is degenerative arthritis of her hip. The patient's noninflammatory symptoms, physical examination, unremarkable laboratory test results, and radiographs support this diagnosis. Hip radiographs are significant for joint space narrowing in the area of maximal stress accompanied by sclerosis and osteophyte formation. Hand radiographs reveal the classic "seagull" sign in the PIP and DIP joints. Physical examination would show Heberden's and Bouchard's nodes. (See Chapter 55.)

**4. A 60-year-old woman with long-standing rheumatoid arthritis presents for evaluation of a painful, swollen right knee for the past 2 days. Read the description and determine the diagnosis.**

Her arthritis is moderately well-controlled on methotrexate, prednisone, and naproxen. The examination reveals a temperature of 38.5°C and chronic deformities of rheumatoid arthritis involving the hands, wrists, and feet without active synovitis. The right knee is swollen, warm, and erythematous. There is significant pain with movement, and the knee is held in 30° of flexion. Aspiration of the synovial fluid reveals a synovial fluid white blood cell count of 85,000/mm$^3$ with 95% neutrophils. **What is the diagnosis?**

Whenever a patient with rheumatoid arthritis presents with one joint much more symptomatic ("out of sync") than other joints, the clinician should suspect septic arthritis. The low-grade fever and extremely elevated synovial fluid white blood cell count are also compatible with this diagnosis. The most likely organism in this clinical situation is *Staphylococcus aureus*. (See Chapter 42.)

**5. You are asked to see a 72-year-old woman with right knee pain. She is recuperating from resection of a symptomatic parathyroid adenoma that was performed 3 days earlier. Read the description and make the diagnosis.**

Her initial postoperative course was remarkable for transient hypocalcemia that responded readily to treatment. For over a year, she has had mild right knee pain when she walks more than a block. Last night, she developed pain and swelling of the right knee. Pain steadily worsened over the ensuing 12 hours, and she is quite uncomfortable. There is no history of trauma, and she has no systemic symptoms. She has never had any similar episodes previously. Her examination is normal except for the right knee. The knee is held in flexion. It is warm, swollen, and slightly erythematous. Any further flexion of the knee produces intense pain. A large effusion is present. Laboratory findings include a CBC with a hematocrit of 34%, WBC count of 12,300/mm$^3$, platelets 256,000/mm$^3$, erythrocyte sedimentation rate of 66 mm/hr, normal electrolytes, calcium 8.7 mg/dL, creatinine 1.5 mg/dL, albumin 3.3 mg/dL, and uric acid 8.2 mg/dL. Roentgenogram appears below. Arthrocentesis yields 48 cc of cloudy white fluid. Cell count of synovial fluid shows 28,000 WBC/mm$^3$, with 83% neutrophils. Gram stain is negative with cultures pending. Polarized light microscopy of a specimen of synovial fluid reveals weakly positively birefringent rhomboid-shaped crystals. **What is the diagnosis?**

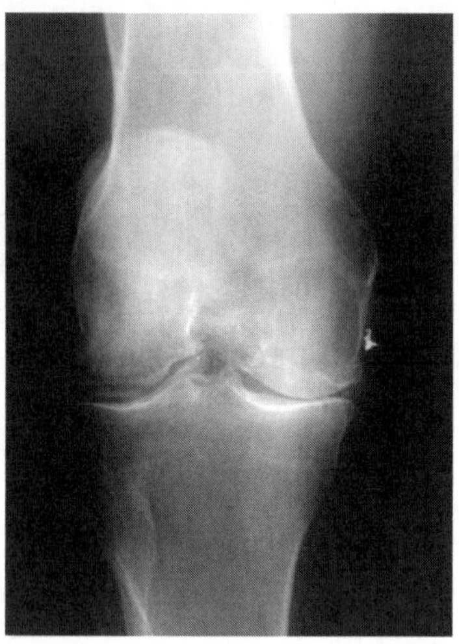

The diagnosis is acute pseudogout caused by calcium pyrophosphate dihydrate (CPPD) crystals. An elderly woman with a history of hyperparathyroidism who is postoperative, has chondrocalcinosis of the meniscus of her knee, and develops an acute monarthritis with weakly positively birefringent rhomboid-shaped crystals in the synovial fluid represents a classic presentation of acute pseudogout. (See Chapter 50.)

**6. A 60-year-old man is referred for evaluation of a rash of 1-month duration. Read the description and formulate the diagnosis.**

The rash is nonpruritic and involves his bilateral lower extremities. Recently, he noted a small ulcer at the left medial malleolus. Review of systems was remarkable for Raynaud's phenomenon, arthralgias of the hands and knees, and severe paresthesias of the lower extremities. Medical and surgical history were remarkable for coronary artery disease treated with bypass grafting 10 years previously and complicated by an episode of "jaundice" postoperatively. Examination revealed palpable purpura of the lower extremities extending to the thighs, with a small ulcer overlying the left medial malleolus. Moderate hepatosplenomegaly was noted. Tenderness of the wrists, MCPs, PIPs, and knees without swelling or warmth was noted. Neurologic examination was remarkable for decreased sensation to pinprick and light touch in the bilateral feet and ankles with absent Achilles reflexes. Laboratory results were remarkable for a normocytic, normochromic anemia with a hematocrit of 34%. Neutrophil and platelet counts were normal. The erythrocyte sedimentation rate was elevated at 70 mm/hr. Serum chemistries revealed a high creatinine (1.4 mg/dL) with mildly elevated liver associated enzymes. Urinalysis revealed 3+ proteinuria with urine sediment containing 5 white cells, 50 red cells, and rare red blood cell casts per high power field. Rheumatoid factor was positive in a titer of 1:2560 with a negative ANA (antinuclear antibody). Serum protein electrophoresis showed a polyclonal gammopathy. Complement levels revealed a markedly low C4 (8 mg/dL) and a normal C3 (85 mg/dL). Biopsy of one of the lower extremity skin lesions showed leukocytoclastic vasculitis. Nerve conduction testing demonstrated a diffuse symmetric sensorimotor polyneuropathy. **What is the diagnosis?**

Symptoms of palpable purpura, arthralgias, and polyneuropathy with liver enzyme transaminitis and an active urinary sediment on laboratory examination in a male is consistent with mixed cryoglobulinemia. Purpura is the most common presenting feature of cryoglobulinemia, with biopsies confirming leukocytoclastic vasculitis. The patient's history of postoperative jaundice and his elevated liver enzymes support a diagnosis of hepatitis C, which may be seen in over 50% of patients with mixed cryoglobulinemia. The positive rheumatoid factor suggests a mixed (type II or type III) cryoglobulin. The marked depression of C4 with normal C3 levels is a common complement profile in cryoglobulinemia. (See Chapter 35.)

**7. A 50-year-old woman is complaining of feeling tired and weak all over. Read the description and make the diagnosis.**

She believes that her symptoms have progressively worsened over the past 2 months. She works in a grocery store where she has had difficulty lifting objects to the top shelves when restocking. Even more concerning to her is that within the past several weeks she has had difficulty brushing her hair and climbing stairs in her home. She relates having little problem walking on flat ground and little trouble performing tasks with her hands. She denies experiencing discomfort in her muscles or joints. Within the past 3 weeks, the patient has noticed a rash over her knuckles. She complains of feeling fatigued but has not experienced fever, chills, or weight loss. Medical history is remarkable only for long-standing hypothyroidism. Her only medications are conjugated estrogens and thyroid hormone replacement. She drinks 2–4 glasses of wine per week. There are no muscle disorders or rheumatic diseases in her family members. Physical examination of the patient reveals symmetric proximal motor weakness quantified at approximately 4/5. Distal strength is normal. No muscle tenderness is noted. Neurologic exam reveals normal and symmetric reflexes and normal cranial nerve function. No fasciculations are noted. Joint exam is normal. Examination of her skin reveals a raised, violaceous rash over the interphalangeal regions of the fingers and presence of periungual erythema. Otherwise, examination is normal. Laboratory studies reveal: AST 100 U/L, ALT 75 U/L, total bilirubin of 0.8 mg/dL, normal creatinine and urinalysis, positive ANA 1:256 in a speckled pattern (ANA profile including anti-SSA, SSB, RNP, Sm, and dsDNA is negative); ESR 25 mm/hour; CPK 1050 U/L (normal < 200 U/L). **What is the most likely diagnosis?**

The patient's complaints of painless symmetric proximal motor weakness is consistent with an inflammatory myopathy. The physical examination confirms the presence of weakness limited to the proximal musculature, and does not reveal findings to suggest a neuropathic etiology. Laboratory results suggest underlying muscle damage with elevated muscle enzymes (CPK, AST, ALT). Other potential etiologies need to be considered in this patient. With a history of hypothyroidism, noncompliance with her medication or under-replacement could result in motor weakness as well as an elevated CPK. Although presence of a positive ANA increases the possibility of an associated connective tissue disease such as SLE, MCTD, or systemic sclerosis, there is no historical, examination, or serologic evidence to suggest such. Myopathies caused by medications must always be a consideration, but this patient is not taking any that would put her at risk. The presence of a rash characteristic of dermatomyositis (Gottron's papules) makes this the most likely diagnosis. Neurodiagnostic studies and/or a muscle biopsy may be necessary to definitively confirm an inflammatory myopathy, although a characteristic presentation, rash, and elevated muscle enzymes may be adequate for diagnosis. Because dermatomyositis in adults is associated with the presence of cancer in approximately 15% of cases, a screen for neoplastic disease is indicated to complete this patient's evaluation prior to embarking upon appropriate therapy. (See Chapter 24.)

**8. A medical student shows you a radiograph of a patient whom he is evaluating for long-standing, severe arthritis. What is the diagnosis?**

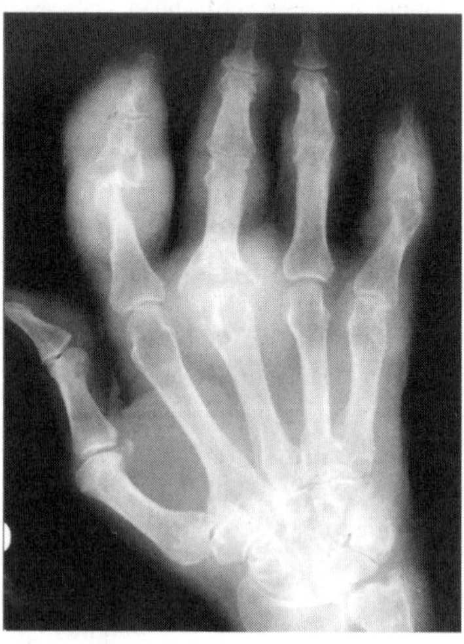

This patient has chronic tophaceous gout. Radiographic findings of erosions with sclerotic margins and overhanging edges (second PIP), cystic changes, expansile joint lesions (third MCP), and soft tissue lumps and nodules (tophi) are all classic for this disease. (See Chapter 49.)

**9. A 38-year-old woman presents with pain and swelling in her right calf. Read the description and decide the diagnosis.**

The pain started 2 days previously in the posterior aspect of her calf and has been associated with increased swelling and edema over the past 24 hours. She denies fever, chills, sweats, any recent trauma to the leg, or changes in physical activity. She has a history of two episodes of similar swelling in her leg—one 7 years and one 3 years previously. The first episode resolved spontaneously, but the second was associated with shortness of breath and required hospitalization. At that time, the diagnosis of thrombophlebitis was made and the patient was given Coumadin for 6 months. The patient has done well with regular checkups and no medical problems until the present episode. The patient denies skin rash, joint pain or swelling, excessive fatigue, hair loss, or photosensitivity. There is no history of kidney problems. There is no known family history of arthritis, connective tissue disease, or bleeding or clotting problems. The patient lives with her husband and one child, age 12. Obstetric history reveals the patient had a normal, healthy child 12 years previously but since that time has had three unsuccessful pregnancies with spontaneous abortions at 28, 14, and 30 weeks.

Examination reveals a healthy-appearing woman with normal vital signs. Skin shows a reticular "lace-like" vascular pattern over her thighs and upper arms. This rash blanches with pressure, and it is not pruritic or painful. The right calf is diffusely swollen and slightly red. It is tender to palpation, and there is a palpable cord extending into the posterior aspect of the distal thigh. Her right foot shows 1–2+ pitting edema. The remainder of the examination is normal.

Laboratory evaluation reveals normal CBC, chemistries, and urinalysis. Chest x-ray is clear. Serologic testing shows a weakly positive ANA (1:40) and negative rheumatoid factor. Clotting tests obtained prior to initiation of heparin therapy shows a prothrombin time of 12.9 seconds (normal 12.8–13.1), aPTT of 47 seconds (normal 33–35); a 1:1 mix with normal plasma yields an aPTT of 44.6 seconds. Anticardiolipin antibodies by ELISA shows an IgG of 48 units (normal < 23) and an IgM of 6 units (normal < 5). **What is the diagnosis?**

This patient has the primary antiphospholipid antibody syndrome (PAPS). She presents now with a deep venous thrombosis of her right leg. In addition to the acute DVT, the patient has a history of DVT and pulmonary embolism, and three fetal losses that occurred relatively late in pregnancy. The clinical constellation of recurrent thrombotic events and fetal loss in the face of clotting abnormalities makes the diagnosis of antiphospholipid antibody syndrome. This patient has a lupus anticoagulant as defined by the presence of a prolonged aPTT that does not correct with a 1:1 dilution with normal plasma. Additional testing should include a platelet neutralization procedure to ensure that the aPTT prolongation is corrected by the addition of frozen platelets, and a Russell viper venom time (RVVT), which should be prolonged. The patient also has anticardiolipin antibodies predominantly of the IgG type, as detected by ELISA. (See Chapter 27.)

**10. A 69-year-old woman presents with a 3-week history of a severe headache and a 30-second transient loss of vision in her right eye. Read the description and make the diagnosis.**

Headache is characterized as a boring pain in her right temporal region. She also has pain and cramping in her jaw muscles when chewing, and arthralgias. Other complaints are low-grade fevers, 5-pound weight loss, and proximal muscle pain and stiffness. Examination reveals a temperature of 38°C, tenderness of her scalp and both temporal arteries, and breakaway weakness of the shoulders due to pain. Funduscopic examination is normal. There is a left carotid bruit. Laboratory findings include hematocrit 35%, white cell count 11,500/mm$^3$, platelet count 522,000/mm$^3$, and erythrocyte sedimentation rate of 110 mm/hr. **What is the diagnosis and initial management of this patient?**

This patient has giant cell arteritis. The new onset of headache, jaw claudication, and polymyalgia rheumatica symptoms coupled with scalp and temporal artery tenderness and an extremely elevated ESR is characteristic of this disease. Diagnosis should be confirmed with a right temporal artery biopsy. Because of the transient visual loss, she should be started immediately on high doses of corticosteroids even before the biopsy is obtained. (See Chapter 31.)

**11. A 40-year-old man presents with nonhealing leg ulcers on the left lower leg of 1-month's duration. Read the case presentation and discuss the diagnosis.**

Review of systems shows he has had chronic sinusitis for the past year that has been worse recently. He also has experienced low-grade fevers, a nonproductive cough, and left hand numbness. Examination shows a temperature 38°C, blood pressure 150/90, left lower leg ulcer (figure), sinus tenderness, normal chest examination, and decreased sensation of the left hand. Radiographs show chronic maxillary sinusitis bilaterally and two nodular lung infiltrates. Laboratory findings include hematocrit 35%, WBC 12,000/mm$^3$, platelets 490,000/mm$^3$, and a sedimentation rate 92 mm/hour. Chemistries are normal, but creatinine is 1.6 mg/dL and urinalysis shows 1+ protein and moderate blood. **What serologic test would help confirm your diagnosis?**

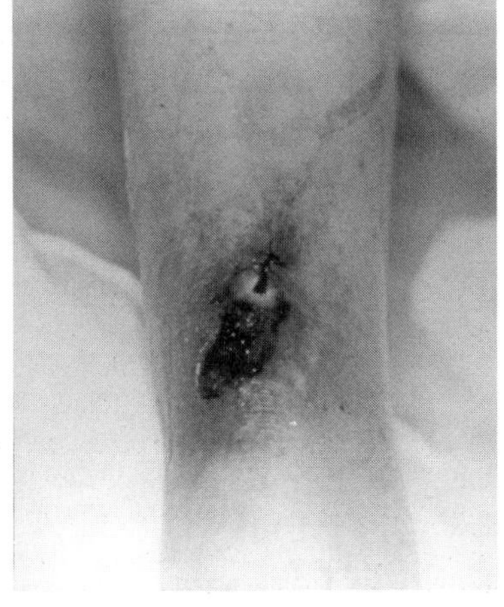

This patient has the triad of sinusitis, lung infiltrates, and glomerulonephritis characteristic of Wegener's granulomatosis. Fever, ulcerative skin lesion, neurologic involvement, and abnormal laboratory findings also may be seen in this disease. The antineutrophil cytoplasmic antibody (C-ANCA) test is likely to be positive and will help confirm the diagnosis. (See Chapter 33.)

**12. A 26-year-old white man comes to your clinic with a 1-year history of low back, buttock, and spine pain. He notes 2 hours of morning stiffness that improves by the afternoon with movement and exercise. Six months previously, he had an episode of sudden pain in his right eye that was diagnosed as acute iritis and resolved after he was placed on steroid eye drops. His father had similar back pain problems. Examination reveals no joint swelling. Back range of motion is limited in flexion, extension, lateral rotation, and lateral bending. His Gaenslen's test is positive. What is the diagnosis?**

This patient has ankylosing spondylitis. Chronic back pain with inflammatory features of prolonged morning stiffness that improves with exercise coupled with a global decrease in back range of motion is characteristic of this disease. Acute anterior iritis can also be a manifestation of this seronegative spondyloarthropathy. This disease occurs most commonly in young, white males, can occur in multiple family members, and is associated with the gene HLA-B27. (See Chapter 38.)

**13. A 65-year-old man was in good health until he developed dysesthesias in both hands. A diagnosis of carpal tunnel syndrome was made, and his symptoms resolved following carpal tunnel release. He returns for evaluation 1 year later because of swelling in his wrists and hands and recurrence of dysesthesias. Read the description and provide the diagnosis.**

The patient denies fever or anorexia but has been fatigued and experienced a 20-pound weight loss since the carpal tunnel release. The wrist swelling is persistent but not painful or associated with prolonged morning stiffness. He has noted some swelling in his hands and more recently his knees and shoulders. Examination reveals a chronically ill-appearing male with normal vital signs. Musculoskeletal examination reveals marked synovitis of both wrists with only minimal warmth and tenderness. There is similar but less marked involvement of bilateral metacarpophalangeal and proximal interphalangeal joints. Tinel's test is positive bilaterally. There is fullness of both shoulders and prominent synovitis of both knees, again with little associated warmth or tenderness. Laboratory studies show normal complete blood count, serum chemistries, and thyroid stimulating hormone. The urine has 2+ protein, the erythrocyte sedimentation rate is 65 mm/hour, and rheumatoid factor and ANA are negative. Serum protein electrophoresis reveals an IgG lambda monoclonal spike. Radiographs of the wrists show cystic changes. **What is the diagnosis?**

Primary systemic amyloidosis. A neuropathic presentation, usually carpal tunnel syndrome, is seen in about 20% of patients with primary amyloidosis. The onset of carpal tunnel syndrome in a male over the age of 40 years should raise the possibility of amyloidosis, as should the recurrence of symptoms following carpal tunnel release. Fatigue and weight loss, though nonspecific, are frequent in amyloidosis. A rheumatoid arthritis–like picture is seen in 7% of patients. Clinical findings that distinguish amyloid arthropathy from rheumatoid arthritis are the relatively mild joint symptoms and mild joint warmth and tenderness despite impressive synovitis, the absence of rheumatoid factor, and the cystic changes (not erosions) of bone seen on radiographs. (See Chapter 77.)

**14. A 45-year-old man returns to see you after your initial evaluation 1 week previously when he presented with a 6-month history of pain and swelling in his hands. Read the description and make the diagnosis.**

At that time, he denied morning stiffness, fever, weight loss, or repetitive trauma to the joints in question. He is otherwise healthy, although he did admit to some increased fatigue over the last 6 months. He is currently taking no medications and denies alcohol or tobacco use. There is a family history of "rheumatoid arthritis" in a brother, and an uncle has hepatic cirrhosis. On physical examination, you identified firm synovial swelling with mild tenderness of the second through fifth metacarpophalangeal and wrist joints bilaterally. Warmth and erythema were absent. The remainder of the physical examination was unremarkable except for mild hepatomegaly. You ordered some routine laboratory tests and hand radiographs. The laboratory results include a normal complete blood count and chemistries. The erythrocyte sedimentation rate is 10 mm/hr. The liver panel reveals that both the SGOT (AST) and SGPT (ALT) are two times normal. The remainder of the liver panel is normal. Hand radiographs are shown below. **What is the diagnosis?**

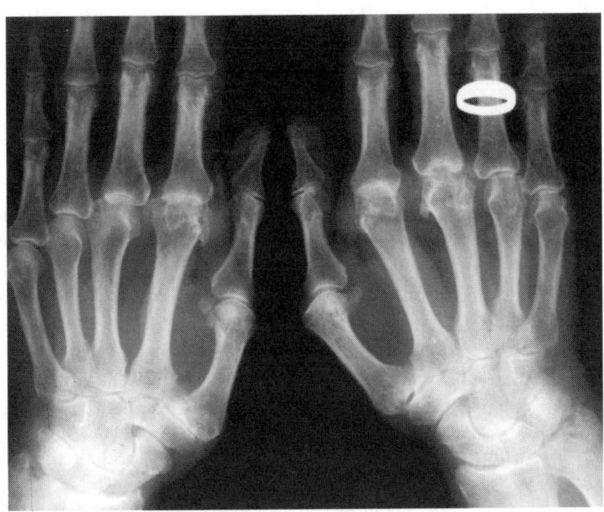

The clinical presentation and radiographs are characteristic for hemochromatosis. There is degenerative arthritis involving the second through fifth metacarpophalangeal joints (MCPs) with prominent joint space narrowing, subchondral cyst formation, sclerosis, and large hook-like osteophytes. Chondrocalcinosis is absent in this case, but can be seen on radiographs in 30–60% of cases, as can degenerative arthritis of the radiocarpal joints.

Hemochromatosis needs to be considered in the differential diagnosis of a seronegative polyarthritis, particularly in middle-aged men with MCP joint involvement. Other joints that may be involved are wrists, knees, ankles, and interphalangeal joints. The typical findings on physical examination are firm joint swelling with only mild tenderness without warmth, erythema, or morning stiffness. The diagnosis in this case is supported by the presence of hepatomegaly, abnormal liver function tests, and the family history of arthritis and cirrhosis; hemochromatosis is inherited as an autosomal recessive trait. Iron studies, genetic testing for HFE gene, and a liver biopsy for iron quantification will confirm the diagnosis of hemochromatosis. (See Chapter 61.)

**15. A 32-year-old woman presents with a 2-year history of pain and color changes in the fingers of her hands when she is exposed to cold weather. The fingers first turn white, then blue and eventually red with pain. Examination shows a few telangiectasias on her face and dilated capillaries with dropout around her nailfolds. What serologic test would help confirm your clinical diagnosis?**

This patient has Raynaud's phenomenon characterized by the classic tricolor changes in her fingers on cold exposure. The facial telangiectasias and abnormal nailfold capillary examination suggest that she may develop limited scleroderma (CREST) in the future. A positive anticentromere antibody would help confirm this clinical diagnosis. (See Chapters 22 and 78.)

**16. A 35-year-old white woman is referred to you for evaluation of diffuse aches and pains of at least 5 years' duration that seem to be getting worse. Read the description and determine the diagnosis.**

The patient also has fatigue, stiffness, headaches, cold intolerance, irritable bowel syndrome, and difficulty sleeping. She is under considerable stress at home with an abusive husband and is chronically behind at work. Examination is completely normal except for bilateral tender points in the occipital region, trapezius muscles, rhomboid muscles, lateral epicondylar area of the elbows, low back and gluteal areas, trochanteric bursal regions, and medial knees. Laboratory and radiographic findings are normal. Specifically a CBC, sedimentation rate, chemistries, thyroid function tests, and creatine phosphokinase are within normal limits. **What is the diagnosis? What further work-up is necessary?**

The patient has fibromyalgia. The prolonged duration of symptoms, multisystem complaints, normal examination except for tender points in characteristic locations, and normal laboratory results help confirm this diagnosis. This is a clinical diagnosis with no specific laboratory test being diagnostic. No further work-up is necessary. (See Chapter 65.)

**17. A 45-year-old woman is referred with a 1-year history of swelling and pain in the MCPs, PIPs, wrists, left knee, ankles, and MTPs. Read the description and make the diagnosis.**

The patient reports hours of morning stiffness, fatigue, and malaise. She has taken ibuprofen, which has provided some help. Physical examination reveals normal vital signs, soft tissue swelling, warmth, tenderness, and limitation of motion of the involved joints. Nodules are seen on the extensor surface of both forearms near the olecranon area. Laboratory findings include a hematocrit of 35%, WBC count 7200/mm$^3$, and platelet count 480,000/mm$^3$. Chemistries, liver enzymes, and uric acid levels are normal. Rheumatoid factor is positive at a titer of 1:640, ANA is negative, and erythrocyte sedimentation rate is elevated at 45 mm/hr. Radiographs of the hands show early MCP and PIP erosions. **What is your diagnosis?**

This patient has rheumatoid arthritis. The gradual onset of a symmetric polyarthritis involving the small joints of the hands, wrists, and feet associated with prolonged morning stiffness and rheumatoid nodules satisfies criteria for this diagnosis. Additional findings of a positive rheumatoid factor and erosions on hand radiographs support this diagnosis. The elevated sedimentation rate, anemia of chronic disease, and elevated platelet count are reflections of the systemic inflammation caused by the rheumatoid arthritis. (See Chapter 19.)

**18. A 44-year-old man is admitted to the hospital complaining of abdominal pain, a 15-pound weight loss, fevers, fatigue, and right foot drop. He has a history of intravenous drug abuse. An abdominal angiogram is obtained. What is your diagnosis?**

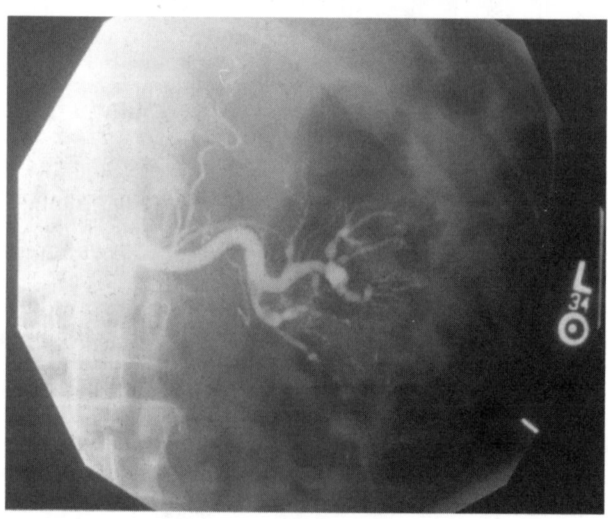

Polyarteritis nodosa. The presentation of multisystem disease coupled with an abdominal angiogram showing aneurysms in the abdominal and renal vessels is characteristic of this vasculitis. Because of his intravenous drug abuse history, you might expect him to be hepatitis B or C antigen positive. (See Chapter 32.)

**19. A 56-year-old woman presents with a complaint of a swollen right cheek. Read the description and formulate the diagnosis.**

She was well until 5 years previously when she experienced a sensation of "sand" in her eyes and a dry mouth that has become progressively worse. She also has had multiple dental caries. Three months previously, she experienced painless swelling of her right cheek as well as diffuse arthralgias. Examination reveals extreme dryness of the eyes and oral mucosa, poor dentition, and a swollen, nontender right parotid gland. A Schirmer's test and rose bengal test are positive. Laboratories are remarkable for hematocrit 35%, white blood cell count of 3,200/mm$^3$, normal urinalysis, erythrocyte sedimentation rate 107 mm/hr, elevated IgG and IgM immunoglobulin levels, a positive rheumatoid factor at 1:640, and a positive antinuclear antibody at 1:256 with a speckled pattern. **What is your diagnosis?**

This patient has primary Sjögren's syndrome, which is the most common autoimmune disease in middle-aged women. The combination of sicca symptoms, dental caries, parotid swelling, and serologic abnormalities is characteristic of this disease. You would expect this patient to have antibodies against SS-A and/or SS-B antigens. (See Chapter 26.)

**20. A 24-year-old male construction worker comes to you for evaluation of a painful, swollen knee and "scabby" feet for over 2 months. Read the description and make the diagnosis.**

There is no history of knee injury, and a review of systems is unremarkable with two exceptions. First, he recalls having a brief bout of "pink-eye" 3 weeks previously that was "hardly noticeable." Second, he remembers having pain with urination on two occasions. He is sexually active with several female partners. As he limps to the examining table, you are told that his vital signs are normal, except for a temperature of 38.2°C. His general appearance is consistent with that of a manual laborer. Inspection of his eyes reveals no inflammation. Examination of his pharynx, however, reveals a desquamated hard palate. The knee is obviously swollen, warm to touch, and flexed at 30°. You are unable to fully extend the knee, and the patella is ballottable. He has two diffusely swollen and tender toes on his right foot. The remainder of the musculoskeletal exam is normal, including the back. On the plantar surfaces of his feet, you observe multiple, papular lesions (figure). Despite their appearance, the lesions are asymptomatic. Inspection of his genitals reveals painless, superficial ulcers on the glans penis and urethral meatus. No discharge is noted. The rectal exam is unremarkable except for a slightly tender and enlarged prostate. Occult blood in his stool is not detected. **What is the diagnosis?**

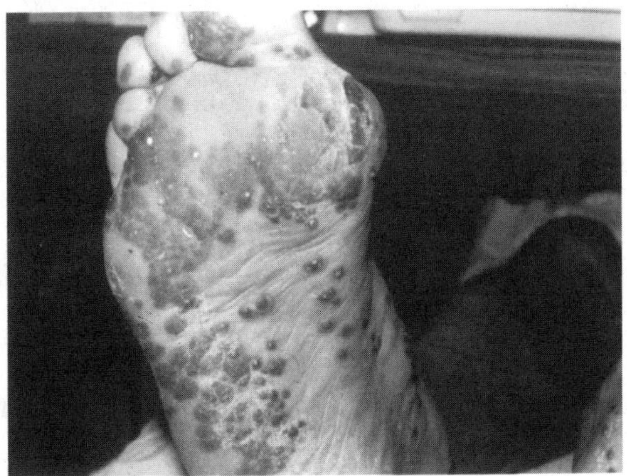

The clinical complex of conjunctivitis (pink-eye), urethritis, and arthritis is classic for Reiter's syndrome. In this patient, the additional features of sausage digits, painless oral ulceration, keratoderma blennorrhagica (see figure), and circinate balanitis confirm the diagnosis. Furthermore, *Chlamydia*-induced urogenital disease is probable, given the history, the mild prostatitis, and the mucocutaneous lesions. (See Chapter 40.)

**21. A 26-year-old black woman presents with a 6-month history of polyarthritis involving the small joints of her hands, wrists, knees, and feet. Read the description and decide the diagnosis.**

Two months previously, she noted she was beginning to lose some of her hair. Four weeks previously, she went to Hawaii on vacation and developed an erythematous rash over her face and upper body with sun exposure. Examination reveals a temperature of 38°C, pulse 120 beats/minute, and blood pressure 140/100 mm Hg. She has an erythematous rash over her cheeks and the bridge of her nose as well as spotty alopecia throughout the scalp without evidence of scarring. The remainder of the examination is normal except for synovitis of MCPs, PIPs, wrists, and MTPs. Laboratory findings include a hematocrit of 32%, white blood cell count 2400/mm$^3$, platelets 110,000/mm$^3$, creatinine 1.8 mg/dL, and a urinalysis with 3+ protein and 5–10 red blood cells and white blood cells per high power field with a few granular casts. **What is your diagnosis?**

This patient has systemic lupus erythematosus. A young black woman presenting with a multisystem disease including polyarthritis, alopecia, photosensitivity, malar rash, nephritis, and hematologic abnormalities including leukopenia and thrombocytopenia is characteristic of this disease. You would expect her antinuclear antibody test to be positive, antibodies against double-stranded DNA to be elevated, and C3 and C4 complement levels to be decreased. (See Chapter 20.)

**22. A 28-year-old woman presents to the emergency room with a 2-day history of joint pain. Read the presentation and make the diagnosis.**

The patient's pain started in her right ankle, migrated to her left knee, and then settled in her right wrist, which became tender, warm, and swollen. She has felt feverish and noted a few painless hemorrhagic skin lesions on her upper and lower extremities. She has no previous history of pelvic inflammatory disease but is sexually active. She began her menstrual cycle 3 days previously. Examination shows a temperature of 38.5°C, a severely swollen and painful right wrist with warmth and erythema along the extensor tendons as well as the true wrist joint. She has scattered discrete hemorrhagic papules over her hands and lower extremities. Laboratory results show a white blood cell count of 13,500/mm$^3$ with 93% neutrophils and 5% band forms. Radiograph of the wrist is remarkable for soft tissue swelling. **What is your diagnosis?**

This patient's presentation of migratory polyarthritis finally settling in one joint associated with fever and skin rash in a sexually active female is characteristic of disseminated gonococcemia. Onset within the first week of menstruation is also common. (See Chapter 42.)

**23. A 72-tear-old grandmother with generalized osteoarthritis complains that she can predict changes in the weather better than the weatherman on television. Can weather changes affect patients with arthritis?**

Yes. It doesn't matter so much whether it is hot, cold, dry, or humid. Many arthritic patients (66%) are affected by changes in barometric pressure and temperature as weather fronts are moving in or out of an area. It is hypothesized that changes in barometric pressure and temperature increase stiffness of joints, which can heighten a nociceptive response. Consequently, the myth that patients with arthritis should move to a warm climate is unlikely to be helpful because changes in weather and barometric pressure occur everywhere.

**24. Who said "The secret of being a bore is to tell everything"?**

Voltaire (1694–1778). This book undoubtedly has left out a "rheumatology secret" that the reader feels should be included in the next edition. Please write the book editor with any suggestions or additional "secrets."

## BIBLIOGRAPHY


1. Hollander J: Environment and musculoskeletal disease. Arch Environmental Health 6:527–536, 1963.
2. Sibley JT: Weather and arthritis symptoms. J Rheum 12:707–710, 1985.
3. Swezey RL, Swezey, SE: The consequences of habitual knuckle cracking. West J Med 122:377–379, 1973.
4. Unger DL: Does knuckle cracking lead to arthritis of the fingers? Arthritis Rheum 41:949–950, 1998.

# INDEX

Page numbers in **boldface type** indicate complete chapters.